# Principles of Medical Pharmacology

## Seventh Edition

Edited by

**Harold Kalant, MD, PhD**
Professor Emeritus
Department of Pharmacology
Faculty of Medicine
University of Toronto

**Denis M Grant, PhD**
Department of Pharmacology
Faculty of Medicine
University of Toronto

**Jane Mitchell, PhD**
Department of Pharmacology
Faculty of Medicine
University of Toronto

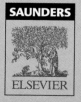

SAUNDERS

ELSEVIER

---

## NOTICE

Pharmacology is an ever-changing field. Standard safety precautions must be followed, but as new research and clinical experience broaden our knowledge, changes in treatment and drug therapy may become necessary or appropriate. Readers are advised to check the most current product information provided by the manufacturer of each drug to be administered to verify the recommended dose, the method and duration of administration, and contraindications. It is the responsibility of the licensed prescriber, relying on experience and knowledge of the patient, to determine dosages and the best treatment for each individual patient. Neither the Publisher nor the editors assume any liability for any injury and/or damage to persons or property arising from this publication.

---

**Library and Archives Canada Cataloguing in Publication**

Principles of medical pharmacology / edited by Harold Kalant, Denis Grant, and Jane Mitchell—7th ed.
Includes bibliographical references and index.
ISBN 0-7796-9945-9
1. Pharmacology. 2. Drugs.
I. Grant, Denis M. (Denis Michael), 1957-
II. Kalant, Harold, 1923- III. Mitchell, Jane, 1954-

RM300.P75 2006      615'.1      C2005-905716-5

*Publisher*: Ann Millar
*Developmental Editor*: Sondra Greenfield
*Managing Developmental Editor*: Martina van de Velde
*Managing Production Editor*: Lise Dupont
*Copy Editor*: Kelly Davis
*Proofreader*: James Leahy
*Cover Design and Some Interior Illustrations*: Imagineering Media Services Inc.
*Interior Design*: Sonya V. Thursby, Opus House Inc.
*Typesetting and Assembly*: Janette Thompson, Jansom
*Printing and Binding*: Courier Companies Inc.
*Cover Printing*: Phoenix

Elsevier Canada
1 Goldthorne Ave., Toronto, ON, Canada M8Z 5S7
Phone: 1-866-896-3331
Fax: 1-866-359-9534

Printed in the United States of America
1 2 3 4 5   11 10 09 08 07

## About the Cover

The cover image is designed to depict two fundamental pharmacological processes. More specifically, the art represents symbolically the permeation of molecules of a drug from the capillary vasculature through intercellular spaces and transient windows or *fenestrae*. The artwork also depicts the binding of a single drug molecule to its intended protein target.

# Contents

# Preface
## to the Seventh Edition

**THIS BOOK** originated over 40 years ago in the form of detailed lecture notes prepared by Drs. H. Kalant, E.A. Sellers, and W. Kalow. The notes were distributed by faculty members of the Department of Pharmacology, University of Toronto, to students in Medicine, Dentistry, and Pharmacy, and later to undergraduate Arts and Science students enrolled in specialist programs in pharmacology and toxicology. The lecture assignments to individual staff members changed from year to year so that the notes gradually came to reflect the combined knowledge and approaches of the whole Department. In addition, as the Department steadily came to include more clinicians with cross-appointments in Pharmacology, the content of the notes acquired a correspondingly improved balance between basic and clinical pharmacological components.

In 1975, the notes were edited to provide greater uniformity of organization and style in all chapters and were combined into the first edition of this textbook. It was intended as a working text for students, not as an exhaustive reference work or as an advanced treatise for senior clinicians or researchers, whose needs are better met by a variety of specialized publications. The illustrations were simple line drawings, and the brief list of suggested readings at the end of each chapter was not intended to provide detailed documentation of every point in the chapter, but only to provide some additional sources of information for those readers who were interested in learning more about the subjects covered in the chapter.

The book has evolved, matured, and expanded through six subsequent editions under the overall supervision of the departmental Book Committee and a succession of editors:

1st edition, 1975: P. Seeman and E.M. Sellers
2nd edition, 1976: P. Seeman and E.M. Sellers
3rd edition, 1979: P. Seeman, E.M. Sellers, and W.H.E. Roschlau
4th edition, 1985: H. Kalant, W.H.E. Roschlau, and E.M. Sellers
5th edition, 1989: H. Kalant and W.H.E. Roschlau
6th edition, 1997: H. Kalant and W.H.E. Roschlau

The first four editions were published by the Department itself, with the technical assistance of the University of Toronto Press. The fifth edition, the first commercially produced one, was published by B.C. Decker, Inc., and later by Mosby-Year Book, Inc. The sixth edition was published by Oxford University Press, New York.

Despite these many changes, *the primary purpose and general character of the book* have remained basically the same. It continues to be a textbook of pharmacology rather than of therapeutics, although the rapid growth of knowledge and the steadily closer interdependence of basic and clinical aspects of the subject have made this distinction less sharp than it formerly was.

The present edition retains this general didactic approach but has undergone some major changes of content and emphasis:

* Most chapters have been extensively or completely rewritten, many by new authors.
* More of the chapters have been written by clinical pharmacologists, with greater emphasis on clinical aspects than in the previous editions.
* A larger number of the authors are from centres other than the University of Toronto, including several Canadian universities and hospitals and one in the United Kingdom.
* Several chapters are completely new, covering for the first time in this book such topics as drugs used in dermatology, herbal remedies and dietary supplements, and clinical pharmacological principles in the pharmacotherapy of hypertension.
* A large amount of new and updated material has been added from recent publications.
* There is expanded use of introductory case histories, which have proven popular and useful for many readers and teachers of pharmacology.
* The Suggested Readings lists that follow all chapters have been considerably enlarged and now include some useful electronic reference sources.

- Most of the illustrations have been revised or are completely new.
- The index is greatly enlarged and should make it easier for readers to locate specific information.

The short case histories at the beginning of most chapters are, as in the previous edition, meant to illustrate the clinical relevance of certain pharmacological principles discussed in the text. They are not meant to serve as primary material for medical curricula built on "case-based learning," for which much longer and more detailed histories would be required. Rather, it is hoped that students encountering these short cases will become motivated to read the basic pharmacology with greater interest and attention and make their own connections between the pharmacological principles and their clinical impact. No questions and answers are provided to accompany these case histories, because we wish to avoid their use as a sort of "catechism." Rather, it is our hope that these cases will stimulate discussions between students and their instructors.

Previous editions of this book have been translated into Italian, Portuguese, and Spanish. We thank the translators in Italy, Brazil, and Mexico for their interest in the book and their excellent renditions of it. We are encouraged to think that this indicates a broad appeal of the didactic approach used in the book, and we hope that readers will welcome its retention in the present edition.

As in previous editions, drugs are referred to by their non-proprietary (i.e., official, approved, or "generic") names, but examples of the most common proprietary ("trade") names are also given in most cases for the reader's convenience. North American spelling and nomenclature are used throughout. In those few instances in which Canadian and U.S. official names differ (e.g., Canadian *adrenaline* and U.S. *epinephrine*), the Canadian name appears first and the U.S. name follows in parentheses.

Every chapter has been read in the manuscript stage by either two or three external reviewers chosen by the publisher for their expertise in the field covered by the chapter. The detailed reviews were made available to the editors and the authors, and most of the suggestions were incorporated into the chapters. The instructors who provided feedback on the seventh edition manuscript are listed alphabetically below. We are greatly indebted to them for their detailed reading and critique of the chapters and the interesting and helpful suggestions they offered.

Jack Bend, University of Western Ontario
Jonathan Blay, Dalhousie University
Ronald Boegman, Queen's University
Deepak Bose, University of Manitoba
Jeff Chan, Thunder Bay Regional Health Sciences Centre
Michael A. Cook, University of Western Ontario
John Downie, Dalhousie University
Helga Duivenvoorden, Thunder Bay Regional Health Sciences Centre
David V. Godin, University of British Columbia
Maurice Hirst, University of Western Ontario
Theodore Hoekman, Memorial University of Newfoundland
Susan Howlett, Dalhousie University
Sam Kacew, University of Ottawa
Ismail Laher, University of British Columbia
Ed Lui, University of Western Ontario
William McLean, University of Ottawa
Mark W. Nachtigal, Dalhousie University
Kanji Nakatsu, Queen's University
Richard Neumann, Memorial University of Newfoundland
Robert J. Omeljaniuk, Lakehead University
William Racz, Queen's University
Kenneth W. Renton, Dalhousie University
Michael J. Rieder, Children's Hospital of Western Ontario
Jane Rylett, University of Western Ontario

Daniel Sitar, University of Manitoba
Zacharias Suntres, Lakehead University
Reza Tabrizi, Memorial University of Newfoundland
Louise Winn, Queen's University

The invaluable organizational and editorial skills contributed by Dr. Walter H.E. Roschlau in the third to sixth editions of this book were greatly missed this time; the present editors extend their very best wishes to him in his retirement.

The editors express their gratitude to the chapter authors for their care, interest, and co-operation in revising, updating, improving, and, in many cases, expanding the text and for their patience during the long and rather complex gestation period of this edition.

We are grateful to the departmental Book Committee for its support of this work and to Ms. Ann Millar of Elsevier Canada for her enthusiastic promotion and encouragement of this project. We thank Elsevier's editorial staff, especially Ms. Sondra Greenfield, Ms. Martina van de Velde, and Ms. Lise Dupont, for their thorough, careful workup of the material and their numerous helpful suggestions to facilitate our editorial handling of the many drafts the book went through.

Finally, the Department wishes to record its gratitude to the authors and editors who, continuing the tradition that has existed since the first edition of this book, have generously donated their efforts for the benefit of the Department and its graduate students. Their royalties from the sale of the book go to a special fund for the support of educational and scholarly activities not covered by the regular departmental budget.

The Editors
*Toronto*
*Spring 2006*

# Contributors

Uwe Ackermann, PhD
Professor
Laboratory of Physiology
University of Oxford
Oxford, United Kingdom

Jonathan D Adachi, MD, FRCP(C)
Professor, Department of Medicine
Director, Hamilton Arthritis Centre
St. Joseph's Healthcare—McMaster University
Hamilton, Ontario

W McIntyre Burnham, PhD
Professor, Department of Pharmacology
Faculty of Medicine
Director, University of Toronto Epilepsy
    Research Program
University of Toronto
Toronto, Ontario

FJ Lou Carmichael, MD, PhD
Medical Director
Amgen Canada Inc.
Mississauga, Ontario

Associate Professor
Departments of Anaesthesia and Pharmacology
University of Toronto
Toronto, Ontario

Vincent WS Chan, MD
Professor, Department of Anaesthesia
Toronto Western Hospital, University Health Network
University of Toronto
Toronto, Ontario

Kenneth R Chapman, MD, MSc, FRCPC, FACP, FCCP
Professor of Medicine
Division of Respiratory Medicine
Department of Medicine
University of Toronto
Toronto, Ontario

Director
Asthma & Airway Centre
University Health Network
Toronto Western Hospital
Toronto, Ontario

Eric X Chen, MD, PhD
Department of Medical Oncology
    and Hematology
Princess Margaret Hospital
Toronto, Ontario

Assistant Professor
Faculty of Medicine
University of Toronto
Toronto, Ontario

Alice YY Cheng, MD, FRCPC
Assistant Professor
University of Toronto
Division of Endocrinology and Metabolism
Credit Valley Hospital and St. Michael's Hospital
Toronto, Ontario

Paul Dorian, MD, MSc, FRCPC
Professor
Departments of Medicine and Pharmacology
Faculty of Medicine
University of Toronto
Toronto, Ontario

Laszlo Endrenyi, PhD
Professor Emeritus
Department of Pharmacology
Faculty of Medicine
University of Toronto
Toronto, Ontario

Subhas C Ganguli, MSc, MD, FRCPC
Assistant Professor
Department of Gastroenterology
McMaster University
Hamilton, Ontario

Michael A Gardam, MSc, MD, CM, FRCPC
Director, Infection Prevention and Control
University Health Network
Toronto, Ontario

Assistant Professor of Medicine
Faculty of Medicine
University of Toronto
Toronto, Ontario

Susan R George, MD, FRCP(C), FACP
Professor and Canada Research Chair
Departments of Medicine and Pharmacology
Faculty of Medicine
University of Toronto
Toronto, Ontario

Head, Molecular Pharmacology
Centre for Addiction and Mental Health
Toronto, Ontario

Denis M Grant, PhD
Professor and Chair
Department of Pharmacology
Faculty of Medicine
University of Toronto
Toronto, Ontario

Larry A Grupp, DSc
Associate Professor
Department of Pharmacology
Faculty of Medicine
University of Toronto
Toronto, Ontario

Research Liaison
Department of Psychiatry
University Health Network
Toronto, Ontario

Daniel A Haas, DDS, PhD, FRCD(C)
Professor and Associate Dean
Faculty of Dentistry
University of Toronto
Toronto, Ontario

Professor
Department of Pharmacology
Faculty of Medicine
University of Toronto
Toronto, Ontario

Patricia A Harper, PhD
Associate Professor
Departments of Pediatrics and Pharmacology
Faculty of Medicine
University of Toronto
Toronto, Ontario

Senior Scientist
Research Institute, The Hospital for Sick Children
Toronto, Ontario

Murray Hong, PhD
Associate Professor
Departments of Surgery (Neurosurgery) and
    Pharmacology
Dalhousie University
Halifax, Nova Scotia

Richard H Hunt, FRCP, FRCP Ed, FRCPC, FACG
Professor of Medicine
Division of Gastroenterology
McMaster University
Hamilton, Ontario

Karen Iverson, MHSc, CIC
Manager, Infection Prevention and Control
University Health Network
Toronto, Ontario

Dezso Kadar, BScPharm, MSc, PhD
Professor Emeritus
Department of Pharmacology
Faculty of Medicine
University of Toronto
Toronto, Ontario

Harold Kalant, MD, PhD
Professor Emeritus
Department of Pharmacology
Faculty of Medicine
University of Toronto
Toronto, Ontario

Director Emeritus
Biobehavioural Research
ARF Division, Centre for Addiction and Mental Health
Toronto, Ontario

Werner Kalow, MD
Professor Emeritus
Department of Pharmacology
Faculty of Medicine
University of Toronto
Toronto, Ontario

Shitij Kapur, MD, PhD, FRCPC
Chief of Research
Centre for Addiction and Mental Health
Toronto, Ontario

Canada Research Chair
Professor of Psychiatry
University of Toronto
Toronto, Ontario

Jay S Keystone, MD, MSc, FRCPC
Professor
Departments of Medicine and Pharmacology
Faculty of Medicine
University of Toronto
Tropical Disease Unit, Division of Infectious Diseases
Toronto General Hospital
Toronto, Ontario

Jatinder M Khanna, MPharm, PhD
Professor Emeritus
Department of Pharmacology
Faculty of Medicine
University of Toronto
Toronto, Ontario

Gideon Koren, MD, FACMT, FRCPC
The Ivey Chair in Molecular Toxicology
University of Western Ontario
London, Ontario

Professor
Departments of Pediatrics, Pharmacology,
    and Medicine
Faculties of Medicine and Pharmacy
University of Toronto
Toronto, Ontario

Director
Division of Clinical Pharmacology & MotherRisk
The Hospital for Sick Children
Toronto, Ontario

A José Lança, MD, PhD
Assistant Professor
Department of Pharmacology
Faculty of Medicine
University of Toronto
Toronto, Ontario

Lawrence A Leiter, MD, FRCPC, FACP
Head, Division of Endocrinology and Metabolism
St. Michael's Hospital
Toronto, Ontario

Professor of Medicine and Nutritional Sciences
University of Toronto
Toronto, Ontario

Peter P Li, PhD
Associate Professor
Departments of Psychiatry and Pharmacology
Faculty of Medicine
University of Toronto
Toronto, Ontario

Sue Lim, MD, FRCPC
Instructor
Division of Infectious Diseases
Faculty of Medicine
University of Toronto
University Health Network
Toronto, Ontario

Laura A Magee, MD, FRCPC, Masc
Department of Medicine
University of British Columbia
British Columbia Women's Hospital
Vancouver, British Columbia

David C Mamo, MD, MSc, FRCP(C)
Assistant Professor of Psychiatry
Department of Psychiatry
University of Toronto
Toronto, Ontario

Staff Psychiatrist
Centre for Addiction and Mental Health
Toronto, Ontario

Jane Mitchell, PhD
Associate Professor
Department of Pharmacology
Faculty of Medicine
University of Toronto
Toronto, Ontario

Gordon Moe, MSc, MD, FRCP(C), FACC
Attending Cardiologist
St. Michael's Hospital
Toronto, Ontario

Associate Professor
Department of Medicine
University of Toronto
Toronto, Ontario

Malcolm J Moore, MD
Professor of Medicine and Pharmacology
Princess Margaret Hospital
University of Toronto
Toronto, Ontario

RI Ogilvie, MD, FRCPC, FACP
Professor Emeritus
Divisions of Pharmacology and Medicine
University of Toronto
Toronto, Ontario

Clinical Pharmacologist
Hypertension Unit
Toronto Western Hospital
Toronto, Ontario

Allan B Okey, PhD
Professor Emeritus
Department of Pharmacology
Faculty of Medicine
University of Toronto
Toronto, Ontario

Cecil R Pace-Asciak, PhD
Professor Emeritus
Departments of Pediatrics and Pharmacology
Faculty of Medicine
University of Toronto
Toronto, Ontario

Senior Scientist Emeritus
Research Institute, The Hospital for Sick Children
Toronto, Ontario

Alexandra Papaioannou, MD, MSc, FRCPC
Associate Professor
Department of Medicine
McMaster University
Hamilton, Ontario

Geriatrician
Hamilton Health Sciences
Hamilton, Ontario

Elizabeth J Phillips, MD, FRCPC
Head, Clinical Pharmacology
British Columbia Centre for Excellence in
    HIV/AIDS
University of British Columbia
Vancouver, British Columbia

Robert MA Richardson, MD
Director of Hemodialysis
Division of Nephrology
Toronto General Hospital
Toronto, Ontario

Professor
Department of Medicine
University of Toronto
Toronto, Ontario

David S Riddick, PhD
Associate Professor
Department of Pharmacology
Faculty of Medicine
University of Toronto
Toronto, Ontario

Eve A Roberts, MD, FRCPC
Professor
Departments of Paediatrics, Medicine, and
    Pharmacology
Faculty of Medicine
University of Toronto
Toronto, Ontario

Myroslava K Romach, MSc, MD, FRCPC
Vice-President, Research and Development
Ventana Clinical Research Corporation
Toronto, Ontario

Andrea Sarkozy, MD
Clinical Fellow in Electrophysiology
Division of Cardiology
St. Michael's Hospital
Toronto, Ontario

Bernard P Schimmer, PhD
Professor
Banting & Best Department of Medical Research
    and Department of Pharmacology
Faculty of Medicine
University of Toronto
Toronto, Ontario

Kerri A Schoedel, BSc, PhD
Research Scientist
Ventana Clinical Research Corporation
Toronto, Ontario

Philip Seeman, MD, PhD, DSc, OC
Professor Emeritus
Departments of Pharmacology and Psychiatry
University of Toronto
Toronto, Ontario

Edward M Sellers, MD, PhD, FRCPC
President and CEO
Ventana Clinical Research Corporation
Toronto, Ontario

Professor
Departments of Pharmacology, Medicine,
    and Psychiatry
Faculty of Medicine
University of Toronto
Toronto, Ontario

John W Semple, PhD
Professor
Departments of Pharmacology, Medicine, and
    Laboratory Medicine and Pathobiology
Faculty of Medicine
University of Toronto
Toronto, Ontario

Senior Staff Scientist
St. Michael's Hospital
Toronto, Ontario

Neil H Shear, MD, FRCPC
Helen & Paul Phelan Professor and Director of
    Dermatology
Departments of Medicine, Pharmacology, and Pediatrics
Faculties of Medicine and Pharmacy
Sunnybrook & Women's College Health Sciences Centre
University of Toronto
Toronto, Ontario

Daniel S Sitar, BScPharm, PhD
Professor and Head, Department of Pharmacology
    and Therapeutics
Professor, Department of Internal Medicine
Faculty of Medicine
University of Manitoba
Winnipeg, Manitoba

Jack Uetrecht, MD, PhD
Professor of Pharmacy and Medicine
Canada Research Chair in Adverse Drug Reactions
Faculty of Pharmacy
University of Toronto
Toronto, Ontario

Sharon L Walmsley, MD
Associate Professor of Medicine
Department of Medicine
Division of Infectious Diseases
Faculty of Medicine
University of Toronto
Toronto, Ontario

Wendy E Ward, PhD
Assistant Professor
Department of Nutritional Sciences
Faculty of Medicine
University of Toronto
Toronto, Ontario

Jerry J Warsh, MD, PhD, FRCP(C)
Head, Laboratory of Cellular and Molecular
    Pathophysiology
Centre for Addiction and Mental Health—Clark Site
Toronto, Ontario

Professor
Departments of Pharmacology and Psychiatry
Institute of Medical Science
University of Toronto
Toronto, Ontario

Peter G Wells, PharmD
Professor
Departments of Pharmaceutical Sciences
    and Pharmacology
Faculties of Pharmacy and Medicine
University of Toronto
Toronto, Ontario

Gavin AE Wong, MBChB, MRCP (UK)
Consultant Dermatologist
Department of Dermatology
Royal Liverpool & Broadgreen University Hospitals
    NHS Trust
Liverpool, United Kingdom

Cindy Woodland, PhD
Senior Lecturer
Department of Pharmacology
Faculty of Medicine
University of Toronto
Toronto, Ontario

Erik L Yeo, MD, FRCP(C), FACP
Head of Laboratory Hematology
Department of Laboratory Medicine
Toronto Medical Laboratories
Toronto, Ontario

Director of Clinical Hemostasis and Thrombosis
Division of Hematology
Department of Medicine
University Health Network
Toronto, Ontario

Associate Professor of Medicine
Faculty of Medicine
University of Toronto
Toronto, Ontario

Yuhong Yuan, MSc, MD, PhD
Research Associate
Division of Gastroenterology
Health Sciences Centre
McMaster University
Hamilton, Ontario

# Part I

# General Principles of Pharmacology

# 1

# Introduction to General Pharmacology

## H KALANT

## WHAT IS PHARMACOLOGY?

The word **pharmacology** is derived from the Greek words *pharmakon* (a drug or poison) and *logos* (word or discourse) and means "the science (discourse) that deals with the fate of drugs in the body and their actions on the body." It overlaps extensively with **pharmacy** (the science of preparation of drugs and the monitoring of their utilization) and with **therapeutics** (the treatment of disease, by drugs and other means). Some of the areas of overlap are mentioned below.

Pharmacology is both a basic and a clinically applied science. As a basic science, it deals with the fate and actions of drugs at various levels (molecular, cellular, organ, whole body, and even large populations in any animal species). It draws on knowledge, concepts, and techniques derived from organic and physical chemistry, molecular biology, biochemistry, physiology, biophysics, genetics, and other divisions of biological science. As an applied science, it deals with the same questions but in the specific context of the human species (in medicine) and domestic animals (in veterinary medicine), and it also deals with the use of drugs in the treatment of disease. This book includes both elements of the subject.

## WHAT IS A DRUG?

No definition of "drug" yet offered is entirely satisfactory. Perhaps the nearest we can come to one is the following: A drug is any substance, other than a normal constituent of the body or one that is required for normal bodily function (e.g., food, water, oxygen), that, when applied to or introduced into a living organism, has the effect of altering body function(s). This alteration may prove useful in the treatment of disease (therapeutic application), or it may cause disease (toxicity), but these outcomes are quite a separate matter from the definition of "drug."

Cold and hay-fever remedies bought off a supermarket shelf, penicillin given by prescription, and MDMA (methyl-

enedimethoxyamphetamine, or "ecstasy") bought illicitly on the street are all drugs. Vitamin C in orange juice is a food, but pure ascorbic acid injected in large doses to alter fibroblast activity is a drug. Hydrocortisone secreted by the adrenal cortex is a hormone, but when administered as replacement therapy in patients with adrenal failure, or in large doses to suppress inflammatory or immune responses, it is a drug. These actions may be useful in treating such diseases as rheumatoid arthritis or asthma, or they may cause Cushing's disease.

*Pharmacology is not concerned primarily with what the drug may be used for, but with what actions it has and what fate it encounters in the living organism.*

## SCOPE AND SUBDIVISIONS OF PHARMACOLOGY

How pharmacology is divided and how it overlaps with pharmacy and therapeutics are best illustrated by showing schematically what happens when a drug enters the body (Fig. 1-1). The processes of drug absorption, distribution, and elimination are described briefly here.

1.  Whether the drug is given as a tablet or capsule by mouth, as a vapour or aerosol by inhalation, or as a crystalline suspension by subcutaneous injection (or in any other form), it must first go into free solution before it can act. This may happen at the site of administration, as in subcutaneous or intramuscular injection, or it may happen downstream from that site, as when a tablet taken by mouth disintegrates and dissolves in the stomach or even further down the gastrointestinal tract. A special formulation of the drug may be needed to protect it against destruction by gastric acid or by other degradative factors or processes elsewhere. Preparation of the drug formulation and adjustment of its physical properties so that it will release the drug into solution at the desired rate, and in the right location, are problems of **pharmacy.**

**FIGURE 1-1** Schematic outline of the fate of a drug in the body. Numbers refer to the successive steps described in this section.

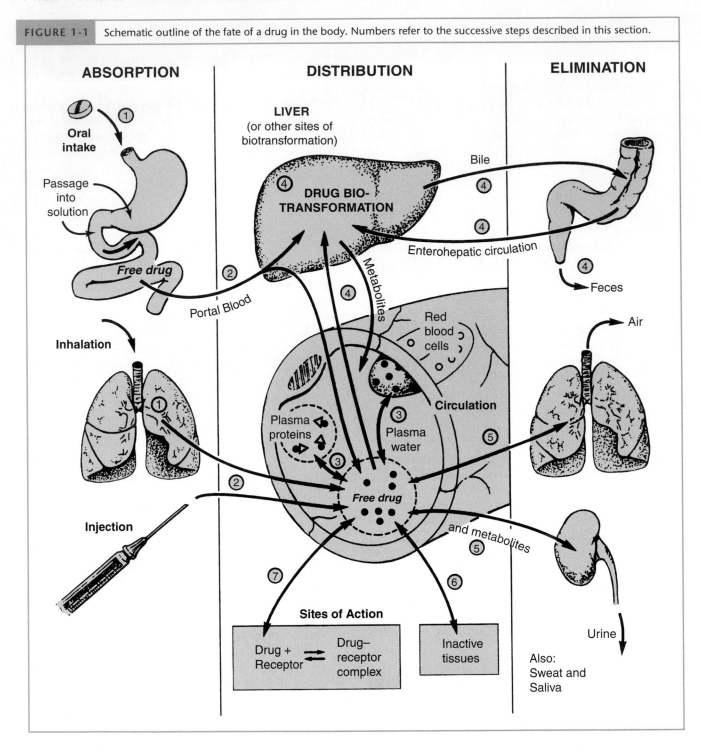

2. The dissolved drug must be absorbed into the portal blood if it is given by mouth; it will be directly absorbed into the systemic circulation if it is given by injection or by inhalation or if it can penetrate skin or mucous membranes. Absorption of the drug can involve a variety of different mechanisms that enable it to cross cell membranes, not only in the gastrointestinal tract but in all tissues. The absorption of a drug is strongly influenced by its molecular size, lipid solubility, ionization, and other physicochemical properties. These questions are discussed in detail in Chapter 2. From the portal blood, some of the drug is taken up by the liver, but some goes on into the systemic circulation. This is considered in detail in Chapter 6. The study of drug absorption and uptake by the liver is part of **pharmacology.**

✓ **Bioavailability** of a drug (i.e., the proportion of an administered dose that eventually reaches the systemic circulation in unchanged form) depends on the factors discussed in both (1) and (2) above and therefore is of concern to **both pharmacy and pharmacology.** It is considered in Chapter 5.

3. Once in the systemic blood, the free drug dissolved in the plasma water may be reversibly taken up into red cells or reversibly bound to plasma proteins.

4. The free drug may be taken up into the liver or other tissues, where it can be converted into metabolites of the original drug. These may be eliminated in the bile, and thus reach the intestine, where they can either be excreted in the feces or be reabsorbed and carried in the portal blood back to the liver (enterohepatic circulation). Alternatively, the metabolites (and the original drug itself) may pass back from the liver into the general circulation and be carried to all other organs and tissues.

5. Among these other organs is the kidney, where both the drug and its metabolites may be filtered by the glomerulus or secreted by the tubule into the urine. However, depending on the concentration, the degree of ionization of the drug at the pH of the urine, and other factors, some of the drug may be reabsorbed from the urine by the tubule and pass back into the blood. This is discussed in greater detail in Chapter 6. Another organ to which the drug is carried is the lung. If the drug or its metabolite is volatile, it can pass from the blood into the alveolar air and be eliminated in the breath. This is particularly important for terminating the action of volatile anaesthetics (see Chapter 20) and is also the basis of the Breathalyzer test for blood alcohol level (see Chapter 22).

6. Some tissues and organs through which the drug passes are not affected by it and therefore simply act as reservoirs that form part of the drug's volume of distribution. This influences the equilibrium concentration of drug in the plasma after administration of a specified dose.

   All of the processes mentioned in (2) to (6) determine the rate at which the concentrations of the drug and its metabolites in the plasma and tissues rise and fall and also determine the maximum concentrations reached after a given dose. Together, these factors influence the speed of onset and duration of action of drug effects. The study of the time course of drug concentration and the factors affecting it is called **pharmacokinetics.** It is discussed in detail in Chapter 5. The pharmacokinetic features of a drug determine the dosage schedule that is used clinically (see Chapter 7) and therefore influence the **therapeutic program.**

7. Most (but not all) drugs bind to relatively specific receptors on the surface or in the interior of the tissue cells on which the drugs act. The binding of a drug to its receptor may initiate biochemical or biophysical changes that lead to its characteristic effects on body functions, and the drug is called an **agonist** at that receptor. In other cases, a drug may bind to a receptor without initiating any change, but it may prevent another substance from gaining access to the receptor where it normally acts; many drugs function in this way as **receptor blockers** or **antagonists.** In a small number of cases, a drug may bind to a receptor and produce changes *opposite* to those produced by other agonists; it is then called an **inverse agonist** (see Chapter 23).

The study of these mechanisms of drug action is called **pharmacodynamics,** and the quantitative study of the relations among drug dose, concentration, and magnitude of effect is called **pharmacometrics.** These topics are discussed in Chapter 7. The ability of a drug to combine with its receptor depends on specific features of the molecular structure of both the drug and the receptor. Therefore, the study of pharmacodynamics overlaps with the field of **pharmaceutical chemistry,** which deals with the design and chemical synthesis of drugs and the study of their **structure–activity relationships.**

In addition to these basic divisions of the subject matter of pharmacology, there are other division schemes based on different criteria. For example, pharmacology may be divided according to the following:

1. The organ system of primary interest (e.g., neuropharmacology, cardiovascular pharmacology, renal pharmacology)

2. The techniques used (e.g., biochemical pharmacology, molecular pharmacology, behavioural pharmacology, immunopharmacology)

3. The purpose or application to which the knowledge is put, for example
   - Clinical pharmacology: the study of pharmacokinetics and pharmacodynamics in patients receiving drugs for the treatment of disease, including the effect of disease on the action and disposition of drugs
   - Genetic factors causing variation in the response to drugs; these studies may relate to variations in the interaction between a drug and a single gene (pharmacogenetics) or between a drug and many different genes (pharmacogenomics)
   - Toxicology: the study of drugs that act as poisons rather than as agents for the treatment of disease; it includes specialized subdivisions such as forensic toxicology, clinical toxicology, industrial and environmental toxicology, and behavioural toxicology
   - Agricultural pharmacology: the use of drugs for pest control

# DRUG CLASSIFICATION

## Classification Based on Origin

Much "drug" use through the centuries has been based on symbolic or magical thinking. For example, a plant with liver-shaped leaves was used to "treat" illnesses thought to arise in the liver. Nevertheless, throughout human history there have been keen observers who, by chance observation or by systematic trial and error, have recognized the interesting or useful drug effects of certain substances. The discovery that curare arrowhead poisons could paralyze a targeted animal, that foxglove plant (digitalis) could relieve fluid retention in certain patients with heart failure, and that the nightshade plant could dilate the pupils of the eyes and dry the mouth are all examples of the accumulation of knowledge by careful observers over the course of centuries or millennia.

With the growth of modern science over the last three centuries, systematic observation of the effects of exogenous substances on the body has given rise to techniques for screening possible new drugs. At first, the substances screened were natural materials gathered by botanists, anthropologists, and explorers. Later, chemists extracted and purified the active ingredients of these natural materials and analyzed their chemical structure, and later still, they synthesized wholly new compounds that did not exist in nature but that, by analogy with natural compounds, might be expected to have drug effects.

On the basis of their origin, drugs may be placed in the following five broad categories.

## Natural preparations, or galenicals

These are relatively crude preparations obtained by drying or extracting plant or animal materials (e.g., digitalis leaf, tincture of belladonna, and desiccated thyroid). This type of medicine, originally prepared by medicine men or priest–physicians, and later by apothecaries or physicians, dates back to prehistoric times. An early careful and systematic description of all known such drugs was written by the Greek physician Galen (A.D. 130–200), who practised in Rome. In Galen's honour, such drugs later became known as "galenicals." Even now, new drugs are found from such materials, but they are no longer likely to be used as galenicals; pharmaceutical chemistry is more likely to carry them immediately to the next stage.

## Pure compounds

These are isolated from natural sources by physical and chemical extraction and purification procedures. A number of classical examples are shown in Table 1-1. The first to be isolated was morphine, which Sertürner purified from opium in 1805. Many important drugs have come from natural sources, even in the last few years. Modern examples include penicillin and numerous other antibiotics that derive from a variety of moulds and fungi, and various anti-cancer and chemotherapeutic drugs such as vinblastine and vincristine, obtained from certain varieties of periwinkle plant, or paclitaxel from the Pacific yew.

## Semi-synthetic substances

These are obtained by chemical modification of pure compounds obtained from natural sources. For example, acetylating two hydroxyl groups in morphine yields diacetylmorphine (heroin), changing a side group in penicillin yields oxacillin, and inserting a fluorine atom in the adrenal steroid hydrocortisone yields fludrocortisone. Many such semi-synthetic modifications result in dramatic improvements of the parent compounds with respect to potency, specificity, and duration of action.

| TABLE 1-1 | Examples of Drugs Derived from Plant Materials in Various Parts of the World | |
| --- | --- | --- |
| **Plant Material or Galenical Preparation** | **Pure Compound** | **Original Source** |
| Tincture of belladonna | Atropine | Orient (ancient) |
| Coca leaves | Cocaine | Peru, Bolivia |
| Curare | *d*-Tubocurarine | Amazon Basin |
| Digitalis leaf, tincture | Digoxin, etc. | England |
| Ephedra | Ephedrine | China |
| Calabar bean | Eserine | West Africa |
| Opium | Morphine | Greece (ancient) |
| Tobacco | Nicotine | North and Central America |
| Cinchona bark | Quinine | Peru |
| Rauwolfia | Reserpine | India |

### Purely synthetic compounds

The first barbiturate was synthesized in 1902. Most drugs are now synthetic. Some of these substances were synthesized for other purposes, and medical uses were discovered accidentally. For example, disulfiram was invented as an agent to vulcanize rubber: the observation that rubber-factory workers underwent very bad reactions when they drank alcohol led to its use as an anti-alcoholism drug. In contrast, other drugs (e.g., dimercaprol [BAL], an antidote for arsenic or mercury poisoning) have been synthesized deliberately on the basis of predicted chemical properties. Still others have been synthesized on the basis of knowledge gained from the study of semi-synthetic modifications of existing compounds. By learning which molecular features are necessary for which drug actions, pharmaceutical chemists are increasingly able to "custom design" a molecule to produce or enhance a desired pharmacological effect while minimizing undesired effects. More recently, dramatic advances in the physical methods of studying the molecular structures of receptors have permitted drugs to be designed to fit a particular receptor and interact with it in a predetermined way, as either an agonist or an antagonist.

### Biological drugs

In the last few years, there has been a rapid development of biological products, such as monoclonal antibodies (see Chapter 40), to be used as drugs with highly selective and potent action. For example, the blood clotting process (see Chapter 38) involves a complex sequence of enzymatic reactions that convert soluble fibrinogen into a fibrin clot. Very small amounts of monoclonal antibodies against the enzymes catalyzing these reactions can interrupt the clotting process very rapidly and selectively, with very low risk of unwanted side effects. If necessary, the interrupted clotting process can then be restored quickly by administering the purified enzyme. Many such immunologically based drugs have been introduced into clinical practice in the last few years.

## Classification Based on Use

Most textbooks of pharmacology, particularly those intended for students and practitioners of medicine, dentistry, pharmacy, nursing, and other health sciences, classify drugs according to the organ system upon which they exert their most prominent actions or the therapeutic use to which they are put. For example, drugs are classed as antibiotics, anti-arrhythmic agents, diuretics, anticonvulsants, and so forth. There are some valid arguments against this method of classification: almost every drug has more than one effect and acts in more than one tissue, and different drugs may produce a similar therapeutic effect by quite different means. Nevertheless, this is still the most commonly used system of classification, and in deference to tradition and clinical usefulness, it is also employed in this book.

## DRUGS AND SOCIETY

Human society comes into contact with drugs in many different ways:

1. **Medical prescription** or therapeutic use. This is the source of exposure that receives the most attention in medical teaching, but it is by no means the most common.

2. **Over-the-counter sale,** without prescription. These drugs are also intended primarily for "therapeutic" purposes, even though their use is most commonly not under medical supervision. A huge range of drugs (cough remedies, analgesics, topical antiseptics, local anaesthetics, antihistamines, hypnotics, and so forth) can be bought in this way. Many are quite potent and are seriously toxic if used improperly.

3. **Dietary supplements and herbal preparations.** These preparations, which may be bought in pharmacies, grocery stores, and herbalist shops, are not classed officially as drugs and are not yet subject to the same strict controls of manufacture and sale as prescription and over-the-counter drugs. Nevertheless, many of these preparations have definite (and sometimes potent) pharmacological actions, and people use them for self-medication of various health problems. These actions are often of considerable medical importance because they can give rise to unrecognized interactions with prescribed drugs that the patient is also taking.

4. **Non-medical use.** Alcohol, cannabis, and a wide range of other psychoactive substances (i.e., that affect mood, perception, psychomotor performance, and emotional responses) dominate this category. Some are legally available, some are diverted from legal production to the illicit market, and some are manufactured illegally. All such use carries the potential risk of abuse, with the attendant problems of toxicity and dependence (see Chapter 70).

5. **Industrial use.** Many preservatives, artificial flavourings, colourings, and fillers are added to processed foods and even to pharmaceutical preparations. Though each is kept to a level considered safe in any individual product, very little is known about cumulative totals, interactions between substances, or how these may contribute to low-grade toxicity in the consumer. Other substances that are used in industrial processes may have toxic effects on the workers who use them (e.g., the effects of disulfiram on rubber workers, mentioned above).

6. **Agricultural use.** Widespread use of pesticides has contributed greatly to increased agricultural productivity in many parts of the world. However, pesticides, weed killers, and herbicides (together with industrial wastes, automobile exhaust fumes, and other prod-

ucts of human industry) contribute to total environmental toxicity.

7. **Accident.** Apart from the obvious cases of accidental poisoning, which come to hospital emergency rooms, and deliberate suicidal or homicidal poisonings, which are dealt with by forensic toxicologists as well as hospitals, there are natural accidents. For example, a certain fungus that grows on peanuts can generate a very potent carcinogen (aflatoxin); a fungus that grows on rye generates ergot alkaloids, which on occasion cause serious poisoning.

Exposure to drugs by all these means has become far more common as a result of population growth, chemical inventions, improved means of communication, and industrialization. Apart from the accident category, the other forms of exposure all carry certain benefits and certain hazards, but the optimum balance of benefits and risks is often hard to define. It depends to a large extent on the scale of social values. This is particularly true of the fourth, fifth, and sixth categories, but is also true of the first and second.

Therefore, most societies control the availability, quality, and permitted uses of drugs. Such controls are generally pragmatic rather than theoretical. To a large extent, they are handled by government administrative regulation, but certain broad principles and policies are laid down in legislation, which differs to some extent from country to country.

## DRUG STANDARDS AND REFERENCES

### Standards of Formulation

The rapid progress in the chemical industry within the past century has altered the nature of pharmacy, pharmacology, and therapeutics. Because most drugs used nowadays are potent pure chemicals, they must be prepared and used under strict controls. Therefore, their definition and standardization are regulated by law in terms of name, purity, potency, and preparation, and so is their distribution to the public.

The active drugs themselves, as well as the forms in which they are dispensed, must be carefully controlled if the effectiveness of drug treatment is to be assured. For application in drug therapy, most chemicals have to be put into tablets, capsules, ampoules, aerosols, ointments, solutions, or suppositories. The drug must have the highest purity possible that is compatible with chemical stability and economic feasibility. It must have appropriate particle or crystal size. It must be compatible with ingredients commonly used to give bulk to a tablet and to regulate its hardness, cohesiveness, and its rate of disintegration in gastric or intestinal juice. The tablet may have to be protected from light and may have to withstand stor-

age in tropical climates. It may require a corrective for taste. It should not explode in the patient's stomach (as have some tablets used in the treatment of tuberculosis). Above all, it must release the drug in such a manner that the drug will be absorbed at a suitable rate. There are equivalent problems in compounding drug vehicles other than tablets. All this falls in the domain of **pharmacy,** and all of it is subject to controls and standards.

The standards are published in **pharmacopoeias** such as the *British Pharmacopoeia (BP)*, the *U.S. Pharmacopeia (USP)*, the *Codex Français,* and the *International Pharmacopoeia (IP)*. These books are revised periodically, and supplements to them may be issued between editions. A drug listed in a pharmacopoeia is termed an "official" drug because it enjoys official recognition by a government. Canada has no pharmacopoeia of its own, but other pharmacopoeias that have official status may be used.

There are also a number of reference books that are widely used in North America (although they do not have official status in every Canadian province). Some examples are listed below.

*Pediatric Dosage Handbook:* American Pharmaceutical Association

*European Pharmacopoeia*

*U.S. National Formulary (NF):* American Pharmaceutical Society

*American Medical Association Drug Evaluations*

*Accepted Dental Therapeutics (ADT):* Published annually by the American Dental Association, this is a convenient and useful reference for dentists. It includes information on (1) drugs of recognized value in dentistry, (2) drugs of uncertain status more recently proposed for use by dentists, and (3) some drugs now generally regarded as obsolete.

*Physician's Desk Reference (PDR):* Published annually by Medical Economics, this reference for American practitioners lists and describes prescribing information approved by the U.S. Food and Drug Administration (FDA), including indications, contraindications, effects, dosages, routes, and methods.

*Compendium of Pharmaceuticals and Specialties (CPS):* Published annually by the Canadian Pharmaceutical Association for use by Canadian practitioners, this publication is very useful. It describes many of the prescription drugs available in Canada, giving their pharmacokinetic features, mechanisms of action, uses, contraindications, adverse reactions, dosage, and available formulations.

## DRUG NOMENCLATURE

Many names given to drugs are often confusing to those who are not familiar with the nomenclature system. When a drug is first synthesized and subjected to initial screening, it is usually referred to, in the scientific literature, by its chemical name or by a code number indicating the manufacturer and test document file number (e.g., R015-4513, EN-2234A). When it reaches the stage of clinical testing, it usually receives a more convenient but unofficial short name. After it comes into general use, it may receive other names indicative of different levels of medical or official approval. When a pharmaceutical company finally receives permission to bring the new drug to market, it is usually given a proprietary (trade, or brand) name, which carries the registered trademark symbol. The use of this name is protected by law and is restricted to the firm that introduces the preparation. Thus, the same drug may be known (unfortunately) under several different names simultaneously. For instance, the drug may be recognized:

1. by its chemical name
2. by its non-proprietary drug name (sometimes called "generic name")
   - by its official names (in pharmacopoeias)
   - by its approved names (not yet in pharmacopoeias)
       U.S. Adopted Name (USAN; Joint Committee of AMA, U.S. Pharmacopeial Commission, and American Pharmaceutical Association)
       Canadian Proper Names
       Approved names, British Pharmacopoeial Commission
3. by its proprietary name: manufacturer's trade name, registered by the owner, somewhat like a copyright
4. by its common name

**EXAMPLES:**
1. *Chemical names:* 1-methyl-4-phenyl-4-carbethoxypiperidine; 1-methyl-4-phenylisonipecotic acid ethyl ester
   *Official names:* pethidine (BP), meperidine (USP), isonipecaine (IP)
   *Proprietary names:* Demerol, Dolantin, Dolantol
2. *Chemical name:* ortho-acetoxybenzoic acid
   *Official names:* acetylsalicylic acid (BP), aspirin (USP)
   *Proprietary names:* Aspirin (in Canada only), Empirin, Entrophen, and many more

It is in the financial interest of the manufacturer to popularize and use the trade name only, because the patent (the exclusive right to sell the drug) will last only 17 years in the United States and 20 years in Canada, but the trade name registration (the right to sell a drug by a given name) lasts for at least 50 years. Even when exclusivity ends, the value of brand-name recognition goes on and may be significant. The time from patenting to marketing is usually 8 to 10 years, and the cost of development is typically in the hundreds of millions of dollars per drug. In addition, the patent may not be valid because someone else may have published an article or may own a patent with close to the same idea. If the drug is really very good, it will also be produced in a country that does not have reciprocal

patent laws (e.g., Italy, Argentina, or Hungary). It is easy to appreciate why a company that has spent hundreds of millions of dollars on drug development will encourage the use of its own brand name. As a rule, the brand name is chosen to be simple and euphonious; the non-proprietary name tends to be difficult and often does not suggest its use or chemical nature. A **Joint Committee on Nomenclature of the American Medical Association, American Pharmaceutical Association, and U.S. Pharmacopeial Commission** has made substantial progress in correcting this situation, and thus, the United States Adopted Name (USAN) is easier to remember and suggests the nature of the drug. The names, chemical structures, and uses of newly introduced drugs are published in the *Journal of the American Medical Association (JAMA)*.

We recommend use of the official, USAN (United States), proper (Canada), or approved (United Kingdom) names, which are used in most reputable journals and which are almost always the same because of international co-operation in naming. If a drug becomes official, the USAN, proper, or approved name will almost certainly become the official name.

The use of trade names can sometimes complicate the exchange of medical information about a patient. The same product is often produced by several reliable manufacturers, all using different brand names, and this can give rise to confusion if different physicians are prescribing drugs for the same patient.

In fairness to pharmaceutical firms, it must be pointed out that some trade name preparations adhere to standards that may be higher than those called for by pharmacopoeial specification. A physician who prefers to use a particular company's product can do so by specifying the brand or the company when writing a prescription. However, generic products now have to conform to high standards of purity and efficacy, as specified in the regulations concerning **bioequivalence** that many governments have put in place. By international agreement, two different drug preparations are considered bioequivalent if equal doses of the two preparations, in the same dosage form (e.g., tablet, capsule), produce very similar pharmacokinetic measures. The measures include the area under the concentration–time curve and the peak concentration. The means of these measures, taking into account their variation, should differ by less than certain pre-specified limits. By these measures, generic products are usually quite reliable and less expensive than brand-name products.

## OTHER SOURCES OF INFORMATION

The material in this book is only a *starting point* in learning about drug actions and drug use. All medical students should consider, and have access to, other reference sources. For anyone with a special interest in drugs or drug research, many scientific journals publish peer-reviewed articles on different aspects of the field. Some cover a broad range of subject matter, for example, *Drugs, Pharmacological Reviews, Journal of Pharmacology and Experimental Therapeutics, British Journal of Pharmacology and Chemotherapy, European Journal of Pharmacology,* and *Canadian Journal of Physiology and Pharmacology.* Others cover much more specialized topics, for example, *Biochemical Pharmacology, Psychopharmacology, Clinical Pharmacokinetics, European Journal of Clinical Pharmacology,* and *Molecular Pharmacology.*

A steadily growing number of journals now appear in both printed and electronic form. The great advantage of electronic journals is that they can be accessed at any hour via the Internet. For some journals, access to some, if not all, of the articles is free to anyone; for others, access is limited to individual subscribers of the journal or to registered staff or student users of a university or hospital library that subscribes to the journal. It is then possible, in most cases, to download a copy of the article one wishes to read.

Other electronic resources include such things as the Cochrane reviews (a series of careful evaluations of the literature on specific topics), various databases, and official reports of government or professional agencies covering specific topics that may be of interest to scientists or to the general public. A number of scientific encyclopedias, such as the *Encyclopedia of Neuroscience*, also have electronic editions.

Most teaching hospitals have drug information centres that can provide useful information to treatment staff, students, and the general public about the nature, actions, and adverse effects of drugs.

Most of the major medical journals continue to present drug information in the form of editorials or reviews.

*The Medical Letter on Drugs and Therapeutics* represents a specialized effort to provide practising physicians and medical students with unbiased data and critical information on newly introduced drugs. It compares new drugs with older agents and critically analyzes claims put forth by manufacturers. The information presented is concise and usually up-to-date. For those who wish to know more about the origins and history of drugs, two very interesting older books and two recent reviews on modern methods of drug discovery are listed in the Suggested Readings below.

## SUGGESTED READINGS

Drug discovery [special section]. *Science.* 2000;287:1960-1973.

Efron DH, Holmstedt B, Kline NS, eds. *Ethnopharmacologic Search for Psychoactive Drugs.* Washington, DC: US Department of Health, Education and Welfare; 1967.

Endrenyi L, Midha KK. Individual bioequivalence–has its time come? *Eur J Pharm Sci.* 1998;6:271-277.

Gray J, ed. *Therapeutic Choices.* 4th ed. Ottawa, Ontario: Canadian Pharmacists Association; 2003.

Holmstedt B, Liljestrand G, eds. *Readings in Pharmacology.* New York, NY: Macmillan; 1963.

Rethinking drug discovery [special section]. *Science.* 2004; 303:1795-1822.

# 2

# Drug Solubility, Absorption, and Movement across Body Membranes

## H KALANT, C WOODLAND, AND P SEEMAN

In Chapter 1, a general outline of the fate of drugs in the body was given, beginning with absorption from the site of administration and going on to distribution throughout the body, including the sites of action, biotransformation, and elimination (see Fig. 1-1). All these processes together determine the speed of onset of drug action, its intensity, and its duration.

When a drug is used therapeutically, it is usually desirable to send an adequate concentration to the site of action as quickly as possible and to maintain that concentration as continuously and evenly as possible. To achieve this, one must understand how the route and rate of administration are chosen and what factors affect the speed with which the drug reaches its sites of action and elimination.

## ROUTES OF DRUG ADMINISTRATION

### Topical

The simplest mode of administration is direct local application of the drug to the place where it must act. Such local application is called "topical" (from the Greek *topos* = a place). This most often means direct application to an accessible body surface. Examples include the use of ointments, creams, lotions, powders, or sprays applied to the **skin** (see Chapter 66); **eye** drops and ophthalmic ointments; **nose** drops and sprays; **ear** drops; and solutions or sprays for use in the **mouth, throat, rectum, vagina,** and **urethra.**

However, drugs applied to mucous membranes can often be absorbed rapidly enough to produce actions in the rest of the body. When cocaine was first used as a local anaesthetic, it was widely adopted in rectal and urological surgery and was used in large amounts that gave rise to many poisonings, including fatal ones. "Topical use" refers to the application of sufficiently small volumes and low concentrations to ensure that the drug acts *only* at that site.

Occasionally, drugs are injected directly into **body cavities** for local action at those sites. For example, cor-ticosteroids may be injected into a joint or a bursa for treatment of a sharply localized arthritis or bursitis not caused by infection. Antibiotics may be injected into the pleural space or into an abscess cavity for treatment of a local pocket of infection surrounded by fibrous tissue that hinders the antibiotic from getting there via the bloodstream. **Intrathecal injection** is employed to administer drugs directly into the cerebrospinal fluid (CSF) bathing the central nervous system, bypassing the blood–brain barrier and the blood–CSF barrier. The doses injected in such cases are enough to produce fairly high local concentrations, but not so large as to produce significant levels in the circulating blood when the drug diffuses away from the site of injection. Therefore, intrathecal injection can properly be considered a form of topical administration.

### Percutaneous

Drug absorption through the intact skin is proportional to the lipid solubility of the drug (the epidermis behaves as a lipoid barrier; the dermis is freely permeable). Absorption can be enhanced by suspending the drug in an oily vehicle. This is generally not an efficient method for delivering drugs to the systemic circulation. However, a number of lipid-soluble drugs are now marketed for percutaneous administration, such as nitroglycerin transdermal patches to treat angina pectoris, scopolamine plasters to prevent motion sickness, nicotine patches to aid cessation of smoking, and patches for administration of male and female sex hormones.

Even though the skin is an effective barrier that hinders the transport of almost all substances, there are very few substances to which it is *totally* impermeable. Even a heavy metal like mercury can be absorbed to some degree through the skin. Indeed, absorption through the skin is an important route of poisoning in humans and animals following accidental exposure to foreign chemicals such as insecticides containing parathion, malathion, or nicotine.

## Gastrointestinal Tract

### Oral mucosa (sublingual)

A number of drugs can be absorbed through the thinner portions of the oral mucosa. A familiar example is nitroglycerin in the form of small tablets that are placed under the tongue (sublingual). The drug is rapidly absorbed, providing fast relief of anginal attacks. Drugs absorbed sublingually or buccally are not exposed to gastric and intestinal digestive juices and are not subject to immediate passage through the liver (i.e., no biotransformation) before entering the systemic circulation. Many drugs, however, are not capable of penetrating the oral mucosa in significant amounts, and others are too irritating to be held in the mouth.

### Stomach and intestine (oral, per os, p.o., PO)

Absorption from the upper gastrointestinal tract depends on many factors, such as pH of the gastrointestinal contents, gastric emptying rate, intestinal motility, solubility of solid drugs, concentration of drug solutions, stability of drugs in gastrointestinal fluids, and binding to other substances in the gastrointestinal contents.

The relatively large blood supply of the stomach and small intestine, combined with the opportunity for prolonged contact of a drug with the relatively large epithelial surface, aids the absorption of most drugs. The length of time a substance remains in the stomach, however, is the greatest variable affecting the extent of gastric absorption. The rate at which the stomach empties its contents into the small intestine is influenced by the volume, viscosity, and composition of those contents, by physical activity and the position of the body, by the secretion of enteric hormones, by the ingested drugs themselves, and by many other factors. Only when a drug is taken with water on a relatively empty stomach is it likely to reach the small intestine fairly rapidly.

### Rectal mucosa (suppositories, enemas)

Drugs that escape absorption in the small intestine may continue to be absorbed during their passage through the colon. Moreover, the terminal segment of the large intestine, the rectum, can serve as a useful site for drug administration, particularly when the oral route is unsuitable because of unconsciousness, nausea, or vomiting or because the drugs have objectionable taste or odour or are destroyed by acid or digestive enzymes. This route also protects susceptible drugs from the biotransformation reactions that would occur on first passage through the liver if they were taken by mouth (see Chapter 4), because the blood draining the lower part of the rectum passes into the inferior vena cava via the internal pudendal veins rather than through the portal vein and liver. However, absorption by this route is often irregular and incomplete, and some drugs cause irritation of the rectal mucosa.

## Pulmonary Epithelium

Gases, vapours, and aerosols can be inhaled and absorbed through the alveolar surface or the bronchial mucosa, giving rapid access to the circulation. The drugs may be intended for local action (e.g., anti-asthmatic agents) or for action elsewhere in the body (e.g., general anaesthetics, amyl nitrite for angina pectoris, nicotine or cannabinoids inhaled by smoking).

## Injection

This is also called "parenteral administration" (from the Greek *para* = beside, i.e., not in, and *enteron* = gut). The main advantages are more rapid and more predictable systemic drug levels, because absorption is bypassed, and more accurate dose selection. General disadvantages are the need for strict asepsis, the possibility of pain, and some difficulty in self-administration of drugs by injection. There is also a higher risk of toxicity because of rapid attainment of high drug levels. Moreover, injectable drugs are usually more expensive than other preparations of the same drugs.

### Subcutaneous injection (s.c., SC, subcut.)

Only non-irritating drugs can be administered in this way. Large volumes may be painful because of tissue distention. This route provides even and slow absorption, producing sustained drug effects. Vasoconstrictors, such as adrenaline, can be added to the drug solution to decrease the rate of absorption from a subcutaneous injection site. Conversely, the enzyme hyaluronidase breaks down mucopolysaccharides in connective tissue and thus aids the spread of drug solutions injected subcutaneously, leading to much faster absorption.

### Intramuscular injection (i.m., IM)

Aqueous solutions are rapidly absorbed from deep intramuscular injection sites. Slow and even absorption becomes possible if the drugs are suspended or dissolved in oil, which forms a depot in the muscle. Irritating substances or large volumes may cause pain, and drugs dissolved in strongly acidic or alkaline solutions can cause sterile abscesses if injected intramuscularly.

### Intravenous administration (i.v., IV)

**Rapid injection** permits the desired blood concentration of a drug to be obtained accurately and immediately, without variation due to irregular absorption or passage through the liver. However, once the drug is injected, its rapid removal is impossible, so there is greater risk of toxicity. Infection, vascular injury, and extravasation of drug into tissues surrounding the injection site are also possible consequences. Moreover, rapid intravenous injection of a small volume of drug solution results in that volume travelling initially as a *bolus* through the vascular system, and it usually takes several complete circuits around the vascular tree before the drug is evenly distributed through the whole blood volume.

Slow infusion (over 20 minutes or more), in addition to the general advantages of intravenous administration, allows the level of the drug in the blood to be "titrated" by proper adjustments of flow rate and drug concentration. Infusions are particularly useful to maintain constant blood levels of drugs over extended periods of time. This lessens the risk of irrevocable administration of an overdose. However, expertise is required to minimize the risk of vascular injury, infection, and accidents (such as severing of infusion lines, bleeding, and air embolism).

### Intra-arterial injection (i.a.)

This method is occasionally employed to direct small volumes of drug solutions at high concentrations to specific target tissues or organs, increasing the drug uptake at those sites but minimizing the effects elsewhere by subsequent dilution of the remaining drug in the general circulation.

### Injection into body cavities

The peritoneum provides a large absorption surface that permits rapid entry of drugs into the circulation. Therefore **intraperitoneal (i.p., IP) injection** is a common laboratory procedure, but it is seldom used clinically because of the risk of infection, intestinal or vascular injury, and adhesions.

### Choice of Route

❧ Regardless of the route of administration, a drug must be absorbed, reach its site of action, and interact in some way with the target tissue. These processes occur at very different speeds depending on the route of administration. This question will be dealt with in detail in Chapter 5, but Figure 2-1 illustrates the order of magnitude of the times required following oral administration.

The choice of route may depend on **therapeutic objectives.** For example, intravenous injection or inhalation may be selected to produce a rapid, intense, but rather short-lived effect, whereas oral dosage may be better and more convenient for long-lasting effects of relatively moderate and even intensity.

The choice of route is sometimes limited by the **properties of the drug.** Thiopental (for induction of anaesthesia), benzodiazepines (anti-anxiety and sedative agents), and phenytoin (anticonvulsant), for example, dissolve only in rather strongly alkaline solution. If they have to be given by injection for rapid effect, they can be injected intravenously (the blood buffers the pH of the drug solution) but not intramuscularly or subcutaneously. EDTA (ethylenediaminetetraacetic acid), a chelating agent for treating heavy-metal poisoning (see Chapter 72), is poorly absorbed from the gastrointestinal tract and is therefore

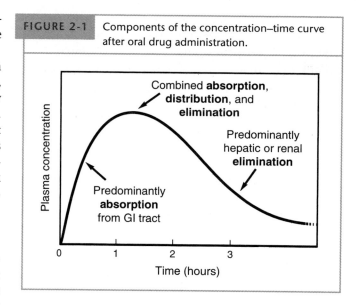

FIGURE 2-1  Components of the concentration–time curve after oral drug administration.

generally given by intravenous injection or infusion. Ordinary penicillin G is rapidly inactivated by gastric HCl. Therefore, if given by mouth, it must be given in huge doses to allow for the high percentage destroyed. In serious infections, this may introduce too much uncertainty, and the penicillin is more likely to be given by intramuscular or intravenous injection to ensure that high enough blood levels are reached.

## MOLECULAR PROPERTIES AND DRUG DISTRIBUTION

Once a drug has been administered, its uptake and distribution depend largely on the physical properties of the drug. It must usually pass from the site of administration across capillary walls into the circulation, and from the circulation it must again cross capillary walls to reach the site(s) of action. Even if the drug is applied topically, it will often have to cross cell membranes to reach specific intracellular sites of action, such as an enzyme or a nuclear receptor.

The ability of the drug to cross capillary walls, cell membranes, and other barriers to free movement depends to a large extent upon its solubilities in aqueous and lipid phases, its type and extent of ionization, and its molecular size and shape.

### Drug Solubility in Aqueous and Lipid Media

To be pharmacologically active, a drug must have some solubility within the aqueous fluids of the body in order to reach its site(s) of action. Although the water molecule as a whole is electrically neutral, it acts as a partial dipole because the O region of the molecule has a slight preponderance of negative charge (i.e., electrons) while the two H regions are preponderantly positive. Drugs that are positively or negatively charged can therefore associate readily with water molecules and are water-soluble (i.e., hydrophilic). In general, any chemical substituent group, when attached to a drug molecule, will affect the electron distribution within the drug and make that molecule either more water-soluble (more hydrophilic, less lipophilic) or more lipid-soluble (less hydrophilic, more lipophilic).

The absolute solubility of a drug is usually less important than its ratio of solubilities in lipid and water. When a drug molecule arrives at the cell membrane, this ratio determines whether it is more likely to stay in the water phase or to permeate into the fatty material of the cell membrane. Relative solubility of a drug is measured by its partition coefficient between oil and water or between water and an organic solvent such as chloroform or hexane. The oil/water partition coefficient ($P$) is the ratio of the drug concentration ($C$) in the oil phase to that in the water phase, as follows:

$$P_{oil/water} = \frac{C_{oil}}{C_{water}}$$

Using a radioisotopically labelled drug, it is also possible to measure the partition coefficient of a drug after equilibration between an aqueous buffer and a cell membrane preparation obtained by homogenizing and fractionating a tissue sample:

$$P_{m/buffer} = \frac{C_{membrane}}{C_{buffer\ or\ water}}$$

The membrane/buffer partition coefficients ($P_{m/b}$) of some basic structures are given in Table 2-1. The partition coefficients of various drugs can also be estimated arithmetically by using the $P_{m/b}$ values of the "parent drug" structures, multiplied by the partition ($P$) factors of common substituent groups shown in Table 2-2. If the $P$ factor for a substituent is greater than 1, this means that the substituent increases the solubility of the drug in the membrane (or in fat, or oil, or octanol) by the factor listed in the table. However, if the $P$ factor of the substituent is less than 1, the substituent reduces the solubility of the drug in the membrane (or oil) phase.

For example, isobutanol is

$$CH_3-CH-CH_2OH$$
$$|$$
$$CH_3$$

and its $P_{m/b}$ will be

$$= P_{m/b}\ (methane) \times (P_{CH_3})^3 \times P_{branch} \times P_{OH}$$
$$= 0.6 \times 3^3 \times 0.63 \times 0.07$$
$$= 0.71$$

This is quite close to the measured $P_{octanol/water}$ of 0.65. The lipid/water partition coefficient is still one of the

**TABLE 2-1** Membrane/Buffer Partition Coefficients of Some Basic Structures

| Parent Chemical | Structure | $P_{m/b}$ |
|---|---|---|
| Methane | $CH_4$ | 0.6 |
| Benzene ring | 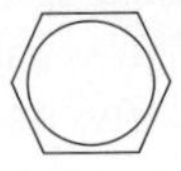 (hexagon with inscribed circle) | 25 |
| Cyclohexane | 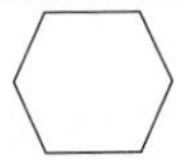 (hexagon) | 16 |

most valuable physicochemical predictors of drug distribution and potency.

## Molecular Size

The mass of a molecule is expressed in daltons (Da), 1 Da being $1/12$ of the mass of a single $^{12}C$ atom. Since there are $6.02 \times 10^{23}$ molecules in 1 g molecular weight of any substance, $1\ g = 1.66 \times 10^{24}$ Da. Most drugs, excluding peptides, have molecular weights of the order of 250 to 450

**TABLE 2-2** Partition Factors of Substituent Groups in Drug Molecules

| Substituent Group | Partition Factor — If on Aromatic Parent | Partition Factor — If on Aliphatic Parent |
|---|---|---|
| –I | × 13 | × 10 |
| –Br | × 7.3 | × 6 |
| –Cl | × 5 | × 2.5 |
| –$CH_2$ or –$CH_3$ | × 3 | × 3 |
| –F | × 1.4 | × 0.7 |
| –SH | × 1.3 | × 0.9 |
| –$OCH_3$ | × 0.95 | × 0.34 |
| –$NO_2$ | × 0.53 | × 0.14 |
| =S=O | × 0.3 | × 0.3 |
| –COOH | × 0.52 | × 0.2 |
| –OH | × 0.2 | × 0.07 |
| –C≡N | × 0.27 | × 0.15 |
| –$NH_2$ or –NH– or –$NH_3^+$ | × 0.06 | × 0.064 |
| –C=O | × 0.09 | × 0.062 |
| = (double bond) | × 0.5 | |
| Branching in C chain | × 0.63 | |
| Ring closure | × 0.9 | |

Da. Among the lightest are the anaesthetic gas nitrous oxide and ethanol, which have molecular weights of 44 and 46 Da, respectively. The muscle relaxant *d*-tubocurarine (curare) is unusually heavy, having a molecular weight of about 700 Da. Small peptides, like ADH (antidiuretic hormone), are in the 1000 to 2000 Da range. Insulin, a small protein, has a molecular weight of 6000 Da; that of albumin is 65 000 Da, while the heavier proteins may range into the hundreds of thousands or the millions of daltons (such as botulinum toxin). Thus, compared to protein molecules, which are the main building blocks of the body, most drug molecules are small. The importance of molecular size is explained in the section on passive diffusion of water-soluble drugs.

## Drug Ionization

Almost all drugs can be classed as uncharged drugs, organic acids, or organic amines (tertiary and quaternary). Organic acids and organic amines are markedly affected by pH (i.e., $-\log[H^+]$).

For example, a tertiary amine type of drug can exist in two forms, with or without a proton attached, that are in equilibrium with each other:

STOMACH  (Low pH)          INTESTINE  (High pH)

(protonated, charged)      (unprotonated, uncharged)

In a medium containing very few free protons (i.e., high pH or low $[H^+]$), such as the fluid in the lumen of the duodenum, the tertiary amine will not be protonated, and it will be uncharged, as shown on the right. This uncharged form of the tertiary amine has a high oil/water partition coefficient and readily permeates membranes. But in a medium containing many free protons (i.e., low pH), such as the gastric juice, the tertiary amine is protonated, resulting in a net positive charge for the molecule. This charged form of the tertiary amine has a low oil/water partition coefficient and, therefore, has a low rate of permeation through the mucosa.

In the case of an organic acid, the same general principles apply. The organic acid molecules also can exist in two forms, as shown below:

STOMACH  (Low pH)          INTESTINE  (High pH)

R – COOH        ⇌          R – COO$^-$

(protonated, uncharged)    (unprotonated, charged)

The protonated organic acid, however, is a neutral molecule and thus permeates the tissues readily, whereas the charged form does not.

The form of the drug (i.e., charged or uncharged) in the tablet, vial, or ampoule does not matter. Rather, it is the degree of ionization of the drug in the gastrointestinal contents or other body fluid that matters, and this depends upon the relation between the pH of the fluid in question and the p$K_a$ of the drug. $K_a$ is the acidic dissociation constant, that is, the equilibrium constant for the dissociation that yields free hydrogen ions:

Acidic drugs

Basic drugs

Obviously, this dissociation will be affected by the concentration of $H^+$ in the medium in which it is occurring (Fig. 2-2). High $H^+$ concentration (low pH) will drive the equilibrium to the left, in accordance with the law of mass action. The higher the pH of the fluid, the higher is the ionization of acidic drugs and the lower that of basic drugs; the lower the pH, the lower is the ionization of

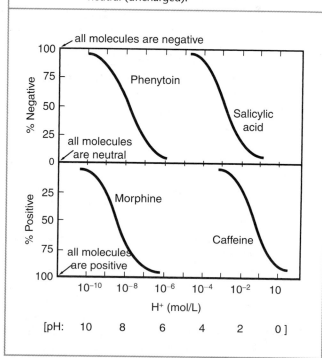

**FIGURE 2-2** Organic amines, such as morphine and caffeine, are positively charged (i.e., protonated) at high concentrations of protons (i.e., high $[H^+]$ or low pH). Organic acids, such as phenobarbital and salicylic acid, are also protonated at high concentrations of protons, which makes them neutral (uncharged).

acidic drugs and the higher that of basic drugs. Put in other terms, basic drugs tend to accept protons and to give them up only when the $H^+$ concentration of the surrounding fluid is very low. Therefore, the $K_a$ of basic drugs is low, and the $pK_a$ (i.e., $-\log K_a$) is high. Conversely, acidic drugs (by definition) give up protons readily, so their $K_a$ values are high and their $pK_a$ values are low. The $pK_a$ of a drug can be calculated from the Henderson–Hasselbalch equation. When the $pK_a$ of a drug equals the pH of the surrounding fluid, equal numbers of ionized and un-ionized molecules of the drug will be present, that is, **the $pK_a$ = pH at which 50% ionization occurs.**

## TISSUE BARRIERS TO DRUG MOVEMENT

Barriers to drug passage across membranes are of two quite different types. *Anatomical barriers* are formed by cells that are linked together in ways which block passage of drug molecules through the intercellular spaces. Examples described below are found in epithelial tissues and various types of endothelium. *Functional barriers* are formed by membrane transport systems that carry drug molecules back out of the cells against a concentration gradient, thus hindering the drug from attaining effective concentrations in tissues in which such transport systems are found. Examples described below include the blood–brain, blood–placenta, and blood–testis barriers. Table 2-3 summarizes the types of tissue barriers to drug permeation.

### Epithelial Barriers

The epithelial membranes of the skin, gastrointestinal lumen, cornea, and urinary bladder all seal off the outside world from the body tissues and fluids. The epithelial cells in these membranes are all joined to one another by occluding zonulae, which are continuous tight junctions somewhat resembling a necklace of pearls, made up of rows of membrane particles of one cell that are fused to rows of membrane particles of the adjacent cell. Thus, these zonulae completely block off the intercellular spaces (Fig. 2-3).

Since drug molecules cannot pass *between* the cells, they are forced to permeate the cell membrane and go *through* the cell. Very large molecules must undergo pinocytosis into the cell in order to traverse the barrier. The basement membrane, adjacent to all epithelial cells, is composed of a loose carbohydrate–protein matrix and offers no resistance to drug permeation.

### Capillary Barriers

There are three types of capillary structures in the body:

- Capillaries with maculae
- Fenestrated capillaries: in the kidney, pituitary, and exocrine glands
- Capillaries with occluding zonulae: all capillaries in the brain except those in the choroid plexus, median eminence, area postrema, pineal gland, and pituitary gland

#### Capillaries with maculae

These include the vast majority of capillaries throughout the body—in muscles, skin, peritoneum, gastrointestinal tract, bone, liver, heart. Their endothelial cells are joined together by macular junctions that do not form a continuous belt but exist only as patches of particles on each cell membrane fused to corresponding sets of particles on adjacent cell membranes (Fig. 2-4). Hence, there are intercellular spaces around these maculae.

| TABLE 2-3 | Summary of Types of Tissue Barriers to Drug Permeation | | |
| --- | --- | --- | --- |
| **Tissue** | | **Barrier** | **Permeability** |
| Epithelial | | | |
| Gastrointestinal mucosa, skin, cornea, lung, urinary bladder | | Occluding zonulae (continuous tight junctions) | Complete blockage of intercellular spaces; drugs must permeate cell membranes |
| Capillaries | | | |
| Most capillaries | | Maculae | Open intercellular spaces |
| Glomeruli, excretory and secretory organs | | Fenestrae | Free passage of drugs with MW <45 000 Da |
| Blood–brain barrier | | Occluding zonulae | Drugs permeate membranes |
| CSF | | | |
| Choroid plexus cells → CSF | | Occluding zonulae | Difficult passage |
| CSF → brain | | No barrier | Very easy passage |
| Placenta | | Limited by blood flow | Slow equilibration |
| Peritoneum | | Maculae | Free passage |

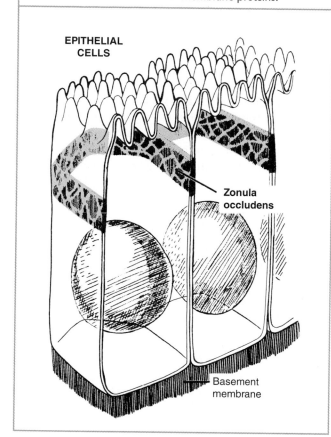

**FIGURE 2-3** The continuous tight junctions between adjacent cells in membranes separating the outside world from the body space are composed of "necklaces" of membrane proteins.

EPITHELIAL CELLS

Zonula occludens

Basement membrane

In addition to the intercellular spaces, these capillaries are rich in pinocytotic vesicles. Some of these vesicles transiently extend through the entire cytoplasm, forming a transient window (fenestra), or open channel, from the capillary lumen all the way to the basement membrane (see Fig. 2-4). Most drugs, regardless of solubility, readily pass through these transient fenestrae and the intercellular spaces. Drug molecules larger than 100 000 Da must be pinocytosed and transported by movement of the vesicles across the cells.

## Fenestrated capillaries

The excretory and secretory organs generally have fenestrated capillaries. Such tissues include the kidney glomeruli (Fig. 2-5), thyroid, pituitary, salivary glands, and pancreas. These fenestrae through the cytoplasm of the cell are longer-lasting, rather than transient as in the macular capillaries. They may be covered by a thin layer (a few angstroms) of non-membrane material, which essentially offers no barrier to any drug or solute existing free and unbound in the plasma. The basement membrane only holds back molecules larger than about 45 000 Da, such as drugs bound to plasma proteins.

## Occluded capillaries: the blood–brain barrier

The only capillaries in the body that have their intercellular spaces completely occluded by occluding zonulae are the brain capillaries. Almost all brain capillary endothelial cells are connected to one another by these occluding zonulae, which thus constitute the anatomical part of the blood–brain barrier (Fig. 2-6). There are five regions of the brain, however, where no occluding zonulae exist; consequently, these regions (listed below) are relatively permeable to drugs present in the blood:

1. Pituitary gland
2. Pineal body
3. Area postrema
4. Median eminence
5. Choroid plexus capillaries

✄ The area postrema contains the vomiting control centre, and since the capillaries there are fenestrated, the vomiting centre is readily accessible to foreign substances such as toxins and drugs circulating in the blood. This arrangement confers a survival advantage by causing the individual to vomit and thus empty the stomach of an ingested toxic material. However, the rest of the brain capillaries with occluding zonulae protect the brain from circulating toxins, drugs, and harmful solutes.

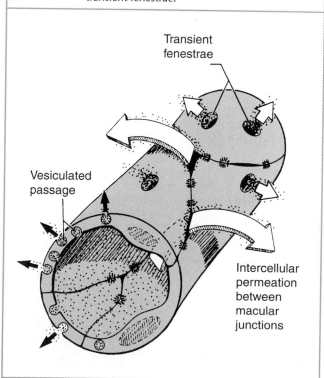

**FIGURE 2-4** Solute and drug permeation across capillary walls occurs via intercellular spaces and transient fenestrae.

Transient fenestrae

Vesiculated passage

Intercellular permeation between macular junctions

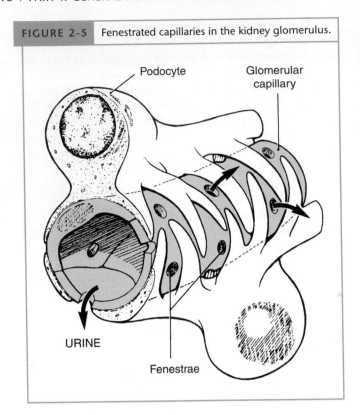

FIGURE 2-5   Fenestrated capillaries in the kidney glomerulus.

## Cerebrospinal Fluid Barriers to Drugs

The CSF is secreted by the epithelial cells of the choroid plexus, which are in contact with the brain ventricular spaces. These epithelial cells are connected by occluding zonulae (see Fig. 2-6, right panel). Therefore, only lipid-soluble drugs normally diffuse into the CSF from the blood (Fig. 2-7), whereas ionizable drugs can enter only if they have appropriate transporters.

The CSF is separated from the brain tissue by epithelial cells lining the ventricles, and these cells are not connected by occluding zonulae (see Fig. 2-6, middle panel). Hence, the CSF–brain barrier is extremely permeable, offering unrestricted passage of drug molecules between the CSF and the brain cells. Clinically, this can be taken advantage of. For example, penicillins are not very lipid-soluble and, therefore, penetrate poorly from the blood into the brain. However, a high concentration of penicillin in the brain (e.g., for treating a brain infection or abscess) can be obtained by intrathecal injections directly into the CSF. Otherwise, a very high oral dose must be administered to compensate for the small percentage that crosses the blood–brain barrier.

Another important feature of the blood–brain barrier is that these brain capillaries have very few vesicles, so there are no transient fenestrae.

## Drug Permeation across the Placenta

Because there is a limited amount of maternal blood flowing into the placenta, the shortest time for equilibration of a drug between mother and fetus is on the order of 10 to 15 minutes (see Chapter 61). This delay can be useful

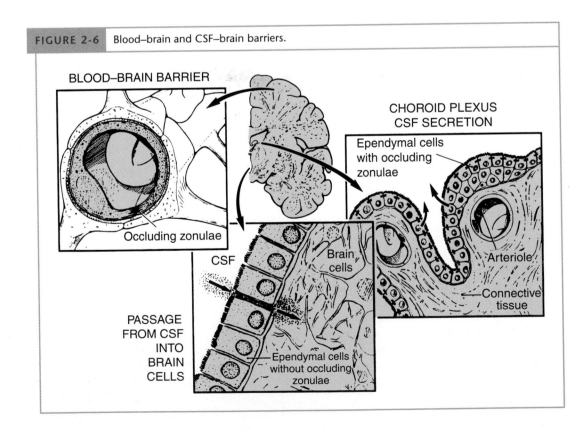

FIGURE 2-6   Blood–brain and CSF–brain barriers.

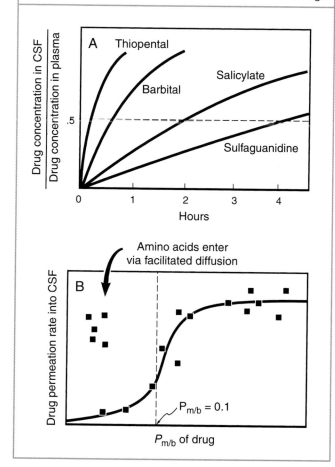

**FIGURE 2-7** (A) Effect of lipid solubility of drugs on rate of equilibration between CSF and plasma. Thiopental is the most lipid-soluble, and sulfaguanidine is the least. (B) General relation between drug permeation rate into CSF and the membrane/buffer partition coefficient. Some amino acids (e.g., L-dopa) have partition coefficients below 0.1 and would not enter the brain were it not for the fact that the brain capillaries have special facilitated diffusion mechanisms for these drugs.

Until proven otherwise, it is safe to assume that all drugs cross the placenta and that all drugs enter the breast milk. Children of opioid-addicted mothers may be born with depressed respiration and pinpoint pupils (see Chapter 19). Antipsychotic drugs are transferred across the placenta, and if the mother is on a rather high dosage, the offspring may be born with extrapyramidal signs (see Chapter 24). Erythromycin and tetracyclines cross the placenta in appreciable amounts and also appear in breast milk.

## Drug Permeation across the Peritoneum

The cells of the peritoneum and of the capillaries in the peritoneum are connected by macular ("spot") junctions. Hence, drugs and other solutes injected intraperitoneally have rapid and unrestricted access to the bloodstream. All drugs, whether lipid-soluble or not, whether charged or uncharged, readily permeate between the cells. Large molecules, however, must be carried across the peritoneum by pinocytosis.

## Drug Permeation across the Lung

As with all epithelial barriers to the outside world, the alveolar cells are also held together by continuous occluding zonulae. The cells are exceedingly rich in vesicles, and the cytoplasm is very thin. Therefore, there are probably many transient fenestrae formed by the momentary fusion of vesicles on both sides of the cell. This would account for the ready alveolar permeation of a water-soluble compound like nicotine.

General anaesthetics have no difficulty crossing the lung barrier since these drugs are quite lipid-soluble.

## MOLECULAR MECHANISMS OF DRUG ABSORPTION

✽The following molecular mechanisms account for most drug passage across membranes:

- Passive diffusion of water-soluble drugs
- Passive diffusion of lipid-soluble drugs
- Active transport
- Pinocytosis/phagocytosis
- Facilitated diffusion
- Passive filtration
- Drug passage via gap junctions

### Passive Diffusion of Water-Soluble Drugs

The passive diffusion of water-soluble drugs into cells largely depends on the molecular size of the drug. This is because the aqueous channels of the cell membrane are only about 8 to 10 Å wide and will restrict passage of any molecules larger than those with molecular weights of

because it permits the mother to be anaesthetized during the final stages of labour, with enough margin of safety (about 10 minutes) to avoid a serious depression of the baby's breathing after birth. (It is also worth noting that newborn babies are more resistant to general anaesthesia, so it takes more than the usual amount of anaesthetic to depress their breathing.)

The following are illustrative half-times for equilibration of various drugs between maternal blood and fetal cord blood:

| | |
|---|---|
| Anaesthetics | 8 minutes |
| Secobarbital | 8 minutes |
| Sulfadiazine | 1 hour |
| Curare | 4 hours |
| Penicillin | 10 hours |
| Streptomycin | 18 hours |

150 to 200 Da. These channels in the cell membrane belong to a family of more than 10 specific proteins (aquaporins), each of which consists of six transmembrane domains surrounding the central pore. Most of them allow only water to pass through, but at least one (aquaporin 3) also permits passage of small water-soluble molecules such as urea, ethanol, and glycerol. Since most drugs are either lipid-soluble or have molecular weights greater than 150 to 200 Da, passive diffusion through these channels is not the major mechanism of drug permeation.

Drugs that are highly water-soluble have low $P_{m/water}$, with values less than 2. Examples of such highly water-soluble drugs that appear to enter cells by simple passive diffusion through aqueous channels are listed in Table 2-4.

The permeation rate of water-soluble drugs falls as the molecular weight of the drug increases (Fig. 2-8). Tetracycline was formerly regarded as a puzzling exception, since the substance is quite water-soluble but has a high molecular weight and yet is able to enter cells readily. However, it is now known to be a substrate for the MDR1 drug transporter (see "Active Transport" and "Facilitated Diffusion" below).

## Passive Diffusion of Lipid-Soluble Drugs

The majority of lipid-soluble drugs permeate cell membranes by passive diffusion between the lipid molecules of the membrane. The permeation rate of a lipid-soluble drug depends on the following factors:

- Concentration (or dose) of drug
- Oil/water partition coefficient of drug
- Concentration of protons (i.e., [H⁺])
- Surface area of the absorbing membrane

Unlike the situation with highly water-soluble drugs, the permeation rate of lipid-soluble drugs does not vary systematically with the size of the molecule. However, extremely large drug molecules of around 1000 Da or more can be absorbed only by pinocytosis.

### Dependence on the concentration (or dose) of the drug

The overall rate of drug permeation increases if the amount of drug administered is increased; this simply means that "the more you give, the more is absorbed." However, the relation between dosage and absorption is not simple. Some drugs are absorbed in direct proportion to the amount given, while other drugs have a non-linear relationship. This may create serious difficulties in trying to regulate the drug dosage for a particular patient.

### Role of the oil/water (or membrane/buffer) partition coefficient

The oil/water partition coefficient of a drug is the principal factor determining the absorption of the drug in the body. In general, the higher the $P_{oil/water}$ or $P_{m/water}$ value of a drug, the more rapidly it will be absorbed across cell

| Drug | Molecular Weight (Da) | $P_{m/b}$ |
|---|---|---|
| Salts (e.g., Li₂CO₃) | ~70 | 0.0002 |
| Caffeine | 194 | 0.17 |
| Ephedrine | 165 | 1.6 |
| Low-molecular-weight diuretics (e.g., furosemide) | ~100 | |
| Ascorbic acid (vitamin C) | 176 | 0.02 |
| Sulfanilamide | 172 | 0.03 |
| Hydrogen peroxide | 34 | 0.02 |
| Nicotinamide (vitamin B₃) | 122 | 0.02 |
| Saccharin | 183 | 1.7 |
| Amino acids | 100–150 | 0.02 |

**TABLE 2-4** Examples of Water-Soluble Drugs That Enter Cells through Aqueous Channels in the Membrane

membranes and tissue barriers. There are many examples of this general rule in homologous series of drugs, such as barbiturates permeating the colon or carbamates permeating the stomach epithelium (Fig. 2-9).

The situation is not simple, however, since the small intestine (where the bulk of drug absorption occurs because of the large surface area involved) shows an optimum $P_{oil/water}$ value for maximum rate of drug absorption (Fig. 2-10). This optimum is explained by the fact that there is a hydrophilic barrier that drugs must pass through before they can permeate across the cell membrane itself. This hydrophilic barrier consists of the unstirred water

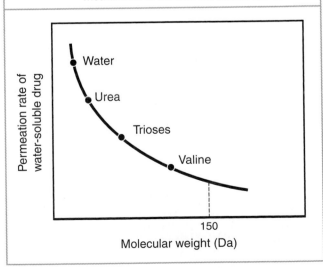

**FIGURE 2-8** Relation between size of water-soluble drugs and rate of permeation. Those above 150 Da permeate extremely slowly and need other mechanisms to traverse the membrane barriers.

FIGURE 2-9  The more lipid-soluble sedatives permeate more easily across the stomach mucosa.

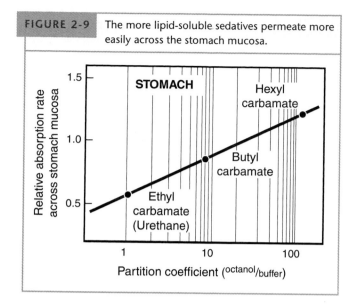

The chemical force that causes lipid-soluble drugs to move readily across membranes is termed the hydrophobic force (or bond). It is not that the membrane and the drug have any particular attraction to one another, but water "repels" the lipid-soluble drug, thus driving it into the membrane. Since the cell membrane is extremely thin (75 Å), it becomes fully loaded with drug molecules in a few milliseconds. Some of the drug molecules in the membrane then spill over into the water on the cytoplasmic side of the membrane, and the permeation process is thus completed.

## Dependence of drug absorption on pH and drug protonation

The net electrical charge on a drug molecule is very important in determining the rate of its absorption across cell membranes and tissue barriers.

The importance of H+ concentration in determining drug absorption is illustrated dramatically by an experiment described by Travell in 1940. He noted that large doses of strychnine (a tertiary amine), given by stomach tube to a cat, produced no toxic effects if the stomach fluid was kept at a high H+ concentration of about $10^{-2}$ mol/L

between the microvilli and immediately next to the surface sugar coat (glycocalyx) at the surface of the cell membrane (Fig. 2-11). In order to permeate a tissue barrier such as the intestinal mucosal epithelium, a drug must therefore have some water solubility as well as some lipid solubility. If it has a very high lipid solubility and very low water solubility, it will be blocked by the water barrier even though its extremely high lipid solubility would otherwise enable it to cross the membrane itself very readily. The point at which this "cut-off" of drug absorption occurs will vary with the cytological features of the membrane involved. For the colon and gastric mucosa, in which the glycocalyx is not nearly as thick as in the small intestine, it does not occur until the partition coefficient of the drug is at least 1000. For human skin, it lies somewhere between 100 and 1000 (Fig. 2-12).

FIGURE 2-11  The cell membrane surface of the small intestine is extensively covered with a rich glycocalyx (i.e., surface sugar coat). The membrane glycophorins (i.e., protein–sugar molecules) are heavily hydrated with water molecules "frozen" to the sugar hydroxyls. The ice-like water forms a hydrophilic barrier that accounts for the existence of a limiting value of lipid solubility for efficient permeation, shown in Figure 2-10.

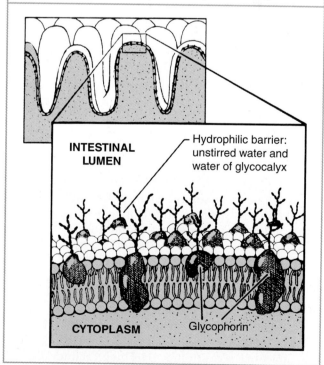

FIGURE 2-10  "Cut-off" phenomenon for lipid solubility as a factor increasing the absorption rate of a drug in the small intestine (see Fig. 2-11 for explanation).

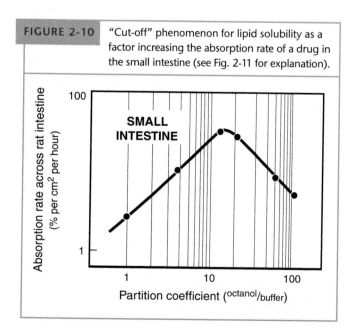

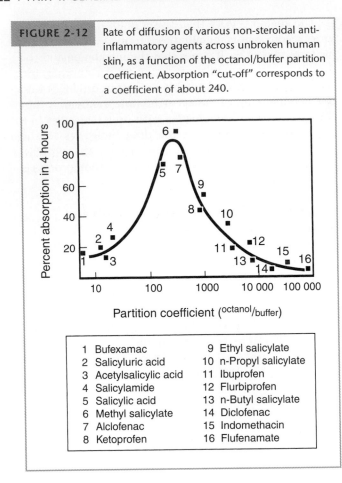

**FIGURE 2-12** Rate of diffusion of various non-steroidal anti-inflammatory agents across unbroken human skin, as a function of the octanol/buffer partition coefficient. Absorption "cut-off" corresponds to a coefficient of about 240.

| 1 | Bufexamac | 9 | Ethyl salicylate |
| 2 | Salicyluric acid | 10 | n-Propyl salicylate |
| 3 | Acetylsalicylic acid | 11 | Ibuprofen |
| 4 | Salicylamide | 12 | Flurbiprofen |
| 5 | Salicylic acid | 13 | n-Butyl salicylate |
| 6 | Methyl salicylate | 14 | Diclofenac |
| 7 | Alclofenac | 15 | Indomethacin |
| 8 | Ketoprofen | 16 | Flufenamate |

**TABLE 2-5** Effect of Local pH on Drug Absorption from Stomach

| Drug | Absorption at pH 1 (%) | Absorption at pH 8* (%) |
| --- | --- | --- |
| Salicylic acid | 60 | 13 |
| Thiopental | 46 | 34 |
| Caffeine | 24 | >24 |
| Morphine | 0 | 16 |
| * In presence of NaHCO₃ | | |

(pH 2). However, when the contents of the stomach were made alkaline (pH 8), the strychnine molecules lost their protons, became uncharged, permeated the mucosa, and killed the cat.

Organic acids such as barbiturates, phenytoin, acetylsalicylic acid, dicumarol, phenylbutazone, sulfonamides, and thyroxine have a higher absorption rate in the stomach, where the $H^+$ concentration is high.

Table 2-5 gives some examples of the effect of the pH of the stomach contents on the absorption of various drugs.

### Dependence on surface area available for absorption

It should be obvious that more drug is absorbed if there is more area available for absorption. For any substance that can penetrate the gastrointestinal epithelium in measurable amounts, the small intestine represents the greatest area for absorption. This is true whether the molecule is charged or uncharged. For example, ethanol can be absorbed to some extent by the stomach, but it is absorbed about ten times faster from the small intestine, and phenobarbital is absorbed 18 times more rapidly from the small intestine than from the stomach (Table 2-6).

The great epithelial area of the small intestine provided by the many villi and microvilli is much larger than the surface of the gastric mucosa. This great intestinal area

more than compensates for the effect of the high pH on the ionization of organic acids. Therefore, the rate at which the stomach empties its contents into the intestine markedly affects the overall rate at which drugs reach the general circulation after oral administration. This is particularly true for the absorption of tertiary amines, which constitute the majority of commonly used drugs. But for almost all drugs, the overall rate of gastrointestinal absorption is directly related to the rate at which the stomach empties. That is why so many agents are administered on an empty stomach with sufficient water to ensure their rapid passage into the intestine.

In certain diseases, such as regional ileitis, the surgeon may have to remove much of the inflamed intestine, thus drastically reducing the surface area available for absorption of nutrients, vitamins, and drugs. This reduction may have an important effect on the therapeutic activity of some drugs in these patients.

## Active Transport

Although the principal mechanism for drug permeation is passive diffusion, more and more examples of active transport of drugs across cell membranes are being discovered. Active transport is defined as a process that moves a drug against its concentration gradient, that is energy dependent and thus can be blocked by inhibiting cellular metabolism or by reducing adenosine triphosphate (ATP) levels, and that can be saturated. It can carry drugs out of the cell or into the cell.

The process involves a membrane protein known as a **drug transporter,** which is usually a transporter for an endogenous molecule or class of molecules (Table 2-7).

**TABLE 2-6** Dominant Role of Surface Area in Drug Absorption

| Drug | Absorbed from Stomach in 1 Hour (%) | Absorbed from Small Intestine in 10 Minutes (%) |
| --- | --- | --- |
| Ethanol | 38 | 64 |
| Phenobarbital | 17 | 52 |

**Uptake transporters,** those that carry drugs across membranes *into* cells, include the transporters for organic anions, organic cations, dipeptides, nucleosides, and monocarboxylates. Drugs which have sufficient structural resemblance to these endogenous substrates can also be carried actively into cells by the corresponding transporters. There is also a large family of ATP-binding cassette (ABC) proteins that act as **efflux transporters,** which carry certain endogenous substances, and drugs which resemble them, *out of* cells. One of these efflux transporters, known as **P-glycoprotein,** is particularly important because it transports a large number of different clinically used drugs, including antibiotics, anti-cancer agents, central nervous system (CNS) drugs, immunosuppressive agents, and cardiac drugs, and it is associated with **multidrug resistance (MDR).**

Drug transporters are often found in intestinal epithelium, renal tubular cells, hepatocytes, bile canaliculi, and various other sites at which drug absorption and excretion are quantitatively important processes. Both influx and efflux transporters play a very important role in the CNS. As noted earlier in this chapter, capillary endothelial cells in most parts of the CNS are held together by tight junctions, which prevent the passage of most drugs. However, there is also a functional, as well as an anatomical, component of the blood–brain barrier. The capillary endothelium and the ependymal lining of the ventricular system contain a variety of transporters that carry drugs either into or out of the brain tissue and therefore determine which drugs do and do not enter the CNS readily. In addition, there are transporters in brain parenchyma itself, which play a major role in the transport of drugs between glial cells and neurons (see Chapter 16).

Among the many examples of drug transport are the following:

- Penicillin by the renal tubule
- 5-Fluorouracil by the intestine
- Nitrogen mustard and melphalan by lymphocytes
- Pravastatin by the liver
- Pentazocine and narcotic antagonists by leukocytes (Fig. 2-13)

| TABLE 2-7 | Examples of Transporters Whose Localization in Healthy Tissues Affects Drug Absorption, Distribution, and Elimination by Active Transport |
|---|---|

These are transporters whose functions are directly dependent upon ATP hydrolysis. Their expression in tumour cells is often associated with resistance to a variety of anti-cancer agents. MDR = multidrug resistance.

| Transporter | Gene | Main Substrates | Predominant Location | Membrane Localization | Functional Roles |
|---|---|---|---|---|---|
| MDR1 | ABCB1 | Amphipathic compounds, organic cations | Kidney, liver, intestine, brain, adrenal cortex, placenta, lung, plus many others | Apical | Efflux of a variety of functionally unrelated and chemically diverse compounds; plays a significant role in drug absorption, distribution (especially in the CNS), and elimination; associated with MDR |
| MRP1 | ABCC1 | Amphipathic organic anions; conjugates of glutathione, glucuronide, and sulfate | Liver, kidney, lung, brain, peripheral blood mononuclear cells, heart, skeletal muscle, testis, and many others | Basolateral | Efflux of compounds, but does not result in decreased drug elimination because of its basolateral localization; associated with MDR |
| MRP2 | ABCC2 | Amphipathic organic anions and anionic conjugates | Liver, kidney, intestine, placenta, brain | Apical | Absence or inhibition impairs bilirubin–glucuronide secretion leading to Dubin–Johnson syndrome; associated with MDR |
| MRP3 | ABCC3 | Amphipathic organic anions and conjugates | Liver, intestine, adrenal gland, pancreas, kidney, colon, gallbladder | Basolateral | Induced in cholestasis; removes amphipathic anions such as bile acids; associated with MDR |
| BCRP | ABCG2 | Large, hydrophobic, charged compounds | Placenta, liver, small intestine, colon, lung, kidney, adrenal gland, sweat glands, endothelium of veins and capillaries | Apical | Efflux of a variety of functionally unrelated and chemically diverse compounds, affecting drug absorption and elimination; associated with MDR |

## Pinocytosis and Phagocytosis

Drugs with large molecular weights, generally 1000 Da or more, enter cells or cross tissue barriers by means of pinocytosis or phagocytosis. Substances normally absorbed in this manner include proteins, various bacterial toxins, milk antigens, and other antigens. Drugs tightly bound to plasma proteins can also enter in the same way. These substances enter the lysosomal system and may be digested within the lysosome (Fig. 2-14). If large amounts of the foreign substance enter, however, it may overwhelm the lysosomal protective mechanism and enter the circulation by exocytosis.

## Facilitated Diffusion

Diffusion along a transmembrane concentration gradient is, for some substances, facilitated by the presence of relatively selective carrier molecules in the membrane. These carrier molecules combine with the substances in question (e.g., glucose entering skeletal muscle cells), forming complexes that can diffuse more rapidly across the membrane than the free substances themselves. These complexes dissociate on the other side of the membrane to release the free substances into the cell. Many transport systems are difficult to classify other than to say that they are not directly energy-dependent, as exemplified in Table 2-8. Compounds that permeate by facilitated diffusion include the following:

- Amino acids into the brain (e.g., L-dopa)
- Bile sats into the liver

**FIGURE 2-14** Endocytosis of proteins results in a secondary lysosome, which in turn fuses with a primary lysosome. After hydrolysis within the fused vesicle, the products may be released by exocytosis.

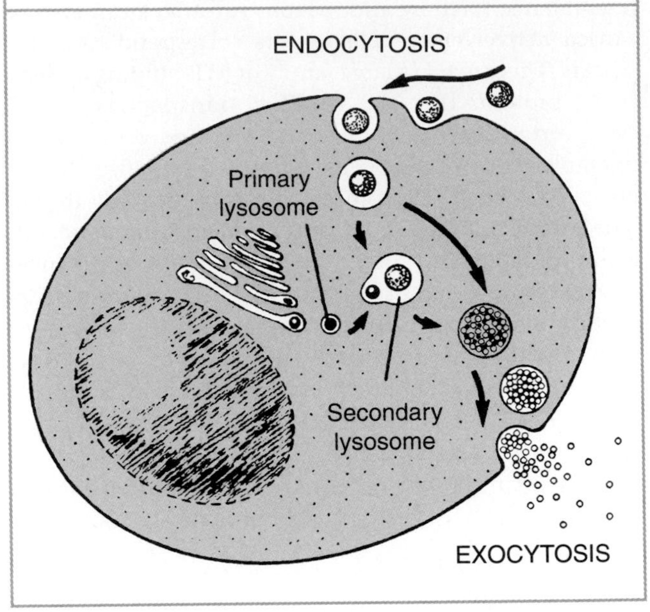

ENDOCYTOSIS

Primary lysosome

Secondary lysosome

EXOCYTOSIS

- Adenosine-like compounds
- Nucleotide anti-metabolites (used in cancer or antiviral chemotherapy)

## Passive Filtration

This is an important mechanism for drug elimination by the kidney glomerulus. Only the free, or unbound, drug and metabolites are available for glomerular filtration. In general, these transporters are still incompletely characterized, particularly with respect to their tissue distribution and cellular localization.

## Drug Passage via Gap Junctions

There are gap junctions between epithelial cells of the same tissue (such as glandular epithelium and neurons), endothelial cells of the same tissue (throughout the vascular system), and mesothelial cells of the same tissue (such as smooth muscle and myocardial cells). Small molecules (<500 Da) can move from cell to cell through these gap junctions. The membranes of the connected cells contain cylindrical protein structures called **connexons** or hemi-channels (analogous to the aquaporins), and aqueous channels run along the centre of the protein coils, across the thickness of the membrane. The **gap junction** is formed by the exact alignment of the connexons of two cells so that their two channels form one continuous passage between the cytoplasmic compartments of the cells (Fig. 2-15).

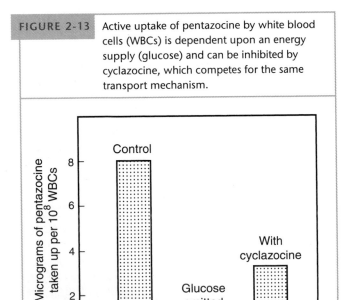

**FIGURE 2-13** Active uptake of pentazocine by white blood cells (WBCs) is dependent upon an energy supply (glucose) and can be inhibited by cyclazocine, which competes for the same transport mechanism.

| TABLE 2-8 | Examples of Transporters Involved in Facilitated Diffusion | | | | |
|---|---|---|---|---|---|
| These are transporters whose functions are *not* directly dependent upon ATP hydrolysis. | | | | | |
| Transporter | Gene | Main Substrates | Predominant Location | Predominant Membrane Localization | Significance |
| OCT1 | SLC22A1 | Organic cations | Liver, brain, intestine | Basolateral | Electrogenic cation transport (usually uptake) |
| OCT2 | SLC22A2 | Organic cations | Kidney, brain | Basolateral | Electrogenic cation transport (usually uptake) |
| OCT3 | SLC22A3 | Organic cations | Liver, skeletal muscle, placenta, kidney, heart, lung, brain | Basolateral | Electrogenic cation transport (usually uptake) |
| OCTN1 | SLC22A4 | Organic cations, carnitine | Kidney, skeletal muscle, placenta, prostate, heart | Apical | $Na^+$-independent organic cation transport; $Na^+$-dependent carnitine uptake |
| OCTN2 | SLC22A5 | Organic cations, carnitine | Kidney, skeletal muscle, heart, prostate, thyroid gland, pancreas, liver | Apical | $Na^+$-independent organic cation transport; $Na^+$-dependent carnitine uptake; mutations in OCTN2 are associated with primary systemic carnitine deficiency |
| OAT1 | SLC22A6 | Organic anions | Kidney, brain, placenta | Basolateral | Organic anion transport (usually uptake) |
| OAT2 | SLC22A7 | Organic anions | Liver, kidney | Basolateral | Organic anion transport (usually uptake) |
| OAT3 | SLC22A8 | Organic anions | Kidney, skeletal muscle, brain | Basolateral | Organic anion transport (usually uptake) |
| OAT4 | SLC22A11 | Organic anions | Placenta, kidney | Apical | Organic anion transport (usually uptake) |
| OATP-1A2 | SLCO1A2 | Amphipathic organic solutes | Brain, liver | Basolateral | Uptake of amphipathic organic solutes including bile salts and hormones |
| OATP-2B1 | SLCO2B1 | Amphipathic organic solutes | Liver, placenta | Basolateral | Uptake of amphipathic organic solutes including bile salts and hormones |
| OATP-1B1 | SLCO1B1 | Amphipathic organic solutes | Liver | Basolateral | Uptake of amphipathic organic solutes including bile salts and hormones |
| OATP-1B3 | SLCO1B3 | Amphipathic organic solutes | Liver | Basolateral | Uptake of amphipathic organic solutes including bile salts and hormones |

The connexons are composed of a family of specific proteins called **connexins,** designated Cx20, Cx36, Cx43, and so forth. These are differentially distributed in the various tissues, so some connexins, for example, are found mainly in the heart (Cx40 and Cx43), others in the CNS (Cx36), and others in glandular tissues (Cx32). They differ in their amino acid composition, charge characteristics, and the diameter of their central channels, and therefore differ functionally with respect to their current-carrying capacity, the maximum size of molecules that can move along the channels, the effect of $Ca^{2+}$ on their patency, and their susceptibility to separation of the two connexons by the actions of drugs.

The gap junctions allow the rapid spread of a wave of depolarization across a mass of tissue, as in the synchro- nous contraction of the whole ventricular myocardium (see Chapter 31), the propagation of an epileptic discharge across the surface of the brain (see Chapter 18), or the combined secretory activity of all the cells in an exocrine gland. Their function can be altered by a variety of different drugs such as ouabain, a cardiac glycoside (see Chapter 32), verapamil (see Chapter 34), angiotensin II (see Chapter 29), quinine, and the anti-ulcer agent carbenoxolone.

# ADSORPTION OF DRUGS TO CYTOPLASM

Most drugs, once having entered the cell, adsorb reversibly to cell proteins and lipids, just as they do to

**FIGURE 2-15** Cell-to-cell passage of drugs through gap junctions as demonstrated in fruit-fly salivary glands.

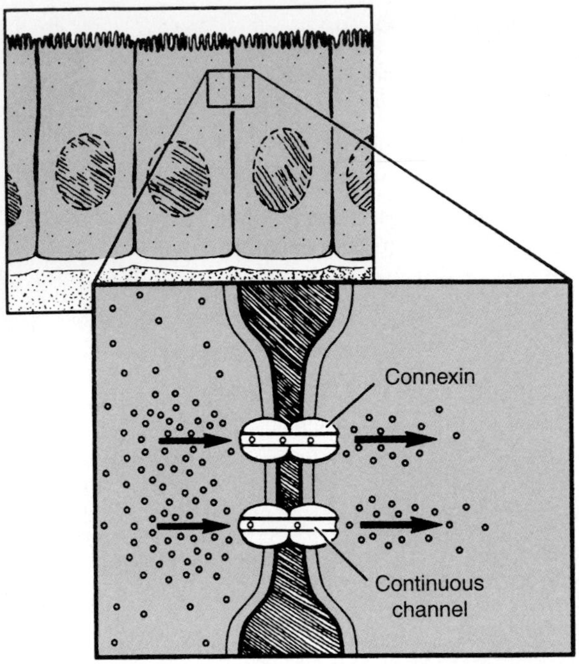

plasma proteins. Since the concentration of cell proteins is very high, the cytoplasmic concentration of the drug can achieve a level many times higher than that in the plasma. Drug adsorption, however, is *not* a drug transport mechanism, but rather, a drug reservoir mechanism. As with plasma proteins, this drug reservoir serves to smooth out the time course of drug action so that the drug is not quickly biotransformed and excreted.

# SUGGESTED READINGS

Alper J. Drug delivery: breaching the membrane. *Science.* 2002; 296:838-839.

Ayrton A, Morgan P. Role of transport proteins in drug absorption, distribution and excretion. *Xenobiotica.* 2001;31:469-497.

Brown D, Katsura T, Kawashima M, et al. Cellular distribution of the aquaporins: a family of water channel proteins. *Histochem Cell Biol.* 1995;104:1-9.

Buchwald P, Boder N. Octanol-water partition: searching for predictive models. *Curr Med Chem.* 1998;5:353-380.

Davson H, Zloković B, Rakić L, Segal MB. *An Introduction to the Blood-Brain Barrier.* London, England: Macmillan; 1993.

de Boer AG, van der Sandt IC, Gaillard PJ. The role of drug transporters at the blood-brain barrier. *Annu Rev Pharmacol Toxicol.* 2003;43:629-656.

Dhein S, Polontchouk L, Salameh A, et al. Pharmacological modulation and differential regulation of the cardiac gap junction proteins connexin 43 and connexin 40. *Biol Cell.* 2002; 94:409-422.

Gerloff T. Impact of genetic polymorphisms in transmembrane carrier-systems on drug and xenobiotic distribution. *Naunyn-Schmiedebergs Arch Pharmacol.* 2004;369:69-77.

Goldberg GS, Valiunas V, Brink PR. Selective permeability of gap junction channels. *Biochim Biophys Acta.* 2004;1662:96-101.

Ho RH, Kim RB. Transporters and drug therapy: implications for drug disposition and disease. *Clin Pharmacol Ther.* 2005;78: 260-277.

Hoffmann U, Kroemer HK. The ABC transporters MDR1 and MRP2: multiple functions in disposition of xenobiotics and drug resistance. *Drug Metab Rev.* 2004;36:669-701.

Houston JB, Upshall DG, Bridges JW. A re-evaluation of the importance of partition coefficients in the gastrointestinal absorption of nutrients. *J Pharmacol Exp Ther.* 1974;189: 244-254.

Lee G, Dallas S, Hong M, Bendayan R. Drug transporters in the central nervous system: brain barriers and brain parenchyma considerations. *Pharmacol Rev.* 2001;53:569-596.

Leo A, Hansch C, Elkins D. Partition coefficients. *Chem Rev.* 1971; 71:525-616.

Li J, Shen H, Naus CC, et al. Upregulation of gap junction connexin 32 with epileptiform activity in the isolated mouse hippocampus. *Neuroscience.* 2001;105:589-598.

Schinkel AH, Jonker JW. Mammalian drug efflux transporters of the ATP binding cassette (ABC) family: an overview. *Adv Drug Deliv Rev.* 2003;55:3-29.

Sohl G, Willecke K. Gap junctions and the connexin protein family. *Cardiovasc Res.* 2004;62:228-232.

Van Lieburg AF, Knoers NV, Deen PM. Discovery of aquaporins: a breakthrough in research on renal water transport. *Pediatr Nephrol.* 1995;9:228-234.

Wright SH, Dantzler WH. Molecular and cellular physiology of renal organic cation and anion transport. *Physiol Rev.* 2004; 84:987-1049.

Yano T, Nakagawa A, Tsuji M, Noda K. Skin permeability of various non-steroidal anti-inflammatory drugs in man. *Life Sci.* 1986;39:1043-1050.

# 3

# Drug Distribution

## L ENDRENYI

The administration of a drug to a patient is often analogous to sprinkling salt all over one's plate in the hope that enough of the salt will land on the potatoes. In fact, most of it will land on other parts of the meal. In understanding drug distribution, one has to consider the pattern of "scatter" of the drug in the body, as indicated schematically in Figure 3-1.

The body fluids act as solvents and carriers for the great majority of drugs so that the drugs reach their sites of action dissolved in the water that bathes the cells. The crudest division of the total body water is into intracellular and extracellular water; extracellular water is further subdivided into plasma water and interstitial fluid. However, some parts of the extracellular water, such as the inaccessible water in bone and the slowly accessible water in tendon and cartilage, are not reached by drugs; therefore, the distribution volumes to be discussed are not necessarily identical to the volumes truly occupied by water in the body. In short, the distribution compartments discussed here are usually physiological rather than anatomical entities (Fig. 3-2).

## TERMINOLOGY

### Actual Volume of Distribution

This is the anatomical volume accessible to the drug. For example, a charged compound, which cannot enter cells, will have as its volume of distribution the extracellular space of about 12 L. A non-polar compound will spread throughout the total body water, a volume of about 40 L (about 60% of the weight of a 70-kg man). Very few therapeutic drugs are confined to such a simply identified space as plasma.

### Apparent Volume of Distribution

The apparent volume of distribution is a calculated value. First, recall the simple relationship between mass (amount of drug), volume, and concentration. Let them be designated by $M$, $V$, and $C$, respectively. Concentration is mass per unit volume:

$$C = M/V$$

Knowing any two of these quantities, one can always calculate the third. For example, to calculate a volume when the mass and concentration of a drug are given, use the following:

$$V = M/C$$

The apparent volume of distribution of a drug can be determined by injecting the drug intravenously. If a plot of the logarithmic concentration versus time yields a straight line, extrapolation to zero time gives the theoretical initial serum concentration of the drug ($C_0$), assuming instantaneous distribution (Fig. 3-3). (For greater detail, see Chapter 5.)

Once an apparent volume of distribution is known for a particular drug, the amount of drug that must be given to achieve a desired concentration can be determined. It is important to realize that this approach is a mathematical convenience that works quite well in practice but says virtually nothing about where the drug really is in the body.

## SITES OF DRUG DISTRIBUTION

### Total Body Water

Ethyl alcohol is the most commonly consumed drug that equilibrates with the total body water. If, for the sake of simple arithmetic, a lean young man weighing 70 kg has a total body water of 50 L (70% of body weight), then a 15-g drink of alcohol (i.e., 0.21 g/kg) would give a concentration of 15 g/50 L of total body water. This is the same as 30 g/100 L, or 0.3 g/L. Since alcohol does not bind significantly to plasma proteins, and plasma is about 93% water, one can therefore expect a concentration in plasma of 0.28 g/L.

However, the body water in an obese elderly female is usually only about one-half of her body weight. If she also weighs 70 kg, she will have only 35 L of body water. There-

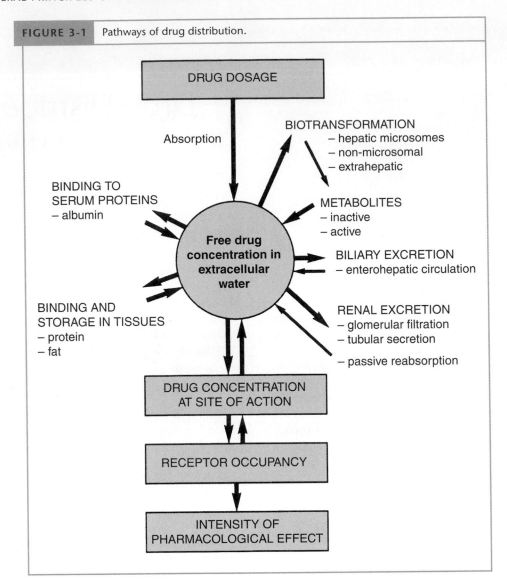

**FIGURE 3-1** Pathways of drug distribution.

fore, the same dose of 15 g of alcohol (i.e., 0.21 g/kg) would produce, in her, an alcohol concentration of 0.40 g/L, more than 40% higher than in the 70-kg lean man.

Antipyrine is another drug that spreads throughout the total body water without concentrating in any one area. It is an old synthetic analgesic, and this drug, as well as some of its derivatives, may be used to determine the volume of total body water. If a known amount of the drug is injected intravenously into the subject and the plasma concentration is measured after equilibrium is reached, the total water in which the drug is now diluted can be calculated.

## Extracellular Water

The cell membrane acts as a diffusion barrier, but most capillary walls are permeable to all but very large molecules (see Chapter 2). For such substances, therefore, the plasma and interstitial fluid can be regarded as a unit called the extracellular fluid (ECF). Since many drugs act at the cell surface but are inert once inside the cell, drug distribution in the ECF is pharmacologically very important.

Mannitol is a sugar alcohol that is often used to measure ECF volume because it does not enter cells and is not transformed in the body, but it is readily excreted through the kidney by glomerular filtration.

In a study of mannitol distribution, 50 g of the substance was administered to a 70-kg man. From repeated observations, referenced to plasma water, an extrapolated initial concentration of 4.46 g/L was measured. Consequently, the apparent volume of distribution was 50/4.46 = 11.2 L, which is 16% of the body weight, or 160 mL/kg. In a series of investigations of healthy adult males, the mannitol distribution volume averaged 160 mL/kg but ranged from 141 to 187 mL/kg. Hence, the concentration of a drug that distributes in extracellular space may vary

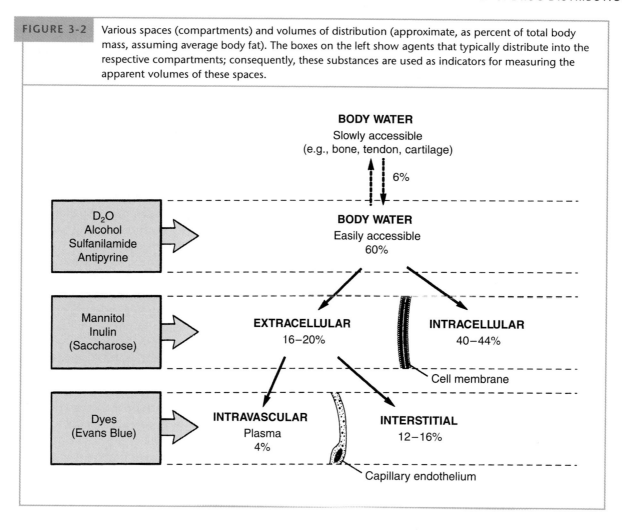

**FIGURE 3-2** Various spaces (compartments) and volumes of distribution (approximate, as percent of total body mass, assuming average body fat). The boxes on the left show agents that typically distribute into the respective compartments; consequently, these substances are used as indicators for measuring the apparent volumes of these spaces.

considerably from person to person, even if all other factors are equal.

Many drugs spread through ECF in less time than it takes them to penetrate cell membranes. There is, therefore, an initial transient period when their extracellular concentration is high compared with their intracellular concentration. If these drugs act on the cell surface, their onset of action will be more rapid than if their site of action is within the cell.

## Blood

Even within the blood, the distribution of a drug could be uneven. While a proportion of the drug molecules could be dissolved in water, others could be attached to various constituents of the blood. These intravascular distribution processes will be considered briefly.

### Intravascular distribution

Drug concentrations are typically measured in plasma and/or serum. Unless the drug is equally partitioned between cells and plasma, drug concentrations will be dependent on the protein concentration and/or the **hematocrit** value (i.e., the proportion, by volume, of red blood cells in the whole blood).

Since the distribution of ethanol between plasma and cells is a passive one, it follows that the ethanol content of tissue is determined by its water content. This has important consequences for blood analysis as cells contain less water than plasma. The average water content of cells and plasma is about 68% and 94%, respectively. Since cells occupy about half of the blood volume (hematocrit approximately 0.5), the whole blood contains about 81% water. The commonly accepted conversion factor for calculating plasma ethanol from blood ethanol is 1.16 (= 94/81), although this will obviously vary with the hematocrit value. Hence, a whole blood alcohol value of 50 mg/100 mL implies a plasma ethanol concentration of about 58 mg/100 mL.

The situation becomes even more complex if variations in plasma composition are taken into account. A volume of 100 mL of human blood plasma contains 4 to 9 g protein, about 0.1 g sugars, and 0.4 to 0.6 g lipids, which, after a fatty meal, may rise to over 1 g. Hence, the

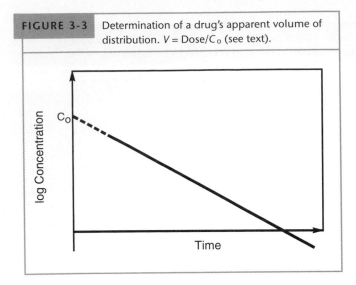

**FIGURE 3-3** Determination of a drug's apparent volume of distribution. $V = Dose/C_0$ (see text).

normal variation in plasma water is from about 89% to about 96%.

### Serum and plasma protein binding

Most drugs are carried from their sites of absorption to their sites of action and elimination by the circulating blood. Although some drugs are simply dissolved in serum water, most others are at least partly associated with blood constituents such as albumin, globulins, lipoproteins, and erythrocytes. For the great majority of drugs binding to serum constituents, **albumin** is quantitatively the most important macromolecule and often accounts for almost the entire drug binding. For example, intravenously injected Evans Blue binds so strongly to plasma albumin that almost the whole dose is retained in the plasma, so its plasma concentration provides a measure of plasma volume. Some basic drugs bind extensively to $\alpha_1$-acid glycoproteins.

Misleadingly small distribution volumes can be obtained for highly bound drugs when their total concentration (bound plus unbound) is measured in the plasma. However, it is the free drug in the plasma water that equilibrates with the rest of the body. Consequently, for meaningful interpretation, the volume of distribution should be evaluated from the concentration of the unbound drug.

### Consequences of serum and plasma protein binding

Plasma protein binding influences the fate of drugs in the body. Only the unbound, or free, drug can diffuse through capillary walls, leave the circulation, distribute throughout the body, reach the sites of drug action, and be subject to elimination from the body. Since drug binding to albumin is readily reversible, the albumin–drug complex serves as a circulating drug reservoir that releases more drug as free drug is biotransformed or excreted.

Thus, albumin binding decreases the maximum intensity but increases the duration of action of many drugs.

The binding of a drug to plasma proteins can slow down its elimination by processes that are controlled by **passive diffusion**. These include hepatic biotransformation when a drug enters hepatocytes by simple diffusion, and renal excretion by glomerular filtration (see Chapter 6 for more details). In contrast, **active, enzymatically mediated transport mechanisms** are more rapid and are not (or only slightly) affected by protein binding. These processes include renal tubular secretion and active hepatic transport and biliary secretion (see Chapter 6).

If a drug has high affinity for a protein molecule, then, at low concentrations, most of the drug is in bound form and only a small fraction is unbound. Thus, for highly albumin-bound drugs, the free drug concentration in serum is only a small percentage of the total concentration. For example, during phenylbutazone therapy, the total serum concentration of the drug is nearly 100 times higher than its concentration in serum water and ECF. At high concentrations, however, the binding sites on the protein will become saturated and the free fraction of the drug rises.

Therefore, the **consequences** of binding to plasma proteins are most important for drugs that are highly bound at comparatively low therapeutic concentrations (for a partial list, see Table 3-1). It is for these drugs that protein binding may decrease the concentration of the drug that is available for pharmacological activity, extend the duration of action, slow down diffusion-controlled elimination, and affect the unbound concentration by the competitive displacement of other highly protein-bound drugs.

## Body Fat

Adipose tissue is capable of storing large amounts of lipid-soluble drugs. Since blood flow to fat is relatively low per gram of tissue, a long period of time will be required for equilibrium to be achieved between the concentrations of unbound drug in plasma and in fat. Conversely, drug stored in fat may require a long time to be removed completely from the body. Thus, body fat generally becomes an important site of storage after prolonged exposure to a highly lipid-soluble drug or chemical. For example, the insecticide DDT can be stored in the body fat of living creatures. Some wild animals have died suddenly from the DDT released when their fat deposits were depleted by starvation.

## Tissue Binding

If the tissue concentration of a drug is higher than its concentration in the plasma free water, tissue localization has occurred, usually to a tissue-specific binding site. If the binding site has a large capacity for the drug, this results

| TABLE 3-1 | Approximate Drug Binding in Human Serum (Examples of Highly Bound Drugs) |
|---|---|
| **Drug** | **Free Drug (%)** |
| Anticoagulants | |
| Warfarin | 0.5 |
| Bishydroxycoumarin | 1 |
| Anti-infectives | |
| Cloxacillin | 5 |
| Oxacillin | 8 |
| Doxycycline | 10 |
| Sulfisoxazole | 10 |
| Anti-inflammatory agents | |
| Fenoprofen | 1 |
| Phenylbutazone | 3 |
| Oxyphenbutazone | 3 |
| Indomethacin | 10 |
| Salicylic acid | 18 |
| Cardiovascular agents | |
| Digitoxin | 5 |
| Propranolol | 13 |
| Diazoxide | 9 |
| Quinidine | 15 |
| Nifedipine | 4 |
| Verapamil | 10 |
| Central nervous system agents | |
| Diazepam | 1 |
| Amitriptyline | 4 |
| Imipramine | 10 |
| Chlorpromazine | 4 |
| Chlordiazepoxide | 3 |
| Nortriptyline | 6 |
| Desipramine | 8 |
| Phenytoin | 10 |
| Thiopental | 15 |
| Valproic acid | 7 |
| Diuretics and uricosurics | |
| Probenecid | 1 |
| Furosemide | 1 |
| Chlorothiazide | 5 |
| Sulfinpyrazone | 5 |
| Ethacrynic acid | 10 |
| Oral hypoglycemics | |
| Tolbutamide | 5 |
| Tolazamide | 6 |
| Chlorpropamide | 13 |
| Miscellaneous | |
| Clofibrate | 5 |

in an increase in the apparent volume of distribution of the drug. The end result can be a marked prolongation of the half-life of the drug in the body. For example, radioactive strontium ($^{90}$Sr) is so strongly bound to sites in the bone (which is relatively poorly perfused anyway) that it has a tissue half-life of years.

## Enterohepatic Circulation as a "Reservoir"

Enterohepatic circulation is another potential site of drug distribution. Imipramine and morphine, for example, are rapidly extracted from the body by the liver, excreted via the biliary system into the gut, and then reabsorbed across the intestinal mucosa back into the blood. The recirculating quantities of these drugs thus act as reservoirs, and they stay in the body for a much longer period than they would without recirculation. As another illustration, some drugs excreted as glucuronide conjugates pass back to the intestine and are then hydrolyzed back to the parent drug by enzymes that are present in the intestinal bacteria. Unfortunately, however, little is known of the relative rates of biliary excretion and intestinal reabsorption of drugs, so the general significance of the enterohepatic cycle as a drug reservoir is difficult to assess. Enterohepatic circulation is discussed further in Chapter 6.

## DRUG DISTRIBUTION FOLLOWING RAPID INTRAVENOUS INJECTION

The general conditions described above apply to the distribution of a drug some time after its administration (say, at steady state). The following considerations apply to the *time course* for approaching these conditions.

The concentration of a drug in blood following a rapid intravenous injection is at its highest value initially and then falls ultimately to zero (Fig. 3-4). The time course of drug concentrations can be divided into three stages: initial dilution and distribution, redistribution, and elimination (renal and metabolic). (See also Chapter 5.)

## Initial Dilution and Distribution

A drug rapidly injected in a small volume will, for approximately two or three circulation times, be distributed as a "bolus" within the circulation (Fig. 3-5). If the drug has a very narrow margin of safety and acts on receptors within sensitive vital systems, serious toxicity may occur if the injection is too rapid (e.g., isoproterenol and cardiac arrhythmias; thiopental and medullary respiratory depression). Generally, drugs should be injected slowly (e.g., diazepam is injected at less than 2.5 mg/min). Conversely, for a few drugs with a high concentration threshold for the onset of action, rapid bolus injection may be required to initiate a response. A special situation applies

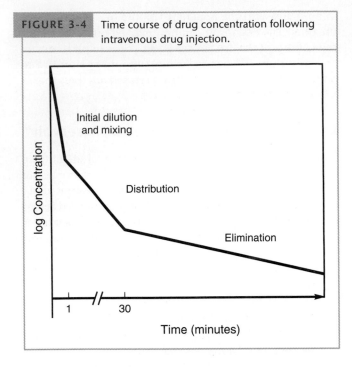

**FIGURE 3-4** Time course of drug concentration following intravenous drug injection.

## Redistribution

If the drug is injected rapidly, the total dose is distributed in only a small volume of blood. As this blood moves through the lungs and out into the body, the drug mixes in a larger volume of blood, and when this blood reaches the capillaries, the drug is distributed by diffusion to the extracellular space (and into cells if it can cross the cell membrane). After about 15 minutes or so, the drug will be distributed fairly evenly throughout the ECF space. There are some exceptions to this—for instance, the drug will not reach the average concentration within this time in poorly perfused tissues.

Different tissues in the body have different blood perfusion rates; hence, drugs reach equilibrium quickly in some tissues and more slowly in others. This effect can be illustrated by inhaling a constant concentration of halothane (a general anaesthetic) and measuring the time course for the amount taken up by the whole body. As shown in Figure 3-6, the uptake of halothane by the whole body generally can be subdivided into three phases: (1) a rapid-uptake phase, which reflects the uptake of halothane by the **vessel-rich group (VRG) of tissues**, the brain, heart, and liver; (2) an intermediate phase, which shows the uptake of halothane by the **muscle group (MG) of tissues**; and (3) a very slow phase, which reflects the uptake of halothane into the **vessel-poor group (VPG) of tissues**, the fat, skin, bone, ligaments, teeth, and hair. After exposure to the drug is stopped, the rates for the declining amount of halothane again demonstrate the presence of the three tissue groups. (Note the qualitative similarity of the graph shown in Fig. 3-6 to that in Fig. 3-4.)

It is the organs and tissues of the vessel-rich group that are the targets in most drug therapy, and the rate of onset of drug action in them can be very fast. But it is important to remember that blood flow can be different in various parts of the same organ. For example, the blood flow to

if the rapidly injected drug is highly protein-bound. During the "bolus" phase, drug binding sites on albumin will be saturated, and free drug concentration will be much higher relative to total drug concentration than after complete redistribution has occurred. Highly protein-bound drugs for which such kinetics may be important include quinidine, phenytoin, and diazoxide.

**FIGURE 3-5** Mixing of drug after rapid intravenous injection (i.e., dissipation of bolus over two or three circulation times).

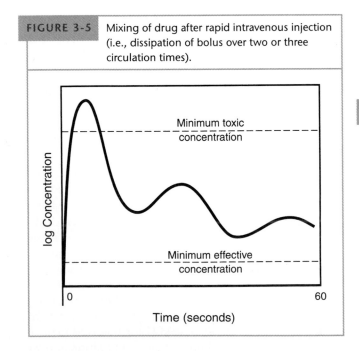

**FIGURE 3-6** Uptake and distribution of a drug (halothane) in various tissue groups depending on blood perfusion rates (see text). VRG = vessel-rich group; MG = muscle group; VPG = vessel-poor group.

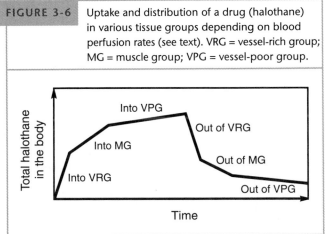

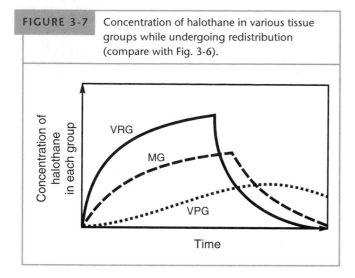

FIGURE 3-7   Concentration of halothane in various tissue groups while undergoing redistribution (compare with Fig. 3-6).

the grey matter of the brain is almost four times as high as to the white matter, so drugs that are able to cross the blood–brain barrier reach the cortex and brain nuclei much faster than the rest of the brain.

The muscle group fills up with drug more slowly than the vessel-rich group, and because of relative concentrations, drugs that have initially gone to vessel-rich organs can be carried out of them by the circulation and relocated in the muscle and fat groups of tissues. This **redistribution** is shown in Figure 3-7 in a general way, and various specific examples are given in succeeding chapters.

## SUGGESTED READINGS

Buxton IL. Pharmacokinetics and pharmacodynamics: the dynamics of drug absorption, distribution, action, and elimination. In: Brunton LL, Lazo JS, Parker KL, eds. *Goodman & Gilman's The Pharmacological Basis of Therapeutics*. 11th ed. New York, NY: McGraw-Hill; 2001:1-39.

Oie S. Drug distribution and binding. *J Clin Pharmacol*. 1986;26: 583-587.

Shargel L, Wu-Pong S, Yu ABC. *Applied Biopharmaceutics & Pharmacokinetics*. 5th ed. New York, NY: McGraw-Hill/Appleton; 2004.

Winter ME. *Basic Clinical Pharmacokinetics*. 4th ed. Philadelphia, Pa: Lippincott Williams & Wilkins; 2004.

# 4

# Drug Biotransformation

## DS RIDDICK

We live in a chemically hostile world in which we are exposed daily to a wide variety of foreign chemicals via inhalation, ingestion, and percutaneous absorption. These foreign chemicals, or xenobiotics, include therapeutic and recreational drugs, environmental contaminants, and dietary constituents. Fortunately, we possess a diverse array of enzymes that are able to act on xenobiotics in a manner that hastens their elimination from our bodies. **Drug biotransformation** refers to the chemical transformation of a xenobiotic within a living organism, usually by enzyme-catalyzed reactions.

## BIOLOGICAL SIGNIFICANCE OF BIOTRANSFORMATION

All foods that animals eat contain traces of potentially toxic chemicals. This is particularly true of plants, which lack excretory mechanisms and therefore accumulate metabolic excretory products in vacuoles inside their cells. Many plants produce alkaloids that are potent pharmacological agents. When the plants are eaten as food, those toxic or pharmacologically active materials that have high lipid solubility are the most likely to be absorbed from the gastrointestinal tract and the least likely to be excreted in their original form. They may be filtered at the glomerulus and reabsorbed from the renal tubule, or excreted in the bile and reabsorbed from the intestine, thus remaining in the body for long periods of time. The same is true for drugs and environmental contaminants.

The kidneys of terrestrial animals conserve water by producing highly concentrated urine. This favours reabsorption of lipid-soluble chemicals in the renal tubule by increasing the concentration gradient from lumen to blood. These animals also possess enzymatic machinery that converts lipid-soluble xenobiotics into more polar and, hence, more water-soluble products. This permits more efficient excretion in a limited volume of water in the urine or bile.

Drug biotransformation reactions have three potential consequences with respect to pharmacological activity, as outlined below.

1. **Activation.** An inactive precursor may be converted into a pharmacologically active drug (e.g., the insecticide parathion [inactive] is converted into the toxic agent paraoxon [active]; the prodrug L-dopa [inactive] is converted to dopamine [active] in the basal ganglia).
2. **Maintenance of activity.** A pharmacologically active chemical may be converted into a different, but still active metabolite (e.g., diazepam [active] is converted to oxazepam [active]).
3. **Inactivation.** An active drug may be converted into inactive products (e.g., pentobarbital [active] is converted to hydroxylated metabolites [inactive]).

The only feature common to all of these reactions is that the products of biotransformation are usually more water-soluble than the original drugs.

It is important to point out that, in many cases, the same enzymes that biotransform xenobiotics are also involved in the biotransformation of endogenous chemical substances. For example, the synthesis and/or degradation of steroid hormones, cholesterol, eicosanoids, bile acids, and bile pigments utilize enzymes that are also involved in drug biotransformation. Thus, there is a close relationship between drug biotransformation and fundamental homeostatic processes.

## DRUG BIOTRANSFORMATION REACTIONS

Drug biotransformation reactions are commonly grouped into **phase I** and **phase II reactions**. Phase I processes include oxidation, reduction, and hydrolysis reactions that may increase, decrease, or not alter the pharmacological activity of a drug. In general, phase I reactions introduce or unmask a functional group (e.g., hydroxyl, amine, sulfhydryl) that makes the drug more polar. Phase II processes consist of synthetic or conjugation reactions in which an endogenous substance (e.g., glucuronic acid, glutathione) combines with the functional group derived from phase I reactions to produce a highly polar drug conjugate. Most phase II reactions result in a decrease in the pharmacological activity of the drug. Although many drugs undergo the sequential process of phase I reaction followed by phase II reaction, there are numerous exceptions. For instance, the product of phase I biotransformation may be sufficiently polar to be eliminated directly without the need for a phase II reaction, or a drug may possess a functional group that can be conjugated directly via a phase II reaction without the need for a phase I reaction. In some cases, phase II reactions may precede phase I reactions. Finally, a parent drug may be eliminated unchanged without the need for any biotransformation. These relationships are summarized in Figure 4-1. In some cases, biotransformation processes appear to be coordinated with active transporters that can efflux drugs and/or metabolites across cellular membranes. Although not strictly a biotransformation event, transporter-mediated efflux is sometimes referred to as a phase III reaction.

Virtually every tissue has some ability to carry out drug biotransformation reactions. However, the most important organ of biotransformation is the **liver.** The gastrointestinal tract, lungs, skin, and kidneys also display substantial drug biotransformation activity. The fact that the gastrointestinal tract and liver are major sites of drug biotransformation means that many drugs that are administered orally will be extensively biotransformed before they reach the systemic circulation. This **first-pass effect** can severely limit the systemic bioavailability of some drugs taken by the oral route. In addition, intestinal microorganisms are capable of catalyzing drug biotransformation reactions. For example, a glucuronide conjugate of a drug may be excreted via the bile into the intestine, where gut bacteria may convert the conjugate back into free drug. The free drug may then be reabsorbed from the intestine and re-enter the liver via the portal vein. In the liver, the free drug may once more be conjugated with glucuronic acid and secreted into the bile, and this process of **enterohepatic circulation** may begin again.

At the subcellular level, various enzymes of drug biotransformation may be located in the endoplasmic reticulum, mitochondrion, cytosol, lysosome, and, to a limited extent, the nuclear envelope and plasma membrane. A major site of drug biotransformation within hepatocytes and other cells is the membranes of the smooth endoplasmic reticulum. When a tissue is homogenized and subjected to differential centrifugation, the membranes of the endoplasmic reticulum form vesicles called **microsomes.** The microsomal fraction is able to carry out many drug biotransformation reactions in vitro.

## Phase I Reactions

### Oxidation

Oxidations are the most important category of drug biotransformation reactions in quantitative terms. The microsomal mixed-function oxidase (MFO) system is capable of catalyzing a wide variety of oxidation reactions. This microsomal drug-oxidizing system requires the participation of two distinct proteins embedded in the phospholipid bilayer of the endoplasmic reticulum membrane. First, a member of a hemoprotein superfamily termed the **cytochromes P450** functions as the terminal oxidase in this pathway. The name cytochrome P450 is

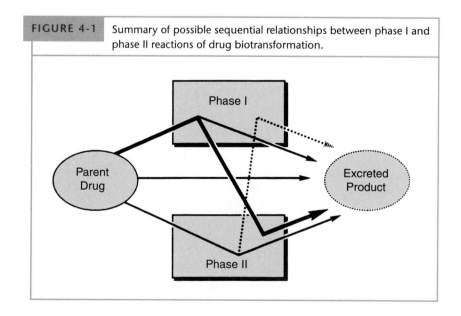

**FIGURE 4-1** | Summary of possible sequential relationships between phase I and phase II reactions of drug biotransformation.

derived from the fact that the reduced (ferrous) form of this hemoprotein binds carbon monoxide, forming a complex that has a unique absorption spectrum with a maximum at 450 nm. Second, a flavoprotein termed **NADPH–cytochrome P450 reductase** serves to transfer reducing equivalents from the reducing cofactor NADPH (reduced nicotinamide adenine dinucleotide phosphate) to the hemoprotein. The activity of this enzymatic system also requires molecular oxygen. Typically, this system functions as a monooxygenase in that one atom of oxygen is incorporated into the drug substrate and the other atom of oxygen contributes to the formation of water. The overall balanced equation for a typical monooxygenase reaction is as follows:

$$RH + O_2 + NADPH + H^+ \rightarrow ROH + H_2O + NADP^+$$

In this scheme, RH represents an oxidizable drug substrate, and ROH represents the hydroxylated product of the reaction.

A simplified scheme of the cytochrome P450–catalyzed oxidative cycle is shown in Figure 4-2. The numbers in the cycle correspond to the major steps described below:

1. The drug (RH) binds to cytochrome P450 to form a binary complex. Initially, the hemoprotein is in its oxidized ferric form ($Fe^{3+}$). The binding of substrate to cytochrome P450 results in specific changes in the hemoprotein absorption spectrum. Depending on the nature of the spectral change, drugs can often be classified as "type I" or "type II" substrates. Type I substrates bind to a lipophilic substrate pocket of the cytochrome P450 protein and tend to shift electron distribution of the hemoprotein in a way that permits subsequent easy electron transfer between the reductase and the cytochrome. However, type II substrates bind directly to the heme iron of cytochrome P450, resulting in an interaction that tends to retard the subsequent reduction of cytochrome P450.

2. The reducing cofactor NADPH donates an electron to the flavoprotein NADPH–cytochrome P450 reductase, which in turn reduces the substrate-bound cytochrome P450 to its ferrous form ($Fe^{2+}$). The reductase utilizes both flavin adenine dinucleotide (FAD) and flavin mononucleotide (FMN) as electron-shuttling prosthetic groups.

3. Molecular oxygen binds to the ferrous iron of the cytochrome P450–substrate complex to generate a ternary product.

4. An electronic rearrangement is thought to occur, although the precise oxidation states of the oxygen and iron in these intermediates are not well characterized.

5. A second electron transfer occurs. There are at least two possible sources of this reducing equivalent. The flavoprotein NADPH–cytochrome P450 reductase can transfer an electron from NADPH as in step 2. Alternatively,

**FIGURE 4-2** The catalytic cycle for a cytochrome P450–mediated hydroxylation reaction. Fe = the heme iron; RH = substrate; ROH = hydroxylated product.

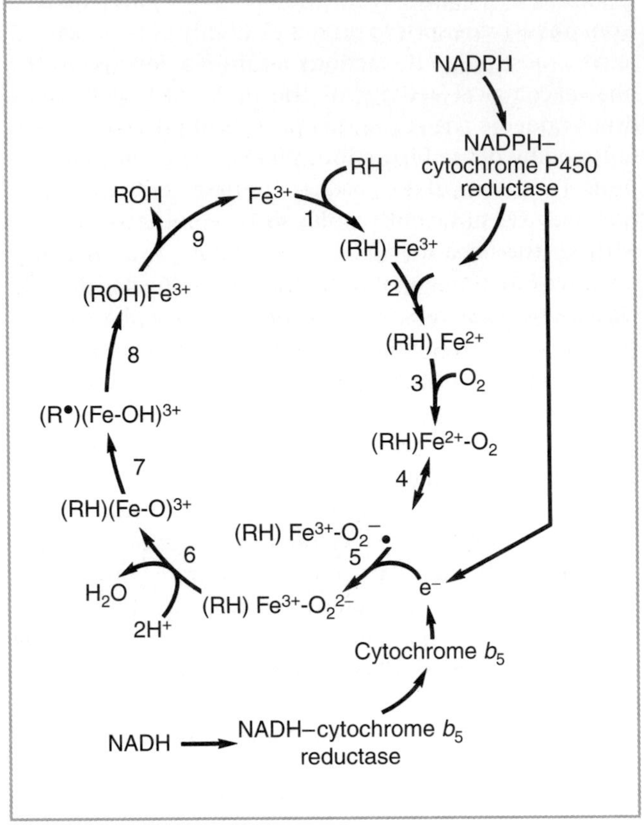

an electron may be donated by the cofactor NADH and shuttled via the flavoprotein NADH–cytochrome $b_5$ reductase and the hemoprotein cytochrome $b_5$ to cytochrome P450. This second electron is required to activate the bound oxygen.

6. In a poorly understood step, the oxygen–oxygen bond is split with the uptake of two protons. The result is the release of water and the generation of an "activated oxygen," perhaps an iron-oxo or iron-oxene species ($Fe-O)^{3+}$. Recent evidence suggests that cytochromes P450 can use multiple electrophilic oxidants in the catalytic cycle.

7. Hydrogen abstraction from the substrate is thought to occur, resulting in the production of transient hydroxyl and substrate carbon radical species.

8. Recombination of the hydroxyl and carbon radicals occurs to give the product (ROH).

9. Dissociation of ROH restores the cytochrome P450 to its initial oxidized (ferric) state.

The cytochrome P450 catalytic cycle does not function with perfect efficiency. In the presence of particular drug substrates that are "difficult" to biotransform, such as ethanol, the catalytic cycle becomes "uncoupled." That is, the utilization of reducing equivalents is dissociated from product formation. As a result, potentially toxic reactive oxygen species (superoxide anion, hydrogen peroxide) can be liberated in the process of cytochrome P450 catalysis (see Chapters 22 and 67).

The phospholipid of the endoplasmic reticulum membrane is a key component in the monooxygenase reaction. The precise function of the lipid is not clear, but it has been suggested that the lipid is required for substrate binding, electron transfer, or facilitating the interaction between cytochrome P450 and its reductase. There appear to be between five and 20 molecules of cytochrome P450 per molecule of reductase in liver microsomes, and in many cases, processes of electron transfer to the active site heme moiety can be the rate-limiting step in drug oxidation reactions. However, determination of the rate-limiting step is greatly influenced by the specific enzyme, substrate, cofactor concentrations, and experimental conditions under examination.

The cytochromes P450 appear to be the most versatile biological catalysts known to date, being capable of catalyzing over 60 different types of reactions on literally hundreds of thousands of substrates. This has prompted the suggestion that they be called "diversozymes" in recognition of this catalytic promiscuity. Although the initial reaction product of most cytochrome P450–catalyzed reactions is the corresponding hydroxylated derivative, a wide range of products is formed from many drug substrates. In many cases, the initial hydroxylated derivative is unstable and promptly breaks down into the recognized end product. Figure 4-3 illustrates some of the diverse oxidation reactions that can be carried out by cytochromes P450.

The cytochrome P450 system can handle a diverse array of chemical substrates for two reasons. First, there are multiple molecular forms of cytochrome P450 present in any given species. Second, many cytochrome P450 species are capable of biotransforming a large number of substrates.

**FIGURE 4-3**  A limited sample of the diverse oxidation reactions catalyzed by cytochromes P450.

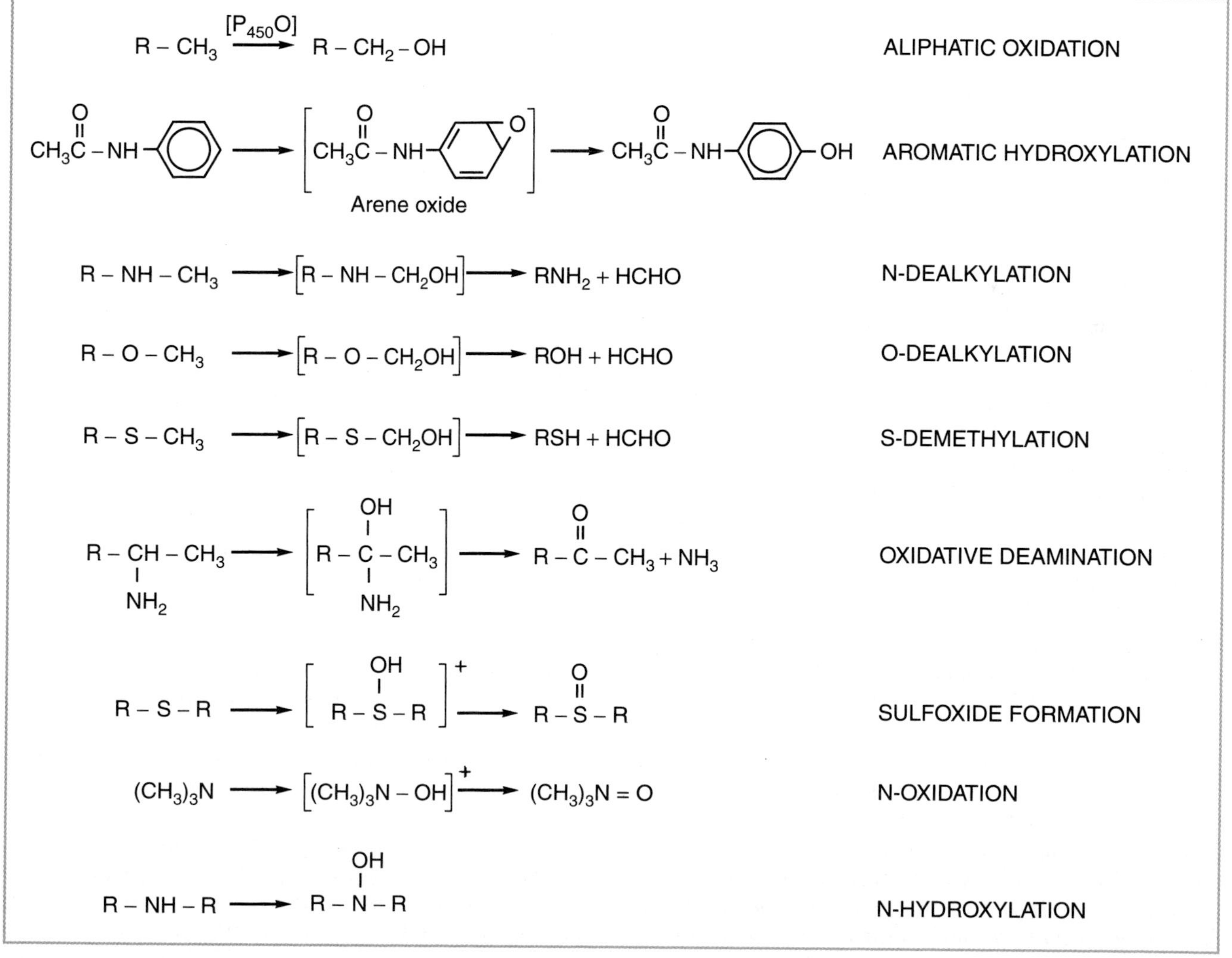

Thus, the microsomal cytochrome P450 system combines the properties of **enzyme multiplicity** and **broad substrate specificity.** The existence of multiple forms of cytochrome P450 was firmly established during the 1970s and 1980s by classical protein biochemistry techniques. Individual purified cytochromes P450 were distinguished on the basis of spectral properties, molecular masses as determined by electrophoretic mobilities, substrate selectivities, and immunoreactivities with polyclonal and monoclonal antibodies. During the 1980s and 1990s, cDNA clones encoding multiple forms of cytochrome P450 proteins were isolated and sequenced. Molecular cloning techniques have led to the adoption of a standardized nomenclature system based on amino acid sequence similarity and divergent evolution. Each cytochrome P450 protein is identified by the root symbol "CYP" followed by an Arabic number denoting the gene family, a capital letter designating the gene subfamily, and an Arabic number representing the individual gene (e.g., CYP1A1).

In general, cytochrome P450 proteins with greater than 40% sequence identity are included in the same family, and those mammalian sequences with greater than 55% identity are included in the same subfamily. With the completion of various genome sequencing projects, we now have a clearer picture of the extent of cytochrome P450 enzyme multiplicity in humans and several other important organisms. The human genome appears to encode 57 cytochrome P450 proteins, and these are distributed among 18 families. Pharmacologists are mainly interested in families 1, 2, and 3; fortunately, a relatively small number of enzymes from these families carry out the biotransformation of the majority of drugs in clinical use (Fig. 4-4). Enzymes from the other gene families play important roles in the biotransformation of endogenous chemical substances. It is informative to compare the estimated numbers of cytochrome P450 genes in eukaryotic organisms whose genomes have been sequenced: the yeast *Saccharomyces cerevisiae* has 3, the nematode worm *Caenorhabditis elegans* 74, the fruit fly *Drosophila melanogaster* 84, the plant *Arabidopsis thaliana* 249, the mouse *Mus musculus* 102, and the rat *Rattus norvegicus* 84.

The molecular cloning approach has led to an increased understanding of the evolutionary relationships among members of the cytochrome P450 superfamily. The cytochromes P450 display a wide phylogenetic distribution: these enzymes have been detected in organisms ranging from bacteria to humans. The steroidogenic cytochromes P450 are probably among the "oldest" members of the superfamily. They are necessary in early organisms for maintenance of membrane integrity. Xenobiotic-transforming cytochromes P450 probably evolved from the steroidogenic enzymes as an adaptive response to detoxify dietary chemicals. Much of the diversification of cytochrome P450 forms may have been driven by "animal–plant warfare," in which animals evolved a battery of

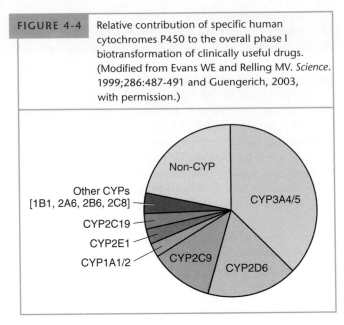

**FIGURE 4-4** Relative contribution of specific human cytochromes P450 to the overall phase I biotransformation of clinically useful drugs. (Modified from Evans WE and Relling MV. *Science.* 1999;286:487-491 and Guengerich, 2003, with permission.)

enzymes to handle the array of toxic chemicals produced by the various plant species upon which they fed.

A major distinction between cytochromes P450 relates to the nature of the electron transport process utilized. As described earlier, the eukaryotic microsomal system utilizes the flavoprotein NADPH–cytochrome P450 reductase to transfer electrons directly from NADPH to the hemoprotein. However, most bacterial and eukaryotic mitochondrial cytochromes P450 utilize a ferredoxin reductase and a non-heme iron–sulfur protein to transfer electrons from NADPH to the hemoprotein. Unlike the eukaryotic cytochromes P450, which are integral membrane proteins, the bacterial cytochromes P450 are soluble, and thus it has been possible to obtain X-ray crystallographic data from several bacterial enzymes. These crystal structures were instrumental in generating the first proposed three-dimensional models of mammalian cytochromes P450. More recently, the successful determination of crystal structures for various mammalian cytochromes P450 (rabbit CYP2C5 and CYP2B4; human CYP2C9, CYP2C8, CYP3A4, and CYP2A6) has provided particularly useful insights into the mechanisms of action of these proteins.

Not all oxidation reactions are catalyzed by cytochromes P450. The microsomal **flavin-containing monooxygenases** (FMO) catalyze NADPH-dependent oxygenation of nucleophilic phosphorus, nitrogen, and sulfur atoms present in a wide variety of xenobiotics, including thioether- and carbamate-containing pesticides and numerous therapeutic agents (e.g., ephedrine, phenothiazines, *N*-methylamphetamine). Molecular cloning has identified a single gene family composed of six genes *(FMO1 to FMO6)* that have been identified in a variety of mammalian species including human, pig, rabbit, rat, and guinea pig.

Another important drug-oxidizing system appears to involve **prostaglandin synthase–dependent co-oxidation.** In the normal process of eicosanoid turnover (see Chapter 27), prostaglandin $G_2$ is reduced to prostaglandin $H_2$ by the hydroperoxidase activity of the enzyme prostaglandin synthase. Along with this reduction reaction, many xenobiotics, including acetaminophen, phenytoin, and benzo[a]pyrene, can be co-oxidized. This pathway appears to be of considerable toxicological importance as it often leads to the generation of toxic reactive metabolites. Other enzymes that can catalyze the oxidation of xenobiotic chemicals include **alcohol dehydrogenase, aldehyde dehydrogenase, xanthine oxidase, monoamine oxidase,** and **diamine oxidase.**

## Reduction

Several drugs are biotransformed by reductive pathways. Microsomal and cytosolic enzymes catalyze the reduction of **azo** linkages (RN=NR'; e.g., Prontosil), **nitro** groups ($RNO_2$; e.g., chloramphenicol), and **carbonyl** groups (RCOR'; e.g., haloperidol). Although these pathways have been recognized for several years, our understanding of the enzymes that catalyze these reactions is limited. However, there has been considerable recent progress in characterizing the aldo–keto reductase gene superfamily, which includes the aldehyde reductase subfamily (AKR1A), the aldose reductase subfamily (AKR1B), and the dihydrodiol/hydroxysteroid dehydrogenase subfamily (AKR1C).

Interestingly, the cytochrome P450 and NADPH–cytochrome P450 reductase enzymes that catalyze oxidation reactions may also participate in reduction reactions. The examples of doxorubicin and halothane biotransformation illustrate this point. Doxorubicin and many other anti-neoplastic agents contain a quinone moiety that can undergo a one-electron reduction catalyzed by NADPH–cytochrome P450 reductase, resulting in the formation of a semiquinone free radical (Fig. 4-5). The semiquinone radical can be oxidized back to the quinone with concurrent generation of superoxide anion. The production of superoxide anion and other reactive oxygen species promotes oxidative stress, lipid peroxidation, and DNA damage; these effects contribute to the cytotoxic properties of the drug. Quinone-containing drugs can also undergo a two-electron reduction catalyzed by the enzyme **NAD(P)H–quinone oxidoreductase** (also known as **DT-diaphorase**), resulting in the production of the hydroquinone derivative. This process generally, but not always, represents a detoxification pathway.

Biotransformation of the anaesthetic halothane under hypoxic conditions involves a cytochrome P450–catalyzed reductive dehalogenation reaction. This pathway is thought to be responsible for the hepatotoxicity of this drug. The reaction mechanism is distinct from the cytochrome P450–catalyzed oxidation pathway in the following way: under hypoxic conditions, limited oxygen is present, and as a result, the electrons derived from NADPH are not utilized to activate oxygen, but, rather, contribute directly to the formation of halothane radical species. This type of reduction reaction may be of particular importance in centrilobular hepatocytes and in cells in the centre of solid tumours that display very low oxygen tensions.

## Hydrolysis

Drugs containing ester functions (RCOOR'; e.g., procaine, succinylcholine) are hydrolyzed by a variety of non-specific **esterases** in liver, plasma, gastrointestinal tract, and other tissues. Amides (RCONHR'; e.g., procainamide, lidocaine) are hydrolyzed by **amidases**; most of this biotransformation occurs in the liver. Finally, **peptidases** in plasma, erythrocytes, and many other tissues biotransform polypeptide drugs (e.g., insulin, growth hormone).

A number of olefins and aromatic compounds can undergo phase I oxidative biotransformation to an epoxide intermediate, in which an oxygen atom is inserted across a carbon–carbon double bond. Drugs such as carbamazepine and carcinogens such as benzo[a]pyrene are biotransformed by cytochromes P450 to epoxide derivatives. Epoxides are reactive electrophilic species that can bind covalently to proteins and nucleic acids, leading to

**FIGURE 4-5** Pathways of biotransformation of quinone-containing drugs (e.g., doxorubicin). One-electron reduction initiates the process of "redox cycling," leading to oxidative stress and cytotoxicity. Two-electron reduction is a detoxification pathway leading to the formation of the hydroquinone derivative. Doxorubicin can also be reduced at a side-chain position (catalyzed by carbonyl reductase) to yield its major metabolite, doxorubicinol.

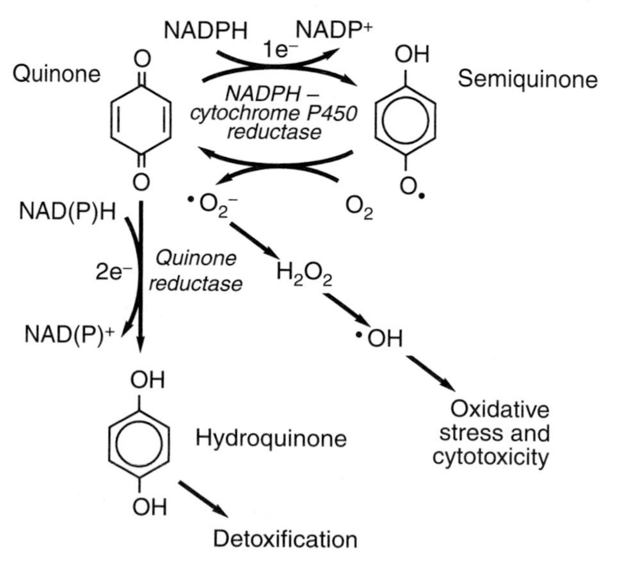

cytotoxicity. One means by which epoxides can be detoxified is via the nucleophilic attack of water on one of the electron-deficient carbon atoms of the oxirane ring, a reaction catalyzed by the enzyme **epoxide hydrolase**. The product of this enzymatic reaction is a dihydrodiol derivative, while non-enzymatic rearrangement of aromatic epoxides leads to the production of phenols. As noted for other drug biotransformation enzymes, there is more than one molecular form of epoxide hydrolase. Both microsomal and cytosolic (soluble) forms of this enzyme have been characterized in liver and other mammalian tissues. Although this can be categorized as a hydrolysis reaction, epoxide hydrolase is sometimes identified as a phase II enzyme (see below), since it can be viewed as catalyzing the conjugation of an endogenous substance (water) to a drug metabolite (epoxide).

## Phase II Reactions

In general, phase II reactions involve the coupling of a drug or drug metabolite with an endogenous substance. These reactions require the participation of specific transferase enzymes that are localized in the microsomal or cytosolic fractions and of high-energy activated endogenous cofactors. Most conjugation reactions result in detoxification; however, several examples of bioactivation by phase II enzymes are now known. The most important phase II reactions are described below.

### Glucuronidation

One of the most important phase II reactions involves conjugation of drugs with the endogenous substance glucuronic acid. Many functional groups are subject to glucuronidation, including hydroxyl (e.g., morphine, acetaminophen), carboxyl (e.g., clofibrate, benzoic acid), amine (e.g., meprobamate), and sulfhydryl (e.g., 2-mercaptobenzothiazole) groups. The reaction mechanism for the formation of a glucuronide conjugate with benzoic acid is shown in Figure 4-6. Free glucuronic acid will not couple with drugs; however, uridine diphosphate glucuronic acid (UDPGA) will. UDPGA is formed from glucose-1-phosphate in a two-step process that occurs in the cytoplasm. The conjugation of glucuronic acid to the drug substrate is catalyzed by a member of the **UDP-glucuronosyltransferase** superfamily. In the glucuronide conjugate of the drug, the C-1 atom of glucuronic acid now has the β configuration. Glucuronide conjugates can be excreted via the bile or urine; intestinal microorganisms that contain the enzyme β-glucuronidase may hydrolyze the conjugate and initiate the process of enterohepatic circulation. Many endogenous substances including bilirubin, bile acids, and steroids are also subject to glucuronidation.

Multiple forms of UDP-glucuronosyltransferase exist. These enzymes are present in highest concentrations in the liver, but are also found in the kidney, small intestine, lung, skin, adrenal gland, and spleen. The enzymes are located in the endoplasmic reticulum. There are at least 16 human UGT enzymes, classified into three gene subfamilies: *UGT1A, UGT2A,* and *UGT2B.*

### Glutathione conjugation

The **glutathione *S*-transferases** catalyze the enzymatic conjugation of xenobiotics with the endogenous tripeptide glutathione (glutamylcysteinylglycine, or GSH). Xenobiotics such as ethacrynic acid and bromobenzene that have a suitably electrophilic centre (e.g., epoxides, arene oxides, nitro groups, hydroxylamines) can be subject to nucleophilic attack by glutathione. Indeed, glutathione conjugation reactions can proceed non-enzymatically. The products of glutathione conjugation reactions undergo further modification (Fig. 4-7) to yield mercapturic acid derivatives as final elimination products. In most cases, glutathione conjugation represents an important detoxification process; however, some xenobiotics (e.g., 1,2-

---

**FIGURE 4-6**    Reaction sequence for glucuronic acid conjugation of benzoic acid. UDPGA = uridine diphosphate glucuronic acid; UGT = UDP-glucuronosyltransferase; PP = pyrophosphate.

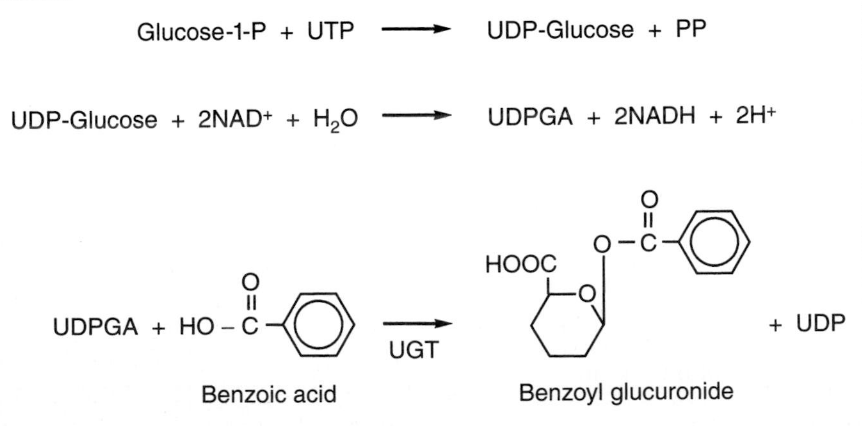

Glucose-1-P + UTP ⟶ UDP-Glucose + PP

UDP-Glucose + 2NAD$^+$ + H$_2$O ⟶ UDPGA + 2NADH + 2H$^+$

UDPGA + HO–C(O)–C$_6$H$_5$ (Benzoic acid) →(UGT)→ Benzoyl glucuronide + UDP

**FIGURE 4-7** Glutathione conjugation catalyzed by glutathione S-transferase. (A) Structural formula of glutathione. (B) Pathways of mercapturic acid formation. X = an electrophilic drug metabolite or epoxide reacting with glutathione; AA = amino acid; GST = glutathione S-transferase; GGTP = γ-glutamyl transpeptidase; CG = cysteinyl glycinase; AT = acetyltransferase; Acetyl-CoA = acetyl-coenzyme A.

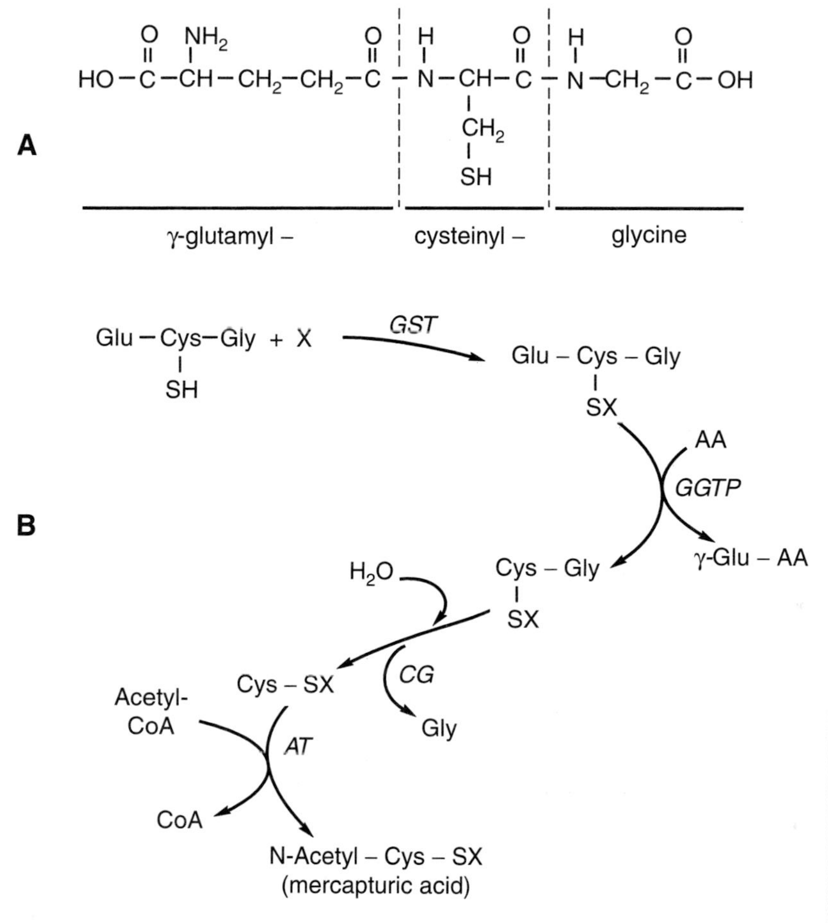

dihaloalkanes and halogenated alkenes) are toxic only after conjugation with glutathione or cysteine.

Both soluble and microsomal forms of glutathione S-transferase exist. Most of the soluble forms are localized in the cytosol. The catalytically active cytosolic enzymes are homo- or heterodimers consisting of two protein subunits derived from the same subfamily. The family of soluble human glutathione S-transferases currently consists of at least 16 different gene products, distributed among six subfamilies. Each gene product is given a capital letter designation for the subfamily (A, M, P, T, Z, O for alpha, mu, pi, theta, zeta, omega, respectively) and an Arabic numeral indicating the order in which the protein subunits were characterized within a subfamily (e.g., GSTA1). Any two members within a subfamily generally display greater than 50% amino acid identity.

The glutathione S-transferases appear to be of particular interest in the field of cancer chemotherapy. The increased and/or differential expression of one or more glutathione S-transferases in tumour cells has been implicated as a contributing factor in the resistance of those cells to drugs such as doxorubicin and melphalan (see Chapter 57).

## Sulfation

Many phenols, alcohols, and hydroxylamines can undergo sulfation reactions catalyzed by **sulfotransferases.** Inorganic sulfate must first be activated to 3'-phosphoadenosine-5'-phosphosulfate (PAPS) in a two-step process (Fig. 4-8). A member of the sulfotransferase superfamily then catalyzes the formation of the sulfate ester. Compounds that undergo sulfation reactions include acetaminophen, salicylamide, methyldopa, ethanol, and many steroid hormones.

The sulfotransferases are cytosolic enzymes found in many tissues, including liver, kidney, gut, and platelets. At least 10 human sulfotransferases are known. To date, the

FIGURE 4-8    Reaction sequence for sulfate conjugation of an alcohol. PP = pyrophosphate; ROH = substrate for the sulfation reaction; ST = sulfotransferase.

$$\text{ATP} + \text{SO}_4^{2-} \xrightarrow{\text{Sulfurylase}} \text{Adenosine-5'-phosphosulfate (APS)} + \text{PP}$$

$$\text{APS} + \text{ATP} \xrightarrow{\text{APS kinase}} \text{3'-Phosphoadenosine-5'-phosphosulfate} + \text{ADP}$$
$$\text{(PAPS)}$$

$$\text{PAPS} + \text{ROH} \xrightarrow{\text{ST}} \text{RO} - \text{SO}_3\text{H} + \text{3'-Phosphoadenosine-5'-phosphate}$$

sulfotransferases have been classified into five major groups, mainly on the basis of substrate selectivity: phenol sulfotransferases (SULT1A1, 1A2, 1A3), estrogen sulfotransferases (SULT1E1), thyroid hormone sulfotransferase (SULT1B1), hydroxysteroid sulfotransferases (SULT2A1), and others (SULT1C1, 1C2, 2B1). The phenol sulfotransferases have been the most extensively studied from the viewpoint of drug biotransformation. Humans possess at least three forms of phenol sulfotransferase, one of which is thermolabile and catalyzes the conjugation of dopamine and other phenolic monoamines (SULT1A3), whereas the other forms (SULT1A1, 1A2) are thermostable and carry out the sulfation of simple phenols.

## Acetylation

Cytosolic enzymes known as **N-acetyltransferases** catalyze the transfer of acetate from acetyl-coenzyme A (acetyl-CoA) to primary aromatic amine and hydrazine functional groups to yield acetamides and hydrazides (Fig. 4-9). Examples of chemicals that undergo acetylation include sulfonamides, isoniazid, procainamide, p-aminobenzoic acid, caffeine, as well as a variety of aromatic amine carcinogens such as 4-aminobiphenyl and 2-naphthylamine,

which are present in cigarette smoke. In humans, only two functional drug-acetylating enzymes exist, NAT1 and NAT2, and these display 81% amino acid identity.

N-Acetylation of aromatic amine procarcinogens is generally thought to be a detoxification pathway. However, acetyltransferases may also play an important role in the bioactivation of potentially carcinogenic aromatic amines by virtue of their ability to also catalyze the O-acetylation of hydroxylamines produced by cytochrome P450–catalyzed N-oxidation of the primary amino group. The product is an unstable acetoxy ester that spontaneously decomposes to a nitrenium ion, which can bind covalently to DNA and produce mutations that result in malignant transformation.

## Methylation

A variety of drugs and endogenous chemicals are biotransformed by **methyltransferase** enzymes that utilize S-adenosylmethionine as the methyl donor (Fig. 4-10). Most of the methyltransferases are cytosolic enzymes. Catechol O-methyltransferase catalyzes the methylation of phenolic hydroxyl groups found in endogenous and exogenous catecholamines (see Chapter 11). N-Methylation of numerous

FIGURE 4-9    Acetylation of an exogenous amine with endogenous acetate catalyzed by N-acetyltransferase (NAT). CoA–SH = coenzyme A.

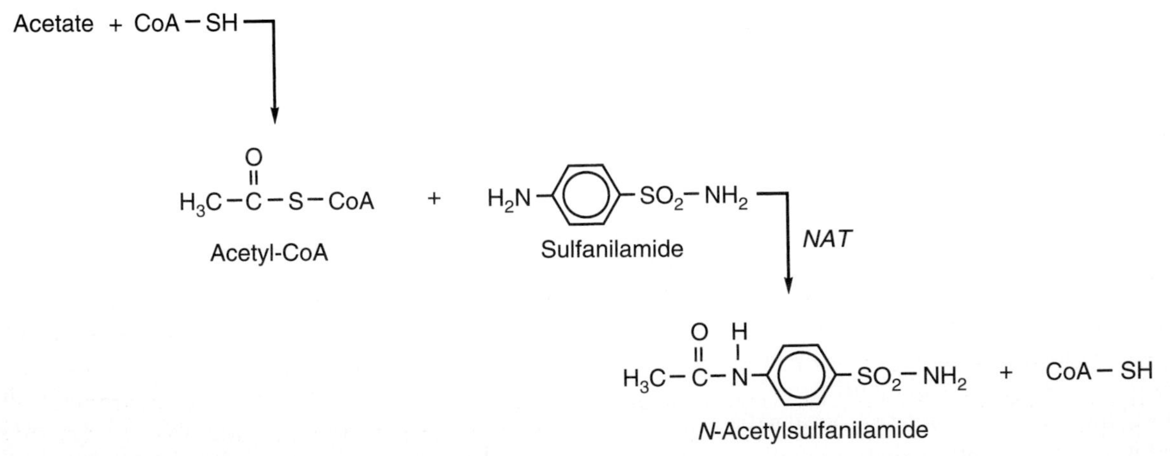

**FIGURE 4-10** Reaction sequence for the methylation of 6-mercaptopurine catalyzed by thiopurine S-methyltransferase (TPMT). PP = pyrophosphate.

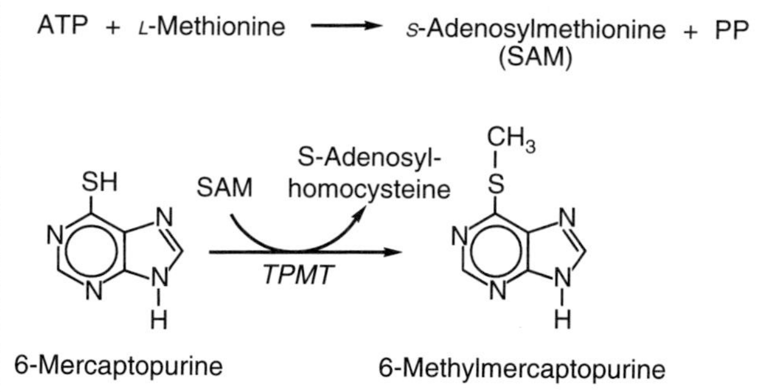

ATP + L-Methionine $\longrightarrow$ s-Adenosylmethionine + PP
(SAM)

6-Mercaptopurine → 6-Methylmercaptopurine

amines occurs. Histamine *N*-methyltransferase catalyzes the methylation of histamine and related compounds in the liver, whereas phenylethanolamine *N*-methyltransferase carries out the methylation of noradrenaline in the adrenal gland. Nicotinamide *N*-methyltransferase catalyzes the methylation of nicotinamide and other pyridine compounds to produce pyridinium cations. At least two *S*-methyltransferases have been characterized in humans: thiopurine *S*-methyltransferase catalyzes the methylation of purine derivatives such as 6-mercaptopurine (see Fig. 4-10) and azathioprine, whereas thiol *S*-methyltransferase acts on non-purine agents including captopril and D-penicillamine.

Thiopurine *S*-methyltransferase displays genetic polymorphism in human populations, and this is responsible for very important individual variations in the efficacy and toxicity of drugs such as 6-mercaptopurine (see Chapter 10). This is a striking example of how predictive testing of patients for a genetic polymorphism can be used in the clinic to enhance drug safety.

### Glycine conjugation

Aromatic carboxylic acids such as benzoic acid (Fig. 4-11) and salicylic acid can be inactivated by conjugation with the endogenous amino acid glycine. In this scheme, the inert carboxylic acid is activated to its acyl coenzyme A derivative prior to amide formation with the amino function of the donating amino acid. Such reactions are commonly catalyzed by **transacylases** found in hepatic mitochondria. Other amino acids, including glutamine and taurine, can also be utilized for conjugation.

## DRUG BIOTRANSFORMATION AND ADVERSE DRUG REACTIONS

Many adverse drug reactions (see Chapter 59) can be traced to an **improper balance between bioactivation and detoxification reactions.** A classic example involves hepatic necrosis caused by the analgesic acetaminophen

(see Fig. 43-3 for details). When used at normal therapeutic doses, acetaminophen undergoes glucuronidation and sulfation, reactions that terminate the actions of the drug and hasten its elimination. Some acetaminophen is bioactivated to *N*-acetylbenzoquinonimine via a cytochrome P450–catalyzed reaction. Under normal circumstances, this reactive intermediate can be detoxified by conjugation with glutathione. Thus, a favourable balance exists between bioactivation and detoxification. However, when acetaminophen is administered in excessive doses, the glucuronidation and sulfation pathways become saturated. More acetaminophen biotransformation is channeled through the cytochrome P450–mediated bioactivation pathway. Detoxification of the reactive metabolite depends on the presence of adequate levels of glutathione. With time, glutathione becomes depleted faster than it can be regenerated. At this point, detoxification cannot keep pace with bioactivation. The reactive metabolite is able to bind covalently to cellular protein thiols and initiate hepatotoxicity. It is possible to prevent hepatotoxicity and death by the administration of *N*-acetylcysteine within 8 to 16 hours following acetaminophen overdose. The antidote serves to increase intracellular glutathione stores and thus re-establish a favourable balance between bioactivation and detoxification.

Many adverse drug reactions that were previously labelled "idiosyncratic" (to indicate that they occurred in a small fraction of the population for no apparent reason) now appear to be caused by genetic deficiencies in various enzymes of drug biotransformation, such as CYP2D6, CYP2C19, and NAT2 (see Chapter 10). Several adverse drug reactions also appear to have an immunological component. For instance, certain drugs (such as dihydralazine, tienilic acid, and some aromatic anticonvulsants) may be bioactivated by cytochromes P450 to reactive metabolites that bind covalently to proteins. The drug–protein adduct may be perceived by the host as "foreign," leading to the production of auto-antibodies that may play a role in toxicity.

## INDUCTION AND INHIBITION OF DRUG BIOTRANSFORMATION

### Induction

Many drug-biotransforming enzymes are known to increase in amount in response to chemicals known as inducers, in a process referred to as **enzyme induction.** In many cases, an inducer is also a substrate for the enzyme that it induces; however, some substrates are not good inducers and some inducers are not good substrates. In the field of drug biotransformation, most is known about the induction of members of the cytochrome P450 superfamily, although individual forms of epoxide hydrolase, UDP-glucuronosyltransferase, and glutathione *S*-trans-

**FIGURE 4-11** Conjugation of the endogenous amino acid glycine with exogenous benzoic acid catalyzed by a transacylase (TA). PP = pyrophosphate; CoA–SH = coenzyme A.

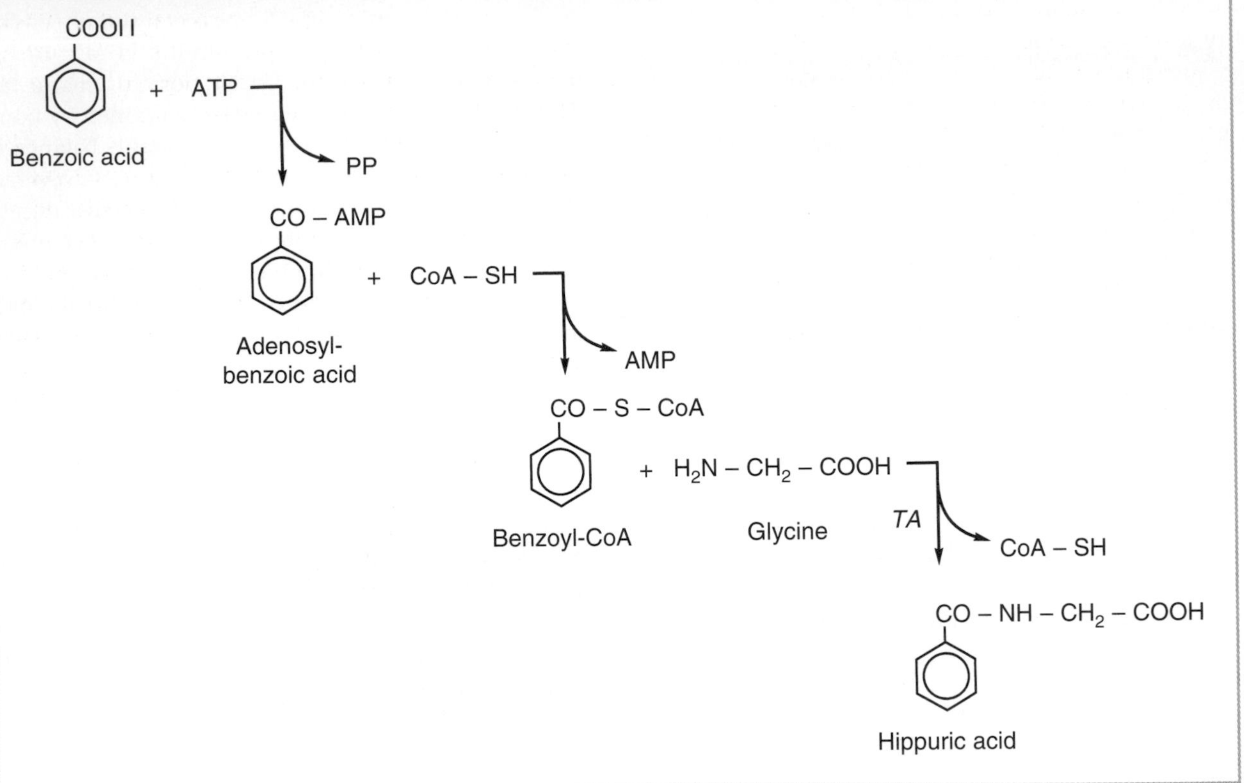

ferase are also inducible. Many molecular mechanisms for enzyme induction have been characterized. The most common means of regulation is **increased DNA transcription;** however, post-transcriptional mechanisms such as RNA processing, mRNA stabilization, translational efficiency, and protein stabilization have also been identified as important in the regulation of expression of cytochromes P450.

CYP1A1 and CYP1A2 are induced by halogenated aromatic hydrocarbons (e.g., dioxins, polychlorinated biphenyls [PCBs]) and polycyclic aromatic hydrocarbons (e.g., 3-methylcholanthrene, benzo[a]pyrene), many of which are present in cigarette smoke. These types of chemicals bind to a cytosolic receptor protein known as the aryl hydrocarbon (AH) receptor, which mediates an increase in the rate of transcription of the genes encoding CYP1A1 and CYP1A2 (see Chapter 67). Exposure of humans to hydrocarbon inducers has been shown to increase the clearance of antipyrine, acetaminophen, phenacetin, caffeine, and theophylline, and it can be expected to influence the biotransformation of many other substrates for these enzymes as well. This induction process also has great toxicological significance since CYP1A1 and CYP1A2 play important roles in the bioactivation of aromatic hydrocarbons and aromatic amines to toxic, mutagenic, and carcinogenic metabolites. This may be of particular importance in extrahepatic sites such as the lung.

A broader spectrum of induction of hepatic drug-biotransforming enzymes is produced by barbiturates such as phenobarbital. Phenobarbital causes proliferation of the hepatic endoplasmic reticulum and increases in NADPH–cytochrome P450 reductase, several phase II enzymes, and several forms of cytochrome P450 (e.g., CYP2A1, 2B1, 2B2, 2C6, 3A1, and 3A2 are all induced in the rat). CYP2B1 is the classical phenobarbital-inducible enzyme in rat liver. The constitutive androstane receptor (CAR) is involved in mediating the increase in the rate of transcription of *CYP2B* genes caused by barbiturates and various other xenobiotics. Phenobarbital increases the biotransformation of many drugs in humans, including such diverse agents as phenytoin, warfarin, chlorpromazine, digitoxin, and cyclophosphamide.

Isoniazid or chronic ethanol administration increases the levels of CYP2E1, an enzyme that plays a role in the oxidation of alcohols and is important in the bioactivation of carcinogenic nitrosamines. Induction of CYP2E1 by these chemicals occurs mainly via protein stabilization.

Glucocorticoids, macrolide antibiotics, anticonvulsants, and rifampin induce members of the CYP3A subfamily. This is of tremendous importance as species of CYP3A are the major contributors to the hepatic biotransformation of a broad array of therapeutic agents in humans (such as cyclosporin A, erythromycin, nifedipine, diazepam, and ketoconazole). The pregnane X receptor (PXR) plays a key role in increasing the rate of transcription of *CYP3A* genes.

The hypolipidemic drug clofibrate induces CYP4A enzymes that are involved in the hydroxylation of several fatty acids and eicosanoids. A member of the nuclear receptor superfamily, termed the peroxisome proliferator–activated receptor α (PPARα), mediates the induction of *CYP4A* genes by clofibrate and several other chemicals. Interestingly, CAR, PXR, and PPARα were all originally considered "orphan" nuclear receptors (i.e., without any known function), and they have subsequently turned out to play key roles in the regulation of drug-biotransforming enzymes via interaction with the retinoid X receptor (RXR).

Induction of drug-biotransforming enzymes can be an important cause of drug interactions. Phenobarbital and ethanol serve as two important examples. Phenobarbital and phenytoin are both used in the treatment of epilepsy. Phenobarbital can induce the enzymes responsible for phenytoin biotransformation, thus lowering the steady-state plasma concentrations of phenytoin and altering the ability of phenytoin to control seizures. Chronic ethanol consumption induces CYP2E1 and leads to enhanced biotransformation of acetaminophen, isoniazid, and carcinogenic nitrosamines. Chronic ethanol users are at greater risk for acetaminophen-induced hepatotoxicity because of the increased rate of generation of reactive metabolites of acetaminophen. Some examples of drugs that are known to induce drug biotransformation in humans are listed in Table 4-1.

## Inhibition

In view of the large numbers of drugs that share the same enzymatic sites of biotransformation, it is not surprising that interactions among them are very common. In general, acute interactions tend to be inhibitory (i.e., two drugs may simply compete for the same enzyme binding site, and each drug thus inhibits the biotransformation of the other). Several mechanisms are available for the inhibition of cytochromes P450 by xenobiotics, as follows:

- Imidazole-containing drugs such as cimetidine and ketoconazole coordinate tightly to the heme iron and thereby inhibit the biotransformation of other drugs and endogenous chemicals.
- Macrolide antibiotics and several other drugs are biotransformed by cytochromes P450 to intermediates that form a tight complex with the heme moiety and thus prevent the further participation of the enzyme in drug biotransformation reactions.
- Many other drugs function as mechanism-based or suicidal inactivators of cytochromes P450 in that the chemical is biotransformed by the enzyme to a reactive intermediate that irreversibly inactivates the enzyme via a covalent interaction with the protein (e.g., chloramphenicol) or heme (e.g., ethinyl estradiol, secobarbital, spironolactone) moiety.

The number of such inhibitory drug interactions is extremely large, and cytochrome P450 inhibition is a leading contributor to clinically significant drug interactions. In some cases, these interactions can be life-threatening. **Oral contraceptives** containing estrogens and progestins inhibit the hepatic biotransformation of several drugs. Consumption of **ethanol** together with certain drugs can decrease the clearance of the drug and lead to an exaggerated pharmacological effect. **Ketoconazole** or **erythromycin** can inhibit the CYP3A4-mediated biotransformation of the antihistamine terfenadine, leading to elevated plasma levels of terfenadine and increased risk of developing a life-threatening ventricular arrhythmia termed torsades de pointes. A final interesting example involves the interaction between dihydropyridine calcium-channel blockers and **grapefruit juice**. Grapefruit juice contains certain bioflavonoids and furanocoumarins that can inhibit the CYP3A-mediated biotransformation of drugs such as felodipine, thereby increasing the systemic bioavailability of these drugs. Some examples of drugs that inhibit biotransformation of other drugs in humans are listed in Table 4-1.

## OTHER FACTORS AFFECTING DRUG BIOTRANSFORMATION

### Species and Strain

Species differ with respect to biotransformation reactions, both qualitatively and quantitatively. Cats are deficient in UDP-glucuronosyltransferase activity, and as a result, they are very susceptible to the pharmacological actions of morphine. A bromocyclohexenyl derivative of barbituric acid that was developed in an attempt to generate a short-acting barbiturate was indeed rapidly biotransformed in

| TABLE 4-1 | Examples of Xenobiotics that Function as Inducers or Inhibitors of Cytochrome P450–Mediated Drug Biotransformation in Humans |
|---|---|
| **Inducers** | **Inhibitors** |
| Barbiturates [CYP2C9, 2C19, 3A4] | Disulfiram [CYP2E1] |
| Carbamazepine [CYP3A4] | Fluconazole [CYP2C19] |
| Cigarette smoke [CYP1A1/2] | Fluvoxamine [CYP1A2] |
| Dexamethasone [CYP3A4] | Furafylline [CYP1A2] |
| Ethanol [CYP2E1] | Gestodene [CYP3A4] |
| Isoniazid [CYP2E1] | Grapefruit juice [CYP3A4] |
| Omeprazole [CYP1A2] | Ketoconazole [CYP3A4] |
| Rifampin [CYP2C9, 2C19, 3A4] | Methoxsalen [CYP2A6] |
| St. John's wort [CYP3A4] | Quinidine [CYP2D6] |
| | Sulfaphenazole [CYP2C9] |

dogs; however, when administered to human volunteers, it was found to be very slowly biotransformed and to produce a prolonged hypnosis. Species differences in drug biotransformation emphasize the problems that may be encountered in drug development because of the fact that experimental animals may be poor models for human drug biotransformation.

Differences in biotransformation between various strains of the same animal species are also common. For example, the Gunn rat is deficient in the UDP-glucuronosyltransferase responsible for bilirubin conjugation, making this strain a valuable experimental model for clinical conditions characterized by jaundice due to unconjugated hyperbilirubinemia. Certain inbred mouse strains (e.g., C57BL/6N) respond to 3-methylcholanthrene with an induction of CYP1A1, whereas other strains (e.g., DBA/2N) are highly resistant.

## Age

Drug-biotransforming enzymes display interesting developmental patterns of changing expression both before and after birth. The implication is that individuals may be at increased risk of drug toxicity or suboptimal therapy at particular ontogenic stages. In general, neonates and geriatric patients display reduced drug biotransformation capacity and increased susceptibility to the toxic effects of some drugs (see Chapters 61 and 62). For example, in premature infants and during the first week or two of life in full-term infants, there is a deficiency in glucuronidation and renal function. Chloramphenicol is eliminated in the urine mainly as a monoglucuronide conjugate; therefore, when chloramphenicol is administered to newborns without proper dose adjustments, life-threatening hematological toxicity can occur. The result is often a combination of pallor and cyanosis, the hallmarks of the "grey baby syndrome." Caffeine elimination is also markedly impaired in newborns due to low expression of CYP1A2 at birth. Although it is more difficult to make generalizations about elderly populations, age-related decreases in hepatic biotransformation have been documented for many drugs, especially those biotransformed by cytochromes P450.

## Genetic Factors

Individuals differ in their ability to biotransform many drugs, and part of this variation may be due to genetic factors. Pharmacogenetics is the study of unusual drug responses that have a hereditary basis (see Chapter 10 for details). Briefly, mutations in genes coding for drug biotransformation enzymes may be important causes of variation in drug responses in human populations. For example, variant alleles at the *NAT2* gene locus account for the slow acetylation of drugs such as isoniazid and procainamide in about 50% of the individuals in Caucasian popula-

tions. Similarly, genetic variation at the *CYP2D6* locus results in impaired biotransformation of numerous therapeutic agents, including dextromethorphan, codeine, several β-adrenoceptor antagonists, and tricyclic antidepressants. Variant *CYP2C19* alleles account for impaired hydroxylation of the proton pump inhibitor omeprazole, and defects in CYP2C9 affect the clearance of the anticoagulant warfarin and the anticonvulsant phenytoin.

## Sex and Hormonal Factors

Many enzymes of drug biotransformation are under strict control by specific endocrine factors. Sex differences in drug biotransformation are pronounced in rats; adult male rats show higher rates of biotransformation of many drugs than females do. Many of these differences are due to the fact that rats express sex-specific forms of cytochrome P450. Gonadal steroids contribute to these sex differences, but the major hormonal determinant appears to be the sex-dependent patterns of growth hormone secretion from the pituitary gland. Sex differences in drug biotransformation in humans are not as pronounced as in the rat, but male and female patients have been found to biotransform many drugs (e.g., propranolol, benzodiazepines, salicylates) at different rates. Pregnancy, adrenal insufficiency, diabetes, and hypothyroid conditions have all been shown to alter drug biotransformation capacity.

## Diet

Both macronutrient and micronutrient dietary components affect drug biotransformation. It is difficult to make generalizations about the effects of diet on drug biotransformation because individual enzymes may display unique responses to dietary factors. For example, fasting causes a characteristic increase in CYP2E1 levels and activity, but diets that are low in protein or deficient in essential fatty acids generally result in decreased cytochrome P450–mediated biotransformation. Many vitamins (e.g., vitamins A, $B_1$, $B_2$, C, E, K) and minerals (e.g., calcium, magnesium, iron, copper, zinc, iodine) can also have complex effects on drug biotransformation capacity.

In addition, many non-nutrient dietary components may affect drug biotransformation. Polycylic aromatic hydrocarbons found in charcoal-broiled meats are inducers of CYP1A1 and CYP1A2 and are also potential carcinogens. There is also evidence that the ability of specific compounds found in vegetables to prevent chemical carcinogenesis is related to their effects on procarcinogen biotransformation. For example, chemicals found in broccoli and Brussels sprouts (e.g., indole 3-carbinol) and in garlic (e.g., diallyl sulfide) display potentially beneficial cancer chemopreventive properties that are at least partially based on modulation of drug-biotransforming enzymes. As discussed above, the inhibition of cytochrome P450 enzymes by grapefruit juice is an extremely important dietary influence on drug biotransformation.

## Disease States

Liver cirrhosis and liver cancer are associated with decreased hepatic biotransformation capacity, particularly with respect to cytochrome P450–dependent pathways. Such effects may be due to decreased expression of drug-biotransforming enzymes, as well as to alterations in liver architecture that decrease and alter hepatic blood flow. Many tumour cells display reduced cytochrome P450 content and increased levels of phase II biotransformation enzymes, making them particularly resistant to chemical insult, including the action of cytotoxic antineoplastic agents (see Chapter 57).

Infectious diseases and inflammatory conditions are often associated with reduced hepatic drug biotransformation. Interferons and cytokines that are produced after activation of host defence mechanisms appear to mediate the suppression of drug biotransformation. By limiting blood flow to the liver, the condition of congestive heart failure can impair the biotransformation of several therapeutic agents (e.g., alprenolol, meperidine, verapamil).

## METHODS FOR THE STUDY OF DRUG BIOTRANSFORMATION

Modern investigations of drug biotransformation are conducted in experimental systems that range in complexity from an isolated enzyme to an intact animal or human subject.

Studies of drug pharmacokinetics in vivo provide valuable information about the overall fate of a drug in an intact biological system, but measurement of the disappearance of parent drug from plasma cannot distinguish between processes of distribution, biotransformation, and renal elimination. It can be very informative to identify and measure specific biotransformation products (i.e., metabolites) in plasma, urine, and/or bile. If the rate of disappearance of parent drug equals the rate of appearance of metabolites, this is good evidence that drug disappearance is due to biotransformation. However, this in vivo approach does not reveal the sites and mechanisms of drug biotransformation. With the use of non-invasive probe drug assays, it is possible to phenotype human subjects with respect to the function of specific hepatic enzymes of drug biotransformation. For example, the measurement of specific metabolites of caffeine in urine can be used as an indication of both CYP1A2 and NAT2 catalytic functions in humans. This is possible because CYP1A2-mediated caffeine 3-demethylation is a major pathway for caffeine elimination in humans, while a sub-

sequent pathway mediated by NAT2 produces an additional urinary metabolite.

Transgenic and "knock-out" mouse models now play a prominent role in research on drug biotransformation. The conventional approach to generating a mouse that is null for a specific gene product (i.e., a "knock-out") is gene targeting via homologous recombination in embryonic stem cells. This has resulted in the production of several mouse lines, each lacking a specific drug-biotransforming enzyme (e.g., CYP1A2- or NAT-null mice) or a specific receptor responsible for the regulation of such enzymes (e.g., AH receptor–null mice). Such animal models have been instrumental in helping to define the physiological function of these enzymes and receptors and the roles that they play in adaptive and toxic responses to xenobiotics. It has also become possible to create "humanized" mouse lines, in which a specific mouse enzyme or receptor is replaced by the corresponding human protein.

At the organ level, most interest in drug biotransformation has focused on the liver. Liver perfusion studies have yielded important information concerning the kinetic and spatial aspects of drug biotransformation. Within the liver, hepatocytes contain the highest concentrations of drug-biotransforming enzymes, and it is possible to study drug biotransformation in freshly isolated and cultured hepatocytes. A problem with the use of cultured hepatocytes is that the cells tend to show a loss of differentiated hepatocyte functions (including cytochrome P450–mediated drug biotransformation) during in vitro culture. Similarly, many immortal hepatoma cell lines are deficient in cytochrome P450 function.

Biotransformation of drugs is commonly studied in subcellular fractions, especially microsomes and cytosol. For example, hepatic microsomes supplemented with exogenous NADPH contain all the enzymatic machinery required to carry out the oxidative biotransformation of numerous drugs. Using protein biochemistry techniques, it is also possible to purify a specific drug-biotransforming enzyme and study its function in isolation. An individual cytochrome P450 enzyme can be reconstituted with purified NADPH–cytochrome P450 reductase and phospholipid to yield a functional monooxygenase system. Using molecular biology techniques, one can express the cDNA for a single drug-biotransformation enzyme in a variety of cellular systems, including mammalian and insect cells, yeast, and bacteria that do not normally contain that enzyme. This approach can be particularly powerful as it allows the study of a single enzyme in isolation within a cellular environment.

It must be kept in mind, however, that in vitro drug biotransformation reactions are usually studied under optimal conditions of substrate and cofactor concentrations, temperature, pH, and so forth. The rate of reaction may therefore be quite different from that seen under the influence of rate-limiting factors in vivo.

## DRUG BIOTRANSFORMATION IN THE DRUG DEVELOPMENT PROCESS

During the process of developing a new therapeutic agent for clinical use, it is essential to characterize the routes and rates of biotransformation of the compound. Traditionally, this has involved the characterization of the metabolites produced in experimental animals. However, species differences in drug biotransformation render rodents poor experimental models for human biotransformation. Therefore, the biotransformation of new drugs by human enzymes should be studied before the drug is administered to patients. It is of considerable interest to identify the human enzyme(s) responsible for the biotransformation of a drug so that adverse reactions resulting from drug interactions or genetic defects can be understood and predicted.

Using the cytochromes P450 as an example, it is possible to use four major in vitro approaches in combination in order to determine which particular enzyme carries out the biotransformation of a drug. First, studying the drug biotransformation by a purified or cDNA-expressed human enzyme can tell whether that enzyme has the inherent capability to transform the drug. Second, using a human liver microsomal preparation, it is possible to determine the effect of cytochrome P450 isozyme–selective chemical inhibitors on the reaction of interest. For example, furafylline will inhibit the biotransformation of the drug if CYP1A2 is involved in the reaction. Third, many antibodies that are directed against a drug-biotransformation enzyme can serve as isozyme-selective inhibitors. Thus, if anti-CYP1A2 antibody inhibits the reaction to a large extent, then this is good evidence that CYP1A2 makes an important contribution to this reaction in human liver. Finally, if a panel of human liver microsomal samples is available from a number of donors, it is possible to perform correlation analyses. For example, if the rate of biotransformation of the drug of interest correlates with the level of CYP1A2 protein or catalytic activity in a number of human liver samples, then it would appear that CYP1A2 is an important contributor to this reaction. In this manner, advances in protein biochemistry and molecular biology are having an impact on the development of therapeutic agents and improvement in human health.

## SUGGESTED READINGS

Conney, AH. Induction of drug-metabolizing enzymes: a path to the discovery of multiple cytochromes P450. *Annu Rev Pharmacol Toxicol.* 2003;43:1-30.

Elizondo G, Gonzalez FJ. Understanding molecular mechanisms of toxicity and carcinogenicity using gene knockout and transgenic mouse models. *Handbook of Experimental Pharmacology.* 2004;159:639-660.

Gibson GG, Skett P. *Introduction to Drug Metabolism.* 3rd ed. Cheltenham, United Kingdom: Nelson Thornes Publishers; 2001.

Glatt H, Boeing H, Engelke CE, et al. Human cytosolic sulphotransferases: genetics, characteristics, toxicological aspects. *Mutat Res.* 2001;482:27-40.

Guengerich FP. Cytochrome P450, drugs, and diseases. *Mol Interv.* 2003;3:194-204.

Handschin C, Meyer UA. Induction of drug metabolism: the role of nuclear receptors. *Pharmacol Rev.* 2003;55:649-673.

Hayes JD, Flanagan JU, Jowsey IR. Glutathione transferases. *Annu Rev Pharmacol Toxicol.* 2005;45:51-88.

Hein DW. Molecular genetics and function of NAT1 and NAT2: role in aromatic amine metabolism and carcinogenesis. *Mutat Res.* 2002;506-507:65-77.

Morisseau C, Hammock BD. Epoxide hydrolases: mechanisms, inhibitor designs, and biological roles. *Annu Rev Pharmacol Toxicol.* 2005;45:311-333.

Nebert DW, Russell DW. Clinical importance of the cytochromes P450. *Lancet.* 2002;360:1155-1162.

Nebert DW, Vasiliou V. Analysis of the glutathione S-transferase (GST) gene family. *Hum Genomics.* 2004;1:460-464.

Nelson DR, Zeldin DC, Hoffman SMG, Maltais LJ, Wain HM, Nebert DW. Comparison of cytochrome P450 (*CYP*) genes from the mouse and human genomes, including nomenclature recommendations for genes, pseudogenes and alternative-splice variants. *Pharmacogenetics.* 2004;14:1-18.

Oppermann UC, Maser E. Molecular and structural aspects of xenobiotic carbonyl metabolizing enzymes: role of reductases and dehydrogenases in xenobiotic phase I reactions. *Toxicology.* 2000;144:71-81.

Ortiz de Montellano PR, ed. *Cytochrome P450: Structure, Mechanism, and Biochemistry.* 3rd ed. New York, NY: Kluwer Academic/Plenum Publishers; 2005.

Parkinson A. Biotransformation of xenobiotics. In: Klaassen CD, ed. *Casarett and Doull's Toxicology: The Basic Science of Poisons.* 6th ed. New York, NY: McGraw-Hill; 2001:133-224.

Riddick DS, Lee C, Bhathena A, Timsit YE. The 2001 Veylien Henderson Award of the Society of Toxicology of Canada. Positive and negative transcriptional regulation of cytochromes P450 by polycyclic aromatic hydrocarbons. *Can J Physiol Pharmacol.* 2003;81:59-77.

Ross D. Quinone reductases multitasking in the metabolic world. *Drug Metab Rev.* 2004;36:639-654.

Tukey RH, Strassburg CP. Human UDP-glucuronosyltransferases: metabolism, expression, and disease. *Annu Rev Pharmacol Toxicol.* 2000;40:581-616.

Weinshilboum RM, Otterness DM, Szumlanski CL. Methylation pharmacogenetics: catechol O-methyltransferase, thiopurine methyltransferase, and histamine N-methyltransferase. *Annu Rev Pharmacol Toxicol.* 1999;39:19-52.

Ziegler DM. An overview of the mechanism, substrate specificities, and structure of FMOs. *Drug Metab Rev.* 2002;34:503-511.

## ONLINE RESOURCES

ASPET Division for Drug Metabolism:
http://www.aspet.org/public/divisions/drugmetab/

Cytochrome P450 drug interaction table:
http://medicine.iupui.edu/flockhart/

Extensive databases of cytochrome P450 nomenclature and
    diversity:
http://drnelson.utmem.edu/CytochromeP450.html

Human cytochrome P450 allele nomenclature:
http://www.imm.ki.se/CYPalleles/

International Society for the Study of Xenobiotics:
http://www.issx.org/

N-Acetyltransferase nomenclature:
http://www.louisville.edu/medschool/pharmacology/NAT.html

Sulfotransferase nomenclature:
http://www.fccc.edu/research/labs/blanchard/sult/

UDP-glucuronosyltransferase nomenclature:
http://som.flinders.edu.au/FUSA/ClinPharm/UGT/

# 5

# Pharmacokinetics: Principles and Clinical Applications

## L ENDRENYI

### Aims of Pharmacokinetics

Pharmacokinetics describes quantitatively the rates of the various steps of drug disposition. These steps include (1) the absorption of drugs, which enables them to reach the systemic circulation, (2) their distribution to various organs and tissues in the body, and (3) their elimination by biotransformation and excretion.

The rates of these processes have two main applications. First, they are in themselves of great interest to pharmacologists because they characterize in some detail the fate of a drug in the body and thus permit the factors that determine this fate to be studied. Second, physicians use pharmacokinetic data for calculating and selecting the routes, doses, and frequencies of drug administration.

Such pharmacokinetic assessments are particularly essential for clinicians when, for a given drug, the doses eliciting toxic side effects are not much higher than those required for therapeutic action. Care must also be exercised when there is large variation in the responses of different patients to a given dose of a drug. The variability can appear in several forms: there may be a wide spread among the responses of different people; the responses to some drugs may be separated into two or more distinct groups, based on genetic differences; and rare idiosyncratic responses may occur. In all these cases, a pharmacokinetic study of an individual patient is desirable to optimally adjust the drug dose.

### Relation of Dose, Plasma Drug Concentration, and Effect

A particular amount (dose) of an administered drug will produce an effect according to the following sequence:

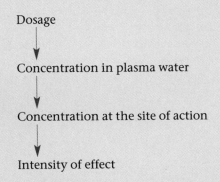

Dosage

↓

Concentration in plasma water

↓

Concentration at the site of action

↓

Intensity of effect

The intensity of drug action is most often related to the concentration of the drug at the site of action ("receptor"). Similarly, the duration of the drug effect is related to the greater or lesser persistence of its presence at this site. The concentration at the receptors changes, in turn, as the drug enters, is distributed in, and leaves various parts of the body and as it undergoes biotransformation (metabolic degradation) reactions.

**Pharmacodynamic** investigations examine the intensity and the time courses of responses to drugs. Unfortunately, some clinical responses (e.g., effectiveness of sleep induction, or decrease in chronic skeletal pain) are difficult to characterize quantitatively. Therefore, we frequently assume that the intensity of pharmacological action correlates better with the concentration of free drug in plasma than with the dose, and in **pharmacokinetic** studies, we evaluate the time course of drug concentrations in the plasma (and in other body fluids) following various routes of drug administration. As an important application, the efficacy of drug therapy can be improved and toxicity can be decreased by using plasma drug concentrations as an aid in adjusting drug dosage.

In some situations, however, the relation between plasma concentration and effect is difficult to interpret—for example, in the case of irreversibly acting drugs (phenoxybenzamine); acute, chronic, or cross-tolerance (opiates); combinations of drugs with synergistic (morphine and ethanol) or antagonistic actions (morphine and naloxone); and the presence of active metabolites (e.g., diazepam and desmethyldiazepam).

## DRUG CONCENTRATIONS FOLLOWING INTRAVENOUS INJECTION

Since first-order drug disposition is the most common (and simplest) pattern, we shall assume it in this model. This means that the rate of the process at any given time is proportional to the concentration at that time. Consequently, after the intravenous administration of a drug, its concentration ($C$) in the plasma decreases at a rate that is proportional to the concentration itself at all times ($t$). This statement is described mathematically by

$$Rate = (-dC/dt) = kC$$

where $k$ is the proportionality, or rate, constant. If the initial concentration is $C_0$, the solution of this differential equation is

$$C = C_0 e^{-kt}$$

where $e$ is the base of the natural logarithm. The exponentially moderated decrease of the plasma concentration is shown in Figure 5-1.

In practice, a more convenient form of this equation is obtained by using logarithms:

$$log\ C = log\ C_0 - kt$$

Here, *log* refers to natural logarithm. Thus, if we plot the logarithm of the concentrations (*log C*) against the times of their observation ($t$), we should obtain a straight line (Fig. 5-1B). The plot provides the values of $k$ and $C_0$ at once since the slope of the line equals $-k$ and the vertical intercept is *log* $C_0$.

From the estimated $C_0$ and the injected dose ($D_0$), the **volume of distribution** ($V$) can be calculated:

$$V = D_0/C_0$$

Another important quantity, the **half-life of elimination** ($t_{1/2}$), can also be evaluated from the elimination rate constant ($0.693 = log\ 2$):

$$t_{1/2} = 0.693/k$$

This is the time period during which the concentration decreases to one-half of its previous value.

**EXAMPLE:** A 100-mg dose of a drug was injected intravenously, and its concentration (in milligrams per litre) in the plasma was observed repeatedly. The natural logarithms of the concentrations were plotted against the times (in hours) of their observation. A straight line could be drawn through the points, which had a slope of –0.173 and an extrapolated intercept of 3.00. Consequently,

$$k = 0.173\ hr^{-1}$$

and

$$C_0 = e^{3.00} = 20\ mg/L$$

From these, the half-life of elimination is

$$t_{1/2} = 0.693/0.173 = 4.0\ hours$$

and the volume of distribution is

$$V = 100\ /\ 20 = 5.0\ L$$

The half-life of 4.0 hours means that, 4 hours after the injection of the initial 100 mg, only 50 mg is left in the plasma (and in those parts of the body in which the concentration of this drug is in constant proportion to that in the plasma). After 8 hours, 25 mg is left; after 12 hours, 12.5 mg remains; and so on. With a distribution volume of 5.0 L, this is equivalent to concentrations of 20, 10, 5, and 2.5 mg/L at 0, 4, 8, and 12 hours after injection, respectively.

After intravenous injection, curvature can often be detected in the early part of the semi-logarithmic elimination plot. This is reasonable because, as already indicated, it takes some time for the drug to be redistributed from the circulating plasma to the extracellular space. During this period, the logarithmic concentration in plasma decreases more rapidly than in the later, linear, steady-state section of the curve (Fig. 5-2).

## Total Body Clearance

Clearance is a quantitative measure characterizing the rate of removal of endogenous or exogenous substances, including drugs, from the body or from a specific part of the body. Hepatic biotransformation, excretion by the kidneys and bile, exhalation by the lungs, and fecal excretion are the usual routes of drug elimination. The corresponding specific clearances are considered in Chapter 6. Here, we will deal with their sum, the total body clearance (TBC), a measure of the overall rate of disappearance or elimination of a substance from the whole body.

Clearance is expressed as *the volume of body fluid from which a substance (drug) is removed in unit time*. Consequently, when concentrations are measured in plasma, the volume of this fluid from which the drug is apparently removed (cleared) in unit time is referred to as the *plasma clearance*.

In terms of kinetic parameters, that is, the first-order elimination rate constant ($k$) and the apparent volume of

| FIGURE 5-1 | Time dependence of a drug concentration in blood after an intravenous injection. The drug concentration is plotted on a linear (A) and a logarithmic (B) scale. In the former, the area under the curve is shaded. |
|---|---|

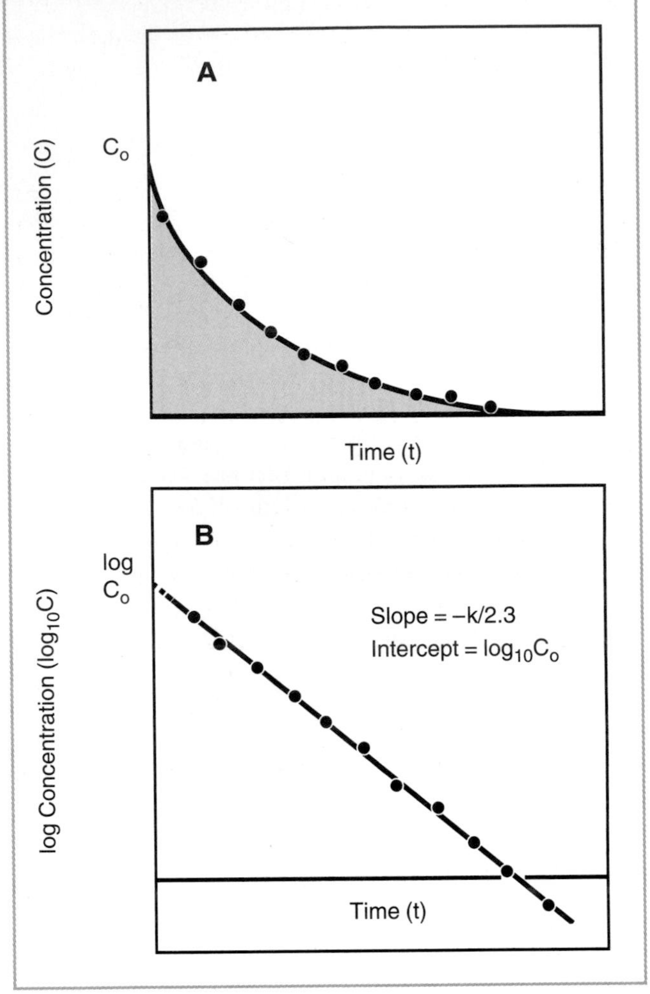

distribution ($V$), the total body clearance can be expressed as the following:

$$Cl = kV \ [mL/min] = [min^{-1}] \times [mL]$$

(Dimensions, given as illustration, of the various quantities in this and all following equations are in square brackets.)

This simple calculation is in agreement with the definition of clearance given above since, as seen earlier, the rate constant is defined numerically as the fraction of a substance eliminated (cleared) in unit time; its product with the apparent volume of distribution yields the volume from which the drug is apparently removed in unit time.

The volume defined by clearance is often measured by dividing the amount of drug removed in unit time by the concentration of the drug in the relevant body fluid. Usually, however, evaluation of the total body clearance is based on a different kinetic principle. It can be shown that clearance is inversely proportional to the area under a curve (AUC) fitted to concentration readings obtained at different times. If the drug is completely absorbed following its administration, such as after intravenous injection, then

$$Cl = Dose / AUC \ [mL/min] = [mg]/[(mg/mL) \times min]$$

When only a fraction (F) of the dose is absorbed, as is often the case following oral administration, then

$$Cl = F \cdot Dose / F \ AUC$$

For measuring the AUC, the concentrations should be plotted on a linear scale, not a logarithmic one (see Fig. 5-1A). Also, AUC refers to the complete area under the curve evaluated between the times of zero and infinity following drug administration. Therefore, the curve fitted through the observed values must be extrapolated to the time of infinity by an algebraic procedure.

*The concept of clearance is biologically meaningful and important.* Its study enables pharmacologists to reach conclusions about the effect of hepatic blood flow, renal processes, and protein binding on drug elimination. This is discussed in other chapters.

Furthermore, the steady-state concentration of a drug, which is reached when the rate of intake equals the rate of elimination, is determined by the total body clearance. This question is discussed below in some detail (see "Dosage for Intravenous Infusion").

## Duration of Drug Action

It is usually assumed that a drug evokes some demonstrable effect when its plasma concentration is higher than a minimal therapeutically effective plasma concentration ($C_{ther}$). Detectable drug action is maintained as long as the drug concentration exceeds this minimum effective level.

A useful guideline characterizing the duration of drug action can be established on the basis of this principle. This states that **the duration of drug effects is proportional to the half-life of elimination and to the logarithm of the dose,** provided that the absorption and distribution of the drug are rapid in comparison with its elimination (including biotransformation and excretion) and that these are first-order processes.

Therefore, it is very difficult to obtain increased duration of drug action by increasing the dosage, since the latter must be raised exponentially to attain only a linear increase in the duration.

In order to demonstrate these proportionalities, let us assume elimination without a distribution phase. If different doses of a drug are introduced by a given route of administration, the semi-logarithmic concentration–time profiles will be parallel lines (Fig. 5-3). Furthermore, if the ratios between the consecutively higher doses (i.e., the differences between their logarithms) are constant, then the lines are equally distanced. In the horizontal direction, equal distances between lines, particularly at the concentration level $C_{ther}$, imply the uniformly gradual increase in the duration of drug action ($t_D$). Thus, equal

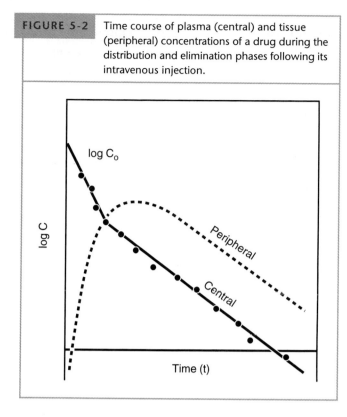

**FIGURE 5-2** Time course of plasma (central) and tissue (peripheral) concentrations of a drug during the distribution and elimination phases following its intravenous injection.

increments of duration are paralleled by uniform increments of the logarithm of the dose, and, therefore, the two quantities are linearly related.

An important application of this rule states that **the duration of drug action is extended by one half-life when the dose is doubled.** This conclusion can be formalized as follows:

$$t_{2D_0} = t_{D_0} + t_{1/2}$$

**EXAMPLE:** Let us assume that for the drug considered earlier, with a half-life of 4 hours and an apparent volume of distribution of 5 L, the therapeutically effective concentration $C_{ther}$ is 5 mg/L. We have already seen that the plasma concentration has fallen to this level 8 hours after the intravenous injection of a dose of 100 mg. If the dose is doubled to 200 mg, then, according to our rule, the duration of effective drug action is extended to 8 + 4 = 12 hours.

The proportionality of duration and elimination half-life can be similarly illustrated. After all, shallower lines in the semi-logarithmic plot indicate longer half-lives (shallow dashed line in Fig. 5-3). Consequently, for a given intercept (initial concentration), the minimal effective concentration is reached after a longer time, and thereby the duration of drug action is also longer.

The guidelines characterizing the duration of drug action can also be applied, with very good approximation, in the presence of fast absorption and distribution because these alter the concentration profile only slightly. However, caution must be exercised when non-linear kinetics or extended absorption and/or distribution

causes substantial curvature in the semi-logarithmic concentration–time plot.

The above considerations are not applicable when the effects of a drug or chemical are not proportional to its plasma concentration. For instance, organophosphate insecticides destroy certain enzymes in the body. Consequently, their effect is prolonged well after their elimination, until the enzymes are re-synthesized.

## Concentration Dependence of Rates

We have assumed that the rates of various processes are proportional to the drug concentration. This is usually a reasonable assumption. For example, it is valid for diffusion-controlled processes since the rate of diffusion is proportional to the concentration gradient (the difference of concentrations on the two sides of a membrane or other barrier), and the concentration of the "receiving" side is usually negligibly small in comparison with the concentration in the "donating" compartment. Similarly, the rate of urinary excretion is usually proportional to the concentration of the free drug in the systemic circulation. Certainly, this is true for excretion by glomerular filtration, but in practice, it is often valid even for active transfer processes such as tubular secretion or reabsorption when the drug concentration in the relevant compartment is low enough that the carrier system is not close to being saturated.

However, carrier systems can become saturated at high concentrations. The rate of urinary excretion is then constant, independently of the plasma concentration, and thereby conforms to the features of a *zero-order process*. A linear plot for the time course of concentrations (Fig. 5-4A) shows a constant rate of decline; in contrast,

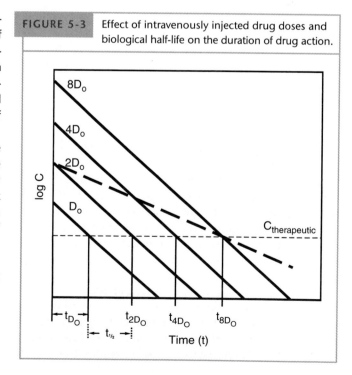

**FIGURE 5-3** Effect of intravenously injected drug doses and biological half-life on the duration of drug action.

the slope in the semi-logarithmic plot of concentrations (Fig. 5-4B) is not constant in this region but gets gradually steeper. Eventually, the concentration decreases sufficiently so that the carrier system is no longer saturated. After passing through an intermediate region, the concentration reaches, at its lower levels, the range of first-order removal.

Some drugs act therapeutically in the transitional range between the regions of purely zero-order and purely first-order kinetics (e.g., phenytoin, dicumarol, salicylic acid). Other substances are physiologically effective within the range of zero-order kinetics (e.g., ethanol). Similar considerations apply to biotransformation reactions or to the binding to plasma proteins. At high drug concentrations, the catalyzing enzyme or the binding protein (albumin) becomes saturated with substrate (drug) molecules, and, therefore, the rate of the appropriate process is independent of the drug concentration. However, at much below saturating concentrations, these rates also become proportional to the concentrations.

As mentioned earlier, the rate of absorption is also proportional to the amount of the unabsorbed drug. This is, of course, not so when drug tablets are specially coated to form slow, sustained-release preparations that are absorbed at a rate independent of the amount of drug remaining in the intestinal lumen.

## DRUG CONCENTRATIONS DURING INTRAVENOUS INFUSION

### Concentration Profiles

If the drug is introduced at a constant rate, in the form of intravenous infusion, its concentration in the plasma increases at a gradually diminishing rate. After a while, fairly constant concentration is reached. The infusion may be discontinued either before or after reaching the plateau. This is indicated by arrows in Figure 5-5, showing a curve obtained at high infusion rate that is continued to steady state at the plateau and, with identical kinetic constants, another curve that characterizes a lower-rate infusion that is interrupted before reaching the plateau.

After interruption of the infusion, the time course of drug concentrations follows principles described earlier. If redistribution of the drug is essentially complete, then its elimination is characterized by a descending straight line in the semi-logarithmic plot (Fig. 5-5B).

In the plot of concentration against time (Fig. 5-5A), the accumulation curve is the inverted mirror image of the elimination pattern.

### Dosage for Intravenous Infusion

Let us consider the rates of input and output processes involving the whole body.

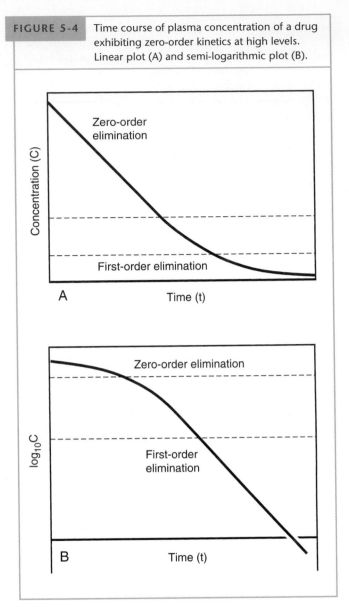

FIGURE 5-4 Time course of plasma concentration of a drug exhibiting zero-order kinetics at high levels. Linear plot (A) and semi-logarithmic plot (B).

Input could refer to the sum of endogenous production and exogenous intake of a substance. We shall be concerned mainly with the latter. Initially, we shall assume that a drug is administered at a constant rate, $Q$ (e.g., by intravenous infusion). The rate is the amount administered per unit time and has units of, say, milligrams per minute.

The amount of drug in the body at any time is $VC$, where, as before, $V$ is the apparent volume of distribution and $C$ the concentration in the plasma. The fraction of this amount that is being removed in unit time is given by the elimination rate constant ($k$). Consequently, the amount eliminated per unit time is $kVC$.

At steady state, the rate of input is equal to the rate of elimination, therefore,

$$Q = kVC_{ss}$$

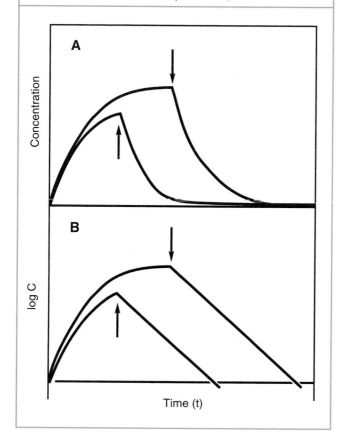

**FIGURE 5-5** Time course of drug concentration during and following intravenous infusion. The arrows indicate the cessation of drug administration. Linear plot (A) and semi-logarithmic plot (B). (See text for additional explanations.)

Thus, it is possible to calculate the rate of drug administration (Q) that is required to maintain a desired steady-state concentration ($C_{ss}$).

In terms of clearance,

$$Q = Cl \cdot C_{ss}$$

Consequently, the steady-state concentration is

$$C_{ss} = Q / Cl \; [\text{mg/mL}] = [\text{mg/min}]/[\text{mL/min}]$$

This is reasonable since, according to this expression, the steady-state concentration is determined by the ratio of inflow and outflow rates.

We could consider the analogy of water in a tub (Fig. 5-6) in which both the inflow and outflow faucets are open. The *level* of water finally attained depends on the rates of both inflow and outflow. However, if the faucets are adjusted, the *rate* at which the new water level is reached depends only on the setting of the faucet for outflow but not of that for inflow. Try it out!

Since an immediate effect is desired, a **loading dose** of the drug is given by rapid administration (e.g., by injection) to fill the body stores and establish the effective,

steady-state plasma concentration. As we have seen, at steady state, the amount of drug in the body is $VC_{ss}$. This is the amount that the loading dose (L) should introduce at once. Consequently,

$$L = VC_{ss} \; [\text{mg}] = [\text{L}] \times [\text{mg/L}]$$

(The relationships between infusion rate, clearance, and steady-state concentration are used for the convenient evaluation of the clearance. This can be done because the infusion rate is set by the physician or the investigator, and the steady-state concentration can be easily measured. If, in addition, the elimination rate constant or the related half-life is observed, the apparent volume of distribution can also be calculated. This is often the preferred approach.)

**EXAMPLE:** lidocaine infusion
Besides being a local anaesthetic agent, lidocaine is effective in the treatment of certain cardiac arrhythmias (see Chapter 33). Continuous infusion is indicated in patients in whom the arrhythmia tends to recur and to whom oral therapy cannot be given.

Let us assume the following characteristics of the drug in a 70-kg man:

$C_{ther} = 2.0$ mg/L (therapeutically effective concentration)
$t_{1/2} = 80$ minutes (biological half-life) [where $t_{1/2} = 0.693/k$]
$V_w = 0.70$ L/kg (apparent distribution volume as a proportion of body weight)

Consequently,

$$k = 0.693/80 = 0.0087 \; \text{min}^{-1}$$
$$V = 0.70 \; [\text{L/kg}] \times 70 \; [\text{kg}] = 49 \; \text{L}$$

which indicates that lidocaine is distributed throughout the total body water.

Therefore, the desired infusion rate is

$$Q = kVC_{ss}$$
$$= 0.0087 \times 49 \times 2.0 = 0.85 \; \text{mg/min}$$

Incidentally, the total body clearance is

$$Cl = kV$$
$$= 0.0087 \times 49 = 0.43 \; \text{L/min}$$

The corresponding loading dose is

$$L = VC_{ss}$$
$$= 49 \times 2.0 = 98 \; \text{mg}$$

In practice, a loading dose of 100 mg could be given. The steady-state infusion rate would be about 1 mg/min, and the resulting $C_{ss}$ would be just slightly higher than the target value of 2.0 mg/L.

## Time to Steady-State Concentration: Plateau Principle

Let us assume again that a drug follows first-order kinetics, and, for now, that it is administered by continuous intra-

FIGURE 5-6 Hydrodynamic analogy for drug kinetics: water in the tub.

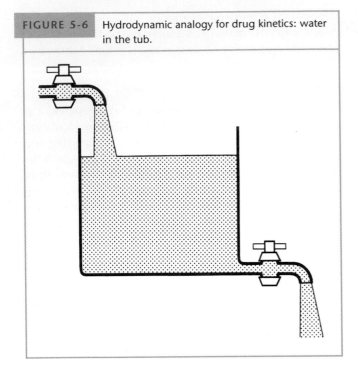

venous infusion. We have seen that the steady-state concentration ($C_{ss}$) depends on the rates of both administration and removal of the drug. In contrast, the rate of approach to the steady-state level depends only on the elimination rate constant. Thus, according to the so-called plateau principle, *the time to reach a given fraction of the steady-state concentration is determined only by the elimination rate constant.* In the example of the partially filled tub in Figure 5-6, if a constant level had previously been reached (this could be any level, including an empty tub), and then either of the two faucets is adjusted, the rate at which the new water level is approached depends solely on the setting of the outflow tap.

(The sense of the plateau principle can be appreciated by recalling that the plasma concentration of a drug changes at a rate determined by two simultaneously occurring processes. A constant rate of inflow is assumed by maintaining steady infusion. Thus, the rate of outflow, or elimination, completely determines the overall rate of concentration change and, with it, the time course of plasma concentration. The elimination rate, in turn, is defined again by the elimination rate constant.)

The time required to reach a given fraction (*f*) of the steady-state concentration can be calculated from the plateau principle. This time depends only on *kt,* and therefore, the time to reach this fraction depends only on the elimination rate constant, *k.* The principle applies to all shifts from one steady state to another.

The time required to reach a given fraction, $f = 1 - e^{-kt}$, of the steady-state level can be evaluated from the formula or from the diagram depicting it (Fig. 5-7). The fraction *f* is called the *fractional attainment.*

For instance, the time required to reach 90% of a steady state is $3.3t_{1/2}$. This can be seen from the graph in Figure 5-7, where, at $f = 0.90$, we find $kt = 2.3$.

But also,

$$k = 0.693/t_{1/2}$$

and therefore

$$t = 2.3/0.693 \times t_{1/2} = 3.3t_{1/2}$$

Consequently, 90% of the steady-state, plateau concentration is indeed reached during a period of 3.3 half-lives.

Analogous calculations show that

time to reach 95% plateau = $4.3 \times t_{1/2}$
99% plateau = $6.6 \times t_{1/2}$
99.9% plateau = $10.0 \times t_{1/2}$

For most practical purposes, a useful "rule of thumb" to remember is the following:

**The time to plateau is roughly 5× half-life.**

This approach is quite simplified but nevertheless will give a good ballpark estimate for most drugs.

Two comments should be made at this point about assumptions and applications. First, the plateau principle itself is based on the supposition of first-order kinetics. The quantitative implementation also assumes a simple description of physiological processes with either intravenous administration or rapid absorption. In spite of these simplifications, the quantitative conclusions can be usefully applied under most practically occurring conditions. Second, the principle and its quantitative consequences can be utilized not only for the simple case of drug infusion but also for other conditions of accumulation and elimination, both in the absence and presence of endogenous substances.

FIGURE 5-7 Relationship of fractional attainment of the plateau to *kt*. Recall that $kt = 0.7(t/t_{1/2})$. Consequently, the diagram also depicts the dependence of the fractional attainment on the number of elapsed half-lives.

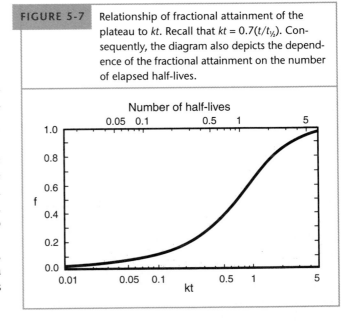

## Application of the plateau principle

1. Lidocaine, as mentioned in the example above of calculation of loading dose and infusion rate, has a $t_{1/2}$ of 80 min, or 1.33 hours. If a continuous infusion were started, it would take $6.6 \times t_{1/2} = 8.8$ hours before plasma concentrations reached 99% of the maximum. This would explain the late appearance of toxicity of the drug.
2. Phenytoin has a $t_{1/2}$ of 22 hours; therefore, the time to plateau is 110 hours (by rule of thumb).
3. For drugs administered orally, the same calculations allow us to estimate when a given proportion of maximum cumulation of drug has taken place (e.g., phenytoin by mouth will take 3 days for 90% cumulation).

*It will also take this long to eliminate these drugs.* Several examples one may wish to think about are tetrahydrocannabinol, $t_{1/2} = 50$ hours; diazepam (Valium), $t_{1/2} = 35$ hours; and phenobarbital, $t_{1/2} = 4.1$ days.

*If the dose (or rate of administration) of a drug is changed, the time to reach the new plateau is calculated in exactly the same way as if one started from zero concentration.*

# REPEATED DRUG ADMINISTRATION

## Dosage Regimens

The aim of approximately constant plasma concentration levels can also be reached by repeated applications of the drug. We would like the concentration to stay above the threshold level for effective therapeutic action ($C_{ther}$) but safely below the toxic concentration ($C_{tox}$) that would begin to cause harmful side effects. This aim is achieved when appropriate maintenance doses are given repeatedly at the proper dosing intervals.

Figure 5-8 illustrates the time course of drug concentrations following repeated intravenous administrations. The discontinuation of drug administration is indicated by arrows.

In the semi-logarithmic plot (Fig. 5-8A), the descending segments are linear and parallel since all of them are characterized by the same elimination rate constant and half-life. In the concentration–time plot (Fig. 5-8B), the vertical (ascending) lines are of equal length, on the assumption that identical maintenance doses are used; the descending sections are exponential and not linear. When the initial dose equals the maintenance doses, the final desired concentration range is reached not immediately, but only after several dosage intervals. But the patient is probably sickest and in greatest need of reaching the proper therapeutic drug concentration in the initial phase of the medication. Therefore, it is very desirable to initially administer a high, so-called **loading or priming dose** ($L$) and to continue later with the small **maintenance doses** ($D_m$). These are generally given at regular dosing intervals, or **maintenance intervals** ($T_m$) (Fig. 5-9).

A systematic dosage schedule involving repeated drug administration is referred to as a **dosage regimen**. Its components are the loading dose, maintenance doses, and dosing intervals.

## Quantitative Determination of the Ideal Dosage Regimens

The principles described for determining doses with intravenous infusion apply also to the situation when the drug is given intermittently. The main difference is that now we cannot *exactly* maintain the steady-state concentration. Rather, the concentration will fluctuate around an

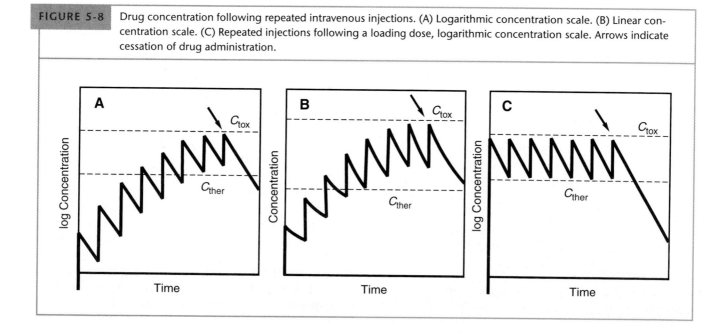

**FIGURE 5-8** Drug concentration following repeated intravenous injections. (A) Logarithmic concentration scale. (B) Linear concentration scale. (C) Repeated injections following a loading dose, logarithmic concentration scale. Arrows indicate cessation of drug administration.

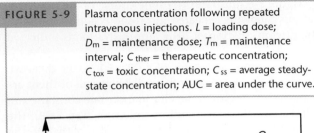

FIGURE 5-9    Plasma concentration following repeated intravenous injections. $L$ = loading dose; $D_m$ = maintenance dose; $T_m$ = maintenance interval; $C_{ther}$ = therapeutic concentration; $C_{tox}$ = toxic concentration; $C_{ss}$ = average steady-state concentration; AUC = area under the curve.

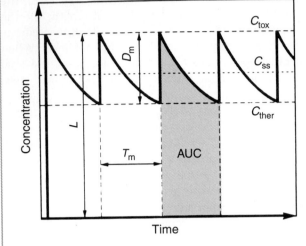

*average* steady-state value. This average concentration is brought about by the balance of the outflow rate (represented by the clearance) and the average inflow rate.

Consequently, the relationships described earlier remain applicable as long as we consider average concentrations and input rates. When **maintenance doses** of $D_m$ are administered following each **maintenance interval** of $T_m$, the average rate of drug intake is $D_m / T_m$. Therefore, the average steady-state concentration is

$$\bar{C}_{ss} = (D_m/T_m)/Cl$$

Thus, in order to sustain this concentration, a maintenance dose of

$$D_m = Cl \cdot \bar{C}_{ss} \cdot T_m$$
$$= kV\bar{C}_{ss} \cdot T_m$$

is required.

(Rather incidentally, it can be shown that for the calculation of total body clearance, AUC can be also calculated as the area under the plasma concentration curve segment that is obtained, at steady state, between the administrations of consecutive maintenance doses [see Fig. 5-9].)

The maintenance dose is proportional to the maintenance interval. This implies that plasma concentrations show larger *fluctuation* when a drug is administered less frequently.

The proportionality between maintenance dose and maintenance interval raises an important question: How should these two quantities be chosen? The answer will be the result of a compromise between two considerations: the **safety** and the **convenience** of drug administration.

The drug concentration fluctuates around its steady-state average value proportionately to the maintenance dose (see Fig. 5-9). Thus, when the maintenance intervals are shortened and the maintenance doses are correspondingly reduced, the changes in concentration also become smaller. As a result, the safety of drug administration is improved.

However, larger maintenance doses permit longer maintenance intervals (i.e., less frequent administration of the drug). Beyond the obvious convenience, it may increase the probability of a patient's co-operation and compliance with the schedule.

The **maintenance dose** keeps the plasma concentration safely between the minimum therapeutically effective concentration ($C_{ther}$) and the concentration above which toxic effects would begin ($C_{tox}$). Therefore,

$$D_m = (C_{tox} - C_{ther})V$$

The **maintenance interval** can then be obtained from

$$T_m = D_m/(D_m/T_m)$$

that is, by dividing the maintenance dose by its ratio to the maintenance interval.

The **loading dose** ($L$) aims to reach the maximum value of the therapeutic steady-state concentration range immediately following drug administration. Therefore,

$$L = VC_{tox}$$

## Two Frequently Applied Dosage Regimens

Two dosing procedures deserve particular consideration. In the first dosing approach, *maintenance intervals equal the half-life* ($T_m = t_{1/2}$). At steady state, the maximum plasma concentration is twice the minimum concentration ($C_{max} = 2C_{min}$); this implies a substantial fluctuation amounting to 100%. It can be demonstrated that the maximum concentration reached at steady state is twice the maximum concentration obtained after a single drug administration. It follows that *the loading dose should be twice the maintenance dose* ($L = 2D_m$).

The second interesting dosing strategy administers the drug relatively frequently, at maintenance intervals that are less than the half-life of the drug, say, by a factor of at least three ($T_m < t_{1/2}/3$). With this regimen, the plasma concentration at steady state shows only moderate fluctuation. These concentrations are much higher than those seen following a single administration, thereby indicating *substantial accumulation* of the drug. As a result, the loading dose should substantially exceed the maintenance dose. Their relationship is approximately given by ($L = 1.44 \, (t_{1/2}/T_m)D_m$). This condition describes the effect of many environmental chemicals.

## Practical Dosage Regimens

The calculated ideal maintenance interval should be reduced to a practically manageable value such as 24, 12, 8, 6, or 4 hours, for giving the drug once, or two, three, four, or six times a day. The maintenance dose is adjusted correspondingly. It will be set by taking into account the available dosage forms and the desirability of staying below the toxic and above the minimum therapeutically effective concentration levels (see Fig. 5-9).

Thus, drugs that have long half-lives, exceeding 24 hours, will be ingested once daily. Consequently, the dosing interval is less than the half-life, and the initial dose is more than double the maintenance dose.

Drugs having reasonably high safety margins and intermediate half-lives of between 6 and 24 hours could be ingested at intervals approximating their half-lives. Ideally then, the loading dose is twice the maintenance dose. With drugs having a low margin of safety, more frequent administration of lower maintenance doses is required. Occasionally, prolonged-release formulations can be used satisfactorily.

If a drug has a half-life shorter than 6 hours, then it must have a very high safety margin if we wish to consider its repeated administration. The initial dose will equal the maintenance dose. Drugs having a low margin of safety must be administered by continuous infusion.

**EXAMPLE:** repeated intravenous administration of aminophylline, a bronchodilator
Let us assume the following characteristics of the drug in a 50-kg, 32-year-old woman:

$C_{ther}$ = 5 mg/L (therapeutically effective plasma concentration)
$C_{tox}$ = 20 mg/L (toxic plasma concentration)
$\bar{C}_{ss}$ = 10 mg/L (approximate average steady-state plasma concentration)
$t_{1/2}$ = 4.5 hours (biological half-life)
$V_w$ = 0.56 L/kg (apparent distribution volume relative to body weight)

Consequently,

$$k = 0.693 / 4.5 = 0.154 \text{ hr}^{-1}$$
$$V = 0.56 \times 50 = 28 \text{ L}$$

Therefore, to get a ballpark figure, the desired approximate rate of drug administration is

$$D_m / T_m = kV\bar{C}_{ss}$$
$$= 0.154 \times 28 \times 10 = 43.1 \text{ mg/hr}$$

where the total body clearance is

$$Cl = kV = 0.154 \times 28 = 4.31 \text{ L/hr}$$
$$= 4.31 \times 1000 / 60 = 72 \text{ mL/min}$$

The maintenance dose is

$$D_m = (C_{tox} - C_{ther}) \, V$$
$$= (20 - 5) \times 28 = 420 \text{ mg}$$

The maintenance interval is then evaluated from

$$T_m = D_m / (D_m / T_m)$$
$$= 420 / 43.1 = 9.7 \text{ hours}$$

Finally, the loading dose is

$$L = VC_{tox}$$
$$= 28 \times 20 = 560 \text{ mg}$$

For a **practical dosing** schedule, the maintenance interval should be lowered from 9.7 hours. If we choose 8 hours, then the maintenance dose would be approximately

$$D_m = 420 \times (8 / 9.7) = 346 \text{ mg}$$

However, in this example, preparations for intravenous administration are available in either 250- or 500-mg forms. Therefore, we should consider a maintenance interval of

$$T_m = 6 \text{ hours}$$

This would lead to an approximate maintenance dose of

$$D_m = 420 \times (6 / 9.7) = 260 \text{ mg}$$

which is close to the actually available dose of

$$D_m = 250 \text{ mg}$$

The loading dose, immediately establishing the steady-state levels, is

$$L = VC_{max}$$
$$= 28 \times 14.8 = 414 \text{ mg}$$

In practice, therefore, a loading dose of 500 mg would be given. (This yields an initial maximum concentration of 500/28 = 17.9 mg/L, still below the minimum toxic level.) This would be followed by the administration, four times a day, of 250 mg of the drug in 10 mL diluent, which is injected over a 10-minute period.

Note that we have ended up with a dosage schedule in which the maintenance interval (6 hours) was somewhat higher but fairly close to the half-life of the drug (4.5 hours). As a result, the plasma concentration was expected to show over two-fold fluctuation. The loading dose (500 mg) was twice the maintenance dose (250 mg).

## DRUG CONCENTRATIONS FOLLOWING ORAL ADMINISTRATION

After the oral intake of a solid, immediate-release drug product (e.g., a capsule or tablet), it will first disintegrate into small particles. These then dissolve in the surrounding aqueous medium. Finally, the drug should get absorbed from the gastrointestinal lumen by passing through the gut wall and through the liver into the systemic circulation. Some of the drug may be decomposed in any of the stages of absorption, and thereby only a fraction of the administered dose could reach the general circulation. Thus, the *bioavailability* of the drug could be lower, at times substantially lower, than 100% (see also Chapters 3 and 6).

If a drug is administered not intravenously but, for example, orally, intramuscularly, or subcutaneously, then generally its concentration in the plasma will rise during the initial absorption phase and will decrease when (1) the absorption is complete, (2) the drug is in steady state between the plasma and the peripheral compartments, and (3) the rate of concentration decrease is dominated by the elimination processes (Fig. 5-10). In a semi-logarithmic scale, the terminal descending part of the curve is linear (Fig. 5-10B).

Absorption and distribution processes alter the concentration profiles only very slightly if they are fast in comparison with elimination. Slower absorption and/or distribution distort the curves in a manner similar to that seen with a single drug administration: in the semi-logarithmic concentration–time plot, curvatures downward and upward, respectively, are introduced. In particular, after intramuscular or oral drug intake, the multiple peaks of the concentration profile do not rise suddenly, and are not sharp, in contrast to those seen in the intravenous examples.

If equivalent doses of a drug are given to a person by single intravenous and oral drug administrations (when the concentrations recorded after oral administration are multiplied by the bioavailability, $F$), the maximal concentration ($C_{max}$) attained by the oral route is lower, and the time taken to get down to the minimum therapeutically effective concentration ($C_{ther}$) is usually longer. The latter statement is equivalent to saying that, from about the time of reaching $C_{max}$ by the oral route, the corresponding concentration remains higher than that seen following the equivalent intravenous administration.

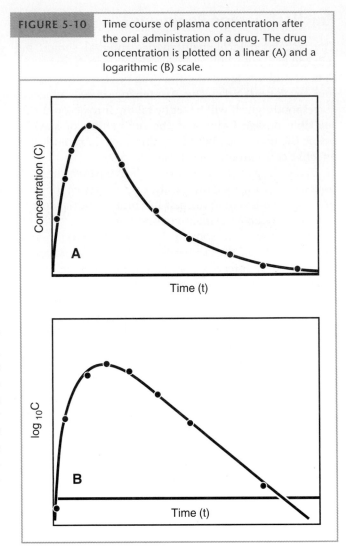

**FIGURE 5-10** Time course of plasma concentration after the oral administration of a drug. The drug concentration is plotted on a linear (A) and a logarithmic (B) scale.

## Dosing after Repeated Oral Administrations

The expressions evaluating dosage regimens for repeated oral administration are almost the same as those discussed for repeated intravenous injections when these aim at reaching an *average* steady-state concentration. The only difference is that, for oral administration, *all dosing equations must be multiplied on the right-hand side by the bioavailability (F)* (i.e., by the fraction of a drug dose reaching the systemic circulation). This is the reason for talking about "equivalent doses" for the two routes of drug administration.

If we aim again at remaining between the therapeutic and toxic concentration levels, the exact formulae for calculating dosage regimens for repeated oral administration are more complicated and require kinetic information about the relative rates of absorption and elimination.

Fortunately, in many cases, it is quite sufficient to apply the expressions given for repeated intravenous administration, since the resulting loading dose and also the maintenance interval and maintenance dose are generally conservative. Indeed, we may recall the following pharmacokinetic observations: after repeated oral drug administrations, $C_{max}$ is lower and $C_{min}$ is higher than the equivalent quantities calculated for repeated intravenous dosing. Consequently, we maintain the plasma concentration safely within the desirable range between $C_{tox}$ and $C_{ther}$ when dosage regimens described earlier are calculated.

## Bioavailability

### Definitions

**Bioavailability:** The percentage of a drug contained in a drug product that enters the systemic circulation in an unchanged form after administration of the product. This concept includes not only the amount of drug that enters the body, but also the rate of entry.

**Bioequivalence:** Comparable bioavailability between related drug products.

**Therapeutic equivalence:** Comparable clinical effectiveness and safety between similar drug products.

**Bioinequivalence:** Statistically determined difference in bioavailability between related drug products.

**Therapeutic inequivalence:** Clinically important difference in bioavailability between similar drug products.

## Measurement of bioavailability

After a **single oral dose** of drug, serial measurements of plasma concentration are obtained (see Fig. 5-10A). Three parameters of importance are derived from such a procedure:

1. Peak drug concentration ($C_{max}$)
2. Time to peak concentration ($T_{max}$)
3. Area under the concentration–time curve (AUC; in mg · hours/L)

The first two quantities are simple indicators for the **rate** of absorption. An increased rate is suggested by a higher peak concentration and a shorter time required to reach the peak concentration. In contrast, AUC reflects the **extent** of absorption. Consequently, after oral or intramuscular administration of a drug, the *absolute bioavailability* can be evaluated by comparing the measured AUC with the AUC determined after intravenous injection (i.e., 100% absorption) of the same dose of the drug:

$$\text{Bioavailability} = \frac{\text{AUC (oral)}}{\text{AUC (intravenous)}}$$

Repeated doses of most drugs result in accumulation, and the mean steady-state plasma drug concentrations are a good index of drug bioavailability. Again, it is not the steady-state concentration ($C_{ss}$) itself, but the ratio of $C_{ss}$ (oral) to $C_{ss}$ (intravenous) that provides the estimate of the absolute bioavailability after oral ingestion.

## Relative bioavailability

The *relative bioavailability* of one orally administered drug product (generally a new formulation of an existing drug) is compared with that of an existing reference drug product. It is usually expressed as the ratio of the AUCs for the two preparations.

After the patent of a drug expires, new formulations are often made available. The minimum requirement for the regulatory approval of these so-called "generic" drugs involves a demonstration that their bioavailabilities are identical to that of the original drug (i.e., that their relative bioavailability is 1.0, or that they are bioequivalent).

## Therapeutic importance of bioavailability

Fluctuations and differences in the completeness of absorption can be of major therapeutic importance if a drug exhibits at least one of the following characteristics:

* A given (e.g., twofold) variation in the attained concentration evokes a large change in the response in the therapeutic range (e.g., warfarin).
* The relationship between effect and concentration is clearly non-linear at the recommended doses (e.g., phenylbutazone, phenytoin, salicylate in high anti-inflammatory doses).
* The difference between concentrations eliciting therapeutic effects and those associated with toxicity is small, resulting in a narrow margin of safety (e.g., digoxin; see Chapter 7).

## SUGGESTED READINGS

Birkett DJ. *Pharmacokinetics Made Easy.* Revised. New York, NY: McGraw-Hill; 2005.

Ritschel WA. *Handbook of Basic Pharmacokinetics—Including Clinical Applications.* 5th ed. Washington, DC: American Pharmaceutical Association; 1999.

Rowland M, Tozer TN. *Clinical Pharmacokinetics: Concepts and Applications.* 3rd ed. Philadelphia, Pa: Lippincott Williams & Wilkins; 1995.

Shargel L, Wu S, Yu ABC. *Applied Biopharmaceutics and Pharmacokinetics.* 5th ed. New York, NY: McGraw-Hill; 2005.

Winter ME. *Basic Clinical Pharmacokinetics.* Philadelphia, Pa: Lippincott Williams & Wilkins; 2004.

# 6

# Drug Clearance by Specific Organs

## L ENDRENYI

## ADDITIVITY OF ORGAN CLEARANCES

In Chapter 5, *total body clearance* was defined as the volume of body fluid (usually blood) from which the drug is completely removed in a unit time. *Clearance by an individual organ* (e.g., the liver or kidney) *refers to the volume of body fluid from which that organ completely removes the drug in a unit of time.*

The total *amount* of a drug eliminated from the body is the sum of the amounts eliminated by the various routes. Correspondingly, the overall *rate* of elimination is the sum of the specific rates of elimination of the drug through the various routes. (This is because the rate of elimination is the amount of a drug removed in unit time.) For first-order processes, the respective specific organ clearances are also additive and sum to the total body clearance (*Cl* or TBC; see Chapter 5). This can be seen from the additivity of the corresponding elimination rate constants. The clearances can be thought of as products of the apparent volume of distribution and the respective rate constants.

As an example, consider a drug eliminated in part by hepatic (H) biotransformation and in part by renal (R) excretion. Then, the total amount of the eliminated drug can be considered as a sum of its components:

Amount eliminated = amount transformed in
the liver + amount excreted by the kidney

The overall rate of elimination can be regarded in the same way:

Rate of elimination = rate of hepatic transformation
+ rate of renal excretion

Since first-order rate constants are additive, the hepatic and renal constants sum to the elimination constant:

$$k = k_H + k_R$$

The corresponding clearances are obtained by multiplying both sides of this expression by $V$ (the apparent volume of distribution):

$$kV = k_H V + k_R V$$

Consequently, the following equation illustrates the additivity of the organ clearances:

$$Cl = Cl_H + Cl_R$$

In the following sections, drug elimination by various organs, and the corresponding clearances, will be considered briefly.

Organ clearance can also be obtained by *dividing the amount of a drug removed by the organ during a unit time by the concentration of the drug entering the organ.* This second definition is demonstrated below under "Perfusion Model."

## CLEARANCE BY THE LIVER

### Perfusion Model

Consider an organ such as the liver, into which the drug enters at an arterial concentration of $C_a$, and from which it exits at a smaller venous concentration of $C_v$ (Fig. 6-1). The blood flow through the organ is $Q$ (mL/min). Then, at steady state during 1 minute, the following applies:

Amount of drug entering the organ = $Q \cdot C_a$
Amount of drug leaving the organ = $Q \cdot C_v$
Amount of drug removed in the organ = $Q \cdot (C_a - C_v)$

The fraction of drug removed or extracted by the organ from the blood is $(C_a - C_v)/C_a$. This fraction is called the (steady-state) **extraction ratio,** $E$, which characterizes the effectiveness of the process of removing the drug:

$$E = (C_a - C_v)/C_a$$

A value close to 1 (unity) suggests that most of the drug is quickly and efficiently cleared by the organ; a small extraction ratio, approaching 0, indicates a slow, ineffective process of removal by that organ.

If the blood flow, $Q$, is multiplied by the fraction of drug extracted by the organ, $E$, one should obtain the volume of blood from which the organ removes the drug in unit time. This is the organ clearance as defined earlier. As an example, the hepatic clearance is

$$Cl_H = Q \cdot E$$

In the liver, $Q$ = total hepatic blood flow; $C_a$ = mixed portal venous and hepatic arterial drug concentrations; and $C_v$ = hepatic venous drug concentration. Notice that hepatic clearance can be written as

$$Cl_H = Q \cdot (C_a - C_v) / C_a$$

The numerator is the amount of drug cleared by the liver from the blood in 1 minute. This is divided by the concentration of the drug entering the organ. When expressed thus, the clearance is indeed calculated by following the second definition given in the previous section.

For an effectively extracted drug ($E = 1$), the hepatic clearance approaches the blood flow ($Cl_H \approx Q$). The liver is admirably set up for extracting large amounts of drugs because of its large size (1500 g), high blood flow (approximately 1 mL/g tissue/min), and unique architecture that brings blood into contact with many cell surfaces. It follows that the hepatic clearance of highly extracted drugs approaches 1500 mL/min. Conversely, low extraction is indicated by hepatic clearance much below 1500 mL/min.

## First-Pass Effect

Following oral intake of a drug, only a fraction ($F$) of the administered amount may reach the systemic circulation. Losses may occur by decomposition or by biotransformation in the gastrointestinal lumen. From there, the drug passes across the membranes of the gastrointestinal tract into the portal vein, then through the liver, and finally into the general circulation. During this so-called "first pass," enzymes may transform some of the drug either in the membranes and cells of the gut wall, in the liver, or perhaps in both locations. For instance, lidocaine is extensively extracted by the liver, while salicylamide undergoes extraction and biotransformation in both the intestinal wall and liver.

A substantial loss of a drug can be expected during its first pass through the liver if its hepatic biotransformation is fast and efficient (i.e., if its hepatic extraction ratio is high). Generally, the availability after first passage through the liver can be obtained from

$$F_H = 1 - E$$

For example, the hepatic extraction ratio of lidocaine, an anti-arrhythmic drug, is 0.7. Consequently, the oral bioavailability of the drug is only 30%. This is an upper limit for the oral bioavailability of the drug since losses during the first pass can occur not only by hepatic biotransformation but also by other processes. This is one reason for administering the drug by intravenous injection or infusion.

There are a number of **important properties of first-pass drug extraction**:

- It is drug-specific, ranging from zero to complete removal.
- The first-pass effect is often saturable.
- For some drugs, it is so effective that at low doses no drug may reach the systemic circulation.
- In liver disease, drugs with high first-pass extraction will become systemically available in higher-than-expected concentrations. This can happen as a result of either impaired function of liver parenchymal cells or intrahepatic shunts bypassing the sinusoid and carrying blood directly from the hepatic artery and portal vein to the terminal hepatic vein. Therefore, the drug dose may need to be decreased to prevent toxicity.
- Pharmacological effects may be markedly different after intravenous than after oral administration. For instance, if it is a drug metabolite that is active, oral administration of the drug may be more effective (or toxic) than intravenous injection of the same dose, provided that the biotransformation occurs in the liver.
- Low systemic bioavailability (see Chapter 5) often (but not always) indicates a first-pass effect.
- Complex and unpredictable drug kinetics can be expected as a consequence of the first-pass effect, depending on the relative contribution of intestinal or hepatic binding and/or biotransformation.

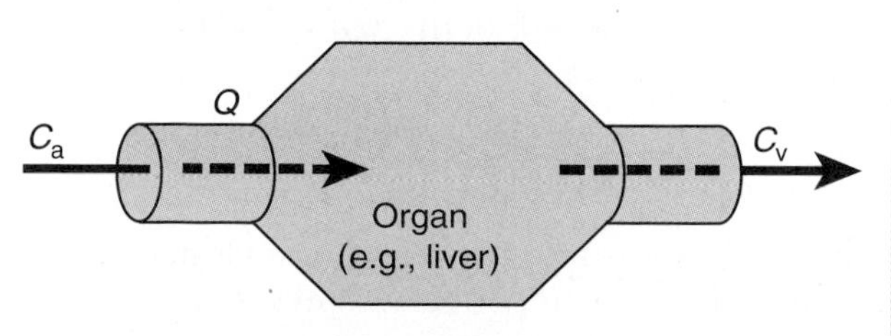

## Factors Affecting Hepatic Clearance

Two main factors contribute to the efficiency of hepatic drug clearance:

1. The amount extracted by the liver is expected to increase along with the blood supply, that is, when the **blood flow** ($Q$) is higher.
2. Transformation in the liver is assisted when the molecular relationships and conditions in the organ are favourable to biotransformation. These conditions can be characterized by a parameter that is called the **intrinsic clearance of the free (unbound) drug**

**FIGURE 6-1** Model for organ clearance of drugs. As applied to the liver, $Q$ = total hepatic blood flow; $C_a$ = mixed portal venous and hepatic arterial drug concentration; and $C_v$ = hepatic venous drug concentration (see text).

($Cl_{intr,f}$). The intrinsic clearance increases together with (1) a larger concentration and amount of the catalyzing enzyme in the liver and (2) a larger affinity between the drug molecule and the enzyme.

If one of the two components, blood flow or intrinsic clearance, is much smaller than the other, then it has controlling influence on the extraction ratio and, therefore, on the hepatic clearance. For instance, if the intrinsic clearance is much lower than the blood flow ($Cl_{intr,f} << Q$), the blood supply is quite ample and its change would, in practice, not affect the hepatic extraction. Alteration of the intrinsic clearance, however, directly modifies the hepatic clearance in such cases. (Low intrinsic clearance can be a consequence of a drug entering the hepatic cells relatively slowly, by simple diffusion. Drugs with low intrinsic clearance include antipyrine and the anticoagulant warfarin.)

In the reverse condition, if the intrinsic clearance substantially exceeds the blood flow ($Cl_{intr,f} >> Q$), the available enzymic activity is relatively in excess and does not limit the overall rate of biotransformation. Hepatic clearance is now dependent on blood flow; a change in the blood flow causes a corresponding alteration of the clearance. (Drugs having high intrinsic clearance are often concentrated in the hepatocytes and thereby allow the enzymatic reactions to be carried out efficiently. Examples of drugs with high intrinsic clearance include acetylsalicylic acid, morphine, and propranolol.)

For drugs exhibiting a low extraction ratio, the hepatic clearance is modified by various factors that affect the intrinsic clearance of the free drug, including the following:

- The binding of a drug to plasma proteins and other constituents in the blood: Binding reduces the concentration of the free drug and its intrinsic clearance.
- Conditions modifying the activity of the catalyzing enzyme: Inhibitors reduce this activity, and enzyme inducers increase it.

These factors lose importance for drugs having a high intrinsic clearance. In fact, binding to plasma proteins may have, to some extent, an opposite effect. Since proteins efficiently carry the drug molecules within the circulation, binding to them may actually facilitate clearance. Drugs with high intrinsic clearance show a substantial first-pass effect.

Table 6-1 summarizes factors involved in, and influencing, the hepatic clearance of high- and low-extraction drugs.

## CLEARANCE BY THE KIDNEY

Urinary excretion is a major route for the elimination of many drugs from the body. Generally, the kidney efficiently removes polar (hydrophilic) but not lipophilic drugs. Consequently, before being excreted, many of

| TABLE 6-1 | Features of, and Representative Drugs with, High and Low Hepatic Extraction | |
|---|---|---|
| | **High Extraction** | **Low Extraction** |
| **Features** | Hepatic clearance controlled by rate of blood flow | Hepatic clearance controlled by intrinsic clearance (hepatic biotransformation processes) |
| | Strong first-pass effect | Biotransformation limited by diffusion |
| | Plasma protein binding may facilitate clearance | Plasma protein binding reduces clearance |
| | | Sensitive to enzyme inhibition, induction |
| **Representative Drugs** | Amitriptyline | Antipyrine |
| | Imipramine | Diazepam |
| | Chlorpromazine | Digitoxin |
| | L-Dopa, lidocaine | Phenylbutazone |
| | Morphine, methadone, heroin | Phenytoin |
| | Propoxyphene | Theophylline |
| | Propranolol, alprenolol | Tolbutamide |
| | Tyramine | Warfarin |

these drugs undergo either conjugation or hydroxylation reactions that yield more polar products (see Chapter 4).

The functional anatomical units of the kidney are the nephrons (see also Chapter 37). Arterial blood passes first through the glomerulus, which filters some of the plasma water and its contents. Many, but not all, substances are also secreted in the proximal tubules. Most of the water is reabsorbed all along the nephron, in sequence, from the proximal, distal, and collecting tubules. Consequently, only 1 to 2 mL/min of the filtered water remains in the form of urine for elimination. Many solutes can also be reabsorbed by the tubular epithelium and passed into the renal interstitial fluid and from there back into the plasma.

Thus, renal excretion of drugs is the result of three processes: glomerular filtration, tubular secretion, and tubular reabsorption:

$$\text{Rate of renal excretion} = \text{rate of filtration} + \text{rate of secretion} - \text{rate of reabsorption}$$

The renal clearance of a substance can be calculated, in accordance with the definition given earlier, by measuring the amount of a drug excreted during a time period and dividing it by the length of the period and by the average plasma concentration observed during this interval:

$$Cl_R = \frac{\text{excreted amount/time interval}}{\text{mean plasma concentration}}$$

Similarly to the rate of excretion, the clearance can be subdivided into components representing filtration, secretion, and reabsorption.

## Glomerular Filtration

Glomerular filtration is limited by the size of the pores in the capillary endothelium and the ultrafiltration membrane (400 to 600 Å diameter). Thus, only small molecules are readily filtered by the glomeruli into the tubular fluid. Large macromolecules, including most proteins, either cannot pass through the filter or, if some passage does occur, are reabsorbed farther down the tubule. Consequently, only free drugs, not bound to plasma proteins, are found in the final filtrate. Farther down the tubule, most of the filtered water is reabsorbed together with variable amounts of free drug, which re-associate with proteins in the capillary blood. The end result is that the binding equilibrium remains almost unchanged.

The filtration process is *passive* (i.e., it proceeds *in the direction of the concentration gradient*) and relatively slow; it is limited by the rate of diffusion to and across the filter. Plasma water is filtered at a rate of about 120 mL/min. This is called the *glomerular filtration rate (GFR)*. Inulin, an exogenous polysaccharide, and creatinine, an endogenous nitrogen-containing substance, do not bind to plasma proteins and do not undergo tubular secretion or reabsorption to any significant degree. Therefore, they are widely used as indicators of the GFR. An observed inulin or creatinine clearance of substantially less than 120 mL/min suggests impairment of renal glomerular function.

The GFR of about 120 mL/min is also used as a marker of excretion processes in healthy subjects. Renal clearance in excess of 120 mL/min points to tubular secretion of a substance in addition to its glomerular filtration. A renal clearance less than 120 mL/min indicates net tubular reabsorption (following, or in addition to, filtration and secretion).

## Tubular Secretion

The cells of the proximal convoluted tubules *actively transport* certain substances from the plasma to the tubular urine. The transfer of drugs here occurs *against the concentration gradient,* and the drugs become relatively concentrated within the tubular lumen.

**Active transport** processes are characterized by the following:

1. **Energy requirement.** Active transport processes do not occur if the cell metabolism is impaired. Uncouplers of oxidative phosphorylation, such as dinitrophenol, which inhibit the synthesis of ATP by the cell, block active transport.
2. **Saturation kinetics.** In most cases, the process can be described by simple Michaelis–Menten–type kinetics in which the combining of the molecule to be transported (*D*) and the carrier system (*C*) occurs first; *CD* is translocated and dissociation occurs afterward. As in enzymatic reactions, the carrier system recognizes the transported molecules in a stereospecific fashion.

When all carrier molecules are in the *CD* form, maximal velocity of transport, called $T_m$, is attained. Since the cell membrane contains limited amounts of carrier molecules, in the presence of two substances ($D_1$ and $D_2$) transported by the same carrier, $D_1$ acts as an inhibitor of the transport of $D_2$ and vice versa. In general, the more slowly a substance is transported (i.e., the longer it occupies the carrier), the more effectively it inhibits the transport of another.

Active tubular secretion is a relatively fast process that clears practically all the drug, either bound to plasma proteins or free, from the blood. Actually, only the unbound drug is transported across the tubular epithelium; however, as the free drug is removed from the plasma, its equilibrium with the protein-bound entity is disturbed, and the complex dissociates, replacing some of the unbound substance. The result is the apparent (but not physically simultaneous) removal of nearly all the drug during the passage of the blood along the peritubular capillaries.

There are at least two transport mechanisms, one for acidic, the other for basic substances (Table 6-2). It is the ionized molecules that are transported.

Para-aminohippuric acid (PAH), an exogenous organic acid, is virtually completely filtered and secreted but not reabsorbed. Since, following ingestion, it is located in the plasma (partially bound to proteins), its renal excretion provides a measure of renal plasma flow. Typically, it is around 600 mL/min.

## Tubular Reabsorption

The importance of renal tubular reabsorption of organic substances as a homeostatic process is clear when one considers that most nutrients and vitamins present in plasma gain access to the glomerular filtrate. Consider, for example, the case of glucose. Under normal conditions, virtually all the glucose filtered is reabsorbed, so no glu-

| TABLE 6-2 | Examples of Drugs and Metabolites Actively Secreted into the Renal Tubules |
|---|---|
| **Acids** | **Bases** |
| Penicillin | Quaternary ammonium |
| Chlorothiazide | compounds (e.g., choline, |
| Salicylic acid | tetraethylammonium, |
| Phenolsulfonphthalein | N-methylnicotine, |
| Diodone (urographic medium) | N-methylnicotinamide) |
| Carinamide | Guanidine derivatives |
| Probenecid | Tolazoline |
| Cinchophen | Quinine |
| Para-aminohippuric acid | Pseudoephedrine |
| and other glycine conjugates | Trimethoprim |
| Glucuronic acid conjugates | Lamivudine |
| Sulfuric acid conjugates | |

cose appears in the urine unless the capacity of the transporting mechanisms is exceeded, as occurs in the advanced diabetic state or after large infusions of glucose. The fact that glucose, an uncharged substance, is reabsorbed into the blood against a large concentration gradient (tubular fluid to plasma) indicates that an **active transport process** is responsible for the absorption.

Not all the reabsorption of organic molecules is accomplished by active transport processes. Many compounds undergo **passive reabsorption.** These substances leave the filtrate to enter the tubular cells and should be able to leave the cell again, in the direction of the blood. Thus, at least two lipidic cell membranes have to be crossed. As described in Chapter 2, lipid-soluble substances are able to cross cell membranes and are thus passively reabsorbed. Charged molecules, in general, are not able to cross the tubular epithelial cell membranes and are thus excreted in the urine. (Note, however, that this does not mean that all uncharged molecules will be reabsorbed. Molecules such as sucrose, which are not charged but are not lipid-soluble either, are not passively reabsorbed.)

Factors that have to be considered in the passive reabsorption of substances from the tubular filtrate are the volume of the filtrate formed per minute (and thus the rate of movement down the tubule and the degree of probability of contact with the membrane) and, most importantly from the clinical point of view, the pH of the tubular fluid. Acidification of urine by different means results in a greater proportion of an acidic molecule, $A^-$, being in the uncharged HA form, thus increasing its passive reabsorption at the tubular level. The reverse will occur for basic molecules, which, in an acidic medium, will tend to shift to the $BH^+$ (charged) form. The $pK_a$ of the substance (i.e., the pH of the aqueous phase at which the numbers of ionized and non-ionized molecules are equal) will of course determine the relative proportions of the charged and uncharged forms at any pH. Changes in the pH of the tubular fluid are known to markedly affect the urinary excretion of phenobarbital and salicylate (Table 6-3). Some types of diuretics will render the filtrate acidic or alkaline (see Chapter 37). For a large variety of drugs, conjugation with strong acids occurs in the liver. Conjugates that are strong acids, such as glucuronic acid conjugates and sulfuric acid conjugates, will remain dissociated at most physiological pH levels attained in the kidney and are therefore readily excreted in the urine.

## Competitive Inhibition of Renal Tubular Transport

Some drugs act by interfering with the active transport of other drugs or endogenous substances. For example, probenecid competes with penicillin for active secretion by the tubular acid secretion system, thus lengthening the

| TABLE 6-3 | | Effect of Degree of Ionization on Rate of Urinary Excretion of Drugs | |
|---|---|---|---|
| | | Urinary Clearance Ratios* | |
| Drug | pKₐ | Acidic Urine | Alkaline Urine |
| Basic drugs | | (more ionized) | (less ionized) |
| Quinacrine | 7.7 | 3.0 | 0.5 |
| Procaine | 8.95 | 2.25 | 0.25 |
| Mecamylamine | 11.2 | 4.6 | 0.06 |
| Acidic drugs | | (less ionized) | (more ionized) |
| Phenobarbital | 7.4 | 0.1 | 0.7 |
| Salicylate | 3.0 | 0.02 | 1.6 |

*Clearance ratio $= \dfrac{\text{Clearance of substance}}{\text{Clearance of inulin}}$

Ratios higher than 1 imply net tubular secretion; ratios less than 1 imply net reabsorption.

half-life of penicillin and raising its plasma concentration (see Chapter 50). Sulfinpyrazone competitively inhibits the active reabsorption of uric acid and thus increases its elimination from the body (see Chapter 28). In other instances, adverse drug reactions can occur as a result of unintended interactions at the renal transport systems (see Chapter 60).

## BILIARY EXCRETION

The biliary excretion of substances involves two steps: (1) transfer from the plasma across the hepatic cell membrane into parenchymal cells of the liver, and (2) active transport across the membrane separating the liver cell from the bile canaliculus. After transient storage in the gallbladder, the compounds enter the small intestine. From here, they are either excreted into the feces or reabsorbed into the portal circulation. In the latter case, by returning to the plasma, they complete the **enterohepatic cycle,** which can substantially extend the duration of their presence in the body.

The active secretion of drugs into the bile takes place against a concentration gradient and results in the elevation of their biliary concentration. As in the kidney, acids and bases have separate transport systems, and two substances transferred by the same system can inhibit each other's secretion.

The biliary clearance can be calculated by dividing the amount of drug excreted in unit time by the plasma concentration. The amount excreted in unit time is the product of the concentration in bile and the bile flow, hence

$$Cl_B = \frac{\text{concentration in bile}}{\text{concentration in plasma}} \times \text{bile flow}$$

The bile flow is typically 0.5 to 0.8 mL/min. Consequently, biliary clearance is sizeable only when the drug concentration in the bile is much higher than that in plasma. For example, with a concentration ratio of 1000, the biliary clearance is about 500 to 800 mL/min.

Generally, polar compounds are able to undergo biliary excretion. Often, such substances are formed in the liver when a drug is transformed to a polar conjugate such as a glucuronide, glycine, or sulfate conjugate. A substantial fraction of the conjugates can be re-hydrolyzed upon reaching the gut to re-form the original drug, thus allowing it to be reabsorbed under certain conditions.

Another limitation on substances undergoing biliary excretion is their size. Only those having molecular weights of at least 250 Da appear in the bile. The explanation for this phenomenon is not well understood.

## SUGGESTED READINGS

Bekersky I. Renal excretion. *J Clin Pharmacol.* 1987;27:447-449.

Morgan DJ, Smallwood RA. Clinical significance of pharmacokinetic models of hepatic elimination. *Clin Pharmacokinet.* 1990;18:61-76.

Plaa GL. The enterohepatic circulation. In: Gillette JR, Mitchell JR, eds. *Handbook of Experimental Pharmacology.* Vol 28. Berlin, Germany: Springer-Verlag; 1975:130-149.

Rowland M, Benet LZ, Graham GG. Clearance concepts in pharmacokinetics. *J Pharmacokinet Biopharm.* 1973;1:123-136.

Rowland M, Tozer T. *Clinical Pharmacokinetics: Concepts and Applications.* 3rd ed. Philadelphia, Pa: Lea & Febiger; 1995.

Sirianni GL, Pang KS. Organ clearance concepts: new perspectives on old principles. *J Pharmacokinet Biopharm.* 1997;25:449-470.

Wilkinson GR. Clearance approaches in pharmacology. *Pharmacol Rev.* 1987;39:1-47.

Winter ME. *Basic Clinical Pharmacokinetics.* 4th ed. Philadelphia, Pa: Lippincott Williams & Wilkins; 2004.

# 7

# Dose–Response Relationships

## L ENDRENYI

## LOG-DOSE–RESPONSE CURVES

A central question of drug therapy is "What is the proper dose of a drug that will produce the desired therapeutic action without harmful side effects?" To answer this question, an analysis of the relationship between dose and response is required.

It is customary to contrast these quantities (doses and responses) in diagrams that plot the effect of the drug against the logarithm of the corresponding dose. These diagrams yield **log-dose–response (LDR) curves**. Figure 7-1 provides an example. Raising doses of histamine causes gradually increasing contraction of the guinea pig ileum. Very low doses of histamine have practically no effect, and responses can be observed only beyond a threshold dose of about 20 ng. Very high doses of more than about 50 μg have no additional effect, and the response remains constant at this maximal (≥50 μg) level.

The effect of using a logarithmic dose scale is very important. First, notice that in the example of the histamine response, the horizontal dose scale is indeed logarithmic since the distances between 1 and 10 μg, or 10 and 100 μg, are identical. Second, Figure 7-1 indicates that there are only small differences between the responses that are produced by doses of, for instance, 1.0 and 1.1 or even 1.5 μg histamine. The physician is often too concerned about such minute differences. Rather, one should want to know the effects of double, fivefold, tenfold dosages.

## Properties of Log-Dose–Response Curves

1. These curves describe the LDR relationship over a wide range of doses.
2. LDR curves are typically S-shaped, or sigmoidal. Their middle section is approximately straight; this facilitates their statistical analysis. This property is used to good advantage in the analysis of bioassays when drug concentrations (doses) are evaluated from the corresponding responses observed in biological samples.

3. Frequently, the same effect is produced by different drugs acting with an identical, or at least similar, mechanism. In such cases, the LDR curves of the drugs may be expected to run parallel to each other. For example, let us assume that drug A is twice as potent as drug B. Then, in comparison with A, twice as much B is needed to produce some given identical response. This is true throughout the full range of concentrations. Consequently, in a plot contrasting a response with the corresponding dose, points on the curve characterizing drug B will always lie the same distance to the right of the curve for drug A (Fig. 7-2).

Furthermore, at a given height (i.e., response) of the plot, the dose of drug B will be twice as large as that of drug A (Fig. 7-2B). In a plot having a linear dose scale (i.e., 20-, 40-, 60-, and 80-mg/kg doses are spaced with equal distance), the response curves for the two drugs are not parallel (see Fig. 7-2A). In contrast, in the LDR plot (with the logarithmic dose scale), the distance between the curves is constant and equals log 2 = 0.30 (see Fig. 7-2B). Thus, curves of similarly acting drugs are expected to be parallel in the LDR plot.

## Comparison of Log-Dose–Response Curves

The strengths of drugs A and B, in the example above, can be compared quantitatively. In this case, when the potency of drug A is double the potency of drug B, we would say that the **relative potency** of drug A with respect to drug B is $R = 2.0$. Of course, this can be stated in other ways, for example, that drug B is only one-half as potent as drug A, or that the relative potency of drug B with respect to drug A is $R = 0.50$.

In general, if different drugs have parallel LDR curves (as when they act by identical mechanisms), the relative potencies can be evaluated from the horizontal distance between them. The horizontal concentration scale is logarithmic, and therefore the horizontal distance between two curves equals the corresponding value of log $R$.

Relative potencies are customary measures for comparing relative strengths of different drugs or drug prepa-

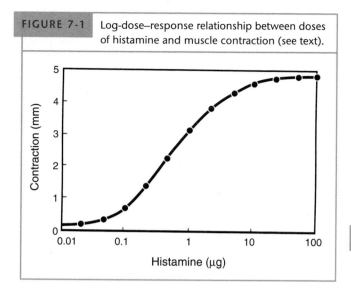

FIGURE 7-1 Log-dose–response relationship between doses of histamine and muscle contraction (see text).

plementarity; that is, the molecular shapes and the locations of their binding groups must fit with each other.

The requirement for complementarity of binding groups between drug and receptor means that minor alterations of the drug molecule drastically alter the ability of the drug to bind to its receptor. This is reflected in the relative potencies of a series of related drugs, as shown in Table 7-1. It can be seen that addition or removal of a single carbon atom alters the potency of acetylcholine analogues by a factor of 10 or more at both muscarinic and nicotinic acetylcholine receptors. Similarly, specific recep-

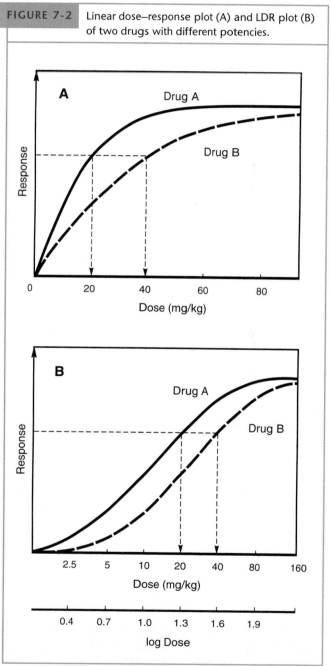

FIGURE 7-2 Linear dose–response plot (A) and LDR plot (B) of two drugs with different potencies.

rations. Their use implies parallelism of LDR curves. In contrast, parallelism is not assumed when the strengths of drugs are compared on the basis of their **equipotent doses.** These are doses of drugs that give rise to the same magnitude of the designated response. For instance, in Figure 7-2, 20 mg/kg of drug A and 40 mg/kg of drug B are equipotent doses.

## DRUG BINDING

### An Interpretation of the LDR Curve: Receptor Occupancy

According to the most common theory of drug action, the drug molecules must **bind specifically** to receptors in the body before initiating the process of response. Thus, the intensity of drug action is proportional to the occupancy of the receptors or, in other words, to the concentration of the drug–receptor complexes, $[DR]$:

$$\text{Response} = \alpha[DR]$$

The proportionality constant $\alpha$ is also referred to as **intrinsic activity.** Drugs with intrinsic activity higher than zero (i.e., that produce a detectable degree of response) are called **agonists.**

### Specific Binding of Drugs to Receptors

The interaction of a drug with a receptor involves various types of chemical forces. Although there are examples of drugs that form covalent bonds with receptors, most drugs bind reversibly to receptors through a combination of electrostatic forces, hydrogen bonds, and van der Waals forces. To permit these weak, short-range binding forces to act, the ligand and receptor must show **molecular com-**

| TABLE 7-1 | Relative Potencies of Acetylcholine Analogues | |
|---|---|---|
| Analogue | Muscarinic Receptor of Guinea Pig Ileum (%) | Nicotinic Receptor of Frog Rectus Abdominis (%) |
| Formylcholine | 25 | 10 |
| Acetylcholine | 100 | 100 |
| Propionylcholine | 5 | 400 |
| Butyrylcholine | 0.5 | 150 |

tors are also **stereoselective**, showing preference for one optical isomer of a drug. Thus, *l*-noradrenaline is 100 times as potent as *d*-noradrenaline.

## Quantitative Characterization of Specific Binding

The first step in the mechanism that gives rise to a drug response is the specific binding of a small drug molecule, *D*, to its unoccupied receptor, $R_f$. The complex forms and decomposes in a dynamic steady state:

$$D + R_f \underset{k_2}{\overset{k_1}{\rightleftharpoons}} DR \rightarrow Effect$$

The bound form of the drug (*DR*) is formed with an onset rate constant, $k_1$, dissociates into its components with an offset rate constant, $k_2$, and elicits a pharmacological response equal to α*DR*.

The mechanisms for specific drug binding and for the subsequent development of a drug response are analogous to the Michaelis–Menten description of simple enzyme reactions, in which an enzyme–substrate complex is in dynamic steady state with its components and forms the reaction product at a rate proportional to the concentration of the complex. It is not surprising, then, that the mathematical descriptions of the processes are also similar. The dependence of the concentration of the drug–receptor complex, [*DR*], and of the subsequent response, on the concentration of unbound drug, [*D*], is characterized by expressions representing a hyperbola. In binding studies in which equilibrium is reached, the equation is as follows:

$$[DR] = [D][R]/(K_d + [D])$$

Here, the ratio of the offset and onset rate constants is the *dissociation constant,* with units of molar concentration:

$$K_d = k_2/k_1$$

$K_d$ is an index of binding affinity and numerically equals the drug concentration at which 50% of the receptors are occupied. [*R*] is the total receptor concentration.

The hyperbolic relationship between the concentrations of bound, [*DR*], and free drug, [*D*], predicts that all specific binding sites become saturated at high drug concentrations so that no additional drug molecules can attach to receptors. This is illustrated by the specific binding curve in Figure 7-3A.

Such relationships are determined by performing binding assays, which are quite simple in principle. Samples of tissue homogenate are mixed with different concentrations of radiolabelled drug in the presence of a physiological buffering system. After incubation of the mixture in order to reach equilibrium (the time required will depend on the temperature), each sample is processed to separate unbound drug from drug bound to the tissue. This is often performed by filtering the binding assay mixture through a glass-fibre filter such that the tissue will be retained on the filter and the unbound drug will pass through. After sufficient washing to remove unbound drug, the amount of drug bound to the tissue can be measured by counting the radioactivity retained on the filter.

Typical results of a binding assay are shown in Figure 7-3A, where it can be seen that binding increases with the addition of increasing concentrations of labelled free ligand. The lack of apparent saturation in this reaction is the result of ligand binding not only to the *specific receptors* in the tissue but also to *non-specific components* such as membrane lipids and other proteins. To distinguish specific binding to the receptor from the non-specific binding sites, a second set of tissue samples is assayed with the same concentrations of labelled drug but now in the presence of excess unlabelled ("cold") drug. The distinction between specific and non-specific binding sites is based on the higher affinity of the ligand for the specific receptors and the low abundance of these receptors. This means that in the presence of excess cold ligand, the specific sites will be saturated and the residual binding of radioligand will be, for all practical purposes, only to the relatively unlimited number of non-specific sites. As seen in Figure 7-3A, the radioactivity bound to the filters in the presence of cold drug is diminished (dashed line) compared with the total binding seen in the absence of cold ligand (solid line). Specific binding of radioligand to the receptors (dotted line) is then calculated by subtracting non-specific binding from total binding, and the hyperbolic relationship between this specific binding and the free concentration of the drug becomes obvious.

The hyperbolic relationship between bound and free drug concentrations can be rearranged to yield a convenient linear form. The so-called *Scatchard plot* contrasts the ratio of bound and free drug concentrations with just the bound concentration (Fig. 7-3B). The slope of the straight line gives the negative reciprocal of the dissociation constant ($-1/K_d$), whereas the horizontal intercept yields the overall concentration of the specific binding sites, [*R*].

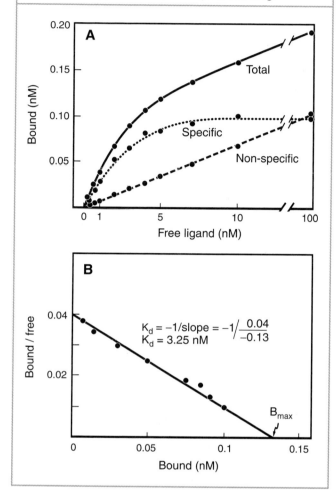

FIGURE 7-3 — Measurement of the binding of radiolabelled ligand to tissue homogenate. (A) Total binding (solid line), non-specific binding in the presence of excess unlabelled ligand (dashed line), and specific binding calculated by subtracting non-specific from total binding (dotted line). (B) Scatchard plot of specific binding.

## Quantitative Characterization of the Intensity of Drug Effects

It was noted earlier that, according to the occupancy theory of drug action, the intensity of drug effects is proportional to the concentration of drug–receptor complexes:

$$\text{Response} = \alpha[DR]$$

Consequently, the relationship between the magnitude of a drug effect and the concentration of the unbound drug is characterized by a hyperbola:

$$\text{Response} = \alpha[D][R]/(K + [D])$$

(Equilibrium does not prevail now. Therefore, $K$ is not the dissociation constant here but is related to it.)

The hyperbolic relationship between drug response and free drug concentration is similar to that shown in Figure 7-3A for specific drug binding. The same picture is often typical for the contrast of drug effect and linear dose, which was illustrated earlier in Figure 7-2A. And as was noted previously, applying the logarithmic scale to the horizontal axis converts the curves to an *LDR relationship* (see Fig. 7-2B).

## MEASUREMENT OF ANTAGONIST POTENCY

Not all drugs that bind to specific receptors elicit a pharmacological response. Some drugs bind to their receptors but have zero intrinsic activity and produce no demonstrable effect. However, such drugs are able to prevent active drugs (agonists) from binding to the receptors and producing their effects, and therefore the inactive drugs are called **antagonists** or **receptor blockers**. Many of the drugs used in clinical medicine are antagonists that are designed to prevent the excessive action of endogenous substances such as histamine, noradrenaline, acetylcholine, opioid peptides, and so forth. Since such antagonists produce no demonstrable effects when they bind to receptors, their activity can be measured only by the extent to which they interfere with the actions of agonists.

Drug antagonism is quantified by the use of the pA scale, which is an empirical measure of the activity of an antagonist that is not dependent on its mechanism of action. The $pA_2$ is defined as the negative logarithm (base 10) of the molar concentration of antagonist that reduces the effect of a known concentration of agonist to that of one-half the concentration or, in other words, causes a parallel displacement of the concentration–effect curve of a given agonist twofold to the right without changing the maximum response.

This expression is derived from the Gaddum equation

$$D_2/D_1 = 1 + [A]k_2$$

which, when transposed, gives

$$D_2/D_1 - 1 = 1 + [A]k_2$$

where $D_2$ and $D_1$ are the drug concentrations needed to produce the same effect in the presence and absence, respectively, of a competitive reversible antagonist $A$, $[A]$ is the molar concentration of $A$ that makes the drug concentration ratio $D_2/D_1$ equal to 2, and $k_2$ is the dissociation constant of the antagonist–receptor complex. If the second equation above is converted to logarithms, it becomes the following:

$$\log (D_2/D_1 - 1) = \log [A] + \log k_2 \text{ (the Schild equation)}$$

The $pA_2$ can then be determined by measuring the value of the concentration ratio of agonist at three or more antagonist concentrations. A graph of log $(D_2/D_1 - 1)$ against log $[A]$ yields a line with a slope of unity, and the x-intercept equals the $pA_2$ for true competitive antagonism (Schild plot).

Antagonists are never completely receptor-specific. The pA scale can also be used to assess the degree of specificity.

## ALL-OR-NONE EFFECTS

The example of histamine, discussed at the start of the chapter, described a typical graded drug effect: a slight increase in the dose should bring about a small increase in the response. There are occasions when the available information indicates only that a given dose of a drug either has or has not evoked a certain effect in the various subjects under investigation. Examples of such **quantal**, or **all-or-none**, responses are the presence or absence of convulsion, death, anaesthetic effect, and improvement in a disease state. Usually, either the proportion (the percentage) or the actual number of subjects responding to a given dose of the drug is recorded.

Thus, actually only a fraction of the subjects respond to certain drug dosages, while the remaining proportion fails to react. The reason lies in biological variation (i.e., the differing sensitivity of the individual subjects to drug action). Individuals range from the very sensitive (hyperreactive) to the least sensitive (hyporeactive), in whom the drug produces its usual effect at unexpectedly low or uncommonly high doses, respectively.

## HISTOGRAMS AND CUMULATIVE FREQUENCY PLOTS

When the dosage is varied, the number (or better, the fraction or percentage) of subjects responding can be plotted against the dose or, preferably, its logarithm. Consider the following example: In each of 60 dogs, an investigator gradually increased the rate of intravenous adrenaline infusion until a 35% enhancement of the heart rate was observed. Up to 10 ng/kg/min, this end point was reached in one dog; between 10 and 13 ng/kg/min, it was reached in two additional dogs; between 13 and 17 ng/kg/min, it was reached in six more; and so on. These data are displayed in a histogram that illustrates the distribution of sensitivities to adrenaline induction of heart rate increases in the various dogs (Fig. 7-4). The histogram is characteristically bell-shaped, in similarity to curves describing the so-called **normal distribution** (see next paragraph).

The data can be rearranged to give the cumulative number (or fraction) of subjects responding to *all* doses that are lower or equal to the dose under investigation. For example, as before, a 35% increase in heart rate was recorded in one dog (1.7%) *up to* an adrenaline infusion rate of 10 ng/kg/min; it was recorded *in a total of three* dogs

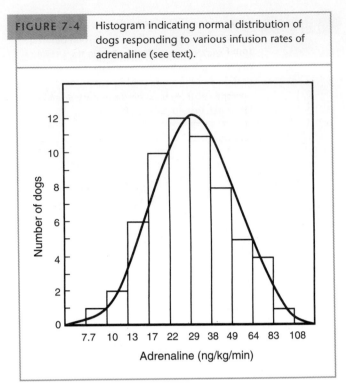

**FIGURE 7-4** Histogram indicating normal distribution of dogs responding to various infusion rates of adrenaline (see text).

(5.0%) *up to* 13 ng/kg/min; was recorded *in a total of nine* dogs (15.0%) *up to* 17 ng/kg/min; and so on. The data characterize the **cumulative distribution** of the sensitivities (Fig. 7-5). A curve fitted to them describes the cumulative rearrangement of the normal distribution; the shape of this distribution is very similar to that of an LDR curve.

It is important to notice that all-or-none responses are observed in individual subjects (or experimental animals) and that the recorded quantity (proportion, percentage, or actual number of subjects reacting) is not identical to the response itself. On the other hand, as illustrated in the example of the response to adrenaline, graded effects (e.g., an increase in heart rate) can be converted to quantal responses by selecting a given level of the effect (e.g., 35% increase) and observing the number (or fraction, or percentage) of subjects affected to that degree by certain doses of the drug.

In the example, the doses corresponding to consecutive class limits were increased by a constant ratio, about 30%. An equivalent statement is that the observations are pooled into groups (classes) defined by limits with logarithmically uniform increments (i.e., that the horizontal dose scale is approximately logarithmic).

## MEDIAN EFFECTIVE AND MEDIAN LETHAL DOSE

It is possible to evaluate doses to which 20%, 70%, 84%, or any other percentage of the subjects respond. It is customary to calculate such **effective doses,** abbreviated as $ED_{20}$,

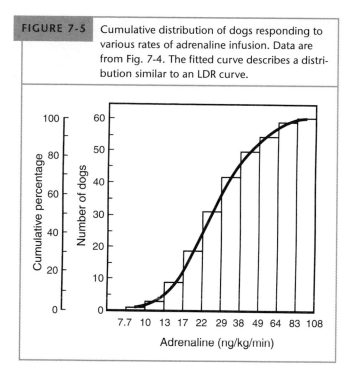

**FIGURE 7-5** Cumulative distribution of dogs responding to various rates of adrenaline infusion. Data are from Fig. 7-4. The fitted curve describes a distribution similar to an LDR curve.

$ED_{70}$, and $ED_{84}$, and especially to calculate the **median effective dose,** or $ED_{50}$, which is, of course, the dose that gives rise to the designated response in 50% of the subjects. When drugs have parallel LDR curves, their potencies can be compared through their $ED_{50}$ values; the more potent the drug, the lower its $ED_{50}$.

If the response is mortality (e.g., in animal experiments designed to evaluate potency or toxicity), then, instead of effective doses, we speak of **lethal doses.** For instance, we characterize a dose that gives rise to the death of 50% of the subjects as the **median lethal dose,** or **$LD_{50}$.** A harmful side effect is manifested in one-half of the subjects at the **median toxic dose,** or **$TD_{50}$.** Anaesthetists talk about an anaesthetic dose, or $AD_{50}$, which has the same interpretation as the $ED_{50}$.

The strict definition of effective doses, and specifically the $ED_{50}$, involves quantal responses: the dosage is that at which a given percentage (frequently 50%) of the subjects are affected. A looser, less rigorous definition, which is often used in the pharmacological literature, extends to graded responses. According to this interpretation, the $ED_{50}$ is the dose giving rise to one-half of the asymptotic, maximum (continuous) effect.

# EVALUATION OF DRUG SAFETY

In addition to its therapeutic effect, a drug is likely to have one or more kinds of harmful side effects. Higher doses may even cause death. Each of these responses can be characterized by an LDR curve. In general, the drug is considered to be safe if the dose range of the harmful side effects is much higher than the therapeutic dose range. This idea is expressed by the therapeutic index

$$TI = TD_{50}/ED_{50}$$

which should be as high as possible for maximal safety.

However, this frequently used index does not sufficiently characterize the *relative safety* of different drugs. Figure 7-6 shows all-or-none LDR curves for the therapeutic response and one toxic effect of two drugs, A and B. (For convenience only, the responses are illustrated using the so-called probit scale, in which straight lines are obtained. For further convenience, parallel lines for therapeutic and toxic responses are assumed. However, the following arguments could also be pursued with non-parallel responses depicted in any diagram.)

The two drugs shown in Figure 7-6 have identical $ED_{50}$ and identical $TD_{50}$ values; consequently, they have identical therapeutic index values. The relative safeties of the two drugs, however, are quite different: a comparatively high dose of drug B may be beneficial to many or even most patients, but it will also be toxic to some of them (indicated by the solid triangles). Drug A, on the other hand, which has a steeper probit line, does not involve such risks: an almost completely curative dose has nearly none of the toxic effects (indicated by solid circles). Such differences in drug behaviour are characterized by the certain safety factor:

$$CSF = TD_1/ED_{99}$$

It will be low for drug B and much higher for the "safer" drug A. Such quantitative considerations of drug safety apply equally to side effects and to lethality: in the latter case, $CSF = LD_1/ED_{99}$.

Two further remarks can be made. First, a drug may have several therapeutic indices and certain safety factors, one for each comparison of a toxic or lethal response with

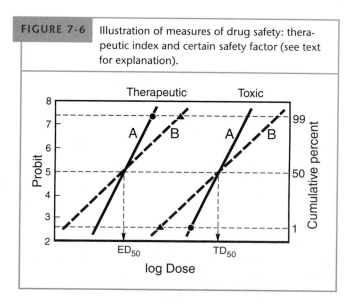

**FIGURE 7-6** Illustration of measures of drug safety: therapeutic index and certain safety factor (see text for explanation).

a therapeutic response. Second, the LDR curves for various responses to a drug, whether therapeutic, toxic, or lethal, need not be parallel. Indeed, evaluation of therapeutic indices and certain safety factors does not require any assumption of parallelism.

There is an additional complication. The therapeutic and side-effect LDR curves vary from patient to patient. So it is possible, and occurs with alarming frequency, that a dose which is therapeutic in one patient causes ill effects in another. The physician must be alert to such variations.

## SUGGESTED READINGS

Kenakin TP. *Pharmacologic Analysis of Drug-Receptor Interaction*. 3rd ed. Philadelphia, Pa: Lippincott Williams & Wilkins; 1997.

Tallarida RJ. *Drug Synergism and Dose-Effect Data Analysis*. Boca Raton, Fla: Chapman Hall/CRC Press; 2000.

# 8

# Drug Receptors

## J MITCHELL

Many drugs initiate their actions by binding to specific receptors on target cells in the body. Although knowledge of the molecular structure of receptors is recent, the concept that drugs elicit their effects by binding to molecular receptors was formulated more than a century ago. Paul Ehrlich, working in the late 1800s in the rapidly developing synthetic pharmaceutical industry, experimented with arsphenamine (Salvarsan), which he attempted to develop into a specific anti-syphilis drug. To explain the apparent structural specificity of drug action, he introduced the idea that a drug might act as a "magic bullet" directed at a vulnerable "receptor." Although Ehrlich's concepts were not entirely realized, they eventually led to the discovery, by Domagk in 1935, of sulfonamides for the systemic treatment of bacterial infections and to the further refinement of the receptor concept as it is presently understood.

The direct identification of receptors for drugs, hormones, and neurotransmitters by means of radiolabelled ligands began in the mid-1960s. It had become apparent that most receptors have such high affinity for their respective "ligands" (i.e., neurotransmitter, hormone, or drug) that they become saturated when the ligand concentration is in the nanomolar range. Hence, it was necessary to develop methods for preparing radioactive ligands with specific activities sufficiently high to permit detection of the very small amounts of receptors that are present in body tissues. This development was instrumental in both the identification of receptors and the development of many new drugs over the last 30 years.

## NATURE OF BIOLOGICAL DRUG RECEPTORS

Regardless of the route of administration, drugs interact with multiple components of the body, but not all of these interactions elicit an effect. Therefore, a functional distinction can be made between these components. A **non-specific binding site** is defined as any body component that a drug binds to without leading to an effect.

Drug binding to serum albumin is an example of non-specific binding. If binding of the drug to the component leads to an effect on the cell or the organism, that component is said to be a **drug receptor.**

Most drug receptors are protein in nature, and many of them are proteins that bind endogenous ligands such as the neurotransmitters, hormones, and growth factors. This chapter deals with the structure and characterization of such receptors; their role in regulatory signalling systems is discussed in Chapter 9.

Not all drugs act on receptors of endogenous ligands; in fact, a range of different biological components may serve as binding sites that mediate the actions of drugs. Some of these sites are also proteins, such as the many enzymes that are targets of drug action. These include enzymes in the cells of our own bodies as well as those in the cells of pathogens that infect us. A number of examples of these drugs and their sites and mechanisms of action are given in Table 8-1. There are also many targets of drug action that are not protein in nature, and these include components such as lipids, ions, and water. For example, sterols in fungal and bacterial cell membranes are the targets of polyene and polymyxin antimicrobial agents (see Chapter 51). Chelating drugs have divalent metal ions as their targets, such as dimercaprol for $Hg^{2+}$ or $As^{2+}$ poisoning (Chapter 72), penicillamine for $Cu^{2+}$ in Wilson's disease (Chapter 43), and EDTA for $Pb^{2+}$ poisoning (Chapter 72). Body water may be considered as the target for osmotically active drugs, such as bulk laxatives (Chapter 42), osmotic diuretics (Chapter 37), and plasma expanders, which all act to change the water content of various body compartments.

The use of biochemical and molecular biological techniques over the past decade has led to the purification of many receptors and, more recently, to the molecular cloning of literally hundreds of specific receptor genes. Currently, we know the molecular sequences of several hundred cell surface and intracellular receptors with which a significant number of therapeutic drugs interact. With this knowledge, it is now possible to gain more precise information about how drugs bind to specific receptors and to design drugs with highly specific binding characteristics.

| TABLE 8-1 | Examples of Enzymes as Drug Targets |
|---|---|
| **Drug** | **Receptor and Mechanism of Action** |
| β-Lactam antibiotics (penicillins and cephalosporins) | Bind to penicillin-binding proteins on bacteria and inhibit transpeptidase reaction required for synthesis of bacterial cell wall |
| Cardiac glycosides (digitalis) | Inhibit membrane $Na^+/K^+$-ATPase; increase force of contraction in cardiac muscle |
| Rifampin | Binds to bacterial DNA-dependent RNA polymerase and inhibits RNA synthesis |
| Fluorouracil | Competes with uracil and becomes incorporated into RNA, blocking RNA processing; also metabolized to ribose and deoxyribose derivatives that inhibit thymidylate synthetase and thus block thymine nucleotides |
| Sulfonamides | Bind to a bacterial condensing enzyme necessary for the formation of folic acid from para-aminobenzoic acid; bacterial growth is consequently inhibited by lack of folic acid |

# G PROTEIN–COUPLED RECEPTORS

This is the largest family of cell surface receptors comprising approximately 1000 members that respond to a diverse array of stimulants such as hormones, neurotransmitters, prostaglandins, light, and olfactory stimuli. The G protein–coupled receptors have a number of common structural features that have facilitated the identification of this large family of proteins primarily by molecular cloning techniques. Each receptor has seven stretches (domains) of hydrophobic amino acids within the receptor polypeptide. These hydrophobic domains represent membrane-spanning segments embedded in the membrane in such a manner that the receptor snakes back and forth through the membrane, with the amino terminus of the protein protruding outside the cell and the carboxyl terminus inside the cytoplasm (Fig. 8-1). For this reason,

these receptors are often referred to as "seven transmembrane" receptors. A large number of biochemical studies of different G protein–coupled receptors have confirmed this basic structure, and we now have the X-ray crystal structure of rhodopsin, which has revealed the spatial relationship between the transmembrane domains of this receptor as depicted in Figure 8-1.

The endogenous ligands for G protein–coupled receptors bind to the extracellular side of the receptor. Small ligands, such as the catecholamines, bind to sites within the various transmembrane domains of the receptor, while the larger polypeptide ligands, which are less able to penetrate the hydrophobic regions, bind to sites on the amino terminus and extracellular loops of the receptor. One subfamily of these receptors that binds very small ligands, such as glutamate and calcium ions, has its ligand binding sites entirely within the very large amino-terminal domains.

FIGURE 8-1    Structure of G protein–coupled receptors. Each membrane-spanning domain is numbered sequentially from I to VII, with their orientations depicted according to the X-ray crystal structure of retinal rhodopsin. (From Filipek et al., 2003. Reprinted with permission.)

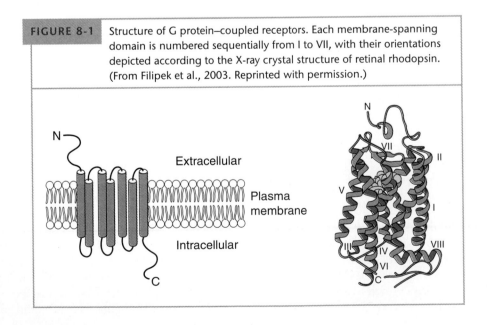

The G proteins bind to intracellular segments of the receptors, especially the third intracellular loop between the fifth and sixth transmembrane domains and carboxyl-terminal tail. The effect of agonist binding to the receptor is still poorly understood, but it is likely to stabilize the receptor in a conformation that permits efficient interaction between the receptor and the G protein trimer. These interactions result in stimulation of the G protein and subsequent regulation of a number of intracellular signalling systems (see Chapter 9).

Generally, there are more types of receptors than of endogenous extracellular ligands because multiple subtypes have been found for most of the G protein–coupled receptors. Multiple receptor subtypes for a single ligand were predicted in some cases from pharmacological studies. For example, the differential effects of nicotine and muscarine on cholinergic receptors predicted that there are two distinct classes of acetylcholine receptor, which were named nicotinic and muscarinic receptors. With the application of molecular cloning techniques to the field of receptor pharmacology, an even greater number of receptors has been revealed than was anticipated by the pharmacology. For example, five different muscarinic acetylcholine receptors are now known, and nine different genes encode adrenergic receptors. In some cases, the complex physiological responses to a single ligand have been associated with specific receptor subtypes by gene deletion studies in mice. For example, $\beta_1$-adrenergic receptors are responsible for cardiac inotropic effects, while the $\alpha_{2A}$-adrenergic receptors are the primary presynaptic feedback autoreceptors. In many cases, however, we still do not understand the physiological roles of many receptor subtypes. There are also a number of G protein–coupled receptors that have been identified by molecular cloning methods for which we do not know the endogenous ligands. These receptors are known as **orphan receptors,** and they are being used to identify new ligands in a process called **reverse pharmacology.**

When an agonist stimulates a receptor, the effect is usually of limited duration. The limitation of receptor stimulation involves a number of processes. Most G protein–coupled receptors have a number of serine and threonine residues in the cytoplasmic loops and carboxyl-terminal tail of the receptor. These residues can be phosphorylated by several kinases, including the family of **G protein receptor kinases (GRKs)**, as well as the second messenger–activated kinases, **protein kinase A** and **protein kinase C.** Receptor phosphorylation has been shown to facilitate the binding of members of a group of intracellular proteins known as **arrestins** to the receptors. Arrestin binding to the receptors results in diminished interaction between the receptor and G protein. This process, known as receptor desensitization, allows the receptor to respond to a large range of extracellular concentrations of stimuli. After prolonged activation, a process of receptor internalization occurs that can regulate the number of receptors in the plasma membrane. This **receptor down-regulation** appears to be regulated by the binding of arrestin to proteins within **clathrin-coated pits.** Once internalized from these pits within vesicles, the receptors may be dephosphorylated and recycled back to the cell surface or catabolized by cellular protein degradation pathways.

# ENZYME-LINKED RECEPTORS

## Receptor Tyrosine Kinases

This group of receptors mediates signals from a group of endogenous compounds known as **growth factors,** which includes **insulin, epidermal growth factor (EGF), and platelet-derived growth factor (PDGF).** The receptors are composed of single polypeptide chains that traverse the plasma membrane, creating three domains: an extracellular ligand-binding domain, a transmembrane domain, and an intracellular domain that contains the portion responsible for the kinase activity of the receptor (Fig. 8-2). Some members of this group of receptors, such as the insulin receptor, exist as dimers of two receptors coupled together by non-covalent disulfide bonds. Others, such as the EGF receptor, exist as monomers within the membrane and only come together to form dimers in response to ligand binding. In either case, the binding of the growth factor to the receptor results in allosteric activation of the tyrosine kinase activity in the cytoplasmic domains of the receptor. The first step in the activation process appears to involve cross-phosphorylation of the receptor subunits on multiple tyrosine residues within the intracellular domains. This autophosphorylation of the receptor acts as a signal for binding other intracellular proteins, which themselves may become phosphorylated on tyrosine residues by the receptor and thereby activated.

## Receptor Serine/Threonine Kinases

The **transforming growth factor β (TGFβ)** family of cytokines controls a diverse array of cellular processes, including cell proliferation, differentiation, and apoptosis. The 42 members of this family of ligands are divided into two subfamilies, the TGFβ/activin/nodal subfamily and the bone morphogenic protein (BMP)/growth and differentiation factor subfamily. The active forms of all TGFβ ligands are dimers.

TGFβ cytokines bind to the receptor serine/threonine kinase family. This family of receptors comprises 12 members in humans, seven type I and five type II receptors, each of which has a similar structure. These receptors comprise an amino-terminal extracellular ligand-binding domain, a single transmembrane domain, and an intracellular serine/

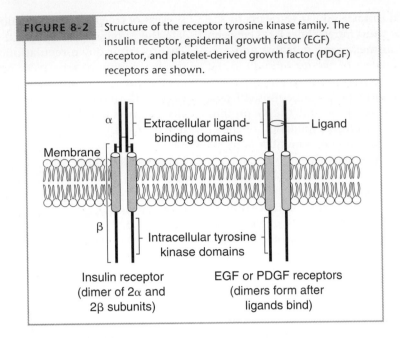

**FIGURE 8-2** Structure of the receptor tyrosine kinase family. The insulin receptor, epidermal growth factor (EGF) receptor, and platelet-derived growth factor (PDGF) receptors are shown.

threonine kinase domain. Ligand binding brings together a type I receptor and a type II receptor, allowing receptor II to phosphorylate receptor I in the kinase domain. This phosphorylation stimulates the binding and subsequent phosphorylation of intracellular receptor substrates and initiation of signal transduction (see Chapter 9).

## Receptor Guanylyl Cyclases

Members of this class of receptors can be divided into three groups. The receptors for a family of peptide hormones known as the natriuretic peptides constitute one group. Atrial natriuretic peptides (ANPs) are peptides secreted by cardiac atrial muscle cells in response to increases in blood pressure. ANPs bind to their receptors in the kidney, where they induce natriuresis (increased Na$^+$ and water excretion), and in smooth muscle cells of the vasculature, where they induce relaxation. The ANP receptor (Fig. 8-3) is a dimer of two polypeptides that contain extracellular ANP-binding domains, single transmembrane domains, intracellular ATP-binding regulatory domains, and guanylyl cyclase catalytic domains. Activation of the receptor by ligand binding to the extracellular domains results in increased production of cyclic GMP from GTP by the guanylyl cyclase.

There are also two groups of intracellular guanylyl cyclases that are regulated by intracellular compounds. The soluble guanylyl cyclases in the photoreceptors of the retina are constitutively active enzymes and are physiologically regulated by calcium-mediated inhibition. The heme-containing soluble guanylyl cyclases are more widely expressed and are composed of two subunits joined by a heme group (Fig. 8-3). This group of enzymes is expressed in vascular smooth muscle and activated by nitric oxide (NO) binding

to the heme group. NO is produced by nitric oxide synthases in endothelial cells in response to increased blood pressure. The NO has a very short half-life but can freely diffuse into the adjacent smooth muscle cells. The cyclic GMP produced as a result of NO stimulation goes on to induce smooth muscle relaxation and vasodilation. These enzymes are the targets of vasodilator nitrates, such as nitroglycerin, that are metabolized to NO (Chapter 34).

# ION CHANNELS

## Ligand-Gated Ion Channels

The synaptic neurotransmitters bind to a group of receptors on postsynaptic membranes known as the ligand-gated ion channels. Neurotransmitters that bind to this class of receptors/ion channels include acetylcholine, γ-aminobutyric acid (GABA), glycine, and glutamate. Ligand-gated ion channels are important targets for drugs. Indeed, many of the drugs used in the treatment of mental illness as well as the sedative–hypnotic drugs act on this group of receptors.

These various ion channels are structurally similar in that each of them is composed of multiple subunits that together form the ion channel through the plasma membrane. Each subunit of the channel is a polypeptide that contains four membrane-spanning domains. The neurotransmitter-binding specificities and ion selectivity are quite distinct for each channel (Table 8-2). The best characterized of this class of receptors is the nicotinic acetylcholine receptor depicted in Figure 8-4. This ion channel is composed of five subunits (two α, one β, one γ, one δ) that together form an aqueous pore passing through the

**FIGURE 8-3** Structure of natriuretic peptide receptor guanylyl cyclase and a heme-containing soluble guanylyl cyclase.

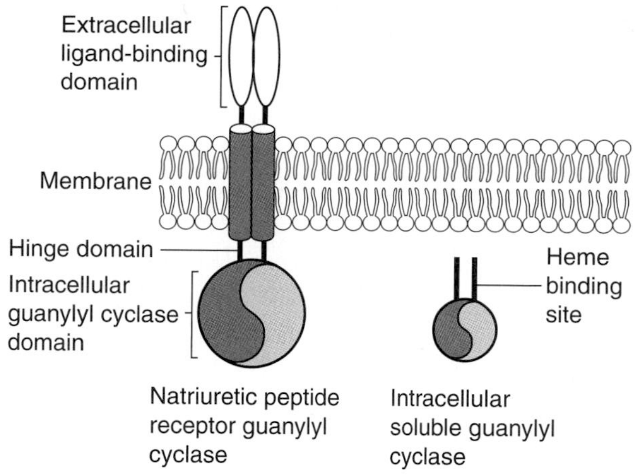

plasma membrane. The close apposition of the two α subunits within the membrane forms a gate that prevents ions from flowing through the channel. Acetylcholine binds to extracellular sites on the two α subunits, causing a conformational change in these two proteins such that the gate is opened and cations (particularly $Na^+$) flow down their chemical gradient into the cell.

## Voltage-Gated Ion Channels

Voltage-gated ion channels are also transmembrane proteins that selectively allow the passage of $Na^+$, $Ca^{2+}$, $K^+$, or $Cl^-$ ions across cellular membranes. The channels are composed of an α subunit that has multiple transmembrane domains. The α subunit, either as a monomer, dimer, or tetramer, forms the channel pore. There are also a variety of accessory subunits that regulate channel activity (Table 8-3). Channels exist in multiple molecular states than can be classified as open, closed, or inactivated. In the closed state, no ions can flow through the channel. Opening of the channels occurs in response to changes in membrane potential that are "sensed" by elements in the transmembrane domains of the channel. The voltage-dependent conformational change in channel structure opens a pore and allows for the flow of selective ions across the cell membrane. A second conformational change then occurs, resulting in an inactive state that does not allow the flow of ions but is distinct from the closed state. The channel must revert to the closed state upon membrane repolarization before it can be re-opened.

Voltage-dependent ion channels are the receptors for a number of important pharmacological agents such as local anaesthetics and some of the anti-arrhythmic, antihypertensive, and anticonvulsant agents. All of these agents bind to sites in the transmembrane domains of the channel and reduce the cellular excitability or contraction by inhibiting channel activity.

## NUCLEAR HORMONE RECEPTORS

Ligands that are sufficiently lipid soluble to cross the plasma membrane of cells exert their actions by binding to a group of intracellular proteins known as the nuclear hormone receptor superfamily. Activation of each of these receptors results in increased transcription of particular genes within the target cell, and therefore, they have been called **ligand-responsive transcription factors**. The genes regulated by these receptors are involved in a wide variety of cellular processes, including metabolism, growth, and differentiation.

**FIGURE 8-4** (Left) Structure of a principal subunit of a ligand-gated ion-selective membrane channel. M1 through M4 are the membrane-spanning domains. (Right) Cross-sectional view of a complete channel, the nicotinic acetylcholine receptor, consisting of five principal subunits surrounding the aqueous pore through which the ion passes.

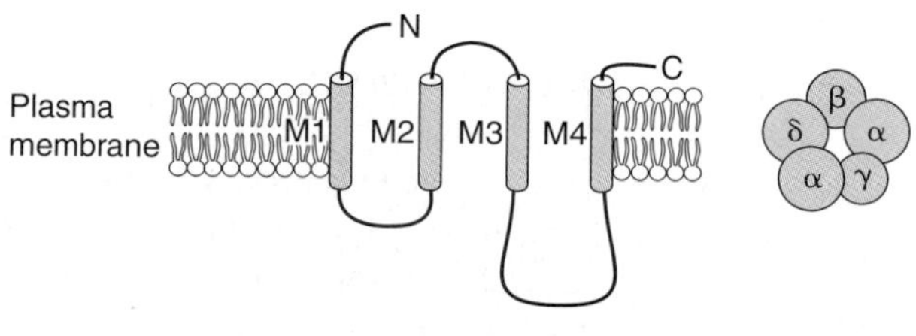

| TABLE 8-2 | Ligand-Gated Ion Channels | | |
|---|---|---|---|
| Neurotransmitter | Channel (Receptor) | Ion Selectivity | Effect |
| Acetylcholine<br>Serotonin<br>Glutamate | Nicotinic<br>5HT$_3$<br>NMDA,* non-NMDA | Cations,<br>primarily Na$^+$ | Excitatory |
| GABA<br>Glycine | GABA$_A$<br>Gly | Anions,<br>primarily Cl$^-$ | Inhibitory |

*$N$-Methyl-D-aspartate; this receptor channel also has an important Ca$^{2+}$ selectivity.

The general structure of a nuclear hormone receptor, as depicted in Figure 8-5, is that of a single polypeptide that can be divided into three functional domains. The amino-terminal region of the receptor is the least conserved domain. The DNA-binding domain of the receptor is in the middle of the protein and contains a structural motif, known as "zinc fingers," that is common to DNA-binding proteins. Ligands bind to the receptor within a hydrophobic cavity in the ligand-binding domain in the carboxyl terminus, which results in receptor activation. Within the ligand-binding domain, activation function (AF-2) sites bind co-regulatory factors. Co-regulatory factors function as adaptors that either increase (co-activators) or decrease (co-repressors) transcriptional responses to the receptor when activated by ligand.

Nuclear hormone receptors have been divided into three groups. Class I receptors bind steroid ligands such as **glucocorticoids, mineralocorticoids,** and the **sex steroids.** These receptors form homodimers in the absence of DNA binding. In the absence of hormone, steroid receptors associate with a chaperone complex composed of heat shock proteins, immunophilins, and other factors. The chaperone complex inhibits receptor binding to DNA and helps to maintain the receptor in a conformation that can bind ligand. When a ligand binds to the receptor, the chaperone complex dissociates and the receptor can bind to

DNA. The amino terminus of steroid receptors contains a second transcriptional activation domain, termed AF-1, that binds co-regulatory factors. Class II receptors are those receptors for **vitamin D, thyroid hormone, retinoic acid,** and **peroxisome proliferator.** Class II receptors form heterodimers with retinoid X receptors and bind to DNA in the absence of ligand binding. Binding of ligand results in the activation of receptors and stimulation of DNA transcription. Class III receptors are orphan receptors whose ligands have yet to be identified.

Because the actions of ligands that bind to nuclear hormone receptors require changes in gene transcription, translation, and subsequent protein synthesis, responses are slow, often taking many hours before the onset of action. Similarly, the slow turnover of most proteins regulated by these ligands results in a persistent effect following withdrawal of the ligand. Consequently, there is no simple temporal correlation between the plasma concentration of hormones or therapeutic agents acting on intracellular receptors and their effects.

## EFFECT OF DRUGS ON RECEPTORS

Drugs that act on specific receptors can be classified by their effect on the receptor. **Agonists** are drugs that mimic

| TABLE 8-3 | Voltage-Gated Ion Channels | | | |
|---|---|---|---|---|
| Ion Selectivity | Name | Number of Transmembrane Domains in α Subunit | Number of α Subunits Forming Functional Channel | Accessory Subunits |
| Potassium | K$_v$ 1–11 (voltage-gated K$^+$ channels)<br>K$_{ir}$ 1–6 (inwardly-rectifying K$^+$ channels) | 2, 4, or 6 | Tetramer | β subunit |
| Sodium | Na$_v$ 1.1–1.9 | 24 | Monomer | β subunits |
| Calcium | Ca$_v$ 1.1–1.4 (L type)<br>Ca$_v$ 2.1 (P/Q type)<br>Ca$_v$ 2.2 (N type)<br>Ca$_v$ 2.3 (R type)<br>Ca$_v$ 3.1–3.3 (T type) | 24 | Monomer | β, γ, α$_2$δ |
| Chloride | ClC | 12 | Dimer | |

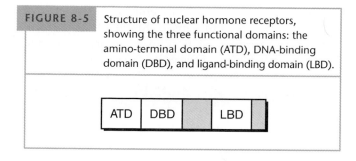

FIGURE 8-5 Structure of nuclear hormone receptors, showing the three functional domains: the amino-terminal domain (ATD), DNA-binding domain (DBD), and ligand-binding domain (LBD).

the effects of the endogenous ligands and evoke a response when bound to the receptor. Depending on their ability to induce the active state of the receptor, agonists may be considered **full agonists,** those drugs that can elicit a maximal response through the receptor (drugs A and B in Fig. 8-6), or **partial agonists,** those that cannot elicit a maximal response even at very high drug concentrations (drug C in Fig. 8-6). A partial agonist is said to have reduced **efficacy** compared with full agonists (i.e., the $E_{max}$ of the partial agonist is lower than that of the full agonists). Efficacy should not be confused with drug **potency,** which is the relationship between the concentration of the drug and its ability to elicit an effect (i.e., the $EC_{50}$ for the drug). In the example given in Figure 8-6, drugs A and C are equipotent (they have the same $EC_{50}$) and more potent than drug B, whereas drug C has lower efficacy than drugs A and B.

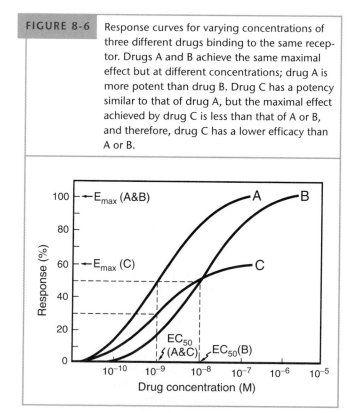

**FIGURE 8-6** Response curves for varying concentrations of three different drugs binding to the same receptor. Drugs A and B achieve the same maximal effect but at different concentrations; drug A is more potent than drug B. Drug C has a potency similar to that of drug A, but the maximal effect achieved by drug C is less than that of A or B, and therefore, drug C has a lower efficacy than A or B.

Since it is often desirable to inhibit rather than mimic the actions of endogenous ligands, many therapeutic agents that act on specific receptors are **antagonists.** Antagonists bind to the receptor but do not induce the active state and can therefore be considered to have zero efficacy. They do not elicit a response themselves but block the response elicited by the endogenous agonists and can therefore be considered to have **clinical utility.** Antagonists may be divided into two major classes depending on the type of chemical bonds formed between the drug and the receptor. **Reversible competitive antagonists** bind reversibly to the same site on the receptor as the agonists do and thus compete for the receptor binding site. The presence of a competitive antagonist will result in a shift of the dose–response curve for an agonist at that receptor (Fig. 8-7A). An example of reversible competitive antagonism is the effect of the β-adrenergic receptor antagonist propranolol, which attenuates increases in heart rate and force of contraction caused by adrenaline (Chapter 13). **Irreversible antagonists** may also compete with agonists for receptor binding, but either by forming covalent bonds or by virtue of their extremely high affinity for the receptor, they effectively bind irreversibly. Phenoxybenzamine is an example of an irreversible antagonist that forms covalent bonds with α-adrenergic receptors (Chapter 13).

The effect of an irreversible antagonist on the dose–response relationship of an agonist is dependent on the quantitative relationship between receptor occupancy and response. In the case of a linear relationship between receptor occupancy and response, in which $K_d$ is the same as $EC_{50}$, addition of even small doses of an irreversible antagonist will decrease the maximal response that can be elicited by the agonist (Fig. 8-7B). In many cases, however, not all receptors on a cell must be occupied in order to elicit the maximum response of an agonist. This phenomenon, that is, the existence of **spare receptors,** can be seen in many tissues and means that the $K_d$ measured for an agonist will be higher than its $EC_{50}$. If there are spare receptors, then the effect of a very small dose of an irreversible antagonist on the dose–response curve of an agonist will appear to be much the same as seen for the reversible antagonist (i.e., the dose–response curve for the agonist will be shifted to the right). Only when the dose of an irreversible antagonist is increased to a level that occupies enough receptors to overcome the spare receptors will the effect of the antagonist be to decrease the maximal response elicited by the agonist.

Drugs may also act by exhibiting allosteric effects on the response to an endogenous agonist. This effect may be positive or negative, and it results from drug binding either to a site on the receptor that is distinct from the agonist binding site or to an adjoining component of the cell distinct from the receptor. If the effect of the drug is inhibitory, then it is classified as a **non-competitive**

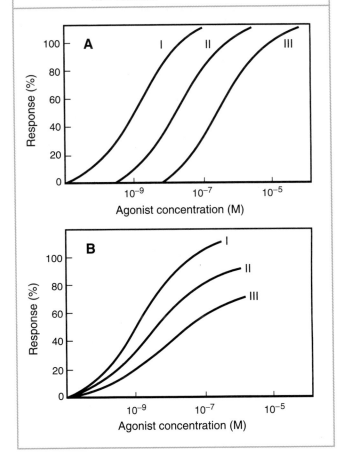

**FIGURE 8-7** Response curves for varying concentrations of an agonist. (A) Response curves for agonist alone (I), and in the presence of two concentrations (II, III) of a *reversible* competitive antagonist. As the concentration of the antagonist increases, the response curve for the agonist is shifted progressively to the right, increasing the $EC_{50}$ for the agonist, but the maximal effect of the agonist is unchanged. (B) Response curves for the same agonist alone (I), and in the presence of two different concentrations (II, III) of an *irreversible* antagonist. Because the antagonist can "permanently" occupy the receptors that it binds to, the maximal effect of the agonist is now reduced.

but their action is mediated by enhancing the effect of GABA on $GABA_A$ receptor–linked chloride channels, causing hyperpolarization of postsynaptic membranes and hence decreased firing of the postsynaptic neurons.

## DEFINING THE BINDING SITE AS A BIOLOGICALLY RELEVANT RECEPTOR

In order to establish the relationship between a radio-labelled ligand binding site in vitro and the physiological or pharmacological actions of that ligand in vivo, a number of parameters must be compared in the two systems. To define the site, the types of drugs that compete with that labelled ligand for binding need to be determined. These competition experiments result in a list of $K_i$ values for the competing drugs ($K_i \simeq IC_{50}$), the concentration of competing drug required to inhibit 50% of specific binding of the labelled ligand.

In this type of assay, the binding site should demonstrate stereoselectivity: the active enantiomer should have a much lower $K_i$ than the pharmacologically inactive enantiomer. Similarly, a series of related congeners should demonstrate good correlation between their relative potencies in vivo and their $K_i$ values in competition assays. For example, in the case of α-adrenergic receptors, the $K_i$ values should increase in the following order: (–)adrenaline, (–)noradrenaline, (+)adrenaline, dopamine, (–)isoproterenol. If the binding site is a β-adrenergic receptor, the order of increasing $K_i$ values should be the following: (–)isoproterenol, (–)adrenaline, (–)noradrenaline, dopamine, (+)isoproterenol.

These criteria are equally relevant whether one examines a drug binding site in a tissue homogenate or in cloned receptor DNA expressed in a cell system. In either case, it is the order of the drug $K_i$ values that characterizes the receptor; the absolute values are not important.

## CONCLUSION

Much has been learned about the targets of drug action in the body since the early use of synthetic compounds as drugs a century ago. In particular, the molecular cloning of receptors for many hormones, neurotransmitters, and cytokines, which are the targets of many of our therapeutic agents, has brought a new understanding of drug receptors at the molecular level. Many of the soluble protein receptors, such as enzymes, are being co-crystallized with their respective drugs, illustrating the precise binding interactions between drug and receptor. This information allows the medicinal chemists to design new drugs with very specific binding characteristics. Methods to crystallize membrane-bound receptors have now been developed and make possible similar studies for these types of receptors.

**antagonist.** An example of this type of drug action is seen with some gaseous anaesthetics that increase the stimulus threshold required to elicit firing by neurons in the CNS by stabilizing the closed state of ion channels linked to nicotinic cholinergic receptors (see Chapter 20). This effect is mediated by drug interactions with sites on the channels that are distinct from the acetylcholine binding site. Other examples of drugs that have allosteric effects on a receptor are the benzodiazepines and barbiturates (Chapter 23). These two groups of sedative–hypnotic drugs also decrease the firing rate of neurons in the CNS,

## SUGGESTED READINGS

Carpenter G. Receptors for epidermal growth factor and other polypeptide mitogens. *Annu Rev Biochem.* 1987;56:881-914.

Claesson-Welsh L. Mechanism of action of platelet-derived growth factor. *Int J Biochem Cell Biol.* 1996;28:373-385.

Filipek S, Teller DC, Palczewski K, Stenkamp R. The crystallographic model of rhodopsin and its use in studies of other G protein-coupled receptors. *Annu Rev Biophys Biomol Struct.* 2003;32:375-397.

Friebe A, Koesling D. Regulation of nitric oxide-sensitive guanylyl cyclase. *Circ Res.* 2003;93:96-105.

Hulme EC, ed. *Receptor-Ligand Interactions: A Practical Approach.* Oxford, United Kingdom: IRL Press; 1990.

Lucas KA, Pitari GM, Kazerounian S, et al. Guanylyl cyclases and signaling by cyclic GMP. *Pharmacol Rev.* 2000;52:375-414.

Mangelsdorf DJ, Thummel M, Beato P, et al. The nuclear receptor superfamily: the second decade. *Cell.* 1995;83:835-839.

Massagué J. How cells read TGF-β signals. *Nat Rev Mol Cell Biol.* 2000;1:169-178.

Myers MG Jr, White MF. Insulin signal transduction and the IRS proteins. *Annu Rev Pharmacol Toxicol.* 1996;36:615-658.

Palczewski K, Kumasaka T, Hori T, et al. Crystal structure of rhodopsin: a G protein-coupled receptor. *Science.* 2000;289:739-745.

Pierce KL, Premont RT, Lefkowitz RJ. Seven-transmembrane receptors. *Nat Rev Mol Cell Biol.* 2002;3:639-650.

Ullrich A, Schlessinger J. Signal transduction by receptors with tyrosine kinase activity. *Cell.* 1990;61:203-212.

# 9

# Signal Transduction Systems

## J MITCHELL

## SIGNALLING MECHANISMS

There are a number of basic mechanisms by which extracellular ligands regulate intracellular processes. The molecular components of each of these signal transduction systems are quite distinct. The **G protein–coupled receptor** systems are composed of a transmembrane receptor that binds a ligand on its extracellular surface and couples to a guanine nucleotide–binding protein (G protein) on its intracellular surface. The G protein, in turn, regulates effector enzymes to generate intracellular second messengers or modulates ion channel activity. The **receptor tyrosine kinases, receptor guanylyl cyclases,** and the **transforming growth factor β receptor** systems are composed of transmembrane receptors in which the intracellular portion has enzymatic activity that is allosterically regulated by ligand binding to the extracellular portion of the receptor. These transduction systems are described in more detail below.

## G PROTEIN–COUPLED SIGNAL TRANSDUCTION SYSTEMS

Most hormones and a few neurotransmitters act by regulating G protein–coupled receptors. Examples of the ligands that act by this mechanism and the signalling systems that they regulate are shown in Table 9-1. The three primary components of each system—receptor, G protein, and effector—are either embedded in the plasma membrane or tightly associated with it. The second messengers that are produced by the effector enzyme systems are, for the most part, water-soluble compounds that are freely diffusible in the cytoplasm.

Before examining each component of these systems in detail, it is useful to consider some of their general properties. If we look at even a partial list of distinct receptors and compare it with the number of systems they regulate (see Table 9-1), it is clear that many different first messengers regulate a common signal transduction system, yet

the physiological effect of each first messenger on its target cells is very different. For example, glucagon stimulates cyclic adenosine monophosphate (cAMP) production in liver cells and results in increased carbohydrate breakdown, whereas vasopressin stimulates cAMP in kidney cells, which results in increased water resorption from the nephron. This specificity of a first messenger's actions is the result of two processes: (1) receptors for a ligand are only present on specific cells, and (2) the expression of proteins that are regulated by the G protein subunits or second messengers is also specific to each cell type.

## G Proteins

The family of G proteins that transduce signals from the membrane G protein–coupled receptors (see Chapter 8 for the structure of these receptors) to effector enzymes and ion channels are known as the heterotrimeric G proteins. Each of these proteins is composed of three distinct subunits termed α, β, and γ in order of decreasing molecular weight. The α subunit of the trimer binds guanine nucleotides and is the major mediator of the G protein's actions on its effector. The β and γ subunits of the trimer function to support α subunit interactions with the plasma membrane and receptors, but like α subunits, they may also regulate effectors directly (Table 9-2).

The G proteins that participate in transmembrane signalling are all regulated by common mechanisms. The cycle of activation and inactivation of these proteins is depicted in Figure 9-1. In the resting, or basal, state, the three G protein subunits, α, β and γ, are bound together with guanosine diphosphate (GDP) within the guanine nucleotide–binding region of the α subunit. When an agonist binds to its receptor, the associated G protein is altered in some way that causes the release of the GDP. Guanosine triphosphate (GTP), which is present in high concentrations in the cytoplasm, then occupies the empty guanine nucleotide–binding site on the α subunit. GDP–GTP exchange on the α subunit changes the structure of the protein in three areas known as the switch regions I to III. These regions are intimately involved in the interaction of

**TABLE 9-1** Examples of G Protein–Coupled Receptor Systems

| Type of Ligand | Receptor | G Protein | System | Effect |
|---|---|---|---|---|
| **Neurotransmitters** | | | | |
| Adrenaline | $\beta_1$ | a) $G_s$ | AC | Stimulated |
| | | b) $G_s$ | $Ca^{2+}$ channel | Opened |
| | $\beta_2$ | $G_s$ | AC | Stimulated |
| | $\alpha_1$ | $G_{q/11}$ | PLC-$\beta$ | Stimulated |
| | $\alpha_{2a,2b}$ | $G_i$ | AC | Inhibited |
| Serotonin | 5-HT$_{1a}$ | a) $G_i$ | AC | Inhibited |
| | | b) $G_i$ | $K^+$ channel | Opened |
| | 5HT$_{1c}$ | $G_{q/11}$ | PLC-$\beta$ | Stimulated |
| | 5HT$_2$ | a) $G_s$ | AC | Stimulated |
| | | b) $G_o$ | $Ca^{2+}$ channel | Closed |
| **Peptide hormones** | | | | |
| Angiotensin II | AT$_{1a,1b}$ | a) $G_i$ | AC | Inhibited |
| | | b) $G_q$ | PLC | Stimulated |
| | | c) $G_i$ | $Ca^{2+}$ channel | Opened |
| Glucagon | | $G_s$ | AC | Stimulated |
| **Prostanoids** | | | | |
| Prostaglandins | PGE$_{1,2}$ | $G_i$ | AC | Stimulated |
| | PGF$_{2\alpha}$ | $G_q$ | PLC | Stimulated |
| Prostacyclin | PGI$_2$ | $G_s$ | AC | Stimulated |

AC = adenylyl cyclase; GABA = γ-aminobutyric acid; PDE = phosphodiesterase; PLA = phospholipase A; PLC = phospholipase C; PLD = phospholipase D.

GTP on the α subunit of a G protein regulates signal transduction from both the α and βγ subunits. Similarly, acceleration of GTPase activity by RGS proteins inhibits both α and βγ subunit activity.

Functional diversity among the different members of the G protein family is primarily the result of different α subunits, of which 20 are now known (see Table 9-2). The nomenclature for G proteins was originally based on their function. Thus, $G_s$ indicates the stimulatory protein and $G_i$ the inhibitory protein for adenylyl cyclase, and $G_t$ was so named because it was originally called transducin when it was first identified as the stimulatory protein in the retina. This system very quickly broke down, however, when G proteins were isolated and cloned without knowledge of their function, so we also have $G_o$ (G other), $G_q$, and more recently, $G_{11}$, $G_{12}$, and so on. Some G proteins are only expressed in defined cell types and have very specialized functions; for example, $G_t$ is found only in rods and cones of the retina and activates a cGMP-specific phosphodiesterase. Other G proteins such as $G_s$, $G_i$, and $G_q$ are widely expressed in most tissues of the body, where they regulate adenylyl cyclase and phospholipase C.

The effect of most G proteins on their effectors is stimulatory, but a few act to inhibit their effectors. For exam-

**TABLE 9-2** Families of Mammalian G Proteins

| Family | G Protein | Function | Expression |
|---|---|---|---|
| $G_s$ | $G_s\alpha$ | AC stimulation<br>$Ca^{2+}$ channel opening | Ubiquitous |
| | $G_{olf}\alpha$ | AC stimulation | Olfactory, brain |
| $G_i$ | $G_{i-1}\alpha$ | AC inhibition | Ubiquitous |
| | $G_{i-2}\alpha$ | AC inhibition | Ubiquitous |
| | $G_{i-3}\alpha$ | AC inhibition | Ubiquitous |
| | $G_i\beta\gamma$ | $K^+$ channel opening | |
| | $G_{oA,B}\beta\gamma$ | $Ca^{2+}$ channel closing | Brain, heart, endocrine |
| | $G_{t1,2}\alpha$ | cGMP PDE stimulation | Retina rods, cones |
| | $G_z\alpha$ | AC inhibition | Brain |
| $G_q$ | $G_q\alpha$ | PLC-$\beta$ stimulation | Ubiquitous |
| | $G_{11}\alpha$ | PLC-$\beta$ stimulation | Ubiquitous |
| | $G_{14}\alpha$ | PLC-$\beta$ stimulation | |
| | $G_{15}\alpha$ | PLC-$\beta$ stimulation | Myeloid and B cells |
| | $G_{16}\alpha$ | PLC-$\beta$ stimulation | Myeloid and T cells |
| $G_{12}$ | $G_{12}\alpha$ | Rho GEF stimulation | Ubiquitous |
| | $G_{13}\alpha$ | Rho GEF stimulation | Ubiquitous |

AC = adenylyl cyclase; cGMP = cyclic guanosine monophosphate; NHE = sodium/hydrogen exchanger; PDE = phosphodiesterase; PLC = phospholipase C; Rho GEF = GTP exchange factor for Rho protein.

Gα with Gβγ, effectors, and regulatory proteins. The effect of GTP binding is stimulatory to the G protein, and the α subunit dissociates from the receptor and G protein βγ subunits and binds to the effector. The G protein βγ subunits remain associated with each other at all times, and when dissociated from α-GTP they can also bind to their effector.

After a few seconds, the intrinsic GTPase activity of the α subunit hydrolyzes the bound GTP to GDP, thereby inactivating itself. The rate of Gα GTPase activity is enhanced five- to a hundredfold by interaction with proteins known as **regulators of G protein signalling (RGS)**. RGS proteins are a family of more than 20 proteins that all contain a 130-amino-acid motif known as an RGS domain. Specific RGS proteins can regulate one or more G protein α subunits. In some cases, such as the $G_q$ family of G proteins, interaction of the α subunits with their effector phospholipase C proteins also enhances the GTPase activity of Gα and increases the rate of G protein inactivation. Following GTP hydrolysis, the GDP-bound α subunit dissociates from the effector, re-associates with the G protein βγ complex, and is then available for another cycle of activation by the receptor. In this way, the hydrolysis of

| FIGURE 9-1 | G-protein activation–inactivation cycle. α, β, γ = subunits of G proteins; GDP = guanosine diphosphate; GTP = guanosine triphosphate; $P_i$ = phosphate; $R_H$ = high-affinity receptor; $R_L$ = low-affinity receptor; E = effector; RGS = regulator of G protein signalling. |
|---|---|

are the most common targets of hormone and neurotransmitter receptors (see Table 9-1). These two systems are well understood, and their components are detailed in Figures 9-2 and 9-3.

### Adenylyl cyclases and cAMP as a second messenger

The study of second-messenger systems began with the pioneering studies of Sutherland and Rall in the late 1950s. They found that stimulating cardiac membranes with adrenaline increased the concentration of a water-soluble nucleotide, cyclic adenosine monophosphate (cAMP), and they proposed that the cAMP acted as an intracellular messenger. We now know that cAMP is synthesized from ATP by the adenylyl cyclase enzymes embedded in the plasma membrane. These enzymes are large polypeptides thought to contain two clusters of six transmembrane segments (M1 and M2) separating two similar catalytic domains (C1 and C2). The C1 and C2 domains interact with each other to form a catalytic enzyme. $G_s\alpha$ activates adenylyl cyclase by binding to the C2 domain, while $G_i\alpha$ inhibits cyclase activity by binding to the C1 domain. The effects of these two G proteins on cyclase enzyme activity appear to result from either increasing ($G_s\alpha$) or decreasing ($G_i\alpha$) the stability of the two C domains in their active conformation. The diterpene

ple, the βγ subunits from $G_o$ or $G_i$ inhibit $Ca^{2+}$ channels in the brain and heart, and some types of adenylyl cyclase are inhibited by $G_i\alpha$. Simultaneous activation of receptors coupled to $G_s$ and $G_i$ results in an attenuated adenylyl cyclase response in that cell. This dual regulation, in addition to interaction of signal transduction components distal to the G proteins (see "Effector Enzymes Regulated by G Proteins" below), allows for an integrated response to multiple stimuli on the same cell.

Some G proteins are also targets for pathological agents. A toxin produced by the bacterium *Vibrio cholerae* modifies $G_s\alpha$ by addition of adenosine diphosphate–ribose (ADP-ribose) to the $\alpha_s$ subunit. ADP ribosylation of $\alpha_s$ inhibits the GTPase activity of the G protein, resulting in persistent activation of $G_s\alpha$. When the bacterium infects the intestinal cells, the resulting activation of $G_s\alpha$ elevates intracellular cAMP and causes the cells to secrete large amounts of water into the gut, resulting in severe diarrhea characteristic of cholera infection. The bacterium *Bordetella pertussis,* which causes whooping cough, secretes a similar toxin that ADP-ribosylates $G_i\alpha$ and $G_o\alpha$, preventing their activation by receptors. With the inhibitory effect of $G_i$ on adenylyl cyclase disrupted by the toxin, cAMP accumulation also increases in cells infected by the pertussis bacterium, resulting in the characteristic cough and immune responses associated with the disease.

## Effector Enzymes Regulated by G Proteins

Of the three components that constitute the G protein–coupled signal transduction systems, the effectors were the most difficult to study at the molecular level. The adenylyl cyclases and the phospholipase C enzymes

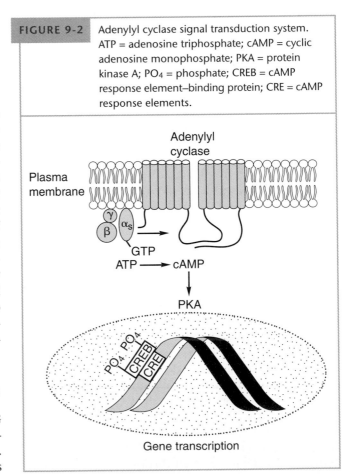

| FIGURE 9-2 | Adenylyl cyclase signal transduction system. ATP = adenosine triphosphate; cAMP = cyclic adenosine monophosphate; PKA = protein kinase A; $PO_4$ = phosphate; CREB = cAMP response element–binding protein; CRE = cAMP response elements. |
|---|---|

**forskolin,** a potent activator of most types of adenylyl cyclase, binds to each of the C domains, stabilizing their interaction and increasing adenylyl cyclase activity.

There are at least nine forms of membrane adenylyl cyclase. All are stimulated by $G_s\alpha$ and all except type IX are stimulated by forskolin, but they differ in their sensitivity to inhibition by $G_i\alpha$, stimulation by calcium/calmodulin, and effect of G protein subunits and protein kinases (Table 9-3). These additional regulators allow for the integration of many signals acting on different second-messenger systems within the same cell.

cAMP exerts most of its effects in cells by activating the cAMP-dependent protein kinases, **protein kinases A (PKAs).** These tetrameric enzymes are composed of two regulatory and two catalytic subunits. The enzymes are activated when two molecules of cAMP bind to each of the regulatory subunits, releasing the catalytic subunits from the tetramer. The released subunits then catalyze the transfer of the terminal phosphate group from ATP to specific serine and threonine residues on their target proteins. Among these target proteins are enzymes that participate in cellular metabolic pathways and proteins that regulate gene transcription. A well-studied example of a cAMP-activated metabolic pathway is the cascade of enzyme activation leading to breakdown of glycogen in the liver. Activated PKA phosphorylates phosphorylase kinase, which in turn phosphorylates glycogen phosphorylase, the enzyme that breaks down glycogen. The effect of cAMP on gene transcription is primarily mediated by PKA-catalyzed phosphorylation of a protein known as the **cAMP response element–binding protein (CREB).** CREB binds to specific short DNA sequences known as **cAMP response elements (CRE).** CREB is bound to the CRE and, when phosphorylated by PKA, it stimulates transcription of genes containing the CRE in their regulatory region (see Fig. 9-2).

## Phospholipase C and phospholipid second messengers

Members of the $G_q$ family of proteins (see Table 9-2) couple various receptors to a group of enzymes known as **phospholipase C beta (PLC-β).** These enzymes belong to a larger family of phospholipases that all use membrane inositol phospholipids as substrates. Signal transduction through this pathway follows a sequence of molecular events similar to that for the activation of adenylyl cyclase. Receptor occupation by an agonist activates the $G_q$ proteins, which in turn bind to the PLC-β on the inner surface of the plasma membrane. Once activated, the lipase rapidly breaks down phosphatidylinositol 4,5-bisphosphate (PIP2) to **inositol 1,4,5-trisphosphate (IP3)** and **diacylglycerol.** Both of these molecules can act as second messengers by two different pathways (see Fig. 9-3).

IP3 is a small water-soluble molecule that can rapidly diffuse through the cytoplasm and bind to an IP3 receptor (IP3-gated $Ca^{2+}$ channel) in the smooth endoplasmic reticulum, resulting in release of stored $Ca^{2+}$ into the cytoplasm. The rise in cytoplasmic calcium concentration initiates a wave of calcium-dependent reactions in the cell. Many of these reactions are mediated by specific $Ca^{2+}$-binding proteins, the most ubiquitous being **calmodulin.** $Ca^{2+}$/calmodulin regulates a number of enzymes, including plasma membrane $Ca^{2+}$-ATPase, which pumps calcium out of the cell; myosin light-chain kinase, which regulates myosin phosphorylation and muscle contraction; and, as we have seen, some types of adenylyl cyclase (see Table 9-3). Some of the effects of calcium in the cell are the result of activation of a group of protein kinases known as **$Ca^{2+}$/calmodulin-dependent protein kinases.** These kinases phosphorylate serines and threonines on a variety of proteins. Once again, the physiological response of any given cell to activation of the phospholipid second messengers is dependent on the $Ca^{2+}$/calmodulin kinase target proteins expressed in that cell.

The other molecular product of PIP2 hydrolysis by phospholipase C is diacylglycerol. This lipid molecule remains in the plasma membrane, where, in concert with phosphatidylserine, it activates some members of another family of serine/threonine kinases known as **protein kinase C** (Table 9-4). Once activated, these kinases phosphorylate a cell-specific array of substrate proteins that include many ion channels, receptors, and other kinases that eventually result in increased gene transcription, which can lead to changes in cell proliferation, differentiation metabolism, and cellular death by apoptosis.

## Ion Channel Regulation by G Proteins

G proteins have been shown to modulate the activity of many of the voltage-gated ion channels. This modulation occurs either directly by G-protein subunit interaction with ion channel proteins or indirectly through the acti-

| TABLE 9-3 | | Regulation of Cloned Mammalian Adenylyl Cyclases | |
|---|---|---|---|
| Group | Isoforms | Activators | Inhibitors |
| 1 | I | $G_s\alpha$, Fsk, $Ca^{2+}$/CaM | $G_i\alpha$, Gβγ, CaM kinase IV |
| | III | $G_s\alpha$, Fsk, $Ca^{2+}$/CaM | CaM kinase II |
| | VIII | $G_s\alpha$, Fsk, $Ca^{2+}$/CaM | |
| 2 | II | $G_s$, Fsk, Gβγ, PKC | |
| | IV | $G_s\alpha$, Fsk, Gβγ | PKC |
| | VII | $G_s\alpha$, Fsk, Gβγ, PKC | |
| 3 | V | $G_s\alpha$, Fsk, PKC | $G_i\alpha$, PKA, $Ca^{2+}$ |
| | VI | $G_s\alpha$, Fsk | $G_i\alpha$, PKA, $Ca^{2+}$, PKC |
| 4 | IX | $G_s\alpha$ | Calcineurin |

Fsk = forskolin; CaM = calmodulin; CaM kinase = $Ca^{2+}$/calmodulin-regulated kinase; PKA = protein kinase A; PKC = protein kinase C.

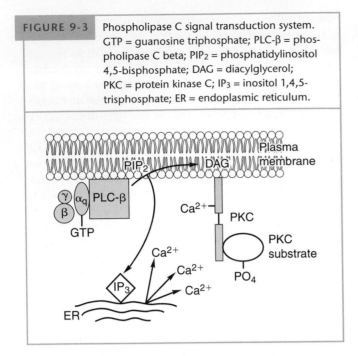

FIGURE 9-3 | Phospholipase C signal transduction system. GTP = guanosine triphosphate; PLC-β = phospholipase C beta; PIP₂ = phosphatidylinositol 4,5-bisphosphate; DAG = diacylglycerol; PKC = protein kinase C; IP₃ = inositol 1,4,5-trisphosphate; ER = endoplasmic reticulum.

vation of kinases such as PKA and PKC that phosphorylate sites on the intracellular side of ion channel proteins and alter their rates of activation or inactivation. As can be seen from Table 9-1, many hormones and neurotransmitters regulate both a second messenger and an ion channel by activating a single G protein; for example, $G_s$ stimulates both adenylyl cyclase and some types of $Ca^{2+}$ channels. G protein βγ subunits mediate the inhibition of some types of voltage-gated $Ca^{2+}$ channels by G protein–coupled receptors, and $G_i$ proteins stimulate some types of $K^+$ channels, also through the G protein βγ subunits.

## Termination of Second-Messenger Signalling

In addition to the mechanisms of inactivation of G protein–coupled receptors discussed in Chapter 8, and the regulation of G protein subunits by RGS and effector proteins discussed above, second-messenger signalling is limited by breakdown of the second messengers themselves. A large family of phosphodiesterases (PDEs) limits the

activity of cAMP and cGMP by catalyzing their hydrolysis to 5'AMP and 5'GMP. The PDEs are divided into groups based on their selectivity for cAMP and cGMP (Table 9-5). Some of the PDEs are targets for therapeutic agents. For example, **sildenafil**, which is used to treat erectile dysfunction (see Chapter 34), acts as a vasodilator by inhibiting PDE-5, thereby inhibiting the breakdown of cGMP.

# ENZYME-LINKED RECEPTOR SIGNAL TRANSDUCTION SYSTEMS

## Receptor Tyrosine Kinases

The receptor tyrosine kinases are stimulated by a group of endogenous compounds known as **growth factors,** which includes **insulin, epidermal growth factor (EGF), and platelet-derived growth factor (PDGF).** The structure of these receptors was discussed in Chapter 8. The autophosphorylation of these receptors when occupied by their ligands acts as a signal for binding of other intracellular proteins, which themselves become phosphorylated on tyrosine residues by the receptor and are thereby activated. Once again, different combinations of proteins that bind to each growth factor receptor determine the specificity of cellular responses to different growth factors.

| TABLE 9-4 | Regulation of Protein Kinase C Enzymes | |
|---|---|---|
| Group | Isoforms | Activators |
| Classical | α, β, γ | $Ca^{2+}$, PS, DAG |
| Novel | δ, ε, η, θ | PS, DAG |
| Atypical | ι, ζ | $PI_3$ kinase |

PS = phosphatidylserine; DAG = diacylglycerol; $PI_3$ = phosphoinositide 3 phosphate.

| TABLE 9-5 | Regulation of Mammalian Phosphodiesterases | | |
|---|---|---|---|
| Family | Substrates | Activators | Inhibitors |
| 1 | cAMP and cGMP | $Ca^{2+}$/CaM | PKA, CaM kinase II, theophylline |
| 2 | cAMP and cGMP | cGMP, PKC | Theophylline |
| 3 | cAMP > cGMP | PKA, PKB | cGMP, milrinone, theophylline |
| 4 | cAMP | PKA, PA, ERK | Caspases, rolipram, theophylline |
| 5 | cGMP | cGMP, PKA, PKG | Caspases, zaprinast, theophylline, sildenafil |
| 6 | cGMP | $C_t α$ | cGMP |
| 7 | cAMP | | Theophylline |
| 8 | cAMP | | |
| 9 | cGMP | | |
| 10 | cGMP > cAMP | | cAMP |
| 11 | cAMP and cGMP | | |

cAMP = cyclic adenosine monophosphate; cGMP = cyclic guanosine monophosphate; CaM = calmodulin; CaM kinase = $Ca^{2+}$/calmodulin-regulated kinase; PKA = protein kinase A; PKB = protein kinase B; PKC = protein kinase C; PKG = protein kinase G; PA = phosphatidic acid; ERK = extracellular signal–regulated protein kinase.

Activated insulin and insulin-like growth factor receptors bind a group of proteins known as the **insulin receptor substrates (IRS).** Four mammalian IRS proteins have been identified, with IRS-1 and IRS-2 co-expressed in most tissues. The IRS proteins contain two functional regions: (1) the highly conserved amino-terminal region contains a pleckstrin homology (PH) domain and a phosphotyrosine binding domain that binds to the activated receptor, and (2) the carboxyl-terminal region contains multiple tyrosine residues that are phosphorylated by the receptor and also contains an SH2 domain (see next paragraph) that can bind and activate a number of proteins that mediate the many actions of insulin on cells. The molecular pathways that mediate some of the actions of insulin in its target tissues are well known. For example, stimulation of glucose uptake into muscle and adipose cells is mediated by IRS protein activation of the enzyme phosphoinositide 3 (PI3) kinase, which, in turn, increases the translocation of glucose transporters from intracellular stores to the plasma membrane.

A large number of proteins that bind to activated growth-factor receptors other than the insulin receptor have been identified. These proteins have varied structures, but they share two highly conserved domains known as **SH2 and SH3** for *Src homology regions 2 and 3* because they were first identified in the proto-oncogene–encoded *Src* protein. The SH2 domain recognizes the phosphotyrosines on the growth-factor receptors, and the SH3 domain binds other proteins. Characterization of the

many proteins containing SH2 and SH3 domains has been the subject of intense research efforts, and the roles of some of these proteins are now clear. For example, one mechanism by which growth factors regulate cellular growth or differentiation is by activating a cascade of protein kinases known as the **mitogen-activated protein (MAP) kinases pathway.** There are four distinct MAP kinase (MAPK) pathways in mammalian cells: (1) the extracellular signal–regulated kinases (ERK1,2) pathway, (2) the c-Jun amino terminal kinase also called the stress-activated protein kinases (JNK/SAPK) pathway, (3) the p38 MAPK pathway, and (4) the most recently characterized ERK5 pathway (Fig. 9-4). In general, it is the ERKs that are activated by growth factor regulation of receptor tyrosine kinases. Activation of ERK1,2 is initiated by tyrosine phosphorylation of Grb2 (a protein containing SH2 and SH3 domains). The SH3 domain on Grb2 binds another protein known as mSOS, and together with a third protein, Sch, the Sch/Grb2/mSOS complex activates Ras, a monomeric G protein. Ras has a structure similar to the α subunits of heterotrimeric G proteins that interact with the G protein–coupled receptors, and it is activated and inactivated by similar mechanisms (see Fig. 9-1). Hence, the interaction of Ras with Sch/Grb2/mSOS promotes exchange of GDP for GTP on Ras, thus promoting its activation. The next step in this cascade involves Ras activation of a serine/threonine kinase known as Raf-1. Raf-1 then activates (by phosphorylation) another set of kinases, MEK1,2 (also known as MAP-kinase kinases), which in turn phosphory-

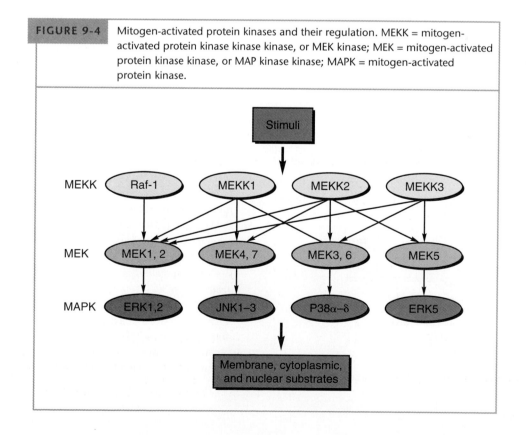

**FIGURE 9-4** Mitogen-activated protein kinases and their regulation. MEKK = mitogen-activated protein kinase kinase kinase, or MEK kinase; MEK = mitogen-activated protein kinase kinase, or MAP kinase kinase; MAPK = mitogen-activated protein kinase.

late the ERK1,2 MAP kinases. All MAP kinases can traverse the nuclear membrane, and in the nucleus, they phosphorylate a variety of transcription factors. The consequent regulation of gene transcription initiates processes resulting in cellular proliferation or differentiation.

Other proteins that interact with growth-factor receptors are known to regulate intracellular second messengers. For example, members of the **phospholipase C gamma (PLC-γ)** family of proteins, which regulate intracellular IP3 and diacylglycerol levels in a similar manner to that of the PLC-β family discussed above, contain SH2 and SH3 domains and are known to be activated by tyrosine kinase receptors.

The only member of the family of growth-factor receptors that is currently a target for pharmacological agents is the insulin receptor in diabetic patients (see Chapter 47). However, the role of receptor tyrosine kinases in cellular growth, and the association of uncontrolled signalling through these receptors with neoplastic and inflammatory diseases, has created a great interest in the development of agents that will block their activity. For example, mutated *ras* proteins have been found in more than 30% of human cancers. Various agents are being developed to inhibit the activity of mutated *ras* and other proteins in the MAP kinase pathway, as potential therapeutic drugs. Several of these are undergoing clinical trials for use in the treatment of tumours.

## Transforming Growth Factor β Receptors

The transforming growth factor β (**TGFβ**) family of cytokines control a broad range of cellular processes by binding to receptor serine/threonine kinases (see Chapter 8). Upon binding the TGFβ dimer, the type II receptor phosphorylates the type I receptor kinase domain, which in turn phosphorylates its intracellular target, **Smad** protein. There are three different groups of Smad proteins: (1) R-Smads (Smads 1,2,3,5,8) that bind to the receptors, (2) co-mediator Smad (Co-Smad 4), and (3) inhibitory Smads (I-Smads 6,7). Activated TGFβ receptors bind and phosphorylate R-Smads, causing them to undergo trimerization and formation of complexes with Smad 4. These Smad complexes are then translocated into the nucleus, where they regulate the transcription of target genes (Fig. 9-5). The I-Smads play an inhibitory role in TGFβ signalling by competing with R-Smads for receptors and targeting receptors for degradation.

## SUGGESTED READINGS

Berridge MJ. Inositol trisphosphate and diacylglycerol: two interacting second messengers. *Annu Rev Biochem.* 1987;56:159-193.

Birnbaumer L, Abramowitz J, Brown AM. Receptor-effector coupling by G proteins. *Biochem Biophys Acta.* 1990;1031:163-224.

Bourne HR, Sanders DA, McCormick F. The GTPase superfamily: conserved structure and molecular mechanism. *Nature.* 1991;349:117-127.

Dolphin AC. G protein modulation of voltage-gated calcium channels. *Pharmacol Rev.* 2003;55:607-627.

Ing NH, O'Malley BW. The steroid hormone receptor superfamily: molecular mechanisms of action. In: Weintraub BD, ed. *Molecular Endocrinology: Basic Concepts and Clinical Considerations.* New York, NY: Raven Press; 1995:195-215.

Mellor H, Parker PJ. The extended protein kinase C superfamily. *Biochem J.* 1998;332:281-292.

Michell RH. Inositol lipids in cellular signaling mechanisms. *Trends Biochem Sci.* 1992;17:274-276.

Pearson G, Robinson F, Beers Gibson T, et al. Mitogen-activated protein (MAP) kinase pathways: regulation and physiological functions. *Endocr Rev.* 2001;22:153-183.

Shi Y, Massague J. Mechanisms of TGF beta signaling from cell membrane to the nucleus. *Cell.* 2003;113:685-700.

Sunahara RK, Dessauer CW, Gilman AG. Complexity and diversity of mammalian adenylyl cyclases. *Annu Rev Pharmacol Toxicol.* 1996;36:461-480.

Taylor SS, Buechler JA, Yonemoto M. cAMP-dependent protein kinase: framework for a diverse family of regulatory enzymes. *Annu Rev Biochem.* 1990;59:971-1005.

Ullrich A, Schlessinger J. Growth factor signaling by receptor tyrosine kinases. *Neuron.* 1992;9:383-391.

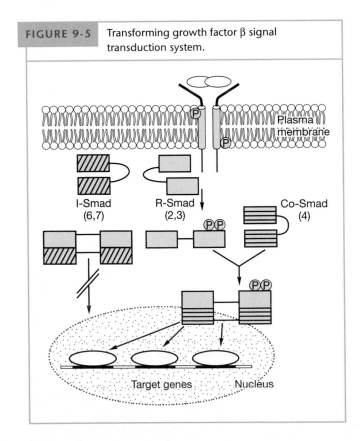

**FIGURE 9-5** Transforming growth factor β signal transduction system.

# 10

# Pharmacogenetics and Pharmacogenomics

## DM GRANT AND W KALOW

### CASE HISTORY

A woman receiving the anticoagulant warfarin at a dose of 5 mg/day was hospitalized for gastrointestinal bleeding. Her prothrombin time—a measure of the time required for blood to clot—was found to be drastically elevated, with an international normalized ratio (INR) of 32.6. The usual INR value in an appropriately anticoagulated patient is 2 to 3. Warfarin was discontinued, and her INR fell to 2.8 after transfusion of fresh-frozen plasma, but it rose again spontaneously to 8.3. Twenty-six days after the last dose of warfarin had been administered, the drug was still detectable in the patient's plasma.

## INTRODUCTION AND HISTORICAL PERSPECTIVE

The concept that therapeutic and toxic responses to exogenous chemicals may vary significantly among the individuals in human populations is by no means a new one. Indeed, inter-individual variation in drug response has been commented on by clinicians since the late nineteenth century. Such variation may occur due to differences in pharmacological processes related to drug disposition (pharmacokinetics) or drug–target interactions (pharmacodynamics), either intended or not. Moreover, the basis of such observed variations may lie in the contribution of environmental and disease-related factors, as well as in the differing genetic constitutions of the individuals who make up human populations. The purpose of this chapter is to focus on an overview of **pharmacogenetics**, defined as **the study of the contribution of genetic factors to variation in drug response and toxicity;** the equally important role of non-genetic factors as sources of variable drug response is discussed in detail in Chapter 58.

Although, in the broadest sense, pharmacogenetics includes phenomena such as genetically based bacterial resistance to antibiotics and strain differences in response to exogenous enzyme inducers in mice, this chapter will deal exclusively with human pharmacogenetics and pharmacogenomics. **Pharmacogenomics** is an applied discipline, largely arising as a consequence of technological advances in our ability to interrogate the human genome. It can be defined as **the use of genomic information and technologies to optimize the discovery and development of drug targets and drugs.** Although the experimental approaches used in pharmacogenetics and pharmacogenomics research differ (see "Pharmacogenetics and Pharmacogenomics: Experimental Approaches" below), the ultimate goal of both these fields of study is to explain, predict, and control variation in the response to drugs so that, at the level of the individual patient, the right dose of the right drug is more likely to be used.

Notwithstanding a tremendous upsurge in recent interest in pharmacogenetics and pharmacogenomics among the scientific, medical, and business communities within the past decade, pharmacogenetics is not a new field of investigation. For instance, as early as the 1930s, it was observed that individuals could be distinguished as "tasters" or "non-tasters" of particular bitter substances, a phenotypic trait that followed Mendelian inheritance. The 1950s and 1960s witnessed a number of clinical observations documenting genetically controlled unexpected or adverse responses to therapeutic agents. These included drug-induced hemolytic anemias related to defects in glucose-6-phosphate dehydrogenase (G-6-PD), prolonged muscle paralysis from succinylcholine caused by deficient plasma cholinesterase activity, malignant hyperthermia from general anaesthetics, and increased risk for neuronal and liver toxicity from the tuberculostatic drug isoniazid due to its impaired metabolism.

In the years since the first use of the term "pharmacogenetics" in 1957 and the publication of the first monograph on the topic in 1962, a large number of observations of pharmacogenetic variants affecting drug disposition and drug effects have accumulated (Tables 10-1 and 10-2).

Examples from these lists have been chosen for more detailed discussion in later sections of this chapter because of their historical significance, clinical impact, or the level of our mechanistic understanding of the underlying biochemical and molecular mechanisms producing the observed traits in human populations.

## VARIATION IN THE HUMAN GENOME

An understanding of pharmacogenetics naturally requires knowledge of basic principles of both pharmacology and genetics. The principles of pharmacology are covered extensively throughout this book and need not be recapitulated here, but a brief description of some key principles of molecular and population genetics is in order.

The human genome is composed of over $3 \times 10^9$ nucleotide bases, strung together in linear polymers of DNA. It is organized into 23 *pairs* of chromosomes (i.e., humans are *diploid* organisms), with one member of each chromosome pair in any individual being derived from each of the *haploid* parental germ cells at the time of sperm–egg fusion. A small proportion of the total DNA complement is organized into genes, which encode the transcription of messenger RNA that is ultimately translated into proteins. Hence, the DNA code contains all of the necessary information to produce the proteins that make up the organism's cellular components, including structural proteins, regulatory factors, and catalytic enzymes. Because of the diploid nature of the human genome, with some exceptions, humans possess two copies of every nucleotide and hence of every gene.

Variation in the human genome is by definition a population concept: it is observed by comparing DNA nucleotide sequences among individuals in populations. Such genetic variation, which is observable as variable diploid *genotypes* at any particular location on the DNA, produces variation in *phenotypes,* or physically distinguishable traits in individuals. Variations that occur with a frequency greater than 1% in populations are arbitrarily defined as *polymorphisms* in order to distinguish them from rare variants. DNA variations may have a variety of genetic causes, ranging from the deletion of entire segments of chromosomal DNA to the substitution of single nucleotide bases. The latter type of DNA sequence variant, when present in more than 1% of a population, is thus termed a *single nucleotide polymorphism,* or SNP. Recent human genome re-sequencing efforts have produced a database of over 10 million putative SNP locations across the human genome where at least 1% of the population possesses a sequence divergent from that of the rest of the population. Thus, SNPs are the most abundant type of DNA sequence variation. SNPs are of particular importance not only because they may be useful markers for the mapping of new disease gene loci, but also because they have been shown to be causally related to a variety of genetic diseases and drug response polymorphisms.

| TABLE 10-1 | Monogenic Variants Affecting Drug Biotransformation and Pharmacokinetics |
|---|---|
| Plasma cholinesterase | |
| Serum paraoxonase | |
| Monoamine oxidase B | |
| Catalase | |
| Alcohol dehydrogenase | |
| Aldehyde dehydrogenase | |
| Dihydropyrimidine dehydrogenase | |
| Dopamine β-hydroxylase | |
| Cytochromes P450<br>CYP1A1<br>CYP1A2<br>CYP1B1<br>CYP2A6<br>CYP2C8<br>CYP2C9<br>CYP2C19<br>CYP2D6<br>CYP2E1<br>CYP2J2<br>CYP2R1<br>CYP2S1<br>CYP3A4<br>CYP3A5<br>CYP4B1 | |
| Arylamine N-acetyltransferase<br>NAT1<br>NAT2 | |
| UDP-glucuronosyltransferase<br>UGT1A1<br>UGT2B4<br>UGT2B7<br>UGT2B15 | |
| Sulfotransferase<br>SULT1A1<br>SULT1A3 | |
| Thiopurine S-methyltransferase | |
| Catechol O-methyltransferase | |
| Glutathione S-transferase<br>GSTM1<br>GSTM3<br>GSTP1<br>GSTT1 | |
| P-glycoprotein ABCB1 | |

| TABLE 10-2 | Monogenic Variants Affecting Intended or Unintended Drug Targets |
| --- | --- |
| Hypoxanthine–guanine phosphoribosyltransferase deficiency | |
| Glucose-6-phosphate dehydrogenase deficiency | |
| Malignant hyperthermia | |
| NADH methemoglobin reductase deficiency | |
| Uroporphyrinogen I synthetase deficiency | |
| Coproporphyrinogen oxidase deficiency | |
| $\alpha_1$-Antitrypsin deficiency | |
| Angiotensin-I converting enzyme | |
| $\beta_1$-Adrenergic receptor | |
| $\beta_2$-Adrenergic receptor | |
| Angiotensinogen | |
| Angiotensinogen-II receptor type 1 | |
| 5-Lipoxygenase | |
| Bradykinin receptor | |
| Human growth hormone receptor | |
| Cholesterol ester transfer protein | |
| Dopamine $D_2$ receptor | |
| Dopamine $D_3$ receptor | |
| Dopamine $D_4$ receptor | |
| Estrogen receptor $\alpha$ | |
| Glycoprotein IIIa subunit | |
| Inotropic glutamate receptor | |
| Serotonin 2A receptor | |
| Apolipoprotein E4 | |
| Hepatic lipase | |
| Methylene tetrahydrofolate reductase | |
| Methylguanine methyltransferase | |
| Dopamine transporter | |
| Serotonin transporter | |
| Stromelysin-1 | |
| Tryptophan hydroxylase | |
| Thymidylate synthetase | |
| Prothrombin | |
| Factor V | |
| Potassium channels<br>    HERG<br>    KvLQT1<br>    hKCNE2 | |

From a mechanistic perspective, DNA sequence variation may have a number of functional consequences that ultimately affect protein function. DNA alterations may produce changes in upstream promoter regions that alter gene transcription, transcript processing, or transcript stability. Mutations may also alter transcript secondary structure so as to alter the efficiency of translation. Each of these will ultimately affect the quantity of protein produced. Alternatively, mutations may directly affect the protein-coding sequence of the transcript, resulting in the production of proteins with altered amino acid sequences and consequent changes in structure, stability, and/or substrate–ligand binding properties.

## PHARMACOGENETICS AND PHARMACOGENOMICS: EXPERIMENTAL APPROACHES

Although numerous definitions have been put forward in an attempt to distinguish pharmacogenetics and pharmacogenomics, it may be most practical to simply apply an operational distinction in terms of the focus of the experimental approaches taken in each instance. Classical pharmacogenetic studies usually begin with the clinical observation of an unexpected drug response, such as that observed in the patient in the case study at the beginning of this chapter, which may be subsequently investigated at the mechanistic level using biochemical and molecular genetic approaches. This may thus be considered a "phenotype-to-genotype" approach to scientific investigation, which uses a focused hypothesis-testing paradigm. On the other hand, the newer discipline of pharmacogenomics takes advantage of the essentially complete nucleotide sequence of the entire human genome and its identified sequence variants among human populations, combined with high-throughput assay technologies for genotyping isolated genomic human DNA samples, in order to uncover relationships between DNA sequence variation and phenotypic variation in drug response. Pharmacogenomic methods are therefore effective means of utilizing advanced genomic technologies to generate hypotheses regarding variable drug action, which can then be further tested with focused studies. Thus pharmacogenetic and pharmacogenomic approaches are complementary means to investigate the relationship between pharmacological variation and genetic variation, with the same ultimate goal of optimizing the effective use of drugs in individual patients.

## CLASSIFICATION OF PHARMACOGENETIC VARIANTS

As suggested from the above discussions, pharmacogenetic variation may be classified according to either pharmacological principles or genetic principles. From a pharmacological perspective, variation may affect drug pharmacokinetics via alteration of drug transport channels or of enzymes involved in drug biotransformation, or it may directly affect drug pharmacodynamics via alteration of the function of drug targets, such as neurotransmitter or hormone receptors.

From a genetic perspective, pharmacogenetic variants may first be distinguished according to the multiplicity of genes contributing to the phenotype. Phenotypic variants that are determined primarily by the action of allelic variants at a single gene locus are termed *monogenic,* whereas traits that are determined by the action of multiple genes are termed *multigenic.* In monogenic inheritance, which is often called Mendelian inheritance, one can further distinguish traits according to the frequency with which they occur, that is, between polymorphic and rare variants, as defined above. Monogenic inheritance is often detectable on the basis of an observable phenotype that deviates from a normal distribution, becoming, in some cases, trimodal (in the absence of dominance of one trait over the other), with three different phenotypic groups derived from the possible combinations of homozygous and heterozygous variants—the $pp$, $pq$, and $qq$ diploid genotypes, derived from the $p$ and $q$ haploid allelic variants—at the single gene locus.

Monogenic traits that segregate in an expected fashion in populations are also characterized by the Hardy–Weinberg law and equation. In the case of two possible allelic variants at a single gene locus in which the population frequency of one variant allele is $p$ and the other is $q$, then $(p + q) = 1$. The Hardy–Weinberg law states that the frequencies of the three possible genotypes $pp$, $pq$, and $qq$ are determined by the equation $p^2 + 2pq + q^2 = 1$. For example, if the frequency of the $p$ allele is 0.8 and that of the $q$ allele is 0.2, then the genotype frequencies are 0.64, 0.32, and 0.04, adding to a total of 1.0 (100%). Monogenic traits can be verified by family pedigree studies that demonstrate expected segregation of the phenotypes from parents to offspring according to Mendelian laws of inheritance.

Multigenically determined phenotypes, on the other hand, often display a normal unimodal distribution as a result of the contribution of multiple genetic factors, and often significant environmental factors. Possible genetic contributions to multigenic phenotypes have generally been identified by deriving heritability values in studies comparing the trait in monozygotic versus dizygotic twins. As genomic technologies continue to advance, studies of multigenic traits will increasingly utilize either candidate gene (i.e., genes selected on the basis of a predicted effect) or genome-wide association studies (see "New Drug Target Discovery" below) to attempt to identify specific genes that contribute to a given phenotype.

# SELECTED EXAMPLES OF PHARMACOGENETIC VARIANTS

Tables 10-1 and 10-2, while not exhaustive, serve to illustrate the extensive knowledge that is currently available regarding the influence of genetic variation on drug action as a consequence of alterations in drug pharmacokinetics and target interactions, respectively. Although not detailed here, it should also be mentioned that a number of statistically significant associations between drug effects and genetic variants have been reported, for which mechanistic models and causal mechanisms have yet to be established. The following examples demonstrate the depth and diversity of the field, as well as highlight some notable clinical correlates. Although early studies of pharmacogenetic variants suggested that genetic variation occurred only in certain genes, the vast extent of genetic variation across the human genome indicates that considerable DNA sequence variation of some form is likely to be detectable in essentially every human gene.

## Variants Affecting Drug Biotransformation and Pharmacokinetics

### Atypical plasma cholinesterase

Although not a polymorphic trait in the clinical sense (since the clinically significant cholinesterase variants occur in about one in 2000 people in Caucasian populations), atypical plasma cholinesterase has particular historical significance as one of the early examples of a clinically dramatic genetic alteration in drug action. The plasma cholinesterase is capable of hydrolyzing a number of drugs, including cocaine, but its inactivation of the muscle relaxant succinylcholine (see Chapter 15) is of greatest clinical importance. This drug is often used to facilitate surgery done under general anaesthesia by relaxing the skeletal muscles. Since succinylcholine paralyzes respiratory as well as other muscles, the patient requires artificial respiration until the drug effect wears off.

Succinylcholine is given intravenously, and it is therefore immediately and fully exposed to plasma cholinesterase. The fate of the drug thus depends directly on esterase activity. In the presence of atypical cholinesterase, the muscle relaxant action of an ordinary dose of succinylcholine lasts for about an hour instead of only a few minutes (Fig. 10-1). The biochemical basis of the defect is a very low affinity (i.e., high $K_m$) of the enzyme for succinylcholine, so the two combine inefficiently. The underlying nucleotide alterations in the cholinesterase gene that lead to the production of the atypical variant, and several other mutant forms, have recently been defined. However, in spite of these advances, the physiological role (if any) of the plasma cholinesterase remains unknown. Occasionally, there are

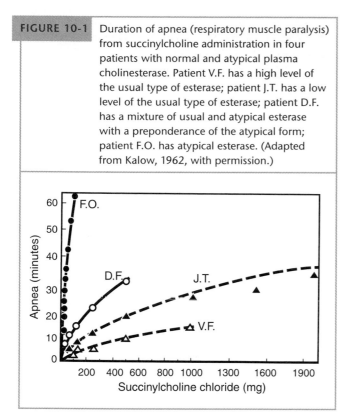

**FIGURE 10-1** Duration of apnea (respiratory muscle paralysis) from succinylcholine administration in four patients with normal and atypical plasma cholinesterase. Patient V.F. has a high level of the usual type of esterase; patient J.T. has a low level of the usual type of esterase; patient D.F. has a mixture of usual and atypical esterase with a preponderance of the atypical form; patient F.O. has atypical esterase. (Adapted from Kalow, 1962, with permission.)

families with cholinesterase activities about threefold higher than average. In these cases, ordinary doses of succinylcholine have little or no effect.

## Acetylation polymorphism

Genetic control of acetylation was first observed for isoniazid almost 50 years ago, and it has since been shown to affect the elimination of many aromatic amine and hydrazine drugs and environmental chemicals. Simplified tests for "acetylator phenotype" have been developed that employ measurements of urinary ratios of *N*-acetylated metabolite to parent drug for a variety of compounds, including sulfamethazine, dapsone, and caffeine. Marked inter-ethnic differences in phenotype frequencies can be observed: Caucasian populations comprise more than 50% slow acetylators, whereas in Asians and North American Aboriginals, the proportion of rapid acetylators approaches 90%.

The genetically variable enzyme responsible for producing these phenotypic differences is one of two arylamine *N*-acetyltransferases (NATs) found in human liver (see Chapter 4). This enzyme, known as **NAT2**, catalyzes the *N*-acetylation of isoniazid, many other drugs (phenelzine, hydralazine, sulfamethazine, sulfapyridine, sulfamethoxazole, procainamide, and dapsone), drug metabolites (nitrazepam and caffeine), and several amine carcinogens (benzidine, 2-aminofluorene, 4-aminobiphenyl, and β-naphthylamine). However, the *N*-acetylation of para-aminobenzoic acid (PABA), para-aminosalicylic acid (PAS), and some of the antibacterial sulfonamides is mediated by the structurally related yet independently expressed **NAT1** enzyme; thus the disposition of these compounds, while also subject to genetic variation, is unaffected by the classically defined isoniazid acetylator phenotype. Both NAT1 and NAT2 are also capable of *O*-acetylation of hydroxylamine metabolites of aromatic amines to produce highly reactive acetoxy esters that can bind covalently to intracellular macromolecules (DNA, proteins) and lead to cellular toxicity or mutations.

Several mutant alleles at the *NAT2* gene locus on human chromosome 8 have been cloned and characterized. Each allele possesses between one and three SNPs relative to the "wild-type" (high activity) allele. Defective acetylation in most cases is caused by single amino acid changes that reduce protein stability and lead to reductions in the quantity of NAT2 enzyme in the livers of slow acetylators.

A number of adverse drug reactions or chemical toxicities have been associated with the slow acetylator phenotype. These include peripheral neuropathy while taking isoniazid, drug-induced lupoid reactions during hydralazine and procainamide therapy, hemolytic reactions to sulfapyridine or dapsone, and bladder cancers in factory workers exposed to benzidine. On the other hand, it has been reported that rapid acetylators may be at higher risk for colorectal cancer, possibly due to increased bioactivation of diet-derived heterocyclic amine procarcinogens.

## Cytochrome P450 polymorphisms

Since the most abundant class of drug biotransformation reactions are oxidations catalyzed by the microsomal mixed-function monooxygenases having a cytochrome P450 as their terminal element (see Chapter 4), it is not unexpected that intensive study over the past three decades has been aimed at investigating the basis for observed variations in the functions of the isoforms in this gene superfamily. Indeed, a vast amount of allelic variation in cytochrome P450 genes has now been documented and, in many instances, causally linked with variation in drug pharmacokinetics, response, and side effects (see Chapter 4).

## CYP2D6

A polymorphic oxidation defect severely affecting the fate of several drugs was first discovered in the mid-1970s. The discovery arose from independent studies of two drugs that are metabolized by a specific isozyme of P450 now referred to as CYP2D6: (1) In Germany, it was found that about 5% of the population was incapable of metabolizing sparteine, an alkaloid with anti-arrhythmic and oxytocic properties. In "poor metabolizers," sparteine had a long half-life and accumulated in the body upon repeated administration. (2) In an English study of the metabolism of debrisoquine (an antihypertensive drug of the guanethidine class), a severe deficiency in the formation of the main metabolite, 4-hydroxydebrisoquine, was found in about 8% of the British population. This explained why the dose of the drug required by different patients during therapy could vary as much as thirtyfold. It was later shown that the failures to biotransform sparteine and debrisoquine have an identical genetic basis and that the disposition of numerous additional drugs from a variety of therapeutic classes is affected by the same defect.

Assignment of a given individual to the poor or extensive group of metabolizers of debrisoquine or sparteine can be achieved by giving a small test dose of the drug and measuring the ratio of drug and metabolite excreted in urine during the following 8 hours. More recently, the cough suppressant dextromethorphan has been increasingly used as a safe and widely available alternative substrate for phenotype discrimination studies.

Biochemical and molecular genetic studies performed in the past decade have provided a wealth of information concerning the mechanisms underlying the debrisoquine/sparteine oxidation defect in humans. The poor metabolizer phenotype is usually characterized at the protein level by the absence of **CYP2D6**, which is normally encoded from a gene in the *CYP2D* gene cluster located on human chromosome 22. At the genetic level, cloning and expression studies have so far revealed the existence of at least 90 allelic variants at the *CYP2D6* gene locus. A variety of gene mutations, including point mutations in the amino acid coding region, exon/intron splice-site disruptions, and even deletion of the entire *CYP2D6* gene have been associated with the poor metabolizer phenotype in human populations. In addition, the existence of certain novel gene duplication alleles results in the occurrence of "ultra-rapid" metabolizers in whom therapeutic failure on standard drug doses may be more likely to occur.

The potential clinical consequences of defective CYP2D6 function have been widely discussed and debated. For instance, debrisoquine itself is more likely to cause fainting in poor metabolizers because of excessive lowering of blood pressure; however, this drug is no longer widely used. Sparteine also fell into disuse as an oxytocic agent when it was found that about 7% of women receiving it had severe side effects. In retrospect, it is likely that these 7% were the ones with the oxidation defect. There are also clinical consequences with a variety of other drugs. Anti-arrhythmic agents, β-adrenergic receptor antagonists, neuroleptics, selective serotonin reuptake inhibitor antidepressants, and tricyclic antidepressants are among the therapeutic classes containing currently used drugs that have been claimed to show relevant variations in clinical outcome as a result of defective oxidation by CYP2D6. Codeine presents an interesting example of variable clinical effect caused by ineffective prodrug activation. The analgesic effects of administered codeine (see Chapter 19) are due to its partial conversion to morphine by CYP2D6. Thus, CYP2D6 poor metabolizers do not experience codeine analgesia and, therefore, are also unlikely to become dependent.

Interestingly, the fate of some drugs is biochemically affected by the CYP2D6 defect but without any clinically important consequence. The reasons for this may vary. For instance, since the β-adrenoceptor blocker propranolol undergoes biotransformation by several parallel pathways, including oxidation by CYP2D6, other reactions and effective renal elimination can compensate for the CYP2D6 defect. The experimental β blocker bufuralol, on the other hand, is metabolized almost exclusively by CYP2D6, but its metabolite has a pharmacological potency similar to that of bufuralol itself; hence, the clinical consequences of a defect in metabolite formation are minor.

The tricyclic antidepressant desipramine is another example of a drug whose pharmacokinetics is clearly affected by genetically variable CYP2D6 function (Fig. 10-2A), yet this variation has no consistent impact on clinical response (Fig. 10-2B). In this case, possible reasons include a generally poor concentration–response relationship with desipramine, heterogeneity in the diagnosis and severity of the disease, the possible contribution of hydroxylated desipramine metabolites to its pharmacological effect, and the confounding effects of including placebo responders in such studies.

## CYP2C19

Another polymorphic defect of drug oxidation by a cytochrome P450 isozyme was discovered in the early 1980s. This defect was first shown to impair the 4'-hydroxylation of the *S*-enantiomer of mephenytoin, an anticonvulsant drug that is no longer widely used. However, the metabolism of a number of other currently used drugs is also affected by this defect, including omeprazole, diazepam, the biguanide anti-malarials, and some barbiturates. About 3 to 5% of the individuals in Caucasian populations are phenotypically poor metabolizers of mephenytoin, while the frequency of this phenotype approaches 20% in Asian populations.

The cytochrome P450 isozyme now known to be altered in the *S*-mephenytoin hydroxylation defect is one of those within the CYP2C subfamily, specifically termed CYP2C19. Livers from individuals of the poor-metabolizer phenotype display reduced levels of CYP2C19 protein in the microsomal fraction. The molecular defects that produce this phenotype in the majority of cases have been determined for both Caucasian and Asian population groups. A total of 20 allelic variants at the *CYP2C19* gene locus have been detected. Of these, the *CYP2C19*2* variant accounts for about 80% of all defective alleles in both populations and possesses an SNP at the intron–exon splice junction of exon 5, which produces a premature stop codon. This results in production of a truncated cytochrome P450 protein lacking the heme-binding region that is necessary for its catalytic function. A second variant allele, *CYP2C19*3*, accounts for much of the remaining defective phenotype in Asians but is very rare in Caucasians. It also contains an SNP that creates a pre-mature stop codon and thus yields a truncated and nonfunctional enzyme.

Variable CYP2C19-dependent metabolism of the proton pump inhibitor omeprazole has a marked influence on the efficacy of this agent in the treatment of gastrointestinal ulcers. The degree of inhibition of gastric acid secretion (Fig. 10-3), and the resulting effectiveness of combined omeprazole and amoxicillin in treatment of gastric ulcers, is markedly improved in CYP2C19 poor metabolizers. This suggests that extensive metabolizers may require larger doses for effective therapy because of excessively rapid drug clearance.

## CYP2C9

CYP2C9 is important for the metabolism of certain clinically important drugs, including warfarin, phenytoin, and tolbutamide. Since the original cloning of the *CYP2C9* gene in the early 1990s, a total of 20 allelic variants at this locus have been described. Of these, the most frequently occurring, *CYP2C9*2* and *CYP2C9*3*, possess characteristic diagnostic SNPs that alter single amino acids in the enzyme and result in decreased catalytic function. Individuals who possess two defective CYP2C9 alleles experience more frequent bleeding complications during therapy with the anticoagulant warfarin, and they require drastically reduced doses to achieve appropriate therapeutic responses. The patient in the case study outlined at the beginning of this chapter possessed two defective alleles of CYP2C9. This led to an impairment of warfarin elimination and the accumulation of drug above safe therapeutic levels following repeated dosing, resulting in excessive anticoagulation and bleeding complications. Such individuals also have dramatically impaired phenytoin clearance and, as a result, are more prone to central nervous system toxicity.

## CYP2A6

This P450 isoform is important for the metabolism of nicotine and therefore for influencing the duration of the central stimulant effects of this alkaloid during cigarette smoking. Again, over the past decade, extensive allelic variation has been detected at the *CYP2A6* gene locus. A number of studies have suggested that smokers with genetically defective CYP2A6 function may smoke fewer cigarettes and thereby be at lower risk for smoking-related diseases.

## Thiopurine *S*-methyltransferase

Thiopurine *S*-methyltransferase (TPMT) is a methyl-conjugating enzyme that is involved in one of the pathways of biotransformation of 6-mercaptopurine and azathioprine. These agents are used in the treatment of childhood acute lymphoblastic leukemia and rheumatoid arthritis, and for immunosuppression (see Chapter 40). The action of TPMT on these prodrugs serves to inactivate them, while their intended cytotoxic action requires activation to thiogua-

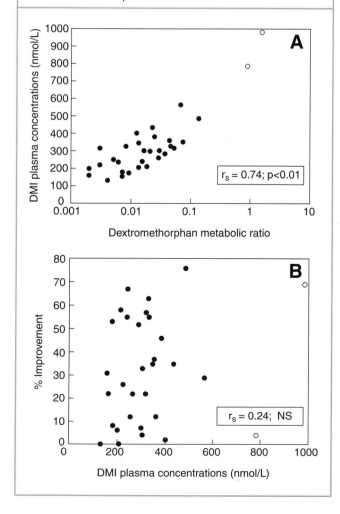

**FIGURE 10-2** (A) Relationship between CYP2D6 metabolizer phenotype (determined by using the urinary dextromethorphan metabolic ratio, x-axis) and desipramine (DMI) plasma concentration (y-axis). The two measures are highly correlated, suggesting that DMI plasma pharmacokinetics is governed largely by CYP2D6 function. Open circles indicate CYP2D6 poor metabolizer individuals. (B) Relationship between DMI plasma concentrations (x-axis) and percentage clinical improvement (y-axis). Since no correlation between plasma concentration and improvement is observed, predicting outcome from CYP2D6 metabolizer status would not be useful. Adapted from Spina E, Gitto C, Avenoso A, Campo GM, Caputi AP, Perucca E. Relationship between plasma desipramine levels, CYP2D6 phenotype, and clinical response to desipramine: a prospective study. *Eur J Clin Pharmacol.* 1997;51:395-398, with permission.

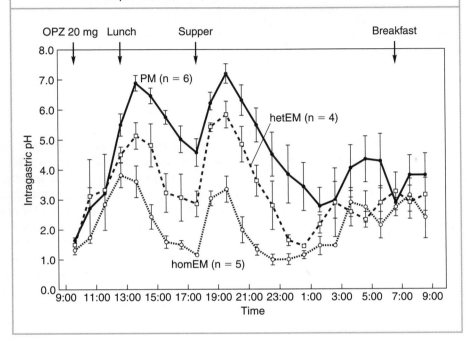

**FIGURE 10-3** Effect of CYP2C19 metabolizer phenotype on the therapeutic efficacy of omeprazole for the inhibition of gastric acid secretion. The graph represents a comparison of 24-hour measurements of intragastric pH determined following the single-dose administration of omeprazole in patients genotyped as homozygous extensive metabolizers (homEM), heterozygous (hetEM), and homozygous poor metabolizers (PM) at the *CYP2C19* gene locus. Patients with increasing numbers of PM alleles show progressive improvements in clinical efficacy (increases in intragastric pH). Adapted from Furuta T, Ohashi K, Kosuge K, Zhao XJ, Takashima M, Kimura M, Nishimoto M, Hanai H, Kaneko E, Ishizaki T. CYP2C19 genotype status and effect of omeprazole on intragastric pH in humans. *Clin Pharmacol Ther.* 1999;65:552-561, with permission.

nine nucleotides by an alternate pathway. Genetic variation in the gene encoding TPMT can lead to production of a defective product. About 1 in 300 individuals in Caucasian populations have two copies of defective alleles, resulting in marked impairment in enzyme function. Heterozygous individuals, making up about 10% of the population, show intermediate levels of enzyme function. Three allelic variants at the *TPMT* gene locus account for about 95% of all intermediate or low activity individuals.

In individuals with defective TPMT, an imbalance between inactivation and bioactivation pathways leads to excessive formation of the cytotoxic species and to blood toxicities that can be life-threatening. Moreover, leukemia patients who are deficient in TPMT function are at higher risk for the occurrence of a second malignancy, presumably due to somatic mutations caused by the excessive cytotoxicity of the bioactivated drugs. As a result of these findings, a number of pediatric hospitals have instituted predictive testing for TPMT status prior to the initiation of chemotherapy for childhood leukemia in order to set appropriate drug dosing levels, and they have observed improved long-term patient outcomes.

### Drug transporter variants

Another mechanism that plays a role in drug absorption, distribution, and excretion involves the participation of membrane-bound drug transporter proteins (see Chapter 2). For instance, P-glycoprotein, a member of the ATP-binding cassette family of membrane transporters, mediates the energy-dependent cellular efflux of endogenous compounds as well as of several drugs, including the cardiac glycoside digoxin and the HIV protease inhibitor nelfinavir. Recent evidence suggests that SNPs in the *ABCB1* gene, which encodes P-glycoprotein, influence the bioavailability of digoxin and nelfinavir, as reflected by differences in plasma concentrations of these agents among individuals of different genotypes. Further work will be required to determine the clinical impact of these and other findings regarding drug transporters on drug efficacy and/or toxicity.

### Variants Affecting Drug Pharmacodynamics and/or Drug Targets

With the few notable exceptions of variants of drug targets discussed below, much of the early work in pharmacogenetics investigated monogenic defects in drug biotransformation capacity, as described above. The reason for this is twofold: (1) parameters of variable drug pharmacokinetics, such as plasma drug levels or urinary metabolite ratios, are analytically simple to measure in patients presenting with variable drug response or toxicity, and (2) genetic variants of enzymes that are primarily responsible for xenobiotic biotransformation may be less likely to produce functional disturbance in the absence of exogenous chemical challenge, so more severely defective variants can be maintained in populations during the course of human evolution. On the other hand, variants of targets for drug action—which are often mediators of important physiological processes—are likely to exhibit more subtle phenotype changes since any severe defects that arose by mutation would be expected to suffer strong evolutionary pressure and be weeded out by negative selection. Nonetheless, in recent years, many investigations have uncovered significant genetic variations in drug targets (see Table 10-2) that show clinical relevance.

### Glucose-6-phosphate dehydrogenase deficiency

The most intensively investigated early examples were hemolytic drug reactions related to a deficiency of glucose-6-phosphate dehydrogenase (G-6-PD) and a resulting inability to maintain the necessary intracellular concentration of reduced glutathione. Oxidant drugs form $H_2O_2$ in the red blood cell, which oxidizes glutathione. The oxidized disulfide form of glutathione may be attached to hemoglobin in an unstable mixed disulfide complex that results in hemoglobin oxidation and denaturation (Heinz bodies). These changes result in damage to the erythrocyte membrane and subsequent hemolysis.

Approximately 400 million people carry the trait for G-6-PD deficiency, and about 300 allelic variants are known. All of these variants are inherited as sex-linked traits, and many are associated with specific biological sequelae. Several variants are classified as "normal," one variant has increased enzymatic activity, and some variants cause such severe deficiencies of activity that they lead to hemolytic disease even in the absence of drugs. The role of drugs has been most closely investigated with respect to two G-6-PD variants. The A⁻ variant, present in Black Americans, is an unstable enzyme. Young erythrocytes have about the normal level of enzyme activity, but it diminishes more rapidly than normal during the lifespan of the red cell. Drug-induced hemolytic reactions are therefore self-limited because they cease once the older erythrocytes have been eliminated. On the other hand, the Mediterranean variant has low G-6-PD activity even in young erythrocytes. As a consequence, hemolytic crises, when they occur, are much more severe since they do not tend to be self-limiting. A number of agents (e.g., quinine, acetylsalicylic acid) in high doses cause hemolysis in the presence of the Mediterranean G-6-PD deficiency but do not do so in the A⁻ variant.

The different frequencies of G-6-PD deficiency in different populations are determined by elements of Darwinian selection. G-6-PD deficiency favours survival by increasing resistance to *Plasmodium falciparum* malaria (see Chapter 54), a factor beneficial only in countries where malaria is endemic, so the gene tends to accumulate in such countries.

### Malignant hyperthermia

Malignant hyperthermia is a serious but rare complication of general anaesthesia that occurs in genetically predisposed patients. Failure of muscles to relax after succinylcholine, and an unexplained tachycardia, often herald the onset. There is a rise in body temperature, which can rapidly reach extreme levels. In most cases, there is rigidity of skeletal muscles. During the episode, muscle enzymes and proteins (including myoglobin) are released into the plasma, there is profound hypoxia and metabolic and respiratory acidosis, and the plasma potassium level rises. Early death is often due to cardiac failure, while delayed death may be due to renal failure as a consequence of myoglobinemia.

The cause of the condition is an unusual effect of halothane or other general anaesthetics on skeletal muscle. This was originally proven by pharmacological tests in which muscle biopsy samples obtained from survivors showed high in vitro susceptibility to caffeine-induced contracture, an effect that was potentiated and partially mimicked by halothane. Since caffeine affects intracellular calcium metabolism by enhancing calcium-induced calcium release from the sarcoplasmic reticulum of muscle cells, halothane was thought to initiate hyperthermic attacks by also causing excessive calcium release. The increased calcium concentrations in the sarcoplasm during a hyperthermic attack would be expected to have a number of biochemical effects, such as increasing ATPase activity by actomyosin, the reticulum, and the mitochondria. Muscular contracture and a hypermetabolic state with lactic acidosis are the consequences, and the resulting huge increase in heat production probably explains the sharp rise in body temperature. Early recognition of the attack, speedy termination of surgery and anaesthesia, cooling of the patient, and correction of the acidosis are among the indicated measures. Intravenous infusion of the muscle relaxant dantrolene has saved lives by terminating the attack.

Recent molecular studies have now indeed established that a majority of malignant hyperthermia cases are related to molecular defects in the RyR1 ryanodine receptor, which is the major sarcoplasmic reticulum calcium-release channel in skeletal muscle that is required for excitation–contraction coupling.

### β-Adrenergic receptor variants

Much recent attention in pharmacogenetics has shifted to the study of genetic variants of the components of cellular signal transduction pathways, including the proteins of cell surface receptors for neurotransmitters and hormones. Polymorphisms of the β-adrenergic receptors provide several examples of variations with demonstrated physiological and pharmacological effects. For instance, the β2-adrenergic receptor, a member of the 7-transmembrane domain G protein–coupled receptor superfamily (see Chapters 8, 9, and 11), is a catecholamine-responsive cell surface signal transducer that also acts as a target for a variety of medications used in the treatment of cardiovascular and airway disorders. SNPs in the *ADRB2* gene produce single amino acid changes at positions 16 and 27 within the cytoplasmic N-terminal tail of the β2-adrenergic receptor. These alterations, which occur very commonly in human populations (allele frequencies of about 0.4 and 0.6, respectively), produce marked changes in receptor function and response to exogenously applied agonists (Fig. 10-4). Individuals homozygous for the amino acid glutamic acid at position 27 show an increased venodilatory response to isoproterenol when compared with individuals who are homozygous for glutamine at that position. On the other hand, amino acid differences at position 16 affect the process of agonist-induced receptor desensitization: individuals homozygous for arginine at position 16 show dramatic desensitization of the venodilatory response to isoproterenol over time, whereas those possessing at least one copy of the receptor with glycine at that position are completely resistant to desensitization.

## Human growth hormone receptor variants

A striking example of drug target variation leading to alterations in therapeutic efficacy has recently been provided from studies of the efficacy of exogenous human growth hormone in the treatment of short stature. In two separate studies, patients possessing a shortened variant form of the human growth hormone receptor showed twofold greater growth acceleration following growth hormone administration than did patients with the full-length form of the receptor.

## Tumour genetics and targeted cancer chemotherapy

The concept of targeting drug use to specific patient subgroups has started to be applied in the field of cancer chemotherapy. In this field, the genetic constitution of the growing tumour rather than of the patient can be used to predict the effectiveness of particular agents (see Chapter 57). In this regard, trastuzumab (Herceptin) has been shown to be effective for the 25 to 30% of metastatic breast cancers that over-express the HER-2/neu receptor, a member of the ErbB family of signal transduction factors that plays a role in the development of certain solid tumours. Thus, pre-screening of tumours for HER-2/neu over-expression is used to determine which patients are likely to benefit from trastuzumab treatment. Similarly, gefitinib is an inhibitor of the epidermal growth factor

**FIGURE 10-4** Effect of polymorphisms in the β2-adrenergic receptor on in vivo responses to agonist stimulation. (A) Individuals homozygous for the amino acid glutamic acid (Glu) at position 27 show an increased venodilatory response to isoproterenol when compared with individuals who are homozygous for glutamine (Gln) at that position. (B) Individuals homozygous for arginine (Arg) at position 16 show increased acute airway responsiveness to agonist stimulation. (C) Individuals homozygous for Arg at position 16 show marked desensitization of the venodilatory response to isoproterenol over time, whereas those possessing at least one copy of the receptor with glycine (Gly) at that position are completely resistant to desensitization. (Adapted from Evans and McLeod, 2003, with permission.)

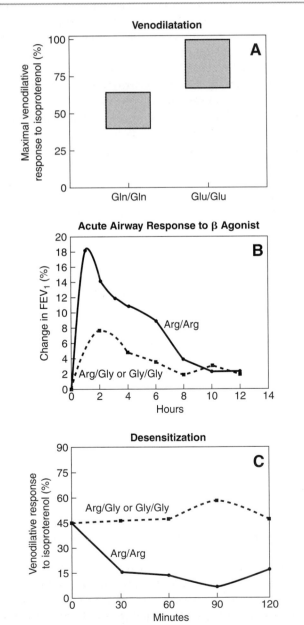

receptor tyrosine kinase domain (EGFR-TK), and its efficacy has recently been shown to correlate with activating mutations in the EGFR-TK in non-small-cell lung cancer.

## PHARMACOGENETICS AND MULTIPLE GENE EFFECTS

All of the examples above deal with the examination of monogenic pharmacogenetic defects. Such studies are methodologically straightforward since they require only the identification, isolation, and functional characterization and correlation of phenotypes with genotypic variants of a single gene locus. However, as noted earlier, many so-called complex disorders, as well as the responses to therapies used in their treatment, may have contributions from multiple independent genes, including those involved in the disease process itself, those functioning as both intended and unintended drug targets, and those responsible for clearing the active drug from the body. Thus, a challenge for pharmacogenetics in the future will be to devise effective experimental designs and data analysis strategies for the simultaneous investigation of multiple contributory genetic factors in drug response, while at the same time recognizing the degree to which environmental factors may be capable of obscuring genetic associations.

Nonetheless, a number of studies have begun to explore the analysis of multiple gene contributions to drug response phenotypes. For instance, preliminary association studies between multiple candidate genes and the response to the atypical antipsychotic agent clozapine (see Chapter 24) yielded a 77% success for prediction of clozapine response by combining six polymorphisms in neurotransmitter receptor genes. In another study, investigators screened 74 polymorphic SNPs in 25 candidate genes related to blood pressure regulation and observed significant associations between multiple gene variants and the blood pressure lowering effects of the angiotensin II type I receptor blocker irbesartan and the $\beta_1$-adrenergic receptor antagonist atenolol (see Chapter 34). Studies of this type are clearly still at an early stage and require much further confirmation of positive associations, which will be aided by further refinement of genetic and data analysis methods.

## PHARMACOGENETICS AND PHARMACOGENOMICS IN DRUG DEVELOPMENT

There is considerable current interest and debate within the pharmaceutical and biotechnology sectors regarding the utility of pharmacogenetics and pharmacogenomics in the drug development process. Clearly, there is now widespread appreciation that genetically based, and therefore potentially predictable, population variation in drug effects is the norm rather than the exception. With this understanding comes the realization that conventional drug development paradigms, embracing a "one-drug-fits-all" philosophy aimed at the development and marketing of "blockbuster" drugs, may no longer be appropriate under many circumstances. On the one hand, the segmentation of market share that will occur as a consequence of individualizing therapy for patient subgroups may be a disincentive to adoption of such approaches in the multinational pharmaceutical industry. An alternative consequence may be industry's use of information about potential pharmacogenetic variation in a drug target or a promising new compound to make early-stage strategic decisions on termination of drug or drug target development.

### New Drug Target Discovery

Genomic approaches may be of particular value in the identification of disease-related genes whose protein products may be suitable molecular targets for the development of novel drug therapies. In such approaches, panels of either genome-wide or candidate gene mapping markers, composed of sets of assays to measure the genotypes of location-specific DNA markers, are applied to matched groups of diseased patients and healthy subjects. Statistically significant differences in genotype frequencies between the two groups at any locations in the genome are thus predictive for the locations of genes that associate with the disease phenotype. Genes in the vicinity of these markers may then each be isolated, characterized, and compared in detail between diseased patients and healthy controls to search for possible causative mutations that contribute to disease pathology and to better understand the pathophysiology of the disorder itself. In the best-case scenario, the disease-causing gene itself can be isolated, and its expressed protein product may be used in high-throughput small-molecule screening procedures to identify chemicals that can alter the protein's function to therapeutic benefit.

### Patient Stratification in Clinical Trials

A hypothetical future application of pharmacogenetics in improving the drug development process arises later during the clinical trials phase. In this phase, the efficacies of a new chemical entity and currently existing therapies or placebo controls are compared in patient populations in the hope that the new agent shows statistically significant benefit when compared with the reference group. Often a great deal of within-group variation in clinical effect is observed, resulting in substantial overlap in treatment groups and thus the need for very large patient sample sizes in order to achieve statistical significance. This makes studies very costly and time-consuming. Assuming that a significant portion of the within-group variation may be due to known genetic factors, pharmacogenetics could be of practical benefit in clinical trials by allowing for the prior genetic stratification and pre-selection of treatment groups according to these factors. As a result, within-group variation could be reduced, and patient sample sizes could be significantly reduced, reducing also the time and cost of the clinical trials.

However, a practical consequence of this approach would be that a drug whose approval was guided by clinical trials using genetically stratified patient selection would, in all likelihood, require its post-marketing prescribing to be linked to the same genetic stratification method. Such a procedure is not yet a practical reality.

## THE FUTURE OF PHARMACOGENETICS: PERSONALIZED MEDICINE

As mentioned above, the ultimate goal of pharmacogenetics is to aid in the more appropriate use of medications among the individuals in populations. The prescribing of drugs and doses based upon mean response in a population tends to ignore the existence of variation within populations and our expanding appreciation of the genetic factors that can contribute to this variation. Current evidence suggests that for many important classes of therapeutic drugs, a significant proportion (often ranging from 30 to 60%) of patients do not show any clinically significant therapeutic effect. This is perhaps not surprising when one considers that, historically, new medications have been developed and marketed on the basis of clinical trials that compare population means in clinical response parameters between two treatment groups. Statistical significance between mean responses may result in drug approval, despite the fact that within a given treatment group, individual patient responses may range from profound effect to a complete lack of response. Thus there is an ongoing need for better targeting of therapies to individuals who are most likely to respond appropriately to them.

Recent studies have also suggested that the morbidity, mortality, and economic costs associated with the occurrence of adverse drug reactions represent a very significant burden on the healthcare system. With continuing improvements in our understanding of both the genetic and environmental factors that can contribute to such variation in response and toxicity (see also Chapter 58), it is hoped that both the development and use of drugs tailored for genetically defined subgroups of the population may be practically feasible.

### When Does Pharmacogenetic Variation Matter?

However, a reality check is appropriate at this time in order to counterbalance a significant amount of recent hype in both the scientific literature and the popular press concerning the current and future potential of pharmacogenetics to improve the use of medications. A recent editorial review of pharmacogenetics is welcome in this regard:

> The pharmacogenetic learning curve is not particularly steep—experience of the principles has been gathering slowly over the past half-century—but it will be long and grinding for all sides. The stakes are high and the future is uncertain. There is no doubt that pharmacogenetics will improve therapeutics, but it will arrive gradually, and will not provide a panacea.
>
> *Nature.* 2003;425:759.

Quite apart from many of the technological, logistical, ethical, and political challenges associated with incorporating pharmacogenetic testing into routine clinical practice (discussed further below), it is important to recognize from a purely clinical perspective those instances where knowledge of pharmacogenetic variation may be of practical benefit at the population level. Possible instances for consideration may include the following:

1.  The genetically variable protein plays a quantitatively major role in determining the disposition or effect of the drug (for monogenically determined response phenotypes).
2.  A major proportion of a drug's disposition or effect can be accounted for by known drug targets or drug-clearing enzymes (for multigenically determined response phenotypes).
3.  The contribution of environmental factors to drug response is either minor or quantifiable.
4.  The drug in question is widely used clinically.
5.  The drug has a narrow therapeutic index—relatively small alterations in plasma levels significantly alter efficacy or toxicity.
6.  The clinical indication (disease to be treated) for the therapeutic agent is significant.
7.  Therapeutic drug monitoring of plasma levels is not feasible or useful.
8.  Therapeutic alternatives are not available.

### Practical Challenges for Pharmacogenetics and Pharmacogenomics

As pointed out earlier, it is important to note that many of the most compelling historical examples of pharmacogenetic variation represent monogenic variants of drug biotransformation, in which pharmacokinetic effects of allelic variation at a single gene locus may be readily observed for particular drugs. A practical challenge from the research perspective will be to accurately identify and quantify the relative contributions of multiple genetic factors, acting on a background of environmental influences, that produce response phenotypes for complex disorders. This will be technologically challenging since it will require the ability not only to generate large quantities of genetic data at multiple gene loci, but also to handle the data analysis and statistical methods required to gain usable knowledge from the data generated. Subsequently, technological advances would then be required to devise simple, accurate, rapid, and highly predictive genetic testing procedures that would provide clinicians with timely information for making appropriate prescribing decisions for individual patients.

Further work will also be required from a cost–benefit perspective in order to determine under what circumstances the determination of a responder phenotype will be practically feasible from the point of view of the economics of the healthcare system. Possible ethical concerns regarding the use of genetic testing and the privacy of genetic information will need to be addressed on an ongoing basis, although many of the ethical concerns of genetic diagnostics may not apply to the analysis of pharmacogenetic variants, which are usually silent until drug challenge occurs and thus are used only to guide therapeutic options. Finally, ongoing and improved education of clinicians, patients, and regulatory bodies will be necessary before pharmacogenetic testing can realistically be expected to arrive in the physician's office for use in routinely optimizing patient care.

## SUGGESTED READINGS

Daly AK. Pharmacogenetics of the major polymorphic metabolizing enzymes. *Fundam Clin Pharmacol.* 2003;17:27-41.

Evans WE, McLeod HL. Pharmacogenomics—drug disposition, drug targets, and side effects. *N Engl J Med.* 2003;348:538-549.

Evans WE, Relling, MV. Pharmacogenomics: translating functional genomics into rational therapeutics. *Science.* 1999;286: 487-491.

Goldstein DR, Tate SK, Sisodiya SM. Pharmacogenetics goes genomic. *Nat Rev Genet.* 2003;4:937-947.

Ingelman-Sundberg M. Pharmacogenetics: an opportunity for a safer and more efficient pharmacotherapy. *J Internal Med.* 2001;250:186-200.

Kalow W. *Pharmacogenetics: Heredity and the Response to Drugs.* Philadelphia, Pa: WB Saunders; 1962.

Kalow W, Grant DM. Pharmacogenetics. In: Scriver CR, Beaudet AL, Sly WS, Valle D, eds. *The Metabolic and Molecular Bases of Inherited Disease.* New York, NY: McGraw-Hill; 2001:293-326.

Kalow W, Meyer UA, Tyndale RF, eds. *Pharmacogenomics.* 2nd ed. Boca Raton, Fla: Taylor & Francis; 2005.

Lindpaintner K. The impact of pharmacogenetics and pharmacogenomics on drug discovery. *Nat Rev Drug Discov.* 2002;1: 463-469.

McLeod HM, Evans WE. Pharmacogenomics: unlocking the human genome for better drug therapy. *Annu Rev Pharmacol Toxicol.* 2001;41:101-121.

Roses AD. Genome-based pharmacogenetics and the pharmaceutical industry. *Nat Rev Drug Discov.* 2002;1:541-549.

Service RF. Going from genome to pill. *Science.* 2005;308: 1858-1860.

Weinshilboum R. Inheritance and drug response. *N Engl J Med.* 2003;348:529-537.

# Part II

# Autonomic Nervous System and Neuromuscular Junction

# 11

# Functional and Neurochemical Organization of the Autonomic Nervous System

## AJ LANÇA

The autonomic nervous system regulates the physiological activities that are mainly involuntary and not under conscious control. It is responsible for the integration and processing of primarily visceral afferent information that reaches the brain (inputs) and for the outputs (efferents) that play a major role in the maintenance of homeostasis in the body (i.e., it controls the steady states of the internal environment by coordinating physiological processes). It regulates the rate and force of contraction of the heart, the calibre of blood vessels, and the muscle tone in the gastrointestinal tract, genitourinary tract, and bronchioles. It adjusts accommodation of the eye for near and distant vision, and it controls pupil size. It can also modify the secretions of both exocrine and endocrine glands.

Transmission of nerve impulses across synapses and neuroeffector junctions occurs by release of small amounts of chemical messengers that diffuse across to the target cell and bind to selective receptor molecules on its surface. Receptor activation on the target cell can mediate either an excitatory or an inhibitory response.

Autonomic pharmacology is the study of those drugs that act either on the autonomic neurons or on target organ cells that are innervated by the autonomic nervous system. Some drugs act directly on receptors, located on either pre- or postsynaptic neurons or on the effector targets, whereas other drugs act indirectly by altering synthesis, storage, release, and inactivation of neurotransmitters. Practical examples are pharmacotherapy of hypertension, bronchial asthma, and angina pectoris. The actions of an autonomic agent can often be predicted if the responses to nerve stimulation are known. In order to understand the selective actions of drugs on the autonomic nervous system, it is essential to have an understanding of its anatomy and physiology.

## ANATOMY OF THE AUTONOMIC NERVOUS SYSTEM

The afferent fibres of the autonomic nervous system (ANS) are mostly non-myelinated and reach the central nervous system (CNS) as an important component of peripheral nerves. The vagus nerve carries information from the abdominal and thoracic organs, and the glossopharyngeal nerve carries information from the head and neck. This information reaches the nucleus of the solitary tract in the brainstem and is subsequently distributed to different central regions, including the hypothalamus, the main locus of autonomic integration. Other centres, including the amygdala and some regions of the cerebral cortex (see Chapter 16), are also part of the circuitry responsible for the interface of the ANS with the limbic system.

The various control centres, however, are not purely autonomic, and there are no important physiological differences between visceral and somatic afferent (sensory) fibres. By convention, the term "autonomic nervous system" is used only in reference to the efferent (motor) neurons supplying the peripheral effector organs. The efferent autonomic nervous system has its origin in nerve cell bodies within the CNS, which give rise to pre-ganglionic fibres (usually myelinated) that are outside the CNS. These fibres synapse in peripheral ganglia with the cell bodies (ganglionic neurons) that give rise to the non-myelinated post-ganglionic fibres that innervate the effector organs.

Structurally and functionally, the ANS is further divided into sympathetic and parasympathetic systems. The main pathways of autonomic innervation are shown schematically in Figure 11-1.

In the **sympathetic division**, the cells of origin lie in the lateral horns of the thoracic and lumbar portions of the spinal cord, from T-1 to L-3. There are two major groups of sympathetic ganglia—namely, the paravertebral ganglia that lie in a chain close to and on each side of the vertebral column (sympathetic trunk), and the prevertebral ganglia that lie in the abdomen at some distance from the vertebrae (e.g., the celiac, or "solar plexus," and mesenteric ganglia). The adrenal medulla resembles a sympathetic ganglion in that it is innervated by typical pre-ganglionic fibres and is also functionally, anatomically, and embryologically related to the sympathetic ganglia. The sympathetic innervation of the head and neck

**FIGURE 11-1** Schematic representation of the principal pathways by which organs of the body receive parasympathetic and sympathetic innervation. CelG = celiac ganglion; CilG = ciliary ganglion; ICeG = inferior cervical ganglion; IMG = inferior mesenteric ganglion; MCeG = middle cervical ganglion; OG = otic ganglion; SCeG = superior cervical ganglion; SMaG = submaxillary ganglion; SMeG = superior mesenteric ganglion; SPG = sphenopalatine ganglion.

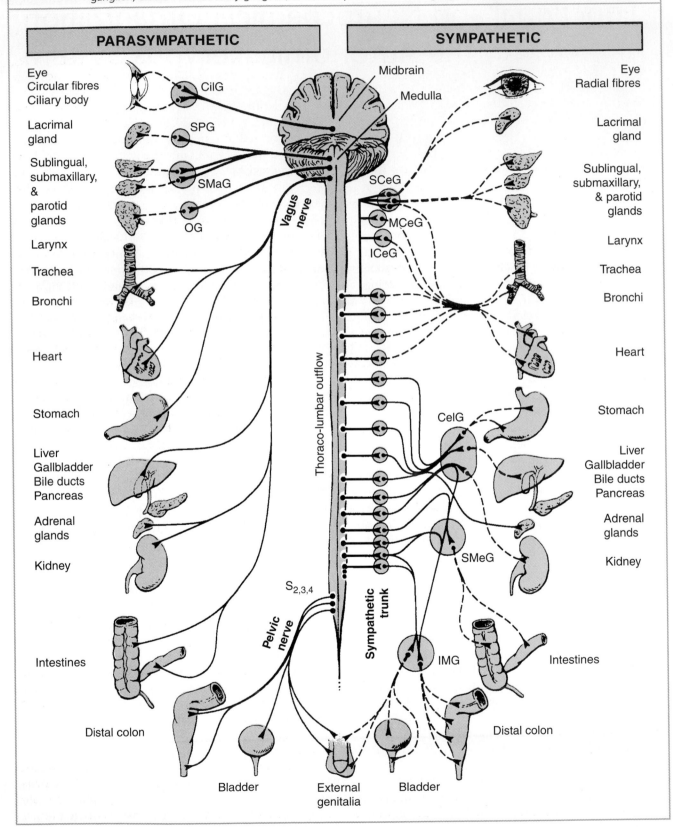

arises from the superior, medial, and inferior cervical ganglia, which receive pre-ganglionic input from the upper thoracic levels of the spinal cord.

The **parasympathetic division** comprises the cranial and sacral outflow of the ANS. The cells of origin are located in the lower brainstem (midbrain and medulla oblongata) and in the sacral portion of the spinal cord from S-2 to S-4. In contrast to the sympathetic ganglia, the parasympathetic ganglia are located very close to, on, or within the innervated organs (e.g., the heart and gastrointestinal tract). Therefore, the pre-ganglionic branch of the parasympathetic system is much longer than its sympathetic counterpart.

There are important exceptions to most generalizations about autonomic innervation. Nevertheless, in general, sympathetic pre-ganglionic fibres tend to synapse with large numbers of ganglionic neurons, but parasympathetic, with few. Sympathetic post-ganglionic fibres tend to have diffuse distributions, while parasympathetic distribution is more limited and discrete.

There is no true synapse between post-ganglionic autonomic nerves and their effector organs. The nerve terminals have a characteristic bead-like appearance, the beads or "varicosities" being the sites at which the neurotransmitter is released. The released neurotransmitter diffuses 20 to 100 nm to reach the effector cell, and effector cells may be simultaneously under the influence of neurotransmitters originating from more than one type of nerve terminal.

## PHYSIOLOGY OF THE AUTONOMIC NERVOUS SYSTEM

Most organs are innervated and controlled by both sympathetic and parasympathetic nerves. There are, however, organs that are innervated and controlled by only one division of the ANS.

In organs with both sympathetic and parasympathetic nervous control (e.g., heart, bronchi, gastrointestinal tract, bladder, and eye), the effects of the two divisions are usually opposite. Both systems are normally active at all times. The basal rate of their activity is referred to as sympathetic tone or parasympathetic tone. Thus, the level of function usually depends upon the balance between the tonic activities of two opposing innervations. In certain organs, such as the heart and intestines, there is also an intrinsic control that persists even when the dual external control by the ANS is absent. The parasympathetic and sympathetic nerves can override and adjust the activity of the organ to a level above or below that established by the intrinsic mechanisms.

Many organs have dual innervation of individual cells with opposing effects. For example, in the sinoatrial node of the heart, sympathetic stimulation increases heart rate whereas parasympathetic stimulation of the same cells lowers the rate. However, in some instances, the opposing effects of the sympathetic and parasympathetic divisions arise from the fact that they innervate different and functionally opposing cells. In the iris of the eye, for example, the parasympathetic fibres control mainly the circular muscles, whereas the sympathetic fibres control mainly the radial muscles. As a result, increased parasympathetic tone causes constriction of the pupil, and increased sympathetic tone causes dilatation.

In a few organs with dual autonomic control, such as the salivary glands, the effects of the sympathetic and parasympathetic divisions are believed to be complementary. For example, parasympathetic stimulation increases the secretion of the water, electrolyte, and enzyme components of saliva, whereas sympathetic stimulation increases secretion of the mucinous components.

Each division of the ANS can exert either an inhibitory or an excitatory effect upon a given organ. The effect upon a particular organ is determined by the characteristic responses of the effector cells in that organ. In many cases, all the cells respond in the same manner; however, in the intestine, the smooth muscle cells of the outer muscular layers relax in response to sympathetic impulses, whereas those of the sphincters contract. These differential effects are determined by the presence of different subtypes of adrenergic receptors in the various regions.

Arteriolar smooth muscle provides examples of three possible responses related to the location of the vessel: sympathetic impulses cause constriction of the arterioles in the skin and viscera, but dilatation of some vessels, particularly in skeletal muscle, and essentially no effect on cerebral arterioles. Again, these differences are due to the presence of different receptor subtypes in the different structures.

## CHEMICAL NEUROTRANSMITTERS IN THE AUTONOMIC NERVOUS SYSTEM

Fibres in the ANS are either cholinergic or adrenergic, depending on which transmitter is synthesized, stored, and released by the particular fibre (Fig. 11-2).

**Cholinergic fibres:** (1) All pre-ganglionic fibres to all ganglia in the ANS and to the adrenal medulla store and release acetylcholine (ACh) as a chemical transmitter. (2) All post-ganglionic parasympathetic fibres to effector organs are cholinergic. (3) Post-ganglionic sympathetic fibres to sweat glands and a few fibres to blood vessels in skeletal muscle are also cholinergic.

**Adrenergic fibres:** All other post-ganglionic sympathetic fibres store and release noradrenaline. Noradrenaline and its immediate precursor, dopamine, are also found in certain brain areas, where they act as neurotrans-

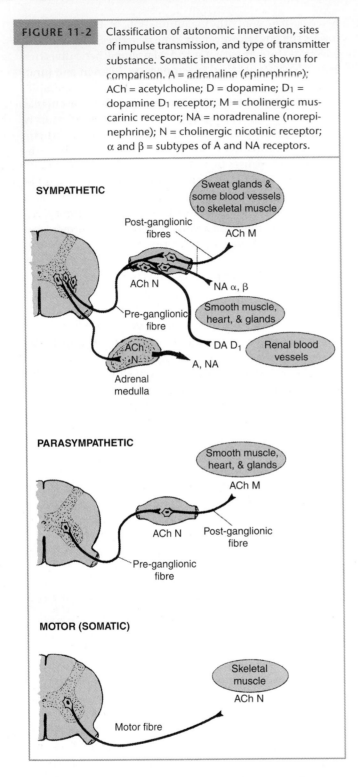

**FIGURE 11-2**  Classification of autonomic innervation, sites of impulse transmission, and type of transmitter substance. Somatic innervation is shown for comparison. A = adrenaline (epinephrine); ACh = acetylcholine; D = dopamine; $D_1$ = dopamine $D_1$ receptor; M = cholinergic muscarinic receptor; NA = noradrenaline (norepinephrine); N = cholinergic nicotinic receptor; α and β = subtypes of A and NA receptors.

## Other Autonomic Neurotransmitters

Although the organization of the ANS into cholinergic and adrenergic divisions is still functionally and pharmacologically valid, it is now well established that most neurons in both the central and peripheral nervous system contain more than one chemical neurotransmitter. Other chemical messengers, including peptides, purines, and eicosanoids, are present in ANS neurons and have been shown to play functionally significant roles. The co-localization of vasoactive intestinal polypeptide (VIP) in cholinergic neurons and of neuropeptide Y in adrenergic neurons is well established, and the future development of drugs capable of regulating these chemical transmitters may present more selective pharmacotherapies.

## Criteria for Designation as Chemical Neurotransmitters

A substance that is present in the brain or the spinal cord is not necessarily located in neurons. Non-neural elements (the neuroglia) outnumber neurons about tenfold and may well contain pharmacologically active substances. The fact that an active substance is released (usually under non-physiological conditions) does not provide true evidence for its postulated transmitter status. The latter becomes more likely if it can be shown that the amount released by stimulation at a physiological intensity is adequate to stimulate or inhibit neighbouring neurons or effector cells.

A set of general criteria must be satisfied before a particular chemical compound can be classified as a neurotransmitter (see also Chapter 16). These criteria apply throughout the nervous system:

1. Transmitter substances must be present and synthesized in neurons and must be released primarily by the presynaptic terminals as a result of stimulation.
2. Exogenous application of the presumed transmitter substance must produce changes that are characteristic of those that occur when the neuron is excited or inhibited by physiological stimuli.
3. The pharmacological actions of the putative transmitter can be either potentiated or inhibited by other chemical compounds (i.e., direct agonists or direct antagonists, respectively). These chemical compounds also interact with the same molecule (e.g., receptor) that is targeted by the natural transmitter.
4. All enzymes responsible for the synthesis and degradation of the transmitter must be present in the relevant neurons and neuroanatomical structures. These mechanisms can be altered by chemical compounds that either increase or decrease the amount of transmitter available (i.e., indirect agonists or antagonists).

mitters. Adrenaline is produced from noradrenaline in the chromaffin cells of the adrenal medulla and may also be present in some areas of the brain. Both adrenaline and noradrenaline (known in the United States as epinephrine and norepinephrine, respectively) are released into the circulation from the adrenal medulla.

## AUTONOMIC CHOLINERGIC TRANSMISSION

### Biosynthesis of Acetylcholine

Acetylcholine is synthesized in the axon terminals of cholinergic nerves (Fig. 11-3). Acetyl coenzyme A (readily available within the cytoplasm) and choline (transported into the nerve terminal from the synapse, as well as from cytoplasmic sources) undergo an acetyl transfer reaction, catalyzed by the enzyme choline acetyltransferase, to form acetylcholine, which is transported into and stored in membrane-bound vesicles known as synaptic vesicles. Transport into the vesicles is inhibited by **vesamicol**, which thus depletes the nerve terminals of acetylcholine. Each vesicle normally contains about 10 000 molecules of acetylcholine. It is not certain whether all neuronal acetylcholine is packaged within the vesicles, but it is clear that most of the acetylcholine released from the nerve terminal is from the vesicular pool. Also, for reasons unclear, the most recently synthesized acetylcholine is likely to be the first to be released upon stimulation. When the turnover of acetylcholine is high, the transport of choline into the nerve terminal can become the rate-limiting step. Blockage of choline transport by **hemicholinium** leads to acetylcholine depletion in the nerve terminal.

| FIGURE 11-3 | Biosynthesis of acetylcholine (ACh) in cholinergic neurons. Presynaptic $\alpha_2$-adrenergic receptors are found in only some cholinergic neurons (see Table 13-2). |
| --- | --- |

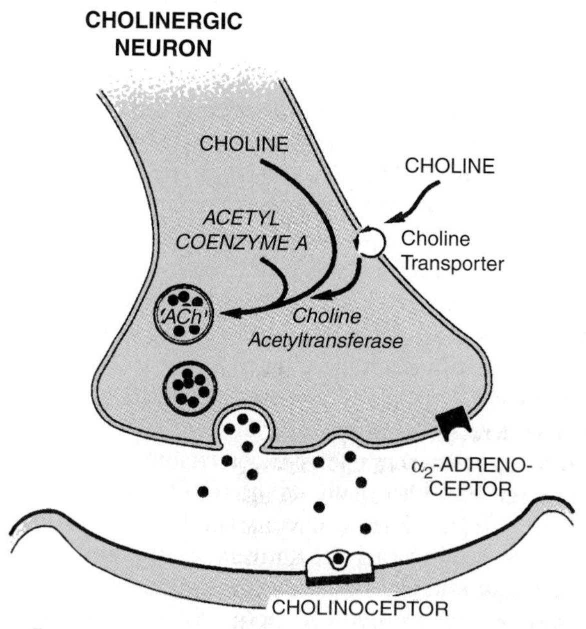

### Release of Acetylcholine

A calcium-dependent sequence of events is initiated when an action potential arrives at the nerve terminal. The vesicles migrate towards the membrane of the presynaptic terminal, fuse with it, open to the synaptic cleft, and release their contents (acetylcholine, vesiculin, and ATP). This process of vesicular emptying into the synapse is known as exocytosis. After exocytosis, the vesicle membrane is recycled by invagination and sealing off of the membrane, and the reconstituted vesicle moves back into the nerve terminal, where it can be replenished with new acetylcholine. The membrane of the synaptic vesicle contains specific proteins that regulate transmitter release. For example, **synapsin I** anchors the vesicle to the cytoskeleton and thus prevents mobilization, while **synaptobrevin** regulates vesicle fusion with the cell membrane and exocytosis. Some toxins, such as **tetanus and botulinum toxins**, cause proteolysis of synaptobrevin and *inhibit* exocytosis, whereas α-**latrotoxin**, the black widow spider venom, *promotes* exocytosis. However, it should be noted that the main neuronal target of the tetanus toxin is the spinal inhibitory GABAergic neurons. Inhibition of the release of γ-aminobutyric acid (GABA) therefore disinhibits the spinal motoneuron and causes spastic paralysis.

### Breakdown of Released Acetylcholine and Choline Reuptake

Acetylcholine is broken down extremely rapidly, in less than 1 msec after its release, by the specific enzyme acetylcholinesterase (AChE), and 90% of the acetylcholine released may be hydrolyzed before it reaches the postsynaptic receptor to produce the biological effect. AChE is found in high concentrations wherever acetylcholine acts as a neurotransmitter (i.e., on both pre- and postganglionic membranes within the autonomic ganglia, on the membranes of parasympathetic nerve terminals, and on pre- and postsynaptic membranes of neuromuscular junctions). Acetic acid, which is produced during hydrolysis, is rapidly removed into various biochemical pathways (e.g., the Krebs cycle) within the cytoplasm. The choline is actively transported back into the nerve terminal, where it can be used to re-synthesize acetylcholine.

## AUTONOMIC ADRENERGIC TRANSMISSION

### Biosynthesis of Catecholamines

Phenylethylamine, the parent compound of the catecholamines, consists of a benzene (phenyl) ring and an ethylamine side chain. A phenyl ring with two adjacent hydroxyl groups is called catechol. Therefore, phenylethylamine derivatives having hydroxyl groups at C-3 and C-4 on the phenyl ring, such as the endogenous sympathetic neurotransmitters, are termed catecholamines.

The primary precursor for the catecholamine biosynthetic pathway is the amino acid L-tyrosine, which is actively transported from the blood into the adrenergic neuronal cell bodies and the chromaffin cells (see Chapter 16). In the cytoplasm of the adrenergic neuron, L-tyrosine is converted to L-dopa (dihydroxyphenylalanine) by the enzyme tyrosine hydroxylase. This is the rate-limiting step in the biosynthesis of catecholamines (Figs. 11-4 and 11-5). The essential requirements for tyrosine hydroxylase activation are a tetrahydropteridine cofactor, oxygen, and ferrous ion ($Fe^{2+}$).

L-Dopa is the substrate for another cytoplasmic enzyme, dopa decarboxylase (L-aromatic amino acid decarboxylase), which converts it to dopamine (dihydroxyphenylethylamine), a true catecholamine. Dopa decarboxylase exhibits a rather low substrate specificity; for example, it can produce 5-hydroxytryptamine from 5-hydroxytryptophan. In addition, this enzyme can also convert α-methyldopa to α-methyldopamine, which in turn forms α-methylnoradrenaline, a "false" neurotransmitter in the sympathetic system. The essential cofactor for the enzyme is pyridoxal phosphate. Once formed,

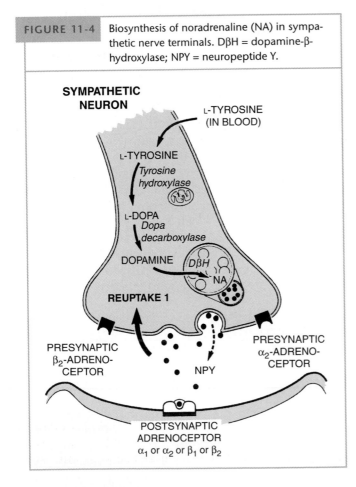

**FIGURE 11-4** Biosynthesis of noradrenaline (NA) in sympathetic nerve terminals. DβH = dopamine-β-hydroxylase; NPY = neuropeptide Y.

**FIGURE 11-5** Biosynthesis of catecholamines. Essential cofactors are shown in parentheses. MAO = monoamine oxidase.

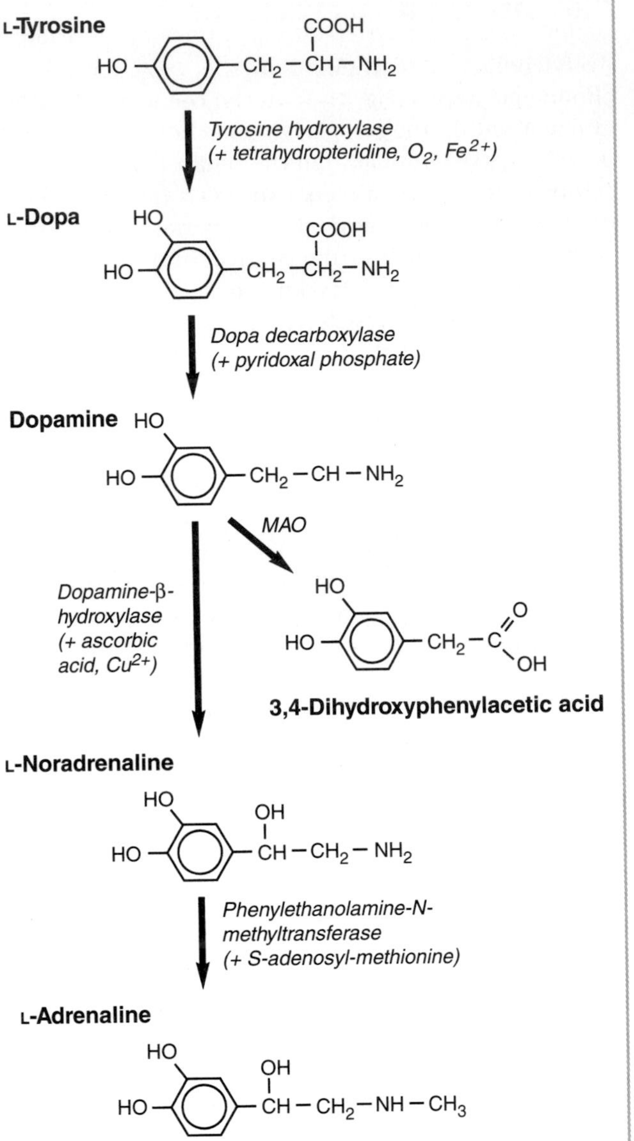

dopamine is either actively taken up by storage vesicles within the nerve terminal or deaminated to 3,4-dihydroxyphenylacetic acid (DOPAC). In the vesicles, dopamine is converted to noradrenaline by the action of dopamine-β-hydroxylase (DβH). The essential cofactors for DβH are ascorbic acid and cuprous ion ($Cu^{2+}$; see Fig. 11-5).

Each progressive step in the conversion of L-tyrosine to noradrenaline has been evaluated by using known inhibitors of the various enzymes (Table 11-1). Noradrenaline itself also inhibits the conversion of L-tyrosine to L-dopa by a negative feedback mechanism involving competition with the tetrahydropteridine cofactor. This process of "end-product" inhibition controls the rate of its own synthesis and also that of dopamine. During increased sympathetic neuronal activity, end-product inhibition is decreased and the synthesis of noradrenaline is enhanced.

In the adrenal medulla, noradrenaline is methylated in the cytoplasm by the enzyme phenylethanolamine-*N*-methyltransferase (PNMT) to form adrenaline. The rate of synthesis of adrenaline in the chromaffin cells is dependent on glucocorticoids secreted by the adrenal cortex, which are carried in high concentrations directly to the chromaffin cells of the adrenal medulla, where they induce PNMT. In the adult human, adrenaline constitutes approximately 80% of the total catecholamines of the adrenal medulla.

## Storage of Noradrenaline and Adrenaline

The most important sites for storage of noradrenaline are granular vesicles, which are highly concentrated in the varicosities of the nerve terminals. There is evidence to suggest that storage vesicles are actually formed in the cell bodies of the neurons and carried down the length of the axon to the terminal varicosities.

Noradrenaline is stored in high concentrations in these granules as a molecular complex with ATP in a 4:1 ratio. The granules also contain specific proteins (chromogranins) as well as DβH and dopamine. Noradrenaline is also present in free form outside the ATP complex, with which it is in tight equilibrium. Outside the granule, there is some free cytoplasmic noradrenaline that probably plays a role in the regulation of synthesis by means of end-product inhibition.

Within the granules, noradrenaline is present in at least two different metabolic pools. Pool I contains material with a rapid turnover: it probably functions as the neurotransmitter. Pool II turns over slowly and contains material of limited physiological significance. Specific transporters located in the vesicular membrane have a high affinity for catecholamines and are responsible for the storage of dopamine in the synaptic vesicles. These ATP- and magnesium-dependent vesicular monoamine transporters (VMATs) use proton transmembrane gradients to transport the neurotransmitter from the cytoplasm into the more acidic vesicular compartment. This transport system can concentrate noradrenaline against a 200-fold gradient across the vesicular membrane. VMATs are proteins of approximately 500 amino acids, and they have 12 hydrophobic transmembrane domains, as cell membrane transporters do. They are inhibited by reserpine, which thus prevents the vesicular storage of dopamine and its subsequent intravesicular conversion into noradrenaline (see Chapter 14).

In the chromaffin cells, most of the noradrenaline leaves the granules and is methylated in the cytoplasm to adrenaline, which then re-enters the storage granules and remains there until it is released.

## Release of Catecholamines

When a nerve impulse is propagated along the axon of a post-ganglionic adrenergic neuron, it initiates the calcium-dependent exocytotic release of noradrenaline from the storage granules. The entire contents are released following fusion of the granule membrane with that of the neuronal membrane. A similar process for adrenaline release occurs in the adrenal medulla. There is also evidence that neuropeptide Y (NPY) is released together with noradrenaline and acts as a co-transmitter. The ratio of released NPY to noradrenaline differs in different pathological states and may, therefore, be a key factor in various pathophysiological events.

After release from the axon terminal, the actions of the neurotransmitter can be terminated by (1) reuptake by the presynaptic terminal (neural uptake; or uptake 1), (2) diffusion in the intercellular space and uptake by some non-neural elements (glial and smooth muscle cells; uptake 2), or (3) metabolic transformation.

Following noradrenaline release, most (approximately 80%, depending on the distance from the target site) is retrieved by reuptake into the cytoplasmic pool of the presynaptic neuron (Fig. 11-6). This process involves the active transport of L-noradrenaline by a selective noradrenaline transporter (NAT). This is the most important mechanism by which the action of noradrenaline is terminated. A similar process takes place in dopaminergic neurons, where the selective dopamine transporter (DAT) is responsible for the reuptake of dopamine into the presynaptic terminal. Inhibition of the catecholamine transporters by cocaine strongly increases the synaptic availability and effects of the transmitter. After presynaptic reuptake, the recycled transmitter is then transported into the vesicle by a VMAT. Both processes are susceptible to drug action (see Chapters 13 and 14).

Some of the released noradrenaline can also bind to presynaptic $\alpha_2$-adrenoceptors that mediate feedback inhibition of further noradrenaline release. Only a small percentage of released noradrenaline goes directly to the cir-

| TABLE 11-1 | Inhibitors of Enzymes Involved in the Biosynthesis of L-Dopa, Dopamine, and Noradrenaline |
|---|---|
| **Enzyme** | **Inhibitor** |
| Tyrosine hydroxylase | Alpha-methyl-*p*-tyrosine Noradrenaline and dopamine (negative feedback mechanism) |
| L-Aromatic amino acid decarboxylase (dopa decarboxylase) | α-Methyldopa Benserazide (RO4-4602) |
| Dopamine-β-hydroxylase | Disulfiram (Antabuse) |

FIGURE 11-6 Fate of intraneuronal and extraneuronal noradrenaline (NA). The relative importance and order of each step are indicated by differently sized arrows and by numbers, respectively. COMT = catechol-*O*-methyltransferase; DHMA = dihydroxymandelic acid; DHPEG = dihydroxyphenylethylene glycol; MAO = monoamine oxidase; MHPEG = methoxyhydroxyphenylethylene glycol; VMA = vanilmandelic acid.
(1) Noradrenaline reuptake 1. (2) Intraneuronal metabolism by MAO. (3) Diffusion of DHEPG into circulation. (4) Combination with presynaptic $\alpha_2$-adrenergic receptor. (5) Combination with postsynaptic adrenergic receptors. (6) Circulating NA. (7) Extraneuronal metabolism of DHPEG by COMT to MHPEG. (8) Extraneuronal metabolism of DHMA by COMT to VMA. (9) Extraneuronal metabolism by COMT to normetanephrine, followed by MAO (10) to form an intermediate that may be converted to either VMA or MHPEG. (11) Very-low-potency combination with presynaptic $\beta_2$ receptor.

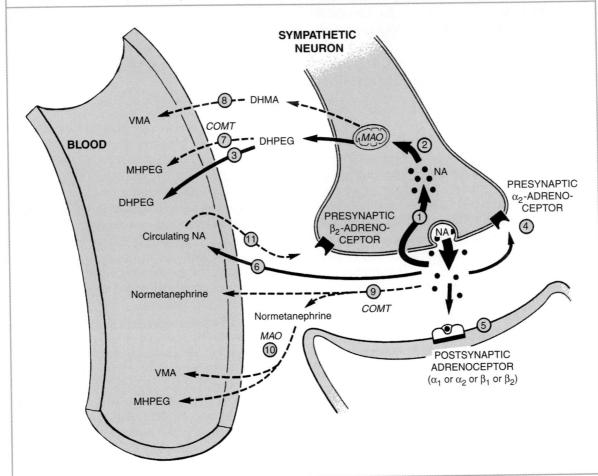

## Degradation of Catecholamines

culation. Therefore, the measured concentration of circulating noradrenaline does not correlate with its actual concentration within the sympathetic nervous system or with the amount of noradrenaline released from sympathetic nerve terminals. The released noradrenaline is further metabolized or acts on specific post-junctional adrenoceptors to mediate an effect (see "Adrenergic Receptors (Adrenoceptors)" below).

Two enzymes are responsible for the degradation of catecholamines: monoamine oxidase (MAO) and catechol-*O*-methyltransferase (COMT). Both enzymes are widely dis-

tributed throughout the body. MAO is chiefly associated with the outer surface of mitochondria, in particular, those within sympathetic nerve terminals, whereas COMT is located primarily in the synaptic cleft. This distinction is of great importance with respect to the primary metabolic pathways followed by catecholamines. MAO exists in two isoforms, MAO-A and MAO-B; their pharmacological significance is discussed in Chapter 25.

Noradrenaline entering or already in the cytoplasmic pool (but not in the vesicles) is deaminated by MAO. Furthermore, noradrenaline released from the vesicles by drugs such as reserpine is also deaminated by MAO. The product initially formed by the action of MAO is 3,4-dihydroxyphenylglycol aldehyde (DHPGAL), which is subsequently reduced to dihydroxyphenylethylene glycol (DHPEG). DHPEG subsequently enters the plasma or is further metabolized by COMT to 3-methoxy-4-hydroxyphenylethylene glycol (MHPEG), which is excreted in the urine.

Noradrenaline that is released into the synapse is rapidly O-methylated by COMT, either directly in the synaptic cleft or in adjacent tissue (glial or smooth muscle activity; uptake 2) to form normetanephrine. Finally, normetanephrine may be metabolized by MAO, via 3-methoxy-4-hydroxyphenylglycol aldehyde, to 3-methoxy-4-hydroxymandelic acid (MHMA, also called vanilmandelic acid, VMA). The enzymatic degradation of the catecholamines is illustrated in Figure 11-7.

# RECEPTORS IN THE AUTONOMIC NERVOUS SYSTEM

In order to elicit a biological response, a drug or neurotransmitter must bind to, and interact with, specific receptors situated on the cell membrane. This interaction produces a drug–receptor or neurotransmitter–receptor complex that mediates a series of cellular events leading to a characteristic cellular response (see Chapter 8). Neurotransmitter receptors can be characterized by means of specific agonists that stimulate the receptor, or by antagonists that block or inhibit the response to the specific neurotransmitter.

## Cholinergic Receptors (Cholinoceptors)

Although acetylcholine is the neurotransmitter both in autonomic ganglia and at post-ganglionic parasympathetic nerve terminals, two different types of acetylcholine receptor are involved. Dale (1914) was the first to describe the dual function of acetylcholine and to recognize that these separate effects were similar to those of either nicotine or muscarine. Additional evidence for the dual nature of acetylcholine receptors came from studies with d-tubocurarine, a nicotinic antagonist, and with atropine, a selective muscarinic antagonist. To date, these differential effects remain the primary basis of classification of cholinergic receptors.

## Nicotinic Receptors

The nicotinic receptors are ligand-gated ion channels formed by five subunits arranged around a central pore; the pore becomes permeable to $Na^+$ and $Ca^{2+}$ when the receptor is activated by acetylcholine, resulting in depolarization and excitation of the cell. There are two main types of nicotinic receptors, the neuronal type and the muscular type. These receptors have a heteromeric composition, with two $\alpha$ subunits (of which there are nine types designated $\alpha_1$ to $\alpha_9$) and three $\beta$ subunits (of which there are four types, $\beta_1$ to $\beta_4$). The $\alpha_1$ and $\beta_1$ subunits are found only in the muscular type of nicotinic receptors, whereas different combinations of the various $\alpha$ and $\beta$ subunits are found in different brain regions. The difference in subunit composition is responsible for the distinct pharmacological actions of various agonists and antagonists. The neuronal receptor is selectively antagonized by agents such as **hexamethonium** and **trimethaphan**, and the selective agonist is **dimethylphenyl piperazinium** ion (DMPP). These receptors are located in all autonomic ganglia and on cell bodies of sympathetic and parasympathetic post-ganglionic fibres. The muscle nicotinic receptor (see Chapter 15) is selectively blocked by agents such as **d-tubocurarine**, **vecuronium**, and **decamethonium** and is selectively activated by **phenyltrimethyl ammonium**.

## Muscarinic Receptors

Muscarinic receptors are activated non-selectively by acetylcholine, muscarine, carbachol, and (+)-cis-dioxolane. Muscarinic receptors are blocked by atropine and scopolamine. To date, five different subtypes of muscarinic receptors (designated $M_1$ to $M_5$) have been identified, which have distinct anatomical locations and distinct molecular and pharmacological characteristics. This diversity was first recognized when the pharmacological actions of **pirenzepine** were examined. Pirenzepine is unique in that it is the only muscarinic antagonist that selectively inhibits gastric acid secretion.

The activation of muscarinic $M_1$, $M_3$, and $M_5$ receptors results in their interaction with G proteins. They are coupled to $G_{q/11}$ protein, which in turn stimulates phospholipase C. This causes the immediate hydrolysis of phosphatidylinositol phosphates to produce inositol trisphosphate ($IP_3$), which causes release of intracellular $Ca^{2+}$ and hence an excitatory cellular response (e.g., contraction of smooth muscle). In addition, this process also causes the production of diacylglycerol (DAG), which activates protein kinase C (PKC), which in turn modulates many ionic and cellular events. $M_1$ receptors are located in ganglia and in some glands; they are selectively activated by a compound known as McN A343 and are antagonized by pirenzepine and telenzepine. $M_3$ receptors are located in smooth muscle and secretory glands; they are blocked rather selectively by **4-DAMP**, a piperidine derivative. $M_5$ receptors are present in the endothelium of blood vessels, where their activation increases intracellular calcium concentration, promoting the release of the endothelium-derived relaxing factor, nitric oxide, which causes relaxation of the smooth muscle fibres and vasodilatation.

$M_2$ and $M_4$ receptors are coupled to the $G_{i/o}$ protein, which results in inhibition of the adenylyl cyclase/cAMP transduction pathway and inhibition of the target cell (see also Chapter 9). $M_2$ receptors are abundant in the myocardium, and their activation accounts for the negative cardiac chronotropic and inotropic responses to acetyl-

**FIGURE 11-7** Steps in the metabolic degradation of noradrenaline and adrenaline. MAO = monoamine oxidase; COMT = catechol-*O*-methyltransferase; VMA = vanilmandelic acid.

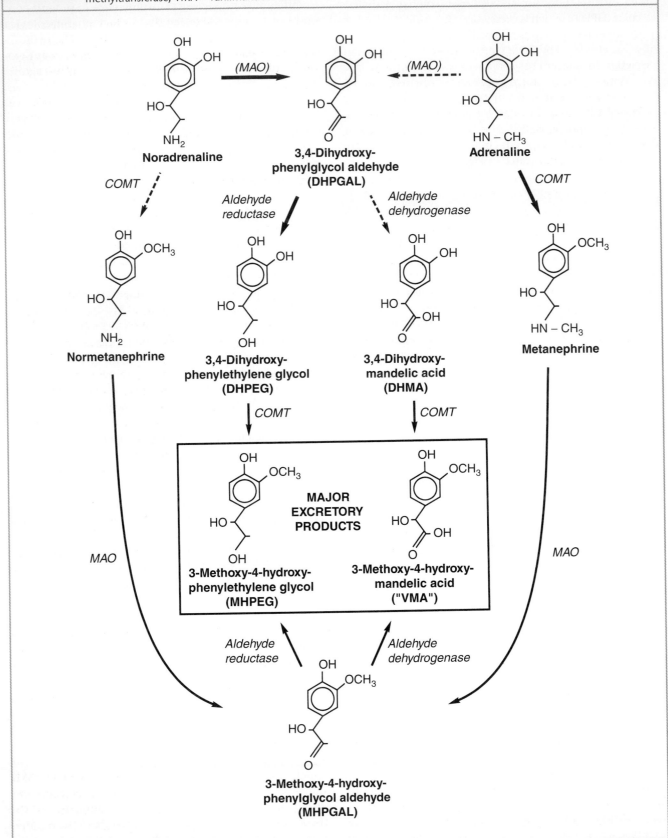

choline; they are selectively antagonized by **gallamine** and **methoctramine**. $M_4$ receptors are located in the myenteric plexus and muscle layers, but not on smooth muscle cells.

## Adrenergic Receptors (Adrenoceptors)

There are two major classes of adrenergic receptors ($\alpha$ and $\beta$), which were first proposed by Ahlquist (1948) on the basis of the ability of adrenaline, noradrenaline, and iso-proterenol (a synthetic catecholamine) to regulate various physiological processes (e.g., smooth muscle contraction). The rank order of potency for agonists at $\alpha$-adrenergic receptors is adrenaline, noradrenaline, isoproterenol, and for $\beta$ receptors it is isoproterenol, adrenaline, noradrenaline. The later finding that certain antagonists act selectively on the different types corroborated this initial classification. Whereas **phentolamine** is a selective antagonist for $\alpha$ receptors, **propranolol** selectively blocks $\beta$ receptors.

More recent pharmacological and molecular studies have shown that there are two main subtypes of $\alpha$-adrenergic receptors ($\alpha_1$ and $\alpha_2$) and three main subtypes of $\beta$-adrenergic receptors ($\beta_1$, $\beta_2$, and $\beta_3$). All known adrenergic receptors are coupled to G proteins that regulate different transduction pathways. Stimulation of the $\alpha_1$-adrenergic receptors causes depolarization (i.e., excitation) through $G_q$ activation of the phospholipase C pathway and increases intracellular $Ca^{2+}$, whereas stimulation of the $\alpha_2$-receptors causes hyperpolarization (i.e., inhibition) through $G_i$ inhibition of the adenylyl cyclase pathway. All $\beta$ receptors activate adenylyl cyclase through $G_s$ and have an excitatory effect (see Table 16-4).

### $\alpha$-Adrenergic receptors

The first suggestion that there were different subtypes of $\alpha$-receptors came from the observation that noradrenaline, in high doses, can inhibit its own release from pre-synaptic terminals. This feedback mechanism is mediated through pre-junctional $\alpha$ receptors that are pharmacologically distinct from post-junctional adrenergic receptors. The pre-junctional receptors are termed $\alpha_2$, and the post-junctional receptors, $\alpha_1$. When exogenous noradrenaline is administered as a drug, the effects of $\alpha_2$ stimulation may not be observed because the large excess of drug can act directly on the $\alpha_1$ receptors, bypassing the release of endogenous transmitter. **Clonidine** was one of the first compounds to be described as being a more potent agonist at pre-junctional receptors ($\alpha_2$), whereas **phenylephrine** was a more potent agonist at post-junctional sites ($\alpha_1$). Subsequently, selective antagonists were also found for the two types: **prazosin** for $\alpha_1$- and **rauwolscine** for $\alpha_2$-adrenergic receptors. The antagonist affinity for $\alpha_2$ receptors occurs in a very narrow concentration range.

However, it is now evident that $\alpha_2$-adrenergic receptors are also present at post-junctional sites. Activation of these post-junctional $\alpha_2$ receptors has different results depend-ing on the type of cell on which the receptors are located. In vascular smooth muscle, it causes inhibition and thus produces vasodilatation, indirectly caused by release of nitric oxide from the vascular endothelium. Activation of $\alpha_2$ receptors on platelets causes platelet aggregation. In addition, it may also result in contraction of some types of smooth muscle through the activation of the phospholipase $C_{\beta 2}$-mediated increase in intracellular $Ca^{2+}$.

Both $\alpha_1$- and $\alpha_2$-adrenergic receptors have been further subdivided. The various subtypes, their selectivity for binding different ligands, and their functional significance will be highlighted in Chapters 13 and 14.

### $\beta$-Adrenergic receptors

Classically, the $\beta$-adrenergic receptors are classified into $\beta_1$ and $\beta_2$ on the basis of their differential responses to noradrenaline and adrenaline. Noradrenaline is equally potent on $\beta_1$ and $\beta_2$ receptors and is slightly more potent than adrenaline on $\beta_1$, whereas adrenaline is some 100 times more potent than noradrenaline on $\beta_2$ receptors. Recently, a third subtype of $\beta$-adrenergic receptor has been identified that was at first termed "atypical" but is now named $\beta_3$. This receptor is about 10 times more sensitive to noradrenaline than to adrenaline. Further characterization of these subtypes by their differential binding of other ligands is described in Chapters 13 and 14.

All three $\beta$-adrenergic receptors are coupled to a stimulatory G protein ($G_s$). Agonist binding stimulates adenylyl cyclase, leading to an increase in cyclic AMP, activation of cAMP-dependent protein kinase A (PKA), and phosphorylation of specific cellular proteins. In skeletal and myocardial myocytes, $G_s$ also activates voltage-sensitive L-type $Ca^{2+}$ channels and elicits contraction. The $\beta_1$ receptor is located primarily in cardiac tissue, where it mediates the inotropic and chronotropic effects of catecholamines. Activation of the $\beta_1$ receptor enhances phosphorylation of troponin and phospholamban, which in turn raises intracellular $Ca^{2+}$ and thus contributes to the inotropic response. Activation of $\beta_1$ receptors in the cardiac pacemaker cells decreases their firing threshold and thereby increases conductivity (i.e., chronotropy).

The $\beta_2$-adrenergic receptor mediates smooth muscle relaxation in many organs, causing such effects as bronchodilatation and vasodilatation (Table 11-2). In smooth muscle, accumulation of cyclic AMP accelerates the phosphorylation of myosin light-chain kinase (MLCK), thus preventing contraction (see Chapter 13).

### Distribution of adrenoceptors

This varies from organ to organ, as listed in Table 11-2. The receptor distribution determines the characteristic response because the endogenous release of noradrenaline and adrenaline stimulates all adrenergic receptors, and the effects in any given organ will depend on the balance between $\alpha$ and $\beta$ receptors and their respective subtypes.

**TABLE 11-2**  Response of Effector Organs to Autonomic Transmitters

| Effector Organs | Adrenergic | | Muscarinic Cholinergic Responses |
|---|---|---|---|
| | Receptors* | Responses | |
| **Eye** | | | |
| Radial muscle of iris | $\alpha_1$ | Contr (mydriasis) | — |
| Sphincter muscle of iris | | — | Contr (miosis; strong) |
| Ciliary muscle | $\beta_2$ | Relax (slight)† | Contr (strong)‡ |
| **Heart** | | | |
| Heart rate | $\beta_1$§ | ↑ | ↓ |
| Atrial contractility/conduction | $\beta_1$ | ↑ | ↓ |
| AV conduction | $\beta_1$ | ↑ | ↓ (block) |
| Ventricular contractility/conduction | $\beta_1$ | ↑ | ↓ |
| **Blood vessels‖** | | | |
| Coronary | $\alpha_1, \beta_2, \alpha_2$‖ | Constr; dilat ($\beta_2$) | |
| Skin and mucous membranes | $\alpha_1, \alpha_2$ | Constr (strong) | ? |
| Skeletal muscle | $\alpha_1, \beta_2$ | Constr; dilat ($\beta_2$) | Dilat |
| Cerebral | $\alpha_1$ | Constr (slight) | |
| Pulmonary | $\alpha_1, \beta_2$ | Constr; dilat ($\beta_2$) | |
| Abdominal viscera | $\alpha_1, \beta_2$ | Constr; dilat ($\beta_2$) | |
| **Lung** | | | |
| Bronchial smooth muscle | $\beta_2$ | Relax | Contr |
| Bronchial glands | | Inhibition (?) | Stimulation |
| **Stomach and intestine** | | | |
| Motility and tone | $\alpha_1, \beta_2, \alpha_2$¶ | ↓ | ↑ (strong) |
| Sphincters | $\alpha_1$ | Contr (?) | Relax (usually) |
| Secretion | | Inhibition (?) | Stimulation |
| **Gallbladder and ducts** | | Relax | Contr |
| **Urinary bladder** | | | |
| Detrusor muscle | $\beta_2$ | Relax (usually) | Contr |
| Trigone and sphincter | $\alpha_1$ | Contr | Relax |
| **Ureter** | | | |
| Motility and tone | $\alpha_1$ | ↑ (usually) | ↑ (?) |
| **Uterus** | $\alpha_1, \beta_2$ | $\alpha_1$ = Contr# <br> $\beta_2$ = Relax | Variable |
| **Skeletal muscle** | $\beta_2$ | ↑ contractility; glycogenolysis | — |
| **Sex organs, male** | $\alpha_1$ | Ejaculation | Erection |
| **Skin** | | | |
| Sweat glands | $\alpha_1$ | Slight secretion | Profuse secretion |
| Pilomotor muscles | $\alpha_1$ | Contr | |
| **Spleen capsule** | $\alpha_1, \beta_2$ | Contr (strong) | |
| **Adrenal medulla** | | — | Secretion of adrenaline and noradrenaline (*nicotinic* effect) |
| **Pineal gland** | $\beta$ | Melatonin synthesis | — |
| **Posterior pituitary** | $\beta_1$ | ADH secretion | — |
| **Fat cells** | $\beta_3$ | Lipolysis | — |
| **Liver** | $\alpha, \beta_2$ | Glycogenolysis and gluconeogenesis | Glycogen synthesis |

*continued*

**TABLE 11-2**    continued

| Effector Organs | Adrenergic Receptors* | Adrenergic Responses | Muscarinic Cholinergic Responses |
|---|---|---|---|
| Pancreas | | | |
|   Acini | $\alpha_1$ | ↓ Secretion | Secretion |
|   Islet cells | $\alpha_2$, $\beta_2$ | $\alpha_2$ = ↓ Secretion <br> $\beta_2$ = ↑ Secretion | — |
| Salivary glands | $\alpha_1$ | Potassium and water secretion (slight) | Potassium and water secretion (profuse) |
| Lacrimal glands | | — | Secretion (profuse) |
| Nasopharyngeal glands | $\alpha_1$, $\beta_2$ | ↓ (moderate) | Secretion |
| Kidneys | $\alpha_1$, $\beta_1$ | $\alpha_1$ = ↓ Renin release <br> $\beta_1$ = ↑ Renin release | — |
| Adrenergic nerve terminals | $\alpha_2$ (presynaptic) | ↓ Release of noradrenaline | |
| Cholinergic nerve terminals | $\alpha_2$ (presynaptic) | ↓ Release of acetylcholine at some sites | |

*Where known.

†For far vision.

‡For near vision.

§$\beta_2$- and $\alpha$-adrenoceptors are present in the heart also, but they are less important than $\beta_1$ receptors.

‖Renal and mesenteric blood vessels have dopamine receptors, which cause dilatation when stimulated. $\alpha_2$-Adrenoceptors in blood vessels cause contraction when stimulated.

¶$\alpha_2$-Adrenoceptors in the myenteric plexus inhibit acetylcholine release when stimulated.

#$\alpha_1$-Adrenoceptor stimulation contracts the uterus during pregnancy.

↑ = increase; ↓ = decrease; – = No effect; Constr = constriction; Contr = contraction; Dilat = dilatation; Relax = relaxation.

## MODULATION OF AUTONOMIC NERVOUS SYSTEM ACTIVITY

At least three different levels of control interact to modulate activity in the ANS.

### Physiological Interaction of Sympathetic and Parasympathetic Innervation

At central sites (e.g., the medulla oblongata), cholinergic and adrenergic systems can interact with each other by reflex mechanisms to maintain homeostasis. A drug-induced elevation of mean arterial pressure causes a baroreceptor-mediated negative feedback response that results in marked bradycardia. This is due to increased acetylcholine release at the sinoatrial node, causing a compensatory decrease in heart rate. Bradycardia occurs even when the pressor drug is a potent myocardial stimulant that normally increases the heart rate (e.g., noradrenaline; see Chapter 13). In this way, the parasympathetic nervous system becomes dominant and overrides sympathomimetic effects on both the sinoatrial and atrioventricular nodes.

### Presynaptic Control of Transmitter Release

This is another mechanism by which one system may be inhibited or stimulated relative to the other. Presynaptic receptors may respond either to the neurotransmitter substance released by the nerve terminal itself (i.e., autoreceptors) or to neurotransmitters released from axons that synapse with the nerve terminal (i.e., heteroreceptors).

Presynaptic $\alpha_2$ receptors, when stimulated by released noradrenaline, exert a negative feedback control that diminishes further noradrenaline release from nerve endings. Conversely, noradrenaline release can be enhanced by stimulation of $\beta_2$ receptors. However, this latter mechanism may be more sensitive to circulating adrenaline.

Presynaptic $\alpha_2$-adrenergic receptors located on parasympathetic nerve endings can also reduce the amount of acetylcholine released at certain sites. In the mesenteric plexus, for example, the release of acetylcholine is decreased to an extent that causes relaxation and reduced motility of the intestine.

Other endogenous substances (e.g., prostaglandins and enkephalins) also inhibit noradrenaline release by interacting with specific presynaptic receptors. Contrasting with this is the effect of angiotensin II (see Chapter 29), which enhances the release of catecholamines.

## Changes in Postsynaptic Receptors

At postsynaptic adrenergic receptor sites in target organs, the response of the organ to neurotransmitters may be altered by a decrease in receptor numbers (e.g., desensitization due to down-regulation of receptors following periods of excessive stimulation). Up-regulation (i.e., increased receptor numbers) may occur in other circumstances (e.g., when a drug acts on neurons to inhibit transmitter release).

## SUGGESTED READINGS

Arner P, Hoffstedt J. Adrenoceptor genes in human obesity. *J Intern Med.* 1999;245:667-672.

Bunemann M, Lee KB, Pals-Rylaarsdam R, et al. Desensitization of G protein-coupled receptors in the cardiovascular system. *Annu Rev Physiol.* 1999;61:169-192.

Burnstock G, Hoyle CHV. *Autonomic Neuroeffector Mechanisms.* Philadelphia, Pa: Harwood Academic; 1992.

Bylund DB, Eikenberg DC, Hieble JP, et al. International Union of Pharmacology nomenclature of adrenoceptors. *Pharmacol Rev.* 1994;46:121-136.

Cooper JR, Bloom FE, Roth RH. *The Biochemical Basis of Neuropharmacology.* 8th ed. New York, NY: Oxford University Press; 2003.

Esler M, Lambert G, Brunner-La Rocca G, et al. Sympathetic nerve activity and neurotransmitter release in humans: translation from pathophysiology into clinical practice. *Acta Physiol Scand.* 2003;177:275-284.

Gand P, Vita JA. Testing endothelial vasomotor function. *Circulation.* 2003;108:2049-2053.

Gonçalves J, Bueltmann R, Driessen B. Opposite modulation of cotransmitter release in guinea-pig vas deferens: increase of noradrenaline and decrease of ATP release by activation of prejunctional β-receptors. *Naunyn-Schmiedebergs Arch Pharmacol.* 1996;353:184-192.

Grahame-Smith DG, Aronson JK. The drug therapy of cardiovascular disorders: hypertension. In: *Oxford Textbook of Clinical Pharmacology and Drug Therapy.* 3rd ed. New York, NY: Oxford University Press; 2002:226-233.

Kiss JP, Vizi ES. Nitric oxide: a novel link between synaptic and nonsynaptic transmission. *Trends Neurosci.* 2003;24:211-215.

Langer, SZ. 25 years since the discovery of presynaptic receptors: present knowledge and future perspectives. *Trends Pharmacol Sci.* 1997;18:95-99.

MacDermott AB, Role LW, Siegelbaum SA. Presynaptic ionotropic receptors and the control of transmitter release. *Annu Rev Pharmacol.* 1999;22:442-485.

Marder E. Neural signaling: does colocalization imply cotransmisssion? *Curr Biol.* 1999;9:R809-R811.

Mathias CJ. Autonomic diseases management. *J Neurol Neurosurg Psychiat.* 2003;74(suppl III):iii42-iii47.

Nestler E, Hyman SE, Malenka RC. Autonomic nervous system. In: *Molecular Neuropharmacology: A Foundation for Clinical Science.* New York, NY: McGraw-Hill; 2001:255-276.

Pang CC. Autonomic control of the venous system in health and disease. *Pharmacol Ther.* 2001;90:179-230.

Pellizzari R, Rossetto O, Schiavo G, Montecucco C. Tetanus and botulinum neurotoxins: mechanism of action and therapeutic uses. *Philos Trans R Soc Lond B Biol Sci.* 1999;28:259-268.

Takeuchi T, Fujinami K, Goto H, et al. Roles of M2 and M4 muscarinic receptors in regulating acetylcholine release from myenteric neurons of mouse ileum. *J Neurophysiol.* 2005;93: 2841-2848.

Turton K, Chaddock JA, Acharya KR. Botulinum and tetanus neurotoxins: structure, function and therapeutic utility. *Trends Biochem Sci.* 2002;27:552-558.

Waldeck B. Beta-adrenoceptor agonists and asthma—100 years of development. *Eur J Pharmacol.* 2002;445:1-12.

# 12

# Cholinergic Agonists and Antagonists

## M HONG

**CASE HISTORY**

A 55-year-old man who operates a small farm and garden centre was found unconscious by his son in the chemical storage room. During the past week, he had been spending much of his time spraying trees and shrubs with his new formula of plant food and had also been complaining of abdominal cramps and tightness in his chest similar to having an "asthmatic attack." Since he did not suffer from asthma and was usually of remarkably good health, his son suspected that he might have poisoned himself with his new plant food mixture while spraying. The ambulance was called and he was taken to the hospital at once.

Upon arrival at the hospital emergency room, the patient was unconscious, he was salivating profusely, and his breathing was shallow. His skin was warm and moist. Blood pressure was 140/90 mmHg, pulse was 45 beats/min and regular, respiration rate was 30/min, and temperature was normal. There was no evidence of trauma. Both pupils were constricted and did not respond to light. Auscultation of the chest revealed moderate wheezing and numerous rhonchi. The heart sounds were normal. Palpitation of the abdomen revealed no abnormalities, but hyperactive bowel sounds were heard. The rectal examination revealed nothing remarkable, and an occult blood test of the stool was negative. The extremities showed subcutaneous muscle fasciculations at the time of admission. These disappeared during the course of the examination, but muscle tone decreased and breathing became shallower during this time. The neurological examination revealed no response to painful stimuli, no localizing signs, and no abnormal reflexes.

During this examination, the son reported that his father had mild hypertension, controlled by salt restriction (about 5 years' duration) and non-insulin-dependent diabetes, controlled by diet (about 10 years' duration). He had no history of mental illness, he did not smoke or drink, and he was not taking medication.

The signs and symptoms of excessive cholinergic activity, together with the patient's occupation, allowed a provisional diagnosis of poisoning by organic phosphate insecticides to be made. When questioned directly, the son confirmed that they had recently experimented with such chemicals for use on the farm.

An airway and intravenous line were inserted, followed at once by intravenous injections of 2 mg atropine sulfate, repeated every 10 minutes until signs of atropinization appeared, shown by dry, flushed skin and tachycardia of 140 beats/min. Atropinization was continued for 24 hours with intramuscular injections of 2 mg of atropine sulfate every 4 hours.

At the same, time the patient was given a slow intravenous infusion of pralidoxime, 1 g in 250 mL saline, over a 30-minute period. This dose was repeated 1 hour later because of persisting muscle weakness, which then disappeared, and respiration strengthened. No further treatment with pralidoxime was indicated. The patient slowly began to recognize his surroundings and regained consciousness about 6 hours after being admitted to hospital. He felt very weak and confused. His respiration and the effects of atropinization continued to be monitored for the next 24 hours, and he remained under observation for an additional 3 days. He was discharged with the admonition to avoid strenuous activity and with instructions in the handling of organophosphate insecticides and the early recognition of signs of poisoning.

## ACETYLCHOLINE

As described in Chapter 11, acetylcholine acts as the principal neurotransmitter at distinct cholinergic sites of innervation of the parasympathetic nervous system. In order to understand cholinomimetic drug actions, it is important to recognize that acetylcholine can act at the following sites: (1) ganglionic synapses, (2) post-ganglionic parasympathetic terminals, (3) central cholinergic synapses, and (4) neuromuscular junctions. In addition, acetylcholine also acts on part of the sympathetic nervous system (i.e., sweat glands and adrenal medulla) and at sites that lack direct innervation, such as endothelial cells of blood vessels and cardiac ventricles.

The synthesis and release of acetylcholine and the characteristics of the receptor systems on which it acts, namely the muscarinic receptors and the nicotinic receptors, are described in Chapter 11. Currently, five distinct subtypes of the muscarinic receptor ($M_1$ to $M_5$) have been identified using molecular cloning studies of the genes (*m1* to *m5*) that encode for the binding proteins of the receptor subtypes. The muscarinic receptors belong to the family of G protein–linked receptors with a structure that includes seven transmembrane domains (see Chapter 8). These receptor subtypes are widely distributed throughout the body and can be broadly classified as follows: (1) $M_1$ receptors are found in secretory glands, autonomic ganglia, and the central nervous system (CNS); (2) $M_2$ receptors are present in the heart, autonomic ganglia, smooth muscle, and CNS; (3) $M_3$ receptors are located in smooth muscle, secretory glands, endothelial cells of the vessels, and the brain; (4) $M_4$ receptor subtypes are found in the autonomic ganglia and brain; and (5) $M_5$ receptors are found mostly in the CNS. The $M_1$, $M_3$, and $M_5$ subtypes have been demonstrated to use both the inositol trisphosphate ($IP_3$) and diacylglycerol (DAG) cascades as second messengers. The $M_2$ and $M_4$ subtypes inhibit adenylate cyclase activity and decrease cyclic adenosine monophosphate (cAMP) levels. The $M_2$ subtype can also activate potassium channels, resulting in membrane hyperpolarization and thus decreasing cell excitability; this is the principal action at the sinoatrial and atrioventricular nodes to cause slowing of the heart.

In contrast, the subtypes of the nicotinic receptor are diverse due to the complex receptor structure. Thus, the nicotinic receptor subtypes are classified according to the actions of classical nicotinic agonists and antagonists that interact with the receptor and according to the location of the receptor in skeletal muscle, autonomic ganglia, or the CNS. The nicotinic receptor is a pentameric ligand-gated ion channel composed of four distinct subunits in different stoichiometric configurations. The receptor found on skeletal muscle ($N_M$) is different from that found on autonomic ganglia ($N_N$). Acetylcholine stimulates both of these receptor subtypes, which are referred to as the nicotinic-cholinergic receptors.

## Principal Actions of Acetylcholine

### Muscarinic actions

The principal action of acetylcholine on the major organ systems occurs through stimulation of muscarinic receptors located on effector cells to produce the following effects:

1. Eye: Contraction of the circular muscles of the iris (iris sphincter), resulting in constriction of the pupil (miosis) and of the ciliary muscles of the lens to accommodate for near vision
2. Secretory glands: Stimulation of secretion by exocrine glands, such as sweat, salivary, mucous, and lacrimal glands. Gastric, intestinal, and pancreatic secretions are also increased, although they depend only partly on parasympathetic innervation. Where both sympathetic and parasympathetic innervation are involved, parasympathetic (muscarinic) stimulation produces a watery secretion, while sympathetic stimulation produces a more concentrated one. Both may be required for copious production of a "quality" secretion.
3. Heart: Decrease in the rate and force of contraction of the heart and a reduction in conduction velocity
4. Lungs: Contraction of the smooth muscles of the bronchi to produce bronchoconstriction, and stimulation of bronchial glands to secrete mucus
5. Stomach and intestines: Stimulation of smooth muscle to increase propulsive motility and tone, stimulation of gastric secretions, and relaxation of sphincters
6. Gallbladder: Contraction of the gallbladder to empty its contents
7. Urinary bladder: Contraction of the detrusor muscle and relaxation of the sphincters to allow for voiding of its contents

### Nicotinic actions

The stimulatory action of acetylcholine on nicotinic receptor subtypes produces the following effects:

1. Autonomic ganglia: Stimulation of sympathetic and parasympathetic ganglia (i.e., stimulation of postsynaptic neurons within the ganglia so that the postganglionic fibres release their respective transmitters at their peripheral endings)
2. Adrenal medulla: Stimulation to release adrenaline and noradrenaline
3. Skeletal muscles: Contraction of skeletal muscles

### Acetylcholine as a drug

Acetylcholine is an ester of choline and acetic acid that acts with little selectivity at the different cholinergic receptors. It is poorly absorbed following oral or subcutaneous administration and is rapidly degraded by a group of enzymes called cholinesterases that are present in both the plasma and the liver. When given intravenously, acetylcholine is rapidly hydrolyzed by plasma cholinesterase to choline and acetic acid. In order to produce an observable effect following intravenous administration of acetylcholine, it is necessary to administer a rather large dose.

The pharmacological effects of intravenous acetylcholine include a transient fall in blood pressure; bradycardia; partial or complete heart block or cardiac arrest; flushing, sweating, salivation, lacrimation, and increased bronchial mucus secretion; and, as secondary consequences, nausea, coughing, and dyspnea. These effects are all due to muscarinic actions; no nicotinic actions are noted. The effects on skeletal muscle can be observed only after intra-arterial injection. Exogenously administered acetylcholine will not produce effects on the CNS since the molecule is a quaternary ammonium compound that cannot cross the blood–brain barrier (Fig. 12-1).

Although there is no cholinergic innervation to blood vessels, acetylcholine produces an effect by acting directly on the endothelial cells. It produces dilation of blood vessels by stimulating the release of an endothelium-derived relaxing factor (EDRF) that has been identified as nitric oxide (NO). This activates guanylyl cyclase to increase production of cGMP, which then relaxes smooth muscle.

## CHOLINERGIC DRUGS

The usefulness of acetylcholine as a therapeutic agent is limited because of its poor absorption, rapid degradation, and lack of receptor selectivity. In order to avoid these limitations, at least in part, substitutes for acetylcholine are used to produce parasympathetic effects for diagnosis or therapy. All cholinergic drugs mimic the effects of stimulation of the parasympathetic nervous system. They may do so either by direct action, in the same way as acetylcholine, or by inhibition of acetylcholinesterase, thereby preventing the degradation of endogenous acetylcholine.

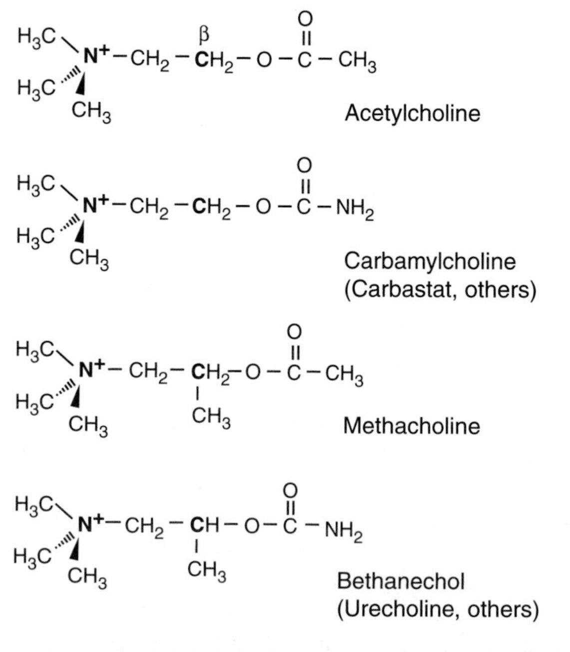

Agents that stimulate the mechanism that releases endogenous acetylcholine are not used therapeutically.

The contraindications are essentially the same for all the cholinergic drugs. They are contraindicated in patients with intestinal or urinary obstruction because the increased peristaltic movement of the bowel or contraction of the bladder would exacerbate the effects of the obstruction. These agents should be used cautiously in patients with bronchial asthma for similar reasons.

## Cholinergic Agonists

### Naturally occurring alkaloids
**Muscarine** is found in the mushroom *Amanita muscaria* (Fly agaric) and related species. It was the alkaloid agent first used to characterize the muscarinic receptor. Its actions are solely muscarinic, but it has no therapeutic use. Excessive cholinergic stimulation is frequently seen following ingestion of these mushrooms by uninformed mushroom pickers. This type of poisoning can readily be treated with specific muscarinic antagonists (e.g., atropine) to block cholinergic stimulation.

**Pilocarpine** is found in the leaves of *Pilocarpus*, a South American shrub. It has predominantly muscarinic action but also produces some nicotinic actions. The effects of pilocarpine on glands, such as the sweat and salivary glands, are particularly pronounced; therefore, it has been used to increase salivation and to induce sweating. Because pilocarpine is readily absorbed by the cornea of the eye, it is used mainly in ophthalmology to treat glaucoma (by opening the drainage canals for the intraocular fluid and thereby reducing the intraocular pressure), to produce miosis, and to counteract the mydriatic and cycloplegic actions of drugs such as atropine and the ganglion-blocking agents.

### Synthetic analogues of acetylcholine
In order to prevent or reduce the enzymatic degradation of acetylcholine, choline ester derivatives have been developed (see Fig. 12-1). When the acetyl group in acetylcholine is replaced by a carbamyl group, the resulting compound (carbamylcholine) is much more resistant to cholinesterase hydrolysis. Substitution of a methyl group at the β-carbon results in analogues (e.g., methacholine and bethanechol) that have a greater selectivity for muscarinic receptors and a somewhat reduced susceptibility to cholinesterase hydrolysis.

**Carbamylcholine** (carbachol) has both muscarinic and nicotinic properties, but at usual therapeutic doses it produces mainly muscarinic actions. It selectively stimulates the urinary and gastrointestinal tracts, but it is not used for this purpose because of its concomitant ganglion stimulant effects. It is available for use in ocular surgery to produce miosis and thus reduce intraocular pressure. It may also be used in the treatment of open-angle glaucoma resistant to pilocarpine therapy.

**FIGURE 12-1** Structural formulae of acetylcholine and analogues.

**Methacholine** has a resistance to hydrolysis similar to that of carbachol but possesses much less nicotinic action. It has marked effects on the cardiovascular system that limit its therapeutic use. The main application of methacholine is by inhalation in the diagnosis of bronchial hyper-reactivity and asthma.

**Bethanechol** (carbamyl-β-methylcholine) demonstrates selectivity for the smooth muscle of the intestine and bladder. Thus, it is mainly used to increase gastrointestinal motility and to overcome urinary retention consequent to anaesthesia or vagotomy. It has also been used to test pancreatic function since it increases secretion but constricts the sphincter of Oddi. This results in an increase in plasma amylase, because the secreted amylase cannot reach the intestine and is reabsorbed into the blood. Pancreatic function can thus be correlated with plasma amylase levels.

## Cholinesterase Inhibitors

All clinically used cholinesterase blockers inhibit both acetylcholinesterase and plasma cholinesterase, although not always to the same extent, depending upon the chemical interaction between the drug and enzyme. Chemically, there are two main classes of compounds that inhibit acetylcholinesterase: carbamate derivatives, which are reversible inhibitors, and organophosphates, which inhibit acetylcholinesterase irreversibly by forming stable complexes with it. The main pharmacological effects of cholinesterase inhibitors are the result of an increase in endogenous acetylcholine due to inhibition of degradation by the enzymes.

These agents are considered more selective than the directly acting agents (i.e., cholinergic agonists) because they increase acetylcholine levels only at cholinergic sites that actively release the neurotransmitter. Since the mechanism of action of cholinesterase inhibitors is dependent upon there being active release of acetylcholine, in organs (e.g., endothelial cells) that do not receive cholinergic innervation and in which no acetylcholine is released, inhibition of acetylcholinesterase does not produce a pharmacological effect.

Following a lethal overdose of most acetylcholinesterase inhibitors, a characteristic sequence of reactions results from the rapid accumulation of acetylcholine at the various receptor sites. Restlessness usually develops early and reflects the central actions of acetylcholine. This is accompanied by increasing abdominal distress, with more and more severe pain due to intestinal spasm. There is frequent, involuntary defecation and urination. The pupils of the eyes become constricted (miosis). The skeletal muscles show fasciculation (i.e., small groups of muscle fibres twitch but produce no coordinated movement), so there is virtual paralysis. There is also increased glandular activity with salivation, lacrimation, sweating, and increased bronchial secretion. At the

same time, there is a bronchiolar constriction that, with the accumulation of bronchial secretions, results in stertorous, difficult breathing. Later, there are usually convulsions, during which the breathing ceases. The heart, although slowed, continues to beat for some time after breathing stops. Ultimately, death is due to respiratory failure.

### Acetylcholinesterase structure

The active site of acetylcholinesterase consists of an anionic site, which interacts with the quaternary nitrogen on the choline moiety of acetylcholine, and an esteratic site, which interacts with and hydrolyzes the ester grouping of acetylcholine (Fig. 12-2). A serine hydroxyl group at the esteratic site accepts the acetyl group and becomes acetylated but is subsequently regenerated by interaction with water.

Plasma cholinesterase shows genetic variation, and some individuals have an atypical variant that has very low hydrolytic activity. This will influence the pharmacokinetics of many drugs with ester linkages (see Chapter 10). Acetylcholinesterase variants have not been observed, probably because "atypical" acetylcholinesterase would be lethal in the first hours of life.

### Reversible cholinesterase inhibitors

These agents are competitive inhibitors of the cholinesterases (Fig. 12-3). They are a chemically heterogeneous group of substances. The earlier ones have carbamyl ester linkages that are slowly hydrolyzed by the enzyme, resulting in a reversible carbamylation of the enzyme. The newer ones include pyridine and acridine derivatives that act by quite different mechanisms. These various agents have mainly muscarinic side effects that can be blocked by atropine.

*Physostigmine (eserine).* This is an alkaloid extracted from the Calabar bean; its effects were utilized in many African "trial-by-ordeal" ceremonies. It is lipid-soluble and can therefore cross the blood–brain barrier and produce CNS side effects. Its main use is in the treatment of glaucoma. It is readily absorbed locally from eye drops

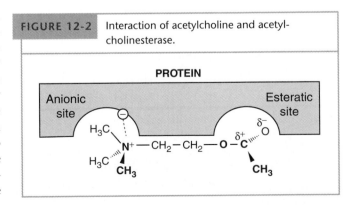

FIGURE 12-2  Interaction of acetylcholine and acetylcholinesterase.

**FIGURE 12-3** Structural formulae of some reversible cholinesterase inhibitors.

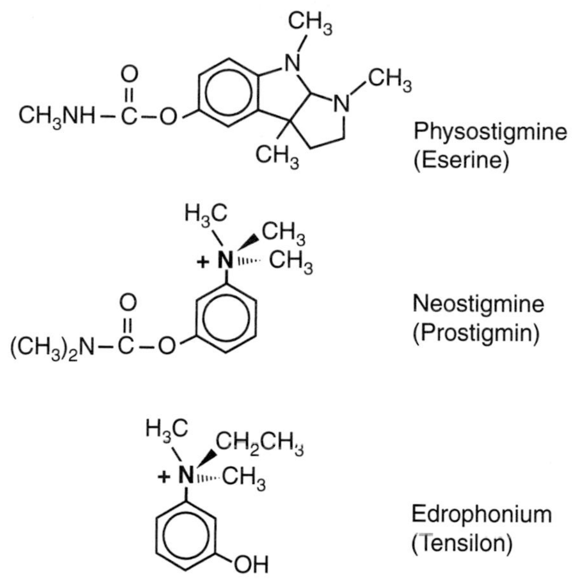

and, by increasing the availability of acetylcholine, reduces intraocular pressure, mainly by facilitating the outflow of aqueous humor.

*Neostigmine, pyridostigmine, ambenonium.* These anticholinesterases are all quaternary ammonium compounds and therefore do not readily cross the blood–brain barrier. They also have some direct nicotinic agonist actions in skeletal muscle, which makes them very suitable for the treatment of myasthenia gravis (see Chapter 15). Ambenonium has the longest duration of action, whereas neostigmine has the shortest. They are taken orally for the treatment of myasthenia gravis. Some CNS side effects are observed with ambenonium because it does appear to cross the blood–brain barrier to some extent, although slowly.

In addition to the common muscarinic side effects found with cholinesterase inhibitors, all of the reversible inhibitors described above, as well as the irreversible inhibitors described in the next section, can produce a potentially fatal cholinergic crisis as a consequence of excess acetylcholine producing a depolarizing block at the neuromuscular junctions. The major symptom is muscle paralysis resembling myasthenia gravis, the disease these agents are being used to treat.

*Edrophonium.* This is a short-acting, reversible cholinesterase inhibitor that is given by intravenous injection to diagnose myasthenia gravis and to differentiate between it and a cholinergic crisis. It has a brief duration of action (3 to 4 minutes). The myasthenic patient will experience transient improvement; a patient in a cholinergic crisis will become transiently worse.

*Donepezil, rivastigmine, and galantamine.* These newer reversible cholinesterase inhibitors are used mainly to improve or maintain cognitive function in the treatment of Alzheimer's disease, which is characterized by the loss of central cholinergic function. Donepezil (Aricept), rivastigmine (Exelon), and galantamine (Reminyl) readily cross the blood–brain barrier and exhibit relative specificity for inhibition of acetylcholinesterase and low activity for the plasma cholinesterases. These drugs have been shown to improve cognitive function in mild to moderate stages of Alzheimer's disease and certain other forms of dementia, including that associated with some cases of parkinsonism. They are well tolerated and have fewer peripheral side effects (nausea, vomiting, diarrhea) than the older agents. These drugs do not share the hepatotoxic effects of **tacrine**, which was the first cholinesterase inhibitor used in the treatment of Alzheimer's, but was non-specific.

## Irreversible cholinesterase inhibitors

This class of cholinesterase inhibitors, which consists of hundreds of active organophosphorus chemicals, is important more for toxicological than for therapeutic reasons. These agents include nerve gases for biological warfare and insecticides (Fig. 12-4). They produce phosphonylation or phosphorylation of the esteratic site of acetylcholinesterase, and once this covalent interaction is complete, it cannot be reversed. The reaction takes place in three stages, as shown in Figure 12-5.

1. The reversible phase in which the irreversible inhibitor competes with acetylcholine for binding to the acetylcholinesterase. This stage may be symptom-free.
2. Phosphorylation of the serine residue occurs in the esteratic site. At this stage, the acetylcholinesterase can be reactivated by pralidoxime (2-PAM; see Fig. 12-4), which binds close to the esteratic site and has a hydroxyl side chain that can lead to dephosphorylation at a higher rate than the free water present.
3. This is an "aging" process in which there is loss of an alkyl group or migration of the phosphoryl group to a histidine. The enzyme is now irreversibly inhibited, and restoration of cholinesterase activity requires *de novo* synthesis of acetylcholinesterase.

*Nerve gases.* These inhibitors are volatile liquids that have been studied since World War II as potential chemical weapons to be used as sprays or aerosols. Being very highly lipid-soluble, they rapidly penetrate intact skin and mucous membranes, enter the circulation, and quickly reach all central and peripheral cholinergic synapses. Accidental contact with these agents has occurred through incautious handling in laboratories, storage depots and so forth, and during poorly controlled

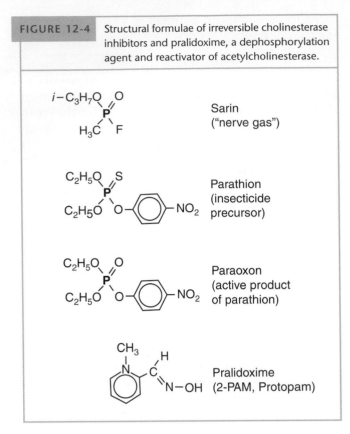

FIGURE 12-4  Structural formulae of irreversible cholinesterase inhibitors and pralidoxime, a dephosphorylation agent and reactivator of acetylcholinesterase.

Sarin ("nerve gas")

Parathion (insecticide precursor)

Paraoxon (active product of parathion)

Pralidoxime (2-PAM, Protopam)

testing in the field. Incidents of deliberate use as chemical weapons during armed conflicts in various parts of the world have occurred in recent years. High concentrations kill almost instantaneously; low concentrations are more insidious because symptoms may develop slowly and resemble mental or neurological illness. The fluorine-containing organophosphate cholinesterase inhibitors, such as sarin, have also been shown to induce a delayed neurotoxicity even when present in trace amounts. Reactivation of the enzyme with 2-PAM (see "Cholinesterase reactivators" below) can be achieved only within the first few minutes following exposure.

*Insecticides.* These are organophosphate cholinesterase inhibitors that have been designed to be more toxic to insects than to mammals. They are all thiophosphates that must be converted to phosphates (by replacement of the sulfur with oxygen) to become activated. This occurs very rapidly in insects but more slowly in humans. The commercially available insecticides are developed to be readily inactivated by mammalian metabolism, thus minimizing toxicity to humans and domestic animals.

However, these compounds do cause human toxicity through accumulation from repeated exposure of persons handling them in their daily work. Mild poisoning may produce only nausea, headache, and weakness. This may lead to unusual neurological symptoms that may not be

recognized as being due to poisoning. Since these agents are also very lipid-soluble, they may concentrate in body fat, which will form a reservoir from which the insecticide may leak slowly back into the circulation where it can be activated. Atropine can be used to block muscarinic side effects, and unless the level of inhibitor is very high, careful support of the patient and the use of artificial respiration may allow survival until *de novo* synthesis of acetylcholinesterase returns the patient to normal.

### Cholinesterase reactivators

The phosphorylated acetylcholinesterase can be reactivated before the "aging" process occurs (see Fig. 12-5). The drug used for this purpose is pralidoxime (pyridine-2-aldoxime, 2-PAM; see Fig. 12-4).

The ability of 2-PAM to reactivate the enzyme is a function of the phosphoryl group and the rate at which stage III of the inhibition process occurs, which is also a function of the organophosphate structure. 2-PAM does not influence carbamylation of acetylcholinesterase, and because it has some anticholinesterase activity of its own, it is contraindicated in the presence of overdose of a reversible cholinesterase inhibitor.

### Therapeutic use

Echothiophate (Phospholine Iodide) is one of the few organophosphates used clinically. It is a thiocholine analogue that is fairly stable and has a long duration of action (100 hours). It is the only one of these compounds used mainly in the treatment of open-angle glaucoma, but with caution even in pilocarpine-resistant cases since there is a risk of developing cataracts following use of these compounds. Topical application of this long-lasting cholinesterase inhibitor can present a risk of systemic effects since it causes a reduction in the total body content of acetylcholinesterase. It should therefore not be used within 4 to 6 weeks before surgery because of possible complications with muscle relaxants. Muscarinic side effects can be overcome with atropine, or they may be reversed with 2-PAM. Other organophosphate cholinesterases are used in veterinary medicine.

## Dopamine Antagonists

Incompetence of the gastroesophageal sphincter that results in lower esophageal sphincter pressure can lead to reflux of acidic gastric contents into the lower esophagus, producing irritation of the esophageal mucosa and reflux esophagitis. Although direct-acting cholinergic drugs can increase sphincter tone, they also increase gastric secretion. Indirectly acting agents such as metoclopramide are therefore preferred.

**Metoclopramide** (Fig. 12-6) increases gastroesophageal sphincter pressure, increases the force of esophageal peristalsis, increases the rate of gastric emptying without

**FIGURE 12-5** The steps of acetylcholinesterase inhibition by organophosphorus compounds, and enzyme reactivation with pralidoxime (pyridine-2-aldoxime, 2-PAM).

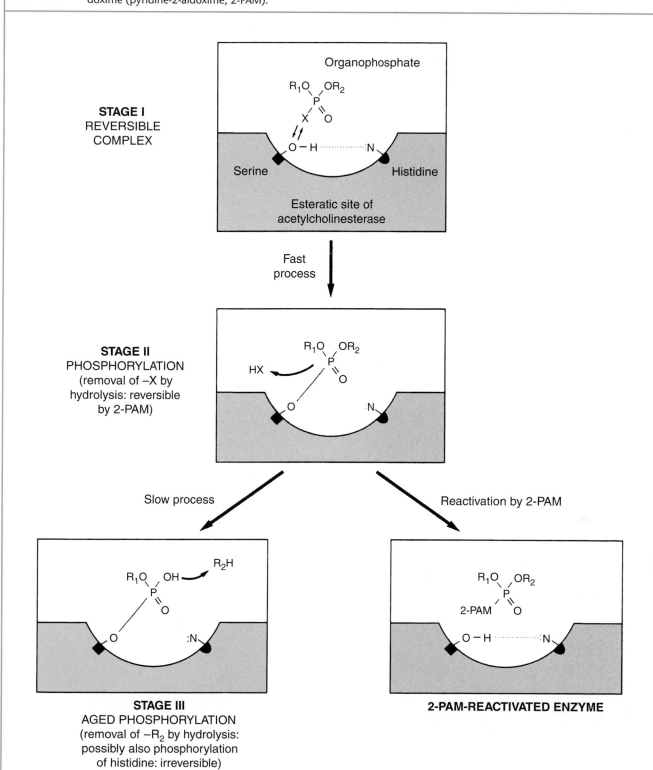

STAGE I
REVERSIBLE
COMPLEX

Organophosphate

Serine

Histidine

Esteratic site of
acetylcholinesterase

Fast
process

STAGE II
PHOSPHORYLATION
(removal of –X by
hydrolysis: reversible
by 2-PAM)

HX

Slow process

Reactivation by 2-PAM

2-PAM

STAGE III
AGED PHOSPHORYLATION
(removal of –R$_2$ by hydrolysis:
possibly also phosphorylation
of histidine: irreversible)

2-PAM-REACTIVATED ENZYME

FIGURE 12-6 Structural formula of metoclopramide.

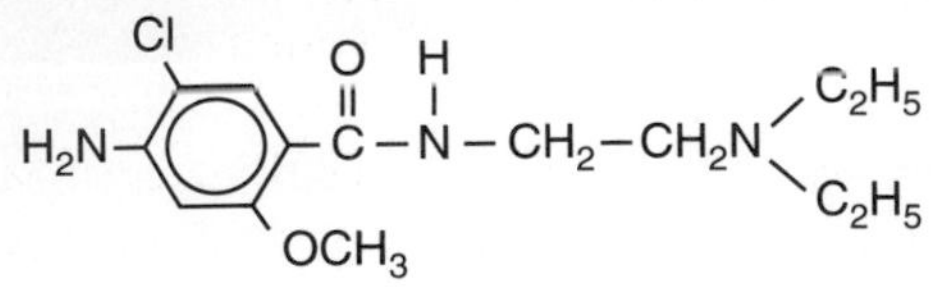

influencing the rate of acid secretion, and increases small intestinal motility. It has been shown to markedly reduce reflux esophagitis, but it has not proven to be effective in the treatment of gastric ulcer (see Chapter 41).

Metoclopramide is a dopamine $D_2$ receptor antagonist with some neuroleptic properties; it is used extensively as a centrally acting antiemetic. Its effects on gastrointestinal motility (see Chapter 42) are employed to speed up the absorption of drugs that are taken up in the lower intestine or to hasten the passage of barium contrast medium through the small intestine. It is also used to facilitate gastrointestinal intubation.

Its mode of action is not clearly understood. It may work by reducing the dopaminergic inhibitory tone on the cholinergic ganglia of the myenteric plexus. This is analogous to the dopaminergic/cholinergic interaction in the basal ganglia (see Chapters 16 and 17) and is consistent with the fact that parkinsonian side effects occur in some patients receiving metoclopramide. It has also been reported to increase the sensitivity of intestinal smooth muscle to acetylcholine. Anticholinergic drugs diminish the effects of metoclopramide.

In spite of its structural resemblance to procainamide, metoclopramide is only a poor local anaesthetic.

# NICOTINE, LOBELINE, AND ARECOLINE

## Nicotine

Nicotine (Fig. 12-7) is of significant medical and pharmacological interest for a number of reasons. First, it is the drug that was initially used to characterize nicotinic pharmacological responses. Second, nicotine is pharmacologically the most active ingredient of tobacco, and the use of the nicotine transdermal patch to reduce tobacco use is now widespread. Third, nicotine is a potent and rapidly acting poison that, when used as an insecticide, can be fatal to human life.

Nicotine is a naturally occurring alkaloid found in the leaves of the tobacco plant. It is a colourless liquid that turns brown upon exposure to air. It is volatile and therefore is easily inhaled with tobacco smoke. It penetrates not only mucous membranes but also intact skin, a property which has permitted the development of the transdermal nicotine patch. In the body, most (80 to 90%) of it is inactivated fairly rapidly (within 2 to 4 hours) by multiple pathways in the liver and lung, but some is excreted unchanged. The major metabolite is cotinine, formed by the sequential action of a P450 enzyme and an aldehyde oxidase. The other primary metabolites are nicotine-1'-N-oxide and 3-hydroxycotinine.

Nicotine is an agonist at the cholinergic receptors located on the autonomic ganglia, and it produces pharmacological effects, in a dose-dependent manner, that are complex and unpredictable. Nicotine intake, in a dose equivalent to the smoking of one or two cigarettes (roughly 0.3 to 1 mg), usually causes a slight increase in heart rate, some rise of blood pressure, and a modest increase in respiratory rate. These effects are comparable to those of mild exercise. Skin temperature and cutaneous blood flow decrease. Secretion of vasopressin (antidiuretic hormone, ADH) is stimulated, with consequent suppression of diuresis; therefore, smoking tests have been proposed for diagnostic distinction between pituitary and other forms of diabetes insipidus. Nicotine-induced release of adrenaline from the adrenal medulla leads to an increase in blood sugar. Effects on mood are difficult to measure; some persons feel stimulated, others sedated. All these effects tend to be qualitatively similar whether the person is a smoker or a non-smoker. In the latter, there may also be nausea and vomiting, an urge to defecate, and sometimes tremor.

The effects of small amounts of nicotine are due to the following actions. The smallest doses stimulate the

FIGURE 12-7 Structural formulae of nicotine, lobeline, and arecoline.

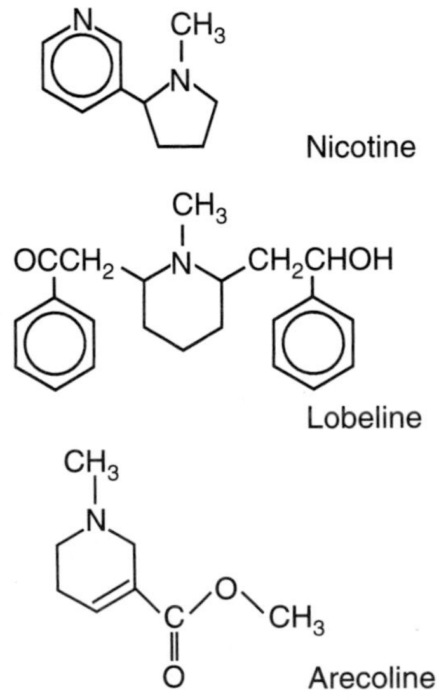

chemoreceptors in the carotid and aortic bodies. This accounts primarily for the effects on respiration. The first circulatory effects are mostly due to noradrenaline release from sympathetic fibres within vascular walls and within the heart muscle. Furthermore, the adrenal medulla is stimulated to release adrenaline, and the supraoptic nucleus is stimulated to release ADH.

Somewhat higher doses of nicotine are necessary to act upon autonomic ganglia. With increasing dosage, there is the following sequence: stimulation of sympathetic ganglia, stimulation of parasympathetic ganglia, blockade of parasympathetic ganglia. These actions account for the gastrointestinal effects and the increasing disturbance of circulation and respiration. Blockade of sympathetic ganglia usually requires very high doses and is seen only during the final stages of intoxication. Tremor and nausea are due to separate actions in the CNS. Radioreceptor assays have demonstrated the presence of nicotinic receptors in the CNS, and nicotine can cross the blood–brain barrier rapidly.

After inadvertent intake of toxic amounts, for example, an insecticide containing 40% nicotine (Black Leaf 40), dyspnea develops rapidly. Gradually, the blood pressure rises exceedingly high (250 to 300 mmHg) while the pulse is very slow. There is diarrhea. Twitching and fasciculation of skeletal muscles are soon followed by paralysis. Death is due to failure of the respiratory muscles and usually occurs within 15 to 30 minutes of nicotine intake. This occurs because, in a very high dose, nicotine behaves like a depolarizing relaxant of skeletal muscle, and paralysis is the usual cause of death in fatal poisoning (see Chapter 15). The emergency treatment of acute poisoning, therefore, is artificial respiration to support the patient over the critical period.

Chronic intoxication is possible. The repeated liberation of noradrenaline in the walls of blood vessels, over long periods of time, leads to vasoconstriction and interference with circulation in susceptible vascular beds. Thus, gangrene and loss of limbs or blindness may occur in predisposed persons. Women who smoke during pregnancy often have smaller-than-average babies. It is not entirely clear whether this represents a retardation of growth or premature delivery, but animal data support the notion of growth inhibition due to nicotine, as well as to high carbon monoxide levels in the blood and tissues.

The effects of tobacco smoke and nicotine are not completely identical. Production of cancer, allergic reactions, and smoking-related impairment of pulmonary function are probably not due to nicotine. More than 260 different chemicals have been identified in tobacco smoke, including potentially toxic amounts of carbon monoxide, cyanide, and oxide of nitrogen. However, the intermittent "puffing" and the dilution of smoke upon inhalation seem to reduce their acute toxicity. (Ingestion of a whole or part of a cigarette would contain a toxic dose of nicotine—up to 22 mg.)

Nevertheless, nicotine self-administration is an important aspect of smoking. Nicotine has reinforcing effects (see Chapter 69) and is the component of tobacco that causes dependence in the tobacco user. The craving for nicotine, and the withdrawal symptoms associated with it, make it difficult to quit smoking "cold turkey." The symptoms of nicotine withdrawal can be reduced by administering nicotine; this is best accomplished with the transdermal nicotine patch. The nicotine patch, by slowly releasing low concentrations of nicotine, can reduce the craving for a cigarette without producing other pharmacological effects. The dose must be adjusted to the individual user. Many reported failures of the nicotine patch result from the side effects of patches that release too much nicotine. A similar principle applies to nicotine-containing chewing gum (Nicorette) used as a smoking-cessation aid.

## Lobeline

Another natural alkaloid that shares similar nicotinic properties is lobeline (see Fig. 12-7). Lobeline, from *Lobelia inflata*, is a nicotinic agonist that was used in the past to ameliorate nicotine withdrawal symptoms during cessation of smoking. Although it is less potent than nicotine, it can increase respiration by stimulating the carotid body, and it was at one time used as a drug for resuscitation.

## Arecoline

Arecoline (see Fig. 12-7) is derived from a seed commonly known as the betel nut (*Areca catechu*). Its peripheral actions are similar to those of the synthetic agent methacholine (see below). Arecoline has no therapeutic use in humans, but it is of interest because the betel nut is habitually chewed by a large part of the world's population for its euphoriant effects. In many countries bordering the Indian and Pacific Oceans, millions of people who do not smoke tobacco show an equivalent addiction to chewing the betel nut. Arecoline produces central effects that are analogous to those of nicotine. When used to excess, however, it can also produce toxicity that includes a variety of peripheral autonomic cholinergic effects on cardiovascular, pulmonary, and other systems. Among these adverse effects are exacerbation of asthma, cardiac arrhythmias, excessive glandular secretions, abdominal cramps, and skeletal muscle weakness.

# AUTONOMIC CHOLINERGIC BLOCKING DRUGS

## Muscarinic Receptor Antagonists

The muscarinic receptor blocking drugs act as antagonists to selectively block the effects of acetylcholine and other cholinergic agonists that stimulate muscarinic receptors at parasympathetic post-ganglionic sites and, if they can cross the blood–brain barrier, in the CNS. This class of drugs was frequently referred to as "cholinergic antagonists" or "anticholinergics" without specific reference to their selectivity for the muscarinic receptors, but it is now commonly referred to as "anti-muscarinics."

## Principles of action

As described in Chapter 11, muscarinic agonists bind to receptor sites with three different levels of affinity. However, the antagonists that have been examined appear to bind with equal affinity to all three states of the receptor. As shown in Table 12-1, the interactions of a number of cholinergic agonists and antagonists with radioactive ligands that label muscarinic receptors have been examined (see Chapter 8). This table shows that the muscarinic antagonists studied have a similar affinity for the receptor regardless of whether it is labelled with an agonist ($^3$H-oxotremorine) or an antagonist ($^3$H-propylbenzilylcholine). It is clear that the antagonist binding site is different from the agonist site, but it does include the agonist site within its binding domain. The antagonists have binding affinities that are much higher (i.e., reflected by the much lower $IC_{50}$ values) than those of agonists (e.g., acetylcholine), even when the radiolabelled compound is an agonist. It is also apparent that nicotinic agonists and antagonists have a very low affinity for the muscarinic receptor, as shown by the very high $IC_{50}$ values.

In this fashion, the radioreceptor binding assay may be used as a predictive indicator of the pharmacological effects of muscarinic antagonists. The higher their affinity in a radioreceptor binding experiment, the more potent they are clinically. Pirenzepine, a muscarinic antagonist, was predicted (and found) to be a more selective inhibitor of gastric secretion than of gastric motility on the basis of its unusual relative selectivity for the "high-affinity" ($M_1$) agonist site over the "low-affinity" ($M_2$) agonist site.

The blockade of muscarinic receptors by these antagonists is competitive and depends on the relative concentrations of the antagonist and acetylcholine and their relative affinities for the receptors. As is the case with most families of antagonists, they are slightly more effective against exogenously applied agonist than against acetylcholine released endogenously as a neurotransmitter. Pre-ganglionic cholinergic nerve stimulation in the presence of a muscarinic antagonist still stimulates autonomic nicotinic ganglia, but only sympathetic effects are elicited since the post-ganglionic parasympathetic effector sites are blocked.

## Pharmacological effects

The muscarinic antagonists possess no intrinsic activity, and the effects seen when they bind to the muscarinic receptor result exclusively from blocking receptor activa-

**TABLE 12-1** Muscarinic Receptor Binding: $IC_{50}$ Values for Various Cholinergic Agonists and Antagonists against Ligands That Label Muscarinic Cholinergic Receptors

| Competing Cold Ligand | $^3$H Ligand | | |
| --- | --- | --- | --- |
| | $^3$H-Propyl-benzilylcholine* (antagonist) (nM) | $^3$H-Oxotremorine* (agonist) (nM) | $^3$H-Quinuclidinyl Benzilate[†] (antagonist) (nM) |
| Muscarinic agonists | | | |
| Acetylcholine | 3300 | 200 | 3000 |
| Oxotremorine | 460 | 38 | 700 |
| Methacholine | 2000 | 350 | 2500 |
| Muscarine | 8300 | — | — |
| Carbachol | 15 000 | 240 | 25 000 |
| Muscarinic antagonists | | | |
| Atropine | 0.59 | 3.0 | 3.0 |
| Benzhexol | 7.10 | 25.0 | — |
| Methylatropine | 0.35 | 0.7 | 0.2 |
| Nicotinic agonists and antagonists | | | |
| Nicotine, d-Tubocurarine, Hexamethonium | >100 000 | >100 000 | >100 000 |

*From Birdsall NJM, et al. Mol Pharmacol. 1978;14:723-736.
[†]Yamamura HI, Snyder SH. Mol Pharmacol. 1974;10:861-867.
— = not measured.

tion by cholinergic agonists or acetylcholine released from the nerve terminal. The effects of the prototypical muscarinic antagonist, atropine (Fig. 12-8), are described below. The effects of atropine are not necessarily used therapeutically in all the sites mentioned below. The list is intended only to show the wide range of functional results of muscarinic receptor blockade. Newer agents are usually preferred because of greater selectivity of action on specific receptors.

*Exocrine glands.* **Salivary** secretion is impaired even after very small doses of atropine, which result in dry mouth and difficulty in swallowing.

**Gastric** secretion is diminished, although gastric pH is unchanged. Therefore, the main contribution of atropine in the treatment of peptic ulcer is relief of spasm (see "Smooth muscle" below).

**Bronchial** secretions are suppressed. This action renders atropine useful as pre-anaesthetic medication for general anaesthesia, to reduce bronchial secretion induced by some inhalation anaesthetics and by intubation.

**Sweating** is impaired. The inability to perspire may interfere with heat regulation, which can be fatal in very hot weather.

**FIGURE 12-8** Structural formulae of natural muscarinic antagonists.

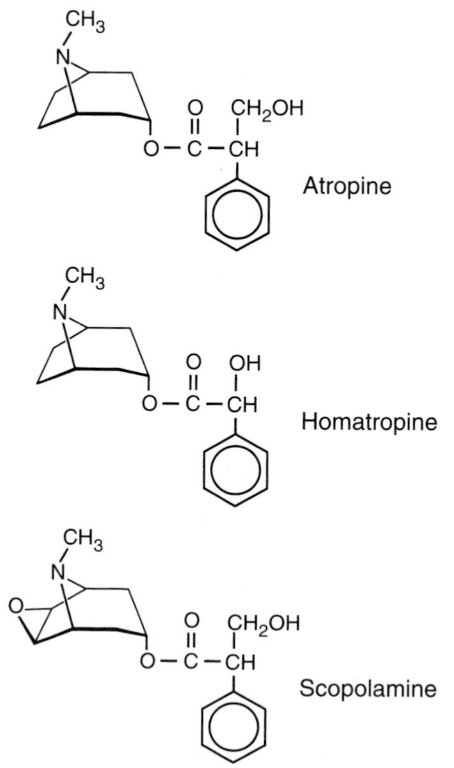

*Smooth muscle.* In the **gastrointestinal tract**, atropine abolishes excessive tone and motility, but it has relatively little effect on normal motility. It is therefore spasmolytic but not constipating. Atropine is particularly effective in relieving spasms of the cardiac sphincter of the stomach, whereas effects on the pyloric sphincter are less reliable.

Atropine has some relaxing action on the **biliary tract** and is moderately effective in relieving biliary colic. It does not influence the formation of bile.

In therapeutic doses, atropine affects the **urinary tract** by diminishing the tone of the fundus of the bladder but increasing the tone of the vesical sphincter. This may cause retention of urine, which can be a serious side effect in patients after surgery and in elderly men with prostatic hypertrophy. This effect is utilized, however, to suppress the frequency and urgency of micturition in cystitis, and it is also exploited in the control of nocturnal enuresis. Atropine also reduces tone and motility of the ureter and thus relieves attacks of renal colic.

*Circulation.* Low doses of atropine (0.2 mg) decrease the heart rate by 10 to 15 beats/min (bradycardia). This decrease is likely a CNS effect due to stimulation of the medullary centres, including the vagal nucleus. In contrast, larger doses (2 mg) of atropine produce the expected effect on the heart rate, which increases by 40 to 50 beats/min (tachycardia) as a result of direct vagal blockade (parasympathetic innervation to the heart). Atropine in therapeutic doses (0.5 to 1 mg) in the adult usually has a dual effect: first a decrease and then an increase of the heart rate. The bradycardia is due to stimulation of the cardioinhibitory centre in the medulla, while the tachycardia is in response to the muscarinic antagonist effects of atropine in the SA node of the heart. There is no major effect on blood vessels, so blood pressure is not affected. Although there is no tonic cholinergic stimulation of the smooth muscle of blood vessels, high doses of atropine can cause selective vasodilatation, including flushing of the face. It is not clear whether this effect is due to direct effects of atropine or is a response to inhibition of sweating and hyperthermia.

There are relatively few therapeutic uses for atropine in relation to cardiovascular function, but intravenous atropine is effective in overcoming excessive bradycardia caused by hypersensitivity to reflexes such as the baroreceptor reflex or the oculocardiac reflex response to traction on the eyeball in pediatric ophthalmologic surgery.

*The eye.* Atropine has two primary effects on the eye— namely, mydriasis (dilatation of the pupil) and cycloplegia (paralysis of accommodation)—which it causes by antagonizing acetylcholine, as shown in Figure 12-9. Both effects can be produced by systemic application of atropine, but they are most prominent after local application, because local application of concentrated solutions produces much

**FIGURE 12-9**    Innervation of the lens and iris of the eye.

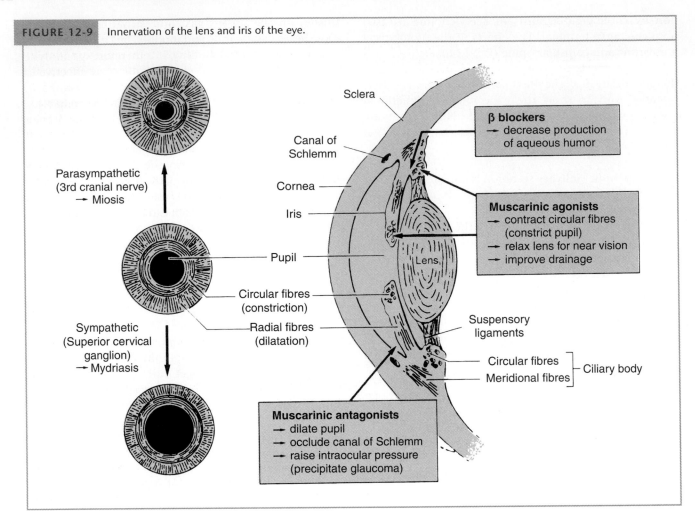

higher intraocular concentrations of atropine than is achieved by systemically tolerable oral or parenteral doses.

This combination of effects makes atropine an important drug in ophthalmology because it permits precise measurements of refraction. The mydriatic effect is utilized in cases of iritis. In eyes with a narrow chamber angle (i.e., the angle between iris and cornea), dilatation of the pupil may cause the iris muscle to block the canal of Schlemm and thereby interfere with the drainage of aqueous humor. In this way, atropine may produce an attack of glaucoma in predisposed persons, which may cause them to lose their eyesight. The effects of atropine applied as eye drops usually disappear in some hours, but occasionally may be noticeable for as long as a week.

*Central nervous system.* Atropine in the usual therapeutic doses has no significant effects upon the CNS because of its limited entry into the CNS. It has few uses here except for its beneficial suppression of tremor and rigidity in Parkinson's disease. This is due primarily to a central action (see Chapter 17), but some effect upon muscle spindles may also contribute to the effect.

In high doses (5 to 10 mg), atropine has profound effects on the brain that have been broadly classified as stimulatory, but disorientation is the most characteristic feature (see Chapter 26). After drug absorption, the subject first becomes restless and confrontational. This state of excitation may be followed by delirium. Usually, there is recovery without recollection; only rarely will the delirium progress into coma with respiratory failure and death.

The central effects of atropine-containing plant extracts differ slightly from those of the pure alkaloid because of the admixture of scopolamine (see "Naturally occurring plant alkaloids" below). Belladonna alkaloids were used as medicines for many centuries, but they also found much disreputable use in witchcraft and quackery. Remnants of these non-medicinal medieval uses are found in the mnemonic jingle on atropine poisoning:

> *Dry as a Bone,*
> *Blind as a Bat*
> *Red as a Beet,*
> *Mad as a Hatter.*

## Naturally occurring plant alkaloids in clinical use

*Atropine.* Atropine (see Fig. 12-8) is *dl*-hyoscyamine extracted from the belladonna (deadly nightshade), hyoscyamus (henbane), or stramonium (jimsonweed) plants, all of which belong to the potato family. *l*-Hyoscyamine is more potent than the racemic mixture atropine, but it is less stable.

Atropine is usually given as the sulfate, subcutaneously in doses of 0.5 to 1 mg. The effects of oral doses are less intense and occur more slowly. In the treatment of anticholinesterase poisoning, atropine may need to be given intravenously. For ophthalmic purposes, atropine is applied directly to the eye in solution or ointment. Narrow-angle glaucoma is a contraindication to its use.

The duration of action varies depending on the dose, route of administration, and respective organ. The systemic effects of atropine, whether it is administered orally or subcutaneously, last only a few hours, so the dose must be repeated every 4 to 6 hours. Following local application of atropine to the eye, however, impairment of accommodation may persist for 3 or 4 days, and dilatation of the pupil even for 6 or 7 days. Application of reversible cholinesterase inhibitors is sometimes used to overcome this problem. However, the half-life of most reversible cholinesterase inhibitors is shorter than that of atropine, and the visual impairment can reappear unexpectedly.

Insofar as the cardiac and ocular effects of atropine are concerned, little or no tolerance develops. However, repeated doses of the drug produce diminishing effects upon the digestive tract and secretions. Appreciable tolerance can develop in patients receiving relatively large doses of atropine, as in the treatment of parkinsonism, so very high doses in the order of 50 mg/day may become necessary to maintain effectiveness. These changes may occur due to up-regulation of muscarinic receptors or because of a change in the conformation of the receptors. Chronic use also tends to cause urinary retention.

*Homatropine hydrobromide, homatropine methylbromide.* Homatropine, an analogue of atropine (see Fig. 12-8), has a more rapid onset and a shorter duration of action. However, it is less potent than atropine. The hydrobromide salt of homatropine is used solely by topical application for ophthalmic purposes; since it has a tertiary N atom, it would be able to enter the CNS if given systemically. The quaternary methyl analogues of homatropine (e.g., homatropine methylbromide) and atropine (methylatropine) are unable to cross the blood–brain barrier and therefore do not have the CNS effects of the parent compounds. Their main use is in the treatment of gastrointestinal disorders.

*Scopolamine.* Scopolamine (see Fig. 12-8) has the same peripheral actions as atropine but has a pronounced sedative action due to easier entry into the CNS. For a long time it was the only drug used to subdue highly agitated mentally ill patients. However, some people get excited after taking scopolamine, rather than sedated.

"Twilight sleep," resulting from a combination of scopolamine and morphine, at one time was very popular in surgery and obstetrics because the anticholinergic action of scopolamine produced amnesia for the events surrounding the surgery or childbirth. Its modern counterpart is the employment of neuroleptanalgesia by a combination of opioid and neuroleptic (see Chapter 20). In most individuals, scopolamine tends to counteract the respiratory depression produced by morphine. For unknown reasons, however, this combination produces in some subjects a pronounced, and potentially fatal, respiratory depression.

Scopolamine in a transdermal patch is used prophylactically to prevent motion sickness. It is not recommended for nausea and vomiting due to non-vestibular causes.

## Synthetic muscarinic antagonists

There are many synthetic substitutes for atropine (Fig. 12-10). Most of these drugs were developed to maximize specific actions of atropine for particular therapeutic uses.

*Suppression of gastric secretion.* The agents used for this purpose are all quaternary ammonium compounds and they exist as two types: those with mixed muscarinic and ganglion-blocking properties (e.g., **propantheline** and oxyphenonium), and those which are purely muscarinic antagonists (e.g., **pirenzepine** and **telenzepine**).

These antagonists all reduce gastric secretions, but the mixed antagonists reduce motility as well. The selectivity of pirenzepine for secretion formerly made it the muscarinic antagonist of choice in ulcer therapy, but it has now been replaced by histamine $H_2$ receptor blockers, proton pump inhibitors, and "cytoprotective" agents (see Chapter 41).

*Suppression of smooth muscle spasm in gastrointestinal tract, biliary tract, and ureter.* The drugs advocated for this purpose (e.g., **dicyclomine**; Bentylol) cause relaxation through their muscarinic antagonist actions as well as through a non-specific relaxant effect on smooth muscle. They are little used in clinical practice, atropine being preferred.

*Ophthalmic use.* For this purpose, use is made of short-acting muscarinic antagonists that are well absorbed from eye drops instilled in the conjunctival sacs (e.g., homatropine). However, they are tertiary amines and, therefore, can have CNS side effects including convulsions, psychotic disorders, and behavioural disturbances.

*Use in respiratory disorders.* Although the use of anticholinergic drugs in the treatment of asthma has been widely replaced by β-adrenergic drugs, the synthetic muscarinic antagonist **ipratropium** has been found useful to treat this disorder. Ipratropium bromide is a quaternary ammonium analogue of atropine that can be topically applied with the use of a metered-dose inhaler. In this manner, little of the drug is absorbed systemically, and thus, systemic antimuscarinic effects are not experienced. Unlike the older anti-muscarinics, ipratropium bromide has little effect on respiratory secretions or mucus transport. Ipratropium bromide is as effective as $\beta_2$ agonists for producing bronchodilatation in patients with chronic obstructive airway disease (COPD), but less effective in asthma. This agent is less suitable for emergencies, when bronchodilatation is required immediately.

*Anti-parkinsonian drugs.* Parkinson's disease, described in Chapter 17, is due to a progressive loss of dopamine innervation in the basal ganglia (important in motor coordination), resulting in an imbalance between cholinergic activity and dopaminergic activity. The drug of choice is L-dopa, which can restore dopamine levels, but unfortunately, it does not affect the progressive loss of dopaminergic neurons. Alternatively, muscarinic antagonists, such as **trihexyphenidyl** (Artane) and **benztropine** (Cogentin), can be used to block cholinergic activity to restore the balance, and thus, they may be useful adjuncts to L-dopa therapy. Occasionally, they are used in patients unresponsive to L-dopa, but they are not drugs of choice since the development of newer dopamine-selective agonists.

The central effects of these synthetic drugs are relatively stronger than their peripheral cholinergic blocking actions, although the latter exist and cannot be disregarded. However, urinary retention and interference with reading ability (caused by cycloplegia) are usually less bothersome than with atropine.

These drugs are used for symptomatic treatment irrespective of the origin of symptoms. Thus, they are not restricted to parkinsonism but are used also in similar disorders induced by phenothiazine antipsychotics and other drugs. The appearance of mental confusion and urinary retention usually indicates that the muscarinic antagonist has reached its limits of usefulness and should be withdrawn.

In addition to the few muscarinic antagonists mentioned above or shown in Figure 12-10, at least 15 other synthetic compounds have been used for this purpose.

## Nicotinic Receptor Antagonists and Ganglion Blockers

The nicotinic receptor blocking agents and ganglion blockers are drugs that competitively inhibit the actions of acetylcholine at autonomic ganglia. Nicotine (an agonist) in high doses can also block these receptors through a desensitization mechanism similar to that described for succinylcholine (see Chapter 15). There is no difference between the nicotinic receptors in sympathetic ganglia

**FIGURE 12-10** Structural formulae of some synthetic muscarinic antagonists.

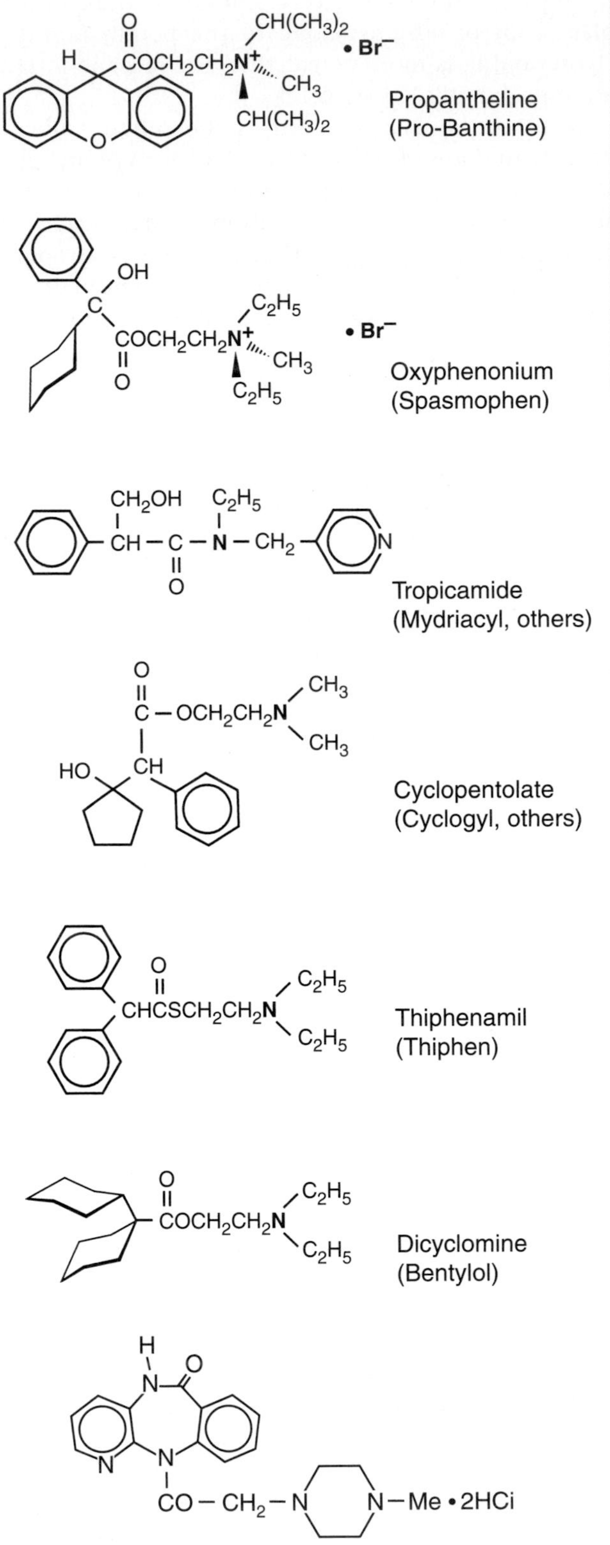

and those in parasympathetic ganglia. Any apparent selectivity in the blockade of sympathetic pathways as distinct from parasympathetic pathways results from the relative importance of the two pathways in controlling the function of a specific organ. Some differences in selectivity may be related to the anatomical location of the sympathetic ganglia a distance away from the innervated organ involved, whereas the parasympathetic ganglia are generally located within that organ. The blood flow through these two locations, and hence the delivery of drug to them, may be quite different.

The nicotinic receptors in autonomic ganglia are not identical to those at the neuromuscular junction. This is illustrated in Figure 12-11, which shows that the optimum carbon-chain length of a compound for ganglion blockade is not the same as for neuromuscular junction blockade. Nevertheless, drugs chosen for clinical use in neuromuscular blockade will have some ganglion-blocking side effects. Historically, ganglion blockers were important in the treatment of chronic hypertension because they lowered vascular sympathetic tone. They are no longer used for this purpose. The reasons become apparent from the description given below of the effects of **hexamethonium** (Fig. 12-12), a prototype of this class of drugs. The physiology of each organ determines its response to ganglion blockade. The wide spectrum of side effects has led to the withdrawal of these drugs from general use.

## Pharmacological effects

What will happen to a person constantly treated with hexamethonium is illustrated by Paton's tongue-in-cheek description of the **"hexamethonium man"**:

> He is a pink-complexioned person, except when he has stood in a queue for a long time, when he may get pale and faint. His handshake is warm and dry. He is a placid and relaxed companion; for instance he may laugh, but he can't cry because the tears cannot come. Your rudest story will not make him blush, and the most unpleasant circumstances will fail to make him turn pale. His collars and socks stay very clean and sweet. He wears corsets and may, if you meet him out, be rather fidgety (corsets to compress his splanchnic vascular pool, fidgety to keep the venous return going from his legs). He dislikes speaking much unless helped with something to moisten his dry mouth and throat. He is long-sighted and easily blinded by bright light. The redness of his eyeballs may suggest irregular habits and in fact his head is rather weak. But he always behaves like a gentleman and never belches nor hiccups. He tends to get cold and keeps well wrapped up. But his health is good; he does not have chilblains and those diseases of modern civilization, hypertension and peptic ulcer, pass him by. He is thin because his appetite is modest; he never feels hunger pains and his stomach

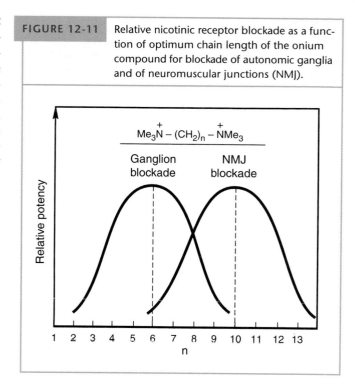

**FIGURE 12-11** Relative nicotinic receptor blockade as a function of optimum chain length of the onium compound for blockade of autonomic ganglia and of neuromuscular junctions (NMJ).

$$Me_3\overset{+}{N} - (CH_2)_n - \overset{+}{N}Me_3$$

Ganglion blockade  NMJ blockade

Relative potency

n: 1 2 3 4 5 6 7 8 9 10 11 12 13

never rumbles. He gets rather constipated so that his intake of liquid paraffin is high. As old age comes on, he will suffer from retention of urine and impotence, but frequency, precipitancy, and strangury will not worry him. One is uncertain how he will end, but perhaps if he is not careful, by eating less and less and getting colder and colder, he will sink into a symptomless, hypoglycemic coma and die, as was proposed for the universe, a sort of entropy death.

The effects of ganglion blockade upon the function of the various systems depend upon the dominant tone, parasympathetic or sympathetic, for each organ. Thus, sympathetic tone predominates in the vasomotor system, and the usual response to hexamethonium is a reduction in blood pressure, particularly in hypertensive subjects. However, the most important feature is the failure of the regulating interplay of vasoconstriction and vasodilatation, which keeps the blood properly distributed in response to exertion or mere changes in posture. After one has taken hexamethonium, one's blood distribution becomes principally determined by gravity. The "hexamethonium man" faints when the blood accumulates in his legs after he has been standing for a while. If the person is lying down and an arm or leg is held up, the limb becomes almost bloodless. Ganglion blockers are therefore used as an aid in special surgical procedures. The same principle is used if ganglion blockers are employed to combat pulmonary edema. While furosemide is the generally accepted drug of choice in

FIGURE 12-12  Structural formulae of the ganglion blockers hexamethonium and trimethaphan.

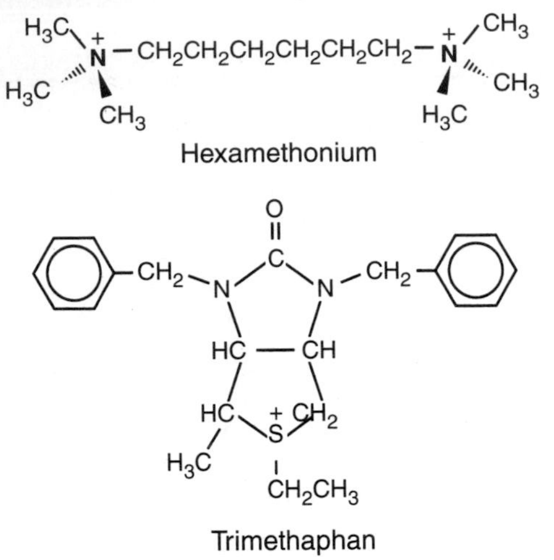

Hexamethonium

Trimethaphan

pulmonary edema, ganglion blockers have the advantage of decidedly faster action.

The iris is predominantly under parasympathetic control, so the response to ganglionic blockade is mydriasis. The gastrointestinal tract responds with partial or complete inhibition of gastric motility, some inhibition of salivary and gastric secretion, and disturbances of intestinal motility, usually constipation. In the respiratory tract, there is sometimes a decrease in nasopharyngeal secretion and some bronchodilatation. The skin becomes dry and flushed because of sympathetic blockade. There are no significant effects upon the CNS.

## Ganglionic blockers in current clinical use

**Trimethaphan camsylate** (Arfonad; see Fig. 12-12) is given only by continuous intravenous infusion. Its action is very rapid but brief, so the reduction of blood pressure can be controlled by varying the rate of infusion. Its main use is to treat acute hypertensive crises (see Chapter 34) and to reduce the circulating blood volume in the emergency treatment of pulmonary edema. It has been known to potentiate neuromuscular blockade in some patients. The drug releases histamine and should be avoided if there is a history of allergy.

## SUGGESTED READINGS

Brown DA, Abogadie FC, Allen TG, et al. Muscarinic mechanisms in nerve cells. *Life Sci.* 1997;60:1137-1144.

Burgen AS. Targets of drug action. *Annu Rev Pharmacol Toxicol.* 2000;40:1-16.

Caulfield MP, Birdsall NJ. International Union of Pharmacology. XVII. Classification of muscarinic acetylcholine receptors. *Pharmacol Rev.* 1998;50:279-290.

Caulfield MP, Robbins J, Higashida H, Brown DA. Postsynaptic actions of acetylcholine: the coupling of muscarinic receptor subtypes to neuronal ion channels. *Prog Brain Res.* 1993;98:293-301.

Coulson FR, Fryer AD. Muscarinic acetylcholine receptors and airway diseases. *Pharmacol Ther.* 2003;98:59-69.

Eglen RM, Chappin A, Watson N. Therapeutic opportunities from muscarinic receptor research. *Trends Pharmacol Sci.* 2001;22:409-414.

Eglen RM, Hedge SS, Watson N. Muscarinic receptor subtypes and smooth muscle function. *Pharmacol Rev.* 1996;48:531-565.

Fryxell KJ. The evolutionary divergence of neurotransmitter receptors and second-messenger pathways. *J Mol Evol.* 1995;41:85-97.

Hegde SS, Eglen RM. Muscarinic receptor subtypes modulating smooth muscle contractibility in the urinary baldder. *Life Sci.* 1999;64:419-428.

Kaneda M. Neuronal nicotinic receptors: molecular organization and regulation. *Neuropharmacology.* 1995;34:563-582.

Lockridge O, Masson P. Pesticides and susceptible populations: people with butyrylcholinesterase genetic variants may be at risk. *Neurotoxicology.* 2000;21:113-126.

Matsui M, Yamada S, Oki T, et al. Functional analysis of muscarinic acetylcholine receptors using knockout mice. *Life Sci.* 2004;75:2971-2981.

McGehee DS. Physiological diversity of nicotinic acetylcholine receptors expressed by vertebrate neurons. *Annu Rev Physiol.* 1995;57:521-546.

Nelson BS, Heischober B. Betel nut: a common drug used by naturalized citizens from India, Far East Asia, and the South Pacific Islands. *Ann Emerg Med.* 1999;34:238-243.

Newmark J. Nerve agents. *Neurol Clin.* 2005;23:623-641.

Paton WDM. The principles of ganglionic block. In: *Lectures on the Scientific Basis of Medicine.* Vol 2. London, United Kingdom: University of London, Athlone Press; 1954.

van Koppen CJ, Kaiser B. Regulation of muscarinic acetylcholine receptor signaling. *Pharmacol Ther.* 2003;98:197-220.

# 13

# Adrenergic Receptor Agonists

## AJ LANÇA

## CASE HISTORY

A 30-year-old man with a history of asthma, which was treated successfully with salmeterol and montelukast, had an anaphylactic reaction as a result of a bee sting. In this emergency, adrenaline 0.3 mg in sterile water was ordered to be given subcutaneously. By error, however, in the emergency room, the adrenaline was given intravenously. It resulted in dangerously high blood pressure (180/125 mmHg) and heart rate (125 bpm), cardiac arrhythmia, and an abnormal ECG (depressed T wave and ST segment deviation from the isoelectric line, both consistent with ischemia). The patient was clearly distressed, tense, and frightened. He had fine tremor of the hands and cold clammy skin, and he complained of a severe headache.

He was immediately given intravenous sodium nitroprusside by continuous infusion at a rate of 0.5 μg/kg/min, as well as propranolol by slow intravenous infusion at a rate of 1.0 mg/min. Continuous monitoring of the blood pressure, ECG, and cardiac function accompanied these interventions. Atropine was available, to be used if bradycardia should become a problem. The hypertension and tachycardia were successfully controlled by these measures. The patient's condition stabilized in a couple of hours without any significant rebound hypertension. However, the patient complained of respiratory difficulty, particularly in exhaling. Propranolol was replaced by atenolol, and within a few minutes, the respiratory symptoms were no longer present. The following day, atenolol was discontinued, the original anti-asthmatic medication was reinstated (i.e., salmeterol and montelukast), and he was able to return home.

On the recommendation of the family physician, in a follow-up visit the patient was given a prescription for a kit containing adrenaline to be administered intramuscularly. He was instructed on how to administer it with the auto-injector and was advised to carry it in case he suffered any subsequent anaphylactic attacks.

The sympathetic nervous system plays a critical role in the regulation of numerous physiological systems (e.g., cardiovascular, respiratory, and endocrine) and a vital role in homeostasis. Its neurotransmitters are the naturally occurring catecholamines (dopamine, noradrenaline, and adrenaline). Pharmacological agents that mimic the effects of these amines activate specific receptors and stimulate the sympathetic nervous system (adrenergic agonists or sympathomimetic drugs). Other compounds (adrenergic antagonists or sympatholytics) inhibit the sympathetic system (see also Chapters 11 and 14). Adrenergic drugs are among the most widely used drugs in medical practice, playing a role in the pharmacological treatment of a variety of disorders including regulation of blood pressure, respiratory functions, neuropsychiatric disorders, and movement control.

## CLASSIFICATION

Drugs acting on the sympathetic system, both agonists and antagonists, can be grouped according to their mechanism of action and specific target.

1. Some drugs, including the catecholamines, bind **directly** to the adrenergic G protein–coupled receptors and activate different G proteins, which trigger different signal transduction pathways (Fig. 13-1; see also Chapter 11). Conversely, though antagonists also bind selectively to the receptor, their binding does not elicit a receptor-mediated response. Instead, occupation of the receptor by the antagonist prevents receptor activation by the agonist and prevents the occurrence of the effects otherwise elicited by the agonist.

**FIGURE 13-1** Effects of substituting OH groups in the phenylethylamine molecule. Increasing the number of substitutions increases the pressor activity and introduces direct adrenergic receptor-stimulant action.

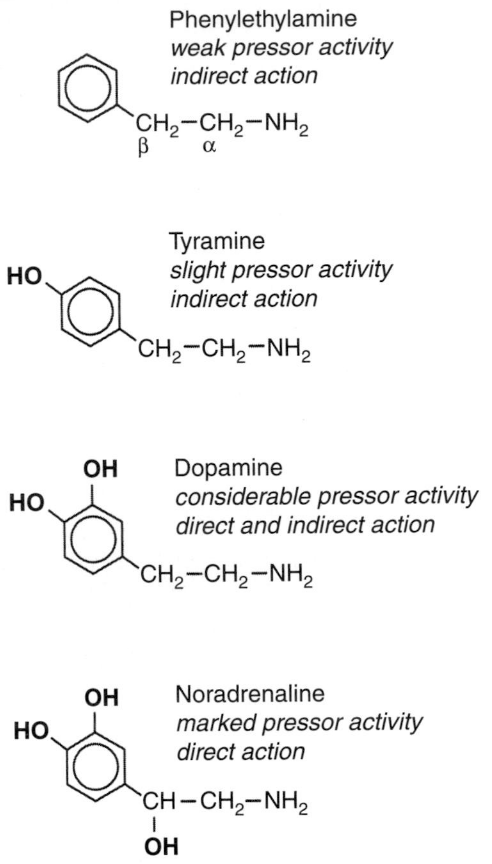

**Phenylethylamine**
*weak pressor activity
indirect action*

$CH_2-CH_2-NH_2$
β     α

**Tyramine**
*slight pressor activity
indirect action*

HO

$CH_2-CH_2-NH_2$

**Dopamine**
*considerable pressor activity
direct and indirect action*

OH

HO

$CH_2-CH_2-NH_2$

**Noradrenaline**
*marked pressor activity
direct action*

OH

HO

$CH-CH_2-NH_2$
|
**OH**

As described in Chapter 11, different adrenergic drugs have different affinities for the various types of receptor. This contributes to their different patterns of pharmacological effects, as described later in this chapter.

2. Some drugs, however, exert their effects not directly through receptor binding, but **indirectly,** as they target a variety of mechanisms involved in the synthesis, storage, release, reuptake, and degradation of catecholamines. Some drugs alter the synthesis of catecholamines by competing for the transport of tyrosine (e.g., α-methyldopa) or by inhibiting the synthetic enzymes tyrosine hydroxylase (e.g., α-methyl-*p*-tyrosine) or dopamine-β-hydroxylase (e.g., disulfiram). Other drugs inhibit the activity of enzymes responsible for the degradation of catecholamines (e.g., pargyline, a monoamine oxidase inhibitor) and therefore increase the availability of bioamines in the synapse. A number of indirectly acting drugs block the monoamine transporter responsible for the vesicular storage of catecholamines (e.g., reserpine) or inhibit the reuptake of catecholamines by the presynaptic terminal (e.g., cocaine).

## CATECHOLAMINES

## Chemical Structures and Structure–Activity Relationships

Substitutions in the catecholamine molecule can be made on (1) the aromatic ring, (2) the α- and β-carbons, and (3) the terminal amino group (Fig. 13-2). These various substitutions yield many compounds with a wide variety of sympathomimetic and sympatholytic activities (Fig. 13-3).

### Substitution on the benzene ring

Many directly acting sympathomimetics have both α- and β-adrenergic activity (Table 13-1), but the ratio of α to β activity varies tremendously from an almost pure α-adrenoceptor agonist (e.g., phenylephrine) to an almost pure β-adrenoceptor agonist (e.g., isoproterenol). Hydroxyl groups in the C-3 and C-4 positions are required for maximal adrenergic activity. Absence of either of these hydroxyl groups decreases the overall potency of an agent and primarily reduces β-adrenergic activity. Phenylephrine, for example, differs chemically from adrenaline in that it has no C-4-hydroxyl group. Although it is an α-adrenergic agonist, it is approximately 100 times less potent than noradrenaline and adrenaline, and it has a negligible activity on β-adrenoceptors.

Hydroxyl groups at C-3 and C-5 positions appear to confer β2-adrenoceptor selectivity (e.g., terbutaline, metaproterenol). Salbutamol (albuterol) is an important exception to this general rule: although it lacks a C-5 substituent, and has a –CH2–OH substituent on position C-3, it has a hydroxyl substituent on C-4, which permits it to exert strong β2 agonist activity. It is interesting to speculate that the C-4-hydroxyl may also confer some properties of α2 receptor activation. Drugs that lack both aromatic hydroxyl groups (e.g., amphetamine, methamphetamine, ephedrine) have a higher oil/water partition coefficient than catecholamines, which increases their distribution in the central nervous system (CNS) due to their increased liposolubility. Also, the absence of one or both of the hydroxyl groups renders these drugs more effective following oral administration and prolongs their half-life, because they have a low substrate affinity for the catecholamine-inactivating enzyme catechol-*O*-methyl-transferase (COMT) expressed in the liver and intestine.

## FIGURE 13-2 · Structural formulae of the catecholamines.

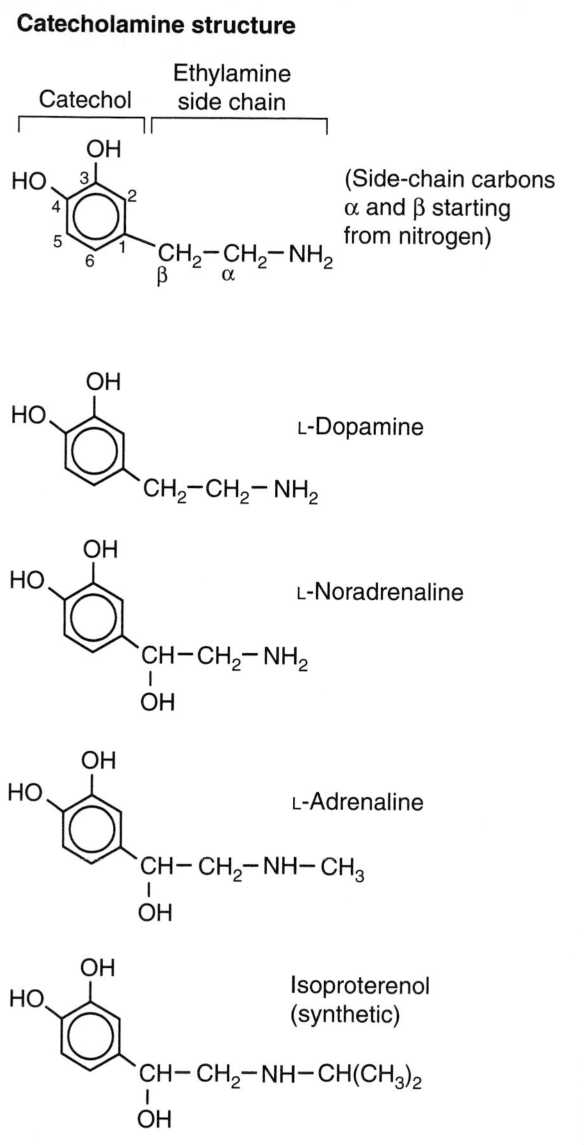

### Catecholamine structure

Catechol    Ethylamine side chain

(Side-chain carbons $\alpha$ and $\beta$ starting from nitrogen)

L-Dopamine

L-Noradrenaline

L-Adrenaline

Isoproterenol (synthetic)

## Substitution on the alpha and beta carbons

Side-chain substitutions also alter the activity of the cate-cholamines. Substitution on the $\alpha$-carbon blocks oxidation by monoamine oxidase and therefore increases the duration of action of the drug. Substitution on the $\beta$-carbon decreases CNS stimulation and increases both $\alpha$- and $\beta$-adrenergic activity. Substitution on either the $\alpha$- or $\beta$-carbon yields optical isomers. Levorotatory substitution on the $\beta$-carbon confers greater peripheral activity, so the naturally occurring $l$-adrenaline and $l$-noradrenaline are 10 times as potent as their unnatural $d$-isomers. Dextrorotatory substitution on the $\alpha$-carbon results in greater CNS activity compared with the $l$-isomer. Thus, $d$-amphetamine is more potent centrally than $l$-amphetamine, but peripherally, the $d$- and $l$-isomers are equipotent.

Interestingly, lack of the OH group on the $\beta$-carbon of indirectly acting phenylethylamines, such as tyramine, decreases their intracellular concentrations. However, $\beta$-hydroxylation of tyramine to octopamine facilitates its

## FIGURE 13-3 · Molecular effects of (A) $\alpha_1$-adrenoceptor agonists and (B) $\alpha_2$-, $\beta_1$-, and $\beta_2$-adrenoceptor agonists. PLC = phospholipase C; $PIP_2$ = phosphatidylinositol bisphosphate; $IP_3$ = inositol trisphosphate; DG = diacylglycerol; $G_i$ = inhibitory G protein for adenylyl cyclase; $G_q$ = stimulatory G protein for phospholipase C; $G_s$ = stimulatory G protein for adenylyl cyclase; GTP = guanosine triphosphate; AC = adenylyl cyclase; ATP = adenosine triphosphate; cAMP = cyclic adenosine monophosphate; + = stimulates; − = inhibits.

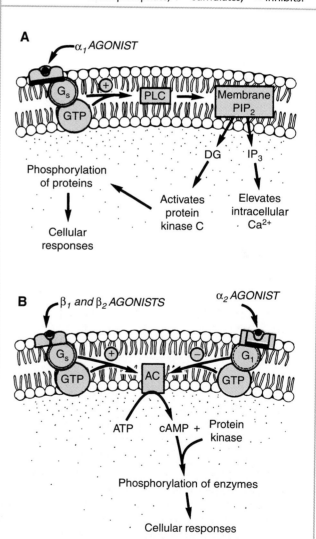

| TABLE 13-1 | Classification of Adrenoceptors with their Respective Agonists, Antagonists, and Effector Pathways* | | |
| --- | --- | --- | --- |
| **Pharmacologically Defined Receptors** | **Agonists** | **Antagonists** | **Effector Pathway** |
| $\alpha_{1A}$ | Noradrenaline<br>Adrenaline<br>Dopamine<br>Phenylephrine<br>Methoxamine | Prazosin<br>Phentolamine, WB 4101<br>Phenoxybenzamine<br>Labetalol<br>*Niguldipine*<br>*5-Methylurapidil* | IP$_3$/DAG<br>Ca$^{2+}$ influx |
| $\alpha_{1B}$ | Noradrenaline<br>Adrenaline<br>Dopamine<br>Phenylephrine | Prazosin<br>Phentolamine<br>Phenoxybenzamine<br>*Chlorethylclonidine*<br>*Spiperone* | IP$_3$/DAG |
| $\alpha_{1D}$ | Adrenaline<br>Noradrenaline<br>Phenylephrine | Prazosin<br>Phentolamine<br>WB 4101<br>*BMY 7378* | IP$_3$/DAG |
| $\alpha_{2A}$ | Noradrenaline<br>Adrenaline<br>Phenylephrine<br>Clonidine<br>BHT 920<br>*Oxymetazoline* | Phentolamine<br>Phenoxybenzamine<br>Rauwolscine<br>Yohimbine | ↓ cAMP |
| $\alpha_{2B}$ | Noradrenaline<br>Adrenaline<br>Phenylephrine<br>Clonidine<br>BHT 920 | Phentolamine<br>Phenoxybenzamine<br>Rauwolscine<br>Yohimbine<br>Prazosin[†] | ↓ cAMP |
| $\alpha_{2C}$ | Adrenaline<br>Noradrenaline | Phentolamine<br>Rauwolscine<br>Prazosin[†] | ↓ cAMP |
| $\beta_1$ | Noradrenaline<br>Adrenaline<br>Dopamine<br>Isoproterenol<br>*d-Dobutamine* | Phentolamine<br>Labetalol<br>*Atenolol*<br>*Metoprolol* | ↑ cAMP |
| $\beta_2$ | Adrenaline<br>Noradrenaline<br>Isoproterenol<br>*(Albuterol)*<br>*Salbutamol*<br>Terbutaline | Propranolol<br>Labetalol<br>*ICI 118551*<br>*Butoxamine* | ↑ cAMP |
| $\beta_3$ | Noradrenaline<br>Adrenaline<br>Isoproterenol<br>*BRL 37344* | — | ↑ cAMP |

*Italics denote the most selective agents. Propranolol is ineffective at $\beta_3$-adrenoceptors. Oxymetazoline is a partial agonist but may show high affinity as an antagonist against $\alpha_{1A}$; it also has been shown to have high agonist affinity at $\alpha_{2A}$.

[†]Prazosin is approximately 100 times less potent at $\alpha_{2B}$- and $\alpha_{2C}$- than at $\alpha_1$-adrenoceptors.

IP$_3$ = inositol trisphosphate; DAG = diacylglycerol; cAMP = cyclic adenosine monophosphate.

intravesicular storage, while concurrently promoting vesicular depletion of noradrenaline through a vesicular exchange process. Continued administration of tyramine leads to chronic noradrenaline depletion. Normally, tyramine is degraded in the periphery by monoamine oxidase (MAO). However, in patients treated with MAO inhibitors, tyramine and octopamine levels are increased, and, although octopamine is less potent than noradrenaline, these patients may experience severe hypertensive crises if they ingest large amounts of tyramine-rich foods such as cheese, beer, or red wine. Severe hypertension is caused by the massive release of noradrenaline elicited by the exceedingly high levels of tyramine.

### Substitution on the amino group

In general, substitutions on the amino N increase $\beta$ selectivity (e.g., isoproterenol). The longer the substituent, the higher the affinity for the $\beta$ receptor. Other structural modifications such as additions of hydroxyl groups at positions 3 and 5 of the benzene ring (e.g., metaproterenol) also contribute to an increased $\beta_2$ affinity.

## Mechanism of Action

The events that follow adrenergic receptor activation by an agonist and lead to production of a biological response are described in Chapter 11. All adrenergic receptors are G protein–coupled receptors with seven transmembrane domains (TM1 to TM7) connected by three extracellular and three intracellular loops, an extracellular amino terminal, and an intracellular carboxyl terminal. Their activation triggers different intracellular transduction pathways and mediates either excitatory or inhibitory cellular responses (see Chapters 8, 9, and 11).

## ADRENERGIC RECEPTORS

### Classification of Adrenergic Receptors

Adrenergic receptors are located throughout the central and autonomic nervous systems, as well as in peripheral tissues (Table 13-2). They are subdivided into distinct receptor subtypes on the basis of their different affinities for a wide range of synthetic agents, as described in Chapter 11. The development of new pharmacological and molecular tools, such as potent and highly selective $\alpha$ and $\beta$ receptor antagonists and in situ hybridization and gene cloning, has contributed to the identification of additional receptor subtypes and their respective tissue distributions (see Table 13-1) and to a better understanding of the mechanisms of action of adrenergic drugs.

### Structural Features

Drug affinity for different adrenergic receptors is determined by structural properties of the ligand (see "Chemi-

cal Structures and Structure–Activity Relationships" above) as well as the molecular structure of the receptor itself. The third intracellular loop, connecting TM5 and TM6, regulates the interaction between the receptor and its G protein. The pocket formed by the transmembrane units TM3, TM5, and TM7 forms the binding site recognized by catecholamines and agonists, whereas the outermost portion of TM2 influences antagonist binding. Only 30 to 40% of the amino acid composition of the TM domains is the same in $\alpha$ as in $\beta$ receptors. Glycosylation of amino terminal residues regulates cell surface expression of adrenoceptors and formation of receptor dimers. Receptor interaction resulting from dimerization has the potential to activate additional signalling mechanisms and may give rise to new patterns of drug action.

## Desensitization

$\beta$-Adrenergic receptors can undergo phosphorylation by specific kinases (e.g., $\beta$-adrenergic receptor kinase, or BARK). Interaction of phosphorylated serine and tyrosine residues in the intracellular C-terminal with the cytosolic protein $\beta$-arrestin inhibits receptor interaction with Gs, thus arresting the activation of the transduction pathway. This accounts for the agonist-induced desensitization of the receptor. Receptor–$\beta$-arrestin interactions also promote receptor internalization, followed by either intracellular degradation of the receptor or its recycling to the cell surface. Repeated exposure to an agonist elicits changes in both the number of receptors (receptor down-regulation and receptor internalization) and their functional state (e.g., receptor phosphorylation), resulting in a decreased cell response. This desensitization process, also known as tachyphylaxis or refractoriness, accounts for the reduction in clinical efficacy of adrenergic agonists when they are administered repeatedly.

## $\alpha$-Adrenergic Receptors

The ability of high-dose noradrenaline to prevent further presynaptic release of noradrenaline can be selectively blocked by yohimbine (an $\alpha_2$ antagonist) or mimicked by clonidine (an $\alpha_2$ agonist). Prazosin (an $\alpha_1$ antagonist) was unable to block the effects induced by clonidine. Genetic studies have identified six genes encoding different subtypes of $\alpha_1$ receptors ($\alpha_{1A}$, $\alpha_{1B}$, and $\alpha_{1D}$) and $\alpha_2$ receptors ($\alpha_{2A}$, $\alpha_{2B}$, and $\alpha_{2C}$) (see Chapters 11 and 16).

$\alpha_1$-Adrenergic receptors activate phospholipase C that catalyses the synthesis of diacylglycerol (DAG) or inositol trisphosphate (IP$_3$) and results in, respectively, the activation of protein kinase C or an increase in the concentration of cytoplasmic calcium. Both mechanisms cause depolarization. In most smooth muscle cells (e.g., blood vessels and myocardium), $\alpha_1$ receptor activation increases calcium concentration, which activates calmodulin-dependent myosin light-chain kinase (MLCK). In turn,

**TABLE 13-2**  Effects of α- and β-Adrenergic Receptor Agonists on the Cardiovascular System*

| Receptor | Drugs | Effects |
|---|---|---|
| $\alpha_1$ | Noradrenaline<br>Adrenaline<br>Dopamine (lower doses)<br>Dopamine (higher doses)<br>Phenylephrine<br>Metaraminol | Large arteries: ↑ tone<br><br>Arteries: ↓ tone (renal, mesenteric, coronary)<br>Arterioles: ↑ tone<br>↑ peripheral resistance<br>↑ diastolic pressure<br>↑ afterload<br>↑ heart rate (reflex)<br>Large veins: ↑ tone<br>↑ venous return<br>↑ preload (↑ ventricular volume) |
| $\alpha_2$ | Noradrenaline<br>Adrenaline | ↑ Tone in large arteries<br>↑ Peripheral resistance (postsynaptic $\alpha_2$-receptors in some<br>  vascular smooth muscle)<br>↑ EDRF (nitric oxide)<br>↑ Coronary vasodilatation<br>↑ Coronary transmitter release |
| $\beta_1$ | Noradrenaline<br>Adrenaline<br>Isoproterenol<br>Dopamine<br>Dobutamine | ↑ Heart rate<br>↑ Automaticity of all pacemaker cells<br>  (arrhythmias can occur)<br>↑ Conduction velocity in atria, AV node, and ventricles<br>↑ Velocity of contraction<br>↑ Force of contraction<br>↑ Stroke volume<br>↑ Cardiac output<br>↑ Oxygen consumption<br>↓ Diastolic time for coronary perfusion and ventricular filling<br>  (with marked tachycardia)<br>↓ Residual (end-systolic) volume<br>↑ Coronary vasodilatation |
| $\beta_2$ | Salbutamol (albuterol)<br>Terbutaline<br>Adrenaline<br>Isoproterenol | ↓ Arteriolar tone<br>↓ Peripheral resistance<br>↓ Diastolic pressure<br>↓ Afterload<br>↓ Heart rate:<br>  (1) reflex<br>  (2) $\beta_1$ stimulation with adrenaline and isoproterenol, and<br>      high doses of selective $\beta_1$ agonists |

*No functional distinction between $\alpha_{1A}$ and $\alpha_{1B}$ receptors has been identified as yet.

active MLCK phosphorylates the light chains of myosin, which initiates the cross-linking with actin and subsequent contraction (Fig. 13-4). However, in other myocytes, such as those in the gastrointestinal system, increased concentrations of intracellular calcium activate $Ca^{2+}$-dependent $K^+$ channels, which then results in hyperpolarization and muscle relaxation.

$\alpha_1$-Mediated activation of protein kinase C (PKC) phosphorylates the insulin receptor and reduces its activity. This results in a reduction in the number of glucose transporter (GLUT4) molecules mobilized to the cell membrane of skeletal muscle fibres and adipocytes, thus decreasing the effect of insulin on glucose uptake.

## $\alpha_1$ Receptor subtypes

Molecular cloning studies, in combination with differential ligand binding patterns and responses, have characterized at least three $\alpha_1$ receptors ($\alpha_{1A}$, $\alpha_{1B}$, and $\alpha_{1D}$) with similarly high affinity for prazosin, but different affinities for other compounds. Selective antagonists for the $\alpha_{1A}$ and $\alpha_{1B}$ receptors have been developed (**5-methylurapidil** and **chlorethylclonidine**, respectively). Functionally, these fur-

**FIGURE 13-4** $\alpha_1$- and $\beta_2$-mediated regulation of smooth muscle contraction. Intracellular increase in calcium concentration activates myosin light-chain kinase (MLCK), which phosphorylates MLC and promotes the formation of the actin–myosin complex and contraction. Cyclic AMP-mediated phosphorylation of MLCK inactivates this enzyme, therefore preventing contraction. $\alpha_1$ R = $\alpha_1$-adrenergic receptor; $\beta_2$ R = $\beta_2$ receptor; AC = adenylyl cyclase; IP$_3$ = inositol trisphosphate; Ca$^{2+}$/calmodulin = Ca$^{2+}$/calmodulin complex; MLC = myosin light chain; MLCK = myosin light-chain kinase; MLCK (PO$_4$)$_2$ = myosin light-chain kinase bisphosphate; MLCK+ Ca$^{2+}$/calmodulin = myosin light-chain kinase bound to the Ca$^{2+}$/calmodulin complex; MLC-PO$_4$ = myosin light-chain phosphate; PKA = protein kinase A; G$_q$ = stimulatory G protein for phospholipase C; G$_s$ = stimulatory G protein for adenylyl cyclase.

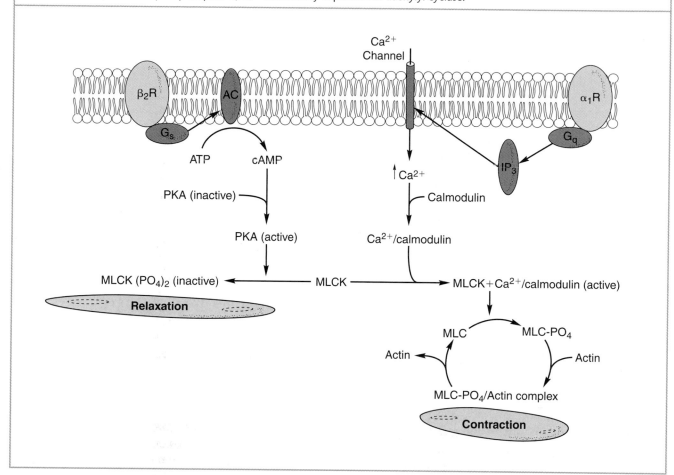

ther subdivisions have been more difficult to characterize, but it is now apparent that definitive functional variations can be accounted for by these distinct receptor subtypes. Tissues with a high population of $\alpha_{1A}$ receptors include prostate, vas deferens, and submaxillary gland, whereas spleen and liver have predominantly $\alpha_{1B}$ receptors.

The $\alpha_{1D}$ receptor has been found on secretory cells in bovine pineal and rat submaxillary glands. It has much lower affinity than $\alpha_{1A}$ and $\alpha_{1B}$ receptors for rauwolscine, as well as low affinity for prazosin.

## $\alpha_2$ Receptor subtypes

$\alpha_2$-Adrenergic receptors differ from $\alpha_1$ in that they are coupled to G$_i$ and inhibit adenylyl cyclase activity. They also activate G protein–gated K$^+$ channels; both of these mechanisms lead to cellular inhibition. Three $\alpha_2$-recep-

tor subtypes ($\alpha_{2A}$, $\alpha_{2B}$, and $\alpha_{2C}$) have been identified to date. Agonist binding to the $\alpha_{2A}$ receptors located in presynaptic sympathetic terminals causes hyperpolarization and thus inhibits release of noradrenaline from these terminals.

All known $\alpha_2$-adrenoceptors can be activated by noradrenaline and adrenaline and blocked by rauwolscine and yohimbine. Subclassification of $\alpha_2$-adrenoceptors was originally based on the ability of prazosin to inhibit [$^3$H]-yohimbine or [$^3$H]-rauwolscine binding. Prazosin, in addition to its high affinity for the $\alpha_1$ receptor, also has some degree of affinity for the $\alpha_{2B}$ and $\alpha_{2C}$ receptors (found in rat lung) but has very low affinity for the $\alpha_{2A}$ receptor (in platelets). Oxymetazoline, a potent $\alpha_1$ receptor agonist used as a topical decongestant of the nasal mucosa, also shows some affinity for the $\alpha_{2A}$ receptor.

In some blood vessels, $\alpha_2$ receptor activation causes vasodilatation due to increased synthesis of nitric oxide.

As in the case of the $\alpha_1$ receptors, the $\alpha_2$ subtypes have now been cloned, and their related genes have been identified and mapped. There is a high degree of structural homology and pharmacological similarity among the corresponding subtypes of $\alpha_2$ receptor in humans, rats, and mice.

## β-Adrenergic Receptor Subtypes

As noted in Chapter 11, three distinct β receptor subtypes ($\beta_1$, $\beta_2$, and $\beta_3$) have been identified on the basis of pharmacological and molecular genetic studies. Isoproterenol is equipotent at all three β receptors, but propranolol, which antagonizes the effects of isoproterenol at $\beta_1$ and $\beta_2$ sites, fails to do so at $\beta_3$.

### $\beta_1$ Receptors
The $\beta_1$ receptor is located primarily in cardiac tissue, where its activation of adenylyl cyclase leads to enhanced phosphorylation of troponin and phospholamban, which in turn raises intracellular $Ca^{2+}$ and thus contributes to the inotropic response. Activation of $\beta_1$ receptors in the cardiac pacemaker cells decreases their firing threshold and thereby increases their rhythmicity (i.e., chronotropy). **Dobutamine** is a selective agonist for the $\beta_1$ receptor, and **atenolol** and **metoprolol** are selective antagonists.

### $\beta_2$ Receptors
**Salbutamol** (known as **albuterol** in the United States) is a selective agonist for $\beta_2$ receptors, and **ICI 118551** and **butoxamine** were more recently found to be selective antagonists.

$\beta_2$ receptors mediate relaxation of bronchiolar, uterine, and vascular smooth muscle (mainly in the coronary arteries) by their action on the regulation of contractility. In smooth muscle cells, unlike in skeletal muscle, contractility is regulated by the phosphorylation state of the myosin regulatory light chain (MLC). In the unphosphorylated state of MLC, there is no contraction, whereas its phosporylation by MLC kinase (MLCK) causes contraction (see Fig. 13-4).

The $Ca^{2+}$-dependent activation of MLCK is regulated by calmodulin. Increased intracellular concentration of $Ca^{2+}$ promotes the formation of the $Ca^{2+}$/calmodulin complex that activates MLCK. On the other hand, an increase in the intracellular concentration of cAMP inactivates MLCK.

In cells that express high amounts of $\beta_2$ receptors (e.g., bronchiolar smooth muscle cells), agonist binding increases intracellular cAMP, thus phosphorylating (i.e., inactivating) MLCK and maintaining MLC in the nonactive state and preventing its cross-linkage with actin.

In other tissues, such as liver hepatocytes, stimulation of the $\beta_2$-receptor activates glycogenolysis.

### $\beta_3$ Receptors
This G protein–coupled receptor has about 50% homology with the $\beta_1$ and $\beta_2$ receptors, and interspecies studies have shown that it is highly conserved. The development of selective agonists (e.g., SR58611, BRL37344) and antagonists (e.g., SR59230) has contributed to a better understanding of its pharmacological profile and physiological roles.

$\beta_3$-Adrenergic receptors are expressed in white and brown adipose tissue in rodents, and in white adipose tissue in humans, where they promote lipolysis and thermogenesis. They are also expressed in the ventricular myocardium, where they produce a negative inotropic effect. This effect, which is selectively elicited by BRL37344 and mediated through the $G_{i/o}$ protein, acts as a counteracting mechanism preventing excessive stimulation of myocardial cells through $\beta_1$ and $\beta_2$ receptors. The potential therapeutic application of selective $\beta_3$ antagonists in the treatment of heart failure is currently being investigated.

Stimulation of $\beta_3$ receptors also causes peripheral vasodilatation, an effect attributed to the activation of nitric oxide synthase (NOS) in endothelial cells.

## EFFECTS OF ADRENERGIC AGENTS ON ORGAN SYSTEMS

The different pharmacological profiles of the various catecholamines result from both their affinities for different adrenoceptors and the diverse expression of adrenoceptors in various tissues and organs.

### Heart

Noradrenaline, adrenaline, and isoproterenol are all potent agonists at $\beta_1$ receptors. The $\beta_1$ effects of noradrenaline on the heart may be observed in vivo after administration of atropine to block vagal inhibitory responses, or in isolated heart preparations. $\beta_1$ Agonists produce the following effects in the heart.

**Tachycardia** results from an increased rate of discharge of pacemaker cells in the SA node. This increases the slope of phase 4 in the action potential (i.e., the rate of diastolic depolarization) because of altered permeability of the cell membrane, allowing a faster influx of $Na^+$ and $Ca^{2+}$. The increase in heart rate is referred to as a *positive chronotropic effect*.

Noradrenaline and adrenaline **increase** both systolic and diastolic **blood pressure**. In larger doses, however, they increase blood pressure to such an extent that baroreceptor stimulation causes increased amounts of acetylcholine to be released by the vagal terminals at the SA node, and reflex slowing of the heart may occur. Although the vagal reflex has a negative chronotropic effect, the cardiac output may be unchanged or decreased, because both **stroke volume** and **peripheral resistance** are increased.

**Automaticity** of latent pacemaker cells is increased, and this may lead to arrhythmias.

**Shortening of the refractory period** of the AV node gives rise to acceleration of impulse conduction between atria and ventricles.

The **force of contraction** of the heart is increased (i.e., there is a *positive inotropic effect*). Increase in **stroke volume** and **cardiac output** is accompanied by **increased oxygen consumption**. There is a decrease in efficiency of the heart; that is, less work is done relative to the amount of oxygen consumed.

Although $\beta_1$ receptors are of major importance in modulating cardiac responses, there are also $\beta_2$ and $\alpha_1$ receptors present in the heart. $\beta_2$-Adrenergic receptors are probably stimulated by circulating adrenaline, resulting in synergism with $\beta_1$ receptor stimulation with respect to increasing the heart rate. Noradrenaline also elicits $\beta_2$-mediated relaxation of vascular smooth muscle and causes coronary vasodilatation.

$\alpha_1$-Adrenergic receptors have a moderate positive inotropic effect and may be an important compensatory mechanism when $\beta$-adrenoceptors are down-regulated, as seen in congestive heart failure.

Isoproterenol or adrenaline may be administered intravenously or directly into the heart for the treatment of complete heart block with slow ventricular response or asystole. The long-term maintenance treatment of heart block may also require isoproterenol.

Selectivity of a drug for a particular receptor is most evident at low doses. At higher doses, the same drug may also act at other receptors for which it has a lower affinity. For example, dopamine at low doses (1 to 5 µg/kg/min, intravenously) exerts its effects selectively through activation of the $G_s$-coupled dopamine $D_1$ receptors (see Chapter 16). $D_1$ receptor–mediated increase in intracellular cAMP causes vasodilatation, especially in the coronary, mesenteric, and renal arteries. At higher doses (5 to 20 µg/kg/min, intravenously), dopamine has a dose-dependent positive inotropic and chronotropic effect on the heart through stimulation of $\beta_1$-adrenoceptors. High doses also stimulate $\alpha_1$-adrenoceptors and cause vasoconstriction.

**Fenoldopam**, a selective agonist at the peripheral $D_1$ receptors, is a potent dilator of peripheral, renal, and mesenteric arteries, with an efficacy identical to that of sodium nitroprusside (see Chapter 34).

## Blood Vessels

The basic difference among the catecholamines is that noradrenaline constricts almost all blood vessels, with only a few exceptions, whereas adrenaline has mixed effects (i.e., it causes vasoconstriction in some vascular beds while dilating blood vessels in skeletal muscle), and isoproterenol is a pure vasodilator. This difference is reflected in the effects of the individual drugs on heart rate.

Noradrenaline causes constriction of arterioles in the skin, skeletal muscle, mucous membranes, and kidneys. In vivo, this is evidenced by an increase in total peripheral resistance, which results in elevation of diastolic blood pressure. Systolic pressure is also increased. Constriction of large veins (capacitance vessels) and larger arteries (conductance vessels) also occurs. The vasoconstrictive response to noradrenaline is mediated predominantly through $\alpha_1$-receptor stimulation, although in some vascular beds, there may be an $\alpha_2$ component. At low doses (e.g., 10 µg/min), noradrenaline has a positive inotropic effect and also increases heart rate (i.e., positive chronotropy). However, at higher doses (e.g., 20 µg/min), the large increase in blood pressure produced by noradrenaline slows the heart by a reflex increase in vagal tone, thus masking the $\beta_1$ receptor effects on heart rate. The $\beta_1$ receptor–mediated inotropic action is maintained (Fig. 13-5).

It is now well established that the vasodilatory effect of noradrenaline on the coronary arteries is mediated by the $\beta_2$ receptor since it is blocked by propranolol (a non-selective $\beta$ antagonist) and butoxamine (a selective $\beta_2$ antagonist), but not by practolol (a selective $\beta_1$ antagonist; see Chapter 14). The net effect of noradrenaline on the coronary bed is vasodilatation, because the vasoconstriction caused by direct activation of the $\alpha_1$ receptors on the smooth muscle cells is overcome by the vasodilatory effects of $\beta_2$ receptors in the myocytes and endothelial $\alpha_1$ receptors.

Noradrenaline is administered intravenously in moderate doses (e.g., 10 µg/min) sufficient to increase cardiac output and raise the arterial blood pressure without causing significant vasoconstriction. Noradrenaline, dopamine, and dobutamine are used in the treatment of **cardiogenic shock** (myocardial infarction).

**Adrenaline** causes vasoconstriction of most blood vessels in the skin, mucous membranes, and kidneys. Dilatation occurs in skeletal muscle vascular beds, which contain $\beta_2$ and $\alpha_1$ receptors. The $\beta_2$ receptors are sensitive to much lower doses of adrenaline than are the $\alpha_1$ receptors. Moreover, adrenaline is much more potent than noradrenaline on the $\beta_2$ receptor. This dilatory response results in a slight decrease in vascular resistance, causing a small decrease in diastolic pressure, and therefore reflex tachycardia may occur rather than reflex slowing of the heart (see Fig. 13-5). Larger doses of adrenaline, however, do stimulate $\alpha_1$ receptors, and the actions of adrenaline become similar to those of noradrenaline, and reflex bradycardia occurs. Adrenaline also causes coronary vasodilatation through activation of multiple intracellular signalling pathways, as reported above for noradrenaline. Adrenaline is traditionally used in the treatment of anaphylactic shock, urticaria, hay fever, and angioneurotic edema because it counteracts the bronchoconstrictor and vasodilator actions of histamine.

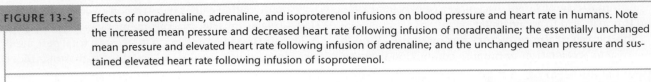

**FIGURE 13-5** Effects of noradrenaline, adrenaline, and isoproterenol infusions on blood pressure and heart rate in humans. Note the increased mean pressure and decreased heart rate following infusion of noradrenaline; the essentially unchanged mean pressure and elevated heart rate following infusion of adrenaline; and the unchanged mean pressure and sustained elevated heart rate following infusion of isoproterenol.

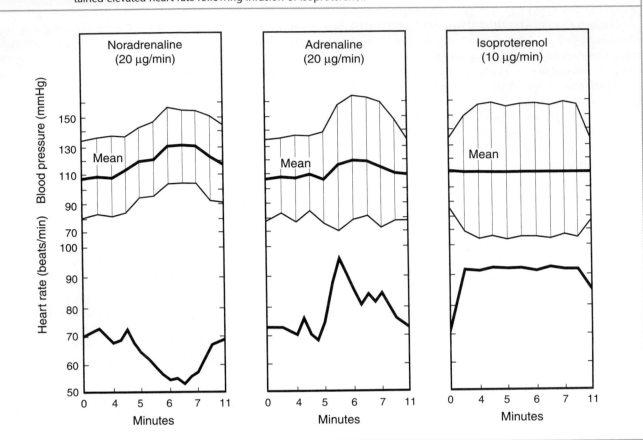

**Isoproterenol** (isoprenaline) is a synthetic catecholamine and powerful non-selective β-adrenergic agonist with a very low affinity for the α receptors (see Chapter 11). It lowers peripheral vascular resistance (β2 stimulation) in renal and mesenteric blood vessels and in skeletal muscle beds, causing a fall in diastolic pressure. Cardiac output is enhanced by an increased force of contraction (positive inotropic action) and tachycardia (positive chronotropic effect), both β1-mediated. Systolic pressure may remain unchanged or rise slightly. Nevertheless, mean arterial pressure typically falls (see Fig. 13-5).

The effects of catecholamines on the cardiovascular system are summarized in Table 13-2.

## Respiratory System

Activation of β2-adrenergic receptors causes relaxation of bronchiolar smooth muscle and decreased airway resistance. Antigen-induced release of asthma mediators is also inhibited.

Activation of α1 receptors causes vasoconstriction in the upper respiratory tract mucosa. This decongestant effect in nasal and bronchiolar mucosa is clinically useful (see "Selective α1 Receptor Agonists" below).

Adrenaline primarily relaxes bronchial smooth muscle. Its powerful β2-mediated bronchodilatory action is most evident when bronchial muscle is contracted, as in bronchial asthma. The beneficial effects may also arise from a decrease in antigen-induced release of inflammatory mediators from mast cells and, to a lesser extent, from diminished bronchial secretions and congestion within the mucosa. Similarly, isoproterenol relaxes bronchial smooth muscle and prevents or relieves bronchoconstriction, but tolerance to this action develops. Isoproterenol also inhibits antigen-induced release of asthma mediators.

## Gastrointestinal Tract

Stimulation of α- and β-adrenergic receptors causes relaxation of gastrointestinal smooth muscle by two different mechanisms:

1. Noradrenaline, by stimulating presynaptic α2 receptors on cholinergic neurons, inhibits the release of acetyl-

choline, causing decreased smooth muscle tone and reduced amplitude of contractions. This is generally accepted as being the primary adrenergic mechanism responsible for the adrenergic inhibition of peristalsis.

2. Stimulation of $\beta_2$ receptors on gastrointestinal myocytes elevates cAMP, resulting in inactivation of MLCK by protein kinase A, which reduces the strength of muscle contraction (see Fig. 13-4).

In addition, $\alpha_2$ receptors stimulate absorption and reduce secretion of water and electrolytes in the intestine, further reducing gastrointestinal motility. $\alpha_2$ Agonists (e.g., clonidine; see Chapter 14) have been used successfully in the treatment of diarrhea in diabetic patients with autonomic neuropathy.

## Genitourinary Tract

The effects of the catecholamines on the uterus are dependent on its reproductive status. Noradrenaline increases the frequency of contraction in the human pregnant uterus. Adrenaline inhibits uterine tone and contractions during the last month of pregnancy and at parturition. On the basis of the latter finding, selective $\beta_2$ agonists (e.g., ritodrine) have been used to delay premature labour, but their use should be under strict control because they may increase maternal morbidity (e.g., pulmonary edema).

$\alpha_1$ Receptors are abundant in the urethral sphincter and prostate. Phenoxybenzamine, a non-selective $\alpha$ antagonist, and more recently, terazocin, a selective $\alpha_1$ antagonist (see Chapter 14), have been successfully used in the treatment of urinary retention caused by benign prostatic hyperplasia.

## Eye

The radial muscle in the iris contains $\alpha_1$-adrenergic receptors that, when stimulated, cause mydriasis (pupil dilatation). This should raise the intraocular pressure by blocking the outflow of aqueous humor. However, stimulation of $\alpha_1$ receptors, unlike anti-muscarinic agents (e.g., atropine), does not cause cycloplegia (i.e., paralysis of the ciliary muscle and subsequent loss of visual accommodation) and consequently does not prevent outflow of aqueous humor. Additionally, $\beta$ antagonists (e.g., timolol) inhibit production of aqueous humor and are commonly used in the treatment of glaucoma.

## Metabolic Effects

The important effects of catecholamines on intermediary metabolism include lipolysis, glycogenolysis, and gluconeogenesis.

**Lipolysis** and **thermogenesis** have been associated with $\beta_1$ stimulation. However, it is now clear that these effects are mediated selectively through the $\beta_3$ receptor.

Receptor-mediated elevation of cAMP levels causes activation of lipase, and the breakdown of triglycerides to glycerol and free fatty acids is enhanced.

**Glycogenolysis** in the liver is increased by $\beta_2$ stimulation (Fig. 13-6), which causes increased glucose release into the circulation, resulting in hyperglycemia. $\alpha$ Receptors may also play a role. **Gluconeogenesis** from lactate and amino acids is also stimulated. Both increased cAMP production and modulation of enzyme formation appear to be involved. Oxygen consumption is increased by both adrenaline and noradrenaline (calorigenic effect).

Adrenaline transiently increases plasma levels of $K^+$; this is followed by a more prolonged fall in $K^+$ plasma levels. This is a $\beta_2$-mediated effect. $\beta_2$ Agonists have been used in the management of hyperkalemic familial periodic paralysis because of their ability to increase uptake of $K^+$ into muscle cells.

## Endocrine Glands

The release of insulin is increased by $\beta_2$ receptor stimulation and inhibited by $\alpha$ receptor activation (see Chapter 47). Moreover, $\alpha_1$-mediated activation of protein kinase C (PKC) phosphorylates the insulin receptor and reduces its activity. Consequently, this results in a reduction in the number of glucose transporter (GLUT4) molecules mobilized to the cell membrane of skeletal muscle fibres and adipocytes, thus decreasing the effect of insulin on glucose uptake and therefore causing hyperglycemia.

Glucagon secretion from $\alpha$-cells in the pancreas is also increased. Renin release from the juxtaglomerular cells in the kidney is increased by $\beta_1$ receptor activation and inhibited by $\alpha$ receptor stimulation.

## Central Nervous System

Catecholamines are potent stimulants of the CNS (see Chapter 16) and mediate the **"fight or flight response"** of the sympathetic division of the autonomic nervous system. The activity of the catecholaminergic system can be stimulated either directly (e.g., selective dopamine or adrenaline receptor agonists) or indirectly (e.g., inhibition of reuptake). The concentration of free catecholamines in the brain is increased by cocaine and amphetamines (via blockade of reuptake of catecholamine neurotransmitters, and enhanced release, respectively). The resulting mood-elevating (euphoriant) effect is the basis for the abuse of these drugs (see Chapter 70). They also enhance alertness and prolong the ability to perform repetitive tasks.

## Skeletal Muscle

Adrenaline and other $\beta_1$ agonists, such as dobutamine, facilitate the release of acetylcholine from cholinergic motor axon terminals, probably by elevating cAMP levels and activating the N-type calcium channel at presynaptic sites. Inhibition of $\alpha_2$-adrenergic receptors on cholinergic neurons in skeletal muscle increases the release of acetyl-

**FIGURE 13-6**   Metabolic pathways by which catecholamines stimulate glycogenolysis.

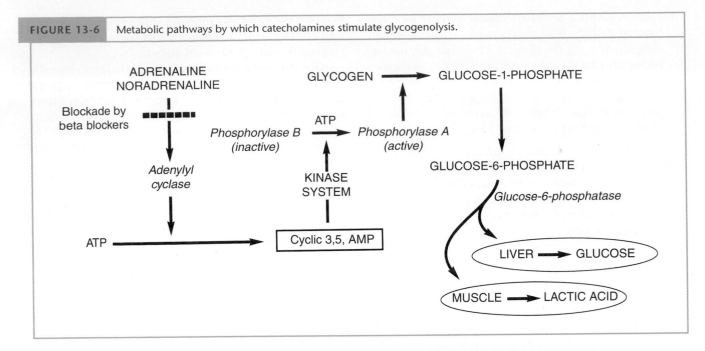

choline. Therefore, in myasthenia gravis, ephedrine and amphetamine can be used to increase the release of catecholamines (in addition to being direct adrenergic receptor agonists), thus increasing cholinergic activity. $\beta_2$ Receptor agonists (e.g., adrenaline, salbutamol) cause muscle tremor that can be prevented by propranolol. The mechanism responsible for tremor induction is associated with $\beta_2$ receptor–mediated hypokalemia and enhancement of muscle spindle discharge.

## ADRENERGIC RECEPTOR AGONISTS

### Selective $\alpha_1$ Receptor Agonists

Figure 13-7 illustrates the structures of some $\alpha_1$-adrenergic receptor agonists, which are discussed below.

### Phenylephrine (Neo-synephrine)

This agent is closely related chemically to adrenaline. Since it is not a catechol, it is not inactivated by COMT, and as a result, it has a much longer half-life than catecholamines (i.e., 2.5 hours vs. just a few minutes). It is a powerful, selective, and directly acting $\alpha_1$-adrenergic agonist that activates $\beta$ receptors only at high concentrations. The pharmacological effects are essentially similar to those of noradrenaline, although it is less potent. The predominant actions are on the cardiovascular system. Intravenous, subcutaneous, and oral administration all cause a rise in systolic and diastolic pressure in humans and other species. Phenylephrine is useful as a vasoconstrictor, decongestant, mydriatic, and anti-allergy agent. It is also used to treat paroxysmal atrial tachycardia by indirectly causing reflex

bradycardia. After repeated administration, both the duration of action and therapeutic efficacy of nasal decongestion are strongly reduced. This desensitization constitutes a typical example of tachyphylaxis.

### Methoxamine (Vasoxyl)

This is another relatively selective $\alpha_1$ agonist. It does not stimulate $\beta$ receptors or the CNS. Its major action on the cardiovascular system is to raise blood pressure; this effect is associated with reflex bradycardia. Like phenylephrine, methoxamine is used to treat hypotensive states and to relieve paroxysmal atrial tachycardia.

### Metaraminol (Aramine)

This agent is both a direct ($\alpha_1$ receptor–stimulating) and an indirect sympathomimetic (it stimulates the release of noradrenaline from sympathetic terminals). It causes an increase in both systolic and diastolic pressure that is due to peripheral vasoconstriction and is accompanied by reflex vagal bradycardia. Its effects, like those of methoxamine, are long-lasting.

Phenylephrine, metaraminol, and methoxamine may be used parenterally to elevate the blood pressure (e.g., in hypotension associated with spinal anaesthesia). The stimulation of $\alpha_1$ receptors leads to an increase in peripheral resistance, which increases diastolic (and systolic) pressure. The use of $\alpha_1$ agonists in hypovolemic shock is controversial since there is already a maximal release of catecholamines causing intense vasoconstriction and resulting in decreased tissue perfusion. The microcirculation may be further impaired by use of $\alpha_1$ agonists. This was the rationale for the proposed use of $\alpha_1$ blockers in treating shock (see Chapter 14). Elevation of the blood

FIGURE 13-7 | Structural formulae of $\alpha_1$-adrenergic receptor agonists.

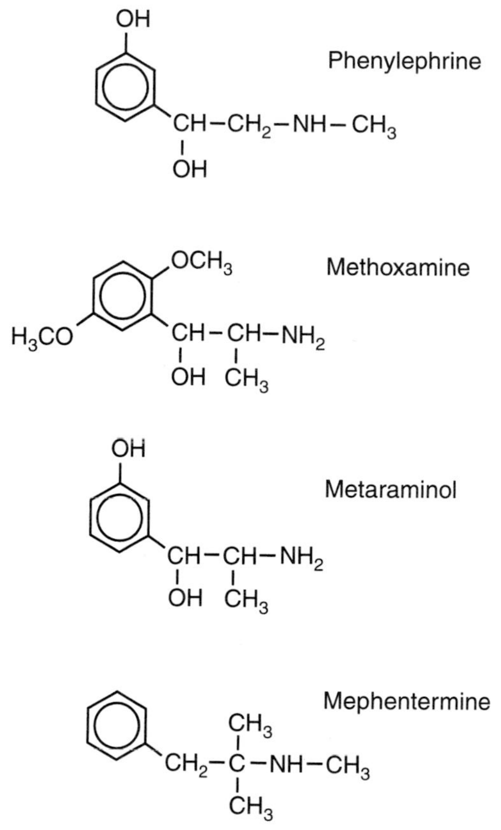

Phenylephrine

Methoxamine

Metaraminol

Mephentermine

pressure is of value only in the absence of hypovolemia and/or electrolyte disturbances.

Other selective $\alpha_1$-adrenergic agonists include **mephentermine, naphazoline,** and **cirazoline.** Oxymetazoline and xylometazoline are less selective for the $\alpha_1$ receptor and also have a lower affinity for the $\alpha_2$ receptor. They are used as nasal and ophthalmic decongestants.

## Selective $\alpha_2$ Receptor Agonists

$\alpha_2$ Agonists are used in the treatment of hypertension. They act on the cardiovascular control centres in the CNS and inhibit sympathetic output.

### Clonidine (Catapres)

When clonidine (Fig. 13-8) was first synthesized, it was found to produce vasoconstriction mediated by $\alpha$ receptors. However, during trials as a nasal decongestant, it was found to cause hypotension, sedation, and bradycardia. The antihypertensive effects of clonidine are produced by a combination of central and peripheral actions. Centrally, clonidine acts on *post*synaptic $\alpha_2$ receptors located on neurons of the cardiovascular regulatory centres in the

medulla oblongata (in the rostral ventrolateral medulla [RVLM] and nucleus of the solitary tract [NTS]) and inhibits their predominantly excitatory outflow. Peripherally, it stimulates the presynaptic $\alpha_2$ receptors and thus inhibits the release of catecholamines from post-ganglionic sympathetic neurons. Functionally, the inhibitory effect of the vagus nerve on the heart is augmented, probably both by increased sensitivity of the baroreceptors and by central actions, further contributing to hypotension.

In the medulla, imidazoline drugs (e.g., clonidine, **moxonidine,** and **rilmenidine**) also produce part of their antihypertensive effects through stimulation of the $I_1$-imidazoline receptors in the RVLM, which activates the $IP_3$/DAG transduction pathway (see Chapter 9). This provides an alternative route of pharmacological manipulation of the central cardiovascular regulatory system, which avoids some of the adverse secondary effects of the adrenergic drugs.

Intravenous administration of clonidine in humans produces an initial brief increase in blood pressure, due to the direct stimulation of post-junctional $\alpha_1$- and $\alpha_2$-adrenoceptors, which is followed by a fall in blood pressure associated with bradycardia.

After oral administration, a decrease in blood pressure is evident within 30 to 60 minutes. The hemodynamic effects of clonidine include bradycardia and a reduced cardiac output, which both contribute to the fall in blood pressure. Oral absorption of clonidine is essentially complete but rather slow, peak plasma levels being reached in about 4 hours. Plasma half-life is about 12 hours, but it is greatly increased by severe renal disease. About 50% of the absorbed drug is excreted unchanged in the urine, the other half undergoing biotransformation in the liver.

Following chronic administration of clonidine, peripheral resistance is also decreased. Clonidine has minor effects on reflex control of blood pressure; therefore, postural hypotension is not a common side effect. A potentially dangerous side effect of clonidine is "rebound" hypertension in patients in whom the drug has been suddenly withdrawn. Prior administration of $\alpha$ receptor antagonists (e.g., phentolamine) will prevent this rebound effect. Renin release is also inhibited by clonidine. Small doses of clonidine are effective in the prophylactic treatment of migraine by reducing the frequency and severity of attacks. Stimulation of $\alpha_2$ receptors found on choliner-

FIGURE 13-8 | Structural formula of clonidine HCl.

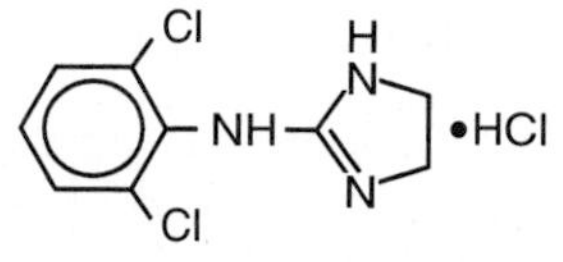

gic fibres innervating salivary glands and the intestine may be responsible for the inhibition of these neurons, thus accounting for the dry mouth and constipation frequently observed in the therapeutic dose of clonidine.

**Apraclonidine** (Iopidine), a more selective $\alpha_2$-agonist, inhibits the formation of aqueous humor and effectively reduces intraocular pressure. It is used as an adjunctive medication in the treatment of glaucoma.

The compounds BHT 920, BHT 933, and S19014, newly developed selective $\alpha_2$ receptor agonists, are useful experimental pharmacological tools for studying $\alpha_2$ receptor mechanisms. The use of selective $\alpha_2$ agonists for the treatment of migraine is currently being evaluated. Results obtained to date suggest that they may have fewer adverse effects than sumatriptan (see Chapter 29).

## Non-selective $\beta$ Receptor Agonist

**Isoproterenol** (isoprenaline; Isuprel), a synthetic catecholamine, is the most potent $\beta_1$- and $\beta_2$-adrenergic agent in use. Peripheral vasodilatation, tachycardia, myocardial stimulation, and bronchial relaxation are the most important effects caused by this drug. Isoproterenol is more potent than adrenaline as a bronchial dilator, but it is not a decongestant. The side effects of isoproterenol, which frequently are very severe, are due primarily to its cardiac action. The tachycardia and myocardial stimulation produce signs of coronary insufficiency by increasing the amount of oxygen required by the heart.

Isoproterenol is metabolized by COMT, just as the endogenous catecholamines are, but it is unaffected by MAO and therefore has a longer half-life.

## Selective $\beta_1$ Receptor Agonist

**Dobutamine** (Dobutrex) is a synthetic derivative of dopamine with the catechol group in its structure (Fig. 13-9). It is known as a selective stimulant of $\beta_1$ receptors. Its action on the heart is unique in that it produces more inotropic than chronotropic effects. The precise reason for this is unclear, but it may be related to the distinct properties of the *d*- and *l*-isomers. While *d*-dobutamine is a pure $\beta_1$ receptor agonist, the *l*-isomer has some $\alpha_1$-stimulant effects, which may contribute to the overall increase in inotropy. At lower doses, dobutamine increases stroke volume while the heart rate remains unchanged. It is used for the short-term treatment of cardiac decompensation in patients with congestive heart failure or acute myocardial infarction, or after heart surgery.

## Selective $\beta_2$ Receptor Agonists

The main problems encountered with $\beta$-adrenergic receptor agonists used for the treatment of asthma are caused by $\beta_1$ receptor stimulation. Therefore, much effort has been put into the development of drugs with high selec-

**FIGURE 13-9** Structural formulae of selective $\beta_1$- and $\beta_2$-adrenergic receptor agonists.

tivity toward $\beta_2$ receptors. **Salbutamol** (albuterol; Ventolin; see Fig. 13-9) and other related drugs are effective bronchodilators because of their action on $\beta_2$ receptors in bronchiolar smooth muscle. Because they stimulate $\beta_2$ receptors preferentially, these agents lack the $\beta_1$ receptor–mediated myocardial stimulating properties of isoproterenol. High doses of salbutamol, however, do stimulate the myocardium. Salbutamol also stimulates $\beta_2$ receptors in the smooth muscle of vessels supplying skeletal muscle, leading to a decrease in peripheral vascular resistance. Since the uterus reacts to $\beta_2$ agonists with relaxation, salbutamol can be used to delay delivery in premature labour. When administered by inhalation, it is effective within 3 to 15 minutes, with a maximum effect reached within 60 to 90 minutes, and persisting for 3 to 6 hours.

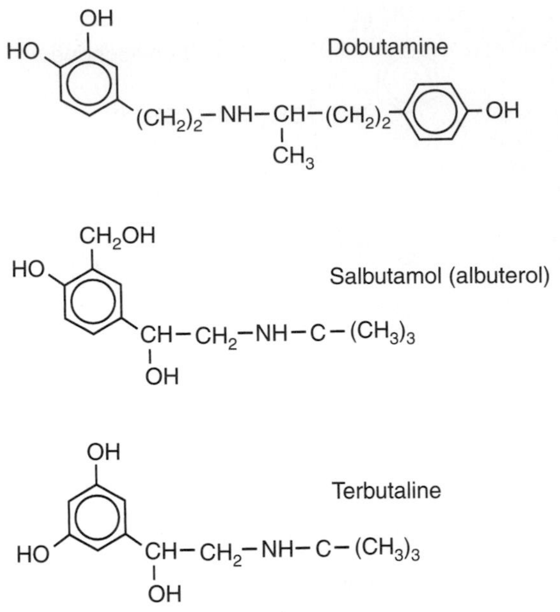

**Salmeterol** (Serevent) and **formoterol** (Oxeze Turbohaler) are newer selective $\beta_2$ agonists with a prolonged duration of action (12 hours). **Fenoterol** (Berotec) has an intermediate duration of action (up to 6 to 8 hours). Although these molecules are highly lipophilic, which may account for their long half-lives, the long-acting bronchodilatory properties of salmeterol are due to the specific interaction of the drug not only with the active site of the $\beta_2$-adrenoceptor, but also with a second locus, known as the exosite, located in TM4. This allows the drug to be anchored to the receptor even in the presence of an antagonist. This mechanism accounts for the high availability of the compound at the receptor site. Other selective $\beta_2$ agonists are **terbutaline** (Bricanyl; see Fig. 13-9) and **orciprenaline** (Alupent), also known as metaproterenol in the United States.

## Selective β3 Receptor Agonists

Selective β3 receptor agonists (e.g., BRL 37344) regulate fat metabolism and ventricular contractility. Recent research indicates that such agents may have a use in the treatment of obesity and heart failure (see "β3 Receptors" above).

# INDIRECTLY ACTING ADRENERGIC AGONISTS

The following sections describe the basic mechanisms of action of drugs that exert their effects not through direct receptor binding but **indirectly** through alterations in the fate of catecholamines, ultimately leading to an increased activity of the sympathetic system. Detailed information on indirectly acting antagonists is presented in Chapter 14. (See also sections on Storage, Release, and Degradation of Catecholamines, Chapter 11).

Indirectly acting agonists target adrenergic neurons by a variety of mechanisms that include the following:

- Stimulation of catecholamine synthesis by increased substrate availability (e.g., L-dopa)
- Stimulation of catecholamine release (e.g., amphetamine)
- Inhibition of the presynaptic transporter responsible for catecholamine reuptake (e.g., cocaine)
- Inhibition of catecholamine degradation by monoamine oxidase (e.g., pargyline)

Due to their non-selective mechanism of action most, but not all, of these drugs act at both central and peripheral sites and cause distinctive, undesirable side effects, many of which are predictable on the basis of the mechanism and site of action of the individual drug.

Some drugs exert their actions through multiple mechanisms. For example, the *mixed* sympathomimetic ephedrine acts both *directly* and *indirectly* (see below).

## Indirectly Acting Amines

Tyramine, amphetamine, and ephedrine, due to their structural similarity with catecholamines, are transported across the adrenergic neuronal membrane into the cytoplasm by monoamine transporters. Then, these drugs are transported into vesicles by vesicular monoamine transporters (VMATs; see Chapter 11) and displace stored noradrenaline from the vesicle into the cytosol. Some of the displaced noradrenaline is metabolized by MAO, while some will be released by the terminal, bind to adrenergic receptors in the effector organs, and produce characteristic responses (e.g., increase in heart rate and elevation of blood pressure). Most of these drugs (e.g., ephedrine) also produce additional sympathomimetic effects by stimulating adrenergic receptors directly. However, the direct stimulation of peripheral receptors by amphetamine is minimal when compared with its noradrenaline-releasing action.

### Ephedrine

Ephedrine (Fig. 13-10) is an alkaloid obtained from the herb Ma Huang (*Ephedra equisetina*) that has been used in Chinese traditional medicine from early times. Both carbon atoms on the aliphatic side chain are asymmetric, resulting in four isomers: (+)- and (–)-ephedrine, and (+)- and (–)-pseudoephedrine. The most potent form in relation to sympathomimetic activity is (–)-ephedrine, which is used clinically.

Ephedrine, a mixed-action drug, exerts its sympathomimetic actions by noradrenaline release from sympathetic nerves (Fig. 13-11C, Table 13-3), as well as by direct action on $\alpha_1$-, $\beta_1$-, and $\beta_2$-adrenoceptors. Tachyphylaxis may occur during chronic administration because of depletion of the intraneuronal pool of noradrenaline.

The change from the catechol ring structure of adrenaline to the phenyl ring structure of ephedrine results in a marked difference in action. Unlike adrenaline, ephedrine is effective orally, has a prolonged action, is a potent central stimulant, but gives rise to tachyphylaxis. Intravenous injection of ephedrine produces a prompt rise in blood pressure. As a vasopressor agent, ephedrine is only 1/1000 to 1/100 as potent as adrenaline, but its duration of action is 7 to 10 times longer, because it is degraded by MAO at a lower rate than adrenaline and is not degraded by COMT. It dilates the coronary vessels, increases the heart rate, and may elevate the arterial blood pressure.

Ephedrine dilates the bronchioles. Although its effect on asthma is not as prompt or pronounced as that of adrenaline, it has the advantages of oral administration and longer duration of action.

Ephedrine increases the tone of skeletal muscle, and for this reason, it may be used as an adjuvant drug in the treatment of myasthenia gravis.

**Pseudoephedrine** (Sudafed) is an active stereoisomer of ephedrine with similar actions and uses.

### Amphetamine and related drugs

These agents are potent stimulants of the CNS; they are described in detail in Chapter 26. The peripheral cardiovascular effects caused by amphetamine are, however, an inherent part of its toxicity.

| FIGURE 13-10 | Structural formula of ephedrine. |

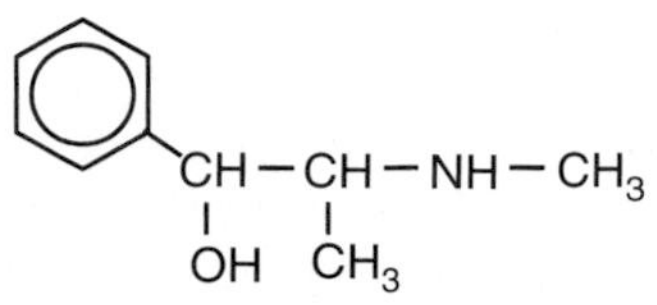

FIGURE 13-11    Schematic representations of various mechanisms of action of drugs on sympathetic nerve activity. NA = noradrenaline; MAO = monoamine oxidase; COMT = catechol-O-methyltransferase; α-CH₃-DOPA = α-methyldopa; α-CH₃-NA = α-methylnoradrenaline. Although not shown in the diagrams, there is a constant resting release of noradrenaline from adrenergic terminals. (This figure and Table 13-3 are summaries of drug effects on adrenergic nerve activity, as variously discussed in Chapters 13 and 14).

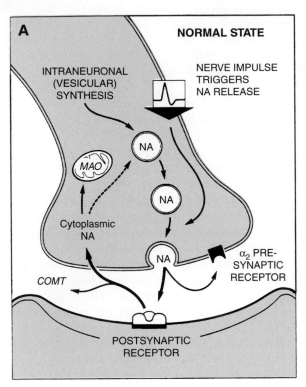

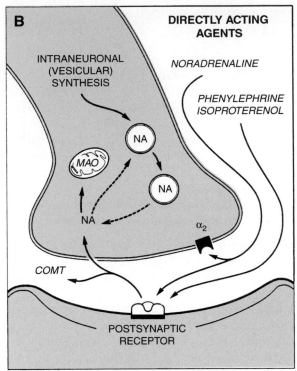

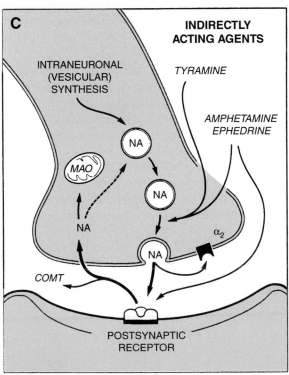

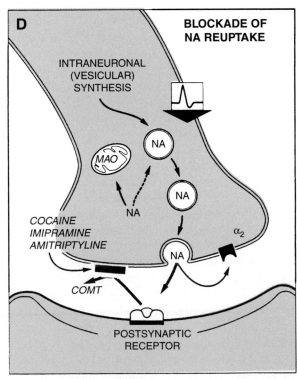

continued

FIGURE 13-11    continued

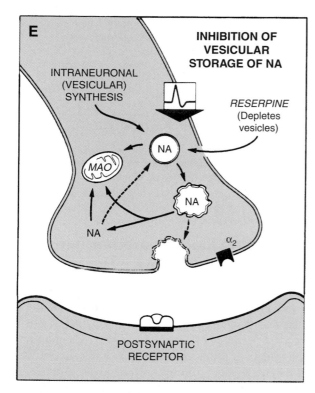

**E**

**INHIBITION OF VESICULAR STORAGE OF NA**

INTRANEURONAL (VESICULAR) SYNTHESIS

*RESERPINE* (Depletes vesicles)

MAO

NA

NA

NA

$\alpha_2$

POSTSYNAPTIC RECEPTOR

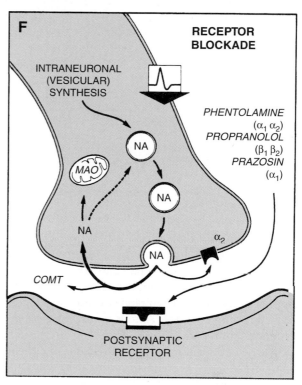

**F**

**RECEPTOR BLOCKADE**

INTRANEURONAL (VESICULAR) SYNTHESIS

*PHENTOLAMINE* ($\alpha_1 \alpha_2$)
*PROPRANOLOL* ($\beta_1 \beta_2$)
*PRAZOSIN* ($\alpha_1$)

MAO

NA

NA

NA

$\alpha_2$

*COMT*

POSTSYNAPTIC RECEPTOR

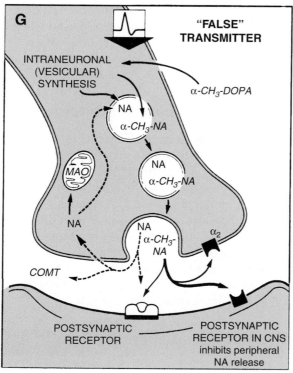

**G**

**"FALSE" TRANSMITTER**

INTRANEURONAL (VESICULAR) SYNTHESIS

$\alpha\text{-}CH_3\text{-}DOPA$

NA
$\alpha\text{-}CH_3\text{-}NA$

NA
$\alpha\text{-}CH_3\text{-}NA$

MAO

NA

NA
$\alpha\text{-}CH_3\text{-}NA$

$\alpha_2$

*COMT*

POSTSYNAPTIC RECEPTOR

POSTSYNAPTIC RECEPTOR IN CNS inhibits peripheral NA release

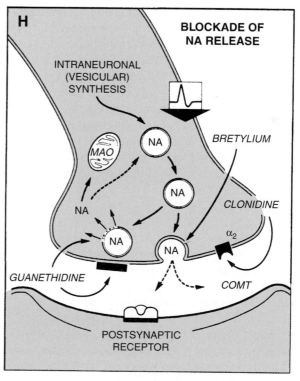

**H**

**BLOCKADE OF NA RELEASE**

INTRANEURONAL (VESICULAR) SYNTHESIS

*BRETYLIUM*

*CLONIDINE*

MAO

NA

NA

NA

NA

NA

$\alpha_2$

*GUANETHIDINE*

*COMT*

POSTSYNAPTIC RECEPTOR

| TABLE 13-3 | Types of Action of Representative Drugs at Adrenergic Neurons, Synapses, and Neuroeffector Junctions | |
|---|---|---|
| **Mechanism of Action** | **Drugs** | **Effects** |
| Blockade of transport system of axonal membrane (i.e., of uptake of noradrenaline) | Imipramine, desipramine Amitriptyline Cocaine | Accumulation of noradrenaline at extracellular sites; potentiation of sympathetic response |
| Displacement of transmitter from axonal terminal | Amphetamine Tyramine Ephedrine | Sympathomimetic (indirect) |
| Mimicry of transmitter at postsynaptic receptor | Phenylephrine Isoproterenol | Sympathomimetic (direct) |
| Inhibition of enzymatic breakdown of transmitter | MAO inhibitors (Pargyline, Clorgyline, Selegiline) | Accumulation of noradrenaline at certain sites; potentiation of tyramine |

**Amphetamine** and derivatives such as MDMA (3,4-methylenedioxymethamphetamine, MDMA, ecstasy) have a euphoriant (mood-elevating) effect and are liable to be abused and to cause drug dependence (see Chapter 70). **Methamphetamine** has a higher ratio of central to peripheral effects than amphetamine. Amphetamine reverses the vesicular monoamine transporter, therefore increasing vesicular release of dopamine and noradrenaline and their subsequent release by the presynaptic terminal. In addition, amphetamine binds to the $Na^+$- and $Cl^-$-dependent presynaptic catecholamine transporters, blocking synaptic reuptake of the transmitters. Together, these mechanisms increase the synaptic amounts of catecholamines and increase synaptic activity. **Methylphenidate** (Ritalin) is used in the treatment of narcolepsy in adults and attention deficit hyperactivity disorder (ADHD) in children. Its abuse potential is similar to that of amphetamine.

Other drugs of this type are **phenmetrazine** and **phentermine**. They are used occasionally as appetite suppressants, although phenmetrazine was withdrawn from the market in Canada because of the risk of abuse, similar to that of amphetamine.

### Tyramine

This compound has no direct adrenergic-agonist activity; its effects are solely due to release of noradrenaline. Tyramine, a naturally occurring phenylethylamine, is abundant in fermented foods (e.g., cheese, wine, and beer). Usually, its intestinal absorption is very limited, and it is readily inactivated by MAO in the gastrointestinal tract and liver. However, MAO inhibitors (e.g., phenelzine, a classical antidepressant) prevent peripheral degradation of tyramine, which is then transported into adrenergic terminals, where it enters the vesicles in exchange for noradrenaline. The massive release of noradrenaline causes a sudden and severe increase in blood pressure, which can cause a stroke or myocardial infarction. Therefore, the prior administration of a drug that depletes intraneuronal stores of noradrenaline (e.g., reserpine) will abolish the effects of tyramine.

## Drugs That Block Neurotransmitter Uptake in the Synapse

**Cocaine,** and some antidepressant drugs (such as **imipramine, amitriptyline,** and **fluoxetine**), belong to this class of drugs. They block the dopamine transporter (cocaine), noradrenaline transporter (desipramine, amitriptyline), and the serotonin transporter (fluoxetine) with different degrees of affinity and selectivity, and they inhibit the presynaptic uptake-1 mechanism responsible for the removal of the neurotransmitter from the synaptic cleft. The increase in availability of the neurotransmitter increases its synaptic activity (Fig. 13-11D). These drugs also prevent the uptake of compounds, such as ephedrine and tyramine, that also require binding to the catecholamine transporters.

## Monoamine Oxidase Inhibitors

These drugs were introduced as antidepressants (see Chapter 25), which is their sole remaining use. MAO is responsible for the intracellular catabolism of catecholamines and therefore regulates the cytoplasmic concentration of noradrenaline in sympathetic nerve terminals. Two MAO isozymes are expressed at different levels in the brain and other organs. Selective MAO-A inhibitors, such as clorgyline, are more effective antidepressants, whereas selective MAO-B inhibitors, such as selegiline, are more effective in the treatment of Parkinson's disease. These drugs irreversibly inactivate MAO.

## SUGGESTED READINGS

Bukcharaeva EA, Kim KC, Moravec J, et al. Noradrenaline synchronizes evoked quantal release at frog neuromuscular junctions. *J Physiol.* 1999;517:879-888.

Collier TJ, Steece-Collier K, McGuire S, et al. Cellular models to study dopaminergic injury responses. *Ann NY Acad Sci.* 2003;991:140-151.

Fowler SJ, Lipworth BJ. Pharmacokinetics and systemic $\beta_2$-adrenoceptor-mediated responses to inhaled salbutamol. *Br J Clin Pharmacol.* 2001;51:359-362.

Gauthier C, Langin D, Balligand JL. $\beta_3$-Adrenoceptors in the cardiovascular system. *TIPS.* 2000;21:426-431.

Gnegy ME. The effect of phosphorylation on amphetamine-mediated outward transport. *Eur J Pharmacol.* 2003;479:83-91.

Green SA, Spasoff AP, Coleman RA, et al. Sustained activation of a G protein-coupled receptor via "anchored" agonist binding. *J Biol Chem.* 1996;271:24029-24035.

He J, Xu J, Castleberry AM, et al. Glycosylation of $\beta_1$-adrenergic receptors regulates receptor surface expression and dimerization. *Biochem Biophys Res Commun.* 2002;297:565-572.

Kapoor K, Willems EW, Maassen van den Brink A, et al. Assessment of anti-migraine potential of a novel $\alpha$-adrenoceptor agonist S19014: effects on porcine carotid and regional haemodynamics and human coronary artery. *Cephalalgia.* 2004;24:425-438.

Lee SP, So CH, Rashid AJ. Dopamine D1 and D2 receptor co-activation generates a novel phospholipase C-mediated calcium signal. *J Biol Chem.* 2004;279:35671-35678.

Lötvall J. The long and short of beta 2-agonists. *Pulm Pharmacol Ther.* 2002;15:497-501.

Mathur VS. The role of the DA-1 receptor agonist fenoldopam in the management of critically ill, transplant and hypertensive patients. *Rev Cardiovasc Med.* 2003;4(suppl 1):S35-S40.

Moniotte S, Balligand JL. Potential use of $\beta_3$-adrenoceptor antagonists in heart failure therapy. *Cardiovasc Drug Rev.* 2002;20:19-26.

Oster JR, Epstein M. Use of centrally acting sympatholytic agents in the management of hypertension. *Arch Intern Med.* 1991;151:1638-1644.

Sun D, Huang A, Mital S, et al. Norepinephrine elicits $\beta_2$-receptor-mediated dilation of isolated human coronary arterioles. *Circulation.* 2002;106:550-555.

Szabo B. Imidazoline antihypertensive drugs: a critical review on their mechanism of action. *Pharmacol Ther.* 2002;93:1-35.

Tsuda K, Tsuda S, Nishio I. Role of alpha 2-adrenergic receptors and cyclic monophosphate-dependent protein kinase in the regulation of norepinephrine release in the central nervous system of spontaneously hypertensive rats. *J Cardiovasc Pharmacol.* 2003;42(suppl 1):S81-S85.

Waugh DJJ, Gaivin RJ, Zuscik MJ, et al. Phe-308 and Phe-312 in transmembrane domain 7 are major sites of the alpha 1-adrenergic receptor antagonist binding. *J Biol Chem.* 2001;276:25366-25371.

Willems EW, Valdivia LF, Villalon CM, et al. Possible role of $\alpha$-adrenoceptor subtypes in acute migraine therapy. *Cephalalgia.* 2003;23:245-257.

# 14

# Adrenergic Receptor Antagonists

## AJ LANÇA

**CASE HISTORY**

A 60-year-old man presented for a routine eye examination. He complained of progressive weakening of vision, and his intraocular pressure was found to be 26 mmHg. His arterial blood pressure was found to be mildly elevated (135/98 mmHg) but was not treated at this stage. Since intraocular pressures of greater than 20 mmHg usually indicate a need for drug therapy, the patient was asked to return to the ophthalmology department for a diagnostic test for glaucoma. The patient's brother (aged 65) and father had also been diagnosed as having glaucoma. After an overnight fast and immediately before the test, the patient was asked to consume 1 L of water. This caused the intraocular pressure to increase by 12 mmHg. The patient had no evidence of trauma, inflammation, or diabetes, and he was not taking any medication. Timolol 0.25% ophthalmic solution was prescribed, to be self-administered at a dose of 1 drop of the solution in each eye, twice daily. On this treatment, the intraocular pressure remained elevated at 24 mmHg, and the concentration of the solution was therefore increased to 0.5%. Following regular treatment for 3 weeks, his intraocular pressure was still elevated. At this point, a combination of timolol 0.5% and dorzolamide 20 mg/mL was prescribed, to be administered at the rate of 1 drop twice daily in each eye. Within a week, the intraocular pressure was within the normal range (10 to 20 mmHg), and the blood pressure was now found to be 130/88 mmHg.

## INTRODUCTORY CONCEPT

The sympathetic nervous system plays a central role in homeostasis and, particularly, in the regulation of cardiovascular functions. Abnormally increased synthesis and release of catecholamines (adrenaline,[1] noradrenaline, and dopamine) increases activation of adrenergic receptors and consequently increases sympathetic activity. Adrenergic antagonists compete with catecholamines at the adrenergic receptors and block receptor activation. Their potency as blockers is expressed in terms of their $pA_2$ (see Chapter 7). The therapeutic effects of these drugs are determined by their selectivity for the $\alpha$ and $\beta$ receptors (for adrenergic receptor classification, see Chapter 11). Adrenergic antagonists, such as selective $\alpha_1$ and $\beta_1$ antagonists, are among the most widely prescribed drugs in clinical practice, and they are used in the treatment of hypertension, coronary heart disease, arrhythmias, and glaucoma.

The response of a given target organ to catecholamines and adrenergic drugs is determined by the types of receptors expressed in that particular organ or tissue. Consequently, the administration of a selective adrenergic antagonist has the potential to specifically block responses elicited by sympathomimetic agents in well-defined tissues or organs. The extent of the blockade obtained in the effector organ is related to (1) the relative concentrations of the agonist and the antagonist present at the receptor sites in the effector organ cells, (2) their relative affinities for these sites, and (3) the level of expression (i.e, the number) of different receptors in the target organs. Selectivity of the antagonist drug for $\alpha$ or $\beta$ receptors is further enhanced by differing affinities of the drugs for the respective receptor subtypes ($\alpha_1$, $\alpha_2$, $\beta_1$, and $\beta_2$).

The development of antagonists with higher affinity for selective receptor subtypes allows for a more discrete targeting of effector organs and a subsequent reduction in adverse effects that result from the unwanted targeting of other receptor subtypes expressed in different tissues. Newer and highly selective antagonists specifically target receptors that are expressed at high levels in a particular organ.

Adrenergic antagonists can also be classified according to their mechanism of action (see also Chapter 13). The molecular targets of directly acting antagonists are the adrenergic receptors, which they block, thus prevent-

[1] In the United States, adrenaline is called epinephrine, and noradrenaline is norepinephrine.

ing activation of the receptor by the agonist. Indirectly acting antagonists decrease synthesis (e.g., $\alpha$-methyl-p-tyrosine), storage (e.g., reserpine), and release (e.g., guanethidine) of catecholamines, thus decreasing catecholaminergic activity.

## $\alpha$-ADRENERGIC RECEPTOR ANTAGONISTS

Binding of an antagonist to the $\alpha$ receptors can be either reversible or irreversible (insurmountable). *Reversible antagonists* (e.g., phentolamine, prazocin) dissociate from receptors and can be competitively displaced by another ligand (e.g., the agonist) that binds at the receptor. The duration of action of a reversible antagonist is determined by the dissociation rate at the receptor and the half-life of the drug. *Irreversible antagonists* (e.g., phenoxybenzamine) form a covalent bond with the receptor, resulting in irreversible blockade. Thus, the effects of receptor antagonism are observed even after the drug is no longer present in the plasma. Reversal of the effect requires *de novo* synthesis of new receptor molecules in the rough endoplasmic reticulum, a process which takes up to several hours.

A further classification distinguishes selective versus non-selective $\alpha$ receptor antagonists; for example, phentolamine and phenoxybenzamine block both $\alpha_1$ and $\alpha_2$ receptors, whereas prazosin selectively blocks $\alpha_1$ receptors. Rauwolscine and yohimbine, plant alkaloids with prominent central nervous system (CNS) effects, are selective $\alpha_2$ antagonists. Tamsulosin and 5-methylurapidil are selective for $\alpha_{1A}$ receptors, whereas chloroethylclonidine is selective for $\alpha_{1B}$ receptors.

## Irreversible $\alpha$ Receptor Antagonist

The haloalkylamine **phenoxybenzamine** (Dibenzyline; Fig. 14-1) is closely related chemically to the nitrogen mustards. It contains a tertiary amine that cyclizes to form a reactive ethylenimonium intermediate. The molecular configuration directly responsible for blockade is a highly reactive carbonium ion formed when the three-member ring breaks. The persistence and completeness of the blockade are caused by covalent bonding to the receptor, which is difficult to reverse. After a single dose of phenoxybenzamine, a progressively decreasing but still significant blockade persists for at least 3 days. With increasing doses of the blocking agent, the dose–response curve for an agonist is shifted progressively to the right, and the maximum possible response is reduced as the number of available receptors becomes decreased. Phenoxybenzamine also binds irreversibly, although with a lower affinity, to histamine $H_1$ receptors, serotonergic, and muscarinic cholinergic receptors. It also blocks the reuptake of noradrenaline and enhances its

release from sympathetic neurons by blockade of presynaptic $\alpha_2$ receptors. This drug also provides a useful pharmacological tool with which to study receptor reserve (spare receptor) characteristics.

In the **cardiovascular system,** blockade of the $\alpha_1$ receptors in smooth muscle decreases peripheral resistance, lowers diastolic blood pressure, decreases venous return to the heart, and, as a result, causes reflex tachycardia. Tachycardia is also caused by blockade of presynaptic $\alpha_2$ receptors, which exert inhibitory feedback control over noradrenaline release. In supine normotensive individuals, the hypotensive effect of phenoxybenzamine is small, whereas in hypertensive patients, the effect is more robust. When the patient assumes an upright posture, a sudden drop in blood pressure causes postural hypotension. Currently, the therapeutic use of phenoxybenzamine is limited to the treatment of pheochromocytoma, a tumour of the adrenal gland that secretes large amounts of catecholamines (see Chapter 34). The drug is usually administered to control severe hypertension and precedes the surgical removal of the tumour.

**Metabolic effects** consist of an increase in insulin secretion and, sometimes, increased lipolysis. The increase in insulin secretion is due both to $\alpha$ receptor blockade, which prevents the inhibitory effects of endogenous catecholamines on insulin secretion, and to the unmasking of the $\beta_2$ receptor activity of endogenous adrenaline, which further enhances the release of insulin.

## Reversible $\alpha$ Receptor Antagonists

**Tolazoline** (Priscoline) and **phentolamine** (Rogitine, Regitine; Fig. 14-2) are competitive inhibitors at both the $\alpha_1$ and $\alpha_2$ receptors, with a higher affinity for the $\alpha_1$ subtype. At high concentrations, phentolamine not only competitively inhibits noradrenaline action, but also blocks that of serotonin. It binds to serotonin (5-HT) receptors, although with an affinity 1000 times lower than for the $\alpha$-adrenergic receptors. The cardiovascular effects of phentolamine are similar to those of phenoxybenzamine but are more transient. The cardiostimulating properties of non-selective $\alpha$ receptor antagonists, result-

FIGURE 14-1 | Structural formula of phenoxybenzamine HCl.

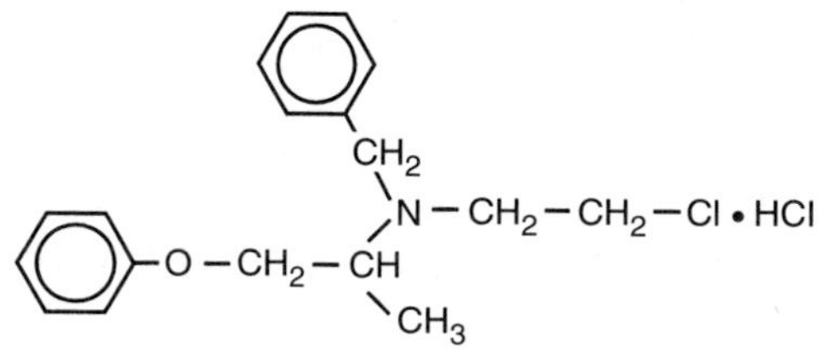

FIGURE 14-2 Structural formulae of tolazoline and phentolamine mesylate.

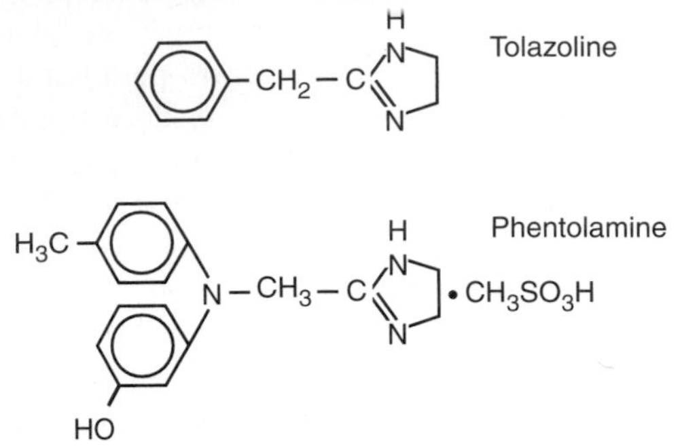

Other selective $\alpha_1$-adrenoceptor antagonists in this family include **doxazosin** and **trimazosin**. These drugs are pharmacodynamically similar to prazosin but differ from it in pharmacokinetic profiles.

Prazosin is well absorbed following oral administration and has a plasma half-life of 3 to 4 hours. It binds extensively to plasma proteins (approximately 97% at therapeutic concentrations) and undergoes biotransformation in the liver. Prazosin is used in the treatment of mild and moderate hypertension, either alone or in conjunction with a diuretic. It has also been used in the treatment of congestive heart failure (CHF). It causes peripheral vasodilatation and decreases venous return, decreases pre- and postload, and therefore decreases pulmonary congestion and increases cardiac output. Although it improves the clinical condition in CHF patients, recent clinical studies failed to demonstrate a beneficial effect on life expectancy in this group.

Terazosin has a higher bioavailability and a longer half-life (10 to 12 hours) than prazosin. It is also used in the treatment of mild to moderate hypertension. It is also effective in the symptomatic treatment of benign prostatic hyperplasia (BPH), an effect related to the $\alpha_1$ antagonism in the smooth muscle of the prostate and sphincter of the urinary bladder, where over 70% of the $\alpha_1$ receptors are of the $\alpha_{1A}$ subtype.

ing from blockade of presynaptic $\alpha_2$ receptors (causing an increased release of noradrenaline from sympathetic nerve endings), can be blocked by atenolol, which is a selective antagonist of $\beta_1$ receptors in the heart. Phentolamine is used in the short-term control of hypertension in pheochromocytoma patients, as well as in the control of hypertension caused by tyramine-rich diet in patients being treated with monoamine oxidase inhibitors.

## Selective $\alpha_1$ Receptor Antagonists

### Prazosin (Minipress) and Terazosin (Hytrin)
At therapeutic dosages, both prazosin (Fig. 14-3) and terazosin competitively inhibit the $\alpha_1$-adrenoceptor, for which they have an affinity 1000 times higher than for the $\alpha_2$ receptor. They have a similar potency at the $\alpha_{1A}$, $\alpha_{1B}$, and $\alpha_{1D}$ receptor subtypes and are therefore unable to selectively target any particular $\alpha_1$ subtype. Selective $\alpha_1$-receptor antagonists are widely used clinically for the treatment of hypertension. The adverse effects that are characteristically observed with non-selective $\alpha$-adrenoceptor antagonists (e.g., tachycardia, positive inotropy, and renin release) are uncommon with prazosin or terazosin treatment.

The selectivity of both drugs for $\alpha_1$-adrenoceptors allows the $\alpha_2$-mediated negative feedback loop for noradrenaline to be retained, thus preventing the occurrence of tachycardia observed with the non-selective $\alpha$ receptor antagonists. However, tachycardia mediated by reflex baroreceptor mechanisms may occur occasionally.

Diastolic pressure falls as a result of decreased venous return, caused by decreased peripheral resistance and reduction of circulating blood volume (due to blood pooling in the large veins) as a result of $\alpha_1$-adrenoceptor blockade in the large veins. Dizziness or syncope, caused by orthostatic hypotension, may occur as a "first-dose phenomenon" and lead to loss of consciousness. This effect may be circumvented by starting with a low dose and increasing it slowly.

### Tamsulosin (Flomax)
This selective competitive antagonist (Fig. 14-4) has a high affinity for the $\alpha_{1A}$ and $\alpha_{1D}$ receptors, but no affinity for the $\alpha_{1B}$. This drug has been successfully used in the symptomatic treatment of BPH, a condition in which the expression of $\alpha_{1A}$ receptors in the prostatic smooth muscle cells is increased. Although its efficacy is the same as that of terazosin, tamsulosin causes less postural hypotension and other cardiovascular side effects, possibly because it does not bind to the $\alpha_{1B}$ receptor, which is the most abundantly expressed in the cardiovascular system.

## Selective $\alpha_2$ Receptor Antagonists

The indolealkylamines **yohimbine** (Fig. 14-5) and **rauwolscine** are competitive antagonists at the $\alpha_2$-adrenoceptor, and they are relatively selective at low doses. At low

FIGURE 14-3 Structural formula of prazosin HCl.

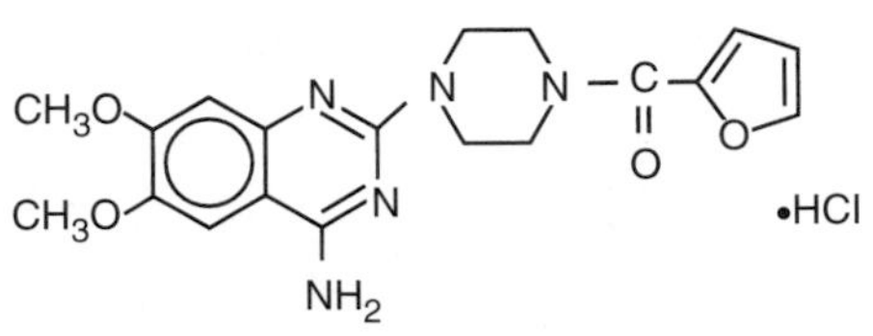

FIGURE 14-4 Structural formula of tamsulosin.

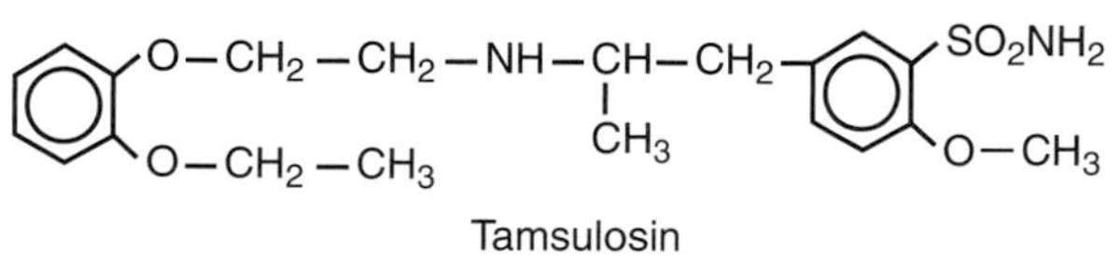

Tamsulosin

doses, yohimbine readily enters the CNS, where it selectively blocks $\alpha_2$ receptors and therefore increases noradrenaline release. As a result, it increases blood pressure and heart rate and causes behavioural excitation, tremor, and increased release of antidiuretic hormone. Yohimbine blocks the cardiovascular and motor actions of clonidine, a selective $\alpha_2$ agonist (see Chapter 13). In contrast, at higher doses, it also blocks peripheral $\alpha_1$-adrenoceptors and produces a short-lived fall in blood pressure, and it also binds to serotonin receptors. Yohimbine has been used to treat impotence, although its benefit in the treatment of male sexual dysfunction is not clearly understood. Other drugs, namely phosphodiesterase inhibitors (e.g., sildenafil, tadalafil) and prostaglandins (e.g., alprostadil), have largely replaced the use of yohimbine in the the treatment of sexual dysfunction.

## Other Agents with $\alpha$-Adrenergic Receptor–Blocking Properties

5-Methylurapidil and niguldipine are selective competitive inhibitors at the $\alpha_{1A}$-adrenoceptor. Chloroethylclonidine is an irreversible $\alpha_{1B}$-adrenoceptor inhibitor.

Other drugs with $\alpha$ receptor blocking activity include neuroleptics (e.g., haloperidol, chlorpromazine), tricyclic antidepressants (e.g., desipramine), and 5-HT receptor antagonists (e.g., ketanserin). In these agents, the $\alpha$ receptor blocking activity is less prominent than their activities at other receptors and is largely related to side effects of these drugs rather than to their primary therapeutic uses.

## Therapeutic Uses of $\alpha$-Adrenergic Receptor Antagonists

$\alpha$ Receptor antagonists are used in the treatment of mild and moderate primary hypertension, either alone or in conjunction with diuretics (e.g., hydrochlorothiazide) or $\beta$-antagonists (e.g., propranolol). Recent studies have shown that prazosin and related compounds have a beneficial effect on plasma lipid concentrations. They lower plasma levels of low-density lipoproteins and triglycerides, and increase high-density lipoproteins, an additional potential benefit in the prevention of atherosclerosis. The side effects of prazosin consist of the "first-dose phenome-

non" (i.e., a rapid and profound fall in blood pressure, faintness, and palpitations shortly after the first dose, or after a significant increase in dose), orthostatic hypotension, edema, and aggravation of pre-existing angina. Other occasional adverse effects are vertigo, headache, depression, vomiting, diarrhea, and constipation.

Formerly, an important use of adrenoceptor antagonists was in the diagnosis of pheochromocytoma, a catecholamine-secreting tumour of the chromaffin tissue of the adrenals. Several agents have been used for this purpose, but phentolamine was the most commonly employed. A significant fall in blood pressure within 2 minutes of administering the drug was considered to be a positive response. With the advent of sensitive chemical methods for the determination of catecholamines and their metabolites in urine and plasma, however, the phentolamine test has declined in importance. $\alpha$ Receptor antagonists are still used in the preoperative management of pheochromocytoma, for the prolonged treatment of cases not amenable to surgery, and to prevent paroxysmal hypertension during operative manipulation of the tumour.

The use of $\alpha$ receptor blocking drugs is occasionally recommended in the treatment of shock, since vasoconstriction is an important feature, with resultant decrease in tissue perfusion. Some $\alpha_1$ receptor blockers may be clinically effective in the treatment of Raynaud's disease, a condition characterized by vasoconstriction due to increased sympathetic nerve activity. However, calcium-channel blockers (e.g., nifedipine, verapamil) are currently the drugs of choice in the treatment of this disorder.

## β-ADRENERGIC RECEPTOR ANTAGONISTS (β BLOCKERS)

Three different types of $\beta$-adrenergic receptors ($\beta_1$, $\beta_2$, and $\beta_3$) have been identified (see Chapter 13). The clinical applications of $\beta$ antagonists are based on their ability to compete with, and prevent receptor activation by, naturally occurring catecholamines or sympathomimetic drugs. A subclassification of $\beta$ antagonists into non-selective and selective became necessary because drugs such as propra-

FIGURE 14-5 Structural formula of yohimbine.

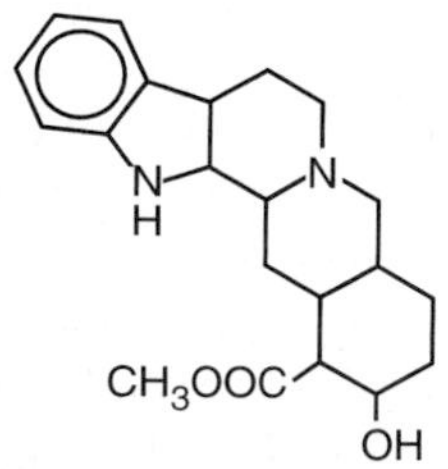

nolol block both $\beta_1$- and $\beta_2$-adrenergic receptors, while other drugs such as metoprolol selectively block $\beta_1$ with only minor effects on $\beta_2$ receptors. The selectivity of a $\beta$ antagonist for a specific receptor subtype is clinically relevant because it will determine the therapeutic efficacy and selectivity of the drug and also decrease the occurrence of adverse effects.

$\beta$-Adrenergic receptor antagonists (Fig. 14-6) are used extensively in the treatment of cardiovascular diseases, including hypertension, angina pectoris, cardiac arrhythmias, CHF, and in the secondary prevention of myocardial infarction and sudden death in patients with coronary thrombosis. They are also used in thyrotoxicosis and glaucoma.

The $\beta$ receptor antagonists differ in their profiles of activity, pharmacokinetics, and adverse effects, and some show greater selectivity for $\beta_1$ receptors in the heart. These "cardioselective" $\beta_1$ antagonists are less likely to cause the adverse effects of bronchospasm, intermittent claudication, and cold extremities. However, at high doses, their selectivity is lost, and they also block $\beta_2$ receptors and must therefore be administered caustiously to patients with asthma and chronic rhinitis. $\beta$ Antagonists block the stimulatory effects of catecholamines on glycogenolysis and glucose mobilization, but they do not block the potentiation of insulin-induced hypoglycemia. Because they reduce the occurrence of tachycardia, they prevent the early symptomatic detection of hypoglycemia in diabetic patients, so their use in diabetic patients with a history of hypoglycemic events should be closely monitored.

When patients are dependent on sympathetic drive because of poor cardiac reserve, a partial agonist at $\beta_1$ receptors is preferred (e.g., pindolol, acebutolol) because it is less likely to cause serious impairment of cardiac output. Conversely, a partial agonist would be less suitable in thyrotoxicosis, which is associated with excessive activity of the sympathetic nervous system.

## Propranolol (Inderal)

Propranolol (see Fig. 14-6), the prototypical $\beta$ antagonist, has an equal affinity for both the $\beta_1$ and $\beta_2$ receptors. It is a racemic mixture of levorotatory and dextrorotatory forms. The $l$-isomer is some 100 times more potent than the $d$-isomer in blocking $\beta_1$ and $\beta_2$ receptors. The two isomers are equally effective as membrane stabilizers. This action, associated with blockade of sodium channels, is seen only at high concentrations of the drug, and therefore, this mechanism is probably not responsible for the anti-arrhythmic and antihypertensive effects of these drugs, although it may play a role in the occurrence of adverse effects at high dosages. Propranolol is a competitive antagonist of endogenous noradrenaline and adrenaline and of all sympathomimetic drugs acting on $\beta_1$- and $\beta_2$-adrenergic receptors. The effects of propranolol antag-

onism of endogenously released catecholamines are dependent upon the extent of the sympathetic tone in a given organ.

### Pharmacokinetics

Because of its lipid solubility, propranolol is quickly and completely absorbed from the gastrointestinal tract, and it undergoes extensive first-pass metabolism in the liver. There is rapid hepatic extraction of the drug from the blood, and systemic bioavailability of an oral dose is less than 30%. Since the hepatic extraction mechanisms are saturable (and vary between individuals), increasing the dose of propranolol may result in disproportionate increases in plasma levels. Hydroxylation of propranolol in the liver produces an active metabolite, 4-hydroxypropranolol, which has a shorter half-life than the parent compound. A large proportion of circulating propranolol is protein-bound, and the plasma half-life is approximately 4 hours. However, the clinical effect may last longer than the reported half-life because of the additive effect of the active metabolite (Table 14-1). Propanolol is also available in a controlled-release formulation, allowing for a single daily administration, better suited for chronic treatment. However, administration of the long-acting formulation should be preceded by titration of the appropriate dosage using the conventional formulation.

### Pharmacological effects

*Cardiovascular.* Propranolol exerts a negative chronotropic action on the heart; that is, it produces bradycardia, particularly when sympathetic discharge to the heart is high, as in hypertensive patients and in normotensive individuals during exercise (Table 14-2). It also has a negative inotropic effect (i.e., it decreases the force of contraction). Consequently, cardiac output (the amount of blood ejected from the heart per minute) is reduced. Oxygen consumption is also decreased because of the decreased work of the heart; this is why it is used in the adjuvant treatment of coronary heart disease. Atrioventricular (AV) conduction velocity is decreased since vagal action on the AV node becomes dominant. Automaticity of pacemaker cells is decreased; this is the basis for the use of propranolol in suppressing ectopic foci and resultant arrhythmias.

Peripheral vascular resistance is increased as a result of vasoconstriction caused by reflex increase in sympathetic tone and by unopposed $\alpha$ receptor stimulation by endogenous noradrenaline in small arteries and arterioles which contain both $\alpha_1$- and $\beta_2$-adrenoceptors (e.g., vessels to skeletal muscles). Nevertheless, hypotension occurs after chronic administration of propranolol, probably because of the decrease in cardiac output, possible central actions (see "Central effects" below), and blockade of renin release from the juxtaglomerular cells in the kidneys, which results in a decreased rate of angiotensin II formation and

**FIGURE 14-6** Structural formulae of β-adrenergic receptor antagonists. (*Acebutolol is a selective antagonist, and partial agonist, that is metabolized to a non-selective antagonist.)

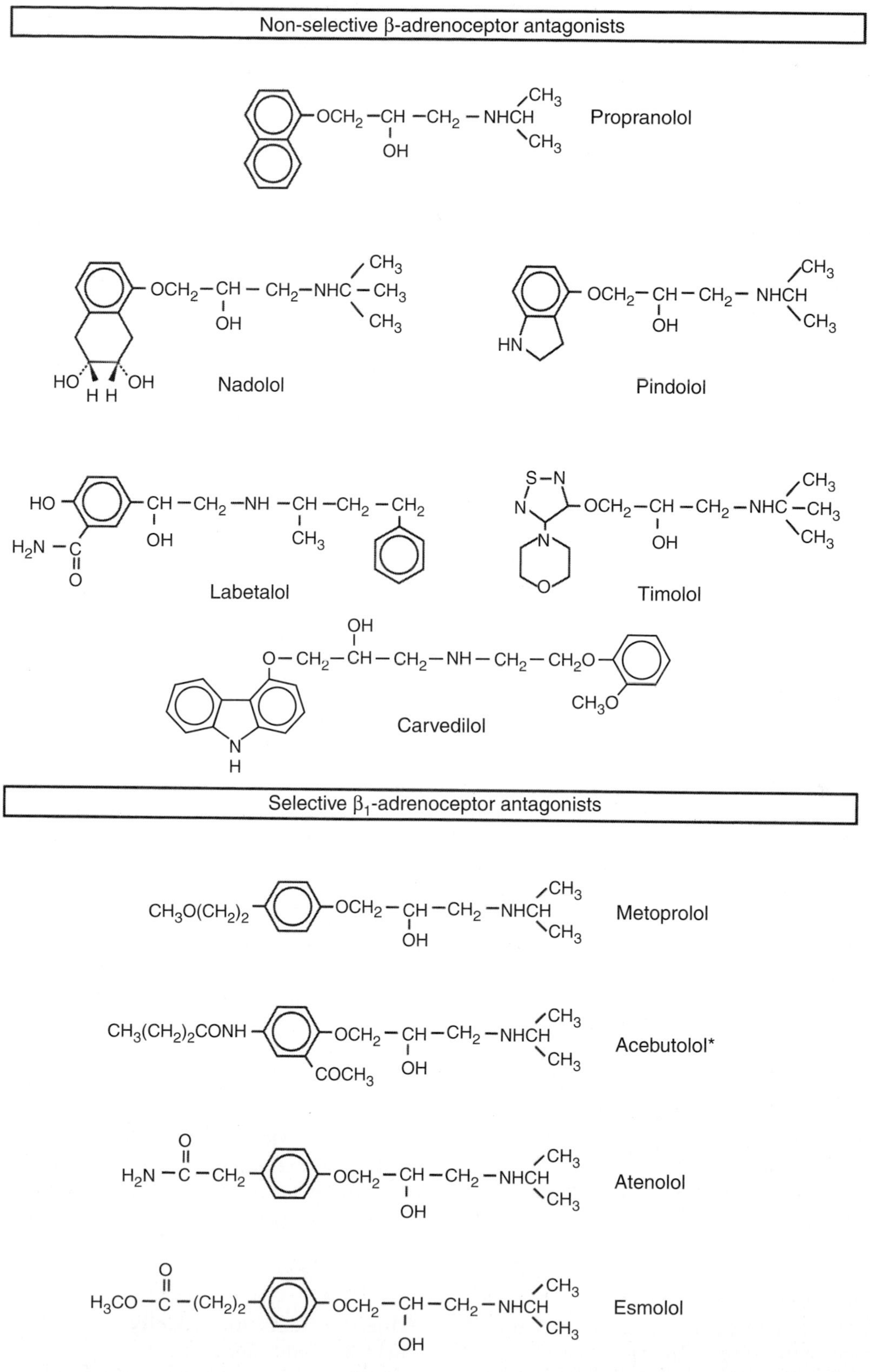

Non-selective β-adrenoceptor antagonists

Selective β₁-adrenoceptor antagonists

| TABLE 14-1 | Pharmacokinetics of Some β Receptor Antagonists | | | | |
|---|---|---|---|---|---|
| | Atenolol | Metoprolol | Pindolol | Propranolol | Timolol |
| Extent of absorption (%) | ~50 | >95 | >90 | >90 | >90 |
| Extent of bioavailability (% of dose) | ~40 | ~50 | ~90 | ~30 | 75 |
| Interpatient variations in plasma levels | 4-fold | 10-fold | 4-fold | 20-fold | 7-fold |
| β-Blocking plasma concentration (ng/mL) | 200–500 | 50–100 | 50–100 | 50–100 | 5–10 |
| Protein binding (%) | <5 | 12 | 57 | 93 | ~10 |
| Lipophilicity | Low | Moderate | Moderate | High | Low |
| Elimination half-life (hours) | 6–9 | 3–4 | 3–4 | 3–5 | 3–4 |
| Predominant route of elimination | Renal excretion (mostly unchanged) | Hepatic biotransformation | Renal excretion (~40% unchanged) and hepatic biotransformation | Hepatic biotransformation | Renal excretion (~20% unchanged) and hepatic biotransformation |
| Active metabolites | No | No | No | Yes | No |

decreased aldosterone release from the adrenal cortex (Fig. 14-7). However, in normotensive individuals, propanolol and other β antagonists do not have negative chronotropic or inotropic properties and do not lower blood pressure. The precise mechanisms underlying these differential responses are not clearly understood.

*Bronchiolar smooth muscle.* Propranolol blocks the bronchodilatation mediated by $\beta_2$ receptor stimulation and potentiates bronchospasm induced by acetylcholine and histamine. Airway resistance is always increased to at least a minor extent by this drug. Bronchospasm following propranolol administration is extremely hazardous in asthmatics.

*Metabolic effects.* The stimulant effects of endogenous catecholamines and sympathomimetic drugs on carbohydrate and fat metabolism are mediated via $\beta_3$ receptors (see Chapter 13). In humans, β antagonists including propranolol also inhibit the increase in plasma free fatty acids induced by catecholamines.

The effects on carbohydrate metabolism are less clear. Propranolol inhibits the secretion of insulin from the pancreas in response to $\beta_2$ receptor agonists, but it also prevents the hyperglycemic response to the action of adrenaline on $\beta_2$ receptors in the liver. Resting plasma glucose concentrations in non-diabetics are usually normal during treatment with propranolol. However, the rate of recovery of blood glucose levels following insulin admin-istration or muscular exercise may be delayed, resulting in hypoglycemia. Propranolol must be used cautiously in diabetics. A cardioselective $\beta_1$ antagonist (e.g., metopro-lol) may be less hazardous, since metabolic effects appear to be more closely associated with $\beta_2$ receptors.

*Central effects.* Propranolol readily crosses the blood–brain barrier and therefore affects central β receptors. It is used for the *prophylaxis* of migraine, although the relevance of β-blockade in treating this condition is questionable, and drugs with intrinsic sympathomimetic properties are clearly not recommended. The exact mechanism underly-ing the prevention of migraine by propranolol is not known, but it may be associated with inhibition of $\beta_2$ receptor–mediated vasodilatation in the brain or with blockade of uptake of serotonin by platelets. This would enhance the vasotonic effects of serotonin on cerebral blood flow. β Antagonists are not effective in the *acute treat-ment* of migraine. The use of propranolol in the treatment of anxiety is no longer recommended (see Chapter 23).

Tremor due to hyperthyroidism, alcohol withdrawal, or nervousness responds successfully to propranolol.

The antihypertensive effect of propranolol may also be related in part to a central adrenergic blocking action that results in enhanced vagal tone in the heart.

### Adverse effects and toxicity

These are predictable on the basis of the action of propra-nolol in producing β-adrenoceptor blockade. Adverse

| TABLE 14-2 | Effects of β-Adrenergic Receptor Antagonists |
|---|---|
| **β1 Receptor Blockade** | **β2 Receptor Blockade** |
| Cardiovascular effects<br>  (effects on cardiac function are more prominent during exercise)<br>Reduced heart rate<br>Delayed conduction velocity at the AV node<br>Decreased rate of diastolic depolarization in all pacemaker cells<br>  (the basis for anti-arrhythmic action)<br>Decreased force of contraction (negative inotropy) leading to:<br>  • reduced stroke volume<br>  • increased residual (end-systolic) volume<br>  • decreased cardiac output (decreased heart rate and stroke volume)<br>Reduced velocity of contraction<br>Decreased cardiac $O_2$ consumption (decreased rate and ventricular<br>  systolic pressure and contractility)<br>Reduced blood pressure<br>Inhibition of renin release from kidneys, causing subsequent<br>  lowering of angiotensin II<br>Edema formation due to sodium retention caused by decreased<br>  cardiac output | Vasoconstriction in some arterioles (e.g., those<br>  supplying skeletal muscle)*<br>Increased airway resistance and precipitation of asthma<br>Decreased glycogenolysis and gluconeogenesis<br>Inhibition of insulin release<br>Antagonism of catecholamine-induced tremor |
| Other effects<br>  Decreased lipolysis | |

*In coronary blood vessels, vasoconstriction would be the predominant effect of β1-adrenoceptor blockade.

effects are also widespread because of the diffuse distribution of sympathetic nerves and adrenergic receptors. Serious reactions include the following:

- Severe bradycardia
- Congestive heart failure
- Depression of AV conduction leading to AV dissociation, especially in patients with conduction defects or in those receiving digitalis
- Bronchoconstriction
- Hypoglycemia, particularly following insulin administration
- Aggravation of peripheral vascular disease, because of unopposed $\alpha_1$ receptor–mediated vasoconstriction by endogenous noradrenaline
- Fatal disturbances of cardiac rhythm or severe anginal attacks as a result of abrupt withdrawal. The dosage should therefore be reduced gradually over 1 or 2 weeks. The effects of propranolol withdrawal may be associated with rapid re-installation of sympathetic drive to the heart or with increased α receptor sensitivity.

## Other Non-selective β-Adrenergic Receptor Antagonists

The properties and relative potencies of some of these drugs are shown in Table 14-3, and their structures are shown in Figure 14-6.

**Nadolol** (Corgard) is one of the longest-acting β blockers, with a half-life of 14 to 24 hours; therefore, it can be administered on a once-daily basis. It is absorbed slowly and therefore is not indicated for the rapid control of hypertensive crisis. It is mainly indicated in the prophylactic treatment of angina pectoris.

**Pindolol** (Visken) and **acebutolol** (Monitan) block the β receptors in the presence of catecholamines. However, in their absence, these drugs have a low intrinsic sympathomimetic activity and act as partial agonists at the β receptors. Because of this property, they cause less reduction in heart rate than propranolol does and are indicated in patients with decreased cardiac reserve or bradycardia.

**Timolol** (Timoptic) has a half-life similar to that of propranolol but is less potent. However, it is only moderately biotransformed in the liver. It is topically administered for the control of elevated intraocular pressure (IOP) in glaucoma. Glaucoma is a chronic and progressive disorder that causes blindness. β Antagonists inhibit the secretion of aqueous humor in the anterior chamber of the eye and decrease IOP. Currently, the topical use of a combination of a β antagonist (e.g., timolol maleate) with a carbonic anhydrase II inhibitor (e.g., dorzolamide; see Chapter 37) is the most effective drug therapy for glaucoma.

## Selective β1 Receptor Antagonists

**Metoprolol** (Betaloc, Lopresor; see Fig. 14-6) and **atenolol** (Tenormin; see Fig. 14-6) are similar in potency

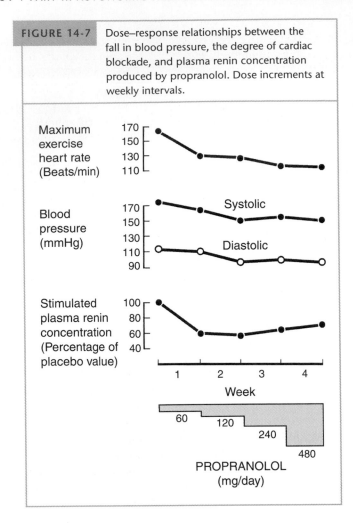

**FIGURE 14-7** Dose–response relationships between the fall in blood pressure, the degree of cardiac blockade, and plasma renin concentration produced by propranolol. Dose increments at weekly intervals.

esterases in erythrocytes. The drug causes a rapid dose-related reduction in blood pressure and heart rate. It is used in the treatment of supraventricular tachyarrhythmias.

**Betaxolol** is a selective $\beta_1$ antagonist that can be administered systemically in the treatment of hypertension or used in an ophthalmic preparation (Betoptic S) either alone or in conjunction with an anti-muscarinic agent, such as pilocarpine, to reduce IOP in acute and chronic glaucoma.

## Other Agents

**Labetalol** (Trandate; see Fig. 14-6) is an antagonist at both $\alpha_1$ and $\beta_2$ receptors. Its β-blocking effects are predominant, with a 3:1 ratio of β to α antagonism. The drug decreases blood pressure without reflex increase in heart rate and cardiac output. For this reason, it is useful in controlling elevated blood pressure associated with pheochromocytoma or hypertensive emergency.

**Carvedilol** (Coreg; see Fig. 14-6) and **bucindolol** are antagonists at both $\alpha_1$ and β receptors, with an affinity about 10 times higher for β than for $\alpha_1$ receptors. These drugs reduce systemic vascular resistance and can improve left ventricular ejection fraction. Because of these properties, carvedilol is used for the treatment of heart failure.

## Drug Interactions with β-Adrenergic Receptor Antagonists

Cimetidine (see Chapter 41) inhibits the hepatic enzymes associated with the first-pass metabolism of propranolol, metoprolol, and labetalol and thus increases bioavailability and plasma levels of these agents. Verapamil (see Chapter 34) may act synergistically to decrease conduction velocity at the AV node and to enhance the negative inotropic effects of propranolol and other β antagonists. Digoxin interacts in a similar manner. Indomethacin and salicylates may decrease the antihypertensive effects of $\beta_1$ receptor antagonists by

to propranolol in blocking $\beta_1$ receptors but much less active in blocking $\beta_2$ receptors. Metoprolol is used in the prophylaxis of angina pectoris and in the treatment of hypertension. Metoprolol also may be useful in some types of heart failure.

**Esmolol** (Brevibloc; see Fig. 14-6) is a short-acting $\beta_1$ antagonist for intravenous use. It is rapidly hydrolyzed by

| TABLE 14-3 | Properties and Approximate Relative Potencies of Some β-Adrenergic Receptor Antagonists | | | | |
|---|---|---|---|---|---|
| Drug | Solubility | Membrane-Stabilizing Effects | Intrinsic Sympathomimetic Activity | Approximate Cardiac Potency Relative to Propranolol | Hypotensive Doses Used (mg/day) |
| Propranolol | Lipid | ++ | 0 | 1 | 160–480 |
| Metoprolol | Aqueous | 0 | 0 | 1 | 100–400 |
| Pindolol | Lipid | ± | ++ | 10 | 15–45 |
| Timolol | Aqueous | 0 | ± | 10 | 30–60 |
| Atenolol | Aqueous | 0 | 0 | 1 | 100–200 |

±, +, ++ = relative degrees of activity; 0 = no activity.

inhibiting the synthesis of vasodilating prostaglandins. The hypoglycemic effect of insulin may be enhanced or prolonged by the non-selective β antagonists.

# INDIRECTLY ACTING ADRENERGIC ANTAGONISTS

## Reserpine

Reserpine (Serpasil; Fig. 14-8) is one of the alkaloids obtained from *Rauwolfia serpentina* (Indian snake root), which grows in India, where it has been used extensively for the treatment of anxiety, insomnia, psychoses, and hypertension. It has been an important tool in pharmacological experimentation because of its action in reducing the concentration of biogenic amines stored in both central and peripheral axon terminals. Clinically, reserpine is now used only occasionally in the treatment of hypertension, usually in conjunction with other drugs such as hydrochlorothiazide (see Chapter 34). Related alkaloids are **deserpidine** and **rescinnamine. Syrosingopine** is a semi-synthetic derivative with less effect on the CNS, but it remains a useful pharmacological tool with which to study the effects of biogenic amines (Table 14-4).

### Mechanism of action

Reserpine depletes central and peripheral stores of noradrenaline, 5-hydroxytryptamine (5-HT, serotonin), and dopamine. Chromaffin cells in the adrenal medulla are also depleted, but at a lower rate and to a lesser extent than the neurons. Reserpine is a potent inhibitor of the active transport system by which noradrenaline (NA) is taken up from the neuronal cell cytoplasm into the storage vesicles within sympathetic nerve endings (Fig. 14-9). The capacity of the storage granules to retain high concentrations of NA within the vesicles against a concentration gradient is also abolished. This allows leakage of NA into the cytoplasm and from there to the mitochondria, where it is deaminated by monoamine oxidase, resulting in depletion of NA stores. The uptake of dopamine from the cytoplasm to the storage vesicle is also impaired, and synthesis of the transmitter is therefore decreased. Noradrenergic and dopaminergic neurons in both the periphery and the brain are affected. The concentration of 5-HT is also significantly lowered in central serotonergic neurons, mast cells, platelets, and in the gastrointestinal tract. Decrease in catecholamine concentration begins within an hour of reserpine administration and is maximal by 24 hours.

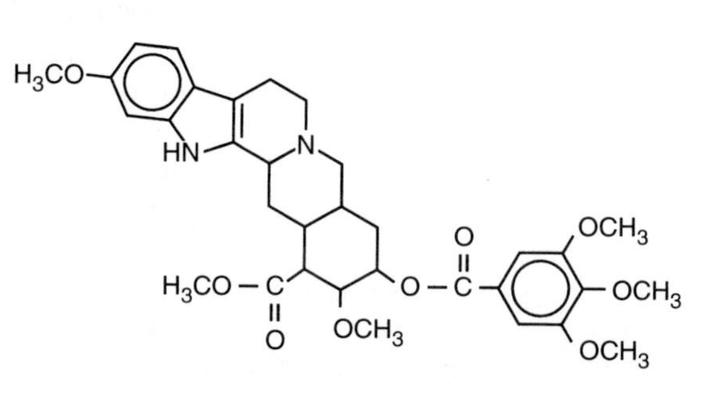

### Pharmacokinetics

Reserpine is well absorbed from the gastrointestinal tract, with a bioavailability of over 80%. At therapeutic levels, about 95% of the drug in plasma is protein-bound. It is highly lipophilic and therefore crosses capillary walls readily, including those in the CNS, and it appears in breast milk. It tends to accumulate in body fat as well as in catecholaminergic and serotonergic terminals. Reserpine is extensively demethylated in the liver and undergoes considerable first-pass biotransformation. However, the slow release from fatty tissues and the high protein binding result in a long half-life of 46 to 168 hours.

### Effects on the cardiovascular system

The antihypertensive actions of reserpine are probably a consequence of the reduced NA levels in peripheral sympathetic nerve endings, although a central action cannot be excluded. The peripheral depletion causes an impairment of responses to sympathetic stimulation. In the vascular system, therefore, there is less transmitter available for stimulation of adrenoceptors, in particular the $\alpha_1$-adrenoceptor. As a result, there is a reduction of tone in arterioles and large veins, resulting in a fall in diastolic blood pressure and venous pooling of blood. Similarly, in the heart, the $\beta_1$-adrenoceptor-mediated excitatory effects of NA are reduced or abolished, allowing acetylcholine to become the dominant transmitter. This results in bradycardia and decreased cardiac output, which also contribute to the reduction in blood pressure.

The fall in blood pressure is progressive and dose-dependent. Pressure begins to fall 3 to 6 days after initial administration of the drug and remains depressed for some time after withdrawal of reserpine. The dose should be as low as possible to avoid suicidal or depressive states. The effects of reserpine are additive with those of other antihypertensive agents including angiotensin-converting enzyme (ACE) inhibitors. Since only small doses are administered in the treatment of hypertension (resulting in less depletion of NA), severe orthostatic hypotension is not frequently observed.

During chronic treatment with reserpine, up-regulation of catecholaminergic receptors occurs, with resulting supersensitivity to the catecholamines and drugs with direct sympathomimetic effects. In contrast, responses to indirectly acting sympathomimetics, which normally increase the amount of NA released (e.g., ephedrine, amphetamine, and the experimental drug tyramine), are

| FIGURE 14-8 | Structural formula of reserpine. |

| TABLE 14-4 | Types of Action of Representative Antiadrenergic Drugs at Adrenergic Neurons, Synapses, and Neuroeffector Junctions | |
|---|---|---|
| Mechanism of Action | Drugs | Effects |
| Interference with synthesis of transmitter | α-Methyl-*p*-tyrosine<br>Disulfiram | Depletion of noradrenaline |
| Metabolic transformation by the same pathway as precursor of transmitter | α-Methyldopa | Displacement of noradrenaline by false transmitter (α-methyl-noradrenaline); blockade of release of noradrenaline |
| Blockade of transport system of storage granule membrane | Reserpine | Destruction of noradrenaline by intraneuronal monoamine oxidase, and depletion of adrenergic terminals; supersensitivity to directly acting amines; subsensitivity to indirectly acting amines |
| Prevention of release of transmitter | Guanethidine<br>Bretylium<br>Clonidine | Antiadrenergic; decreased release of noradrenaline |
| Blockade of endogenous transmitter at postsynaptic receptor | Phenoxybenzamine<br>Propranolol<br>Prazosin | α Receptor antagonism<br>β Receptor antagonism<br>Selective α1 receptor antagonism |
| Selective dopaminergic neurotoxins | 6-Hydroxydopamine<br>1-Methyl-4-phenyl-1,2,3,6-tetrahydropyridine (MPTP) | Irreversible degeneration of dopaminergic neurons |

either decreased or abolished with chronic reserpine treatment, since there is little or no NA to be released.

### Adverse effects

In the presence of reserpine, parasympathetic activity becomes more pronounced because of loss of opposing sympathetic tone. This applies to all organs with dual innervation by sympathetic and parasympathetic systems. Most side effects can be attributed to the unopposed activity of the parasympathetic system in many organs.

*Cardiovascular.* Excessive bradycardia may occur in some patients, as do nasal congestion and flushing of the skin, as well as postural hypotension with larger doses. Nasal congestion in the newborns of mothers treated with reserpine may cause serious respiratory problems. Sodium retention and edema may occur because of decreased perfusion pressure in renal blood vessels. Rapid parenteral injection can release NA initially and cause a transient rise in blood pressure.

The most unpleasant untoward responses to reserpine (and the most important from the point of view of toxicity) are related to the CNS and the gastrointestinal tract.

*Central nervous system.* Decreased concentrations of dopamine in the brain may cause parkinsonism. Lethargy, sedation, nightmares, and depression (occasionally leading to suicide) also may occur. The depression of mood closely resembles the clinical condition of endogenous depression. Hence, reserpine has been used experimentally to induce depression as a model for testing the efficacy of drugs with antidepressant potential.

*Gastrointestinal tract.* Increase in tone and motility gives rise to abdominal cramps and diarrhea. Gastric HCl secretion is increased (possibly by release of gastrin due to enhanced central vagal activity), leading to reactivation or aggravation of peptic ulcer.

*Other effects.* It has been claimed that long-term treatment with reserpine increases the incidence of breast carcinoma in women, but this is uncertain. The secretion of prolactin is also enhanced, probably because of decreased dopamine concentrations in the brain (see Chapter 24). Galactorrhea may occur occasionally.

## Guanethidine

Guanethidine (Ismelin; Fig. 14-10) is actively transported into peripheral sympathetic nerve endings by the uptake system for NA, with which it competes, and accumulates in storage vesicles. As a result, it reduces NA concentration in the sympathetic nerve endings and produces a characteristic, prolonged decrease of NA release, which interrupts transmission of impulses between sympathetic neurons and effector organs.

Other drugs that block the neuronal uptake of NA, such as cocaine and tricyclic antidepressants, also interfere competitively with the uptake of guanethidine. This

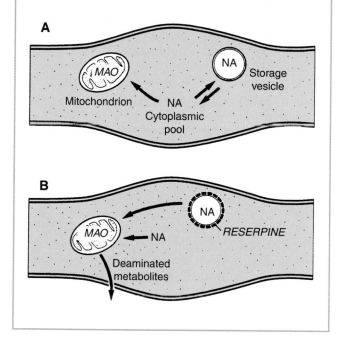

**FIGURE 14-9** Proposed mechanism of noradrenaline depletion from a sympathetic terminal varicosity by reserpine. (A) In the normal state, noradrenaline (NA) is in equilibrium between the cytoplasm and the storage vesicles, controlled by mitochondrial monoamine oxidase (MAO). (B) In the presence of reserpine, the NA uptake into storage vesicles is prevented, and NA from both cytoplasm and storage vesicles is gradually depleted by MAO metabolism.

competitive interference may prevent the onset of action or reverse the neuronal blocking effects of guanethidine.

Blockade of NA uptake by guanethidine causes partial depletion of NA stores, but chronic administration leads to receptor supersensitivity and therefore potentiates the actions of exogenous NA. Responses to indirectly acting sympathomimetic drugs (e.g., tyramine and amphetamine) are reduced in magnitude or blocked.

## Mechanism of action

Following intraneuronal accumulation of guanethidine, NA release (which normally occurs in response to action potentials) is impaired. This effect is associated with a membrane-stabilizing (local anaesthetic) action of guanethidine. Action potentials still occur, but exocytosis is blocked at neuronal membrane sites.

Subsequent and gradual depletion of NA occurs *selectively* in peripheral sympathetic nerve endings and is attributable to the blockade of amine uptake coupled with intraneuronal vesicular NA release and subsequent deamination by monoamine oxidase (MAO). The effects of guanethidine on intraneuronal concentration and release

of NA have been described as "drug-induced sympathectomy." Guanethidine may also act as a false transmitter, since it is released after nerve stimulation but does not act on the receptors.

## Pharmacokinetics

Absorption of orally administered guanethidine varies from 5 to 30%, causing wide inter-individual variations in dose requirements for reliable antihypertensive effects. However, the individually effective dose remains relatively constant in a given patient. The peak effect occurs in 6 to 8 hours, with a duration of action of about 24 hours. Guanethidine is rapidly transported to its intra-neuronal sites of action. It is cleared by the kidney, both in unchanged form (60%) and as two partly inactive metabolites, with an elimination half-life of about 5 days. Because of the long half-life, the effects of a constant daily dose may actually continue to increase for several weeks.

## Effects on the cardiovascular system

Guanethidine is used in patients with severe hypertension. Because it decreases the release of NA, guanethidine reduces sympathetic excitatory effects on the heart and vascular smooth muscle, including reflex compensation for changes in body position. It causes a prolonged fall in blood pressure, particularly in hypertensive patients. As its effect is greater in the erect than in the supine position, it may cause postural hypotension. This is a characteristic response to drugs that block the sympathetic nervous system. The rapid intravenous administration of a large dose of guanethidine can cause a transient, but marked, increase in blood pressure attributable to an initial displacement of NA from the sympathetic nerves. This is then followed by a prolonged fall in blood pressure.

Guanethidine has little effect on the catecholamine content of the adrenal medulla and the CNS; in the latter case, this is probably because the drug does not readily cross the blood–brain barrier.

## Adverse effects

Orthostatic hypotension (postural hypotension, see paragraph above) is aggravated by alcohol, warm weather, and exercise.

Sodium and fluid retention may occur and lead to edema and resistance to the therapeutic effect of the drug if a diuretic is not administered concurrently.

Bradycardia, due to vagal predominance in the heart, may be a decided disadvantage, especially in older patients.

Diarrhea from unopposed activity of the vagus nerve in the gastrointestinal tract is common. Failure of ejaculation may also occur.

Severe hypertensive reactions have been reported in patients with pheochromocytoma and are caused by supersensitivity of the adrenoceptors to catecholamines released from the tumour.

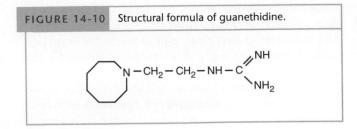

FIGURE 14-10    Structural formula of guanethidine.

## Drug interactions

The uptake of guanethidine into sympathetic neurons, and hence its antihypertensive action, may be blocked by tricyclic antidepressants, cocaine, and amphetamine (Fig. 14-11). Chronic administration of guanethidine also sensitizes the effector cells to catecholamines as much as 100-fold; this effect reaches a maximum in 10 to 14 days. The fact that responses are much reduced or absent in the presence of such sensitization indicates that the amount of transmitter released must be very small indeed.

## Other drugs of this class

**Bethanidine, debrisoquin,** and **guanadrel** are from the same family as guanethidine, with similar mechanism of action, side effects, and interactions. The half-life of bethanidine is much shorter than that of guanethidine (7 to 11 hours versus 43 hours, respectively). Bethanidine is

excreted unchanged in the urine. The biotransformation of debrisoquin shows marked individual differences that are due to genetic variations in the cytochrome P450 species involved; this is discussed in Chapter 10.

## α-Methyldopa

α-Methyldopa (Aldomet, Dopamet) is closely related chemically to L-dopa, which is a precursor in the synthesis of dopamine, noradrenaline, and adrenaline (see Chapter 11).

## Mechanism of action

α-Methyldopa becomes a substrate for dopa decarboxylase (aromatic amino acid decarboxylase) within the brain and in the periphery. It is converted to α-methyldopamine, which is in turn converted to α-methylnoradrenaline by dopamine-β-hydroxylase within the vesicles. α-Methylnoradrenaline acts as a "false" transmitter, which is responsible for the reduction of blood pressure in hypertensive patients (Fig. 14-12).

α-Methylnoradrenaline (formed from α-methyldopa) stimulates presynaptic $\alpha_2$-adrenoceptors, for which it has a high affinity, in the nucleus of the tractus solitarius in the medulla oblongata. Stimulation of these $\alpha_2$-adrenoceptors inhibits synaptic release of NA and thus blocks central sympathetic outflow, which in turn decreases the peripheral release of NA at sympathetic terminals on blood vessels.

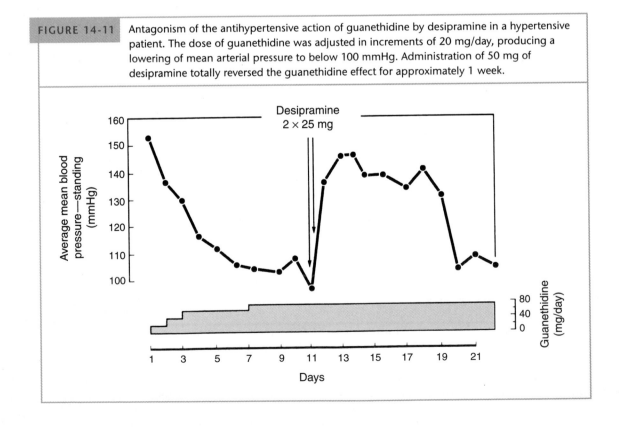

FIGURE 14-11    Antagonism of the antihypertensive action of guanethidine by desipramine in a hypertensive patient. The dose of guanethidine was adjusted in increments of 20 mg/day, producing a lowering of mean arterial pressure to below 100 mmHg. Administration of 50 mg of desipramine totally reversed the guanethidine effect for approximately 1 week.

FIGURE 14-12  Formation of α-methylnoradrenaline from α-methyldopa.

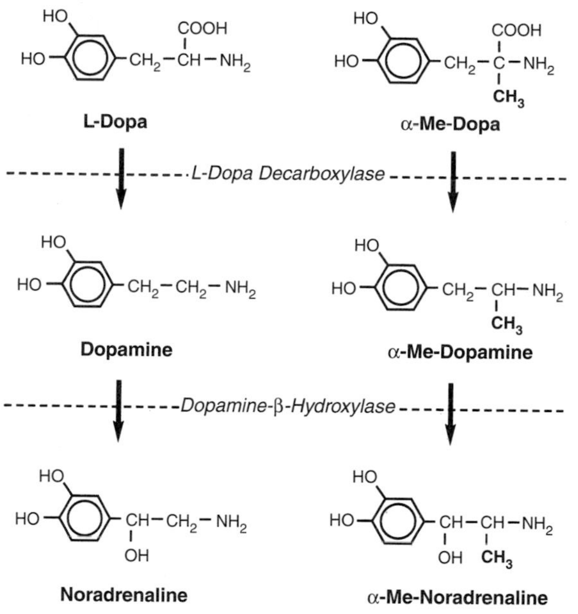

## Adverse effects

Adverse reactions to α-methyldopa include drowsiness, psychic depression, parkinsonism, dryness of the mouth, nasal stuffiness, nausea, and gastrointestinal disturbances. Hypersensitivity reactions include jaundice, pyrexia, and rashes; occasionally, hemolytic anemia may occur. Prolonged treatment may cause a positive Coombs' test. Liver damage may occur in the occasional patient.

## Clonidine

Clonidine (Catapres; Fig. 14-13) is an imidazoline derivative chemically related to the α receptor antagonist tolazoline. Clonidine was originally developed as a nasal decongestant because of its local vasoconstrictor effects, but when tested for this purpose in humans, it produced a marked reduction of blood pressure and heart rate. The fall in blood pressure is due to the $\alpha_2$ receptor stimulant properties of clonidine. Its actions in many respects resemble those of α-methyldopa. Both drugs allow vasopressor centres in the brain to retain some degree of sensitivity to baroreceptor control, thus lowering the incidence of postural hypotension.

Other drugs related to clonidine are **guanfacine** and **guanabenz**.

## Mechanism of action

Clonidine has a marked presynaptic $\alpha_2$ receptor stimulant action, which interferes with the neuronal release of NA at both central and peripheral sites. The central site of action is in the medulla. Stimulation of $\alpha_2$-adrenoceptors in this area (and possibly of $\alpha_1$ receptors on inhibitory interneurons) causes a reduction of efferent sympathetic nerve activity that results in a fall in blood pressure and heart rate. At peripheral sites, stimulation of presynaptic $\alpha_2$ receptors causes a reduction in the release of NA from the terminal varicosities. The inhibitory effect on the vagus nerve of the heart is augmented, probably both by increased sensitivity of the baroreceptors and by central actions.

## Pharmacokinetics

Oral absorption of clonidine is essentially complete but rather slow, peak plasma levels being reached in about 4 hours. Plasma half-life is about 12 hours but is greatly increased by severe renal disease. About 50% of the

In the peripheral nerves, α-methylnoradrenaline is stored in the vesicles and is released by nerve stimulation. It has only weak $\alpha_1$-adrenoceptor agonist properties. The central action of α-methylnoradrenaline prevents the peripheral release of both the false transmitter and NA.

## Pharmacokinetics

α-Methyldopa is poorly and somewhat irregularly absorbed from the gastrointestinal tract, and absorption is decreased by food. Oral bioavailability ranges from 10 to 60% (mean value 25%), due in part to first-pass biotransformation. The peak concentration in plasma is reached in about 2 hours. There is rapid distribution to all organs, especially the kidneys, heart, and brain. The elimination half-life is 1.5 to 2 hours in normal subjects, but it is increased in those with impaired renal function. About 50% of a dose is excreted unchanged in the urine, and 50% is biotransformed to α-methylnoradrenaline and other metabolites.

## Cardiovascular effects

α-Methyldopa produces progressive reductions in blood pressure and heart rate that are maximal in 4 to 6 hours. The fall in blood pressure is greater in hypertensive than in normotensive subjects; it is due to decreases in both cardiac output and peripheral resistance. α-Methyldopa does not produce any major changes in distribution of blood flow. Renal blood flow and glomerular filtration are well maintained in both normotensive and hypertensive subjects.

FIGURE 14-13  Structural formula of clonidine HCl.

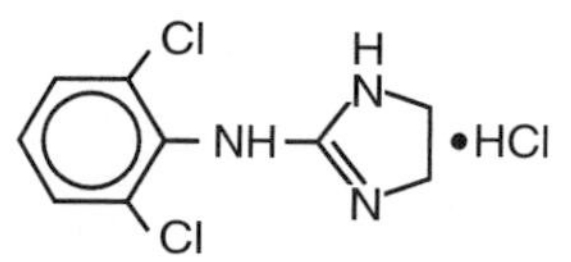

absorbed drug is excreted unchanged in the urine, the other half undergoing biotransformation in the liver.

## Pharmacological effects

Intravenous administration of clonidine in humans produces an initial brief increase in blood pressure followed by a fall in blood pressure associated with bradycardia. The initial increase in blood pressure is caused not only by a transient stimulation of $\alpha_1$-adrenoceptors but also by stimulation of post-junctional $\alpha_2$-adrenoceptors in blood vessels.

After oral administration, a decrease in blood pressure is evident within 30 to 60 minutes. The hemodynamic effects of clonidine include bradycardia and a reduced cardiac output, which both contribute to the fall in blood pressure.

Following chronic administration of clonidine, peripheral resistance is also decreased. Renin release is also inhibited by clonidine.

## Other uses of clonidine

Small doses of clonidine are effective in the prophylactic treatment of migraine, reducing both the frequency and severity of attacks. The drug has been used successfully in alleviating opiate withdrawal symptoms and also has been reported to reduce some of the symptoms of alcohol withdrawal that are attributable to adrenergic overactivity (see Chapter 22).

## Adverse effects

Sedation, dry mouth, and constipation occur frequently in the therapeutic dose range and limit the use of clonidine. It is possible that clonidine stimulation of $\alpha_2$-adrenoceptors found on cholinergic fibres innervating the salivary glands and intestine may be responsible. Central mechanisms also may be involved. Clonidine can also potentiate insulin-induced hypoglycemia.

A potentially dangerous side effect of clonidine is "rebound" hypertension in patients in whom the drug has been suddenly withdrawn. It is associated with overactivity of the sympathetic nervous system, as indicated by elevated plasma and urinary catecholamines. Prior administration of $\alpha$-adrenoceptor antagonists (e.g., phentolamine) will prevent this rebound effect.

## Drug interactions

Desmethylimipramine interferes with the antihypertensive action of clonidine, possibly because of the $\alpha$ receptor blocking activity of the antidepressant. Other tricyclic antidepressants and phenothiazine antipsychotics also may block the cardiovascular responses to clonidine administration and should be used with caution.

## Bretylium

Bretylium tosylate (Bretylate; Fig. 14-14) decreases the amount of NA released per stimulus. Like guanethidine, it inhibits the responses to adrenergic nerve stimulation and to indirectly acting sympathomimetic amines. In contrast to guanethidine, however, a single dose of bretylium produces no detectable reduction in tissue catecholamine levels. The major cardiovascular effects of bretylium are very similar to those of guanethidine, and at one time bretylium was used quite extensively in the treatment of hypertension. However, tolerance to its effects develops quite rapidly. It is used occasionally in the treatment of ventricular arrhythmias.

## α-Methyltyrosine (Metyrosine)

This drug inhibits the biosynthesis of the catecholamines at both central and peripheral sites, including chromaffin cells in the medulla of the adrenal gland. α-Methyltyrosine is a competitive inhibitor of tyrosine hydroxylase, which catalyzes the formation of L-dopa from L-tyrosine, the rate-limiting step in catecholamine synthesis. As a result, the activity of the sympathetic nervous system is reduced. α-Methyltyrosine is sometimes used to treat hypertension associated with pheochromocytoma (see Chapter 34). When this tumour occurs at extra-adrenal sites, it may be surgically less accessible, and therefore drug therapy may be necessary. Surgery may also be contraindicated in some patients. The clinical effectiveness of α-methyltyrosine in the therapy of pheochromocytoma can be determined by measurement of blood and urinary catecholamines.

**Adverse effects** include sedation, extrapyramidal symptoms, and psychic disturbances. Severe diarrhea may also occur. The drug is largely excreted in the urine but is not very soluble at urinary pH. Therefore, there is a risk of urinary crystal formation, and increased water intake is required to prevent this.

## 6-Hydroxydopamine and 1-Methyl-4-phenylpyridinium

6-Hydroxydopamine (6-OHDA) is a potent and selective neurotoxin of the dopaminergic system. In fact, under some in vivo conditions, dopamine itself can also be converted to 6-OHDA. 1-Methyl-4-phenylpyridinium (MPP+) is the active metabolite of 1-methyl-4-phenyl-1,2,3,6-tetrahydropyridine (MPTP), a contaminant produced dur-

FIGURE 14-14  Structural formula of bretylium.

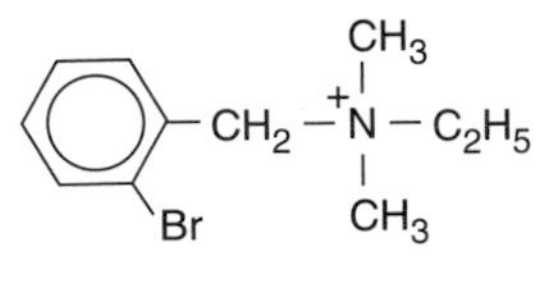

ing the illicit synthesis of "synthetic heroin" (meperidine), that causes selective degeneration of the dopaminergic system (neurons and terminals) in humans as well as in rodents (see Chapter 17). Both of these selective neurotoxins are extensively used as research tools in studies of the cellular and molecular mechanisms underlying Parkinson's disease. 6-OHDA does not penetrate the blood–brain barrier but can be administered intraventricularly in experimental animals. It accumulates within catecholaminergic neurons following its uptake by the amine pump and causes a dramatic reduction in catecholamine synthesis. This can result in a permanent "functional" sympathectomy and in the loss of approximately 80% of all functional adrenergic neurons. It is also used experimentally in order to trace the patterns of dopaminergic innervation in discrete areas of the brain.

## SUGGESTED READINGS

Collier TJ, Steece-Collier K, McGuire S, Sortwell CE. Cellular models to study dopaminergic injury responses. *Ann NY Acad Sci.* 2003;99:140-151.

Curzon G. How reserpine and chlorpromazine act: the impact of key discoveries on the history of psychopharmacology. *TIPS.* 1990;11:61-63.

de la Torre R, Farré M. Neurotoxicity of MDMA (ecstasy): the limitations of scaling from animals to humans. *TINS.* 2004;25:505-508.

Fechtner RD, Realini T. Fixed combinations of topical glaucoma medications. *Curr Opin Ophthalmol.* 2004;15:132-135.

Flordellis CS, Goumenos D, Kourounis G, et al. The shift in the "paradigm" of the pharmacology of hypertension. *Curr Top Med Chem.* 2004;4:487-498.

Holtz WA, O'Malley KL. Parkinsonian mimetics induce aspects of unfolded protein response in death of dopaminergic neurons. *J Biol Chem.* 2003;278:19367-19377.

Hospenthal MA, Peters JI. Long-acting beta(2)-agonists in the management of asthma exacerbations. *Curr Opin Pulm Med.* 2005;11:69-73.

Karamanakos PN, Pappas P, Stephanou P, Marselos M. Differentiation of disulfiram effects on central catecholamines and hepatic ethanol metabolism. *Pharmacol Toxicol.* 2001;88:106-110.

Kenakin TP. Drug antagonism. In: Kenakin TP, ed. *Pharmacologic Analysis of Drug-Receptor Interaction.* New York, NY: Raven Press; 1993.

Khorchid A, Cui Q, Molina-Holgado E, Almazan G. Developmental regulation of alpha 1A-adrenoceptor function in rat brain oligodendrocyte cultures. *Neuropharmacology.* 2002;42:685-696.

Koch WJ. Genetic and phenotypic targeting of beta-adrenergic signaling in heart failure. *Mol Cell Biochem.* 2004;263:5-9.

Lowe FC. Role of the newer alpha-adrenergic-receptor antagonists in the treatment of benign prostatic hyperplasia-related lower urinary tract symptoms. *Clin Ther.* 2004;26:1701-1713.

Magarian GJ. Reserpine: a relic from the past or a neglected drug of the present for achieving cost containment in treating hypertension? *J Gen Intern Med.* 1991;6:561-572.

Roehrborn CG, Schwinn DA. Alpha1-adrenergic receptors and their inhibitors in lower urinary tract symptoms and benign prostatic hyperplasia. *J Urol.* 2004;171:1029-1035.

Taylor MR, Bristow MR. The emerging pharmacogenomics of the beta-adrenergic receptors. *Congest Heart Fail.* 2004;10:281-288.

Wilson TA, Foxall TL, Nicolosi RJ. Doxazosin, an alpha-1 antagonist, prevents further progression of the advanced atherosclerotic lesion in hypercholesterolemic hamsters. *Metabolism.* 2003;52:1240-1245.

Yasuda JM, Schroeder DJ. Guanethidine for reflex sympathetic dystrophy. *Ann Pharmacother.* 1994;28:338-341.

# 15

# Neuromuscular Transmission and Drugs (Muscle Relaxants)

## M HONG

**CASE HISTORY**

A 25-year-old fashion model saw her physician with complaints of diplopia (double vision), dysphagia (problems swallowing), and what she believed to be a mild cold with generalized fatigue that was relieved by bedrest. She had had these problems for a few weeks and was only now seeking medical assistance because of her increasingly hoarse voice and the apparent inability to fully open her eyes, which interfered with on-camera work for TV commercials.

On examination, the patient had normal deep tendon reflexes and no muscle wasting. She had a poor gag reflex and selective weakness of her neck extensor muscles. She had marked bilateral ptosis (drooping of the eyelids) and bilateral ocular paresis that was elicited by sustained lateral gaze. Her thymus gland was swollen and of a tough consistency. Electromyography (EMG) testing revealed a progressive decrease in muscle action potential.

Myasthenia gravis was suspected, and an edrophonium test was ordered. An initial dose of 2 mg of edrophonium was administered intravenously without effect. An additional 8 mg of edrophonium was administered, and within 2 minutes, her muscle strength became normal and was sustained at a normal level for about 5 minutes. There was some salivation and flushing, and a low dose of atropine was administered to reduce the risk of bradycardia.

Her serum IgG antibodies to acetylcholine receptors were measured using a test involving competition with $^{125}$I-$\alpha$-bungarotoxin binding to human acetylcholine receptors. The test was positive. She was also tested with repetitive nerve stimulation, which showed a 20% decline in compound muscle action potential when the nerve was stimulated with surface electrodes six to 10 times at 2 to 3 Hz.

The neurologist decided that the patient's acute symptoms should be treated with pyridostigmine 60 mg three times a day. She also received prednisone 20 mg/day, which was increased to 40 mg/day in increments of 5 mg every 2 or 3 days.

The symptoms of myasthenia improved over the next 6 months but then began to worsen again. Increasing the dose of pyridostigmine appeared to make the symptoms worse, and another edrophonium test was performed. After an intravenous injection of 2 mg of edrophonium, the patient had difficulty breathing, and she lost all muscle tone for a period of about 8 minutes. She subsequently recovered. Her dose of pyridostigmine was then lowered to 40 mg three times a day. This relieved the symptoms, and she remained stable for a further 6 months. At this time, her serum IgG antibodies to acetylcholine receptors started to climb, and it was decided to remove her thymus gland. Over a 6-month period after the surgery, her symptoms gradually abated, and she has remained stable since then.

## CELLULAR EVENTS IN NERVE–MUSCLE TRANSMISSION

Neuromuscular transmission can be loosely described as the events leading from the release of the neurotransmitter acetylcholine at the motor nerve terminal to the production of endplate potentials at the post-junctional site of the neuromuscular synapse. The motor nerve fibres coming from the anterior horn cells of the spinal cord are myelinated up to the point where the fibres enter the muscle. Each nerve fibre then divides into as many as 200 non-myelinated branches that are covered by a Schwann cell. Each nerve terminal branch forms a single endplate region on a single muscle fibre (Fig. 15-1). The portion of the muscle cell membrane (sarcolemma) immediately underlying the nerve terminal forms a specialized structure called the muscle soleplate, characterized by infoldings of the sarcolemma. These are known as junctional folds.

| FIGURE 15-1 | Schema of the nerve–muscle junction. |

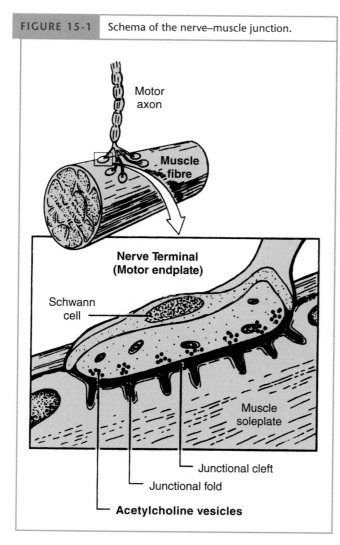

**Nerve Terminal (Motor endplate)**

Motor axon

**Muscle fibre**

Schwann cell

Muscle soleplate

Junctional cleft

Junctional fold

**Acetylcholine vesicles**

1. As with regular action potentials, there is a small influx of $Ca^{2+}$ associated with the action potential of the nerve terminal. This takes place through voltage-gated N-type channels, which have a low sensitivity to the therapeutically used calcium-channel blockers.
2. Since the surfaces of the membranes of the vesicles (and of the cell) are negatively charged, the entering $Ca^{2+}$ neutralizes the charges and causes vesicles to approach the pre-junctional membrane.
3. The vesicle then spontaneously fuses with the presynaptic membrane, releasing the enclosed acetylcholine by exocytosis.
4. The membrane of the vesicle, now incorporated into the presynaptic membrane, is pulled back into the cytoplasm by contractile filaments, which form a basket around the empty vesicle.
5. The basket vesicles lose their baskets and form a cistern. Within this cistern, acetylcholine is formed by the action of choline acetyltransferase on choline and acetyl-CoA (coenzyme A).
6. Vesicles containing acetylcholine then bud off from this cistern.

The entire cycle from (1) to (6) is very fast, taking place in seconds or minutes at most.

## Production of Endplate Potentials

Within 0.1 milliseconds, the released acetylcholine diffuses across the 200-Å junctional cleft and interacts with the acetylcholine receptors in the specialized endplate region of the sarcolemma.

Each vesicle releases about 10 000 molecules of acetylcholine, which act on the nicotinic cholinergic receptors on the outside of the endplate. (Acetylcholine injected inside the muscle has no effect.)

The stimulated receptors then almost simultaneously open up channels in the endplate for $Ca^{2+}$, $Na^+$, and $K^+$. The net result is an endplate potential. If only one (a "quantum" of acetylcholine), two, or three vesicles are released, as occurs spontaneously at a rate of about two pulses per second, only a miniature endplate potential (MEPP) develops, as shown in Figure 15-3. When a nerve impulse invades the nerve terminal, however, about 200 vesicles are released simultaneously, producing a normal endplate potential of 10 to 15 mV.

The endplate potential is a graded event and depends on the number of vesicles of acetylcholine released and the number of acetylcholine molecules interacting with the receptors. The amplitude of the endplate potential becomes greater with repeated stimulation of the nerve; this is called post-tetanic potentiation, or PTP. It is due to an increased concentration of $K^+$ within the synapse, which depolarizes the nerve terminal so that an increased amount of acetylcholine is released. If the endplate potential exceeds 15 mV, the sarcolemmal membrane surround-

The synaptic vesicles within the nerve terminal are clustered immediately opposite the junctional folds of the sarcolemma. The acetylcholine receptors of the sarcolemma are located at the mouths of the junctional folds and constitute at least 90% of the soleplate membrane.

## Impulse Invasion of the Nerve Terminal

The nerve action potential travels along the motor nerve fibre by saltatory conduction between nodes of Ranvier until it arrives at the point where the motor fibre enters the muscle. After this point, the action potential propagates into the terminals in the same fashion as it would in any unmyelinated fibre.

## Release of Acetylcholine

The events related to the release of acetylcholine constitute a cycle that is illustrated in Figure 15-2. (For synthesis of acetylcholine, see Chapter 11.) The distinct steps in this cycle are as follows:

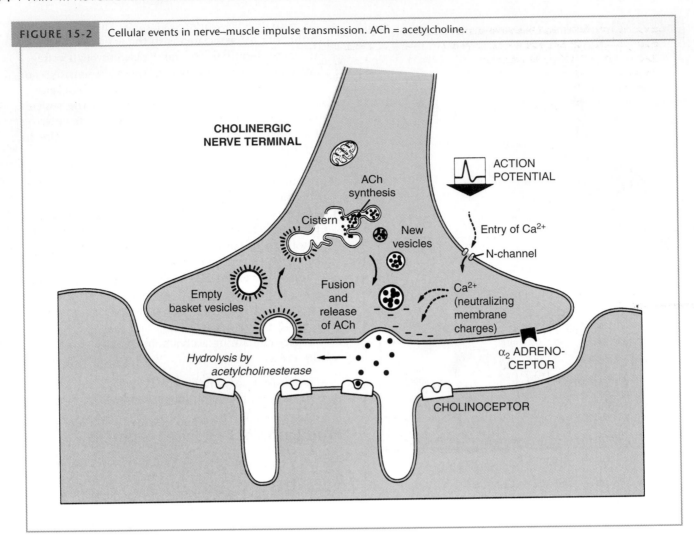

**FIGURE 15-2** Cellular events in nerve–muscle impulse transmission. ACh = acetylcholine.

ing the endplate is raised above its threshold and an action potential is produced (Fig. 15-4). All-or-none action potentials do not originate within the endplate.

## Excitation–Contraction Coupling in Muscle

The action potential travels along the surface membrane and is carried into the central portion of the muscle fibre by the transverse tubular system. The transverse tubules (T-tubules) are invaginations of the plasma membrane and form part of the internal membrane system (also referred to as the triads). Each T-tubule is bounded on either side by the lateral cisternae of the sarcoplasmic reticulum (thus the name triad). Electron microscopic studies have revealed a continuity (appearing as a fuzziness) between the membrane of the transverse tubules and the membrane of the lateral cisternae, and these channels have recently been isolated. Thus, the action potential can depolarize the plasma membrane and the T-tubules, and it can also pass across the junction between T-tubules and lateral cisternae and depolarize the membranes of the sarcoplasmic reticulum. This invasion of the sarcoplasmic reticulum produces a release

of $Ca^{2+}$ from the reticulum. Normally, the $Ca^{2+}$ concentration in the cytosol of the muscle is about $10^{-7}$ M or less. The $Ca^{2+}$ released from the reticulum may bring the cytosol $Ca^{2+}$ level to around $10^{-6}$ M or so, thus triggering the troponin–actin–myosin interactions (discussed in Chapter 31) that result in shortening (contraction) of the fibre.

The sarcoplasmic reticulum continuously pumps $Ca^{2+}$ out of the cytosol, and this pump becomes more active during a contraction. Within a few milliseconds, the $Ca^{2+}$ concentration in the cytosol is reduced below $10^{-7}$ M and the muscle relaxes.

The tension developed during the contraction is a function of the intracellular $Ca^{2+}$ concentration, which in turn depends on the rate of $Ca^{2+}$ release from the sarcoplasmic reticulum and the rate of its reabsorption. As the frequency of stimulation of the muscle increases, the sarcoplasmic reticulum is unable to lower the $Ca^{2+}$ concentration below $10^{-7}$ M between stimuli, so the baseline tension is elevated and there is incomplete relaxation between twitches; this state is called *clonus*. When the rate of stimulation is increased further, there is no significant reduction in $Ca^{2+}$ concentration between stimuli, and a

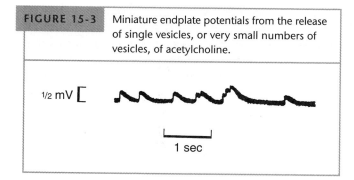

**FIGURE 15-3** Miniature endplate potentials from the release of single vesicles, or very small numbers of vesicles, of acetylcholine.

1/2 mV

1 sec

sustained *tetanic contraction* results. Once this frequency is reached, further increases in frequency can produce graded increases in the tetanic tension (Fig. 15-5). Tetanic stimulation, and not a single twitch, is the physiological state of muscle contraction, and different types of muscles have different intrinsic frequencies at which they are physiologically stimulated (i.e., become tetanic).

## Acetylcholine Breakdown and Reuptake of Choline

Following release and coupling with the nicotinic cholinergic receptor, acetylcholine then dissociates from the receptor and diffuses away into the synaptic cleft. At this point, acetylcholine is broken down by acetylcholinesterase into acetic acid and choline. The choline re-enters the nerve terminal by an active transport process. Up to 90% of the acetylcholine released from the nerve terminal may be broken down by acetylcholinesterase in the synaptic cleft before it even reaches the receptors.

## Cholinergic Nicotinic Receptors at the Neuromuscular Junction

The nicotinic receptors at the neuromuscular junction are distinct from the nicotinic receptors in autonomic ganglia (see Chapter 11) and, as can be seen in Table 15-1, they do not readily bind muscarinic cholinergic agonists or antagonists. This type of nicotinic receptor also has been found in the brain and in the electric organs (electroplax) of certain fish (torpedo) and the electric eel.

From Table 15-1, it is clear that agonists and antagonists bind to the receptor with similar affinities. This receptor does not appear to have separate subsites for agonists and antagonists as was seen with the muscarinic receptor. The receptor has been isolated and purified and even reconstituted into artificial membranes. The availability of antibodies to the pure receptor has been most useful in determining the level of receptors in a number of skeletal muscle diseases and in identifying the genetic determinants of receptor subtypes. The radioreceptor binding assay (e.g., with $^{131}I$ α-bungarotoxin) can also be used to predict the potency of new nicotinic antagonists as neuromuscular blockers.

Binding of acetylcholine to this receptor leads to the opening of ionophores and the resulting ion fluxes that generate the alterations in endplate potential. The more receptors are occupied, the greater the number of ionophores that are "open" and the larger the ion fluxes that move down their electrochemical gradients. This is the basis for the graded endplate potential.

## Desensitization of Acetylcholine Receptors

The interaction of acetylcholine with the nicotinic receptor first leads to an "activated" state of the receptor, which goes to an inactive (desensitized) state when the acetylcholine dissociates from it. This then slowly reverts to the ground state.

Under physiological conditions, because of the high efficacy of acetylcholine, a response can be elicited by occupying only 20 to 30% of the receptors; the rest constitutes a receptor reserve (known as "spare receptors"). This means that, at any time, as many as 10 to 20% of the receptors may be in the inactive state. A situation that would lead to a greater increase in the number of receptors in the inactive state can lead to blockade of the neuromuscular junction.

## SUBSTANCES AFFECTING ACETYLCHOLINE RELEASE

The release of acetylcholine can be modulated by a number of drugs that act at specific sites in the cascade, which can affect neuromuscular transmission.

**Local and general anaesthetics** have varying degrees of blocking action on the pre-junctional nerve terminals, thus preventing nerve impulses from triggering the acetylcholine release sequence (see Chapters 20 and 21).

**Ethanol** at low concentrations (5 to 20 mM) enhances the fusion of acetylcholine vesicle membranes to the pre-junctional membrane. Thus, ethanol can increase the amount of acetylcholine released by an action potential. This also occurs in the spinal cord and possibly in the central nervous system (CNS). In contrast, higher concentrations (40 to 80 mM) of ethanol inhibit the release of acetylcholine.

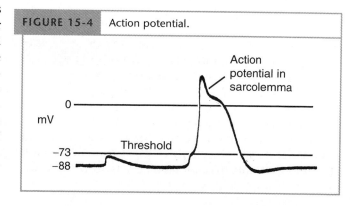

**FIGURE 15-4** Action potential.

Action potential in sarcolemma

0

mV

Threshold

−73
−88

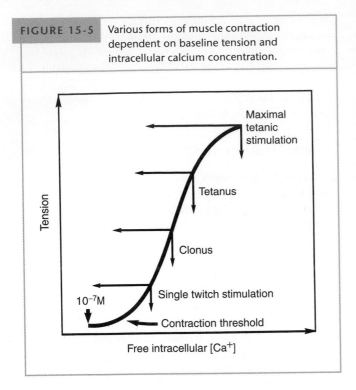

**FIGURE 15-5** Various forms of muscle contraction dependent on baseline tension and intracellular calcium concentration.

**Black widow spider venom** causes a dramatic and almost complete release of all acetylcholine vesicles from the nerve ending. This explains why the victim of such a spider bite initially presents with signs of muscle and abdominal cramps followed by relaxation. The vesicles are not subsequently refilled, and *de novo* synthesis of vesicles is required.

**Botulinum toxin** from the bacterial spores of *Clostridium botulinum* blocks the release of acetylcholine from the vesicles. It kills in very low concentrations by causing paralysis of all muscles, including the respiratory muscles. Paralysis usually occurs 12 to 36 hours following ingestion of the toxin. "Botox" has gained widespread use for cosmetic purposes; injections are made directly into the cutaneous muscles to relax them completely and thus decrease facial wrinkles.

**Calcium** increases the release of acetylcholine, as might be reasoned.

**Magnesium** decreases the release of acetylcholine, probably by modifying the calcium channels.

## NICOTINIC ANTAGONISTS AT THE NEUROMUSCULAR JUNCTION: MUSCLE RELAXANTS

These antagonists selectively block the nicotinic receptors at the neuromuscular junction. They do not affect motor nerves, nor do they block direct stimulation of the muscle. Side effects due to ganglion blockade are occasionally observed. These drugs are used in surgery as muscle relaxants because, while all general anaesthetics are able to cause muscle relaxation, this state is reached only during deep general anaesthesia when most other nervous functions are also severely depressed. By combining muscle relaxants and anaesthetics, one can obtain a surgical plane of anaesthesia with adequate skeletal muscle relaxation at relatively moderate levels of CNS depression.

Some degree of muscle relaxation can also be achieved by the blockade of interneurons with drugs of the benzodiazepine (see Chapter 23) and propanediol carbamate classes. These drugs act at the level of the spinal cord. However, the muscle relaxants of this class lack some of the clinically desirable selectivity. Thus, their use is limited to treatment of acute muscle spasms associated with trauma and inflammation and to certain orthopaedic manipulations.

### Non-depolarizing Competitive Blockers

#### *d*-Tubocurarine

The classical example of the drugs acting in this manner is curare (the generic term for various South American arrow poisons). Claude Bernard demonstrated in 1856 that the site of paralytic action of curare is the synapse between motor nerve and skeletal muscle. The crude extract remained a pharmacological curiosity until the 1940s, when one of the pure alkaloids, *d*-tubocurarine, became available for use as a muscle relaxant in general anaesthesia. The designation "tubo-" indicates that the crude material was used by Indian tribes who carried their arrow poison in hollow bamboo tubes.

The competitive non-depolarizing neuromuscular blocking agents are relatively bulky rigid molecules with two nitrogen groups held apart at a distance of approximately 12 to 14 Å (Fig. 15-6). These drugs compete with acetylcholine for its receptor sites at the endplate. They have zero efficacy; therefore, there is no agonist action and no depolarization, and they act purely as competitive blockers to prevent acetylcholine from binding to its receptors.

The paralytic effects of *d*-tubocurarine can be reversed by increasing the concentrations of acetylcholine at the neuromuscular junction through inhibition of acetylcholinesterase. The drugs used for this purpose are **neostigmine** and **edrophonium** (Fig. 15-7).

Tubocurarine (Tubarine) is inactive by mouth and is always administered intravenously. A typical dose is 0.3 mg/kg. It is distributed widely in body tissues but is concentrated in the neuromuscular junctions. It does not enter the CNS and does not cross the placenta. About one-third of the dose is excreted in the urine over several hours. However, the action on the neuromuscular junctions begins to wear off after about 20 minutes because of redistribution of the drug.

| TABLE 15-1 | Nicotinic Receptor Binding* | | |
|---|---|---|---|
| Competing Cold Ligand | Electroplax Receptors (µM)[†] | Rat Brain Receptors (µM)[‡] | Rat Diaphragm Receptors (µM)[§] |
| Nicotinic agonists | | | |
| Nicotine | 18.0 | 3.1 | – |
| Acetylcholine | 1.5 | 30.0 | 0.47 |
| Carbachol | 40.0 | 90.0 | 3.5 |
| Nicotinic "depolarizing"-type antagonists | | | |
| Decamethonium | 0.8 | 500 | 2.1 |
| Succinylcholine | – | 1 500 | 1.33 |
| Nicotinic "competitive"-type antagonists | | | |
| d-Tubocurarine | 0.17 | 1.9 | 0.24 |
| Gallamine | 0.44 | 3.5 | 1.7 |
| Nicotinic ganglion blocker | | | |
| Hexamethonium | 61 | 900 | 118 |
| Muscarinic agonists | | | |
| Muscarine | – | 10 000 | – |
| Oxotremorine | – | 2 000 | – |
| Muscarinic antagonist | | | |
| Atropine | – | 1 600 | – |
| Cholinesterase inhibitor | | | |
| Physostigmine | – | 2 000 | – |

*$IC_{50}$ values for various cholinergic agonists and antagonists against [131]I α-bungarotoxin, a specific nicotinic antagonist at the neuromuscular junction which labels nicotinic cholinergic receptors at nicotinic sites from various sources. α-Bungarotoxin is a very slowly reversible ligand. These $IC_{50}$ values are therefore obtained from protection experiments and not from competition experiments. They are probably underestimates. The electroplax of the electric eel is a modified nerve–muscle junction in which the response to the binding of acetylcholine leads to energy discharge as an electric shock, rather than energy utilization for contraction.

From [†]Weber M, Changeux JP. *Mol Pharmacol.* 1974;10:15-35.

[‡]Schmidt J. *Mol Pharmacol.* 1977;13:283-290.

[§]Colquhoun D, Rang HP. *Mol Pharmacol.* 1976;12:519-535.

Curare causes progressive paralysis, starting with the muscles of the face, then the limbs, and finally, the respiratory musculature. Cardiac and smooth muscles are not affected, but very high doses will block autonomic ganglia. Rapid intravenous administration of curare causes release of histamine, resulting in transient hypotension. The drug has no analgesic properties, nor does it affect consciousness. Since clinically useful muscle relaxation requires doses that impair or paralyze respiratory muscles, artificial respiration is necessary and must be available whenever curariform drugs are used. With artificial respiration, it is possible to survive without harm doses of tubocurarine that would otherwise be fatal.

Some antibiotics (e.g., aminoglycosides) potentiate curare action, and different general anaesthetics require reduction of the optimal dose of curare to different extents.

*d*-Tubocurarine is used in conjunction with general anaesthesia when prolonged or profound muscle relaxation is required for the purposes of surgery. The drug is also used in the treatment of tetanus (i.e., the disease caused by the tetanus bacillus, not the physiological type of muscle contraction) and may have to be applied for days or weeks in some cases.

## Pancuronium

Pancuronium (Pavulon; Fig. 15-8) is now widely used in place of *d*-tubocurarine. It is five times as potent as tubocurarine and has a faster onset (3 minutes) and a shorter duration of action (110 minutes). It does not release histamine, and in most patients it has no circulatory effects. It is used with caution in patients with impaired cardiovascular function because it can increase the blood pressure, possibly by ganglionic stimulation.

## Atracurium

Atracurium (Tracrium) is a non-depolarizing skeletal neuromuscular blocking agent that has a rapid onset and short duration of action (45 minutes). It is degraded non-enzymatically at pH 7.4 as well as being excreted unchanged by the kidneys. It is of particular usefulness in patients with

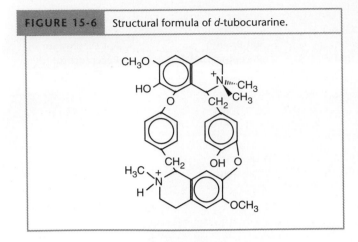

**FIGURE 15-6** Structural formula of *d*-tubocurarine.

renal failure. Atracurium and other neuromuscular blockers such as **vecuronium** (Norcuron), **pipecuronium** (Arduan), and **doxacuronium** (Nuromax) have fewer cardiovascular side effects than other competitive nicotinic receptor antagonists. More recently, **rocuronium** (Zemuron) has been approved. It has a rapid onset (1 minute) and a moderate duration of action (60 minutes) similar to vecuronium. A similar drug, **rapacuronium**, with a rapid onset (1.5 minutes) but much shorter duration of action (20 min-

utes), was formerly available but has been withdrawn from the market because of serious adverse effects.

## Desensitizing (Depolarizing) Blockers: Succinylcholine

These nicotinic receptor ligands produce their effects by first depolarizing and then desensitizing the receptors in the neuromuscular junction. They act to produce effects similar to those of an excess of acetylcholine (either added exogenously or accumulated endogenously after cholinesterase inhibition). There is an initial stimulation of the endplate, which becomes depolarized, resulting in an irregular and uncoordinated contraction of muscle fibres (fasciculation) that generally lasts only 5 to 30 seconds. Its intensity depends somewhat on the speed of intravenous injection of the drug. Some patients complain of sore muscles after succinylcholine, much as an untrained subject does after strenuous exercise. This is known as phase I, or depolarization, block. Subsequently, the endplate remains depolarized (for about 2 to 3 minutes) while the muscle relaxes. Within a further few minutes, the endplate re-polarizes, but the muscle is still relaxed and the endplate is unresponsive to normal acetylcholine release. This is known as phase II, or desensitization, block.

**FIGURE 15-7** The effects of curare on skeletal muscle contraction and their reversal by neostigmine.

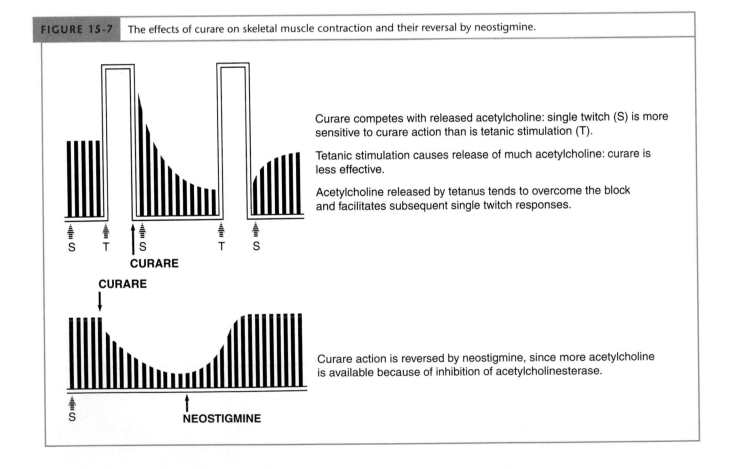

Curare competes with released acetylcholine: single twitch (S) is more sensitive to curare action than is tetanic stimulation (T).

Tetanic stimulation causes release of much acetylcholine: curare is less effective.

Acetylcholine released by tetanus tends to overcome the block and facilitates subsequent single twitch responses.

Curare action is reversed by neostigmine, since more acetylcholine is available because of inhibition of acetylcholinesterase.

FIGURE 15-8    Structural formula of pancuronium.

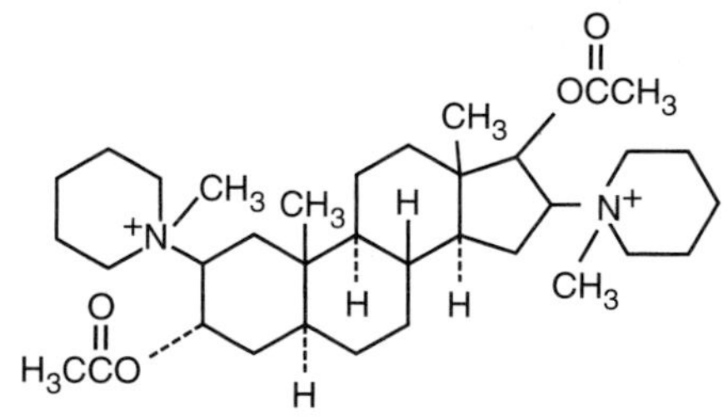

These phenomena can be explained in terms of desensitization of receptors. The depolarization occurs because these "antagonists" have both affinity and efficacy, and the receptors are therefore activated. As an excess of receptors become activated by the sustained high local concentration of succinylcholine, a large fraction of the receptors are converted to the inactive state. Since the endplate membrane is made up largely of receptor protein, the inactivation leads to a change in the membrane properties, and the endplate potential no longer propagates into the sarcolemmal membrane. There are no further action potentials and the muscle relaxes. As more receptors are inactivated, the endplate potential drops and the endplate re-polarizes, but it is now insensitive to acetylcholine or nerve stimulation. The characteristics of desensitizing (depolarizing) block in the neuromuscular junction are illustrated in Figure 15-9.

Since depolarizing blockade is akin to having an excess of acetylcholine at the neuromuscular junction, it is non-competitive with acetylcholine. It cannot be reversed by cholinesterase inhibitors and may actually be made worse by them.

### Succinylcholine

The only blocker of this type in current clinical use is **succinylcholine** (Anectine; Fig. 15-10). It is hydrolyzed by plasma cholinesterase but not by acetylcholinesterase, and therefore when it reaches the neuromuscular synaptic cleft, it acts like an excess of acetylcholine. It cannot cross the blood–brain barrier or placenta.

*Pharmacokinetics.* Succinylcholine has a rapid onset of action (approximately one circulation time) and short duration of action (2 to 3 minutes). The latter is a function of the rapid hydrolysis of the drug by plasma cholinesterase (serum half-life of 2 to 4 minutes). There are rare genetic variants of this cholinesterase that do not readily hydrolyze succinylcholine, as described in Chapter 10. The duration of action may then be greatly prolonged. Therefore, succinylcholine should be used only when facilities are available for giving artificial respiration.

FIGURE 15-9    The effects of succinylcholine on skeletal muscle contraction (compare with Fig. 15-7).

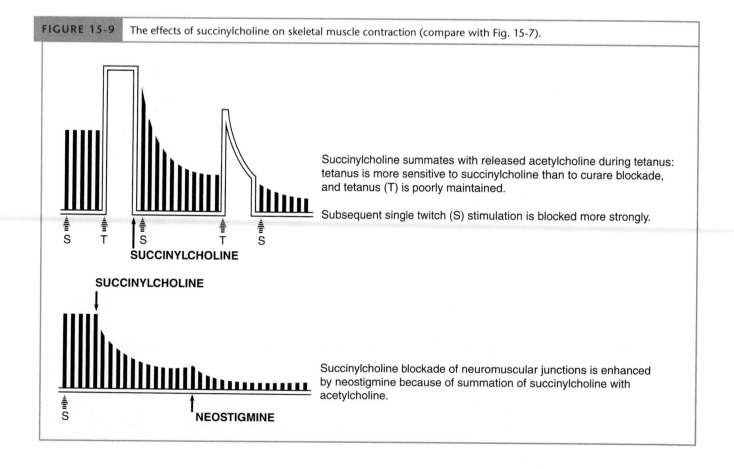

Succinylcholine summates with released acetylcholine during tetanus: tetanus is more sensitive to succinylcholine than to curare blockade, and tetanus (T) is poorly maintained.

Subsequent single twitch (S) stimulation is blocked more strongly.

Succinylcholine blockade of neuromuscular junctions is enhanced by neostigmine because of summation of succinylcholine with acetylcholine.

---

**FIGURE 15-10** Structural formula of succinylcholine.

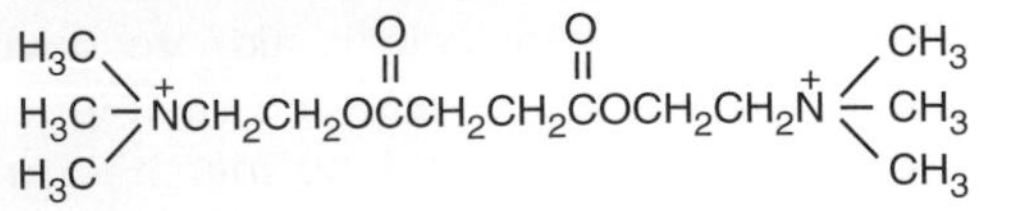

---

Succinylcholine is a double ester (i.e., both carboxyl groups of succinate are esterified with choline); it is metabolized by butyrylcholinesterase to succinylmonocholine. This metabolite is a *competitive* cholinergic nicotinic antagonist. It may accumulate during prolonged use of succinylcholine, and its effect may then persist following the termination of succinylcholine administration. Competitive blockade by this metabolite can be reversed by cholinesterase inhibitors.

*Clinical use.* The clinical use of succinylcholine takes advantage of its rapid and short action. The two main uses are to facilitate tracheal intubation for artificial ventilation during general anaesthesia and to paralyze skeletal muscles during electroconvulsive (shock) therapy of mental disorders.

*Adverse effects.* During depolarizing blockade, the potassium channels in the muscle membrane around the muscle soleplate remain open, so serum potassium rises about 0.5 to 1 mEq/L by 3 to 5 minutes after administration of the drug. This increase is usually of no clinical significance. However, there can sometimes be more severe hyperkalemia, with consequent cardiac arrest. This risk is greatest in patients with many freshly denervated muscles (as after spinal injury) or with extensive burns, because in these situations a proliferation of post-junctional acetylcholine receptors results in an increased $K^+$ release by succinylcholine. The risk is also increased in patients with uremia. Succinylcholine has also been shown to release histamine, so it can sometimes cause allergic-type reactions.

Nicotinic receptors in both sympathetic and parasympathetic ganglia, as well as cardiac muscarinic receptors, are excited by succinylcholine. Therefore, it can produce changes in heart rate, rhythm, or force of contraction, of either sympathetic or parasympathetic type. Pediatric patients are especially at risk of such effects.

*Depolarizing block by other drugs.* The neuromuscular effects of toxic (lethal) doses of nicotine and of anticholinesterases are similar to those of succinylcholine in principle, although not usually in the rate of development. The action of these drugs on the neuromuscular junction is also of the depolarizing type and, therefore, cannot be antagonized by pharmacological means; survival may depend on prompt artificial ventilation.

## DRUGS ACTING ON EXCITATION–CONTRACTION COUPLING IN MUSCLE

### Caffeine

Normally, a muscle does not begin to contract until the membrane potential has been reduced to about –50 mV. But in the presence of caffeine (in vitro), the muscle begins to contract at about –65 mV. It is believed that caffeine produces muscle "sensitization" by releasing $Ca^{2+}$ from either the sarcoplasmic reticulum or the sarcolemmal membrane. In the concentration range of 1 to 5 mM, caffeine (in vitro) produces contracture of muscle, and this may occur without depolarization of the cell membranes.

Caffeine, like theophylline, blocks the phosphodiesterase of tissues, thus enhancing the action of cyclic AMP. It may also inhibit the binding of adenosine to the adenosine receptor, which is involved in the desensitization of the nicotinic receptor in muscle. Thus, caffeine-induced contraction of muscle fibres may result in part from blockade of this action of adenosine. As noted in Chapter 10, the effect of caffeine on muscle contraction can be used as a diagnostic test for carriers of the genetic predisposition to malignant hyperthermia (see below).

### Dantrolene in Malignant Hyperthermia

General anaesthetics such as halothane and other uncharged anaesthetic molecules can make the muscle reticulum "leaky" to $Ca^{2+}$, particularly in genetically vulnerable subjects (approximately one person in 200 000). Such patients exhibit the life-threatening syndrome of malignant hyperthermia. $Ca^{2+}$ stimulates the ATP-dependent contractile mechanism and increases the respiratory quotient of the muscle mitochondria. As a result, the muscles go into intense contracture and enormous amounts of heat are produced (see Chapter 10).

The outcome of an attack of malignant hyperthermia is greatly improved if the patient is cooled quickly and given dantrolene (Dantrium). This drug binds to, and blocks, the calcium channel through which $Ca^{2+}$ is released from the sarcoplasmic reticulum in the course of neuromuscular stimulation. As a result, it uncouples the excitation phase from the contraction phase and prevents the contracture response. At a plasma concentration of 4.2 µg/mL, it decreases the strength of muscle contraction by about 75%. However, the same action also results in decreased strength of muscle contraction during voluntary movement.

Dantrolene (Fig. 15-11) is highly lipophilic and is about 70% absorbed when given by mouth. For intravenous use, it must be given in an alkaline solution and is therefore irritating to the vein unless given via a rapidly running infusion. For the treatment of malignant hyperthermia, it is commonly given as a bolus intravenous dose of 2.5 mg/kg, repeated at 5-minute intervals until the symptoms of hyperthermia disappear. The same dosage is also used in treating the neuroleptic malignant syndrome (see Chapter 24). It has been suggested as a possible therapeutic measure for hyperthermia in "ecstasy" intoxication (see Chapter 26) and in heat stroke, but these uses are not yet supported by proper clinical trials.

**Azumoline** is a new analogue of dantrolene in which the nitrobenzene group is replaced by a bromobenzene group. It is equipotent with dantrolene in malignant hyperthermia but is 30 times more water-soluble and, therefore, may be less irritating to the vein when given by intravenous infusion.

## Local Anaesthetics

Procainamide and other procaine-like local anaesthetics also block the release of $Ca^{2+}$ from muscle reticulum, inhibiting muscle contracture states. These positively charged drugs may simply stop the exit of $Ca^{2+}$ from reticulum by "coating" the reticulum membrane with their positive charges.

## ANTI-SPASTICITY AGENTS

Spasms of skeletal muscle are sustained, painful contractions that can arise from a variety of causes. Occasional spasms do not require treatment, but in some conditions, the spasms are frequent and prolonged and can give rise to serious discomfort, as in upper motor lesions (e.g., in multiple sclerosis) or in sensitization of the stretch reflex by local muscle injury. In the past, such repeated spasms were treated by administration of various sedatives that relieved the discomfort to some degree but produced an unacceptable level of drowsiness. The newer and more selective agents are mainly drugs that enhance the

**FIGURE 15-11** Structural formulae of dantrolene and its more water-soluble analogue, azumoline.

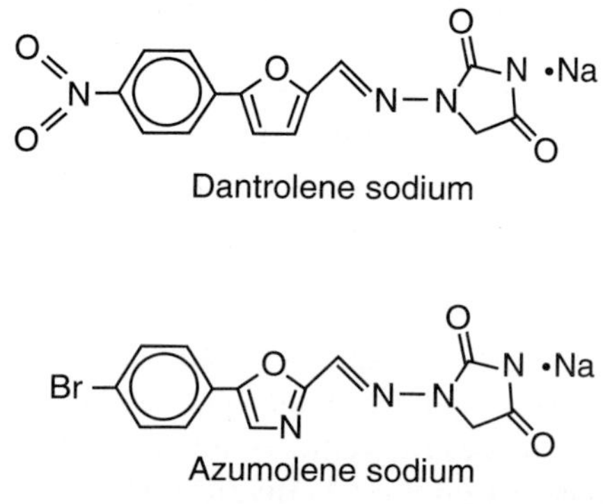

Dantrolene sodium

Azumolene sodium

depressant action of γ-aminobutyric acid (GABA) on presynaptic terminals and postsynaptic neurons in the spinal motor pathways.

## Baclofen

Baclofen (*p*-chlorophenyl-GABA; Lioresal, Liotec, and others) is a selective agonist at the GABA$_B$-receptors located both on presynaptic terminals and on postsynaptic neurons in spinal excitatory motor pathways. At the presynaptic terminals, it inhibits $Ca^{2+}$ influx and thus inhibits release of excitatory neurotransmitters. On the postsynaptic cells, it increases slow $K^+$ conductance and thus depresses neuronal response to excitatory stimulation. Both of these actions decrease muscle tone and contractile responses to reflexes and to motor nerve stimulation. In double-blind controlled clinical trials (mainly in patients with multiple sclerosis), baclofen has been found to reduce the frequency and severity of muscle spasms in about 75% of patients. It is as effective an anti-spasticity agent as diazepam, which facilitates the action of GABA at the GABA$_A$-receptor and exerts an inhibitory effect by increasing $Cl^-$ influx (see Chapter 23). Baclofen has the advantage that it produces less drowsiness than diazepam.

Baclofen (Fig. 15-12) is well absorbed from the gastrointestinal (GI) tract and thus is unaffected by food. In the plasma it is about 30% bound to protein, and it has moderately slow clearance from the plasma with a half-life of 3 to 5 hours. It is mainly excreted unchanged (85%), and a small portion (15%) undergoes hepatic deamination. Baclofen enters the CNS readily and acts throughout the brain and spinal cord. It is also used by slow infusion directly into the spinal intrathecal space for direct local action. Such treatment is very effective in controlling severe spasms in patients with neurological lesions and has been carried on for months or even years.

Overdose effects include muscular hypotonia, respiratory depression, vertigo, coma, seizures (in epileptic patients), and cardiac conduction abnormalities. In patients receiving baclofen by spinal intrathecal infusion, sudden termination of treatment, whether intentional or accidental, can give rise to a severe and potentially life-threatening withdrawal reaction consisting of high fever, mental clouding, and intense muscular rigidity that may lead to lysis of muscle cells, release of myoglobin, and renal failure.

## Tizanidine

Tizanidine (Zanaflex; see Fig. 15-12) is chemically related to clonidine, and like clonidine, it is an $\alpha_2$-adrenergic receptor agonist that exerts an inhibitory effect at both presynaptic and postsynaptic sites in spinal motor pathways (see Chapters 11 and 13) and at the motor axon terminal in the nerve–muscle junction (see Fig. 15-2). It is as effective as baclofen in relieving muscle spasm and causes

**FIGURE 15-12** Structural formulae of the anti-spasticity agents baclofen and tizanidine. Compare the structure of tizanidine with that of clonidine in Figure 14-13.

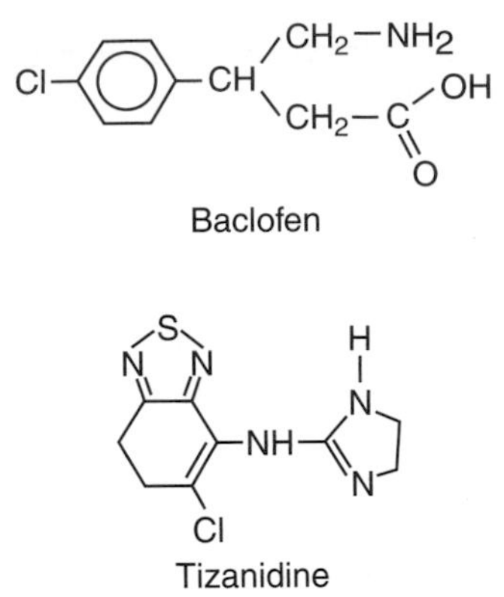

Baclofen

Tizanidine

less drowsiness and weakness than baclofen. It is completely absorbed from the GI tract but undergoes extensive first-pass metabolism in the liver. Tizanidine has a plasma half-life of 2 to 3 hours, and about 95% is metabolized to a variety of inactive metabolites. Clearance is significantly reduced in patients with renal insufficiency.

Adverse effects of tizanidine include dry mouth, hypotension, dizziness, hallucinations, and, rarely, liver damage.

## Other Anti-spasticity Agents

There is a wide range of other drugs that are used mainly to reduce skeletal muscle spasm arising from muscle injury (e.g., neck and lower back pain) rather than from neurological lesions. **Cyclobenzaprine** has been repeatedly demonstrated to be superior to placebo in such cases. The evidence is much less complete for **carisoprodol, chlorzoxazone, metaxolone, methocarbamol,** or **orphenadrine.** Current claims for a beneficial effect of cannabinoids such as **tetrahydrocannabinol** in spasticity and muscle spasms in multiple sclerosis are not yet supported by convincing clinical evidence. Patients report subjective improvement, but objective measures do not confirm any change in muscle tension or movement (see Chapter 26). The reported beneficial effect may be primarily due to analgesic action rather than to a change in muscle spasm.

## DRUGS ACTING ON CHOLINESTERASE

If cholinesterase is inhibited, the effective concentration of acetylcholine in the synaptic cleft is increased. After administration of a cholinesterase inhibitor, the depolarization response to applied acetylcholine is increased.

As described in Chapter 12, cholinesterase inhibitors can be divided into two categories, reversible and irreversible. The reversible inhibitors include **physostigmine, neostigmine,** and **edrophonium.** They are used clinically for the termination of curare-induced block and in the treatment of myasthenia gravis. Clinical use of irreversible cholinesterase inhibitors (organophosphates) is rare, although their prolonged action is occasionally useful in the treatment of glaucoma. However, these compounds are used widely as insecticides and occasionally give rise to accidental poisoning. They have occasionally been employed as chemical warfare agents (the so-called "nerve gases").

## MYASTHENIA GRAVIS

Myasthenia gravis is a chronic disease characterized by muscular weakness of fluctuating intensity. It is aggravated by physical activity and improved by rest. The weakness is not associated with any significant atrophy of the muscles, at least in the earlier stages of the disease.

Myasthenia gravis was first recognized in 1879 by Erb and then later in 1893 by Goldflam, whose clinical characterization of the disorder remains valid. The symptoms are primarily due to dysfunction of the motor system. The muscles of the eyes, the larynx, and of mastication are often first and most seriously affected. As the disease progresses, the muscles of the trunk and extremities may become involved (less often, the symptoms of myasthenia gravis first appear in these muscles). Characteristically, an involved muscle rapidly becomes progressively weaker upon exercise. Most patients are better in the morning than in the afternoon. Remissions and relapses occur. Paralysis of the respiratory muscles may cause the death of some patients.

The similarity between the symptoms shown by laboratory animals treated with curare and those of patients suffering from myasthenia gravis led to the idea of treating a myasthenic patient with physostigmine. This idea was put to the test, and a beneficial therapeutic effect was observed. It became generally accepted that the clinically observed muscular weakness was caused by neuromuscular blockade; this concept was confirmed by the supersensitivity of myasthenia gravis patients to tubocurarine (which can be used as a diagnostic test).

It is now known that myasthenia gravis is an autoimmune disease in which antibodies to nicotinic receptors are produced in the thymus. The antibodies reduce the number of available receptors at the neuromuscular junction. The antibody–receptor interaction also leads to structural damage in the synaptic cleft; the post-junctional membrane loses its characteristic folds, and the cleft itself widens. The consequence of all these changes is that less acetylcholine reaches a smaller number of receptors.

Some patients respond to thymectomy, and treatment with immunosuppressant drugs is now used for long-term management. However, pyridostigmine (Mestinon), a physostigmine analogue, is used as a supplement (30 to 180 mg orally), often in combination with atropine (to reduce cardiovascular complications). This will increase the concentration of acetylcholine reaching the receptors. The action begins within 1 to 2 hours and lasts approximately 5 hours. For diagnostic purposes (myasthenic crisis versus neostigmine excess), a short-acting anticholinesterase such as edrophonium (Tensilon) can be used; remission of symptoms during the test indicates a myasthenic crisis.

## SUGGESTED READINGS

Burry L, HoSang M, Hynes-Gay P. A review of neuromuscular blockade in the critically ill patient. *Dynamics.* 2001;12:28-33.

Chou R, Peterson K, Helfand M. Comparative efficacy and safety of skeletal muscle relaxants for spasticity and musculoskeletal conditions: a systematic review. *J Pain Symptom Manage.* 2004;28:140-175.

Coffey RJ, Edgar TS, Francisco GE, et al. Abrupt withdrawal from intrathecal baclofen: recognition and management of a potentially life-threatening syndrome. *Arch Phys Med Rehabil.* 2002;83:735-741.

Dario A, Tomei G. A benefit-risk assessment of baclofen in severe spinal spasticity. *Drug Saf.* 2004;27:799-818.

Fawcelt WJ, Dash A, Francis GA, et al. Recovery from neuromuscular blockade: residual curarisation following atracurium or vecuronium by bolus dosing or infusions. *Acta Anaesthesiol Scand.* 1995;39:288-293.

Huh KH, Fuhrer C. Clustering of nicotinic acetylcholine receptors: from the neuromuscular junction to interneuronal synapses. *Mol Neurobiol.* 2002;25:79-112.

Krause T, Gerbershagen MU, Fiege M, et al. Dantrolene—a review of its pharmacology, therapeutic use and new developments. *Anaesthesia.* 2004;59:364-373.

McCoy EP. Comparison of the effects of neostigmine and edrophonium on the duration of action of succinylcholine. *Acta Anaesthesiol Scand.* 1995;39:744-747.

Mertes PM, Laxenaire MC. Adverse reactions to neuromuscular blocking agents. *Curr Allergy Asthma Rep.* 2004;4:7-16.

Orebaugh SL. Succinylcholine: adverse effects and alternatives in emergency medicine. *Am J Emerg Med.* 1999;17:715-721.

Perry J, Lee J, Wells G. Rocuronium versus succinylcholine for rapid sequence induction intubation. *Cochrane Database Syst Rev.* 2003;(1):CD002788.

Romi F, Gilhus NE, Aarli JA. Myasthenia gravis: clinical, immunological, and therapeutic advances. *Acta Neurol Scand.* 2005;111:134-141.

Ruff RL. Neurophysiology of the neuromuscular junction: overview. *Ann NY Acad Sci.* 2003;998:1-10.

Slater CR. Structural determinants of the reliability of synaptic transmission at the vertebrate neuromuscular junction. *J Neurocytol.* 2003;32:505-522.

Sparr HJ, Beaufort TM, Fuchs-Buder T. Newer neuromuscular blocking agents: how do they compare with established agents? *Drugs.* 2001;61:919-942.

Thanvi BR, Lo TC. Update on myasthenia gravis. *Postgrad Med J.* 2004;80:690-700.

# Part III

## Central Nervous System

# 16

# Functional and Neurochemical Organization of the Central Nervous System

## AJ LANÇA

In the course of its evolution, the nervous system has developed a highly complex functional and anatomical organization that subserves three main processes: (1) gathering external information (i.e., sensory function or input), (2) storing and processing the information (i.e., integrative function), and (3) triggering an adaptation or response (i.e., motor or secretory function or output).

## ANATOMICAL AND MACROFUNCTIONAL ORGANIZATION OF THE CENTRAL NERVOUS SYSTEM

The anatomical organization of the adult human central nervous system (CNS) reflects the basic organization seen in the embryo. By the fourth week of embryonic development, the caudal portion of the **neural tube** gives rise to the **spinal cord**, while the anterior portion gives rise to the three **primary brain vesicles**: the **forebrain** (prosencephalon), **midbrain** (mesencephalon), and **hindbrain** (rhombencephalon) (Fig. 16-1). The relationship between these structures and their main derivatives in the mature brain is summarized in Table 16-1.

The **cerebellum** is responsible for the coordination of voluntary movements, maintenance of body posture, and coordination of head and eye movements.

The **brainstem** (pons and medulla oblongata) and **midbrain** constitute the primary centres for the coordination of vital functions (such as regulation of respiratory and cardiovascular functions) and reflexes (such as vomiting and swallowing). The **reticular formation** (which regulates the sleep–arousal cycle and coordination of eye movements) and the most important monoamine-producing neuronal groups are also located in the midbrain and brainstem.

The functional organization of the forebrain is more complex. In the **thalamus**, motor, general and special sensory, and visceral information is integrated. The **hypothalamus** receives important ascending input from the spinal cord and brainstem, as well as input from the corti-

cal regions (primarily from the limbic system) and thalamus. The hypothalamus also has sensors that respond to the properties of the circulating blood, such as temperature, osmolarity, and concentrations of different metabolites and hormones. The hypothalamus is responsible for the crucial integration of neural and endocrine functions.

In the **telencephalon,** the final processing and integration of information takes place. The **cerebral cortex,** the convoluted surface layer of the cerebral hemispheres, is divided into different areas, or **lobes,** delimited by well-defined grooves, the **sulci.** Each cortical region is classified according to its anatomical location (e.g., frontal, temporal, occipital) or type of information processed (e.g., motor, sensory, visual). The cerebral cortex has a characteristic histological organization with neuronal cell bodies and fibres arranged in layers. The number and characteristics of the different layers are distinctive in each cortical area.

The components of the **basal ganglia** are the **caudate nucleus** and the **putamen** (together known as the **corpus striatum**) and the **globus pallidus.** The basal ganglia play an important role in the initiation, control, and modulation of movement (see Chapter 17) and are also involved in cognition.

The **hippocampus** and **septum** are involved in learning and memory, while the **amygdala** is involved in the integration of autonomic and endocrine functions. The hippocampus, septum, and amygdala are parts of the **limbic system,** which also includes portions of the hypothalamus, thalamus, and cerebral cortex. The limbic system is involved in the mechanisms of motivation, regulation of mood, emotions, and basic behaviours involving survival of the individual and the species.

## CELLULAR ORGANIZATION OF THE CENTRAL NERVOUS SYSTEM

### Neurons

The morphological and functional unit of the nervous system is the nerve cell, or **neuron,** consisting of a cell

**FIGURE 16-1** The embryonic neural tube forms the brain vesicles and the spinal cord. (A) Three-vesicle stage of the neural tube (fourth week of embryonic development). (B) Five-vesicle stage of the neural tube (fifth week). (C) Mid-sagittal view of the mature central nervous system. (The relationships between developing and mature structures are summarized in Table 16-1.)

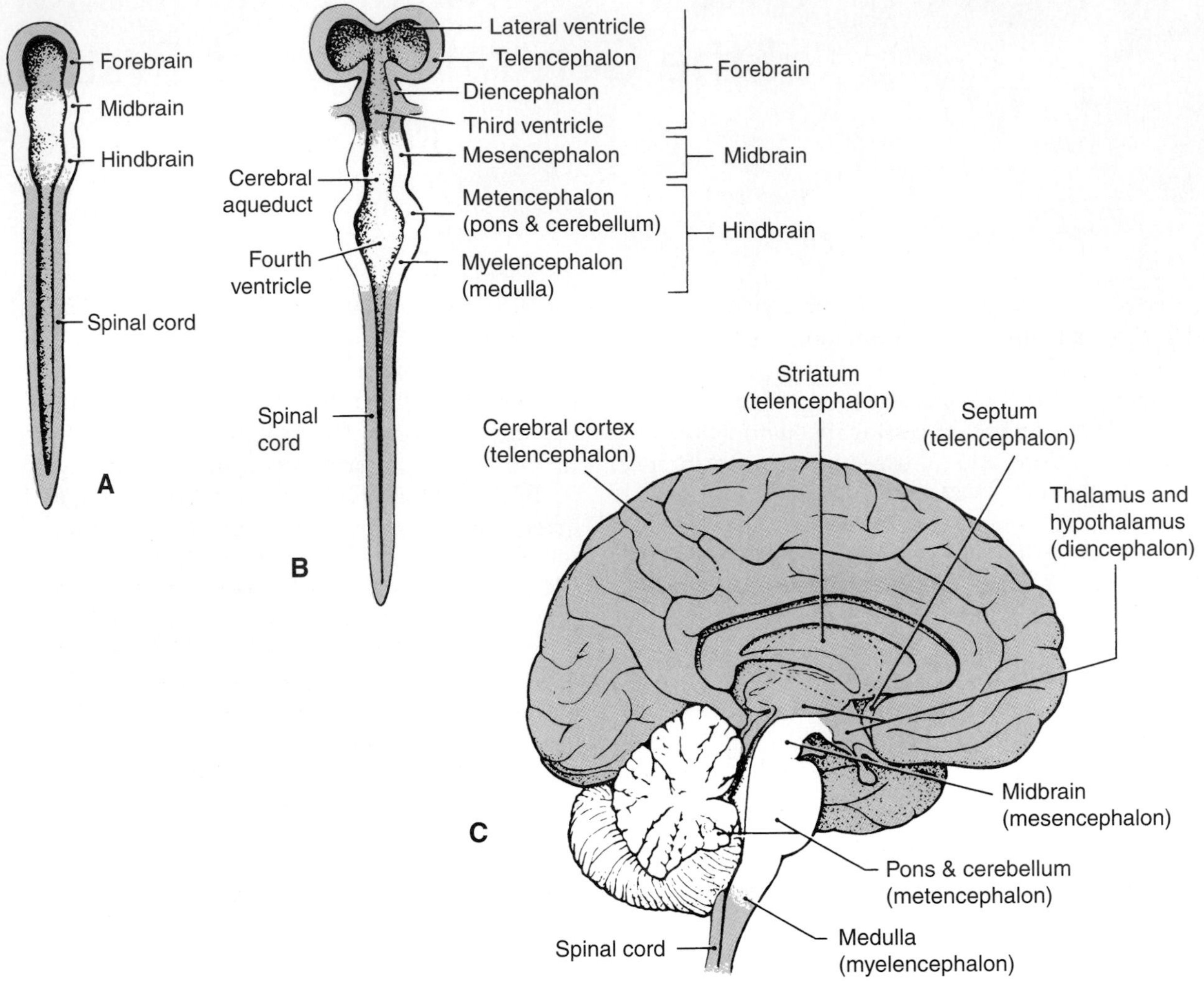

body (**soma**) and its processes. The soma contains a nucleus and surrounding cytoplasm (**perikaryon**), which is packed with **rough endoplasmic reticulum** (Nissl bodies), a network of **smooth endoplasmic reticulum**, a prominent **Golgi complex**, and abundant **secretory vesicles**. These are characteristics of cells active in protein synthesis and secretion.

Neurons have two types of cytoplasmic processes that emerge from the cell body: dendrites and axons. **Dendrites** are usually short, can have highly complex branching patterns, and typically carry signals *toward* the soma (inputs). The **axon** is a long, slender process, usually does not have many branchings, and carries signals *away from* the cell body toward the axon terminals (output).

The neuron has a conspicuous **cytoskeleton** with abundant microtubules, neurofilaments, and microfilaments that maintain the cell shape. **Microtubules** are composed of contractile proteins (tubulin, functionally analogous to myosin) organized in dimers that form elongated strands. Repeated cycles of polymerization and depolymerization of these strands result in the formation (elongation) and disassembly (retraction) of microtubules. Microtubules are also used as tracks along which proteins and organelles such as vesicles are carried along the axon, both toward the axon terminal (anterograde transport) and toward the soma (retrograde transport). Drugs that block polymerization or depolymerization of tubulin, such as colchicine and taxol, respectively, disrupt

| TABLE 16-1 | Organization of the Embryonic Brain Vesicles and Their Mature Counterparts | | |
|---|---|---|
| **Primary Brain Vesicles** | **Secondary Brain Vesicles** | **Mature Brain** |
| 1. Forebrain (prosencephalon) | a. Telencephalon (cerebral hemispheres) | Cerebral cortex Basal ganglia Hippocampus Amygdala Septum Olfactory system |
| | b. Diencephalon | Thalamus Hypothalamus Retinae Optic nerves Optic tract |
| 2. Midbrain (mesencephalon) | Midbrain | Midbrain |
| 3. Hindbrain (rhombencephalon) | a. Metencephalon b. Myelencephalon | Pons, cerebellum Medulla oblongata |

this microtubule-dependent transport and thus prevent axonal transport, release of neurotransmitters, and dynamics of the mitotic spindle in dividing cells.

Unlike microtubules, **neurofilaments** exist in a polymerized and more stable form and are responsible for the maintenance of cell shape and axonal diameter. Neurofilaments are a specific type of intermediate filament composed of three different polypeptides expressed only in neurons. In some neurodegenerative diseases (e.g., Alzheimer's disease), neurofilaments become disorganized and form characteristic neurofibrillary tangles within neurons.

**Microfilaments** are polymers of globular actin organized in double-stranded short filaments. They form a network that is concentrated at the periphery of the cell body and axon terminals, and they play a primary role in the motility of axonal "growth cones" during development and the specialization of pre- and postsynaptic elements. Several naturally occurring toxins, such as cytochalasin and phalloidin, interfere with the process of filament formation and inhibit these actin-mediated events.

In the CNS, neurons are arranged in groups that are connected with each other according to definite patterns. These connective patterns, or **neuronal circuits**, have two types of neurons: (1) large neurons with long axons, which establish synaptic contacts with other neurons located at some distance elsewhere in the nervous system, are known as **projection neurons** or **Golgi type I neurons**; (2) **local circuit neurons**, or **Golgi type II neurons**, are usually small and have short axons that establish synaptic contacts with other neurons located in the same structure or region.

## Synapses

Synaptic contacts between neurons are of two types, electrical and chemical. In **electrical synapses** (also know as gap junctions), the closely apposed membranes of the two neurons, just 2 to 3 nm apart, contain large transmembrane proteins (**connexons;** see also Chapter 2, Fig. 2-15) made of six identical subunits (connexins) arranged around a central pore. Each individual connexin is a transmembrane protein with four membrane-spanning domains. The connexon in the presynaptic membrane is perfectly aligned with its postsynaptic counterpart, so their central pores form a continuous hydrophilic channel through which direct flow of ionic current and small molecules (e.g., second messengers) can occur between the two neurons. Electrical synapses often connect groups of many neurons, synchronizing their activity. Such synapses are also established between neurons and glial cells. Signal transmission between neurons is about 1000-fold faster in electrical synapses than in chemical synapses and can occur in both directions. Electrical synapses between neurons are frequent in the non-mammalian brain but are less frequent in the mammalian brain, though they have been found in the retina and in the cerebellum, hippocampus, and other structures. In mammalian brains, gap junctions between neurons and non-neuronal (glial) cells, and between individual glial cells (see "Neuroglia" below), play an important role in the regulation of extracellular concentrations of ions necessary for the generation of action potentials.

**Chemical synapses** are the typical synapses found in the mammalian brain, and their molecular components (e.g., receptors, transporters) are the major target of neuropharmacological interventions. These synapses are usually unidirectional, and a single synapse establishes connection between only two cells. However, a single presynaptic cell can establish separate synaptic contacts with as many as 100 000 other neurons. This enormous degree of interconnection makes possible the complex circuitry and functional adaptability of the human nervous system.

In chemical synapses, there is no cytoplasmic continuity between the adjacent cells, and the release of a chemical messenger by exocytosis is required to pass the information from one cell to the other. The presynaptic axon ends in an expanded terminal that contains in its cytoplasm a large number of **synaptic vesicles** (with diameters ranging from 40 to 200 nm) clustered near the presynaptic membrane and mitochondria.

The arrival of a nerve impulse causes the voltage-dependent ion channels of the presynaptic terminal to open, allowing extracellular $Ca^{2+}$ to enter the terminal. This calcium entry causes the vesicles to "dock" with the presynaptic membrane, fuse with it, and open to discharge their neurotransmitter content into the **synaptic cleft,** the

20- to 30-nm gap between the pre- and postsynaptic neurons. The functional association of an action potential and exocytosis is known as **action–secretion coupling.**

Fusion of the vesicular membrane to the presynaptic cell membrane and its subsequent retrieval occur by three different processes:

1. In the "kiss-and-run" process, vesicles remain attached to the membrane for just a few hundred milliseconds, during which a pore is formed, allowing the release of neurotransmitter. The empty vesicle is then retrieved.
2. Alternatively, vesicles may remain open for several seconds after neurotransmitter release and are then internalized ("slow" or "compensatory" mechanism).
3. After release of neurotransmitter, the vesicular membrane may fuse with the cell membrane and become part of the presynaptic membrane for tens of seconds. A second stimulus is required for membrane retrieval to take place.

These processes are regulated by the activity of presynaptic potentials, including the activation of presynaptic autoreceptors that exert an inhibitory effect on presynaptic release of neurotransmitter. Recently, it has also been established that the postsynaptic element is also involved in the regulation of presynaptic activity. Postsynaptic activation of certain glutamate receptors increases postsynaptic synthesis of nitric oxide (NO), a highly diffusible gas that easily reaches the synaptic cleft and acts on the presynaptic axon terminal. NO modulates neurotransmitter availability in the synapse by promoting neurotransmitter release and decreasing the effectiveness of neurotransmitter reuptake by the presynaptic terminal; in addition, NO also modulates the efficiency of endocytosis and vesicular recycling.

The released neurochemical messenger diffuses across the cleft and binds to specialized receptor structures on the postsynaptic membrane, initiating the postsynaptic response that completes the process of **synaptic transmission.**

The continuous presence of the neurotransmitter in the synaptic cleft would prevent new signals from getting through and render the synapse non-functional. It is therefore essential for the neurotransmitter to be removed from the synaptic cleft shortly after release. This occurs by three different mechanisms (diffusion, enzymatic degradation, and reuptake) that together remove the transmitter from the cleft in about 1 ms after its release.

In the CNS, conventional synapses can be established between a presynaptic terminal and different parts of the postsynaptic neuron. They can be between an axon and a dendrite (**axodendritic**), an axon and a soma (**axosomatic**), or even between axons (**axoaxonic**). Axodendritic synapses are often excitatory, while the axosomatic are usually inhibitory. Axoaxonic synapses regulate the amount of neurotransmitter released by the postsynaptic axon.

There are also other less common types of synapses, such as **dendrodendritic, dendrosomatic,** and **dendroaxonic.** The physiological properties and relevance of these unconventional synapses are still incompletely understood, but they may take part in intricate local feedback circuits.

## Neuroglia

The CNS contains a large population of small cells that outnumber the neurons. These cells, known collectively as **glial cells,** or **neuroglia** (meaning "nerve glue"), are of two types: the larger-sized, or **macroglial, cells** and the smaller-sized, or **microglial, cells.**

There are two main types of **macroglial cells:** astrocytes and oligodendrocytes. **Astrocytes** are star-shaped cells with cytoplasmic processes rich in cytoskeletal intermediate filaments (made of glial fibrillary acidic protein, or GFAP) and glycogen. Some of their long, slender cytoplasmic processes, known as **pedicels,** or **perivascular end feet,** surround the blood vessels and contribute to the formation of the blood–brain barrier (see Chapter 2). Astrocytes act as structural support for neurons and are also involved in the responses to injury and to immunological challenge. They are also involved in the regulation of extracellular concentrations of potassium, calcium, and small molecules such as γ-aminobutyric acid (GABA) and glutamate. Activation of gap junctions between astrocytes is a major mechanism responsible for the homeostatic regulation of ionic concentrations in the nervous tissue.

**Oligodendrocytes** are present in both white and grey matter, they have a smaller and denser nucleus than the astrocytes, and their cytoplasm displays an abundant, rough endoplasmic reticulum and polyribosomes, which accounts for their conspicuous electron density. These cells typically have large amounts of myelin basic proteins (MBP), which can be easily identified by immunocytochemistry. Their main function is the production of myelin in the white matter of the CNS (equivalent to the role of the Schwann cells in the peripheral nervous system). They also produce and release growth factors and guide the growth of axons during development and regeneration. In oligodendrocytes and Schwann cells, gap junctions are abundant and connect adjacent layers of myelin, and they are possibly involved in the processes of myelination, demyelination, and maintenance of axonal conduction of nerve impulses. In X-linked dominant Charcot-Marie-Tooth disease, a genetically transmitted condition characterized by the breakdown of myelin in peripheral nerves, mutations in connexin-encoding genes result in non-functional gap-junctions in the myelin sheets produced by Schwann cells.

Other macroglial cell types include the **ependymocytes** that form the simple columnar epithelium lining the ventricles and the **epithelial cells of the choroid plexus** that secrete the cerebrospinal fluid (CSF; see Chapter 2).

**Microglial cells** are relatively inactive under normal conditions. They display a moderate phagocytic activity, eliminating cellular debris resulting from neuronal and glial degeneration. Following tissue injury, the microglial cells show greatly increased phagocytic activity. Interestingly, microglia are targeted by the human immunodeficiency virus (HIV), which actively replicates within these cells. Infected microglial cells become a reservoir for HIV in the brain and play a crucial role in the development of neurological symptoms present in advanced stages of acquired immunodeficiency syndrome (AIDS). Unfortunately, little is known about the microglial responses to pharmacological manipulations.

## NEUROCHEMICAL MESSENGERS

### Concept

The neuron is a secretory cell specialized in the production of **neurochemical messengers.** These are molecules that (1) are synthesized by a neuron, (2) are present in the presynaptic terminal and released into a synapse, (3) exert an action on a postsynaptic neuron or effector cell, (4) are removed from the synaptic cleft by a specific mechanism, and (5) when administered exogenously in physiological concentrations, replicate the actions of the endogenously occurring substance.

There are three types of neurochemical messengers: (1) neurotransmitters, (2) neuromodulators, and (3) neurohormones.

1. **Neurotransmitters** are released into the synaptic cleft and cause an electrophysiological change (**postsynaptic potential**) in the postsynaptic cell. This change can facilitate the entry of cations such as $Na^+$ or $Ca^{2+}$ that depolarize the postsynaptic cell membrane, thus producing an **excitatory postsynaptic potential (EPSP).** Alternatively, it can facilitate the entry of anions such as $Cl^-$ that hyperpolarize the membrane, producing an **inhibitory postsynaptic potential (IPSP).**
2. **Neuromodulators** act upon postsynaptic cells but do not themselves produce action potentials. Instead, they change the responsiveness of the postsynaptic cell to the generation of action potentials by neurotransmitters.
3. **Neurohormones** are synthesized in neurons but are released into perivascular spaces rather than into a synaptic cleft. After entering the bloodstream, these substances are carried to remote sites of action either inside or outside the CNS.

The same neurochemical messenger can act as a neurotransmitter, a neurohormone, or a neuromodulator in different brain sites. For example, the neuropeptide vasopressin is synthesized by neurons in the supraoptic and paraventricular nuclei of the hypothalamus, is transported to the neurohypophysis, and is released there into the circulation to act as a hormone. The same hypothalamic neurons also send axonal projections to other brain regions (such as the septum and the spinal cord), where vasopressin is released into synaptic clefts and acts as a classical neurotransmitter.

## Mechanisms of Synthesis and Functional Implications

Two main groups of neurochemical messengers are used in the nervous system: small-molecule neurotransmitters and large-sized neuropeptides (Table 16-2).

**Small-molecule neurotransmitters** are formed in short metabolic pathways from simple and readily available precursors. The pathways of synthesis of the major small-molecule transmitters are summarized in Figure 16-2. Neurotransmitter synthesis occurs in the neuronal cell body, as well as in the presynaptic terminals.

| **TABLE 16-2** | Small- and Large-Molecule Neurotransmitters in the Central Nervous System |
|---|---|
| **Neurochemical Messenger** | **Molecular Weight (Da)** |
| Classical neurotransmitters | |
| Acetylcholine | 146 |
| Serotonin | 176 |
| Histamine | 111 |
| Dopamine | 190 |
| Noradrenaline | 169 |
| Adrenaline | 183 |
| Amino acid neurotransmitters | |
| Glutamate | 147 |
| Aspartate | 133 |
| GABA (γ-aminobutyric acid) | 103 |
| Glycine | 75 |
| Neuropeptides | |
| α-Endorphin | 1746 |
| β-Endorphin | 3438 |
| Dynorphin A | 2147 |
| Dynorphin B | 1571 |
| Leu-enkephalin | 555 |
| Met-enkephalin | 573 |
| Vasopressin | 1084 |
| Oxytocin | 1007 |
| Cholecystokinin 8S | 1143 |
| Angiotensin II | 1046 |
| Neurotensin | 1672 |
| Substance P | 1347 |
| Neuropeptide Y | 4271 |
| Calcitonin gene–related peptide (CGRP) | 3789 |

**FIGURE 16-2** Principal metabolic pathways of biosynthesis and degradation of the main small-molecule neurotransmitters in the mammalian brain. AAA Dec = aromatic amino acid decarboxylase; AAT = aspartate aminotransferase; AChE = acetyl-cholinesterase; ALDH = aldehyde dehydrogenase; CAT = choline acetyltransferase; CoA = coenzyme A; COMT = catechol-O-methyltransferase; DβH = dopamine β hydroxylase; DHMA = 3,4-dihydroxymandelic acid; DHPEG = 3,4-dihydroxy-phenylethylene glycol; DO = diamine oxidase; DOPAC = dihydroxyphenylacetic acid; Dopa Dec = dopa decarboxylase; GABA-T = GABA transaminase; GAD = glutamic acid decarboxylase; GluSyn = glutamine synthetase; 5-HIAA = 5-hydroxy-indoleacetic acid; Hist Dec = histidine decarboxylase; HMT = histamine methyltransferase; HVA = homovanillic acid; α-KG = α-ketoglutarate; MAO = monoamine oxidase; MHPEG = 3-methoxy-4-hydroxyphenylethylene glycol; OAT = ornithine aminotransferase; PNMT = phenylethanolamine-N-methyltransferase; SHMT = serine hydroxymethyltrans-ferase; TH = tyrosine hydroxylase; TryH = tryptophan hydroxylase; VMA = vanilmandelic acid.

**Acetylcholine**

Acetyl-CoA + Choline $\underset{\text{AChE}}{\overset{\text{CAT}}{\rightleftharpoons}}$ ACh + CoA

**Serotonin**

Tryptophan $\xrightarrow{\text{TryH}}$ 5-OH-tryptophan $\xrightarrow{\text{AAA Dec}}$ 5-HT $\xrightarrow{\text{MAO + ALDH}}$ 5-HIAA

**Histamine**

Histidine $\dfrac{\text{Hist Dec}}{\text{AAA Dec}}$ Histamine

$\xrightarrow{\text{HMT}}$ Methyl histamine

$\xrightarrow{\text{DO}}$ Imidazole acetic acid

**Catecholamines**

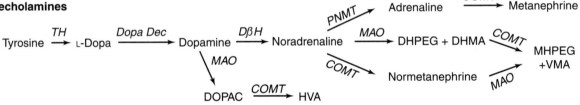

**Glutamate**

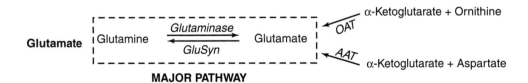

**MAJOR PATHWAY**

**GABA**

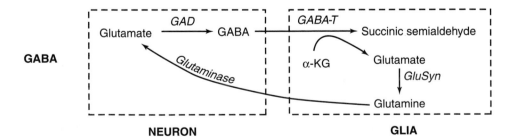

**NEURON**          **GLIA**

**Glycine**   Serine $\xrightarrow{\text{SHMT}}$ Glycine

The precursor molecules required for the synthesis of the neurotransmitter are readily transported across the cell membrane, both in the soma and in the presynaptic terminal. The neurotransmitter locally synthesized in the presynaptic terminal is actively transported into small (40 to 60 nm) synaptic vesicles (**vesicular pool**), where it is stored until released by exocytosis. Enzymes that degrade small-molecule transmitters are also present in the cytosol or mitochondria of the presynaptic terminal and, in some cases, also in the synaptic cleft. The amount of transmitter present in the cytosol (**cytoplasmic pool**) is the result of the balance between synthesis and degradation plus vesicular uptake. Pharmacological agents that inhibit the degradative enzymes disturb this equilibrium and increase the amount of neurotransmitter in the cytoplasmic pool.

The synthesis of **neuropeptides** is a more elaborate process. Initially, **large precursor molecules** (with molecular weights of up to many thousands of daltons) are synthesized by mRNA associated with the rough endoplasmic reticulum (RER) in the cell body. The molecule is transported into the lumen of the RER together with specific **proteolytic enzymes**. The large peptide molecules and proteolytic enzymes are "packaged" in the same secretory vesicles and are carried by anterograde transport along the axon to the presynaptic terminals. During transport, the proteases cleave the large precursor into smaller physiologically active peptides. The same large precursor molecules can be formed in many different parts of the CNS but undergo cleavage by different proteolytic enzymes at different sites, releasing different active peptide products.

The calcium-dependent patterns of release for small-molecule and large-sized messengers differ significantly. First, neuropeptide-containing vesicles are more sensitive to calcium influx than those containing small-molecule neurotransmitters. Second, after stimulation of the neuron, small-molecule neurotransmitters can be rapidly synthesized in the presynaptic terminals and replenish the cytoplasmic and vesicular pools, thus permitting a steady release of the transmitter. Replenishment of the large-sized peptides in a synaptic terminal takes much longer, as a new supply of the peptide has to be synthesized in the cell body and transported to the terminal.

Most, if not all, mature neurons contain more than one chemical messenger. A classical small-molecule transmitter is usually present in association with one or more large-sized neuropeptides in the same neuron. This situation is known as **co-localization** of neurochemical messengers (see examples in Table 16-3). The co-localized chemical messengers are also co-released, and they interact functionally with each other, the peptide acting to modulate the response of the postsynaptic cell to the classical transmitter; this is known as **co-transmission**. Consequently, any given neuronal population is defined not by the existence of a single messenger but, rather, by a specific "profile" or combination of chemical messengers.

The characteristic transmitter profile of any given neuron depends not only on its genetic makeup, but also on factors in its functional environment. Neurotrophic factors released by other cells, such as nerve growth factor (NGF) and brain-derived neurotrophic factor (BDNF), alter the expression of different genes and thus affect which transmitters are produced. In addition, changes in intraneuronal calcium level, as a result of changes in the pattern of stimulation of the neuron by other neurons, alter the profile of transmitters released by that cell.

## Receptors: Concept and Classifications

After release into the synaptic cleft, the neurochemical messenger binds to specific molecules known as **receptors**. The basic criteria for identifying a given molecule as a receptor are discussed in Chapter 8. In addition, exogenous administration of physiological amounts of the naturally occurring transmitter should produce the same physiological response as neuronal release of the transmitter at that receptor and should be blocked by treatment with an antagonist. Receptors show a selective neu-

| TABLE 16-3 | Co-localization of Small-Molecule Neurotransmitters with Neuroactive Peptides |
|---|---|
| **Neurotransmitter** | **Peptide** |
| Acetylcholine | CGRP VIP Substance P Enkephalin Neurotensin |
| Serotonin | Substance P CCK Enkephalin |
| Dopamine | CCK Neurotensin Enkephalin |
| Noradrenaline | Neuropeptide Y Enkephalin Somatostatin |
| Adrenaline | Neuropeptide Y Enkephalin Neurotensin |
| Glutamate | Substance P |
| GABA | Somatostatin CCK Enkephalin Substance P |
| Glycine | Neurotensin |

CCK = cholecystokinin; CGRP = calcitonin gene–related peptide; VIP = vasoactive intestinal peptide.

roanatomical distribution in well-defined neuroanatomical pathways and brain structures where the transmitter in question is found.

Recent advances in molecular techniques have already allowed the isolation and reconstitution of functional receptor molecules, as well as the mapping, isolation, and cloning of **receptor genes.**

Receptor proteins are synthesized in the rough endoplasmic reticulum, transported to different parts of the cell, and inserted into the cell membrane of the soma, dendrites, and axons. Binding of a selective ligand to a **presynaptic receptor** regulates the release of neurotransmitter from the presynaptic cell, while binding to a **postsynaptic receptor** produces a response in the postsynaptic cell. Receptors have also been classified as **autoreceptors** or **heteroreceptors** according to whether they are sensitive to a transmitter released by that same neuron or by another neuron.

There are four classes of receptor molecules: (1) ligand-gated ion channels (ionotropic receptors); (2) G protein–coupled receptors (metabotropic); (3) enzyme-linked (protein-kinase) receptors; and (4) intracellular receptors.

## Ionotropic receptors

Ionotropic receptors are directly linked to ion channels. These large molecules (250 000 to 300 000 Da) consist of four or five subunits embedded in the cell membrane (Fig. 16-3), each subunit containing four membrane-spanning elements. At least one of the receptor subunits has a high-affinity binding site that selectively recognizes the transmitter molecule. The other subunits have low-affinity

binding sites and are primarily involved in regulating the opening and closing of the channel (Fig. 16-4A).

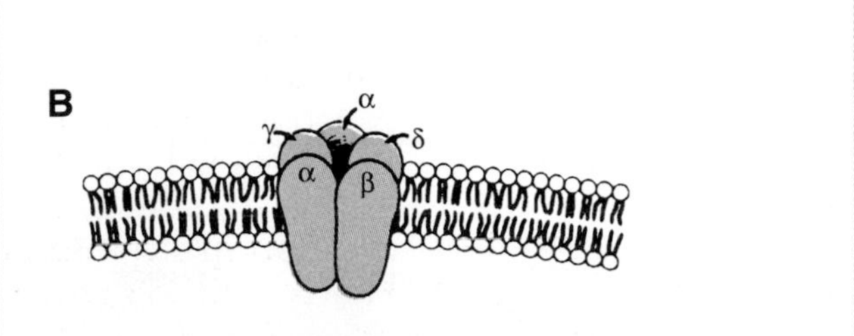

These receptors mediate fast responses (on the order of milliseconds). When activated by the transmitter, they undergo conformational changes that allow ions to pass through the channel. The nicotinic acetylcholine receptor (linked to a $Na^+$ channel) and the $GABA_A$ receptor (linked to a $Cl^-$ channel) are classical examples of ionotropic receptors. Other important examples, including most glutamate receptors, glycine receptors, and the $5-HT_3$ (a serotonin subtype) receptor, are described later in this chapter.

The distribution of ionotropic receptors in different parts of the neuron is not homogeneous. For example, receptors gating $Na^+$ and $K^+$ channels are particularly abundant in the soma and cell processes, whereas receptors linked to $Ca^{2+}$ channels are sparse in those structures but particularly abundant in the presynaptic terminals. Accordingly, inactivation of the $Na^+$ and $K^+$ channels by tetrodotoxin and tetraethylammonium, respectively, prevents the propagation of an action potential along the axon but does not prevent the release of neurotransmitter by the presynaptic terminal. Conversely, inactivation of the calcium channels prevents the release of neurotransmitter by the terminal but does not significantly disrupt the axonal propagation of an action potential.

Ionotropic receptors can mediate either excitatory or inhibitory activity. In the soma and dendritic processes, the transmitter-induced opening of $Na^+$ channels causes an influx of positive charges that depolarizes the membrane and produces an EPSP. Conversely, binding of a transmitter to a receptor that opens a $Cl^-$ channel and allows the influx of $Cl^-$ ions causes hyperpolarization and an IPSP.

Each neuron receives a large number of synaptic contacts; EPSPs are generated in some synapses, IPSPs in others. The changes in net polarity of the neuron are therefore determined by summation of all the EPSPs and IPSPs occurring on the surface of that neuron. If enough EPSPs occur to cancel out the IPSPs, then an action potential will be generated. The inhibitory or excitatory effects of a particular type of transmitter are not determined by the intrinsic properties of the transmitter per se but depend on the type of receptor to which the transmitter molecule binds.

## Metabotropic receptors

Metabotropic receptors are *indirectly* linked to ion channels (Fig. 16-4B). The binding of the transmitter to the receptor is followed by coupling of the receptor to a GTP-binding protein **(G protein).** In turn, the G protein will interact with the ion channel either directly, or indirectly through second-messenger systems. The structural features of metabotropic receptors and the nature of their second-messenger systems are described in Chapters 8 and 9. Functionally, metabotropic receptors mediate slow synaptic actions that last seconds or even minutes. The effects on the neuron can be either excitatory or inhibitory, depend-

**FIGURE 16-3**  Ionotropic receptors (ligand-gated channels) are found in chemical synapses. These receptors have four (A) or five (B) transmembrane subunits.

FIGURE 16-4    (A) In ionotropic receptors, the high-affinity binding site (receptor site), the effector site, and the gating site are all part of the same molecular structure. (B) In metabotropic receptors, the high-affinity binding site (receptor site) and the ion-gating channel are two separate molecules. In this case, the gating of the ion channel is indirectly mediated through the G protein/second-messenger (cAMP) pathway. GTP = guanosine triphosphate.

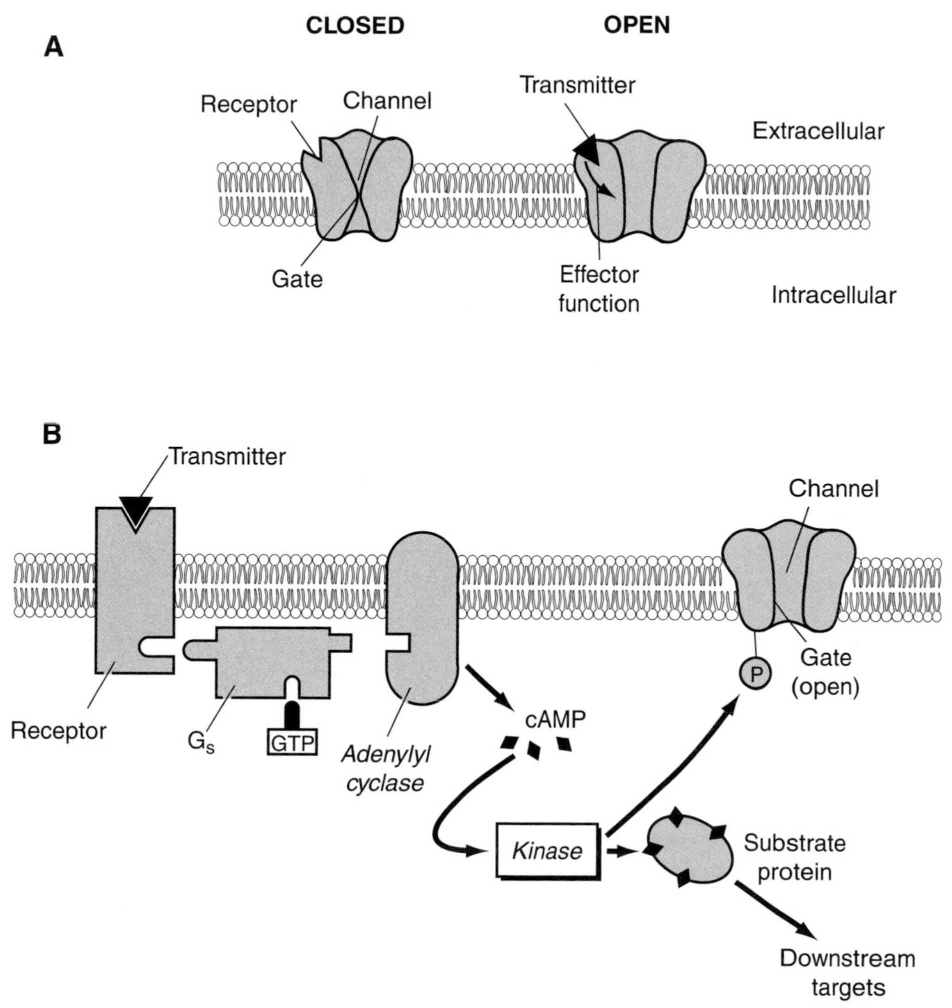

ing on the activation of different G proteins that stimulate or inhibit different transduction pathways and regulate certain ion channels.

One of the most important functional aspects of second-messenger–mediated transmission is that it induces phosphorylation of regulatory proteins, including enzymes involved in neurotransmitter synthesis and proteins that regulate gene transcription. These mechanisms are likely to constitute the basis for long-term cellular changes, as seen in neuronal development and long-term memory.

## Protein-kinase receptors

Enzyme-linked, or protein-kinase, receptors are transmembrane polypeptides that have an extracellular ligand-binding domain, a transmembrane domain, and an intracellular domain that is an enzyme, such as tyrosine kinase or guanylyl cyclase. The effects of insulin and growth factors, including NGF, are mediated by tyrosine kinase receptors, and those of atrial natriuretic peptide, by guanylyl cyclase receptors.

Recently, another subtype of enzyme-linked receptor has been identified that lacks an intrinsic cytoplasmic enzymatic portion. After agonist binding to the extracellular site, the intracellular portion of the receptor binds covalently to a separate, or mobile, protein kinase. This receptor type, also known as **cytokine receptor,** mediates the effects of several groups of molecules including interferons and tumour necrosis factors.

### Intracellular receptors

Intracellular receptors are the targets for highy liposoluble ligands (e.g., steroid and thyroid hormones), which, after crossing the plasma membrane, bind to the receptors located in the cytoplasm. After binding occurs, the hormone–receptor complex is translocated to the nucleus, where it binds to specific DNA sequences (response elements) and regulates gene expression. The effects mediated by activation of these receptors take place only after a long delay of half an hour to several hours after receptor activation because they result from changes in protein synthesis. The elicited effect also persists for a period of hours or days, even after the ligand is no longer present, due to the downstream effect on protein synthesis and the activity of the newly synthesized protein.

## BLOOD–BRAIN BARRIER: STRUCTURE AND PHARMACOLOGICAL IMPLICATIONS

Although the CNS is highly vascularized, the histological and functional properties of its capillary network create a barrier, known as the **blood–brain barrier** (BBB), that severely restricts the passage of most molecules between the bloodstream and the parenchyma of the CNS. The histological basis of the BBB is described in Chapter 2; it consists of continuous tight junctions between the capillary endothelial cells, absence of fenestrations, and marked scarcity of pinocytotic vesicles. Brain capillaries are also surrounded by a prominent basement membrane, limited on the outside by a continuous layer of cellular processes belonging to neurons and glial cells (astrocytes and oligodendrocytes). Consequently, in the CNS, the transport of a molecule from the bloodstream to the perivascular space requires that the molecule either (1) be sufficiently small and lipid-soluble to cross the cell membrane and the cytoplasm of the endothelial cell, or (2) bind to a selective carrier and undergo active (i.e., energy-consuming) transport.

In a few structures surrounding the third and fourth ventricles, such as the area postrema, subfornical organ, and the median eminence, the BBB is weak, or leaky, so these parts of the brain are functionally "outside" the BBB. This fact allows them to act as sensors of the chemical and osmotic properties of the blood. The gathered information is then transferred by neuronal impulses to other brain regions inside the BBB, triggering the appropriate responses. In the case of the median eminence, the existence of a weak BBB permits the hormones and releasing factors produced by hypothalamic neurons to pass readily from the perivascular space into the bloodstream.

The very low permeability of most of the BBB drastically reduces the number of drugs that can effectively cross from the blood into the CNS. With the exception of molecules for which there are specific transport systems (e.g., glucose, amino acids, transferrin, and insulin), only small lipophilic molecules enter the brain. The oil/water partition coefficient of a given molecule (see Chapter 2) can be used as an indicator of its ability to enter the brain.

Several strategies have been developed to facilitate the entry of drugs into the CNS. Molecular changes aimed at increasing liposolubility are the most common approach. Direct delivery of the drug into the brain ventricles or the subarachnoid space is used experimentally to bypass the BBB but is too hazardous for frequent therapeutic use in humans, except for injection into the lumbar spinal subarachnoid space and, occasionally, into the cisterna magna at the base of the brain. One of the most elegant and potentially effective strategies is to bind the drug to a **carrier**, such as an antibody against receptors of molecules known to be actively transported into the CNS (e.g., antibodies against transferrin receptors). The drug–antibody complex binds to the receptor, initiating the active transport mechanisms.

## CLASSICAL NEUROTRANSMITTER SYSTEMS IN THE CENTRAL NERVOUS SYSTEM

### Acetylcholine (ACh)

Cholinergic synapses are found both in the periphery (neuromuscular junction, autonomic ganglia, and parasympathetic postganglionic synapses) and in the brain and spinal cord.

#### Synthesis and degradation

Choline is taken up into neurons by two different transport processes. In the CNS, a carrier-mediated and $Na^+$-dependent high-affinity transport exists only in cholinergic terminals, and 50 to 85% of the choline transported by this mechanism is utilized in ACh synthesis. A low-affinity transport ($Na^+$-independent passive diffusion) is present in cell bodies of cholinergic neurons. **Choline acetyltransferase** is the rate-limiting enzyme in the synthesis of ACh (see Fig. 16-2), and, in the CNS, it is present only in ACh-producing neurons.

After its release, ACh is readily hydrolyzed to acetyl-CoA and choline by cholinesterases in the synaptic cleft. Half of this choline is immediately reutilized in the production of new ACh molecules. There are two types of cholinesterase in the CNS: (1) **butyrylcholinesterase** (also known as non-specific or "pseudo" cholinesterase) and (2) **acetylcholinesterase** (AChE, also called specific or "true" cholinesterase). AChE is by far the more abundant in the mammalian brain. AChE activity can be decreased by inhibitors that compete with ACh for binding to the anionic and esteratic sites of the enzyme. The types of inhibitor are described in Chapters 12 and 15. By increasing the availability of ACh in the synaptic cleft, these inhibitors cause increased binding of ACh to the postsynaptic cholinergic receptors and thus facilitate cholinergic transmission.

## Acetylcholine receptors

There are two classes of cholinergic receptors: muscarinic and nicotinic. **Muscarinic receptors** are metabotropic; they are coupled to G proteins and linked to a variety of ion channels. They have a slow response time (100 to 250 ms). Five different types of muscarinic receptors ($M_1$ to $M_5$) have already been identified (Table 16-4) and are all present in the CNS. $M_1$, $M_3$, and $M_5$ are coupled to $G_q$ and mediate excitatory responses, whereas $M_2$ and $M_4$ are coupled to $G_i$ and mediate inhibitory responses. Autoradiographic studies reveal the highest densities of $M_1$ receptors (those with high affinity for pirenzepine) in the hippocampus, basal ganglia, substantia nigra, and superficial layers of the neocortex; $M_2$ and other subtypes are particularly abundant in the septum, superior colliculus, cerebellum, and brainstem.

**Nicotinic receptors** are ionotropic receptors, and they have a faster response than muscarinic receptors (less than 100 ms). They have a heteromeric structure with five subunits of four different types designated $\alpha$, $\beta$, $\gamma$, and $\delta$ (~250 kDa). Concurrent binding of an agonist molecule to each of the two existing alpha subunits activates the receptor and increases $Na^+$ and $K^+$ permeability, leading to depolarization (i.e., excitation). Different subunit compositions determine the pharmacological profile of different nicotinic receptors. It is now well established that there are several functionally relevant types of nicotinic receptor. Those at the neuromuscular junction have two $\alpha$ subunits and one each of the $\beta$, $\gamma$, and $\delta$ subunits, whereas the neuronal nicotinic receptors do not have either $\gamma$ or $\delta$ subunits, but only have two $\alpha$ and three $\beta$ subunits. In neuronal nicotinic receptors, eight isoforms of the $\alpha$ subunit and three of the $\beta$ have been identified. This variety in the composition of neuronal nicotinic receptors provides a tremendous molecular diversity and raises the possibility of the development of selective pharmacological agents aimed at selective subpopulations of receptors.

In the CNS, high concentrations of nicotinic receptors are found in the periaqueductal grey, cerebellum, dentate gyrus of the hippocampus, and occipital cortex, as well as the perikarya and terminal fields of the nigrostriatal and mesolimbic dopaminergic systems. Cholinergic receptors on spinal Renshaw cells are also nicotinic.

Both muscarinic and nicotinic receptors, when activated by their respective agonists, cause depolarization and excitation of the target neurons. Antagonists of central muscarinic receptors have long-established therapeutic use (see Chapter 12), but central nicotinic receptor antagonists have so far been used only for experimental purposes.

## Central cholinergic pathways

**Local circuit cholinergic neurons** are excitatory interneurons in the caudate–putamen (involved in motor coordination) and in the nucleus accumbens and olfactory tubercle (involved in motivational processes; Fig. 16-5). The **cholinergic projection neurons** are organized into two groups: the basal forebrain (BF) and the pontomesencephalotegmental (PMT) cholinergic complexes (Fig. 16-6A). BF neuron cell bodies are located in the medial septum and related areas with axons that project to the hippocampus, olfactory bulb, and non-striatal forebrain, and they are believed to be involved in mechanisms of learning and memory. PMT neuron cell bodies are located in the ventral midbrain, sending ascending projections to the thalamus and remaining diencephalic and mesencephalic areas and descending projections to the pons and medulla, cerebellum, and vestibular nuclei. These projections are involved in mechanisms of arousal and homeostasis.

## Serotonin

### Synthesis and degradation

Serotonin (5-hydroxytryptamine, or 5-HT) is formed by hydroxylation and decarboxylation of the neutral amino acid **tryptophan** (see Fig. 16-2). Tryptophan, the rate-limiting factor in the synthesis of 5-HT, does not cross the BBB and must be actively transported by a carrier that is also responsible for the transport of other amino acids (e.g., tyrosine, phenylalanine, histidine). Cytoplasmic and membrane-bound pools of tryptophan hydroxylase are present in the cell bodies and axon terminals of 5-HT-producing neurons. Serotonin production can be selectively blocked by inhibitors of tryptophan hydroxylase, such as *p*-chlorophenylalanine; 5-HT produced in the periphery has no central actions, since it does not cross the BBB.

Serotonin is deaminated by **monoamine oxidase** (MAO) to form 5-hydroxyindoleacetaldehyde, which is then oxidized by **aldehyde dehydrogenase** to form **5-hydroxyindoleacetic acid** (5-HIAA). MAO is widely distributed in both nervous and non-nervous tissues. Two types (MAO-A and MAO-B) have been identified on the basis of their substrate affinities, specificity of inhibition by certain MAO inhibitors, and brain distribution in different species. MAO-A has a higher affinity for 5-HT than MAO-B does, and its localization is mainly intracellular, while that of MAO-B is predominantly extracellular. In the human brain, MAO-B is the predominant form. Some drugs, such as pargyline, are irreversible inhibitors of both forms of the enzyme, while other compounds selectively inhibit only one MAO subtype (e.g., MAO-A inhibitor clorgyline, and MAO-B inhibitor deprenyl). However, MAO also participates in the degradation of dopamine and noradrenaline, and inhibition of MAO affects the dopaminergic and noradrenergic systems as well as the serotonergic system (see Chapter 13).

| TABLE 16-4 | Receptor Types and Subtypes for CNS Neurotransmitters: Ligands and Major Effects | | | |
|---|---|---|---|---|
| Transmitter | Receptor Subtypes | Agonists | Antagonists | Cellular Effects |
| Classical Acetylcholine | Muscarinic (M$_{1-5}$) | M$_{1-5}$: Muscarine | M$_1$: Pirenzepine, telenzepine | M$_{1,3,5}$: $\uparrow$ IP$_3$/DG (excitatory) |
| | | | M$_2$: Methoctramine, gallamine | M$_{2,4}$: $\downarrow$ cAMP, $\uparrow$ K$^+$ conductance (inhibitory) |
| | | M$_1$: Oxotremorine M | M$_3$: 4-DAMP | |
| | | | M$_4$: Tropicamide | |
| | Nicotinic | Nicotine | $\alpha$-Bungarotoxin | $\uparrow$ Ca$^{2+}$, $\uparrow$ Na$^+$, $\uparrow$ K$^+$ conductance (excitatory) |
| Serotonin | 5-HT$_{1A,1B,1D}$ | 5-HT$_{1A}$: 8-OH-DPAT | 5-HT$_{1A}$: p-MPPI | $\downarrow$ cAMP, $\uparrow$ K$^+$ conductance (inhibitory) |
| | | 5-HT$_{1B}$: Anpirtoline | — | $\downarrow$ cAMP, $\uparrow$ K$^+$ conductance (inhibitory) |
| | | 5-HT$_{1D}$: L 694247 | 5-HT$_{1D}$: GR 127935 | $\downarrow$ cAMP, $\uparrow$ K$^+$ conductance (inhibitory) |
| | 5-HT$_{1C}$ | — | 5-HT$_{1C}$: Norclozapine | $\uparrow$ IP$_3$/DG (excitatory) |
| | 5-HT$_2$ | — | 5-HT$_2$: Ketanserin, ritanserin | $\uparrow$ IP$_3$/DG (excitatory) |
| | 5-HT$_3$ | 5-HT$_3$: 2-Methylserotonin | 5-HT$_3$: ICS 205930 (Tropanyl) | $\uparrow$ Na$^+$ and $\uparrow$ K$^+$ conductance (excitatory) |
| | 5-HT$_4$ | SC 53116 | — | $\uparrow$ cAMP (excitatory) |
| Histamine | H$_1$ | 2(m-F-Phenylhistamine) | Mepyramine | $\uparrow$ IP$_3$/DG (excitatory) |
| | H$_2$ | Dimaprit | Cimetidine | $\uparrow$ cAMP (excitatory) |
| | H$_3$ | Imetit | Thioperamide | $\downarrow$ cAMP (inhibitory) (autoreceptor) |
| Dopamine | D$_{1,5}$ | D$_1$: SKF 38393 | D$_1$: SCH 23390 | $\uparrow$ cAMP (excitatory) |
| | | D$_5$: High affinity for dopamine | — | $\uparrow$ cAMP (excitatory) |
| | D$_{2,3,4}$ | D$_2$: TNPA | D$_2$>D$_3$: Raclopride | $\downarrow$ cAMP, $\downarrow$ Ca$^{2+}$, $\uparrow$ K$^+$ conductance (inhibitory) |
| | | D$_3$: 7-OH-DPAT | D$_4$>D$_{2,3}$: Clozapine | $\downarrow$ cAMP, $\downarrow$ Ca$^{2+}$, $\uparrow$ K$^+$ conductance (inhibitory) |
| Adrenaline and Noradrenaline | $\alpha_{1A,1B,1C}$ | $\alpha_1$: Methoxamine | $\alpha_1$: Prazosin | $\alpha_{1A}$: $\uparrow$ Ca$^{2+}$ conductance (excitatory) |
| | | | $\alpha_{1A}$: Tamsulosin | $\alpha_{1B,1C}$: $\uparrow$ IP$_3$/DG (excitatory) |
| | $\alpha_{2A,2B,2C}$ | $\alpha_2$: Clonidine | $\alpha_2$: Yohimbine | $\alpha_2$: $\downarrow$ cAMP, $\downarrow$ Ca$^{2+}$ conductance (inhibitory) |
| | $\beta_{1,2,3}$ | $\beta_1$: Isoproterenol>>NA=A | $\beta_{1,2,3}$: Pindolol | $\uparrow$ cAMP (excitatory) |
| | | | $\beta_1$: Atenolol | |
| | | $\beta_2$: Isoproterenol>A>>NA | $\beta_2$: ICI 118551 | $\uparrow$ cAMP (excitatory) |
| | | $\beta_3$: Isoproterenol=NA>A | — | $\uparrow$ cAMP (excitatory) |
| | | $\beta_3$: BRL 37344 | — | $\uparrow$ cAMP (excitatory) |
| Amino acids Glutamate and aspartate | NMDA | cis-ACDA | Dizocilpine (MK 801), kynurenate | $\uparrow$ Na$^+$, $\uparrow$ K$^+$, and $\uparrow$ Ca$^{2+}$ conductance (excitatory) |
| | Non-NMDA: | | | |
| | Kainate | Kainic acid | GAMS | $\uparrow$ Na$^+$, $\uparrow$ K$^+$ conductance (excitatory) |
| | Quisqualate/AMPA | Quisqualate | CNQX | $\uparrow$ Na$^+$, $\uparrow$ K$^+$ conductance (excitatory) |
| | L-AP4 | — | L-AP4 | $\downarrow$ cAMP (inhibitory) (autoreceptor?) |
| | ACPD | ACPD | AP3 | $\uparrow$ IP$_3$/DG (excitatory) |
| GABA | GABA$_A$ | Muscimol | Bicuculline | $\uparrow$ Cl$^-$ conductance (inhibitory) |
| | GABA$_B$ | Baclofen | Phaclofen | $\uparrow$ K$^+$ and $\downarrow$ Ca$^{2+}$ conductance (inhibitory) |
| Glycine | Glycine receptor | $\beta$-Alanine | Strychnine | $\uparrow$ Cl$^-$ conductance (inhibitory) |
| Peptides Opioids | $\mu$ | DAMGO | CTOP | $\downarrow$ cAMP, $\downarrow$ Ca$^{2+}$, and $\uparrow$ K$^+$ conductance (inhibitory) |
| | $\delta$ | DPDPE | ICI 174864 | $\downarrow$ cAMP, $\downarrow$ Ca$^{2+}$, and $\uparrow$ K$^+$ conductance (inhibitory) |
| | $\kappa$ | U 62066 | Binaltorphimine | $\downarrow$ cAMP, $\downarrow$ Ca$^{2+}$, and $\uparrow$ K$^+$ conductance (inhibitory) |
| Vasopressin | V$_1$ | DGAVP | Manning compound | $\uparrow$ IP$_3$/DG (excitatory) |
| | V$_2$ | dVDAVP | DDIAAVP | $\uparrow$ cAMP (excitatory) |

*continued*

**TABLE 16-4** continued

| Transmitter | Receptor Subtypes | Agonists | Antagonists | Cellular Effects |
|---|---|---|---|---|
| Oxytocin | — | Oxytocin | Vasotocin | ↑ IP$_3$/DG (excitatory) |
| Cholecystokinin | CCK$_A$ | CCK-8: CCK$_A$>CCK$_B$ | Devazepide | ↑ IP$_3$/DG (excitatory) |
| | CCK$_B$ | Pentagastrin | CI 988 | ↑ IP$_3$/DG (excitatory) |
| Angiotensin | AII$_\alpha$ | Angiotensin II | AII$_{\alpha,\beta}$: Saralasin | ↑ cAMP, ↑ cGMP (excitatory) |
| | | | AII$_\alpha$: DuP 753 | |
| | AII$_\beta$ | Angiotensin II | AII$_\beta$: PD 123177 | ↑ cAMP, ↑ cGMP (excitatory) |

A = adrenaline; ACDA = 1-aminocyclobutane-*cis*-1,3-dicarboxylic acid; ACPD = (±)-1-amino-1,3-cyclopentanedicarboxylic acid; AMPA = (±)-α-amino-3-hydroxy-5-methylisoxazole-4-propionic acid; AP3 = (±)-2-amino-3-phosphonopropionic acid; cAMP = cyclic adenosine monophosphate; cGMP = cyclic guanosine monophosphate; CNQX = 6-cyano-7-nitroquinoxaline-2,3-dione; CTOP = D-Phe-Cys-Tyr-D-Trp-Orn-Thr-Pen-Thr amide; DAMGO = [D-Ala$^2$, N-Me-Phe$^4$,Gly-ol$^5$]-enkephalin; 4-DAMP = 4-diphenylacetoxy-N-methylpiperidine; DDIAAVP = [d(CH$_2$)$_5^1$,D-Ile$^4$,Ile$^4$,Arg$^8$,Ala$^9$]-vasopressin; DG = diacylglycerol; DGAVP = [des-glycinamide$^9$,Arg$^8$]-vasopressin; DPDPE=[D-Pen$^{2,5}$]-enkephalin; dVDAVP = [deamino-Cys$^1$, Val$^4$, D-Arg$^8$]-vasopressin; GAMS = D-γ-glutamylaminomethanesulfonic acid; IP$_3$ = inositol trisphosphate; L-AP4 = L(+)-2-amino-4-phosphonobutyric acid; Manning compound = [d(CH$_2$)$_5$ $^1$O-Me-Tyr$^2$,Arg$^8$]-vasopressin; NA = noradrenaline; NMDA = N-methyl-D-aspartic acid; 7-OH-DPAT = 7-hydroxy-dipropylaminotetralin; 8-OH-DPAT = 8-hydroxy-dipropylaminotetralin; TNPA = (±)-2,10,11-trihydroxy-N-propylnorapomorphine.

Other abbreviations (e.g., ICI 118551) refer to proprietary codes with the letters standing for abbreviation of the pharmaceutical company's name and the number referring to the product number.

**FIGURE 16-5** Approximate locations of major brain nuclei and structures referred to in subsequent figures.

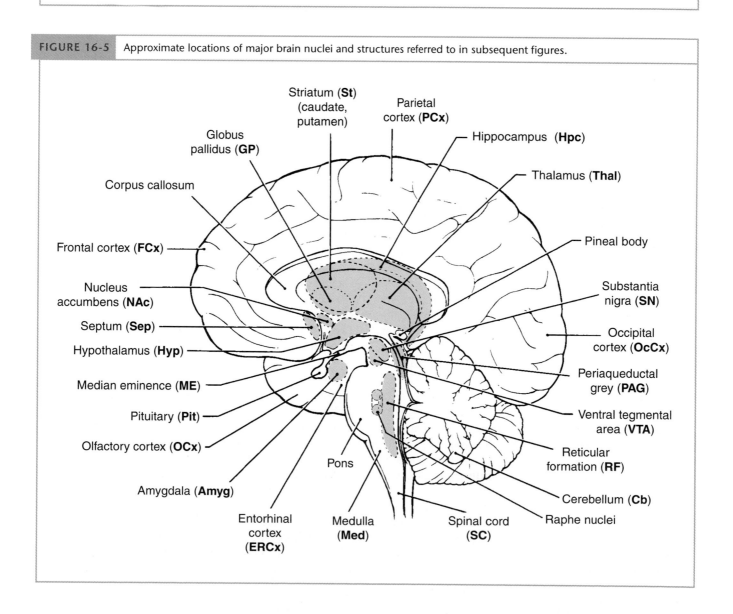

5-HIAA is the most important serotonin metabolite, and its concentration in the CSF is used as a measure of serotonergic activity in the brain. Low CSF concentrations of 5-HIAA have been observed in depressed patients. Drugs that increase the availability of serotonin in the synaptic cleft are used as antidepressants (see Chapter 25). Tricyclics (e.g., imipramine) and non-tricyclic antidepressants (e.g., fluoxetine) act by blocking the reuptake of 5-HT, while MAO inhibitors prevent its degradation.

## Serotonin receptors

The main subtypes of serotonin receptors, defined by their genetic, pharmacological, and electrophysiological properties, are 5-HT$_{1A,1B,1D,1E,1F}$; 5-HT$_{2A,2B,2C}$; 5-HT$_3$; and 5-HT$_4$. Their features are summarized in Table 16.4. All 5-HT$_1$ receptor subtypes are inhibitory and G$_i$-coupled. However, their different isoforms are selectively expressed in different neuronal compartments. Whereas the 5-HT$_{1A}$ isoform is a somatodendritic autoreceptor, the 5-HT$_{1B}$ and 5-HT$_{1D}$ subtypes are presynaptic autoreceptors and postsynaptic receptors. Both 5-HT$_2$ and 5-HT$_4$ receptor subtypes are excitatory. While the former is positively coupled to G$_{q/11}$ and activates phospholipase C, the latter is coupled to G$_s$ and activates adenylylcyclase. The 5-HT$_{2A}$ receptor is the most abundant isoform of the 5-HT$_2$ receptor in nervous tissue. The 5-HT$_3$ receptor subtype is the only ionotropic serotonergic receptor identified thus far. Its activation increases permeability to Na$^+$ and K$^+$ and causes depolarization (excitation). 5-HT$_{5,6,7}$ receptors are G$_s$-coupled, but their complete pharmacological profiles remain to be elucidated.

## Central serotonergic pathways

The classical serotonergic cell nuclei are located in the midline of the pons and upper brainstem (see Fig. 16-5). The more rostral group (RG, mainly the **dorsal and medial raphe nuclei**) send extensive diffuse ascending innervation to the thalamus, hypothalamus, striatal complex, and cortical areas. Limbic brain structures, such as the hippocampus, septum, amygdala, and limbic frontal cortex, receive a very rich serotonergic innervation (Fig. 16-6B). Typically, the 5-HT innervation of each area originates in more than one raphe group. The widespread distribution of ascending serotonergic innervation of the cortical areas contrasts with the well-defined patterns of regional and laminar distribution of the dopaminergic and noradrenergic innervation in the cortex. These findings support the view that the ascending serotonergic innervation exerts a global, but not necessarily uniform, influence upon cortical functions.

A caudal serotonergic cell group (CG) located in the caudal pons and medulla oblongata sends **descending innervation** to the medulla and spinal cord, where serotonin is involved in mechanisms of cardiovascular control and pain perception.

Serotonergic cell groups have also been identified in other structures such as the **area postrema** and functionally related areas, where they are involved in the integration of information concerning gastrointestinal function and respiratory control.

The **pineal gland** contains high concentrations of serotonin, which is locally produced in secretory cells (pinealocytes) and is the precursor in the synthesis of melatonin, a hormone that regulates gonadotropic hormone secretion in some species, and is thought to regulate sleep–wake cycles in humans. High concentrations of serotonin inhibit melatonin activity.

In addition to its role in homeostasis and pain modulation, the serotonergic system also plays a central role in the mechanisms of sleep, feeding, and sexual behaviour. Serotonergic activity is higher in the waking state, decreases during slow-wave sleep, and is almost non-existent during rapid-eye-movement sleep. Finally, hyperactivity of the serotonergic system is involved in the pathogenesis of anxiety, whereas hypoactivity has been implicated in the etiology of depression.

# Histamine

## Synthesis and degradation

Histamine is synthesized by decarboxylation of the amino acid **histidine** (see Fig. 16-2), which is actively transported into the CNS. Pyridoxal phosphate is required as a cofactor for the decarboxylase. Histamine synthesis can therefore be blocked by pyridoxal phosphate antagonists or by α-fluoromethylhistidine, a selective and irreversible inhibitor of histidine decarboxylase.

Histamine can be metabolized either by histamine-$N$-methyltransferase to form methylhistamine or by diamine oxidase to form imidazole acetic acid. Histamine concentrations in the brain are relatively low (except in the hypothalamus), but there is a rapid turnover.

## Histamine receptors

The major types of histamine receptors in the brain are shown in Table 16-4. They are all present in the periphery as well as in the CNS. H$_1$ receptors are G$_q$-coupled and are the site of action of the classical antihistaminic drugs (see Chapter 30). In the CNS, H$_1$ receptors mediate excitatory activity and are abundant in the hypothalamus. First-generation H$_1$ antagonists used to treat allergy and cold symptoms (e.g., diphenhydramine) readily cross the blood–brain barrier (BBB) and cause sedation. Second-generation anti-allergic medications (e.g., loratadine) do not cross the BBB and therefore are free of sedative effects. H$_2$ receptors are G$_s$-coupled and mediate cAMP-dependent activity. They are found in the hippocampus and cortex. In the periphery, activation of H$_2$ receptors increases gastric acid secretion, and selective H$_2$ antagonists are used in the treatment of peptic ulcer (see Chapter 41). H$_3$ receptors are

**FIGURE 16-6** Schematic representation of major cholinergic, serotonergic, and histaminergic pathways in the brain. (A) **Cholinergic:** 1 = local circuit neurons in striatum; 2 = local circuit neurons in nucleus accumbens; BFCC = basal forebrain cholinergic complex; PMT = pontomesencephalotegmental cholinergic complex; OT = olfactory tubercle. (B) **Serotonergic:** RG = rostral group of 5-HT perikarya, including the dorsal and medial raphe nuclei; CG = caudal group, including the nucleus raphe magnus. (C) **Histaminergic:** PH = posterior hypothalamic cell group; RF = reticular formation cell group. For other abbreviations, see Figure 16-5.

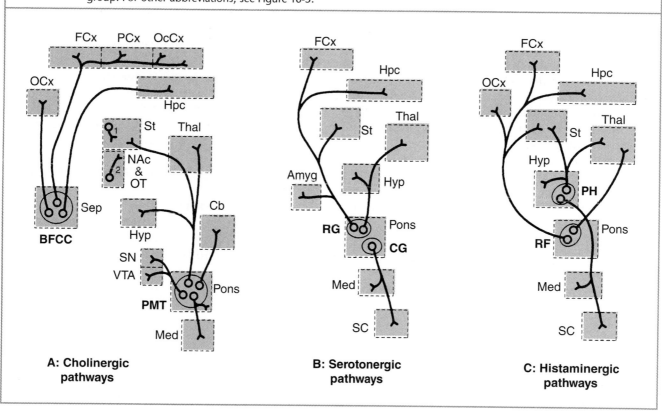

A: Cholinergic pathways

B: Serotonergic pathways

C: Histaminergic pathways

$G_i$-coupled and have the pharmacological profile of inhibitory autoreceptors. They are almost exclusively present in the hypothalamus and regulate the synthesis and release of histamine in histamine-producing neurons.

### Central histaminergic pathways

The two main histaminergic cell groups are located in the brainstem **reticular formation** (RF) and the ventral **posterior hypothalamus** (PH; see Fig. 16-5). The hypothalamus is the CNS region with the highest concentrations of histamine and histamine receptors, because many of the PH histaminergic neurons are local interneurons. **Ascending projection fibres** from both the RF and PH join the **medial forebrain bundle** and diffusely innervate the cerebral cortex, hippocampus, basal ganglia, olfactory tubercle, and thalamus. The PH group also sends **descending fibres** to the brainstem and spinal cord (Fig. 16-6C).

Functionally, the central histaminergic system has been implicated in the mechanisms of arousal (RF-mediated) and regulation of food and water intake (PH-mediated). These central actions have long been suspected since it was well known that systemic administration of the older antihistaminic drugs also caused sedation and loss of appetite.

## Catecholamines: Dopamine, Noradrenaline, and Adrenaline

### Synthesis and degradation

The metabolic routes of synthesis and degradation of **dopamine** (DA), **noradrenaline** (NA), and **adrenaline** (A) are the same in the CNS as in the peripheral autonomic system. They are summarized in Figure 16-2 and described in detail in Chapter 13. The production of DA can be increased by the administration of L-dopa, which readily crosses the BBB and thus bypasses the tyrosine hydroxylase reaction.

The catecholamine neurotransmitters are removed from the synaptic cleft by a combination of degradative reactions and high-affinity binding to membrane-bound **transporters** that carry undegraded transmitters back into the cytoplasm. These uptake mechanisms are blocked by various drugs with strong psychoactive properties, such as amphetamine and cocaine (which block the uptake of DA and NA) and by tricyclic and other antidepressants, such as imipramine and citalopram (which block the reuptake of NA and 5-HT, respectively). Recent studies, triggered by the molecular actions of these drugs on the transporter molecules and their possible implication in the pathology of addiction, depression, and parkinsonism, have identified the molecular stucture and mechanisms underlying the action of neurotransmitter transporters. Transporters for DA, NA, and serotonin are $Na^+/Cl^-$-dependent symporters with 12 transmembrane domains. Although they have 60 to 70% homology, their affinities for the different neurotransmitters are quite different. Selective transporters for other neurotransmitters (e.g., GABA and glutamate) have also been identified.

The concentrations of DA and its metabolites homovanillic acid (HVA) and dihydroxyphenylacetic acid (DOPAc) have been used as indicators of the level of central dopaminergic activity. Stimulation of the DA cells, either by electrical stimuli or by pharmacological means (such as chronic administration of antipsychotic drugs), increases the levels of these metabolites in plasma and CSF. Hypoactivity of the DA system, as in parkinsonism, has an opposite effect.

Similarly, concentrations of NA, A, and their metabolites can be measured in the CSF, plasma, and urine and provide useful biochemical information for the diagnosis of neuropsychiatric disorders (e.g., mania and depression) and endocrine disorders (e.g., pheochromocytoma).

## Dopamine receptors

Classically, two types of DA receptors are recognized: $D_1$-like ($D_1$ and $D_5$; they activate adenylyl cyclase) and $D_2$-like ($D_2$, $D_3$, and $D_4$; they inhibit adenylyl cyclase). Molecular biology techniques have so far identified six different subtypes of DA receptors (**$D_1$, $D_{2(short)}$, $D_{2(long)}$, $D_3$, $D_4$, and $D_5$**) that have been pharmacologically characterized. All the known subtypes are members of the G protein–coupled receptor family (see Chapter 8).

DA excitatory activity is mediated by the $D_1$ and $D_5$ subtypes. The $D_5$ receptor subtype has an affinity for DA ten times higher than that of $D_1$, is found only in nervous tissue, and is particularly abundant in limbic structures (such as the olfactory tubercle and ventral striatum, including the nucleus accumbens). The $D_1$ receptor is abundant in the predominantly motor-related dorsal striatum (i.e., the caudate–putamen; see Chapter 17). Smaller numbers of $D_1$ receptors are present in other limbic structures (e.g., amygdala, frontal cortex, and hypothalamus). In the pituitary gland, $D_1$ binding is restricted to the neural lobe. All $D_1$ receptors appear to be located post-synaptically.

The inhibitory activity of DA is mediated by the $D_2$-like receptors. The $D_{2(short)}$ and $D_{2(long)}$ forms have the same pharmacological properties and originate through alternative splicing of the same gene. In the pituitary gland, $D_2$ binding is very dense in the intermediate lobe, light in the anterior lobe, and absent from the neural lobe. $D_2$ receptors predominate in areas where most of the DA-producing cell bodies are located; they are probably newly synthesized receptors awaiting transport to the axon terminals where they will become autoreceptors.

Unlike the $D_2$ receptor, the $D_3$ and $D_4$ receptors are present in very high amounts in limbic but not in motor structures. This is consistent with the fact that atypical neuroleptics such as clozapine, which have a much higher affinity for the $D_3$ and $D_4$ than for the $D_2$ receptors, have a very low incidence of extrapyramidal (i.e., motor) side effects yet retain their antipsychotic properties (see Chapter 24). The $D_3$ receptor subtype is characterized by its high affinity for the DA agonist quinpirol and for DA autoreceptor inhibitors (such as (+)-AJ76). Very recent evidence suggests that $D_4$ receptors are located mainly on GABA-containing interneurons, which they inhibit.

## Central dopaminergic pathways

There are three types of DA-containing neuronal systems in the CNS. **Ultrashort DAergic** interneurons are found in the retina and the olfactory bulb. **Intermediate-length DAergic** neurons in the hypothalamus project to the hypophysis, where they participate in regulation of the secretion of prolactin and other hormones. The third and largest DAergic system is the **ventral mesencephalic system,** with perikarya located in the substantia nigra pars compacta (SNc) and the ventral tegmental area (VTA; see Fig. 16-5).

The ascending fibres originating in the SNc constitute the **nigrostriatal system,** projecting mainly to the dorsal striatum. They are involved in motor coordination. Massive degeneration of the DA neurons of the substantia nigra, with severe depletion of DA, is the primary lesion in Parkinson's disease (see Chapter 17). The **mesolimbic system** includes primarily the DA neurons of the VTA that project to limbic areas such as the ventral striatum (including the nucleus accumbens), septum, olfactory tubercle, amygdala, and frontal cortex (Fig. 16-7A). This system is involved in the neural mechanisms of motivation and reward and is thought to play an important role in drug addiction (see Chapters 69 and 70). Disturbed activity in this system seems to play an important role in the etiology of schizophrenia (see Chapter 24).

## Adrenergic receptors

Adrenergic receptors are divided into two types: α (antagonized by phentolamine) and β (antagonized by propranolol). NA and A act on both types. Six subtypes of α-**adrenergic** ($α_{1A}$, $α_{1B}$, $α_{1C}$, $α_{2A}$, $α_{2B}$, and $α_{2C}$) and three subtypes of β-**adrenergic** ($β_1$, $β_2$, and $β_3$) receptors have been cloned so far. The $α_1$ receptors are located post-synaptically. Stimulation of the $α_{1A}$ receptor activates a calcium channel and causes increased intracellular concentration of $Ca^{2+}$ and excitation of the postsynaptic cell.

**FIGURE 16-7** Schematic representation of major catecholaminergic pathways in the brain. (A) **Dopaminergic:** 1= hypothalamohypophysial system; SNc = substantia nigra, pars compacta; VTA = ventral tegmental area. (B) **Noradrenergic:** LC = locus coeruleus; LT = lateral tegmental group. (C) **Adrenergic:** LR = lateral reticular group; DMR = dorsomedial reticular group. For other abbreviations, see Figure 16-5.

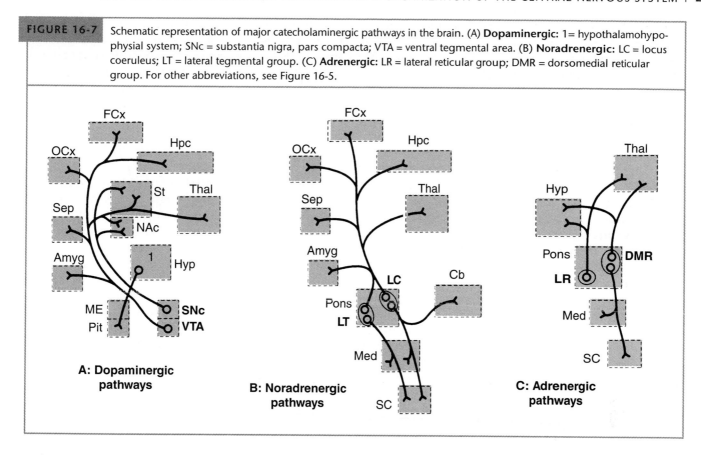

**A: Dopaminergic pathways**

**B: Noradrenergic pathways**

**C: Adrenergic pathways**

The $\alpha_{1B}$ and $\alpha_{1C}$ receptors activate the diacylglycerol/inositol trisphosphate second-messenger system. $\alpha_2$ Receptors are located both pre- and post-synaptically. They inhibit the adenylyl cyclase/cyclic AMP second-messenger system, and stimulation of postsynaptic $\alpha_2$ receptors causes hyperpolarization (i.e., inhibition) of the postsynaptic neuron. Drugs that are agonists at presynaptic $\alpha_2$ receptors (e.g., clonidine) decrease NA turnover in the adrenergic axon terminal, whereas antagonists (e.g., yohimbine) increase the NA turnover.

The $\alpha_1$-adrenoceptors are distributed in the thalamus and neocortex as well as in the dorsal motor nucleus of the vagus nerve (a region involved in blood pressure regulation); the selective $\alpha_1$ antagonist prazosin is an effective centrally acting antihypertensive agent. The $\alpha_2$ receptor concentration is highest in the amygdala, locus coeruleus, and temporal cortex. In the human brain, both $\alpha_1$ and $\alpha_2$ subtypes are also abundant in other cortical areas and the hippocampus and moderately abundant in the basal ganglia and substantia nigra. The $\alpha_{2A}$ type is present in all the regions mentioned above, whereas the $\alpha_{2B}$ type is found only in the basal ganglia.

The $\beta$-adrenergic receptors are members of the G protein–coupled receptor family and share the typical structural properties of this family (see Chapter 8). All three subtypes of $\beta$-adrenergic receptors ($\beta_1$, $\beta_2$, and $\beta_3$) stimulate adenylyl cyclase and cause excitation of the postsyn-

aptic cell. Some of the main features of these receptor types are summarized in Table 16-4. The concentration of $\beta$ receptors in human CNS is highest in the hippocampus and cerebellum, followed by the thalamic nuclei, basal ganglia, and mesencephalon.

The central noradrenergic and adrenergic systems are involved in the regulation of food and water intake. Stimulation of the $\alpha$ receptors induces feeding, while stimulation of the $\beta$ receptors suppresses feeding. Effects opposite to these have been reported in the regulation of water intake. Hypoactivity of noradrenergic and adrenergic systems has also been implicated in the etiology of depression. Chronic treatment with inhibitors of NA and 5-HT uptake, such as desipramine and fluoxetine, respectively, causes alterations in central adrenergic and serotonergic activity that are believed to be responsible for the antidepressant effect of these agents (see Chapter 25).

## Central noradrenergic and adrenergic pathways

*Noradrenergic.* There are two large groups of NA neurons in the CNS (Fig. 16-7B). The **locus coeruleus** (LC) is a large nucleus in the lateral central grey of the pons. The **lateral tegmental group** of NA neurons is diffusely distributed in the caudal brainstem, ventral to the LC. Large-sized NA neurons in both groups have long axons that branch profusely and send widespread innervation to many brain regions. The NAergic ascending projections profusely innervate the brainstem, cerebellum, and most forebrain structures. The descending projections innervate the lower brainstem and the spinal cord.

The NAergic projections have a predominantly inhibitory effect on postsynaptic neurons in the cortex, thalamus, cerebellum, and spinal cord. In the hippocampus, however, the effects of the rich NAergic innervation are more complex, and they vary in different subregions.

*Adrenergic.* Adrenergic neurons are organized into two main groups located in the reticular formation of the brainstem: the **lateral reticular group,** and the **dorsomedial reticular group** (Fig. 16-7C). These groups send ascending projections to the hypothalamus (where they are involved in neuroendocrine regulation), thalamus (pain modulation), dorsal motor nucleus of the vagus nerve and nucleus of the solitary tract (respiratory and cardiovascular control), and locus coeruleus. Descending projections are sent to the central grey matter of the spinal cord. The existence of a rich adrenergic innervation of the locus coeruleus raises the possibility that adrenergic neurons regulate the activity of NA-producing neurons in this region.

## AMINO ACID NEUROTRANSMITTERS

The role of glutamate, aspartate, γ-aminobutyrate, and glycine as neurotransmitters is now well established. However, the amino acid neurotransmitter systems differ from the classical neurotransmitter systems in many respects. Some of the major differences are (1) the high content and ubiquitous distribution of amino acid neurotransmitters in the nervous system, (2) their extensive role in peripheral and central synapses at all phylogenetic levels, and (3) their involvement in multiple metabolic pathways. Glutamate and aspartate are excitatory neurotransmitters, while γ-aminobutyric acid (GABA) and glycine (in most instances) are inhibitory.

## Excitatory Amino Acid Neurotransmitters

### Synthesis and degradation

The amino acids L-**glutamate** and L-**aspartate** are abundant in the adult mammalian CNS. Glutamate does not cross the BBB but is synthesized locally in the CNS, mainly from glutamine but also from a variety of other precursors (see Fig. 16-2).

The calcium-dependent release of aspartate and glutamate into the synaptic cleft is followed by inactivation through the reuptake of the neurotransmitter molecules by a high-affinity sodium-dependent transport system (glutamate transporter), similar to those mediating the reuptake of the catecholamines and serotonin. Aspartate and glutamate share the same reuptake system, located in the terminals of aspartate- and glutamate-producing neurons, as well as in the adjacent glial cells. The glutamate taken up by glial cells is transformed into glutamine by the action of **glutamine synthetase,** which is found only in glial cells. However, the glutamine can diffuse back into glutamate neurons and be reconverted to glutamate by the enzyme glutaminase.

### Excitatory amino acid receptors

The excitatory amino acid receptors have been classified into two main types: the **NMDA** (*N*-methyl-D-aspartate) receptor and the **non-NMDA** receptors, of which there are four subtypes, named for their selective agonists—**kainate, quisqualate/AMPA** (α-amino-3-hydroxy-5-methyl-isoxazole-4-propionic acid), **L-AP4** (L-2-amino-4-phosphonobutyrate, or L-APB), and **ACPD** (1-amino-cyclopentane-1,3-dicarboxylic acid; see Table 16-4). All ionotropic receptors (NMDA, kainate, and AMPA) mediate excitatory effects. The glutamate metabotropic receptors, a family with eight subtypes ($mGluR_{1-8}$), can mediate either excitatory ($mGluR_{1,5}$) or inhibitory effects ($mGluR_{2,3,4,6,7 \text{ and } 8}$).

The **NMDA receptor** is a tetrameric ionotropic receptor linked to a channel that is permeable to monovalent cations and highly permeable to calcium. The NMDA receptor responds rather slowly to glutamate, which is more effective in opening the ion channel when the cell is already depolarized. The increase in intracellular calcium concentration in the postsynaptic cell may lead to the activation of various $Ca^{2+}$-dependent enzymes that mediate the cell responses (e.g., protein kinase C, calcium/calmodulin-dependent protein kinase II, and nitric oxide synthase).

The NMDA receptor complex consists of four different subunits bearing six distinct binding sites of which two are excitatory: (1) the **glutamate binding site** and (2) the **glycine binding site,** both located near the extracellular end of the channel, act as co-agonists to open the channel. (3) The **phencyclidine (PCP) binding site,** located inside the channel; (4) the **voltage-dependent magnesium binding site,** located at the intracellular end of the channel; (5) the **zinc binding site;** and (6) the **polyamine regulatory site** located at the extracellular end of the channel are all inhibitory sites.

**Dizocilpine** (MK-801) and **ketamine** act similarly to phencyclidine as channel blockers. The glycine binding site is selectively blocked by kynurenate and (+)HA-966 and stimulated by D-serine. The NMDA receptor is widely distributed in the CNS, but particularly in the cerebral cortex and hippocampus.

The non-NMDA **kainate** receptor is an ionotropic receptor that regulates a channel permeable to sodium and potassium. This receptor is particularly abundant in the hippocampus.

The **quisqualate/AMPA** receptor also is an ionotropic receptor that regulates sodium and potassium exchange. Its distribution in the CNS is ubiquitous and is similar to that of the NMDA receptor.

L-AP4 binds to the metabotropic presynaptic autoreceptors of the mGluR$_{4,6,7,8}$ types and causes inhibition of the presynaptic neuron.

Finally, the **ACPD** subtype is a metabotropic receptor that activates phospholipase C and the diacylglycerol/inositol trisphosphate second-messenger system.

The excitatory effects of glutamate and structurally related compounds can, if carried beyond physiological limits, give rise to seizure activity and convulsions (see Chapter 18). These substances can also produce neurotoxic effects. For example, kainic acid and ibotenic acid are used experimentally by intracerebral injection to induce selective degeneration and death of neuronal cell bodies at the injection site, while sparing the axons terminating in, or passing through, that area. The neurotoxic effects of glutamate and its analogues are due to prolonged and exacerbated excitation and calcium influx that irreversibly damages the metabolic and functional activity of the neuron. Glycine-binding site blockers, and other NMDA receptor antagonists, are currently being assessed for their therapeutic potential as anti-epileptic agents and as drugs that might prevent ischemic brain damage after stroke or trauma.

Glutamate receptors (especially the NMDA type) are involved in processes of neuronal plasticity, such as long-term potentiation, that are the cellular basis of learning.

## Central pathways containing aspartate and glutamate

These amino acid neurotransmitters are ubiquitously present in the CNS, but glutamate is particularly abundant in certain structures and pathways (Fig. 16-8A). Large populations of glutamate-containing neurons are seen in the **cerebral cortex,** where they provide the major excitatory cortical output, directed heavily to the hippocampus, basal ganglia (caudate–putamen and nucleus accumbens), thalamus, olfactory tubercle, and amygdala.

The **hippocampus** also contains many glutamatergic neurons (pyramidal and granular cells) that project to **limbic structures,** such as the lateral septum and nucleus accumbens. These pathways are thought to be involved in learning.

In the **retina,** glutamate is the major excitatory neurotransmitter and is found in the photoreceptors and bipolar cells.

# Inhibitory Amino Acid Neurotransmitters

## GABA

*Synthesis and degradation.* GABA is the main inhibitory neurotransmitter in the mammalian CNS and is found in concentrations 1000 times higher than those of classical

---

**FIGURE 16-8** Schematic representation of major amino acid neurotransmitter pathways in the brain. (A) **Glutamatergic:** OT = olfactory tubercle. (B) **GABAergic:** 1 = cortical local circuit neurons; 2 = hippocampal local circuit neurons; 3 = cerebellar local circuit neurons; 4 = spinal local circuit neurons; DN = deep nuclei of cerebellum; GP = globus pallidus. (C) **Glycinergic:** RF = reticular formation cell group; RC = Renshaw cells, spinal interneurons. For other abbreviations, see Figure 16-5.

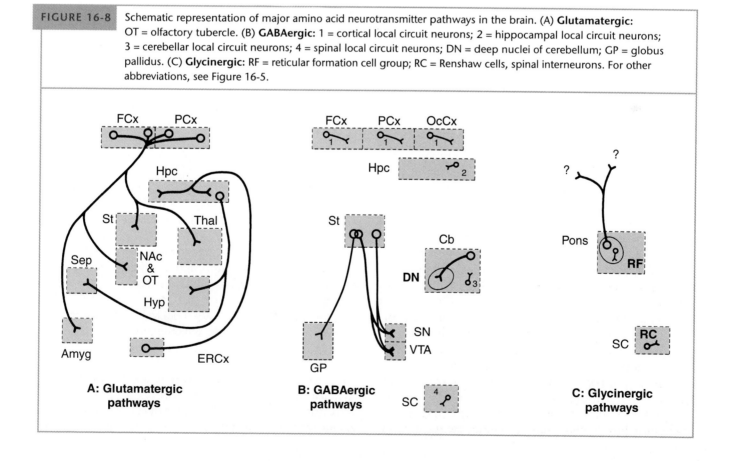

monoamine neurotransmitters. It is synthesized locally by decarboxylation of glutamate (see Fig. 16-2).

After its release into the synaptic cleft, its activity at postsynaptic receptors is terminated through selective reuptake by a glycoprotein, the **GABA transporter,** located in the presynaptic terminals and surrounding glia. To date, four different types of GABA transporters have been cloned. All types are expressed in both neurons and glia. The recaptured transmitter is reused in the nerve terminal or metabolized by GABA transaminase in glial cells. Unlike catecholamine transporters, GABA transporters are also present in postsynaptic cells and are thought to regulate uptake of GABA that is destined to be metabolized.

*GABA receptors.* There are three subtypes of GABA receptors, designated $GABA_A$, $GABA_B$ (see Table 16-4), and $GABA_C$. Both $GABA_A$ and $GABA_C$ receptors are ionotropic receptors. Their stimulation by GABA results in the opening of a chloride channel, influx of $Cl^-$, and hyperpolarization (i.e., inhibition) of the postsynaptic cell. The $GABA_A$ receptor, the most abundant type in the mammalian CNS, is a heteropentamer with five separate binding sites: (1) the **GABA binding site** and (2) the **benzodiazepine binding site** are located at the extracellular end of the channel; (3) the **barbiturate,** (4) the **steroid,** and (5) the **picrotoxinin binding sites** are all located inside the $Cl^-$ channel.

The hyperpolarizing action of GABA exerts an anticonvulsant effect, and specific $GABA_A$ agonists, such as muscimol and tetrahydroxyisoxazolopyridinone (THIP), have anticonvulsant properties, while specific $GABA_A$ antagonists (e.g., bicuculline) produce vigorous convulsions. Binding of benzodiazepines to their selective binding site on the $GABA_A$ receptor facilitates GABA activity by *increasing the frequency* of channel opening. Clinically, benzodiazepines are depressant drugs with anticonvulsant, sedative, and anxiolytic properties (see Chapter 23). Some drugs such as the β-carbolines, which bind to the benzodiazepine binding site but *decrease* GABA activity, are known as **inverse agonists.** It has also been suggested that some of the depressant effects of ethanol may be exerted through the $GABA_A$ receptor, and there is a positive correlation betweeen the potencies of anaesthetic agents and their ability to increase GABA-mediated chloride uptake.

Barbiturates (e.g., phenobarbital and pentobarbital) act by *increasing the opening time* of the chloride channel and are anticonvulsants. Neuroactive steroids, such as alphaxalone, facilitate the binding of agonists to the GABA site and modulate benzodiazepine binding, and in high concentrations they can activate the $GABA_A$ receptor. Picrotoxin and pentylenetetrazol (metrazol) *decrease* the opening time of the $Cl^-$ channel and thus are convulsants.

The **$GABA_B$ receptor** was first identified by its lack of affinity for muscimol and bicuculline and its selective affinity for the agonist baclofen (see Chapter 15) and the antagonist phaclofen. $GABA_B$ receptors are located pre-

synaptically and act through $G_i$ proteins to inhibit cyclic AMP production, open a $K^+$ channel (causing hyperpolarization), and decrease $Ca^{2+}$ influx, thus reducing the presynaptic release of neurotransmitters.

The $GABA_C$ receptor, though it is also an ionotropic receptor, has a pentameric structure different from that of the $GABA_A$ receptor. It is composed of ρ subunits that do not have binding sites for benzodiazepines, barbiturates, steroids, or picrotoxin. It is not blocked by the $GABA_A$ receptor antagonist bicuculline or by the $GABA_B$ antagonist phaclophen or its agonist baclofen. The $GABA_C$ receptor has a higher affinity for GABA than the $GABA_A$ receptor and is more resistant to desensitization. This receptor subtype is highly expressed in the retina and the spinal cord, and current research suggests that different subtypes of this receptor may exist in these two locations.

*Central GABAergic pathways.* Most GABA-containing neurons are inhibitory **local interneurons** located in the retina, cerebral cortex, hippocampus, cerebellum, and spinal cord (Fig. 16-8B). To date, two main inhibitory **GABAergic pathways** have been identified in the CNS: (1) the projections from the **Purkinje cells** to the cerebellar nuclei, and (2) the **striatonigral and striatopallidal pathways,** the descending components of the loop involved in the regulation of motor activity and limbic functions (see Chapters 17 and 69).

### Glycine

*Synthesis and degradation.* Glycine, the smallest amino acid ($CH_2(NH_2)COOH$), is a potent inhibitory neurotransmitter in the mammalian CNS. It is formed from serine by the enzyme **serine hydroxymethyltransferase** (SHMT; see Fig. 16-2). The brain metabolism of glycine is still unclear. After release into the synaptic cleft and binding to the active sites, glycine is removed by a selective reuptake mechanism.

*Glycine receptors.* The glycine receptor, like the $GABA_A$ receptor, is an ionotropic receptor linked to a $Cl^-$ channel in the postsynaptic membrane. It is selectively blocked by the natural alkaloid strychnine and by the synthetic compound RU 5135. Several other amino acids (serine, proline, taurine, and β-alanine) activate the glycine receptor (see Table 16-4). This receptor is distinct from the accessory glycine binding site on the NMDA receptor, which is excitatory in effect and is not blocked by strychnine.

Two different types of selective glycine transporters have been identified (GLYCT-1 and GLYCT-2). Although the two transporters have similar pharmacological profiles, they are expressed in different cellular populations. Whereas the GLYCT-1 is expressed in neurons and glia alike, the GLYT-2 is only expressed in the soma and presynaptic terminal of glycine-containing neurons. It is likely that GLYCT-1 plays an inhibitory modulatory role on NMDA receptor activity.

*Central glycinergic pathways.* The neuroanatomical distribution of glycine in the mammalian CNS is rather restricted (see Fig. 16-8C). In the **ventral spinal cord,** glycine is found in interneurons (Renshaw cells) that exert an inhibitory action on the motor neurons; this action is blocked by strychnine. At supraspinal levels, glycine is found in only a few structures, including the **brainstem, reticular formation,** and **amacrine cells of the retina.**

# NEUROPEPTIDES

In recent years, more than 50 neuropeptides have been identified in the mammalian CNS. An exhaustive presentation of the different peptides is beyond the scope of this chapter. Those for which physiological roles have been best established are the opioid peptides, vasopressin, oxytocin, cholecystokinin, and angiotensin.

## Opioid Peptides

Three different groups or families of opioid peptides are found in the CNS, originating from three different precursors encoded by three different genes. These precursors are **proopiomelanocortin** (POMC, with 267 amino acids), **proenkephalin** (Pro-Enk, 267 amino acids), and **prodynorphin** (Pro-Dyn, 256 amino acids). Pronociceptin/proorphanin (Pro-N/OFQ) is the precursor for a different but related neuropeptide, nociceptin/orphanin Q.

The fragments derived from POMC include the non-opioid peptides α-, β-, and γ-melanocyte-stimulating hormone (MSH) and adrenocorticotropic hormone (ACTH), as well as β-lipoptropin (β-LPH, 91 amino acids). β-LPH is the immediate precursor of the opioid fragments β-endorphin (31 amino acids), γ-endorphin (17 amino acids), and α-endorphin (16 amino acids; see also Chapters 19 and 48). Most neurons expressing POMC-derived peptides, and β-endorphin in particular, are located in the **arcuate nucleus** of the hypothalamus, intermediate and anterior lobes of the **pituitary,** and nucleus of the solitary tract.

The most important opioid fragments derived from Pro-Enk are the pentapeptides methionine-enkephalin (Met-Enk) and leucine-enkephalin (Leu-Enk). Each molecule of Pro-Enk contains six copies of Met-Enk and one copy of Leu-Enk. A heptapeptide, an octapeptide, and two larger fragments (peptide E and peptide F) are also derived from Pro-Enk. The smaller fragments Met-Enk and Leu-Enk are more abundant in nervous tissue, while the larger fragments predominate in the adrenal medulla. Enkephalins are present in interneurons, as well as in projection neurons. A large population of Enk-producing neurons in the striatum sends projections to the globus pallidus, the brain

area with the highest concentration of enkephalins. Enkephalinergic neurons are also present in the hypothalamus, ventral mesencephalon, pons, and cerebellum.

Pro-Dyn contains three copies of Leu-Enk. C-terminal extensions of Leu-Enk form the four peptide fragments α- and β-neoendorphin, dynorphin A, and dynorphin B. The general distribution of Pro-Dyn–derived peptides in the brain overlaps with the distribution of enkephalins. Additionally, high concentrations of dynorphins are also present in the amygdala, septum, and spinal cord (Fig. 16-9).

Pro-N/OFQ is a precursor that encodes three different peptides: nocistatin (110-127 sequence), orphanin-1 (130-146), and orphanin-2 (149-165). These peptides have behavioural and pharmacological profiles distinct from those of the three classes of opioid peptides. They do not bind to opioid receptors and are not blocked by opioid antagonists.

The peptides derived from POMC and Pro-Dyn bind selectively to the three major groups of opioid receptors, μ, δ, and κ (see Table 16-4 and Chapter 19), all of which are metabotropic receptors linked to ion channels via the adenylyl cyclase/cyclic AMP second-messenger system. Binding of opioid peptides to these receptors inhibits adenylyl cyclase activity via an inhibitory G protein. Ultimately, activation of the μ and δ receptors results in opening of a K+ channel, while binding to the κ receptor leads to the closing of a Ca2+ channel, and both actions have

**FIGURE 16-9** Schematic representation of major opioid peptidergic pathways in the brain. CG = central grey. For other abbreviations, see Figure 16-5. In this diagram, St also includes the NAc.

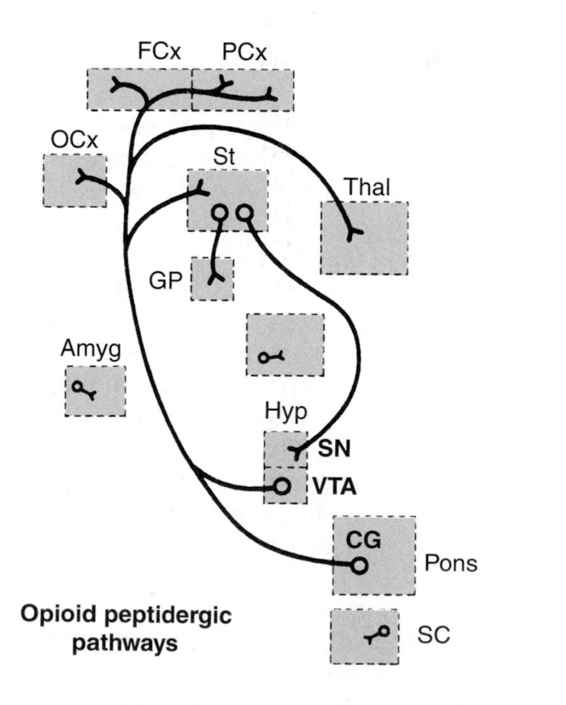

Opioid peptidergic pathways

inhibitory effects on the neuron. The endogenous opioids have different receptor affinities: β-endorphin binds to the μ receptor, the enkephalins have higher affinity for the δ receptor, and dynorphin binds selectively to the κ receptor.

The μ receptor subtype is most abundant in the cerebral cortex, hippocampus, and various sites in the thalamus, hypothalamus, brainstem, and dorsal horn of the spinal cord. This distribution of μ receptors is consistent with their involvement in pain regulation and sensorimotor integration. The δ-opioid receptors are particularly concentrated in the olfactory system, neocortex, and various limbic structures, where they may play an important role in olfaction, motor integration, reward (see Chapter 69), and cognitive functions. Finally, the κ receptors are very abundant in the caudate–putamen, various limbic and hypothalamic sites, and the neural lobe of the pituitary, where they have been implicated in the regulation of food intake and water balance, pain perception, and neuroendocrine function.

## Vasopressin and Oxytocin

The octapeptides arginine vasopressin (AVP) and oxytocin originate from large peptide precursors, the neurophysins, that are normally synthesized in separate populations of hypothalamic neurons located in the supraoptic (SON), paraventricular (PVN), and suprachiasmatic (SChN) nuclei of the hypothalamus (Fig. 16-10). Large axons from the SON and PVN travel through the median eminence and terminate near blood vessels in the neurohypophysis, where the AVP and oxytocin are released into the bloodstream to be carried to their peripheral targets. Other small-sized AVP- and oxytocin-producing neurons send axonal projections to other regions of the CNS. AVP-containing projections are scarce in the cerebral cortex but are abundant in the mediodorsal thalamus and limbic system (including limbic-related cortical areas, septum, and parts of the amygdala). Caudal projections are also present in the brainstem and dorsal horn of the spinal cord. In general, oxytocin-containing fibres have a fairly similar distribution. In the spinal cord, many oxytocin fibres are found in the dorsal horn and central gray.

To date, two different types of vasopressin receptors have been identified: $V_1$ and $V_2$ (see Table 16-4). Both types are metabotropic and G protein–linked. $V_1$ activation leads to cell stimulation via the inositol trisphosphate ($IP_3$) second-messenger system. In the CNS, AVP binding sites are most abundant in the extrahypothalamic limbic structures (septum, amygdala, and ventral hippocampus), but they are also numerous in the hypothalamus, pons, and medulla. The central AVP system has been implicated in mechanisms of learning and memory, including long-term potentiation.

Oxytocin binding occurs predominantly in various limbic structures and ventral hippocampus. The functional role of oxytocin as a central neurotransmitter is still not clear, but recent studies have suggested that it might play an important role in the initiation of maternal behaviours and in the etiology of obsessive–compulsive disorder and related behaviours.

## Cholecystokinin

Pharmacological, behavioural, and neuroanatomical studies have shown that the octapeptide cholecystokinin (CCK) is synthesized in the CNS and acts as a neurotransmitter. CCK-producing neurons have been identified in limbic cortical areas, hypothalamus, amygdala, and ventral mesencephalon (Fig. 16-10C) and are particularly numerous in the nucleus accumbens and median eminence. CCK is co-localized with dopamine and neurotensin in the substantia nigra and ventral tegmental area, and with oxytocin in the paraventricular and supraoptic hypothalamic nuclei.

Two types of CCK receptors ($CCK_A$ and $CCK_B$) have so far been identified (see Table 16-4). Both types are found in many parts of the CNS. Abundant $CCK_A$ and $CCK_B$ receptors are found together, and may have opposing actions, in the caudate–putamen, nucleus accumbens, and ventral mesencephalon. For example, in the nucleus accumbens, stimulation of the $CCK_A$ receptor facilitates the release of dopamine, while stimulation of the $CCK_B$-receptor inhibits it. The central CCKergic system appears to be involved in the regulation of food intake and in the etiology of anxiety.

## Angiotensin

The octapeptide **angiotensin II** (AII) is well known for its effects on water intake and blood pressure. Its metabolism and physiological role in the periphery are described in Chapters 29 and 34. In the brain, AII is produced in neurons that are able to synthesize all the required substrates and enzymes. The larger precursor, **angiotensinogen** (14 amino acids), is converted to the immediate precursor, the decapeptide **angiotensin I**. This is converted to AII by cleavage of the last two amino acids of the carboxylic terminal by **angiotensin-converting enzyme** (ACE). In the diencephalon, the AII-producing neurons are located in the subfornical organ and in the PVN, SON, and SChN of the hypothalamus (Fig. 16-10D). AII-containing perikarya are also found in various sites in the thalamus and brainstem, while angiotensinergic innervation is abundant in limbic forebrain regions and median eminence. In the hypothalamus, AII is co-localized with vasopressin (but not with oxytocin), dynorphin, Leu-Enk, and CCK.

The brain renin–angiotensin system, which is separate from that of the periphery, is involved in the regulation of water and electrolyte balance and neuroendocrine control (stimulation of prolactin, ACTH, and luteinizing hormone release).

**FIGURE 16-10** Schematic representation of other peptidergic pathways in the brain. (A) **Vasopressin:** Hypothalamic nuclei containing vasopressin-synthesizing cells. SON = supraoptic nucleus; PVN = paraventricular nucleus; SChN = suprachiasmatic nucleus; DR = dorsal raphe; NST = nucleus of solitary tract. (B) **Oxytocin:** SON and PVN as above. (C) **Cholecystokinin.** (D) **Angiotensin II:** PVN, SON, SChN, and NST as above; SFO = subfornical organ. For other abbreviations, see Figure 16-5.

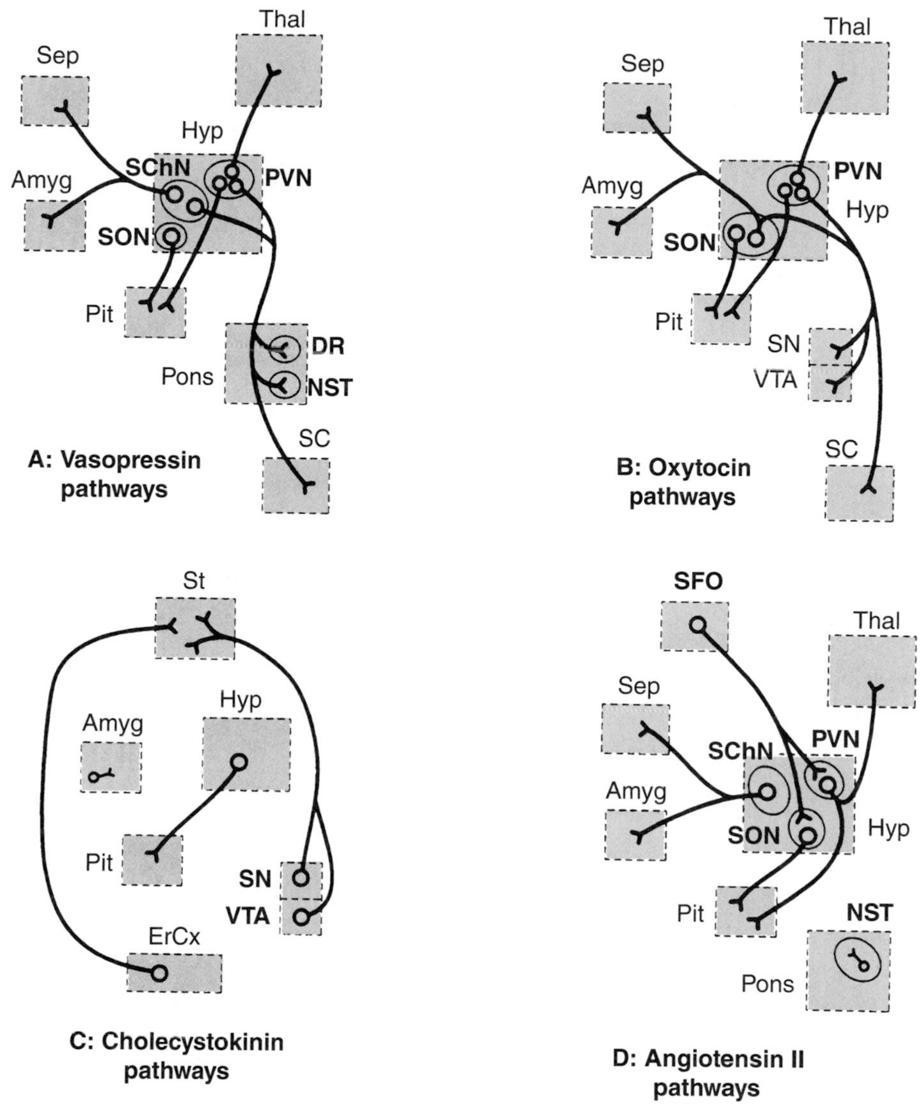

There are two types of AII receptors (see Table 16-4). The AII$_\alpha$ subtype predominates in the areas involved in regulation of water intake and cardiovascular and endocrine function. The AII$_\beta$ receptor is abundant in areas involved in the modulation of sensory input.

# SUGGESTED READINGS

Aghajanian GK, Sanders-Bush E. Serotonin. In: Davis KL, Charney D, Cole JT, Nemeroff C, eds. *Neuropsychopharmacology:*

*The Fifth Generation of Progress.* Philadelphia, Pa: Lippincott Williams & Wilkins; 2002:15-34.

Aravanis AM, Pyle JL, Tsien RW. Single synaptic vesicles fusing transiently and successively without loss of identity. *Nature.* 2003;423:643-647.

Borodinsky LN, Root CM, Cronin JA, et al. Activity-dependent homeostatic specification of transmitter expression in embryonic neurons. *Nature.* 2004;429:523-530.

Chiu AT, Herblin WF, McCall DE, et al. Identification of angiotensin II receptor subtypes. *Biochem Biophys Res Commun.* 1989;165:196-203.

Cooper JR, Bloom FE, Roth RH. *The Biochemical Basis of Neuro-pharmacology.* 8th ed. New York, NY: Oxford University Press; 2003.

Davson H, Zloković B, Rakić L, Segal MB. *An Introduction to the Blood-Brain Barrier.* Boca Raton, Fla: CRC Press; 1993.

Gandhi SP, Stevens CF. Three modes of synaptic vesicular recycling revealed by single-vesicle imaging. *Nature.* 2003;423: 607-613.

Goodenough DA, Paul DL. Beyond the gap: functions of unpaired connexon channels. *Nat Rev Mol Cell Biol.* 2003;4:285-295.

Harrington MA, Zhong P, Garlow SJ, Cianarello RD. Molecular biology of serotonin receptors. *J Clin Psychiatry.* 1992;53 (suppl 10):8-27.

Kandel ER, Schwartz JH, Jessell TM. Elementary interactions between neurons: synaptic transmission. In: *Principles of Neural Science.* 4th ed. New York, NY: McGraw-Hill; 2000: 175-309.

Kandel ER, Schwartz JH, Jessell TM. The generation and survival of nerve cells. In: *Principles of Neural Science.* 4th ed. New York, NY: McGraw-Hill; 2000:1041-1063.

Kiernan JA. *Barr's The Human Nervous System: An Anatomical Viewpoint.* 8th ed. Baltimore, Md: Lippincott Williams & Wilkins; 2005.

Kiss JP, Vizi ES. Nitric oxide: a novel link between synaptic and nonsynaptic transmission. *Trends Neurosci.* 2003;24:211-215.

Lança AJ, Adamson KL, Coen KM, et al. The pedunculopontine tegmental nucleus and the role of cholinergic neurons in nicotine self-administration in the rat: A correlative neuroanatomical and behavioural study. *Neuroscience.* 2000;96: 735-742.

Levitan IB, Kaczmarek LK. *The Neuron. Cell and Molecular Biology.* 3rd ed. New York, NY: Oxford University Press; 2002.

Lodish H, Berk A, Matsudaira P, et al. Cytoskeleton I: microfilaments and intermediate filaments. In: *Molecular Cell Biology.* 5th ed. New York, NY: WH Freeman & Company; 2004: 779-816.

Lodish H, Berk A, Matsudaira P, et al. Cytoskeleton II: microtubules. In: *Molecular Cell Biology.* 5th ed. New York, NY: WH Freeman & Company; 2004:817-852.

Merighi A. Costorage and coexistence of neuropeptides in the mammalian CNS. *Progr Neurobiol.* 2002;66:161-190.

Micheva KD, Buchanan JA, Holz RW, Smith SJ. Retrograde regulation of synaptic vesicle endocytosis and recycling. *Nat Neurosci.* 2003;6:925-932.

Mollace V, Nottet HSLM, Clayette P, et al. Oxidative stress and neuroAIDS: triggers, modulators and novel antioxidants. *Trends Neurosci.* 2003;24:411-416.

Sanes DH, Reh DA, Harris WA. *Development of the Nervous System.* San Diego, Calif: Academic Press; 2000.

Siegel GJ, Agranoff BW, Albers RW, et al. *Basic Neurochemistry. Molecular, Cellular and Medical Aspects.* 6th ed. Philadelphia, Pa: Lippincott Williams & Wilkins; 2000.

Spray DC, Dermietzel R. X-Linked dominant Charcot Marie-Tooth disease and other potential gap-junction diseases of the nervous system. *Trends Neurosci.* 1995;18:256-262.

Woodruff GN, Hill DR, Boden P, et al. Functional role of brain CCK receptors. *Neuropeptides.* 1991;19(suppl):45-56.

Zhang D, Pan Z-H, Awobuluyi M, Lipton SA. Structure and function of GABA$_C$ receptors: a comparison of native versus recombinant receptors. *Trends Pharmacol Sci.* 2001;22:121-132.

# 17

# Drugs That Modify Movement Control

## AJ LANÇA

### CASE HISTORY

Mrs. R.J. was 58 years old when she first consulted her family doctor about motor difficulties that she had begun to experience during the preceding year. While at rest, she noticed a tremor in her hands that seemed to disappear during voluntary movements. Her handwriting became jumbled, and it also became progressively more difficult to walk at a normal pace. After examination by her doctor, a diagnosis of Parkinson's disease was made and L-dopa was prescribed. Although the hand tremor disappeared and she could move more freely, 2 weeks later she returned because she suffered from persistent nausea and occasional vomiting. An accompanying family member also reported that in the last few days the patient often seemed "confused." She was examined by a neurologist, the dose of L-dopa was drastically reduced, and it was combined with carbidopa. A few days later, she was able to return to work, although she did experience temporary dizziness upon standing from a sitting or lying position. Her situation improved for several months, but then gradually she began to display abnormal involuntary movements (dyskinesia) during the time when the drug was effective and sudden loss of mobility as the effects of the drug wore off ("on/off syndrome"). Administration of carbidopa was suspended, the dose of L-dopa was reduced, and pramipexole was also prescribed. The clinical situation improved and she returned to work. At the age of 63, her previous motor symptoms were again noticeable, and her limbs displayed an increased resistance to movement and a typical "cogwheel" rigidity. Her face became less expressive, her speech became slurred and monotonous, and she also began to complain of gradually deteriorating memory. She then retired and withdrew from professional and public activities.

Disorders of motor control, including Parkinson's disease (PD) and Huntington's disease (HD), belong to a larger group of neurodegenerative disorders. These processes are characterized by progressive and irreversible loss of neurons in selective and functionally related brain regions. In PD and HD, loss of neurons in the basal ganglia results in motor disorders, whereas in Alzheimer's disease, neuronal loss in the hippocampus and cerebral cortex account for the loss of memory and cognitive functions. In amyotrophic lateral sclerosis, progressive loss of neurons in different levels of the motor corticospinal (pyramidal) tract, including the cortical and spinal motor neurons, causes muscle weakness and paralysis.

While the exact function of the basal ganglia is not yet clear, pathology of these structures is known to alter motor functions. In some cases, voluntary movement slows or stops, in progressively greater degrees of impairment called bradykinesia, hypokinesia, and akinesia, and the individual freezes into immobility. In other cases, seemingly voluntary-type movements begin to occur even when they are not wanted (dyskinesia, hyperkinesia). However, in both cases, reflex function remains normal.

The pharmacological treatment of PD and HD is aimed at re-establishing the functional balance of neurotransmitters in the basal ganglia. These therapies are limited to the treatment of symptoms and, unfortunately, do not halt the progression of the underlying degenerative processes.

## BASAL GANGLIA

### Neuroanatomical and Functional Organization

The **basal ganglia** and related structures are involved in the initiation and control of movement. Anatomically, the basal ganglia consist of two subcortical forebrain nuclei, the **striatum (caudate–putamen)** and the **globus pallidus** (pallidum), and two nuclei located in the brainstem, the **substantia nigra** (pars compacta and pars reticulata) and the **subthalamic nucleus** (Figs. 17-1 and 17-2). These nuclei neither project to nor receive direct connections from the spinal cord and are not considered part of the motor corticospinal or pyramidal system. However, through abundant reciprocal connections with the cortex, thalamus, and brainstem, the basal ganglia exert a crucial role in the initiation, control, and modulation of motility and are part of the **extrapyramidal system** involved in regulation of muscle tone and posture.

In humans, the **dorsal striatum** is divided into caudate and putamen, which are separated by a bundle of axonal projections (internal capsule) that connects the cortex and the thalamus. In lower mammals, the internal capsule forms discrete bundles that run through the striatum and do not separate the caudate from the putamen.

The striatum receives a profuse innervation from the cortex, thalamus, and substantia nigra (Fig. 17-3), although other brain regions including the hippocampus, amygdala, and the raphe nuclei (the source of the serotonergic input) also innervate the caudate–putamen.

Many cortical regions, including the motor, somatosensory, and limbic areas, send excitatory glutamatergic projections to innervate the striatum in a topographical manner. The striatum also receives a glutamatergic innervation from the thalamus, mainly from the midline and intralaminar nuclei. The rich dopaminergic input of the striatum originates in the substantia nigra and adjacent ventral tegmental area (see Fig. 17-3). Dopamine exerts an excitatory or inhibitory effect in the striatum, mediated through the dopamine $D_1$ and $D_2$ receptors, respectively.

Functionally, the dorsal striatum is involved in motor functions, while the ventral striatum (nucleus accumbens) is part of the limbic system involved in reward and reinforcement (see Chapter 69), and is known to be a pri-

mary target for addictive drugs (e.g., cocaine and amphetamine). The striatum projects to the globus pallidus and substantia nigra, and **all striatal projections are GABAergic** (see Fig. 17-3).

The external segment of the **pallidum** is closely associated with the subthalamic nucleus, whereas the internal segment of the pallidum is associated with the pars reticulata of the substantia nigra (see next paragraph). **All pallidal projection neurons are GABAergic.** The globus pallidus also projects to areas in the thalamus (VA and VL in Fig. 17-3). These thalamic nuclei project back to the cortex, including the frontal and, especially, the motor areas.

The **substantia nigra** (SN) is a nucleus of dopamine-producing neurons located in the ventral midbrain. These neurons contain melanin, a dark pigment chemically related to catecholamines and their metabolites, which accounts for the name of the nucleus (Latin *nigra* = black). The neuronal cell bodies are clustered in the most dorsal portion of the nucleus (SN pars compacta), and their dendrites branch profusely in the most ventral portion (SN pars reticulata), where they receive abundant synaptic inputs. In humans, approximately 200 000 dopaminergic neurons form the pars compacta of the SN, and they are the largest source of striatal dopaminergic input. The medially adjacent **ventral tegmental area** (VTA) also comprises dopaminergic neurons (approximately 150 000). They innervate primarily the ventral striatum, although it is now well established that they also contribute to the dopaminergic innervation of the dorsal striatum. In PD, 70 to 80% of the dopaminergic neurons of the SN are lost, and the concentration of dopamine in the striatum is decreased to the same extent.

The **subthalamic nucleus** is situated between the internal segment of the pallidus and the substantia nigra, located

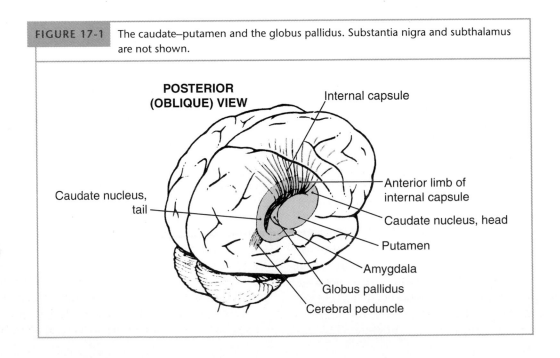

**FIGURE 17-1** The caudate–putamen and the globus pallidus. Substantia nigra and subthalamus are not shown.

**FIGURE 17-2** Coronal section of the human brain showing the basal ganglia and neighbouring structures. (Modified from Kandel ER, Schwartz JH, and Jessell TM, *Principles of Neural Science*. 4th ed. New York: McGraw-Hill; 2000:855, with permission.)

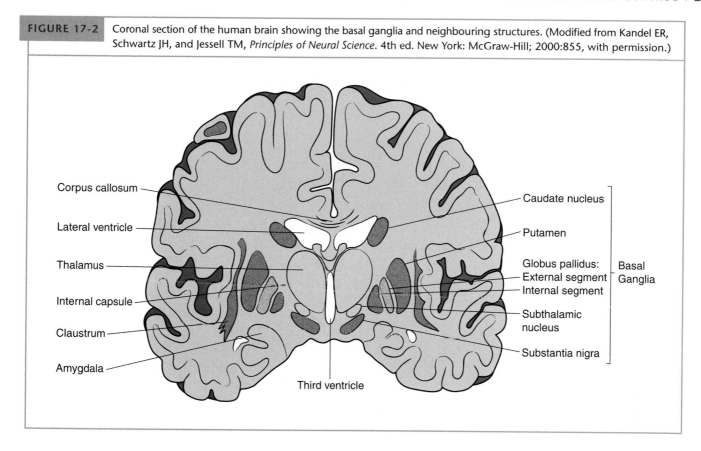

ventrally. It is a more prominent structure in primates than in rodents, and its glutamatergic neurons form the only excitatory projection of the basal ganglia. This neurochemical property is particularly relevant from a physiological and pathological viewpoint (see next section below).

## Neurochemical Organization and Compartmentation of the Striatum

Classically, the striatum was considered a homogeneous structure because it lacks a distinctive visible organization, such as the different layers observed in the cerebral cortex. Histological studies revealed that 90 to 95% of the striatal neurons are medium-spiny and use γ-aminobutyric acid (GABA) as their neurotransmitter. They comprise the output connections of the striatum. Striatal **interneurons** are either large cholinergic non-spiny neurons (1%) or smaller neurons (4%) containing somatostatin, neuropeptide Y, nitric oxide synthase, or parvalbumin. They synapse with GABAergic projection neurons and therefore modulate the striatal output.

Chemical, anatomical, and functional studies revealed that the striatum is further organized into two different compartments characterized by different neuroanatomical connections and differential expression of neurotransmitters and receptors (Fig. 17-4). The two striatal compartments were first identified by the heterogeneous distribution of opioid μ receptors and acetylcholinesterase (AChase).

Whereas small islands (**striosomes**, or **patches**), which cover approximately 15% of the striatum, were rich in μ receptors but poor in AChase, the remaining 85% (**matrix**) was μ receptor-poor but rich in AChase. While the significance of the difference in μ receptors and AChase is not fully understood, this compartmental organization is extremely important with respect to the two output pathways of the striatum.

Thus, neurons in the striosomal compartment form the **direct pathway,** which projects to the internal pallidus and substantia nigra pars compacta (see Fig. 17-4). These GABAergic projection neurons also contain dynorphin and substance P. Striosomal neurons express high levels of dopamine $D_1$ receptors that, when activated by dopamine or dopamine agonists, activate the cell. Striosomes receive limbic input from the cortex. **Stimulation of the $D_1$-mediated direct pathway facilitates movement.**

The matrix compartment forms the **indirect pathway,** which projects to the external pallidum, which in turn projects to the subthalamic nucleus that sends glutamatergic projections to the substantia nigra pars reticulata (see Fig. 17-4). The GABAergic neurons of the matrix are also rich in enkephalins and dopamine $D_2$ receptors. The matrix receives cortical input that originates primarily in the sensorimotor cortex. **Stimulation of the $D_2$-mediated indirect pathway inhibits movement.**

Although several neurotransmitters are present in the striatum, the balance between acetylcholine and dopamine

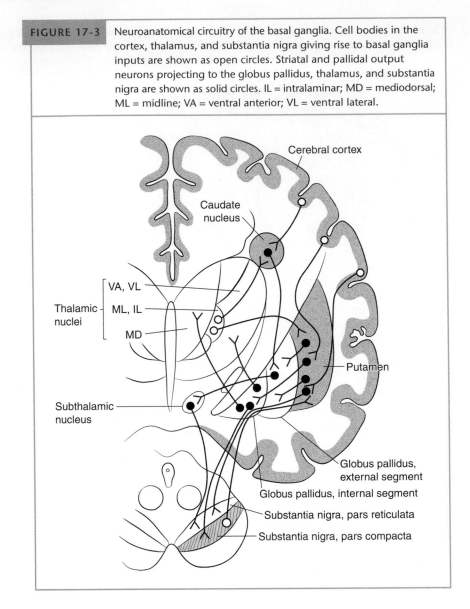

**FIGURE 17-3** Neuroanatomical circuitry of the basal ganglia. Cell bodies in the cortex, thalamus, and substantia nigra giving rise to basal ganglia inputs are shown as open circles. Striatal and pallidal output neurons projecting to the globus pallidus, thalamus, and substantia nigra are shown as solid circles. IL = intralaminar; MD = mediodorsal; ML = midline; VA = ventral anterior; VL = ventral lateral.

plays a central role in the physiology and pathology of the basal ganglia. In terms of the behavioural outcome, dopamine seems to facilitate movement, while acetylcholine inhibits it.

Accordingly, an extensive loss of dopaminergic input from the nigrostriatal pathway, involved in PD, results in decreased or abolished movement (bradykinesia and akinesia). This has also been linked with decreased activity of the direct pathway, which results in a relative overactivity of the $D_2$-mediated indirect pathway and inhibits movement.

Loss of striatal cholinergic neurons, as in HD, creates an imbalance in favour of dopamine influence on the GABAergic neurons of the matrix and results in excessive motor activity, therefore facilitating the occurrence of involuntary movement (e.g., hyperkinesias, chorea).

Although the compartmental organization of the striatum has been crucial for the understanding of its behavioural function, the striatum exerts an integrative role in the modulation of movement. Further understanding of the functional and molecular interactions between the $D_1$ and $D_2$ receptors is necessary for full understanding of striatal physiology and the development of more selective and effective pharmacological tools for the treatment of motor disorders.

# PARKINSON'S DISEASE

## Clinical Syndrome

PD is the most common of the basal ganglia disorders, with a lifetime prevalence of 1 in 400 and an incidence of 1% in the population over the age of 60 years. Clinically, it is characterized by the following: (1) tremor at rest (shaking, which ceases when the affected limb is moved, but which returns when the movement comes to an end);

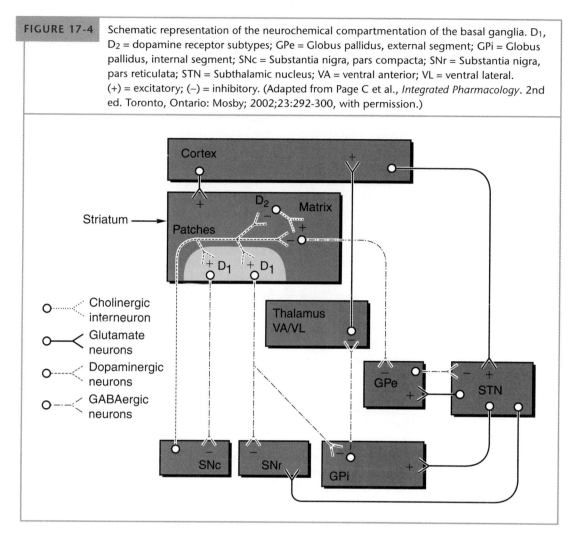

**FIGURE 17-4**  Schematic representation of the neurochemical compartmentation of the basal ganglia. $D_1$, $D_2$ = dopamine receptor subtypes; GPe = Globus pallidus, external segment; GPi = Globus pallidus, internal segment; SNc = Substantia nigra, pars compacta; SNr = Substantia nigra, pars reticulata; STN = Subthalamic nucleus; VA = ventral anterior; VL = ventral lateral. (+) = excitatory; (–) = inhibitory. (Adapted from Page C et al., *Integrated Pharmacology*. 2nd ed. Toronto, Ontario: Mosby; 2002;23:292-300, with permission.)

(2) bradykinesia and akinesia (slowness or inability to initiate voluntary movements); (3) rigidity (stiffness and typical "cogwheel" rigidity of skeletal muscles); and (4) postural abnormalities (stooped posture and mask-like face). Although these motor abnormalities are prevalent in PD, in later stages the disease is also characterized by mood disorders (depression) and cognitive impairments initially manifesting as slow processing of information but that may progress to different degrees of dementia.

## Neuropathology

A number of abnormalities are found in parkinsonian brains. PD is caused by an extensive degeneration of dopaminergic neurons in the SN. Clinical symptoms are observed after massive loss of 70 to 80% of these dopamine-producing neurons. In most cases, the cause of neuronal degeneration in PD is not known (i.e., idiopathic), but it can be caused by exposure to certain chemicals (see below) and post-stroke degeneration. Some cases of PD are associated with genetic disorders, such as the autosomal recessive juvenile PD that causes abnormal expression of specific proteins (e.g., parkin) and intracellular accumulation in degenerating dopaminergic neurons.

Since these dopaminergic neurons of the nigrostriatal system release dopamine from axon terminals in the caudate–putamen, their loss causes a secondary biochemical change: a reduction of dopamine content in the caudate–putamen, eventually to 10% or less of normal. This results in a dopamine/ACh imbalance, which is the actual cause of the parkinsonian syndrome. Since ACh predominates, immobility results. The lack of clinical manifestations during the initial stages of the disease has been attributed to compensatory mechanisms involving the remaining dopaminergic neurons of the SN. Compensatory mechanisms may also involve other neurotransmitter systems of the basal ganglia that result in a compensatory balance between the dopaminergic and other systems (e.g., GABAergic).

Manipulations of the dopaminergic nigrostriatal system further supported its role in the etiology of extrapyramidal motor disorders. A drug-induced parkinsonian syndrome occurs frequently as a reversible side effect of the antipsychotic drugs, which block dopamine $D_2$ receptors (see Chapter 24). Administration of drugs that selectively destroy this dopaminergic system, such as 1-methyl-4-phenyl-1,2,3,6-tetrahydropyridine (MPTP), 6-hydroxy-dopamine, and rotenone, has been used to further elucidate the cellular and molecular mechanisms underlying PD. A permanent and irreversible parkinsonian syndrome is induced by MPTP, a compound originally discovered as a toxic byproduct of the illicit synthesis of meperidine (a synthetic opioid with heroin-like effects). In the early 1980s, in California, a number of drug addicts were seen in hospital emergency services suffering from a severe PD-like syndrome induced by the self-administration of a batch of meperidine contaminated by MPTP. This serious clinical situation had developed only a few days after the drug was taken, even though it resembled the advanced stages of PD. MPTP acts as a protoxin that is biotransformed in glial cells and non-dopaminergic neurons by monoamine oxidase B to MPDP$^+$, which is subsequently oxidized to 1-methyl-4-phenylpyridinium (MPP$^+$). This highly reactive compound is then released to the extracellular space by a still unknown mechanism. Extracellular MPP$^+$, a polar molecule, does not cross membranes efficiently and requires a carrier to re-enter cells. MPP$^+$ has a high affinity for the plasma membrane transporters of dopamine, noradrenaline, and serotonin (see Chapter 16). Once inside the neuron, MPP$^+$ produces its toxicity by inducing mitochondrial dysfunction, oxidative stress, and autoxidation of dopamine. Both MPDP$^+$ and MPP$^+$ cause an overflow of dopamine from dopaminergic neurons, and the free dopamine undergoes a non-enzymatic oxidation to a quinone–semiquinone derivative and free hydroxyl radicals, which cause peroxidation of membrane lipids. This, in turn, increases membrane permeability to calcium, causing a massive influx of Ca$^{2+}$, a mechanism underlying the excitotoxicity responsible for cell death. Lesions of the SN caused by agents that are selectively toxic to the dopaminergic neurons, such as 6-hydroxydopamine (6-OHDA) and the organic pesticide rotenone, are frequently used to create experimental PD and to help elucidate the cellular and molecular mechanisms underlying parkinsonism.

## Non-drug Therapies

Three surgical approaches are sometimes used in the treatment of PD: (1) surgical lesions of the internal thalamus (thalamotomy) or globus pallidus (pallidotomy), (2) placement of microprobes in the subthalamic nucleus, and (3) cellular transplants.

Lesioning of the thalamus or globus pallidus was first done in the mid-1950s, and it is effective in relieving rigidity and tremor but less effective in controlling hypokinesia. These surgical techniques were then virtually abandoned after introduction of the pharmacological treatment with L-dopa. However, the development of accurate means of in vivo visualization of central nervous system (CNS) structures (e.g., computerized axial tomography [CAT] and mag-

netic resonance imaging [MRI]) has lent a much needed accuracy to surgical procedures and has led to the subsequent resurgence of surgical manipulations.

Recently, high-frequency stimulation of the subthalamic nucleus by surgically implanted stimulatory microprobes has resulted in a dramatic decrease in tremor. This amelioration of symptoms also allows a reduction in the dose of L-dopa and hence a reduction of drug-induced side effects. This procedure is less invasive and traumatic than the previously mentioned lesioning techniques, and it is reversible because the probe can be surgically removed if the clinical benefits are no longer observed.

Finally, transplantation of catecholamine-rich tissue containing dopamine-producing cells (from adrenal gland, fetal mesencephalon, or stem cells) into the striatum has been attempted. Transplants have had some success but remain controversial and are not widely practised. Most patients with PD are treated with drug therapy.

## Drug Therapy

The pharmacological manipulations used in the treatment of PD are aimed at re-establishing the functional balance between dopamine and ACh in the striatum.

### L-Dopa

When it was discovered that PD was associated with decreased dopamine in the caudate–putamen, attempts were made to raise dopamine levels. Dopamine itself does not cross the blood–brain barrier, but its precursor, L-dopa (3,4-dihydroxyphenylalanine; Fig. 17-5), crosses via active transport and is taken up by catecholaminergic neurons. In the presence of excess precursor, the surviving dopamine neurons increase their output of dopamine, and most parkinsonian patients quickly return to normal mobility. L-Dopa is the mainstay of therapy for PD.

*Pharmacokinetics.* L-Dopa is well absorbed from the gastrointestinal tract, although presence of food in the stomach delays absorption, and it reaches maximum plasma levels 1 to 2 hours after an oral dose. Most of the drug is rapidly decarboxylated to dopamine by dopa decarboxylase in the periphery, but a small amount is converted by catechol-O-methyltransferase (COMT) to 3-O-methyl-dopa, which has a longer serum half-life than the original compound. Only 1 to 3% of the administered L-dopa remains unaltered, crosses the blood–brain barrier, and reaches the brain. Other important pharmacokinetic parameters of L-dopa are shown in Table 17-1.

*Limitations of therapy.* While the introduction of L-dopa (Larodopa, Dopar, and others) has greatly improved the status of parkinsonian patients, the drug has major drawbacks. **The relief is symptomatic, and the drug does not replace lost neurons or prevent the progression of the disease.** L-Dopa just allows the surviving cells to work with greater efficiency. Thus, relief lasts only while the compound (which has a short half-life) remains in the blood, so the patient must take L-dopa several times a day. As well, the duration of relief is limited as SN cells continue to die even in the presence of L-dopa. Eventually, due to continued cell loss, L-dopa loses its potency in many patients.

*Side effects.* L-Dopa has serious side effects, many of them related to the fact that it raises dopamine levels in the blood and in brain areas outside the caudate–putamen. In the first few months of therapy, nausea is a problem in about 80% of patients; it is due to the effect of circulating dopamine on the chemoreceptor trigger zone. Cardiac arrhythmias

---

**FIGURE 17-5** Drugs used in the treatment of Parkinson's disease. (See Fig. 55-2 for amantadine hydrochloride.)

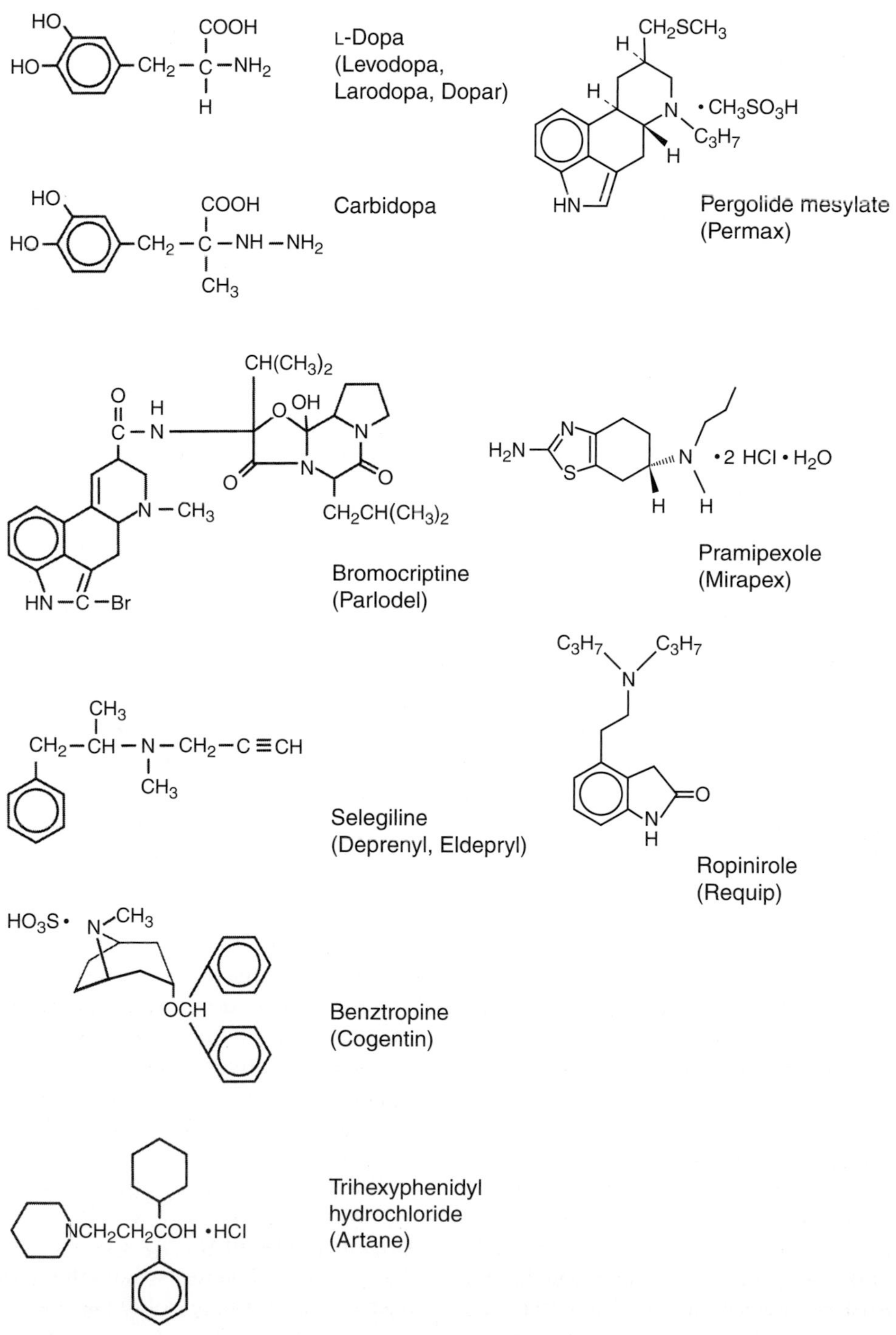

| TABLE 17-1 | Pharmacokinetic Parameters of Drugs Acting on the Basal Ganglia | | | | | |
|---|---|---|---|---|---|---|
| Name | Half-Life (hours) | Oral Bioavailability (%) | Urinary Excretion (%) | Bound in Plasma (%) | Volume of Distribution (L/kg) | Effective Plasma Concentration |
| Amantadine | $16 \pm 3.4$ | 50–100 | 50–90 | 67 | $6.6 \pm 1.5$ | 300 ng/mL |
| Bromocriptine | $7 \pm 5$ | 3–6 | 2 | 93 | $2 \pm 1$ | N/A |
| L-Dopa | $1.4 \pm 0.4$ | $41 \pm 16$ | <1 | unk | $1.7 \pm 0.4$ | $8 \pm 3$ nmol/L |
| Selegiline | $1.9 \pm 0.1$ | negligible | 45 | 94 | 1.9 | N/A |

N/A = not applicable; unk = unknown

appear in about 30% of patients as a result of the effect of circulating dopamine on $\beta_1$-adrenergic receptors in the heart. Orthostatic hypotension is also seen, but the mechanism is unknown. Tolerance to these early effects gradually develops. After 2 to 4 months, however, another set of side effects begins to develop. Paradoxically, these late side effects seem to relate to the development of dopamine hypersensitivity. They consist of hyperkinesias (seen in 80% of patients after 1 year) and psychiatric abnormalities (seen in 15% of patients) such as anxiety, agitation, or psychosis. Tolerance to these late side effects does not develop, although they disappear when L-dopa is discontinued.

## Carbidopa and benserazide

When L-dopa is administered orally, more than 90% of each dose is decarboxylated to dopamine in the periphery, and only 1 to 3% enters the brain. The systemic dopamine circulating in the blood causes side effects but has no therapeutic action since it cannot enter the brain. Carbidopa (see Fig. 17-5) is a peripheral decarboxylase inhibitor that prevents the peripheral conversion of L-dopa to dopamine. Benserazide (available in Canada but not in the United States) has a closely similar action. By increasing the level of L-dopa in the blood, these agents increase the rate of entry of L-dopa into the brain. Neither carbidopa nor benserazide itself enters the brain since these are polar compounds. When carbidopa and L-dopa are given in combination, a much smaller dose of L-dopa is required as approximately 10% of the original dose of L-dopa reaches the brain, and the early peripheral side effects induced by dopamine (nausea, cardiac arrhythmia) are lessened. A combination of carbidopa and L-dopa in a ratio of 1:10 is marketed as a standard commercial preparation (Sinemet). A similar mixture of benserazide and L-dopa in a ratio of 1:4 is marketed in Canada (Prolopa).

*Pharmacokinetics.* Both carbidopa and benserazide are incompletely absorbed from the gastrointestinal tract; their oral bioavailabilities are 40 to 70%. The maximum plasma concentration of carbidopa is reached at 2 to 3 hours after administration, and absorption may be somewhat delayed by food, particularly by dietary protein. The elimination half-life of carbidopa is about 2 hours, and 30% is excreted unchanged in the urine. There are numerous metabolites, all of them pharmacologically inactive. Both carbidopa and benserazide tend to slow the absorption of L-dopa, probably by competing for mucosal transport systems. As a result, they reduce the $C_{max}$ of L-dopa after each dose but prolong its effects and smooth out the plasma peaks and troughs. This mechanism accounts for the reduced fluctuations in the availability of L-dopa in the brain, and it is considered responsible for the regularization of motor activity and decreased occurrence of "on-off" events. Unfortunately, this regulatory effect disappears after long-term treatment.

## Amantadine

Amantadine (Symmetrel; Table 17-1) was originally developed as a synthetic antiviral agent (see Chapter 55). Its usefulness in PD was discovered by chance. Amantadine appears to work by increasing dopamine release from the surviving nigral neurons. Recently, it has been shown that amantadine is an antagonist at the $N$-methyl-D-aspartate (NMDA) glutamatergic receptor. This effect contributes to the re-establishment of a functional balance among the different neurotransmitter systems in the striatum. Amantadine alone is less effective than L-dopa, but it also has fewer side effects. Insomnia and hallucinations may occur, but only at toxic levels. Unfortunately, tolerance to its therapeutic action develops after 6 to 8 months.

*Pharmacokinetics.* Absorption of amantadine from the gastrointestinal tract is essentially complete but slow; maximum plasma levels are reached in 2 to 4 hours after a single dose. It distributes throughout the body, including the brain. The plasma half-life is about 12 to 18 hours but is markedly influenced by the state of renal function because over 90% is eliminated unmetabolized in the urine by a combination of glomerular filtration and tubular secretion. Adverse effects are therefore more common in elderly patients with reduced renal function.

## Dopamine receptor agonists

Recently, a new strategy to enhance dopamine activity has been based on the use of dopamine receptor agonists. A number of these agonists are able to cross the blood–brain barrier and act directly on dopamine receptors (e.g., bromocriptine, pergolide, pramipexole). The advantage of these agents is that, at least in theory, they should be able to act directly on postsynaptic dopamine receptors even if the presynaptic dopamine-releasing neurons have died. Thus, they can be used in all stages of PD, even in advanced cases when there are very few dopamine neurons left. It has also been suggested that these agonists may slow the loss of dopamine neurons by decreasing dopamine turnover and thus reducing the risk of generating oxidative free radicals that can harm the neurons.

In PD, there is a decrease in $D_2$ receptor expression in the striatum, and the balance between $D_1$ and $D_2$ receptors is disrupted. **Bromocriptine** (Parlodel; see Fig. 17-5 and Table 17-1) is a strong $D_2$ agonist and partial $D_1$ antagonist, whereas **pergolide** (Permax; see Fig. 17-5) is an agonist at both receptors. Both drugs are $\alpha_2$-adrenergic receptor antagonists, which accounts for their vasopressor adverse effects. **Pramipexole** (Mirapex; see Fig. 17-5) and **ropinirole** (Requip) are newer non-ergot selective agonists of the $D_2$ receptor with a very high selective affinity for the $D_3$ receptor and no, or very low, affinity for the $D_1$ and the $\alpha_2$ receptor, which accounts for their lower risk of pressor side effects. These drugs are now available for use as an adjunct to L-dopa in the therapy of PD.

The major **side effects** are similar to those of L-dopa, although usually less severe and less frequent. However, a relatively rare but dramatic adverse effect has recently been observed—compulsive gambling with serious financial and social harm to the patient and family. This has been reported most frequently with pramipexole and ropinirole, and it typically begins within a few weeks or months of the start of therapy, occurs even in individuals who have never gambled before, is accompanied in some cases by addictive-like over-eating and sexual appetite, and clears up quickly when the drug treatment is stopped. It has been suggested that the highly selective affinity of these agents for the $D_3$ receptor, which is found in the limbic system, may be related to their special risk of precipitating this aberrant behavioural picture.

### Monoamine oxidase B inhibitors

Another new strategy to raise dopamine levels is to block monoamine oxidase (MAO), the enzyme that breaks down dopamine. Non-specific MAO inhibitors have been used for some time in the treatment of depression (see Chapter 25). However, they must be used with great care because a hypertensive crisis may occur if the patient eats certain foods or takes a drug with pressor effects. Recently, drugs have been developed that specifically block MAO-B, the enzyme responsible for most of the dopamine metabolism in the brain. One of these is **selegiline** (Eldepryl; see Fig. 17-5 and Table 17-1). It is an irreversible inhibitor with a much greater affinity for MAO-B than for MAO-A. Selegi-

line elevates dopamine levels in the brain at doses that do not have the dangerous side effects associated with the traditional MAO inhibitors. It has only a mild therapeutic effect when given alone, but it significantly enhances the effects of L-dopa when the two drugs are given in combination. It has been claimed that selegiline, in addition to its immediate therapeutic effects, may slow the progression of PD, possibly by an antioxidant effect independent of its MAO-inhibitory action. (This is based on the experimental finding that selegiline can block the dopamine cell death caused by MPTP.) To date, however, clinical trials have not provided unambiguous support for this claim.

Selegiline is rapidly absorbed from the gastrointestinal tract and widely distributed into the tissues. The elimination half-life is only about 10 minutes, but the action of selegiline is much longer because it binds irreversibly to MAO-B in the striatum, hippocampus, thalamus, and SN. In the liver, it is biotransformed by the cytochrome P450 system to yield three metabolites: *N*-desmethylselegiline (which is also an irreversible inhibitor of MAO-B) and minor amounts of amphetamine and methamphetamine (which have dopamine-releasing action of their own). Therefore, it is possible that the metabolites contribute to the therapeutic effect of selegiline. The metabolites are excreted mainly in the urine.

### Anticholinergics (muscarinic blockers)

An alternate way to correct the dopamine/ACh imbalance in PD is to lower ACh activity. This can be achieved with muscarinic blockers (see Chapter 12), atropine-like drugs such as benztropine (Cogentin), and trihexyphenidyl (Artane; see Fig. 17-5). Anticholinergic therapy was actually the first pharmacological treatment for PD, having been used (without theoretical basis) for more than a century. The muscarinic blockers, however, are less effective than L-dopa, and they produce unpleasant side effects, including blurred vision, dry mouth, constipation, urinary retention, and ataxia (see Chapter 12). Since the introduction of L-dopa, anticholinergics have been relegated to secondary status because of their modest therapeutic action. However, they may be useful as supplementary agents. Since they work by a different mechanism than L-dopa, combination with L-dopa may increase the maximum therapeutic effect obtained.

## Therapeutic Approaches

The drugs available for PD may be administered in a number of different ways. In each case, L-dopa is the major drug, and the other agents are used as adjuncts. One approach is to start with muscarinic blockers when the syndrome is mild and then add L-dopa and finally carbidopa as the syndrome worsens. Other physicians prefer to use L-dopa from the start. Amantadine may be administered for short periods to help the patient over "flare-ups," and dopamine receptor agonists or selegiline may be used as adjunct therapy. The co-administration of L-dopa and pramipexole is currently seen as a new therapeutic approach, and recent studies suggest that this combination may have a beneficial effect on the irreversible progression of PD.

Whatever the approach, a crucial aspect of therapy is to balance the therapeutic effects of L-dopa against its side effects (e.g., nausea). A good plan is to start with a low initial dose of L-dopa and to increase the level gradually as tolerance develops to the early side effects of the drug.

## Prognosis for Drug Therapy

While impressive results can be achieved in the short term, the long-term prognosis for control of PD is limited. Studies suggest that the average patient obtains relief for up to 5 years and then reverts to pre-treatment conditions because of the continued loss of cells in the SN. Since the disease often occurs late in life, the addition of 5 "good" years may be highly significant. Nevertheless, the present drugs are far from ideal, and the search continues for drugs that not only ameliorate the symptoms of PD, but are also effective is slowing down the neuronal loss.

# HUNTINGTON'S DISEASE (HD)

## Clinical Syndrome

HD, also called Huntington's chorea, occurs with a frequency of 1 in 10 000 people. The predominant symptom is not akinesia but hyperkinesia. The patient makes uncontrolled repetitive and violent movements, which get worse during excitement and cease only during sleep. Since the movements are well coordinated and *appear* to be voluntary, they give a dance-like impression (hence the name *chorea,* Greek for dance). A separate feature is the occurrence of mental symptoms that often appear before the hyperkinesia is observed and range from excess irritability, inappropriate social behaviour and sexual dysfunction, to depression. Cognitive impairments that resemble schizoid psychosis, such as impaired thought processes and difficulty organizing complex tasks, are often present in the later stages of the disease and may progress to outright dementia. Huntington's chorea is an inherited disorder, transmitted by an autosomal dominant gene. Its onset is gradual, occurring in early middle age (age 30 to 50), and after 15 to 20 years of irreversible progression it is invariably fatal.

## Neuropathology

Neuroanatomical examination of the brains of HD patients reveals widespread alterations, including degeneration of the neocortex and caudate–putamen and enlarged ventricular cavities. The caudate–putamen is drastically affected, often being reduced to less than half of its normal mass due to a massive loss of the largest neuronal population of the striatum, the GABA-containing medium-sized projection neurons. Cholinergic interneurons are also reduced in number. These neuropathological changes cause an imbalance in the neurotransmitter systems of the basal ganglia, with severe striatum reductions (over 75%) of GABA and its synthetic enzyme glutamic acid decarboxylase (GAD). The dopaminergic input of the striatum, however, is spared. These processes result in a functional imbalance that favours the role of dopamine, overstimulation of the $D_2$-mediated indirect pathway, consequent hyperactivity that results from the disinhibition of the glutamate projection from the subthalamic nucleus (see Fig. 17-4), and hyperkinesia. Neuronal degeneration is also observed in other brain regions, including the cerebral cortex.

HD is a genetically transmitted dominant autosomal disease caused by an overexpression of the glutamine-encoding trinucleotide sequence CAG in the *IT15* gene on chromosome 4. In normal individuals, there are between 9 and 34 CAG repeats. The number of repeats in HD patients varies from 40 to 100 or more. This mutation results in an abnormally increased expression of the protein *huntingtin,* causing neuronal death. The abnormal CAG repeats in HD patients are expressed not only in neurons but also in peripheral cells, and it is not clear why the striatal neurons are particularly targeted in this disease. Huntingtin interacts with caspases, which are regulatory proteins that participate in excitotoxicity and apoptosis. Recent advances suggest that an increased production of reactive oxygen species and glutamate-mediated neuronal toxicity, as well as reduction in mitochondrial complexes II and IV in the striatum of HD patients, may play an important role in the pathology of HD.

## Drug Therapy

The goal of pharmacological therapy of HD is to restore the functional balance between GABA and the other neurotransmitters in the striatum. Unfortunately, this will not halt the progression of the disease. Four different types of drugs—anxiolytics/hypnotics (barbiturates, benzodiazepines), dopamine antagonists (reserpine, tetrabenazine, phenothiazines, and butyrophenones), GABA agonists (baclofen, muscimol), and cholinergic agonists—have been used.

### Barbiturates

The traditional treatment (without theoretical basis) for Huntington's chorea was barbiturate therapy. This is a symptomatic treatment aimed at keeping the patient quiet and abolishing hyperkinesia. It is now largely abandoned and used only in extreme cases of hyperkinesia.

### Benzodiazepines

Alternatively, benzodiazepines, which enhance the effect of GABA at the GABA$_A$ receptor, have been reported to decrease the choretic movement in a dose-dependent manner, but their long-term therapeutic value is not yet clear.

### Reserpine and tetrabenazine

These indirectly acting drugs (see Chapter 14) deplete dopamine by promoting release and preventing vesicular storage. Their administration has to be closely monitored because their adverse effects include hypotension, depression, and sedation.

### Phenothiazines and butyrophenones

The antipsychotics are dopamine blockers that are usually used in the treatment of schizophrenia (see Chapter 24). More recently, they have also been administered to HD patients on the premise that if ACh is low, dopamine must be predominant. In line with expectations, antipsychotics such as **fluphenazine, bromperidol**, and **clozapine** have proven to be successful at suppressing choretic movements, and neuroleptic therapy is now standard. Unfortunately, these agents do nothing to relieve the dementia that accompanies the chorea. This dementia is believed to result from neuronal degeneration in structures other than the basal ganglia, including the cerebral cortex.

### Baclofen and Muscimol

These drugs are administered to try to increase the activity of the striatal GABAergic system and therefore restore the neurochemical balance disrupted by the loss of medium-spiny neurons in the caudate–putamen. Baclofen is an agonist at the GABA$_B$ metabotropic receptor (see Chapter 16) that is effectively used as a muscle relaxant and spasmolytic in amyotrophic lateral sclerosis, but clinical trials have shown only very limited improvement in HD patients. Muscimol, an agonist at the GABA$_A$ ionotropic receptor, has been used to decrease hyperkinesia and neuroleptic-induced tardive dyskinesia (see Chapter 24), but its therapeutic effectiveness in HD is also limited.

### Acetylcholine agonists

One approach to therapy has been to attempt to raise ACh levels by dietary choline supplements or by use of acetylcholinesterase inhibitors such as physostigmine or neostigmine. So far, the results have been equivocal.

The understanding of the genetic etiology of HD has provided new alternative approaches toward the development of new pharmacological tools aimed at altering the neurotoxic effects of huntingtin. Also, and more importantly, it has shed light on the potential for the repair of the defective gene. Although these developments have not yet provided practical alternatives, there is hope that in the future they will contribute to the possibility of slowing the progression of the disease or preventing its expression before the clinical manifestations occur.

## AMYOTROPHIC LATERAL SCLEROSIS

Amyotrophic lateral sclerosis (ALS, or "Lou Gehrig's disease") is a degenerative disease characterized by progressive wasting and weakness of skeletal muscles that is eventually fatal because of paralysis of the respiratory muscles. Approximately 10% of ALS cases are genetically transmitted in an autosomal dominant pattern, and 20% of these cases are caused by a mutation of the gene for superoxide dismutase (SOD). It has been suggested that increased levels of glutamate, due to decreased reuptake in the synapse, may result in excitotoxic damage to upper and lower motor neurons (i.e., cell death caused by massive calcium influx as a result of excessive action of glutamate at postsynaptic receptors). There is some evidence to suggest that the problem is partly due to defective reuptake of glutamate at presynaptic excitatory terminals. No effective treatment for ALS has been available, but **riluzole**, a drug aimed at decreasing the synaptic availability of glutamate, has recently been approved for this purpose.

Riluzole (2-amino-6-trifluoromethoxybenzothiazole; Rilutek) is believed to inhibit presynaptic release of glutamate. Riluzole also blocks the NMDA and kainate types of glutamate ionotropic receptors and blocks sodium channels. Recent controlled studies have indicated that riluzole produces a dose-dependent prolongation of the mean survival time of patients with this disease, but the effect is of relatively short duration (less than 18 months). However, the drug is well tolerated; the main adverse effects are weakness, dizziness, nausea, and increased serum levels of aminotransferases. Therefore, the drug offers a possibility of some prolongation of life with an acceptably low risk of toxicity. Recently, promising preliminary clinical trials with pramipexole, a dopamine D$_2$ agonist (see "Dopamine receptor agonists" above) that has also been shown to reduce oxidative stress, have shown that it reduced free radical production in patients with ALS.

## SUGGESTED READINGS

Bezard E, Gross CE, Brotchie JM. Presymptomatic compensation in Parkinson's disease is not dopamine mediated. *Trends Neurosci.* 2003;26:215-221.

Borges N. Tolcapone-related liver dysfunction. *Drug Safety.* 2003;26:743-747.

Chiueh CC, Wu R-M, Mohanakumar KP, et al. *In vivo* generation of hydroxyl radicals and MPTP-induced dopaminergic toxicity in the basal ganglia. *Ann NY Acad Sci.* 1994;738:25-36.

Corti O, Hampe C, Darios F, et al. Parkinson's disease: from causes to mechanisms. *C R Biol.* 2005;328:131-142.

DeLong M. The basal ganglia. In: *Principles of Neural Science.* 4th ed. New York, NY: McGraw-Hill; 2000:853-867.

Dodd ML, Klos KJ, Bower JH, et al. Pathological gambling caused by drugs used to treat Parkinson disease. *Arch Neurol.* 2005;62:1-5.

Eriksen JL, Wszolek Z, Petrucelli L. Molecular pathogenesis of Parkinson's disease. *Arch Neurol.* 2005;62:353-357.

Jakel RJ, Maragos WF. Neuronal cell death in Huntington's disease: a potential role for dopamine. *Trends Neurosci.* 2000;23: 239-245.

Juncos JL. Levodopa: pharmacology, pharmacokinetics and pharmacodynamics. *Neurol Clin.* 1992;10:487-509.

Lacomblez L, Bensimon G, Leigh PN, et al. Dose-ranging study of riluzole in amyotrophic lateral sclerosis. Amyotrophic Lateral Sclerosis/Riluzole Study Group II. *Lancet.* 1996;347:1425-1431.

Lewitt PA. Levodopa therapeutics: new treatment strategies. *Neurology.* 1993;43(12 suppl 6):S31-S37.

McMurray CT. Huntington's disease: new hope for therapeutics. *Trends Neurosci.* 2001;24:S32-S38.

Menalled LB, Chesselet M-F. Mouse models of Huntington's disease. *Trends Neurosci.* 2002;23:32-39.

Nestler EJ, Hyman SE, Malenka RC. Control of movement. In: *Molecular Neuropharmacology: A Foundation for Clinical Neuroscience.* New York, NY: McGraw-Hill; 2001:303-326.

Pattee GL, Post GR, Gerber RE, Bennett JP Jr. Reduction of oxidative stress in amyotrophic lateral sclerosis following pramipexole treatment. *Amyotroph Lateral Scler Other Motor Neuron Disord.* 2003;4:90-95.

Perier C, Bové J, Vila M, Przedborsky S. The rotenone model of Parkinson's disease. *Trends Neurosci.* 2003;26:345-346.

Pifl C, Kattinger A, Reither H, Hornykiewicz O. Cellular effects of dopamine—beyond oxidative mechanisms. *Parkinsonism Relat Disord.* 2002;8:433-437.

Poewe W. The role of COMT inhibition in the treatment of Parkinson's disease. *Neurology.* 2004;62(suppl 1):S31-S38.

Przedborsky S, Vila M. MPTP: a review of its mechanisms of neurotoxicity. *Clin Neurosci Res.* 2001;1:407-418.

Storch A, Sabolek M, Milosevic J, et al. Midbrain-derived neural stem cells: from basic science to therapeutic approaches. *Cell Tissue Res.* 2004;318:15-22.

Weiss MD, Weydt P, Carter GT. Current pharmacological management of amyotrophic [corrected] lateral sclerosis and a role for rational polypharmacy. *Expert Opin Pharmacother.* 2004;5:735-746.

# 18

# Anti-seizure Drugs

## WM BURNHAM

### CASE HISTORY

Michael F., an active youngster, was an avid skier and first in his class at a school in rural Manitoba. At age 12, he started to report "visions" and often seemed moody and confused. He began to do poorly in school. A tentative diagnosis of psychosis was made, and he was started on a trial of haloperidol. He began to show tremors and muscular stiffness, and his physician therefore added benztropine to Michael's medication. On this treatment, he became somnolent, non-responsive, and confused, and he was hospitalized for investigation. After 12 days, Michael had a tonic–clonic seizure. His condition was re-diagnosed as complex partial epilepsy, and he was started on carbamazepine. At first, he reacted to this with dizziness and diplopia about 2 hours after each dose. He was therefore changed to a slow-release oral preparation, and these symptoms disappeared. Carbamazepine has prevented further tonic–clonic attacks, but he still experiences occasional complex partial seizures in which he has visual or auditory hallucinations similar to those with which his illness began. He has been able to continue with his schooling but requires careful monitoring of his drug dosage.

# EPILEPSY

## Definitions

**Epilepsy** is a disorder of the central nervous system (CNS) characterized by spontaneous, recurring seizures. It is one of the most common of the CNS disorders, occurring in 1 of every 100 people. Onset is often in childhood, or in old age, although it may occur at any time during life. In many patients, epilepsy is a permanent condition.

**Seizures** are self-sustaining (but self-limiting) episodes of neural hyperactivity. During a seizure, the neurons of the brain cease their normal activities and begin to fire in massive, synchronized bursts. Such synchronized activity produces characteristic "spike" or "spike and wave" patterns in the electroencephalogram (EEG; Fig. 18-1). After a few seconds or minutes, the inhibitory mechanisms of the brain regain control, the seizure stops, and the person returns to normal.

Seizures by themselves do not equal epilepsy. Every brain contains the circuitry necessary to produce seizures, and every brain will do so if subjected to the proper stimuli, such as electric current or convulsant drugs. The essence of epilepsy is a **chronic low seizure threshold**, which leads to the production of **spontaneous attacks**.

## Causes

### Pathology

In 30 to 40% of epilepsy cases, low seizure threshold is associated with some sort of obvious pathology, such as a brain infection, a tumour, or a scar related to a head wound, stroke, or birth injury. These cases are termed "symptomatic" and are more resistant to drug control.

### Genetics

In the other 60 to 70% of cases, there is no obvious pathology in the brain. These cases are termed "idiopathic" and are more responsive to drug therapy. The basic cause of idiopathic epilepsy is assumed to be genetic.

The genetics of idiopathic epilepsy are not yet fully understood. Some types are known to relate to a single mutation, causing, for example, abnormalities in ion channels and GABA receptors. In these "single gene" epilepsies, inheritance follows Mendelian rules. These single gene epilepsies are rare in adults, however. Most idiopathic adult epilepsies seem to relate to the inheritance of several genes. In these multifactorial epilepsies, epilepsy

**FIGURE 18-1** EEG patterns during seizures. (Top) Normal during seizure-free interval. (Middle) 3/sec spike and wave pattern (absence seizure). (Bottom) Poly spike pattern (tonic–clonic seizure).

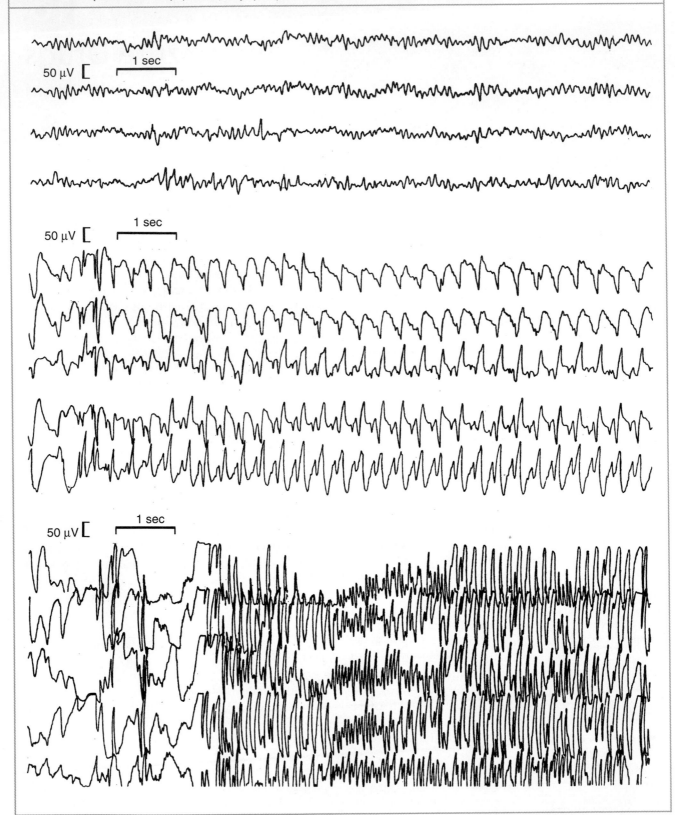

may "run in the family," but inheritance does not follow simple Mendelian rules.

## Seizure Types

There are a number of different types of epileptic seizures. (Because of this, some theorists prefer to talk of "the epilepsies" rather than of "epilepsy.") It is important to distinguish among the seizure types because they respond differently to anti-seizure drugs. The wrong drug may be useless or may even exacerbate a seizure condition.

Four types of seizures commonly seen in adults are described in Table 18-1. The names and characteristics of these seizures should be learned since misdiagnosis of seizure type is one of the most common causes of failure in drug therapy. In particular, mild complex partial seizures tend to be confused with absence attacks.

In addition to the adult seizure types, there are a number of types seen primarily in childhood. Two of these are discussed briefly below, but the others are beyond the scope of this chapter.

## Status Epilepticus

Very long-lasting—or constantly repeating—seizures of any type are called "status epilepticus." This condition is rare, but it is life-threatening when the seizures are of the tonic–clonic variety. Tonic–clonic status epilepticus is a medical emergency that requires immediate treatment in a hospital setting. An ambulance should be called if any tonic–clonic seizure continues for more than 5 minutes.

## Epilepsy Syndromes and Intractable Seizures

In addition to distinguishing different types of seizures, authorities have recently attempted to describe epilepsy syndromes. A "syndrome" is a group of signs or symptoms that occur together as a recognizable entity. An "epilepsy syndrome" will usually include an age of seizure onset (and possibly of offset), a type of seizure (or seizures), a predicted drug response, and possibly other symptoms. Many of the monogenic epilepsies fall into this category.

Seizures are considered to be drug-resistant, or intractable, if they are not under control within 1 year of appropriate therapy. Three epilepsy syndromes are of particular interest to pharmacologists because they involve intractable seizures: West's syndrome, Lennox-Gastaut syndrome, and temporal lobe epilepsy.

**West's syndrome** usually has its onset in the first year of life and its offset a year or two later. It involves generalized myoclonic seizures (infantile spasms), an abnormal

| TABLE 18-1 | Common Seizure Types in Adults* | | |
|---|---|---|---|
| Generalized (appears to involve the whole brain from the outset): | | | |
| Absence (petit mal) | Attack | Brief period of unconsciousness; patient stares blankly, eyelids may flutter; no memory of the period of the attack | |
| | Duration | Less than 30 seconds | |
| | EEG | 3/second spike and wave, whole brain | |
| Tonic–clonic (grand mal) | Attack | Unconsciousness with dramatic tonic–clonic convulsions; may be preceded by an aura;† may involve an "epileptic cry," profuse salivation, tongue-biting, or incontinence; no memory of the period of the attack | |
| | Duration | Less than 5 minutes | |
| | EEG | Constant spiking, whole brain | |
| Partial (at least initially, involves only part of the brain): | | | |
| Simple partial (focal cortical) | Attack | Sensory, motor, perceptual, emotional, or autonomic signs; patient is conscious (will respond to questions); patient will remember the attack | |
| | Duration | Varies | |
| | EEG | Localized spiking in a neocortical or limbic area | |
| Complex partial (psychomotor temporal lobe) | Attack | Patient is out of contact with the environment (will not respond to questions) and may perform automatic movements ("automatisms"); no subsequent memory of the period of the attack; often follows a simple partial attack of temporal-lobe origin (e.g., an olfactory aura, a perceptual aura, [déjà vu, distortion of perspective], or an emotional aura)† | |
| | Duration | Varies | |
| | EEG | Unclear, sometimes spiking in both temporal lobes | |

*Traditional names in parentheses.

†Simple partial seizures may generalize to produce complex partial or tonic–clonic attacks. The simple partial seizure is then called an aura.

EEG between attacks (hypsarrhythmia), and progressive loss of mental function if the seizures cannot be controlled. West's syndrome resists the standard drugs, but it is often responsive to adrenocorticotropic hormone (ACTH) or vigabatrin.

**Lennox-Gastaut syndrome** has its onset in childhood *after* the first year of life. It involves many types of generalized seizures and a progressive loss of mental function if the seizures cannot be stopped. It is often treated with valproate or the benzodiazepines.

West's syndrome and Lennox-Gastaut syndrome are fortunately rare. The syndrome of **temporal lobe epilepsy** is unfortunately very common. The majority of people with complex partial seizures are people with temporal lobe epilepsy. Complex partial seizures are most often treated with carbamazepine, phenytoin, or valproate. These seizures are very drug-resistant, however, and complete seizure control is probably achieved in less than 40% of cases.

## THERAPY FOR EPILEPSY

Most people with seizures are normal between attacks, and seizures themselves are usually brief and relatively harmless. The question arises, "Why treat epilepsy?" The answer is that seizures have an impact on human life that is far out of proportion to their medical significance. Seizures look strange, even frightening, and the public reacts badly to them. People with uncontrolled seizures may face the loss of friends, jobs, and housing. In addition, they are not permitted to drive motor vehicles. Driver's licences are cancelled with the first seizure and reinstated only if the seizures are perfectly controlled for a year. Thus, seizure control becomes a major issue in patients' lives.

## General Principles of Drug Therapy

A large number of drugs suppress seizures (e.g., most hypnotics, sedatives, and anaesthetics). However, a small number of the safest and least toxic drugs are used in the therapy of epilepsy. These are called anti-seizure drugs or, more commonly, anticonvulsants. ("Anticonvulsant" is not an ideal term, since many seizures do not involve convulsions.) Before individual drugs are discussed, a number of general statements can be made about these drugs, their mechanisms of action, and the ways in which they are used.

### Characteristics of anti-seizure drugs

- Anti-seizure drugs do not cure epilepsy; they simply suppress seizures on a temporary basis. Patients must take them once, twice, or three times a day, often for life.

- Anti-seizure drugs are fairly safe, but most of them can cause rare, life-threatening, non-dose-related adverse drug reactions (ADRs), such as liver toxicity or suppression of bone marrow. These rare ADRs, which probably relate to genetic abnormalities in the patient, usually occur within the first few months of therapy. All patients should be closely monitored during this period.

- Most anti-seizure drugs also cause dose-related ADRs, such as stomach upset and/or, at higher doses, sedation. Sedation is a particular problem with the older drugs, which are chemically related to the barbiturates. Thus, the anti-seizure drugs are often perceived as unpleasant to take. Compliance is a problem; abuse is not.

### Mechanisms of anti-seizure drug action

In the past two decades, we have begun to understand the mechanisms of action of the anti-seizure drugs. Three major mechanisms are now proposed:

*Drugs that bind to the voltage-dependent sodium channel.* Several important anti-seizure drugs—including phenytoin and carbamazepine—are believed to bind to the voltage-dependent sodium channel that initiates neuronal action potentials. Each time the neuron fires, the sodium channel cycles through its active, inactive, and resting states. It is believed that these drugs hold the channel a little longer in its inactive state. This means that the neuron can fire at moderate rates (e.g., those involved in normal activity) but not at very rapid rates (those involved in seizures). Newer drugs that bind to voltage-dependent sodium channels include lamotrigine, oxcarbazepine, topiramate, and zonisamide.

*Drugs that enhance activity in the GABA$_A$ system.* A second group of drugs—including the barbiturates and the benzodiazepines—are thought to increase activation in the γ-aminobutyric acid (GABA) system, specifically, GABA$_A$ receptors. This enhances GABA$_A$-mediated Cl⁻ influx, which stabilizes the membrane near its resting potential and results in decreased neuronal excitability (see Chapter 23).

Newer drugs that enhance GABAergic inhibition include tiagabine, topiramate, zonisamide, and (probably) gabapentin. Valproate is also thought to enhance GABAergic inhibition, but by an unknown mechanism.

GABA-enhancing drugs act in several different ways. Topiramate and zonisamide, for instance, are thought to act as agonists at the GABA$_A$ receptor, while the benzodiazepines and phenobarbital bind to the GABA$_A$-related chloride channel and allosterically enhance the effects of GABA. Tiagabine blocks the reuptake of GABA, raising synaptic levels, whereas vigabatrin blocks GABA biotransformation after reuptake, allowing more GABA to be recycled into the vesicles. Gabapentin raises levels of extra-neuronal GABA by an unknown mechanism.

***Drugs that bind to T-type voltage-dependent calcium channels.*** Another group of drugs—including ethosuximide—are thought to bind to T-type voltage-dependent $Ca^{2+}$ channels. These channels are particularly important in the thalamus, where they are thought to contribute to the genesis of absence attacks. Ethosuximide decreases activity in T-type calcium channels. Zonisamide also decreases T-type calcium currents.

As a group, the anti-seizure drugs are relatively weak. With the exception of the benzodiazepines, they work at micromolar blood levels of free drug. At these levels, they tend to attach to several different proteins, and many work by several different mechanisms. The older drugs are effective against either absence seizures or partial and tonic–clonic seizures. Several of the newer drugs, however, are effective against both absence and partial and tonic–clonic seizures. These are termed "broad-spectrum" drugs. It is assumed that they work by **multiple mechanisms**. Among these are lamotrigine, topiramate, and zonisamide. Valproate and the benzodiazepines probably fit into this category as well.

## Principles of clinical therapy

***Whom to treat.*** Before starting therapy, it is important to rule out pseudo-seizures (not uncommon), poisoning, or active pathology. If active pathology is present (e.g., a growing tumour, an infection), it is necessary to treat the pathology, not the seizures. Also, before initiating therapy, it is important to make sure that the seizure problem is chronic. Occasionally, people have a single seizure that is never repeated.

***Choice of drug.*** Before therapy is started, the type of seizure must be carefully established. Different seizure types require different drugs.

***Monotherapy, not polypharmacy.*** Treatment is initiated with a single drug. In most cases, therapy is started at a low dose and is gradually titrated up to normal dose levels. If the first single drug that is tried is not effective, another single drug is tried. Eventually, if the seizures are drug-resistant, polypharmacy is attempted. (Note: The recent advent of new compounds with few side effects or drug interactions has reawakened an interest in "rational" polypharmacy.)

***Drug interactions.*** Anti-seizure drugs interact with each other and also with drugs used for a variety of other disorders. These interactions, which tend to be pharmacokinetic and to involve increases or decreases in blood levels, are too numerous to discuss. (Some of them are discussed in Chapter 60.) A general rule of thumb is that valproate tends to increase blood levels of other drugs by inhibiting hepatic drug-biotransforming enzymes, while phenobarbital, phenytoin, and carbamazepine tend to decrease blood levels of other drugs by inducing these enzymes. Several of the anti-seizure drugs, including phenytoin and carbamazepine, decrease the blood levels (and effectiveness) of oral contraceptives by inducing enzymes of the cytochrome P450 system in the liver.

***Use of blood levels to regulate therapy.*** Therapeutic blood concentrations are now known for all of the older anti-seizure drugs. Monitoring of anticonvulsant blood concentrations is standard practice with these drugs. At the start of therapy, or whenever dosage is adjusted, blood samples are taken to determine whether concentrations are in the therapeutic range. The same blood samples are used to check for the occurrence of ADRs involving liver, kidney, or blood toxicity.

***Compliance.*** Non-compliance is an important cause of failure in anti-seizure drug therapy (see Chapter 58). It is typically revealed by blood samples, which indicate that the patient is not taking the medication. Compliance can often be improved by programs that provide the patient with information about seizure disorders and the ways in which anti-seizure drugs control them.

***Withdrawal of drugs.*** If a patient has no seizures or EEG abnormalities for several years, anti-seizure drugs may be slowly withdrawn. Children outgrow a number of types of childhood seizures (e.g., absence seizures), and even adults occasionally outgrow their attacks. It is important to note that, except in hospital, anti-seizure drugs should never be withdrawn quickly. Rebound seizures may occur, and even status epilepticus. This is particularly true with the barbiturates (phenobarbital) and the benzodiazepines (clonazepam, clobazam).

***Drug therapy during pregnancy.*** Most women taking anti-seizure drugs remain well controlled during pregnancy. It is believed that the risks of seizures to the fetus are greater than the risks related to anti-seizure drugs. There is a slightly increased incidence of fetal malformations in the children of epileptic mothers, however, and this relates in part to the drugs the mothers take. In the general population, the incidence of fetal malformations is about 2%. In women with seizures, it is slightly higher at about 3%. It remains at 3% in women taking only one anti-seizure drug, but rises to 5% in women taking two anti-seizure drugs, to 10% in women taking three, and to over 20% in women taking four anti-seizure drugs. There is hope that some of the new, recently released anti-seizure drugs (see "Role of the New Drugs Recently Introduced in North America" below) will be less teratogenic than the standard compounds.

## Prognosis for seizure control/quality of life

About 60% of patients are greatly helped by the anti-seizure drugs. These drug-responsive patients are completely controlled by low drug doses, and they lead normal lives, experiencing few side effects. If they are compliant, they may never experience another seizure. About 20% of patients are partially responsive to drugs. These patients have fewer seizures when they take anti-seizure drugs, but they do not become seizure-free. They may have significant problems related to driving and employment. The final 20% of patients seem to gain little benefit from anti-seizure drugs. These patients continue to have seizures even when they take high drug doses that are associated with serious side effects. Such patients are said to have intractable seizures. They tend to have major social, economic, and personal problems. Intractable epilepsy—found in about 1 in 500 in the general population—is very hard to live with.

The majority of patients with intractable epilepsy are patients with complex partial seizures, which are often of temporal lobe origin. Complex partial seizures are the most common type of seizures in adults, and they are notoriously resistant to drug therapy. Patients with uncontrolled complex partial seizures are frequent candidates for non-drug therapy (see "Non-drug Therapy for Epilepsy" below).

## SPECIFIC EPILEPSY DRUGS

The drugs most commonly used in North America are discussed below, grouped in terms of their therapeutic applications. Chemical structures are shown in Figure 18-2, and main side effects are summarized in Table 18-2. Pharmacokinetic features appear in Table 18-3. Drugs are presented according to their order of approval in North America. Drugs approved since 1990 are marked with asterisks. Not all of these newer drugs are available in every country.

Discussions of the less common agents, such as acetazolamide, and the older succinimides and hydantoins may be found in medical handbooks.

---

**FIGURE 18-2** Structural formulae of anti-seizure drugs.

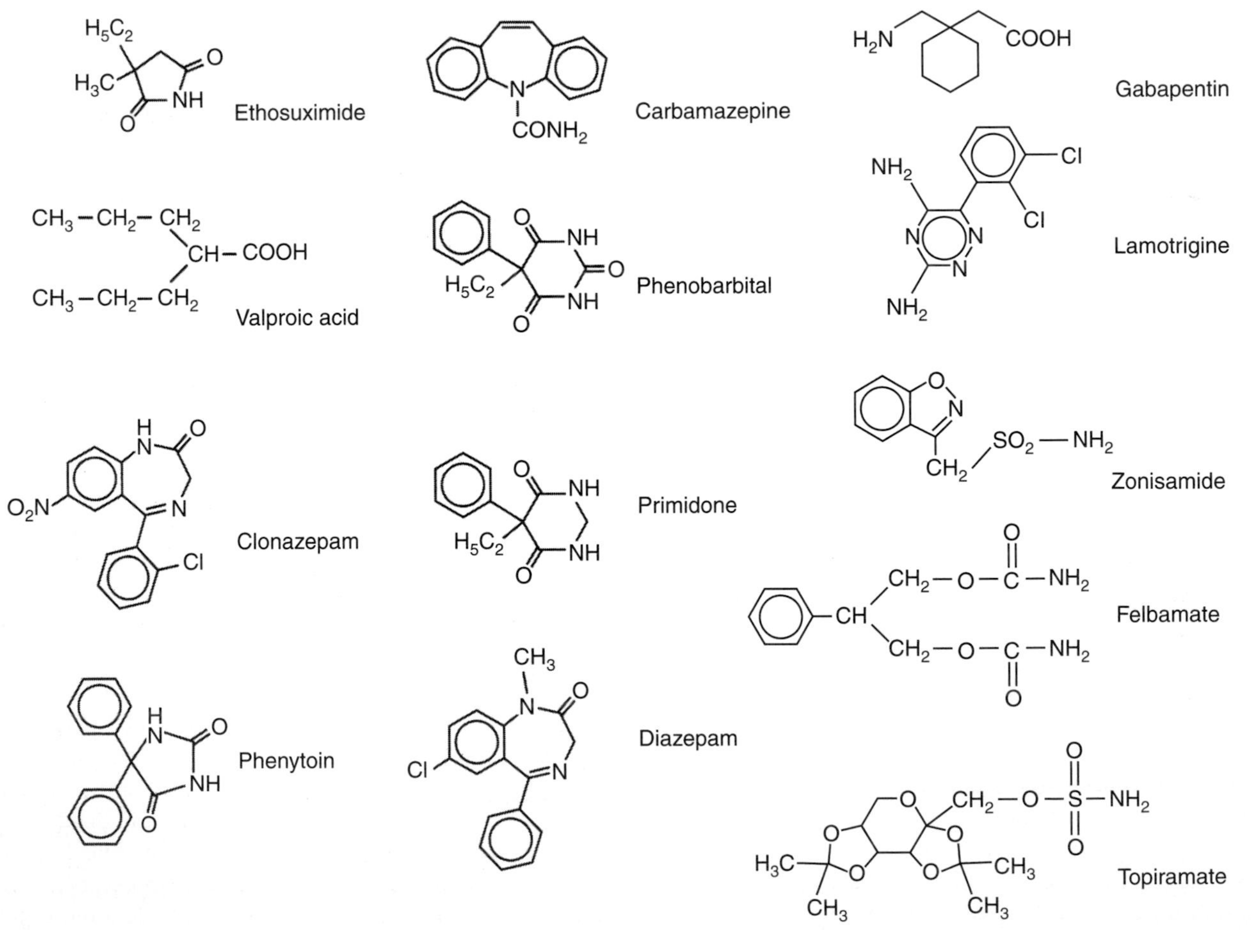

**TABLE 18-2**   Commonly Used Anti-seizure Drugs

| Name (Trade Name) | Chemical Structure (see also Fig. 18-2) | Common Side Effects (at therapeutic blood levels) |
|---|---|---|
| **Drugs for absence seizures:** | | |
| Ethosuximide (Zarontin) | Resembles phenobarbital | GI disturbances, sedation, photophobia |
| **Drugs for tonic–clonic and partial seizures:** | | |
| Carbamazepine (Tegretol) | Resembles tricyclic antidepressants | Diplopia, dizziness, GI disturbances, sedation, transient mild depression of leukocyte count |
| Gabapentin* (Neurontin) | Resembles GABA | Headache, ataxia, fatigue, nausea, somnolence, sedation |
| Oxcarbazepine* (Trileptal) | Resembles carbamazepine | Somnolence, diplopia, rash, hyponatremia |
| Phenobarbital (Luminal) | A barbiturate | Sedation, paradoxical excitement in children (abrupt withdrawal is dangerous) |
| Phenytoin (Dilantin, others) | Resembles phenobarbital | GI disturbances, hirsutism, gingival hyperplasia, acne, sedation (at toxic doses: nystagmus, ataxia) |
| Primidone (Mysoline) | Resembles phenobarbital | Sedation, psychiatric disturbances, decreased libido |
| Tiagabine* (Gabitril) | Novel | Somnolence, nervousness, dizziness, GI upsets (less if taken with meals) |
| Vigabatrin* (Sabril) | Resembles GABA | GI disturbances, sedation, transient psychotic states |
| **Broad-spectrum drugs:** | | |
| Clobazam* (Frisium) | A benzodiazepine | Similar to clonazepam (though milder) |
| Clonazepam (Rivotril) | A benzodiazepine | Sedation, personality change, and/or paradoxical excitement in children (abrupt withdrawal is dangerous) |
| Lamotrigine* (Lamictal) | Novel | Blurred vision, ataxia, diplopia, dizziness, GI upsets, sedation, rash |
| Levetiracetam* (Keppra) | Analogue of piracetam | Dizziness, somnolence, asthenia (weakness); rarely, low hematocrit and leukocyte count |
| Topiramate* (Topamax) | Novel | Fatigue, somnolence, dizziness, tremor, weight gain, GI disturbances, bruising, hair loss |
| Valproate (Depakene) | Fatty acid | Lowered platelet and leukocyte count, weight gain, GI upset, hair loss; rarely, pancreatitis, hepatic failure, neural tube defects |
| Zonisamide* (Zonergan) | A sulfonamide | Somnolence, dizziness, GI upset, rash (less if titrated slowly) |
| **Drugs for status epilepticus:** | | |
| Diazepam (Valium) | A benzodiazepine | Not used in chronic therapy |
| Lorazepam (Ativan) | A benzodiazepine | Not used in chronic therapy |

*Introduced since 1990, these newer drugs may not be available in every country.
GI = gastrointestinal.

## Drugs Used Only for Absence Seizures

### Ethosuximide

Ethosuximide (Zarontin) is the current drug of choice for absence seizures. It has replaced trimethadione (Tridione), a more toxic and less effective drug that has been withdrawn from the market. Ethosuximide is not effective against tonic–clonic or partial seizures.

Ethosuximide binds to and inhibits the T-type voltage-dependent calcium channel.

The drug is relatively effective, safe, and non-sedating. It has a long half-life, allowing once-a-day dosing.

Ethosuximide may cause gastrointestinal disturbances, fatigue, photophobia, and other side effects. Rare, non-dose-related adverse effects include liver and kidney damage, lupus erythematosus, and blood dyscrasias.

## Drugs Used Only for Tonic–Clonic and Partial Attacks

### Phenobarbital

Phenobarbital (Luminal), introduced in 1911, was the first modern anti-seizure drug. It is effective against tonic–clonic and partial seizures, but not against absence attacks. Recently, the use of phenobarbital in adults has declined because of the excessive sedation it causes. It is still used in children, due to its safety, and in patients who are allergic to the other drugs.

Phenobarbital enhances GABA-mediated inhibition by binding to the barbiturate receptor site on the ligand-gated chloride channel associated with the GABA$_A$ receptor (see Chapter 23).

This is one of the cheapest and safest anticonvulsants. Its long half-life simplifies dosing.

Phenobarbital causes serious sedation in many patients at therapeutic dose levels. Its original use, before the discovery of its anticonvulsant effects, was as a daytime sedative. In some patients, particularly the very old or very young, phenobarbital causes "paradoxical excitement." In these cases, the patient becomes restless and agitated, rather than calm and sleepy. Like phenytoin, phenobarbital interacts with many drugs because when given acutely it inhibits the hepatic cytochrome P450 system, and when given chronically it is an inducer of that system.

## Phenytoin

Phenytoin (Dilantin) is an older drug, introduced in 1938. It was formerly known as diphenylhydantoin. It is still widely used in the treatment of tonic–clonic and partial attacks, but it is not effective against absence attacks. Phenytoin replaced phenobarbital as the drug of choice just before World War II because it was less sedating. For many years, it was a mainstay of anti-seizure therapy.

Phenytoin binds to and inhibits voltage-dependent sodium channels, thus preventing the high-frequency discharge typical of seizure activity.

Phenytoin has a long half-life, allowing once-a-day dosing, and it is relatively non-sedating.

This drug causes a number of dose-related ADRs that occur at therapeutic dose levels. These include gastrointestinal disturbances, acne, gingival hyperplasia (excess growth of gum tissue, seen in over 30% of patients), and hirsutism (excess growth of body hair). Sedation is the most frequent nervous system side effect. At toxic doses, ataxia, nystagmus, and impaired motor coordination may occur. A rare non-dose-related ADR is the anticonvulsant hypersensitivity syndrome, indicated by a rash and fever. This ADR necessitates immediate withdrawal of the drug.

Phenytoin also has an unusual metabolism. This complicates dosing and sometimes leads to toxic blood levels. Somewhere in the therapeutic concentration range (10 to 20 µg/mL, or 40 to 80 µmol/L), phenytoin tends to saturate the degradative enzymes in the liver. When this happens, the excess phenytoin that cannot be handled by the normal first-order metabolism is diverted to a "pseudo–zero-order" metabolic pathway, which means that elimination begins to take place much more slowly and is dose-related. The physician who has been gradually raising dose levels may find that the patient suddenly begins to show toxic effects. Phenytoin toxicity (usually nystagmus and ataxia) occasionally presents in idiosyncratic forms that are hard to recognize (pseudo-psychosis, increased seizure frequency). Monitoring of blood levels is particularly important, therefore, when phenytoin dosage is being adjusted.

| TABLE 18-3 | Pharmacokinetic Parameters of Commonly Used Anti-seizure Drugs | | | | | | |
|---|---|---|---|---|---|---|---|
| Drug | Absorption | Half-Life (hours) | Oral Bioavailability (%) | Urinary Excretion (%) | Plasma Protein Binding (%) | Volume of Distribution (L/kg) | Effective Concentration in Plasma |
| For absence seizures: | | | | | | | |
| Ethosuximide | Rapid | 45 ± 8 | 100 | 25 ± 15 | 0 | 0.72 ± 0.16 | 40–100 µg/mL |
| For tonic–clonic and partial seizures: | | | | | | | |
| Carbamazepine | Slow–moderate | 15 ± 5 | >70 | <1 | 74 ± 3 | 1.4 ± 0.4 | 4–10 µg/mL |
| Gabapentin* | Rapid | 6.5 ± 1.0 | 60 | 100 | 0 | 0.80 ± 0.09 | >2 µg/mL |
| Oxcarbazepine* | Rapid | 8–10 | 96–99 | 80 | 40 | 0.76 | 10–35 µg/mL |
| Phenobarbital | Slow–moderate | 99 ± 18 | 100 ± 11 | 24 ± 5 | 51 ± 3 | 0.54 ± 0.03 | 10–25 µg/mL |
| Phenytoin | Slow | 6–24 | 90 ± 3 | 2 ± 8 | 89 ± 23 | 0.64 ± 0.04 | >10 µg/mL |
| Primidone | Slow–moderate | 15 ± 4 | 92 ± 18 | 46 ± 16 | 19 | 0.69 ± 0.18 | 8–12 µg/mL |
| Tiagabine* | Rapid | 5–13 | 90 | 0 | 95 | 1 | 40–100 ng/mL |
| Vigabatrin* | Rapid | 4–9 | 60–80 | 60–70 | 0 | 0.8 | 42 ± 25 µg/mL |
| Broad-spectrum drugs: | | | | | | | |
| Clobazam* | Rapid | 10–30 | 100 | <1 | 85 | "Large" | 50–300 ng/mL |
| Clonazepam | Rapid | 23 ± 5 | 98 ± 31 | <1 | 86 ± 0.5 | 3.2 ± 1.1 | 5–70 ng/mL |
| Lamotrigine* | Rapid | 12–60 | 98 | 70 | 50 | 1.1–1.3 | 1.6 ± 1.3 µg/mL |
| Levetiracetam* | Rapid | 6–8 | 100 | 46–75 | <10 | 1.14 | 5–45 µg/mL |
| Topiramate* | Rapid | 19–25 | 81–95 | 70 | 9–17 | 0.61 | 4–10 µg/mL |
| Valproate | Rapid | 14–30 | 100 ± 10 | 1.8 ± 2.4 | 93 ± 1 | 0.22 ± 0.07 | 30–100 µg/mL |
| Zonisamide* | Slow–moderate | 63 | >95 | 30 | 40 | 1.5 | 10–40 µg/mL |

*Introduced since 1990, these newer drugs may not be available in every country.

Phenytoin is a substrate for the hepatic cytochrome P450 system, for which it can also act as an inhibitor acutely and an inducer during chronic administration. Therefore, it can interact with many other drugs by reciprocal effects on biotransformation with consequent effects on the plasma levels and pharmacological activities, both of phenytoin and of the other drugs involved (see Chapters 4 and 60).

## Primidone

Primidone (Mysoline) is very closely related chemically to phenobarbital. In the body, it is biotransformed into phenobarbital, and most of its therapeutic effect probably depends on this active metabolite.

Primidone is long-acting and fairly safe.

Like phenobarbital, primidone is sedating. For this reason, it has declined in popularity.

## Carbamazepine

Carbamazepine (Tegretol) has fewer side effects than phenytoin and is now widely used for the treatment of tonic–clonic and partial seizures. It is not effective against absence attacks. Carbamazepine is available in a normal and a slow-release formulation (Tegretol CR).

Carbamazepine binds to and inhibits the voltage-dependent sodium channel.

It is as effective as phenytoin and less sedating for most patients. It does not cause acne, gingival hyperplasia, or hirsutism.

Gastrointestinal disturbances and double vision sometimes occur at therapeutic dose levels. Occasionally, patients show sedation, perhaps due to the 10,11-epoxide metabolite of carbamazepine. A mild depression in leukocyte count is often seen early in treatment, but this usually disappears without discontinuation of therapy. Rare non-dose-related ADRs (anticonvulsant hypersensitivity syndrome, severe anemias) occasionally occur and do require withdrawal of the drug.

The half-life of carbamazepine varies from 35 hours (at the start of therapy) to 10 to 12 hours (after prolonged therapy). This change in half-life is due to autoinduction of liver enzymes. It is, therefore, wise to start patients on a low dose of carbamazepine and gradually increase the dose as the liver enzymes are induced. After induction has occurred, the shorter half-life of carbamazepine may make it hard to maintain stable blood levels; therefore, many patients do better on the controlled-release formulation.

## Vigabatrin*

Vigabatrin (Sabril) was approved in the 1990s. It was formerly known as γ-vinyl-GABA. Vigabatrin is effective against tonic–clonic and partial seizures and also against several types of drug-resistant childhood seizures, including the seizures of West's syndrome. It is not effective against absence attacks.

Vigabatrin enhances GABAergic activity by covalently binding to, and irreversibly inactivating, the catabolic enzyme for GABA, GABA transaminase (GABA-T).

The drug has a short half-life, but this is not important because it binds covalently to an enzyme. When drugs bind covalently, their therapeutic effects continue after the blood levels of the drug have declined. It is the drug of choice in treating West's syndrome, particularly when West's syndrome is associated with tuberous sclerosis, an inherited condition.

Vigabatrin sometimes causes dose-related stomach upset and sedation. Up to 6% of patients are reported to experience transient psychotic episodes, which clear when the drug is withdrawn. Non-dose-related ADRs have not as yet been reported. Recently, however, it was discovered that vigabatrin causes serious visual ADRs, including the development of tunnel vision, which does not diminish when the drug is withdrawn. For this reason, the use of vigabatrin has declined greatly.

## Gabapentin*

Gabapentin (Neurontin) is another relatively new drug. It was originally designed to act as an agonist at the GABA_A receptor. It has proved not to be a GABA_A agonist, but it is still a useful anti-seizure drug, effective against tonic–clonic and partial seizures. It is not effective against absence seizures.

The mechanism of action of gabapentin is not yet clear.

Gabapentin has relatively mild side effects and is not associated with any life-threatening ADRs. It has *no* known drug interactions. Because of its mild side effects and lack of drug interactions, gabapentin is an ideal "add on" drug and may eventually find an important role in adjunct therapy.

Gabapentin has a short half-life, requiring three or four doses a day. Some patients experience dose-related somnolence, dizziness, ataxia, and fatigue.

## Tiagabine*

Tiagabine (Gabitril) has recently been approved and is effective in the treatment of tonic–clonic and partial seizures but is ineffective against absence attacks.

Tiagabine inhibits the reuptake of GABA, leaving higher levels in the synapse.

It may be tried against partial seizures that have resisted other medications. Otherwise, it has few special advantages. No non-dose-related ADRs have as yet been reported.

Tiagabine has a short half-life, requiring two, three, or even four doses a day. Dose-related gastrointestinal problems, somnolence, dizziness, and nervousness are sometimes seen. The dosage must be titrated slowly against the effects at the start of administration.

## Levetiracetam*

Levetiracetam (Keppra) has recently been approved. It is useful in the treatment of tonic–clonic and partial seizures. It is not known to be effective against absence attacks, although this question has not yet been settled.

Levetiracetam's mechanism of action is not yet clear.

The major advantages of levetiracetam are that it has no known drug interactions and that it can be started at a full adult dose, without the gradual titration required by most other anti-seizure drugs. No non-dose-related ADRs have as yet been reported.

Levetiracetam has a short half-life, requiring two or three doses a day. Dose-related somnolence, dizziness, and asthenia (feelings of weakness) are sometimes seen.

### Oxcarbazepine*

Oxcarbazepine (Trileptal) is a recently approved drug. It is used in the treatment of tonic–clonic and partial seizures. It is not effective against absence attacks. Oxcarbazepine is chemically related to carbamazepine. It is, in a sense, a prodrug since it is rapidly converted into a 10-monohydroxyl metabolite (MHD) that is primarily responsible for its anti-seizure effects.

Oxcarbazepine (or its MHD metabolite) probably works by binding to and inhibiting the voltage-dependent sodium channel.

Oxcarbazepine is as effective as carbamazepine; however, it causes fewer dose-related ADRs and is associated with fewer drug interactions. No non-dose-related ADRs have as yet been reported.

Like carbamazepine, MHD has a relatively short half-life, requiring two or three doses a day. Dose-related somnolence and double vision sometimes occur at therapeutic dose levels, and a rash is sometimes seen.

## Broad-Spectrum Drugs

Valproate and the benzodiazepines were first used in the treatment of absence seizures. It was later realized that they were also effective against tonic–clonic and partial seizures; hence the term "broad-spectrum." They are also used in several forms of drug-resistant childhood epilepsy. Several of the newly released drugs are also broad-spectrum agents.

### Valproate (valproic acid)

Valproate (Depakene) is a true broad-spectrum drug, effective against absence, tonic–clonic, and partial seizures. It was first used for absence attacks, particularly when they were combined with tonic–clonic attacks. Recently, it has also been used for tonic–clonic seizures, partial seizures, and for a variety of drug-resistant childhood seizures. It has now joined phenytoin and carbamazepine as one of the "big three" drugs in anti-seizure therapy. A slightly different version of the compound, divalproex sodium (Epival), has similar therapeutic effects and is said to cause less gastrointestinal distress.

Valproate enhances GABA-mediated inhibition, but the exact mechanism of enhancement is unknown.

An advantage of valproate is that it is one of the least sedating of the anti-seizure drugs. Because of its broad-spectrum activity, it can be used for patients with mixed seizure types. Traditionally, these patients were given separate drugs for each type, but valproate alone may be sufficient.

Valproate has a short half-life, which necessitates two or more doses every day. Side effects are still being discovered. Known dose-related side effects include gastrointestinal disturbances (frequent in the early stage of therapy), tremor, hair loss, weight gain, and bruising and bleeding. Hepatitis is a rare but potentially fatal non-dose-related ADR, especially in very young children.

### Clonazepam

Clonazepam (Rivotril, Clonopin), a benzodiazepine, is effective against a broad spectrum of seizure disorders. Its usefulness, however, is limited by the sedation and ataxia it often causes. It may be used in absence epilepsy, but, because of its side effects, it is often reserved for other, drug-resistant forms of childhood epilepsy. Tolerance to the CNS-depressant effects, as well as to the anti-seizure effect, may develop when the drug is used chronically to control convulsive seizures.

Clonazepam enhances GABA-mediated inhibition by binding to the benzodiazepine receptor site on the ligand-gated chloride channel associated with the GABA$_A$ receptor (see Chapter 23).

Clonazepam is safe, has a long half-life, and is *not* associated with prominent gastrointestinal disturbances or life-threatening ADRs.

Clonazepam causes sedation or personality change (paradoxical excitement) in up to 50% of the patients who take it. In children, the paradoxical excitement may take the form of impatience, rudeness, or overt aggression. As with other benzodiazepines, the CNS-depressant effects of clonazepam are enhanced by alcohol, opioids, and a variety of sedative and hypnotic drugs.

### Clobazam*

Clobazam (Frisium) is also a benzodiazepine. Most benzodiazepines have nitrogen atoms at positions 1 and 4 (i.e., 1,4-benzodiazepines), but clobazam is a 1,5-benzodiazepine. This difference is said to maximize its therapeutic anti-seizure effects and to minimize its sedative side effects. In some patients, tolerance to the therapeutic effects develops, often within 6 months to a year after starting the drug.

Clobazam, like clonazepam, enhances GABA-mediated inhibition by binding to the benzodiazepine receptor site on the ligand-gated chloride channel associated with the GABA$_A$ receptor.

The advantages of clobazam are the same as for clonazepam, but clobazam is believed to have fewer side effects. Like clonazepam, it has a fairly long half-life, and it has active metabolites that probably prolong its duration of action.

Though side effects may be less than with clonazepam, some patients taking clobazam clearly show sedation or personality changes. Its CNS-depressant effects, like those of clonazepam, are also potentiated by alcohol and other CNS depressants. Tolerance to the drug's anti-seizure effects may develop over time.

### Lamotrigine*

Lamotrigine (Lamictal) is effective against tonic–clonic and partial seizures and, to a lesser extent, absence seizures. It has succeeded in some cases of drug-resistant epilepsy where all other drugs have failed.

Like phenytoin and carbamazepine, lamotrigine is believed to bind to the voltage-dependent sodium channel. It must have other actions as well, since drugs that act on the sodium channel do not usually antagonize absence seizures.

Lamotrigine has a broad spectrum of action, has generally mild side effects, and is not associated with any life-threatening ADRs. It has few known drug interactions other than altered drug metabolism (see next paragraph).

Lamotrigine alone has a half-life of about 24 hours. The concurrent administration of other drugs, however, can make its half-life as short as 12 or as long as 60 hours. Hormonal contraceptive preparations may reduce serum lamotrigine levels enough to require upward adjustment of dosage. Dosing schedules, therefore, vary from two to four times a day. Dose-dependent ADRs include ataxia, dizziness, and blurred or double vision. A rash has been reported in up to 10% of patients. This occurs more frequently in children, particularly if they are also taking valproate. The rash is less likely to occur if patients are started on low doses that are increased gradually, and it may abate without discontinuation of the drug. Due to the occurrence of rash, the drug is titrated slowly, and it may take 4 to 6 weeks to reach a therapeutic dose.

### Topiramate*

Topiramate (Topamax) is a new broad-spectrum drug that is effective against tonic–clonic, partial, and, to a lesser extent, absence seizures. It has been successful in treating some cases of drug-resistant epilepsy that have not responded to any other drugs.

Topiramate appears to have several mechanisms of action, which may explain its broad spectrum of activity. These include binding to and inhibiting voltage-gated sodium channels, acting as an agonist at $GABA_A$ receptors, and acting as an antagonist at non-NMDA glutamatergic receptors.

Side effects of topiramate are generally mild—although it may cause some cognitive impairment—and it is not associated with any life-threatening ADRs.

Dose-related ADRs include fatigue, sedation, and dizziness. Cognitive impairment and word-finding difficulties occur in some patients. These are worse with higher doses or rapid titration. These cognitive effects are perhaps the most serious problem with topiramate. Renal stones occur in about 1% of patients. Topiramate should be used with caution in patients being treated with other therapies that cause renal stones, such as zonisamide, acetazolamide, or the ketogenic diet. Topiramate can also cause dose-related weight loss, which is considered to be a "good" side effect by some patients. Due to the fear of cognitive impairment, topiramate must be titrated slowly.

### Zonisamide*

Zonisamide (Zonegran) has broad-spectrum activity against tonic–clonic and partial seizures and also, to a lesser extent, against absence seizures.

Zonisamide appears to have several mechanisms of action, in keeping with its broad spectrum of activity. These include binding to and inhibiting voltage-gated sodium channels, binding to and inhibiting T-type calcium channels, binding to GABA receptors, and facilitating dopaminergic and serotonergic transmission.

This anti-seizure drug has a long half-life and can be administered once or twice a day. Side effects are generally mild and transient. Its use is rarely limited by side effects. It has few known drug interactions. Slow titration may decrease the incidence of side effects but is not absolutely required.

Dose-related ADRs include gastrointestinal upsets, sedation, and rash. Renal stones have also been reported.

### Felbamate

Felbamate, a broad-spectrum anticonvulsant, was one of the first new drugs to be released. Unfortunately, felbamate proved to have rare but fatal side effects. While it has not been removed from the market, it is used very little, usually in cases of the rare "catastrophic" childhood epilepsies in which it may be the only effective agent.

## Drugs for Status Epilepticus

Drugs for status epilepticus are administered intravenously in hospital. High doses are used, and it is important that the drugs be infused slowly to avoid bolus effects. Mechanisms of action are as noted for similar drugs above.

### Benzodiazepines

Two benzodiazepines, **diazepam** (Valium) and **lorazepam** (Ativan), are the mainstay of therapy for all varieties of status epilepticus. **Diazepam** was the drug of choice for many years. The adult intravenous dose is 10 to 20 mg, and the infusion rate should not exceed 2 mg/min. If necessary, this dose may be repeated after 20 to 30 minutes. While diazepam stops status attacks quickly, its effects may wear off quickly due to redistribution. **Lorazepam** has a shorter $t_{1/2}$ but a slower redistribution and hence a longer duration of initial action. Because of its long duration, it is preferred by many hospitals.

### Fosphenytoin*

Fosphenytoin (Cerebyx) is a recently approved injectable prodrug of phenytoin. After injection, it is quickly broken down into phenytoin by phosphatases in the blood. Phenytoin is very poorly water-soluble; however, fosphenytoin is much more water-soluble, which means that it can be given intravenously or intramuscularly and that side effects related to the phenytoin vehicle are avoided. Fosphenytoin can also be administered more rapidly than intravenous phenytoin. One notable side effect is paraesthesias, which are caused by the phosphates released as fosphenytoin is converted to phenytoin.

### Intravenous valproate*

An intravenous preparation of valproate (Depacon) has also been recently approved. It is somewhat early to forecast, but it seems that it will be another drug useful in controlling status epilepticus.

### Other drugs for status epilepticus

If status epilepticus resists the standard anti-status drugs, intravenous phenytoin or phenobarbital may be tried. If these fail, intramuscular paraldehyde or intravenous lidocaine may be administered. If none of these is effective, general anaesthesia may be required.

## Role of the New Drugs Recently Introduced in North America

Since 1990, nine new anti-seizure drugs have been introduced in North America. (These have been marked with asterisks in the table and in the text above.) As a group, these compounds are felt to have relatively mild side effects, and they are associated with fewer drug interactions. Blood level testing is not yet available.

It is not clear, however, that these new anti-seizure drugs are more effective at controlling seizures than the older drugs. When the new compounds began to come out, it was hoped that the number of patients with intractable seizures would drop from 20% to 0%. It is generally agreed that this has not happened. The new compounds are occasionally successful against seizures that have resisted all past medications. In general, however, the seizures that resisted the old drugs are also resisting the newer drugs. A rough estimate might be that the new drugs have decreased the number of patients with intractable seizures from 20% to 17%.

In assessing the role of the newer drugs, cost must be considered. Generally speaking, the new compounds are far more expensive than the standard drugs. Perhaps because of this, physicians are using the new compounds cautiously, often as adjunct medications in poorly controlled patients. The standard anticonvulsants, and especially ethosuximide, phenytoin, carbamazepine, and valproate, are still dominant in the treatment of epilepsy.

If a patient is well controlled and has few side effects on the standard drugs, there is no particular need to try the newer compounds. If a patient is poorly controlled on the standard drugs or has intolerable side effects, the newer compounds offer an (expensive) alternative.

## Non-drug Therapy for Epilepsy

A number of non-drug therapies are available for epilepsy, including seizure surgery, the ketogenic diet, and vagal stimulation. These are effective, but they all involve certain difficulties and are generally not considered until anti-seizure drugs have failed.

When should non-drug therapies be considered? It is becoming clear that intractable epilepsy can be recognized quite early. If the first appropriate drug fails, there is only about a 15% chance that a second appropriate drug will succeed, and less than a 5% chance that a third drug will succeed. Two drugs can be tried during the first year of therapy. It has recently been suggested, therefore, that epilepsy should be considered intractable if seizures are not controlled within the first year after diagnosis. It is appropriate, therefore, to begin considering non-drug therapies if seizures are not under control by the end of the first year.

## Other Indications for Anti-seizure Drugs

Some of the older, and many of the newer, anticonvulsant drugs are now being used to treat disorders other than epilepsy. These include migraine, neuropathic pain, and bipolar disorder.

## The Comorbidities of Epilepsy

Patients with intractable seizures often suffer from related disorders—disorders that may be more serious than the seizures themselves. These are called the comorbidities of epilepsy and include cognitive, psychiatric, behavioural, and reproductive problems. The most serious of these are probably anxiety and depression and the behavioural problems (attention deficit hyperactivity syndrome). These problems are responsive to drug therapy, but they are often not diagnosed or treated.

The control of complex partial seizures is perhaps the greatest problem in modern therapy for epilepsy. The failure to diagnose and treat comorbidities is perhaps the second-greatest problem.

## SUMMARY

Although the drugs available at present represent a great advance in the therapy of epilepsy, more and better drugs are still needed—most urgently, drugs that are effective against complex partial attacks. Agents with fewer side effects would also be welcome. A second great need is the diagnosis and treatment of epileptic comorbidities. A long-term goal of therapy is to discover drugs that *cure* epilepsy, rather than simply suppressing seizures.

## SUGGESTED READINGS

Bazil CW. New antiepileptic drugs. *The Neurologist.* 2002;8:71-81.

Bialer M, Johannessen SI, Kupferberg HJ, et al. Progress report on new antiepileptic drugs: a summary of the Sixth Eilat Conference (EILAT VI). *Epilepsy Res.* 2002;51:31-71.

Brodie MJ, Dichter MA. Antiepileptic drugs. *N Engl J Med.* 1996; 334:168-175.

Burnham WM. Epilepsy. In: Nadel L, ed. *Encyclopedia of Cognitive Science.* Vol 2. London, United Kingdom: Nature Publishing Group; 2003:1-7.

Burnham WM. Epilepsy: the invisible disability. In: Brown I, Percy M, eds. *Developmental Disabilities in Ontario.* 2nd ed. Toronto, Ontario: Ontario Assoc. Developmental Disabilities; 2003:351-364.

Macdonald RL, Kelly KM. Mechanisms of action of currently prescribed and newly developed antiepileptic drugs. *Epilepsia.* 1994;35(suppl 4):S41-S50.

McNamara JO. Cellular and molecular basis of epilepsy. *J Neurosci.* 1994;14:3413-3425.

McNamara JO. Drugs effective in the therapy of the epilepsies. In: Hardman JG, Limbird LE, Gilman AG, eds. *Goodman & Gilman's The Pharmacological Basis of Therapeutics.* 10th ed. New York, NY: McGraw-Hill; 2001:521-547.

# 19

# Opioid Analgesics and Antagonists

## H KALANT

### CASE HISTORY

A frail 78-year-old woman, looking older than her stated age, was admitted to hospital with a history of severe lower back pain of 3 weeks' duration. Her family physician had made a diagnosis of degenerative arthritis of the lumbar spine and prescribed non-steroidal anti-inflammatory drugs (NSAIDs) for the pain and diazepam as a muscle relaxant and sedative. The pain persisted, however, and radiological examination revealed a compression fracture of the L-4 vertebra.

On admission, the patient was 162 cm (5'4'') in height and weighed 44.5 kg (98 lb.). An order was written for morphine sulfate, 7.5 mg intramuscularly, every 6 hours. The first injection produced a very marked reduction in her pain. However, she felt somewhat nauseated and had no appetite for the meals that were served to her. By the second day on this treatment, she was very drowsy and mentally clouded. Her urine volume fell to 270 mL in 24 hours, and she had no bowel movement. Her colour became greyish, and her respiratory rate fell to 5 to 6/min, with shallow and somewhat irregular breathing.

At this point, an injection of naloxone 100 µg (0.1 mg) was given, and her breathing and colour recovered almost immediately, although her pain also returned. One hour later, she was again very drowsy, with depressed respiration. Another dose of naloxone was given, the order for intramuscular morphine was cancelled, and she was monitored closely until her respiratory rate remained above 10/min. Patient-controlled analgesia (PCA) was initiated with intravenous morphine 1 to 2 mg per injection and a maximum permissible delivery of 7 mg in any 1 hour. Supplementary therapy with oral low-dose NSAIDs was also considered but was held in reserve while the effect of the PCA was assessed.

## OPIATES, OPIOIDS, AND NARCOTICS

The opium poppy (*Papaver somniferum*) has been known and used in Asia Minor and southeastern Europe for over 2000 years. Its juice was known to contain an agent that relieved pain, produced sleep or drowsiness (*somniferum* = bringing sleep), relieved diarrhea, and in low doses, produced a blissful or euphoric state. Only crude preparations were available for medical use until the isolation and purification of morphine by Sertürner in 1805. Other alkaloids with similar properties were isolated from crude opium over the next decades, and by the mid-nineteenth century, these pure compounds (opiates) began to replace opium in medical use. Morphine was named after Morpheus, the Greek god of sleep. The Greek word *narkē* means stupor; therefore, these compounds, which produced drowsiness, analgesia, and a dreamy stuporous state, were called **narcotics.**

In legal terminology, however, a narcotic is any drug included under the Narcotic Control Act in Canada, the Harrison Act in the United States, or equivalent legislation in other countries. Most of these drugs are morphine-like analgesics or synthetic substitutes. However, these acts generally also cover cocaine and cannabis, which have pharmacological properties quite different from those of the opiate analgesics (see Chapter 26). Therefore, the term "narcotic" is no longer used in pharmacology.

In recent years, the term "opioid" was introduced to include not only the opiates with morphine-like action but also substances that are not derived from opium (hence, are not "opiates") and do not have a morphine-like chemical structure but do have morphine-like pharmacological properties. The whole group, including the opiates, is now known as **opioid analgesics.** In 1973, stereospecific receptors for opioid drugs were proven to exist in the central nervous system (CNS). Since it seemed improbable that the animal brain would have evolved receptors for plant alkaloids to which it was never exposed, researchers postulated that these receptors must normally take up endogenous material produced in the brain itself. In 1975, the first such materials were isolated and were found to be short peptides with morphine-like properties, which were named **enkephalins**. Soon afterward, longer peptides with similar properties (**endorphins, dynorphin**) were discovered. These are known collectively as **endogenous opioids**.

## OPIUM ALKALOIDS

Opium is the dry residue of juice from the seedpod of *Papaver somniferum*. It contains a mixture of alkaloids of two main types (Fig. 19-1).

## Benzylisoquinoline Alkaloids

The main example is **papaverine**. This is a smooth muscle depressant that causes relaxation of peripheral arterioles (and therefore lowers blood pressure), coronary arteries, gastrointestinal and other smooth muscle and has a direct quinidine-like effect on the myocardium. Although it is an opiate (i.e., derived from opium), it has no analgesic effect and does not bind to opioid receptors. Papaverine

**FIGURE 19-1** Structural formulae of the two major classes of opium alkaloid. For codeine, CH3O replaces HO at C-3 of morphine. Thebaine has CH3O groups at both C-3 and C-6 of morphine. Heroin is the 3,6-diacetate of morphine.

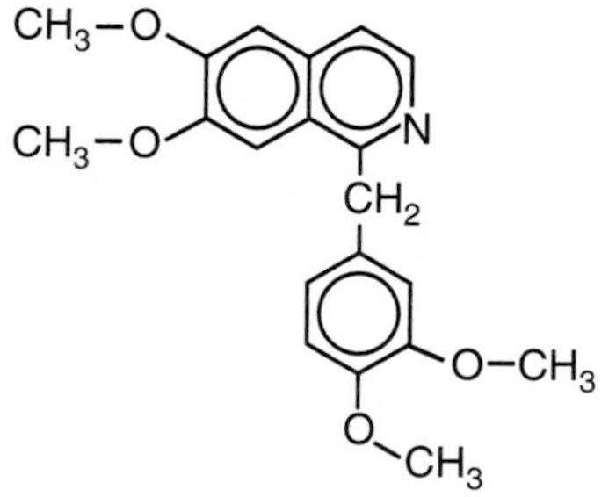

Papaverine – *a benzylisoquinoline alkaloid*

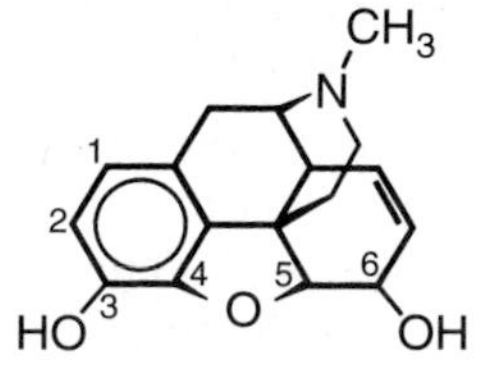

Morphine – *a phenanthrene alkaloid*

HCl is marketed for the relief of cerebral and peripheral ischemia due to arterial spasm, but its therapeutic value in these conditions has been questioned.

## Phenanthrene Alkaloids

These are mainly **morphine, codeine**, and **thebaine**. Morphine is a potent analgesic, but it also has strong excitatory effects in some tissues and some species; **thebaine** has predominantly excitatory rather than analgesic effects and can cause convulsions.

There are **asymmetric C atoms** in the opiates. Hence, all opiates can exist in either the (–), or levo, form (*l*- or levorotatory) or the (+), or dextro, form (*d*- or dextrorotatory).

All morphine synthesized by opium poppy enzymes is the levo isomer. The dextro isomers of the opiates have no analgesic action, except for *d*-propoxyphene and (+) tramadol, which are both weak synthetic codeine-like analgesics.

## PHARMACOLOGICAL ACTIONS OF OPIOIDS

Opioids have a large number of actions, both centrally and peripherally. Although most opioids produce analgesia, they may differ a great deal in their other effects. Morphine, for example, produces euphoria in many people, whereas the opioid ketocyclazocine produces marked dysphoria. The discovery of different classes of opioid receptors has helped to explain this dissociation of effects and the different spectra of effects shown by some of the newer synthetic opioids.

### Opioid Receptors and Endogenous Opioids

#### Properties of opioid–receptor binding
The opioid–receptor binding process has a high degree of structural specificity such that small modifications of the drug molecule cause large changes in drug binding (and in drug effect in vivo). There is stereospecificity: the levo isomers of opioids have much higher binding affinity than the dextro isomers, and only the levo isomers are active as analgesics (with the exception of *d*-propoxyphene). The binding is reversible; bound drug can be displaced from the receptors by an excess of other molecules with binding ability. The affinity of opioids for binding to the receptors is highly correlated with the potency of drug effects, whether as agonist or antagonist, both in vivo and in isolated tissues (Fig. 19-2).

#### Subtypes of opioid receptors and ligands
The major clinical use of opioids is the relief of pain, but all of them have numerous other effects. When they are administered in doses that produce the same degree of

**FIGURE 19-2** Correlation of pharmacological potencies of opiate agonists and antagonists with their affinities for receptor binding in the guinea pig intestine. Potencies refer to $IC_{50}$ for inhibition of electrically induced contraction of isolated gut by agonists or to $K_i$ for inhibition of opioid activity by antagonists. These compounds show the same rank order of potencies for inhibition of contraction of the isolated gut as for in vivo analgesia.

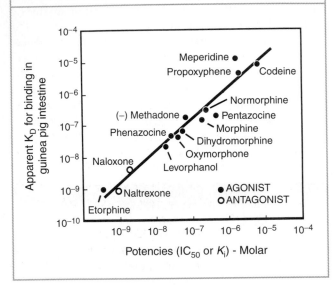

transmembrane regions and the intracellular loops connecting them are quite closely similar in the different opioid receptors, but the extracellular connecting loops and the $NH_2$ and COOH terminals vary in the different types and presumably account for the different ligand affinities and effects. The receptors are linked through G proteins to their second messengers and act to inhibit adenylyl cyclase activity, decrease voltage-gated $Ca^{2+}$ currents, and increase a receptor-gated $K^+$ current. The end result is hyperpolarization of the neuron bearing the receptor, with a reduction in its activity and its transmitter release. Each receptor type interacts with multiple types of G protein to produce the different effects.

Like other G protein–coupled receptors, opioid receptors are able to undergo hetero- or homodimerization, and this process may be related to the ability of opioid ligands to produce analgesia and the development of tolerance.

Opioid ligands can act at these receptors in four different ways:

1. If they activate the receptor and its linked response system, they are **agonists.**
2. If they occupy the receptor but do not activate it, they are **antagonists,** and they can block the activity of agonists.
3. If they activate the receptor incompletely, producing a lower maximum response, they are **partial agonists.**
4. If they have substantial affinity for more than one receptor type and act as an agonist at one type and as an antagonist at another, they are **mixed agonist/antagonists.**

analgesia (equianalgesic doses), the drugs differ with respect to the relative degree of other effects that they produce. This observation led to the current concept of multiple receptor types mediating different effects of the opioids (Table 19-1). The opioids could then be classified according to their relative affinities at the different types of receptor. None of the drugs appear to have absolute specificity for a single receptor type; rather, each drug has a major affinity for one type, with lesser degrees of affinity for the other types (Table 19-2).

Three major classes of opioid receptor are recognized that have different patterns of affinity for the various opioid agonists and antagonists. The prototypic agonist for the μ receptor is morphine, for the κ receptor it is ketocyclazocine, and for the δ receptor it is the enkephalins. However, the synthesis of highly selective opioid agonists and antagonists has permitted the recognition of subtypes with different affinities for various ligands. At present, seven subtypes of opioid receptor have been characterized: μ1 and μ2; κ1, κ2, and κ3; and δ1 and δ2. A fourth class was formerly believed to exist, the σ receptor, but this is no longer considered to be an opioid receptor. The function of the δ receptor is still under investigation.

The various receptor types mentioned above have been cloned from the corresponding cDNA, and their amino acid structures have been determined. They have the structure characteristic of G protein–coupled receptors, with seven membrane-spanning regions (see Chapter 8). These

### Types of endogenous opioid peptides

A possible explanation for the lack of strict specificity of the opiates and synthetic opioids is that the different receptor types evolved as binding sites for various endogenous ligands, not for exogenous drugs. Once the receptors had been identified and isolated, it was possible to search for endogenous materials that would bind to them. To date, three groups of peptides have been discovered in the CNS, with properties similar to those of the opioid analgesics.

**Endorphins** are large peptides that are cleaved enzymatically from known protein hormones of the pituitary and hypothalamus. For example, β-endorphin consists of amino acids 61 to 91 of β-lipotropin (β-LPH).

**Enkephalins** are pentapeptides, and met-enkephalin (Tyr-Gly-Gly-Phe-Met) consists of amino acids 61 to 65 of β-LPH (i.e., 1 through 5 of β-endorphin; Fig. 19-3). Leu-enkephalin is the same as met-enkephalin except that it has a leucine in place of methionine.

**Dynorphin** is an intermediate-length peptide (17 amino acids), of which the first five amino acids are the same as those constituting leu-enkephalin.

These peptides are synthesized within the brain itself as large precursor proteins, which contain the opioid peptides and other neuroendocrine peptides as parts of their

**TABLE 19-1**  Types of Opioid Receptors, Their Prototypic Ligands, and Their Most Important Physiological Effects

| Receptor Type | Ligands Endogenous | Exogenous | Major Effects |
|---|---|---|---|
| **Mu** | | | |
| $\mu_1$ | β-Endorphin | Morphine<br>Hydromorphone<br>Etonitazene<br>Heroin | Supraspinal analgesia<br>Euphoria<br>Prolactin release<br>Miosis |
| $\mu_2$ | β-Endorphin (dynorphin?) | Morphine | Spinal analgesia<br>Inhibition of intestinal motility<br>Respiratory depression |
| **Kappa** | | | |
| $\kappa_1$ | Dynorphin | Ethylketocyclazocine<br>Pentazocine<br>Tifluadom | Hypothermia?<br>Miosis (weak)<br>Sedation<br>Spinal analgesia |
| $\kappa_2$ and $\kappa_3$ | | Nalorphine<br>Ethylketocyclazocine<br>Bremazocine | Supraspinal analgesia<br>Dysphoria<br>Hallucinations |
| **Delta** | | | |
| $\delta_1$ | met-Enkephalin | Etorphine<br>D-Pen$^2$-D-Pen$^5$-enkephalin | Spinal analgesia<br>Inhibition of smooth muscle |
| $\delta_2$ | | D-Ala$^2$-Glu$^4$-deltorphin<br>D-Ser$^2$,Leu$^5$-enkephalin-Thr$^6$ | Supraspinal analgesia |

amino acid sequences. The same precursor may occur at several sites in the brain but be split by different enzymes, thus giving rise to different products at different sites. For example, the precursor protein proopiomelanocortin (POMC) contains within itself the sequences of at least seven different peptide hormones or neuromodulators (see Fig. 19-3). However, enzymatic activity splits it primarily into β-lipotropin and adrenocorticotropic hormone (ACTH) in the anterior pituitary, but into β-endorphin and β-melanocyte-stimulating hormone (β-MSH) in the intermediate lobe of the rat pituitary (see also Chapter 48).

Unfortunately, these peptides have not proven to be specific for individual types of opioid receptors. β-Endorphin, for example, is almost equally active at μ and δ receptors, and somewhat less so at $\kappa_3$ receptors. Therefore, the functional significance of the various categories of receptors and peptides is still under investigation.

During the investigation of the molecular biology of opioid receptors, an "orphan" receptor was found that clearly resembled the opioid receptors in structure, but did not bind the opioid ligands and for which no function could be identified. A different peptide, named **orphanin FQ/nociceptin,** was later discovered that binds to this receptor and is not blocked by naloxone. The binding of nociceptin to its receptor produces neuronal inhibition by mechanisms similar to those of morphine, including inhibition of adenylyl cyclase and $Ca^{2+}$ currents and neuronal hyperpolarization by opening of $K^+$ channels. It was

at first thought to exert these effects on pain pathways (hence the name "nociceptin"), but it is now known to be very widely distributed throughout the nervous system and to exert its effects on a very large number of pathways. Its functional significance is still being studied.

### Regional distribution in the nervous system
The distribution of opioid receptors and opioid peptides is not uniform throughout the nervous system. Autoradiographic and binding data, together with studies of the effects of microinjection of opioids into specific loci in the nervous system, have shown that (1) receptors mediating analgesia are concentrated mainly in the dorsal horn of the spinal cord, the periaqueductal grey matter, and the thalamus; (2) those mediating effects on respiration, cough, vomiting, and pupillary diameter are concentrated in the ventral brainstem; (3) those affecting neuroendocrine secretion are mainly in the hypothalamus; and (4) those producing effects on mood and behaviour are mainly in the limbic structures (e.g., hippocampus, amygdala).

Within the brain, enkephalins are found in highest concentration in the striatum and nucleus accumbens; β-endorphin, in the hypothalamus, pituitary, and periaqueductal grey; and dynorphin, in anterior hypothalamus and substantia nigra. Lesser concentrations of all three are found in many other structures. β-Endorphin and ACTH appear to be released together from the anterior pituitary in response to stress, while dynorphin and vasopressin are co-released from the posterior pituitary by dehydration.

Opioid receptors are also found in the myenteric plexus of small intestine, the vas deferens, the lung, and possibly other peripheral tissues where opiates act. Enkephalins are found in the adrenal medulla and in axon terminals from various parts of the spinal cord, especially in areas with high concentrations of opiate receptors. They appear to be the natural transmitter that binds to the receptors inhibiting transmission of pain stimuli. Met-enkephalin is also found in the myenteric plexus, where it binds to the receptors that inhibit gut contractility by inhibiting release of acetylcholine.

Afferent pain stimuli arriving in the dorsal horn appear to activate ascending neurons of the spinothalamic tract by the release of excitatory amino acids, substance P, and other transmitters. Descending modulatory fibres from the central grey, the locus coeruleus, the nucleus raphe magnus, and other brain loci inhibit the transmission of afferent pain stimuli in the dorsal horn by the release of endogenous opioids, serotonin, noradrenaline, and other transmitters. The complex picture of interactions of the endogenous opioids with each other and with other neurotransmitters and modulators is still being filled in. However, enough is already known to provide a rational basis for the use of exogenous opioids, serotonin reuptake inhibitors, and other agents in the treatment of various types of pain (see also Chapter 25).

## Major Central Effects of the Opioids

### Neuronal activity
Opioids appear to act essentially as inhibitors of neuronal electrical activity, both spontaneous and evoked, and of neurotransmitter release. For example, single-unit recordings from the neocortex show that firing rates, both spontaneous and evoked by the excitatory transmitter glutamate, are reduced after local application of met-enkephalin, β-endorphin, or morphine. The decrease is promptly abolished by naloxone, an opioid-receptor blocker. Hippocampal pyramidal cells show *increased* activity under the influence of morphine, but this is because morphine blocks the inhibitory interneurons that are activated by recurrent collaterals from the pyramidal cell axons (Fig. 19-4). A similar process occurs at the axon terminals of sensory primary afferents entering the spinal cord, where morphine may block transmitter release and thus contribute to the analgesic effect. This locus of action is exploited in the technique of continuous epidural or intrathecal infusion of opioids that is used to maintain smooth, prolonged analgesia in patients while minimizing effects on the brain.

### Analgesia
Morphine relieves pain both by raising the threshold for pain perception and by diminishing the discomfort even if the pain is perceived (i.e., *increasing the pain tolerance*). Increase in pain threshold is readily measured experimentally (e.g., radiant heat, mechanical pressure), but pain tolerance is greatly affected by individual temperament, setting, and other factors. Narcotic analgesics have a greater effect on pain tolerance (which probably reflects action in the limbic system) than on pain threshold (which probably reflects action in the spinal cord and periaqueductal grey), so a patient can still be aware of the presence of pain but not be bothered or distressed by it.

The spinal and supraspinal mechanisms of opioid-induced analgesia interact synergistically. Thus, simultaneous administration of morphine by both systemic and spinal routes produces a marked increase in analgesic effect. Such synergism can also be shown between the actions of morphine at different sites in the brain, such as the periaqueductal grey and the nucleus raphe magnus. The mechanisms underlying these synergistic effects are not yet fully understood.

| TABLE 19-2 | Opioid Receptor Selectivity: Agonist, Partial Agonist, and Antagonist Actions at Different Classes of Opioid Receptor | | | | | |
|---|---|---|---|---|---|---|
| | **Receptor Types** | | | | | |
| Compound | μ1 | μ2 | κ1 | κ3 | δ1 | δ2 |
| Morphine | ++++ | +++ | + | + | 0/+ | 0/+ |
| Buprenorphine | P | | − | | − | |
| Nalorphine | − | − | P | P? | 0 | 0 |
| Nalbuphine | − | − | ++ | + | −? | |
| Pentazocine | −/P | − | +(P) | 0/+ | | |
| Ethylketocyclazocine | + | + | +++ | ++ | + | |
| met-Enkephalin | + | + | 0 | 0 | +++ | +++ |
| Naloxone | − − − | − − − | − − | − − | − | − |
| Naloxonazine | − − − | 0/− | | | | |
| β-Funaltrexamine | − − − | − − − | | | | |
| Naltrindole | | | | | | − − − |
| Naltriben | | | | | | − − − |
| 7-Benzylidene naltrexone (BNTX) | | | | | − − − | |
| Norbinaltorphimine | | | − − − | − − − | | |
| Quadazocine | | | − − − (κ2) | | | |
| Naloxone benzoylhydrazone | | | | − − − | | |

++++ = strongest agonist; + = weakest agonist; 0/−, 0/+ = dubious effect; − − − = strongest antagonist; − = weakest antagonist; 0 = no effect; P = partial agonist.

| FIGURE 19-3 | Schematic diagram of the relationships among the neuropeptides derived from proopiomelanocortin (POMC). (A) POMC contains the amino acid sequences of (1) γ-MSH, (2) ACTH, and (3) β-LPH; ACTH contains the sequence of (4) α-MSH; β-LPH contains the sequences of (5) β-MSH and (6) β-endorphin; β-endorphin contains the sequence of (7) met-enkephalin. All of these are marked off by pairs of basic amino acids (black vertical bars), which theoretically can serve as points of cleavage by various peptidases. (B) β-Endorphin also contains the sequences of γ-endorphin and des-tyrosine-γ-endorphin, but these are not marked off by cleavage points and are probably not formed from β-endorphin (see also Fig. 48-2, Chapter 48). |
|---|---|

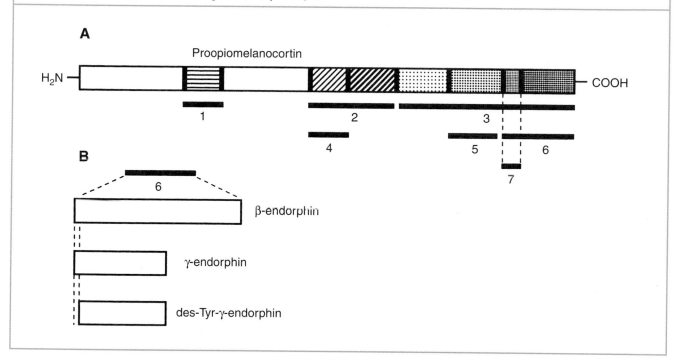

There are a number of other neuronal systems that can modulate the severity of pain by mechanisms distinct from that of the opioid analgesics. Tetrahydrocannabinol ($\Delta^9$-THC), the major psychoactive constituent of cannabis (see Chapter 26), also has significant analgesic activity of its own, and it can interact with morphine either additively or synergistically to improve the analgesic effect. Some of the tricyclic antidepressants (see Chapter 25) and newer anticonvulsants, especially carbamazepine and gabapentin (see Chapter 18), are used as accessory medication in the treatment of chronic neuropathic pain and can also enhance the effect of opioids.

Morphine relieves all types of pain—visceral, somatic, and cutaneous. It is more effective against dull, constant pains than against sharp, severe, intermittent ones.

### Respiratory depression

μ Receptor agonists have pronounced respiratory depressant activity. They cause a decreased sensitivity of the respiratory centre to $CO_2$. The major acute toxicity from morphine and other μ agonists is death from respiratory failure. The blood concentration in a large series of fatal overdoses varied widely, from 50 to 1200 ng/mL, but the modal concentration was 300 ng/mL when morphine was the only drug present, and 200 ng/mL if alcohol was also present. In patients with chronic respiratory disease (e.g., emphysema), morphine may be fatal. In all subjects, increased $P_{CO_2}$ tends to cause cerebral vasodilatation; this leads to an increase in cerebrospinal fluid (CSF) pressure, which may be exaggerated in the presence of head injury. The respiratory depressant effect of opioids is additive with that of alcohol, barbiturates, and other CNS depressants.

Respiratory depression has so far not been separable from the analgesic action of opioids. The two effects increase with dose in parallel fashion, and equianalgesic doses of different μ receptor agonists produce equal degrees of respiratory depression. This appears to be true even of the partial agonists and mixed agonist/antagonists. However, it has recently been reported that serotonin 5-HT$_{4A}$ agonists can reverse opioid-induced respiratory depression without decreasing the analgesic effect.

### Change in mood

Part of the analgesic effect is due to a foggy, unreal feeling of being "detached" from things. For some people, this is alarming or unpleasant; for others, it is a pleasant, relaxed, dreamy state (euphoria). Euphoria is a poor term because it means different things in relation to different drugs; for example, with amphetamines and cocaine, it means a sense of energy, power, and exhilaration; with the opioids, it means the dreamy, pleasant state just mentioned; with heroin and some other opioids taken intravenously, it includes, in addition, an intense visceral sensation of warmth and thrill that may be related to the peripheral actions. Not all opioids produce euphoria in all subjects, but they all produce the clouded state.

## Sedation

Not all opioids produce the same degree of sedation with equianalgesic doses, but most (especially μ agonists) produce some, and it appears to be part of the basic neurophysiological effect. The lesser sedative effect of methadone may possibly be due to protein binding, with slower onset of action; however, with repeated dosage, it causes marked sedation. Even opioids with marked excitatory action may cause convulsions alternating with periods of sedation. The sedative effect of opioids is *at least* additive with that of alcohol and other CNS depressants.

## Separate Central Effects

There are other actions that are not intimately related to the analgesic action. These effects may be produced to varying degrees by non-analgesic opiates such as papaverine or thebaine.

## Excitation

In cats, horses, pigs, cows, and a number of other species, and *in some humans, relatively low doses of morphine cause restlessness,* fright, hyperactivity, and fever. Higher doses may cause convulsions.

## Miosis

Miosis is seen in humans and in most species in which morphine is sedative. In species in which excitation occurs, mydriasis is noted. However, in the monkey, which is sedated by morphine, the pupils nevertheless dilate. Miosis is blocked by atropine and by decortication; therefore, it is thought to be due to removal of cortical inhibitory action on the third cranial nerve nucleus. (**Meperidine**, a synthetic opioid analgesic, is an exception in not causing pupil constriction.)

## Nausea and vomiting

Nausea and vomiting are due to stimulation of the chemoreceptor trigger zone and are aggravated by vestibular stimulation (e.g., turning the head suddenly) and by delayed gastric emptying, which is also produced by opioids. **Apomorphine,** *a non-analgesic derivative of opium, which is an agonist at dopamine receptors and not at opioid receptors, causes a much greater emetic effect than morphine*

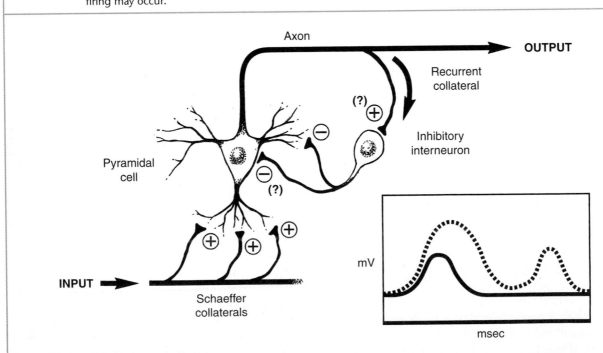

**FIGURE 19-4** Action of morphine on hippocampal pyramidal cell activity. Inhibition of synapse activity occurs either (?) at the excitatory synapse (+) of the recurrent collateral on the interneuron or at the inhibitory synapse (−) on the pyramidal cell. (Inset) As a result, the compound action potential (pyramidal cell output) evoked by excitatory stimulation of the Schaeffer collaterals is increased after morphine (---), compared to control conditions (——), and repetitive firing may occur.

*does,* and it is sometimes used deliberately to produce vomiting in some types of poisoning (see Chapter 72).

### Antitussive action

Direct depression of the cough centre is not related to respiratory depression. *Non-analgesic non-opioid derivatives* (e.g., **dextromethorphan**) can have antitussive action.

### Endocrine effects

Endocrine effects are produced by actions of the opioids in the thalamus and hypothalamus. These agents inhibit the release of luteinizing hormone–releasing hormone (LHRH; see Chapter 46), so the pituitary output of luteotropin (LH) and follicle-stimulating hormone (FSH) is diminished. This, in turn, decreases the secretion of testosterone by the testis and results in decreased libido, reduced volume of ejaculate, and decreased motility of sperm in males; in females, anovulatory cycles or amenorrhea occur. In contrast, serum prolactin level is raised, because the opioids inhibit the release of dopamine by hypothalamic neurons, which normally exert a tonic inhibitory influence on the prolactin secretory cells. In the past, it was thought that morphine stimulated release of vasopressin from the posterior lobe of the pituitary. Recent investigations, however, indicate that the direct effect is to inhibit vasopressin secretion; the antidiuresis caused by morphine apparently results from a peripheral action on the kidney.

### Poikilothermia

Most opioids inhibit the thermoregulatory mechanism centred in the preoptic anterior hypothalamic region. As a result, the ability to maintain a constant body temperature is impaired, and the direction and degree of change in body temperature depend on the ambient temperature. At normal or low room temperature, excessive heat loss to the environment occurs as a result of opioid action, and the body temperature falls. This action is enhanced by alcohol (see Chapter 22).

## Peripheral Effects

### Histamine release

Most opioids provoke the release of histamine, causing peripheral arteriolar and venous dilatation. This results in postural hypotension, cutaneous flushing, and increased loss of body heat.

**Venous dilatation** results partly from histamine release but mainly through neuronal action on vascular smooth muscle. It increases the capacity of the venous bed and decreases the venous return to the heart. This effect of morphine can be very helpful in the emergency treatment of acute left ventricular failure, although it is used much less frequently since the advent of potent loop diuretics such as furosemide (see Chapter 37). There is also evidence for the presence of opioid μ receptors in the alveolar walls, and their activation by morphine may inhibit the release of acetylcholine, thus contributing to relaxation of bronchioles and relief of dyspnea in patients with advanced malignancy. The use of nebulized morphine for this purpose is being investigated.

### Contraction of smooth muscle

Contraction of smooth muscle in the biliary and bladder sphincters is stimulated by morphine and other μ receptor agonists. The tone of the gastrointestinal and biliary tracts and of the ureter is increased, so the intraluminal pressure in these structures increases and there may be spasm. At the same time, inhibition of acetylcholine release from the myenteric plexus causes a marked reduction in propulsive peristaltic movement, resulting in constipation. This is the basis of the anti-diarrheal effect of opioids (see Chapter 42).

### Contact dermatitis and urticaria

Contact dermatitis and urticaria occur occasionally among nurses and pharmacists who handle the drugs frequently.

## Therapeutic Versus Adverse Effects

Most of the effects of opioids noted above can be regarded as therapeutically desirable under some circumstances and adverse under others. For example, the analgesic action is therapeutic when the drug is given for the relief of pathological or post-operative pain, but it may be an adverse effect if it masks the pain of an acute abdominal emergency such as a ruptured appendix or diverticulitis. Similarly, the inhibition of gastrointestinal motility is therapeutic when opioids are given to relieve a severe diarrhea, but it is an adverse effect when an opioid, given for the relief of pain, results in constipation and abdominal distension. Sedation contributes to the therapeutic effect when morphine is given for the relief of immediate post-operative pain, but it is an adverse effect at a somewhat later stage if it interferes with depth of breathing or with early ambulation.

In general, however, the effects most commonly used therapeutically are analgesia, sedation, anti-diarrheal effect, and cough suppression. The effects most often regarded as adverse or undesirable are respiratory depression, nausea and vomiting, hypothermia, constipation, and the effects of histamine release. A troublesome but very infrequent adverse effect is a muscular rigidity resembling that of parkinsonism, apparently resulting from opioid inhibition of dopamine release in the striatum (see Chapters 16 and 17). Some opioids, especially meperidine, produce serious interactions with monoamine oxidase inhibitors (see "Meperidine" below).

## THERAPEUTIC USES

The major therapeutic uses of opioids are consistent with the actions described above. They include the following:

- Relief of pain, both acute (e.g., obstetrical, traumatic, myocardial infarction, post-surgical) and chronic (e.g., musculoskeletal pain of various types, palliative care in metastatic cancer)
- Preoperative sedation, neuroleptanalgesia, and other special procedures
- Severe dyspnea, as in acute left ventricular failure
- Symptomatic treatment of diarrhea
- Suppression of the cough reflex
- Detoxification or maintenance therapy of opioid addiction

Further details of choice of agents and manner of use are given below in the description of individual opioids.

## FATE IN THE BODY

### Absorption

Opioids are generally well absorbed from the gastrointestinal tract as well as from parenteral sites, especially the more lipid-soluble ones such as heroin, which was formerly given by mouth as a cough suppressant. Methadone is normally given by mouth in methadone maintenance therapy of opioid addicts, and codeine, $d$-propoxyphene, tramadol, and others are given by mouth for the relief of mild or moderate pain. However, there is a significant first-pass metabolism in the gastrointestinal tract and liver, so bioavailability is appreciably less after oral administration than after parenteral injection. For example, after a single oral dose of morphine, only 15 to 30% reaches the systemic circulation. As a result, the oral dose required for analgesia is initially about six times as large as the intravenous or intramuscular dose. In contrast, the oral to parenteral ratio for codeine is only 1.5:1. During chronic oral administration of morphine, however, the ratio falls to 3:1 or 2:1. This increase in oral potency may be due to the accumulation of an active metabolite of morphine (see "Metabolism" below).

After intramuscular injection, the rate of absorption is somewhat variable, but peak serum concentration and analgesic response are attained within 10 to 20 minutes. However, because of the short half-life, repeated injections every 3 to 4 hours are required to maintain pain relief. The advantages of oral administration are avoidance of the discomfort of injections and a more prolonged and smooth effect; the disadvantage is slowness of onset. When opioids are being given chronically, however, as for continuous relief of chronic pain in cancer patients, slowness of onset is not really relevant because doses are given frequently enough to produce continuous analgesia. This is facilitated by the use of sustained-release oral preparations, which, combined with the gradual increase in oral potency mentioned above, frequently permit effective analgesia with twice-a-day or once-a-day oral dosage.

### Distribution

Morphine enters all tissues. In adults, relatively little enters the brain because the N is ionized at normal plasma pH. In infants, whose **blood–brain barrier** is less effective, morphine enters more readily, so infants are more susceptible to its action. Morphine also diffuses across the **gastric mucosa** into the lumen of the stomach, where the acidity converts it into the ionized form, which cannot diffuse back across the mucosa into the blood. As a result, morphine accumulates in the lumen, a process known as "ion trapping." For this reason, gastric lavage used to be employed in the emergency treatment of morphine overdose (before naloxone became available), even when the drug had been given parenterally.

Morphine and other opioids also diffuse readily across the **placenta** into the fetal circulation. For example, after administration of meperidine to pregnant women in labour, equilibrium of drug concentration in the maternal and fetal circulations is reached in 6 minutes. Since hepatic drug-metabolizing enzyme activity is very low in the fetus and newborn, the major route of elimination of opioids from the fetus is back-diffusion across the placenta into the maternal circulation. Therefore, if the infant is born too soon after the mother has received meperidine, the drug cannot be eliminated rapidly enough, and severe respiratory depression can occur in the infant.

**Onset of analgesic action** is usually quite rapid after subcutaneous or intramuscular injection, especially with the more lipid-soluble opioids. The time may range from 5 to 15 minutes, depending on the drug, dose, and route. After intravenous injection, the effect begins almost immediately. Continuous subcutaneous or intravenous infusion by means of a portable pump is being tested for the relief of chronic pain, especially in ambulatory cancer patients.

**Protein binding of opioids** in the plasma varies quite markedly from drug to drug. At therapeutic concentrations, morphine is about 30% bound, meperidine about 60%, and methadone about 85%. This difference probably contributes to the disparity of apparent half-life, for example, 2 to 3 hours for morphine and 15 to 22 hours for methadone. However, the dosages for the various opioids are adjusted accordingly, so the usual duration of analgesic effect is about 4 hours for most of them.

## Metabolism

Metabolism also varies with the drug. For morphine, biotransformation is fairly rapid and consists mostly of glucuronic acid conjugation of the 3- and 6-hydroxyl groups by the hepatic smooth endoplasmic reticulum. About 90% of a dose is found as glucuronide in the urine and 7 to 10% in the feces (via the bile). The elimination half-life by all routes ranges from 1.4 to 3.4 hours, and the elimination is first-order over a wide range of concentrations.

The major product is morphine-3-glucuronide, but morphine-6β-glucuronide constitutes a significant fraction of the total. Because of first-pass metabolism in the liver, there is a higher plasma concentration of the 6β-glucuronide after an oral dose of morphine than after the same dose given parenterally. The 6β-glucuronide has a high affinity for the μ receptor and is even more potent an analgesic than morphine itself. Moreover, it has a considerably longer half-life than morphine, so the area under the concentration–time curve is relatively greater for morphine-6β-glucuronide. The fraction of the total analgesic action of a dose of morphine that may be due to the 6β-glucuronide is variable; it may be as high as 66% at low doses but decreases as the total morphine dose increases. Since the glucuronide is more polar than morphine, it crosses the blood–brain barrier into the CNS more slowly than morphine but also leaves more slowly. Therefore, it tends to accumulate gradually, both centrally and peripherally, during chronic morphine treatment, and this is probably an important factor in the increase in oral potency of morphine during chronic administration. Enterohepatic circulation may also play a small role: the glucuronides are excreted in the bile but are partially broken down by bacterial enzymes in the large bowel, releasing free morphine, which can be reabsorbed into the circulation.

With other opioids, *N*-demethylation, hydrolysis, cyclization, and other reactions are quantitatively important, depending on the individual drug. Heroin (diacetylmorphine), for example, is rapidly hydrolyzed to monoacetylmorphine and morphine. Liver disease may reduce the rate of elimination of various opioids and lead to overdose as a result of accumulation of active drug or active metabolite. Renal disease can lead to accumulation of normeperidine, a toxic metabolite of meperidine.

## DOSAGE

There is a huge variation among individual patients in the dosage required for adequate relief of pain. Several studies of large groups of cancer patients have shown that the required dosage may vary from 10 to 1700 mg/24 hours (median dose 80 mg) for oral administration, and from 10 to 1200 mg/24 hours (median 115 mg) for subcutaneous administration. Similar variation is found in the effective steady-state plasma level (oral route: 1 to 2560 nmol/L, median 60 nmol/L; subcutaneous route: 3 to 1680 nmol/L, median 179 nmol/L). These huge variations reflect individual differences in pain intensity, pain tolerance, drug metabolism, other medications used, and so forth. Therefore, there is no recommended dosage or plasma concentration; each patient's dosage must be titrated against the individual requirements and tolerance for the drug.

## Patient-Controlled Analgesia (PCA)

A number of devices that permit such titration have been marketed, consisting essentially of a pump for injecting opioid solution, a switch that the patient can operate to activate the pump, and control equipment by which the physician or nurse can preset the size of the dose, the minimum interval between doses, and the maximum number of doses in a defined period of time. Such equipment can be used for intravenous, subcutaneous, or epidural administration of the drug. It is simple enough that it can be used in children as well as adults. PCA can be used as the sole method of administration of opioid, or it can be used to provide supplementary analgesia on top of a basal level provided in the conventional manner.

The main advantages of PCA are that it permits the patient to titrate dosage against the individual severity of pain and provides a more even and continuous analgesia, avoiding the wide fluctuations between maximum and minimum plasma levels that can occur when successive doses are given at fixed time intervals. Patient satisfaction is correspondingly greater. However, several studies have indicated that the total amount of opioid required may not differ in PCA versus conventional administration, and the frequency of adverse effects does not appear to differ greatly. Indeed, some types of complication, such as adynamic ileus (intestinal paralysis) or urinary retention due to bladder paralysis by opioids, are more common in patients treated with PCA than with conventional opioid therapy. This probably reflects the more constant level of opioid-induced suppression of acetylcholine release, without intervals in which recovery can occur.

## Extended-Release Preparations

While PCA is widely used in hospitals, it is less suitable for home use or for ambulatory patients. To achieve comparably prolonged smooth analgesia in such cases, a variety of oral and other preparations have been developed.

### Oral preparations

These consist essentially of morphine adsorbed onto micropellets of inert material and covered with a synthetic polymer of selected porosity and thickness, which slows the dissolution and diffusion of the morphine. The pellets are incorporated into capsules or tablets, from which the morphine release is slowed and greatly prolonged. Alternatively, the morphine can be bound to small beads of ion exchange resin and suspended in a liquid medium for people who cannot swallow capsules or tablets. The $T_{max}$ (the time required to reach maximum plasma concentration of the drug) is about 1 hour in instant-release preparations, but if it is prolonged to 3 to 4 hours, it permits twice-a-day dosage (MS-Contin and others), and if prolonged to about 9 hours (Avinza, Kapanol, and others) it permits once-daily dosage (Fig. 19-5).

### Rectal preparations

The oral preparations described above can be used rectally, but they are less convenient than a specially formulated suppository in which the morphine is contained in a high-viscosity complex of calcium and sodium alginate that controls the rate of morphine release.

### Percutaneous absorption

The more highly lipid-soluble opioids, such as fentanyl, can be administered as cutaneous patches (see below).

# OTHER ROUTES OF ADMINISTRATION

The most common routes by which opioids are administered to patients by physicians or nurses are the intravenous, intramuscular, and subcutaneous routes; oral administration may also be used by medical or nursing attendants or by the patient or family members. The advantages and disadvantages of these routes have been mentioned above. In recent years, however, epidural or intrathecal administration and percutaneous absorption have become more widely used, and additional routes of administration are being explored.

## Epidural or Intrathecal Administration

Injection and infusion of opioids into the spinal epidural space through which the sensory nerve roots pass, or (much less frequently) directly into the spinal subarachnoid space, are now used in many centres to produce localized analgesia with a reduced risk of respiratory depression, drowsiness, and the other undesired effects. These methods make use of the existence of spinal mechanisms of analgesia noted above. They provide excellent post-operative pain relief, but a small percentage of patients do suffer serious respiratory depression from opioids used in this way.

In the case of intrathecal injection, respiratory depression is usually the result of an overdose. It is more likely to occur if supplementary systemic opioids are given as well. The estimated frequency of this complication is as high as

5% after intrathecal administration but not more than 0.3% after epidural administration. Redistribution of opioid from the injection site toward the brainstem is well demonstrated with morphine but is much less likely with more lipid-soluble opioids that can diffuse more readily into the blood vessels and be carried away from the CNS.

## Percutaneous Absorption

Transdermal patches (see Chapter 2) of fentanyl (Duragesic) provide effective delivery of amounts that are sufficient for sustained analgesia in patients with chronic cancer pain. Drug from the patch forms a depot in the skin, from which it diffuses slowly into the capillary circulation. Therefore, the onset of action is slow (12 to 16 hours), but the half-life is very prolonged (16 to 22 hours after removal of the patch). The effect is evenly sustained, and patch application can be repeated once every 3 days.

Patches containing different doses of fentanyl permit gradation of the opioid effects. This route of administration has a lower incidence of constipation, nausea, vomiting, and drowsiness than oral or parenteral administration and a lower frequency of break-through pain requiring supplementary medication. However, if overdose occurs, the effects are also long-lasting and may require repeated administration of naloxone for a day or more after removal of the patch.

## Nasal Administration

Pharmacokinetic studies of nasal spray administration of a variety of opioids have been carried out in healthy volunteers and in post-operative patients. Onset times for

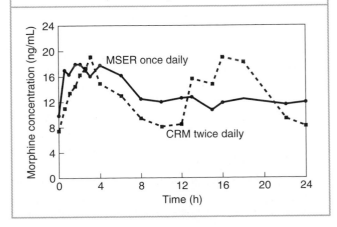

**FIGURE 19-5** Steady-state mean plasma concentration–time profiles of morphine, normalized to a total daily dose of 100 mg, after administration of two sustained-release oral preparations: controlled-release morphine (CRM) twice daily, and morphine sulfate extended release (MSER) once daily. (From Portenoy et al., 2002. Reprinted with permission.)

analgesic effect are fairly rapid but variable. Much developmental work is still required in relation to the spray devices and the formulation of the opioid preparations, but this appears to be a promising route for PCA.

## TOLERANCE AND PHYSICAL DEPENDENCE

Tolerance to the effects of morphine develops rapidly on repeated administration, and larger and larger doses are required for the same effect (see Chapter 70). In animal experiments, continuous slow intravenous infusion of morphine for as little as 4 hours can produce some tolerance. Human addicts can stand many times the normal acute lethal dose without respiratory arrest.

The development of tolerance is usually accompanied by the development of physical dependence. Compensatory changes in the cell are unmasked by removal of opiates and a picture of hyper-excitability is seen: restlessness, extreme anxiety, vomiting and diarrhea, runny nose, muscle twitching, chills, fever and sweating, pupillary dilation, and sometimes circulatory collapse. This picture varies in time of onset and in severity after withdrawal of different opiates, but it can be precipitated almost immediately by opiate antagonists. It can be abolished by giving more narcotic analgesic. (The ability of a new opiate to abolish morphine withdrawal symptoms in human volunteers is used as a method of assessing dependence liability of the new drug; see Chapter 70.)

A number of **hypothetical mechanisms** have been proposed to explain the development of opiate tolerance and physical dependence.

1. If the drug blocks release of a neurotransmitter, postsynaptic receptors for that transmitter might be induced or their sensitivity might be increased, thereby compensating for the drug effect (i.e., tolerance). Withdrawal of the drug would allow normal release of transmitter, but increased receptor numbers and sensitivity would cause excessive postsynaptic effects (i.e., withdrawal reaction). So far, no good evidence of supersensitivity to acetylcholine, catecholamines, or serotonin has been found in opiate-dependent subjects. However, increased sensitivity to noradrenaline following opioid withdrawal appears to be responsible for some of the more obvious and uncomfortable withdrawal symptoms, such as anxiety, gooseflesh (the source of the term "cold turkey"), intestinal cramps, and disturbances in body temperature. These symptoms can be relieved by administration of **clonidine,** an $\alpha_2$-adrenoceptor agonist (see Chapters 13 and 14) that decreases the release of catecholamines from presynaptic terminals.

2. An enzyme that is acutely inhibited by the opiates might undergo compensatory induction. As noted above, opioid agonists acutely inhibit adenylyl cyclase activity and reduce cAMP levels in brain cells. In tolerant animals, the adenylyl cyclase increases and cAMP levels return to normal; in the withdrawal reaction, they are both above normal. However, there is so far no proof that changes in adenylyl cyclase and cAMP cause the tolerance, rather than reflect it.

3. If the drug blocks release of a neurotransmitter, the transmitter might theoretically accumulate intracellularly until its concentration is high enough to overcome the block (tolerance). Withdrawal of the drug would allow massive release of the accumulated transmitter. However, there is no evidence for such a mechanism.

4. More than one neuronal pathway might serve the same physiological function (redundancy). If the major one is inhibited by opiates and the minor one is not, the minor one might hypertrophy and compensate for the drug effect. When the drug is withdrawn, both pathways would function, causing excessive activity. Again, there is no evidence to demonstrate the importance of such a mechanism.

5. High doses of exogenous opioids would lead to a loss (down-regulation) of their receptors, causing tolerance. At the same time, the excessive presence of the drug would cause a feedback inhibition of the biosynthesis and release of endogenous opioid peptides. Withdrawal of the exogenous opioids would leave a deficiency of the endogenous peptides and their receptors (withdrawal reaction) until re-adaptation occurred. A decreased rate of synthesis of β-endorphin has recently been reported in morphine-tolerant rats, but there is no evidence of change in receptors during tolerance, although there is cross-tolerance between morphine and the opioid peptides.

*Tolerance and physical dependence are not the same as addiction.* A normal subject can be made physically dependent but after going through a withdrawal reaction will not resume drug-taking. Addiction also involves a compulsion to take the drug again after going through withdrawal (i.e., a strong psychological dependence on it). Drug dependence is covered in detail in Chapter 70.

## MORPHINE CONGENERS

**Codeine** is a relatively weak analgesic, having one-tenth the potency of morphine and, consequently, shows little respiratory depression and relatively little addiction liability. About 10 to 15% of a codeine dose is metabolically converted into morphine in the human body, and this fraction accounts for the analgesic activity. The conversion is carried out by CYP2D6 (see Chapter 4), and this enzyme is genetically polymorphic with some of the variant forms being deficient in metabolic activity. In about 4 to 10% of Caucasians, both genes for CYP2D6 encode for forms deficient in activity, and these individuals are therefore unable to derive any analgesic effect from codeine, but they also have reduced risk of becoming dependent on it. Most of the antitussive effect is thought to be due to codeine itself rather than to its metabolites. It is used widely in combination with non-opioid analgesics such as acetaminophen and acetylsalicylic acid (ASA), and as a cough suppressant in doses of 10 to 15 mg. Codeine undergoes relatively little first-pass metabolism in the liver, so it is about 60% as potent by mouth as by parenteral injection.

**Hydrocodone** (Hycodan and others), a derivative of codeine, is particularly effective as an analgesic, being as potent as morphine, and it is also commonly used as an antitussive.

Most of the **semi-synthetic morphine derivatives** are fairly old. Of these, **heroin** is twice as potent as morphine in terms of its initial effects. The addict likes heroin because its high lipid solubility enables it to enter the brain much more rapidly than morphine, and its initial action is more intense. However, the later effects are the same as those of morphine, because it is converted to morphine in the body. Because of narcotic control regulations, heroin is no longer available for clinical use in the United States. In Canada, its use is limited to the control of chronic intractable pain in terminal cancer.

**Hydromorphone** (Dilaudid) has strong analgesic and antitussive activity; it is more potent than morphine and codeine, respectively, on a weight basis. It is better absorbed than morphine following oral administration, with an onset of analgesic action in about 15 minutes and a duration of action of more than 5 hours. This drug can therefore be given by mouth as well as by subcutaneous or intramuscular injection, and as rectal suppositories.

**Levorphanol** (Levo-Dromoran) is one of the more potent **synthetic analgesics** presently in wide use; it is four to five times as potent as morphine. It is less constipating than morphine and is longer-acting. This drug has a levo-rotatory structure; its dextro-rotatory isomer, **dextrorphan**, has no analgesic activity but is an effective antitussive. Similarly, **levomethorphan** is an analgesic, whereas **dextromethorphan** is not, but it is widely used in cough mixtures in adult doses of 10 to 30 mg.

**Meperidine** (pethidine; Demerol and others) is the first and perhaps still most widely used synthetic congener. It is a relatively old preparation and has many trade names. The chemical structure resembles that of atropine as well as that of morphine (Fig. 19-6), and it was originally believed to be an anti-spasmodic rather than a constrictor of smooth muscle like morphine. However, this is now known to be false; it does cause spasm. Its action is shorter than that of morphine, and it is less potent by a factor of about 10. In equianalgesic doses, it causes at least as much respiratory depression as morphine. Meperidine does not produce miosis and is, therefore, a favourite of addicted nurses and doctors (it is less likely to be detected). It is quite effective when given by mouth. Normeperidine, a metabolite of meperidine, causes CNS excitatory effects and can produce seizures.

Meperidine is especially likely to interact adversely with monoamine oxidase inhibitors (MAOIs; see Chapter 25) to produce a severe and potentially fatal syndrome characterized by coma, hyperpyrexia, and hypotension. This interaction appears to have two components: (1) the MAOIs inhibit meperidine N-demethylase and thus potentiate the action of meperidine, and (2) meperidine inhibits the neuronal uptake of serotonin and thus potentiates the effect of the MAOIs. The excessive concentration of free 5-HT is probably responsible for the hyperpyrexia. Morphine is much less likely than meperidine to interact with MAOIs in this way.

Two analogues of meperidine, **loperamide** and **diphenoxylate**, are mainly ionized at physiological pH and therefore do not cross the blood–brain barrier readily. They are used for their peripheral effects, principally on μ receptors in the gastrointestinal tract, where they act to inhibit acetylcholine release and thus reduce or arrest peristaltic contractions. They are used to treat diarrhea and fecal incontinence (see Chapter 42).

**Methadone** (Dolophine; see Fig. 19-6) has about the same analgesic potency as morphine but differs from it essentially in two respects. It has a much longer duration of action because it is more slowly eliminated from the body, and in single doses it causes little sedation. The lack of sedative effect did detract from its original popularity. However, because of its much slower clearance from the body, its withdrawal effects are much milder than those of morphine. The main current use of methadone is, therefore, to substitute for morphine in addicts prior to withdrawal.

**FIGURE 19-6** Structural formulae of methadone and meperidine.

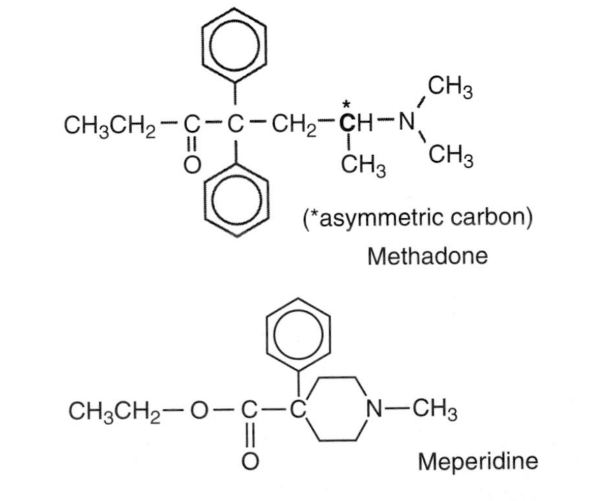

In the 1960s, V. Dole and M. Nyswander began testing the use of **long-term methadone maintenance for the management of opiate addiction.** The purpose is to maintain a sufficiently high level of tolerance that the addict's usual dose of heroin or other opioid produces little or no "high," so there is no inducement to continue taking it. The patients are kept on methadone for months or years while undergoing psychological and social rehabilitation. Between 50 and 80% of patients in well-run methadone maintenance programs continue in treatment and show significant improvement in social and work performance. In the most successful cases, methadone dosage can be gradually reduced and eventually withdrawn, replaced in some cases by naltrexone (see "Opioid Antagonists" below) to prevent a return to heroin.

**Oxycodone** (OxyIR and others) is a semi-synthetic derivative of morphine with a methoxy substituent in place of the hydroxyl on C3 so that it is resistant to 3-glucuronidation. Oral preparations are also available containing oxycodone combined with non-steroidal anti-inflammatory analgesics (Percodan, Oxycocet, and others). Oxycodone is better absorbed orally than morphine, with higher oral bioavailability. Its analgesic and other actions are similar to those of morphine, but its major metabolism is by hepatic CYP2D6, so its toxicity is increased by liver disease. It is widely used orally for chronic pain relief but has also found its way into illicit traffic for non-medical use.

**Propoxyphene** (Darvon) is a commonly used analgesic structurally related to methadone but 12 to 15 times less potent. In equianalgesic doses, it has properties similar to those of the other opioid analgesics.

**Tramadol** (Ultram) is widely used in many countries for oral relief of mild to moderate pain, but it is not available in Canada. It is a synthetic 4-phenyl-piperidine analogue of codeine, which is almost completely absorbed by mouth, with 70% systemic bioavailability and 30% removal by first-pass hepatic metabolism. It is available in oral, rectal, intramuscular, and intravenous formulations; the oral capsules have a $T_{max}$ of 2 hours, the sustained-release oral tablets about 5 hours. The recommended oral dose is 50 to 100 mg every 4 to 6 hours. The drug is metabolized mainly by CYP2D6, forming numerous metabolites that are then conjugated by glucuronidation and sulfation reactions. The elimination half-life is about 5 hours for the parent drug and about 9 hours for the first metabolite. One of the phase 1 metabolites, $O$-desmethyltramadol, is pharmacologically active and may make some small contribution to the analgesic effect.

Tramadol is produced as a racemic mixture, and both isomers contribute to the analgesic effect but by different mechanisms. The (+) isomer is a weak agonist at μ receptors and also stimulates the presynaptic release of serotonin and blocks its reuptake. The (–) isomer blocks presynaptic $\alpha_2$ receptors, thus increasing the release of noradrenaline, and it also blocks its reuptake. The raised synaptic levels of 5-HT and noradrenaline decrease the excitability of spinal pain pathways, and this action is synergistic with the analgesic effect of the μ receptor activation. Tramadol is used for both acute and chronic pain; its analgesic effect is comparable to that of codeine and less than that of codeine–NSAID combinations.

The main adverse effects are also a combination of opioid and monoaminergic symptoms. Its opioid adverse effects include constipation, nausea, potentiation of alcohol and other sedatives, and fatigue (though less than with other opioids); at higher doses, it can give rise to seizures, hallucinations, and confusion. Its monoaminergic side effects include postural hypotension, dizziness, sweating, and dry mouth.

**Fentanyl** (Sublimaze), **sufentanil** (Sufenta), **alfentanil** (Alfenta), and **remifentanil** (Ultiva) are chemically related to meperidine. They are all strong analgesics, with potency ratios (relative to morphine) of about 80:1, 800:1, 20:1, and 800:1, respectively. They produce all the other effects that morphine does in about the same ratio as the analgesia. The main advantages of these agents are that, when given intravenously, they have almost immediate onset of action and a short duration; for example, the half-life of the redistribution phase of fentanyl is only 12.5 minutes, and the effective half-life of remifentanil is 3 to 4 minutes. Therefore, they lend themselves very well to **neuroleptanalgesia** (see Chapter 20). Fentanyl is injected intravenously in a dose of 1 μg/kg mixed with droperidol or a similar neuroleptic, and supplementary doses of 50 to 100 μg are given intravenously every 30 to 45 minutes during surgery. An important advantage of fentanyl is that it causes very little depression of left ventricular function, so it carries only a small risk of hypotension during surgery. However, there is some danger of drug accumulation if doses are repeated too frequently. Because of the short half-life, the patient can wake up rapidly when the surgery is over and have little difficulty with respiratory depression and constipation post-operatively. Sufentanil, alfentanil, and remifentanil are used for the same purpose. Except for remifentanil, these drugs are also used frequently for continuous epidural analgesia in PCA regimens and in transdermal delivery systems.

High doses or rapid infusion of fentanyl and its derivatives tend to produce muscular rigidity, perhaps by action at enkephalin receptors in the striatum, which may inhibit dopamine release there. The effect can be overcome by muscle relaxants, neuromuscular blockers, or by naloxone (see below).

## OPIOID ANTAGONISTS

In the morphine molecule (see Fig. 19-1), the methyl group attached to the N atom is of critical dimensions for agonist activity when the molecule has combined with its receptor. If the CH₃ is changed to an allyl group, or if a cyclopropyl or cyclobutyl group is attached to the methyl, the molecule still binds to the receptor but no longer initiates a typical morphine response. It therefore functions as a receptor blocker, or opioid antagonist. Replacement of the OH at C-6 of morphine by a ketonic oxygen results in a highly specific and powerful blocking action.

**Naloxone** (Narcan; Fig. 19-7) is said to be a pure opioid antagonist since it has no analgesic activity of its own but has the ability to reverse or block the actions of opioid analgesic agonists. It has the greatest affinity for μ receptors, where it prevents or reverses the activity not only of morphine and its congeners but also of β-endorphins and enkephalins. It is less effective as a blocker of κ and δ receptors.

**Naltrexone** (Trexan; see Fig. 19-7) is a related compound that is also a pure blocker, but it has a much longer half-life than naloxone and is well absorbed when given by mouth.

When given together with morphine, these drugs antagonize many of its important actions, including analgesia, respiratory depression, euphoria, increase in CSF pressure, miosis, smooth muscle spasm, and hypotension. Their **clinical uses** are (1) reversal of the respiratory depression caused by morphine-like drugs; (2) diagnostic testing in opioid addicts, in whom they precipitate an acute withdrawal reaction; and (3) treatment of addicts, after they have been withdrawn from opioids, to prevent the "high" from self-administered heroin or morphine and thus to decrease the risk of relapse. They are also used as supplementary therapy to help prevent relapse in alcoholism (see Chapter 22). Overdose effects of tramadol are only partially reversed by naloxone, and blockers of 5-HT and α-adrenergic receptors are required to complete the reversal.

## MIXED AGONISTS/ANTAGONISTS AND PARTIAL AGONISTS

Opioids with allyl or 4- or 5-carbon substituents on the N atom, but that retain the OH group at C-6, display a mixture of agonist and antagonist properties. Examples include nalorphine and nalbuphine. Pentazocine is a synthetic analogue with similar properties (Fig. 19-8).

**Nalorphine** (Nalline) and **levallorphan** (Lorfan) act as μ receptor blockers, preventing the analgesic, respiratory depressant, and euphoriant actions of morphine. However, they are weak agonists at κ receptors and therefore have some analgesic and sedating effects when given by themselves. When given in larger doses, they cause agitation, dysphoria, and hallucinations. Therefore, they carry a lower risk of abuse and dependence than μ receptor agonists do.

**Pentazocine** (Talwin), **cyclazocine**, and **nalbuphine** (Nubain) are also mixed agonists/antagonists that have

some morphine-antagonist (μ receptor–blocking) effect but that exert reasonably good analgesic action through κ receptors. Their mental effects seem to be intermediate between those of morphine and nalorphine. They do not cause severe mental disturbance as nalorphine does, but they are less likely than morphine to produce euphoria (see Table 19-2).

**Buprenorphine** has a cyclopropylmethyl substituent on the N atom, the same as that of naltrexone, and an OCH₃ group like that of codeine in place of the OH on C-6. These offset each other to some extent so that, instead of being a μ receptor blocker, it is a partial μ receptor agonist. This means that it has some morphine-like action, but the maximum response attainable is considerably less than that of morphine, no matter how much the dose is increased. Thus, when it competes with morphine or heroin for μ receptors, it can reduce their maximum effect. It has been suggested that this makes it less attractive to addicts and less likely to be abused. It has been approved for use in the maintenance treatment of heroin addicts (see Chapter 70).

**FIGURE 19-7** Structural formulae of two potent opioid antagonists. Compare these with Figure 19-1. Numbers designate the C-3 and C-6 positions.

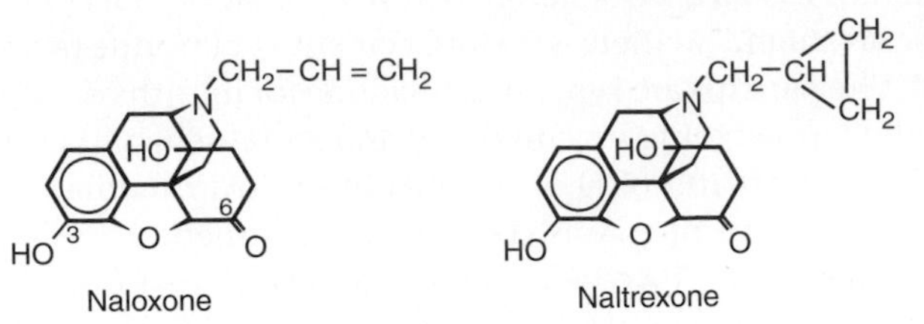

**FIGURE 19-8** Structural formulae of some mixed agonist/antagonist opioids that act as μ receptor blockers, but as agonists at κ and/or σ receptors.

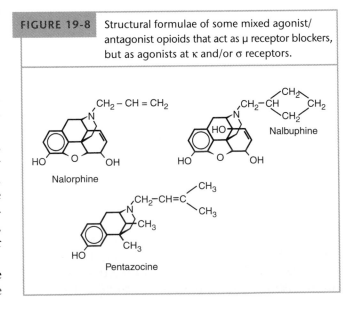

## FINAL COMMENT

The field of opioid peptides, opioid receptors, and synthetic opioids is undergoing rapid change as a result of continuing research. Over the next few years, there will probably be major developments permitting better separation of analgesic, euphoriant, endocrine, and other effects and, therefore, better therapeutic specificity.

## SUGGESTED READINGS

Adler MW, Geller EB, Rogers TJ, et al. Opioids, receptors, and immunity. *Adv Exp Med Biol.* 1993;335:13-20.

Collins SL, Faura CC, Moore RA, et al. Peak plasma concentrations after oral morphine: a systematic review. *J Pain Symptom Manage.* 1998;16:388-402.

Cross SA. Pathophysiology of pain. *Mayo Clin Proc.* 1994;69: 375-383.

Dale O, Hjortkjaer R, Kharasch ED. Nasal administration of opioids for pain management in adults. *Acta Anaesthesiol Scand.* 2002;46:759-770.

Dhawan BN, Cesselin F, Raghubir R, et al. International Union of Pharmacology. XII. Classification of opioid receptors. *Pharmacol Rev.* 1996;48:567-592.

Fowler CJ, Fraser GL. Mu-, delta-, kappa-opioid receptors and their subtypes. A critical review with emphasis on radioligand binding experiments. *Neurochem Int.* 1994;24:401-426.

Gilron I, Bailey JM, Tu D, et al. Morphine, gabapentin, or their combination for neuropathic pain. *New Engl J Med.* 2005;352: 1324-1334.

Heinricher MM. Orphanin FQ/nociceptin: from neural circuitry to behavior. *Life Sci.* 2003;73:813-822.

Klepstad P, Dale O, Kaasa S, et al. Influences on serum concentrations of morphine, M6G and M3G during routine clinical drug monitoring: a prospective survey in 300 adult cancer patients. *Acta Anaesthesiol Scand.* 2003;47:725-731.

Knapp RJ, Malatynska E, Collins N, et al. Molecular biology and pharmacology of cloned opioid receptors. *FASEB J.* 1995;9: 516-525.

Kornick CA, Santiago-Palma J, Moryl N, et al. Benefit-risk assessment of transdermal fentanyl for the treatment of chronic pain. *Drug Safety.* 2003;26:951-973.

Lugo RA, Kern SE. Clinical pharmacokinetics of morphine. *J Pain Palliat Care Pharmacother.* 2002;16:5-18.

Martin WR. Pharmacology of opioids. *Pharmacol Rev.* 1983;35: 283-323.

Mixed agonist-antagonist analgesics [special issue]. *Drug Alcohol Depend.* 1985;14(3-4):221-431.

Murthy BR, Pollack GM, Brouwer KL. Contribution of morphine-6-glucuronide to antinociception following intravenous administration of morphine to healthy volunteers. *J Clin Pharmacol.* 2002;42:569-576.

Payne R. Role of epidural and intrathecal narcotics and peptides in the management of cancer pain. *Med Clin North Am.* 1987;71(2):313-327.

Portenoy RK, Sciberras A, Eliot L, et al. Steady-state pharmacokinetic comparison of a new, extended-release, once-daily morphine formulation, Avinza, and a twice-daily controlled-release morphine formulation in patients with chronic moderate-to-severe pain. *J Pain Symptom Manage.* 2002;23:292-300.

Quigley C, Joel S, Patel N, et al. Plasma concentrations of morphine, morphine-6-glucuronide and morphine-3-glucuronide and their relationship with analgesia and side effects in patients with cancer-related pain. *Palliat Med.* 2003;17:185-190.

Schug SA, Zech D, Grond S. Adverse effects of systemic opioid analgesics. *Drug Safety.* 1992;7:200-213.

Smith AP, Lee NM. Opioid receptor interactions: local and nonlocal, symmetric and asymmetric, physical and functional. *Life Sci.* 2003;73:1873-1893.

Takemori AE, Portoghese PS. Selective naltrexone-derived opioid receptor antagonists. *Annu Rev Pharmacol Toxicol.* 1992;32: 239-269.

Tyndale RF, Droll KP, Sellers EM. Genetically deficient CYP2D6 metabolism provides protection against oral opiate dependence. *Pharmacogenetics.* 1997;7:375-379.

Yaksh TL. Pharmacology and mechanisms of opioid analgesic activity. *Acta Anaesthesiol Scand.* 1997;41:94-111.

Zaveri N. Peptide and nonpeptide ligands for the nociceptin/orphanin FQ receptor OPL1: research tools and potential therapeutic agents. *Life Sci.* 2003;73:663-678.

# 20

# General Anaesthetics

## FJL CARMICHAEL, DA HAAS, AND VWS CHAN

**CASE HISTORY**

A 19-year-old woman was having an operation to remove four impacted wisdom teeth under general anaesthesia. She was fit and healthy, as were her parents and siblings. She had no allergies and was taking no medication.

The patient was given an intravenous injection of fentanyl (50 µg) and a precurarizing dose of *d*-tubocurarine (3 mg). Induction of anaesthesia was carried out with an intravenous injection of propofol (2 mg/kg). Following the administration of propofol, her blood pressure fell to 80/50 mmHg and her heart rate rose to 115 beats/min. When fully unconscious, she was paralyzed with succinylcholine (1.5 mg/kg), and about 45 seconds later, her heart rate was noted to be 44 beats/min. When fully relaxed, she had a nasal endotracheal tube inserted to protect her airway and maintain mechanical ventilation. At this point, her blood pressure was 125/75 mmHg and her heart rate was 82 beats/min. She was given atracurium, an intermediate-acting muscle relaxant, to facilitate ventilation during the dental extraction. Nitrous oxide and isoflurane were started for maintenance of anaesthesia, and gradually over 4 to 5 minutes, her blood pressure fell to 92/60 mmHg and her heart rate remained at about 80 beats/min.

At the time of surgical incision, her blood pressure jumped to 150/95 mmHg and her heart rate increased to 135 beats/min. This was treated with an additional injection of fentanyl (100 µg), and the inspired concentration of isoflurane was increased temporarily. The surgery then proceeded without further incident. At the completion of the procedure, the inhalational agents were discontinued, and neostigmine (2.5 mg) and atropine (0.6 mg) were given intravenously in order to reverse the muscle relaxation. In about 5 minutes, the patient was awake and responding to commands, the endotracheal tube was removed, and the patient was transferred to the post-anaesthetic recovery unit. During recovery, the only problem was that the patient experienced nausea and vomited once.

Anaesthesia can be defined as a reversible, drug-induced loss of sensation in the entire body or in part of it. In *general* anaesthesia, this definition must be extended to include the blocking of sensory responses to painful stimuli; blocking of cardiovascular, respiratory, and gastrointestinal reflexes; blocking of motor functions; and the production of amnesia and unconsciousness.

The proper use of anaesthesia in surgery began in the 1840s, following Morton's successful demonstration of the effectiveness of ether anaesthesia in dentistry. Since that time, new anaesthetic agents have been developed and introduced into clinical practice, and methods for administering these drugs have been improved. The newer agents are safer for the patient in that they are not explosive. Improved methods for delivering anaesthetic drugs and monitoring their effects have allowed the anaesthesiologist to give safer anaesthesia to patients with compromised cardiovascular, respiratory, or central nervous system (CNS) function. Also, these newer agents and methods have contributed immensely to the expansion of the scope of surgery from short operative procedures limited to the extremities or abdomen to the major surgical accomplishments of the present.

## DESIRABLE ACTIONS OF GENERAL ANAESTHETICS

1. **Hypnosis (loss of consciousness):** Although some surgery is conducted on the awake patient, many operative procedures are better carried out with the patient in an unconscious state. Many present-day surgical procedures are done with the patient intubated and perhaps mechanically ventilated. These latter procedures require that the patient be "asleep," or unconscious.

2. **Analgesia (loss of pain):** Surgical procedures, by their nature, are painful, and it is incumbent upon the anaesthetist to alleviate this pain whether the patient is asleep or awake.

3. **Amnesia (loss of recall):** Since surgery can be a frightening ordeal for the patient, it is desirable that there be little or no memory of the event.

4. **Muscle relaxation:** Many surgical procedures are made considerably easier when muscle tone is reduced. Also, when a patient is to be intubated and ventilated, there is a need for relaxation of laryngeal and respiratory muscles.

There is, therefore, a spectrum of separate pharmacological actions required to achieve the various goals of anaesthesia. During anaesthetic administration, one must deal with each of these components and determine the level of these effects separately. The depth of anaesthesia reflects the degree of reduction of these parameters during surgery and, consequently, the degree of unconsciousness, analgesia, amnesia, and muscle relaxation.

No single anaesthetic agent has yet been developed for which these properties are combined in optimal proportions. It is unlikely that any single agent could provide optimal anaesthesia for all patients and all types of procedures. A combination of different anaesthetic agents allows better control of the individual components of the anaesthetic spectrum. Full loss of consciousness and loss of pain-induced reflexes, with good muscular relaxation but minimal disturbance of circulation, are usually obtained with a combination of light anaesthesia together with specific opioid analgesic and muscle-relaxant drugs, a procedure known as *balanced anaesthesia*.

## THEORIES OF ANAESTHESIA

The mechanism by which general anaesthetics exert their effects remains uncertain, although various theories have enjoyed scientific popularity at different times. Most theories of general anaesthesia have attempted to identify a common basis for a reversible interaction between nerve cells and drugs of quite varied physical and chemical properties to explain how such diverse substances can produce closely similar patterns of general anaesthetic effects.

## Metabolic Theories

Early theories attributed the phenomenon of anaesthesia to interference with nerve cell function by the anaesthetic agent through depression of neuronal respiration or metabolism. It is most likely, however, that the metabolic disturbances are the result, rather than the cause, of decreased nerve cell activity.

## Membrane Theories

Most theories of anaesthesia have been based on the concept that the drug interferes with alterations in cell membranes that normally occur during neuronal excitation, impulse conduction, and synaptic transmitter release.

### Lipid solubility theory

The lipid solubility theory was based on the direct correlation between the lipid/water partition coefficients of different substances and their general anaesthetic potencies. This correlation, described by Meyer in 1899 and Overton in 1901, led to the view that the degree of anaesthesia is proportional to the concentration of anaesthetic dissolved in the lipid or lipophilic phase of the cell membrane.

### Thermodynamic activity theory

In 1939, Ferguson proposed this theory to account for exceptions to the Meyer–Overton correlation. He multiplied the concentration of dissolved anaesthetic by its thermodynamic activity coefficient (TAC), which is a correction factor reflecting the degree of physicochemical interaction between the molecules of anaesthetic and those of the phase in which it is located: thermodynamic activity = molar concentration × TAC. Ferguson claimed that equal thermodynamic activity of different anaesthetics in the cell membrane produced equal degrees of anaesthesia.

### Membrane occupancy theory

Since there were still exceptions that did not fit Ferguson's theory, Mullins (1954) introduced a further correction to take account of the molecular size of the anaesthetic agent. At the same thermodynamic activity, a larger molecule would occupy a larger space within the membrane. Mullins proposed that the degree of anaesthesia is proportional to the fractional volume of the cell membrane occupied by the anaesthetic.

### Membrane expansion theory

The membrane expansion theory (suggested separately by Eyring, Seeman, and Miller) extends Mullins' theory by proposing a mechanism of action. According to this hypothesis, the anaesthetic molecules enter hydrophobic regions of the membrane (i.e., in the interstices of membrane proteins and between lipid molecules), expanding and distorting the membrane as well as the proteins associated with the sodium-conductance channel (Fig. 20-1). This expansion would compress ion channels and thus prevent the ion flux associated with the action potential. The effect of this impairment on $Na^+$ influx is seen in a slower rise of the action potential and a correspondingly higher threshold of depolarization before the neuron responds with an action potential. All neurons would be affected in a similar way, but the small neurons in the brain are known to be more sensitive than larger neurons.

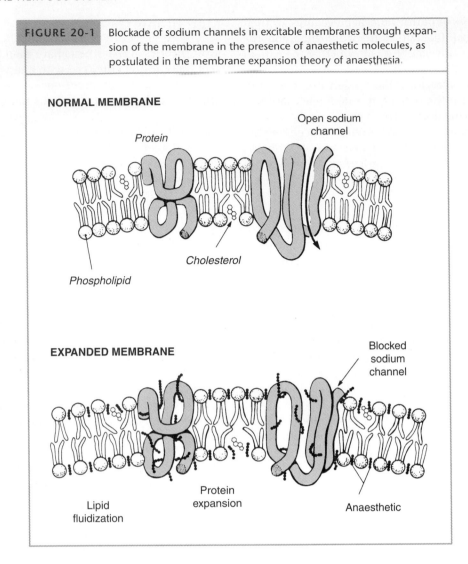

**FIGURE 20-1** Blockade of sodium channels in excitable membranes through expansion of the membrane in the presence of anaesthetic molecules, as postulated in the membrane expansion theory of anaesthesia.

## Membrane receptor theory

Specific drug receptors are known for certain intravenous agents used in anaesthesia, such as CNS opioid receptors for opioid analgesics, the nicotinic receptors at the neuromuscular junction for muscle relaxants, the central dopaminergic receptors for neuroleptic drugs, and the central γ-aminobutyric acid (GABA) receptors for benzodiazepines. The most likely protein targets for anaesthetic agents are ion channels. Indeed, different CNS ion channels display striking sensitivity to various anaesthetic agents.

GABA, the most common inhibitory neurotransmitter in the CNS, increases chloride influx into nerve cells, resulting in CNS depression. There is now a considerable body of evidence that a number of intravenous and inhalational anaesthetics exert their anaesthetic actions in the CNS through specific interactions at the GABA type A receptor (GABA$_A$) associated with the chloride ion channel complex. These agents appear to enhance the effect of the GABA molecule at its receptor, opening the chloride-permeable pore and augmenting the GABA$_A$ receptor–mediated inhibition of postsynaptic neuronal excitability. Barbiturates, benzodiazepines, and propofol, as well as the inhalational anaesthetics, have been suggested to bind to specific sites in the GABA$_A$/chloride channel complex and increase the effect produced when GABA binds to the GABA$_A$ receptor.

Other central ion channels that are sensitive to CNS anaesthetic agents at effective concentrations include those linked to nicotinic acetylcholine receptors, serotonin type 3, glycine receptors and glutamate receptors activated by N-methyl-D-aspartate (NMDA) or α-amino-3-hydroxy-5-methyl-4-isoxazolepropionic acid (AMPA). These findings support the hypothesis that anaesthetic agents exert their physiological and pharmacological effects by enhancing inhibitory postsynaptic ion channel activity (GABA$_A$ and glycine receptors) and inhibiting excitatory postsynaptic channel activity (nicotinic acetylcholine, serotonin, and glutamate receptors). However, considerable work remains to be done with these and other specific anaesthetic targets before the mechanism of action of these various agents is fully known.

## PREMEDICATION

Before a patient undergoes a procedure requiring general anaesthesia, premedication may be required. There are a number of indications for premedication, such as relief of anxiety, induction of sedation, analgesia, amnesia, vagal blockade, reduction of secretions in the upper respiratory tract, lessening of post-operative nausea and vomiting, increase in pH and decrease in volume of gastric contents, and potential reduction of the dose of general anaesthetic agent required for induction. A most effective and simple means to reduce anxiety is the time-honoured preoperative visit to the patient by the anaesthesiologist to provide information and answer questions. In addition, the following classes of drugs are routinely employed by many physicians:

- **Opioids:** Opioid analgesics such as morphine or its synthetic analogues offer analgesia, euphoria, and sedation (see Chapter 19). Complicating problems can be respiratory depression, nausea and vomiting, gastric retention, and reduced sympathetic tone.
- **Benzodiazepines:** These anxiolytics, most notably diazepam, midazolam, and lorazepam, provide a reduction in anxiety without significant effects on respiration or cardiovascular function (see Chapter 23). They are also effective in providing some amnesia and sedation.
- **Anti-muscarinics:** Atropine, glycopyrrolate, and scopolamine may be used as premedicants to block vagal reflexes and inhibit salivary and respiratory tract secretions (see Chapter 12). The resulting dry mouth can be unpleasant for the patient, and therefore, these drugs may be better used during induction rather than as premedication. Scopolamine also has central effects leading to sedation and amnesia. Glycopyrrolate does not cross the blood–brain barrier and is also less likely to induce tachycardia than is atropine.
- **Antihistamines:** Both H$_1$ and H$_2$ antagonists (see Chapter 30) may be given for premedication. H$_1$ antagonists such as hydroxyzine and promethazine offer antiemetic effects as well as some sedation. H$_2$ antagonists such as cimetidine and ranitidine will decrease gastric acidity and reduce the volume of stomach contents. This is important in some patients because general anaesthesia eliminates the usual protective reflexes that prevent aspiration following regurgitation of stomach contents. The dopaminergic antagonist metoclopramide (see Chapter 42) is sometimes administered in order to increase the rate of gastric emptying into the small intestine.
- **Antiemetics:** Post-operative nausea and vomiting are common adverse events following general anaesthesia. In order to minimize these, patients who are predisposed to nausea and vomiting may be given one of a variety of agents, which include the phenothiazines droperidol, prochlorperazine, and promethazine; antihistamines, such as dimenhydrinate and hydroxyzine; selective serotonin 5-HT$_3$ receptor antagonists, such as ondansetron (Zofran) and granisetron (Kytril); and most recently, corticosteroids such as dexamethasone (Decadron).

## SIGNS AND STAGES OF GENERAL ANAESTHESIA

The classical signs of general anaesthesia with diethyl ether were described by Guedel, who divided the process into stages and planes (Fig. 20-2). These classical signs, while still essentially correct, reflect physiological events in response to CNS depression by ether, but they are no longer useful with the modern anaesthetic agents and techniques in current use. Now, depth of anaesthesia is judged by the presence or absence of a response to verbal commands, of the eyelash reflex, of rhythmic respiration, and of the response of heart rate and blood pressure to surgical stimulation. However, the classical signs are given here because they draw attention to some important principles and physiological mechanisms of general anaesthesia.

- **Stage I:** This is the period from the beginning of anaesthetic administration to the loss of consciousness and pain sensation, while motor activity and reflexes remain normal.
- **Stage II:** This period extends from the loss of consciousness, through a stage of irregular and spasmodic breathing, to the re-establishment of regular breathing. The patient may swallow, retch, vomit, or struggle intensely, so this stage of general excitement is not without danger to the patient.
- **Stage III:** This is the stage of anaesthesia during which surgery may be performed. The movements of the eyes gradually stop; the eyelid, corneal, and pupillary reflexes are extinguished; swallowing, retching, and vomiting stop; and skeletal muscles relax. Respiration, which at first is deep and regular, becomes shallower and, in the deeper planes, more diaphragmatic.
- **Stage IV:** In this stage of imminent death, the pupils are completely dilated, and breathing stops as the cardiorespiratory centres in the medulla are depressed. It is the stage of anaesthetic overdose, which is reversible if anaesthetic administration is discontinued and artificial respiration is applied.

Beyond stage IV (medullary paralysis), respiratory arrest is followed by circulatory failure (paralysis of vasomotor centre) and death. These stages clearly demonstrate the progression of depressant effects of the anaesthetic

**FIGURE 20-2** Signs and reflex reactions characterizing the stages and planes of anaesthesia (after Guedel, who devised this scheme with diethyl ether anaesthesia for the training of inexperienced medical personnel during World War I). The wedges indicate the progressive disappearance of signs and reflexes, which may vary somewhat from person to person.

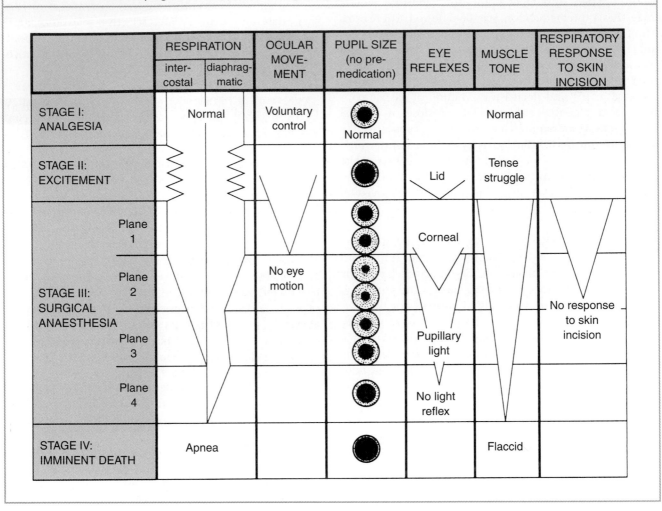

agent on various physiological functions with different levels of sensitivity as the concentration of anaesthetic in the tissues is raised. Different signs are used for the modern agents, but the concept of progressive loss of function remains unchanged.

# INHALATIONAL ANAESTHESIA

## Technique

Anaesthetic gases (such as nitrous oxide) and vapours (of volatile liquids such as isoflurane) are administered to patients at appropriate inspired concentrations, which are achieved by the use of accurate flow meters and other ancillary machinery.

The gases are supplied in compressed form and are passed through pressure reduction valves prior to the delivery of the gas through a flow meter. The gas is then administered to the patient through a mask fitted over the mouth and nose or larynx (laryngeal mask) or through a tube inserted past the larynx directly into the trachea (endotracheal tube).

The volatile anaesthetics (i.e., vapours) are supplied as liquids at room temperature and atmospheric pressure and are delivered in gaseous form from thermocompensated wick vaporizers designed to deliver a precise amount (concentration) of vapour, usually as a percentage of total gas flow.

## General Pharmacokinetics

Anaesthesia results when appropriate concentrations or partial pressures of the anaesthetic agent are present in brain tissue. Between the anaesthetic machine and the brain are a series of diffusion sites as the gas or vapour moves from the machine to the alveoli, into the blood, and finally into body tissues including the brain. At each of these interfaces, there is a partial-pressure gradient that depends on the physicochemical properties of the anaesthetic agent and the body compartments involved.

## Uptake

The rate of rise of anaesthetic concentration in the blood, and therefore in the tissues, is dependent upon a series of clearly defined factors:

1. The *concentration* of the agent in the inspired air
2. The *pulmonary ventilation* (i.e., delivery of the agent to the alveoli): The subsequent transfer from the alveoli to the blood depends upon the solubility of the agent in blood. The more soluble the anaesthetic agent is in the blood, the more important pulmonary ventilation rate is as a limiting factor (Fig. 20-3).
3. *Solubility,* measured as the partition coefficient of the agent between blood and gas phase ($P_{b/g}$): As the concentration in the inspired air rises, the tensions, or partial pressures, of the anaesthetic agents in the blood rise more rapidly with the less soluble agents, such as nitrous oxide, than with the more soluble ones, such as methoxyflurane (see Fig. 20-3). Therefore, the less soluble inhalational agents reach equilibrium more quickly. Yet, even though the tension of the less soluble agents such as nitrous oxide or sevoflurane rises more quickly, less of the agent is transferred and dissolved in blood and tissue when compared with the more soluble agents (Table 20-1 on page 259). The **lipid solubility**, measured as the partition coeffi-

cient of the agent between oil and gas ($P_{o/g}$) at equilibrium, correlates with anaesthetic potency. As the lipid solubility increases, the anaesthetic potency increases (i.e., MAC [minimum alveolar concentration] decreases), as predicted by the membrane theories of anaesthesia. Note that there is virtually no barrier to the movement of anaesthetic agents between the alveoli and blood.

4. *Cardiac output,* which delivers the agent to the tissues: Alterations in cardiac output have opposing effects on uptake. Increases in pulmonary blood flow will result in more rapid transport of anaesthetics from the alveoli; therefore, rate of uptake is increased but the equilibration between the alveolar and arterial partial pressures is delayed. However, increases in cardiac output will increase the delivery of anaesthetic to the brain, increasing the rate of tissue equilibration, and thereby hastening the onset of anaesthesia. Except for extreme conditions of drug solubility or changes in cardiac output, this factor has a minor overall effect.
5. *Transfer of anaesthetic from blood into tissues,* which depends upon the solubility of the agent in tissue and the concentration gradient between blood and tissue: The blood flow (i.e., the rate of delivery) to the tissues is also important. Brain, heart, kidneys, gut, and endocrine glands receive the highest blood flow. This is the vessel-rich group of tissues, and they reach peak concentrations of anaesthetic agents faster than tissues such as muscle or fat (Fig. 20-4).

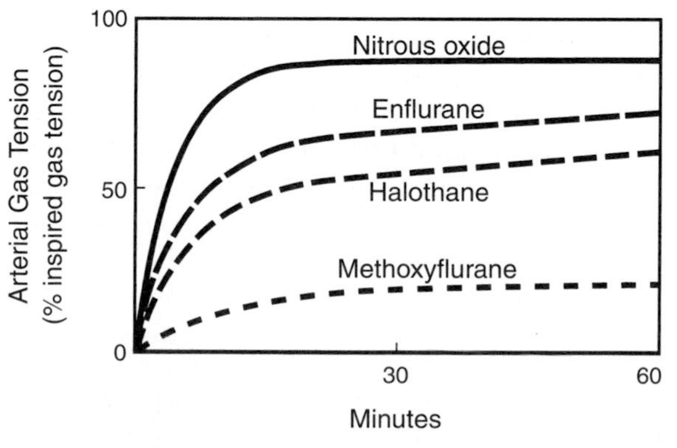

## Distribution

All anaesthetic agents have some degree of lipid solubility, and they will therefore cross cell membranes and distribute into the total body water. They readily cross the blood–brain barrier; otherwise, they would not be able to act as general anaesthetics.

## Biotransformation

Although initially it was thought that the volatile anaesthetics were chemically inert, it is now known that all of them are biotransformed to some degree in the liver. The proportion of anaesthetic agent taken into the body that is biotransformed ranges from as much as 50% for methoxyflurane and 20% for halothane, to 3% for sevoflurane, 2% for enflurane, 0.2% for isoflurane, and 0.02% for desflurane. Biotransformation may continue for a period of 4 to 5 days following the administration of an anaesthetic as the remaining drug is mobilized from muscle and fat stores back into the circulation.

## Elimination

Recovery from a volatile anaesthetic occurs once the administration is stopped and the drug diffuses from the blood into the alveolar gas space and is exhaled. The rate of elimination from the body is dependent upon the following:

---

**FIGURE 20-3** Idealized tensions of inhalational anaesthetics in blood expressed as a percent of the inspired gas tension with time. (Adapted from Eger EI. *Anesthetic Uptake and Action.* Baltimore, Md: Williams & Wilkins; 1974, with permission.)

1. Transfer of anaesthetic from tissue into blood: This can be slow for highly lipid-soluble agents, such as methoxyflurane, coming out of muscle and adipose tissue. This accounts for the prolonged biotransformation of some drugs over 4 to 5 days. Transfer is, however, more rapid from the brain, so a patient is usually awake from the inhalational agents 5 to 10 minutes after administration of the anaesthetic is stopped.
2. Cardiac output, which affects the rate of delivery of the agent to the lungs
3. Relative solubilities of the anaesthetic in blood and in alveolar gas ($P_{b/g}$): As with uptake, elimination of an inhaled anaesthetic from the blood into alveolar air in the lungs is more rapid for the less blood-soluble agents such as nitrous oxide, desflurane, and sevoflurane.
4. Rate of alveolar ventilation

Figure 20-4 shows uptake and elimination phases of a relatively water-insoluble inhalational anaesthetic, nitrous oxide ($N_2O$).

## Minimum alveolar concentration

In order to compare the potencies of the various inhalational anaesthetic agents as well as to give a quantitative basis for their administration, the concept of the minimum alveolar concentration (MAC) was developed. This is the minimal concentration of the inhalational anaesthetic agent (expressed as percent of total gas mixture) in the alveolus that will inhibit purposeful movement of 50% of patients following surgical stimulation, such as a skin incision. Since this is measured at or near steady-state conditions, the concentration of anaesthetic agent in the brain tissue will be about 500 µmoles/100 mL of membrane volume for any inhalational anaesthetic agent used. To achieve this concentration in the neuronal membranes, and thus inhibit purposeful movement by the patient, the inspired concentration must be about 6.6% (v/v) for desflurane, 1.8% (v/v) for sevoflurane, 1.2% (v/v) for isoflurane, 1.6% (v/v) for enflurane, 0.75% (v/v) for halothane, 0.16% (v/v) for methoxyflurane, and 104% (v/v) for nitrous oxide. To achieve such an effect in 95% of patients ($ED_{95}$), 1.3 MAC is required.

Note that MAC is the alveolar concentration at equilibrium and is independent of the time required to reach this. However, the time for induction of anaesthesia and the time required to reach equilibrium depend upon the blood/gas solubility of the agent, being more rapid for the less soluble agents (see "Uptake" above). Also, MAC varies with age.

## ANAESTHETIC GASES

The three best-known anaesthetic gases are $N_2O$, ethylene, and cyclopropane. Of these, only $N_2O$ is in current use. The other agents, which have explosion potential, are of historical interest and can be read about in older textbooks.

## Nitrous Oxide

$N_2O$ (Fig. 20-5, Table 20-1) is a non-irritating, colourless gas with a mildly sweet odour. Its boiling point is –89°C, and its critical temperature is 36.5°C. It is furnished in tanks under pressure, as a liquid in equilibrium with its gas phase. It is non-flammable and non-explosive but does support combustion. Its relevant partition coefficients are shown in Table 20-1.

### Pharmacokinetics

$N_2O$ is characterized by its low solubility in blood ($P_{b/g}$ = 0.47) and tissue. It therefore readily reaches its limiting concentration in blood and tissues, leading to rapid uptake and rapid elimination. It is not biotransformed and is excreted unchanged. In the blood, $N_2O$ is 34 times more soluble than nitrogen. Because of this, $N_2O$ can enter a closed space such as an obstructed bowel, pneumothorax, or middle ear more rapidly than nitrogen can be removed, so the volume of gas contained within that closed space can significantly expand. This expansion raises the pressure within the space and can thus give rise to pain or other disturbances.

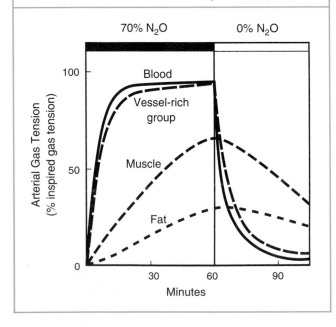

| FIGURE 20-4 | Idealized tensions of inhaled anaesthetic in blood, vessel-rich tissues, muscle, and fat during 60 minutes of nitrous oxide inhalation and 45 minutes elimination. (Modified from Cowles AL, Borgstedt HH, Gillies, AJ. Uptake and distribution of inhalation anesthetics agents in clinical practice. *Anesth Analg.* 1968;47:404-414, with permission.) |

FIGURE 20-5  Structural formulae of some inhalational anaesthetics.

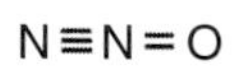

N≡N=O    Nitrous oxide

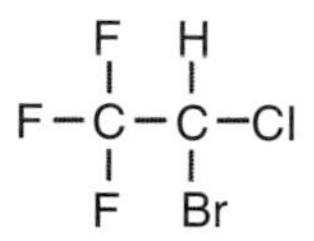

Halothane (Fluothane)

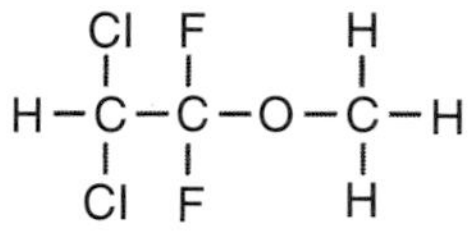

Methoxyflurane (Penthrane)

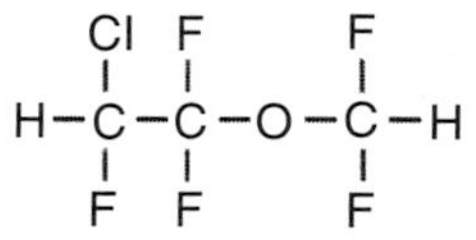

Enflurane (Ethrane)

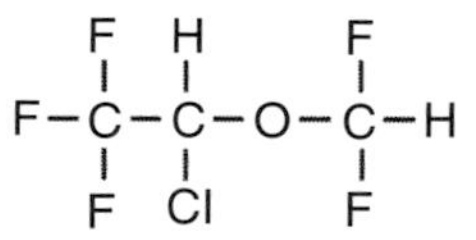

Isoflurane (Forane)

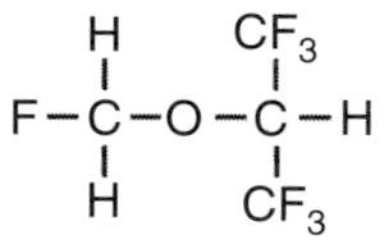

Sevoflurane (Ultane, Sevorane)

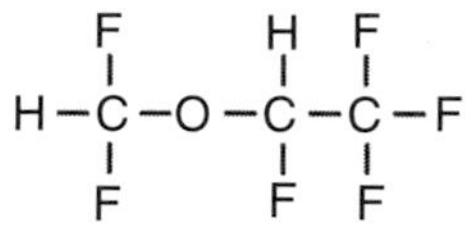

Desflurane (Suprane)

## Pharmacological effects

$N_2O$ has a MAC of 104%, consistent with it being a very weak general anaesthetic and being unable to provide general anaesthesia when administered as the sole agent. It does, however, provide analgesia and sedation even in lower concentrations.

$N_2O$ is used clinically in concentrations up to 70% in combination with oxygen as a supplement to other inhalational or intravenous anaesthetics. Its major advantage is that it will reduce the MAC of volatile agents such as halothane when administered concurrently. This, in turn, allows for a reduction in the dose of volatile agents, with a consequent reduction in their dose-dependent adverse effects.

$N_2O$ on its own has minor effects on respiration, but it will potentiate the respiratory depression produced by other agents such as thiopental, opioids, or other inhalational agents. Its effects on the cardiovascular system include mild myocardial depression, but this is counteracted by a mild sympathomimetic effect.

Short-term administration of $N_2O$ for a few hours is not associated with toxicity, but prolonged exposure may have toxic sequelae. $N_2O$ can oxidize and inactivate vitamin $B_{12}$, the coenzyme for methionine synthase. This can potentially lead to reversible hematopoietic changes such as megaloblastic anemia, leukopenia, and thrombocytopenia, as well as a myeloneuropathy similar to that found in pernicious anemia (see Chapter 39). These changes may assume clinical significance if $N_2O$ is administered continuously for more than 6 hours or is self-administered repeatedly, as occurs when it is used as a drug of abuse. Occupational exposure is of concern for health professionals because chronic, low-dose exposure may cause these toxic effects. (Scavenging of waste gases in operating rooms, which is now applied routinely, has greatly reduced the concerns of occupational exposure.)

## Oxygen

Although not an anaesthetic agent, oxygen is always included as part of the anaesthetic gas mixture and must be considered a drug. It is a clear, colourless, odourless gas, with a boiling point of −182.5°C and critical temperature of −118°C. It supports combustion.

$O_2$ is normally present at a partial pressure of 159 mmHg, or 21.2 kPa, in the atmosphere. Clinically, it is generally used in elevated concentrations during anaesthesia and for patients in intensive care units.

TABLE 20-1  Partition Coefficients and Minimum Alveolar Concentrations for Some Anaesthetic Gases and Vapours

| Agent | $P_{b/g}$* | $P_{br/b}$† | $P_{o/g}$‡ | MAC§ |
|---|---|---|---|---|
| Desflurane | 0.42 | 1.3 | 19 | 6.6 |
| Nitrous oxide | 0.47 | 1.1 | 1.4 | 104.0 |
| Sevoflurane | 0.65 | 1.7 | 47 | 1.8 |
| Isoflurane | 1.46 | 1.6 | 91 | 1.16 |
| Enflurane | 1.9 | 1.4 | 97 | 1.68 |
| Halothane | 2.5 | 1.9 | 224.0 | 0.75 |
| Methoxyflurane | 12.0 | 2.0 | 970.0 | 0.16 |

*Blood/gas partition coefficient at equilibrium.
†Brain/blood partition coefficient at equilibrium.
‡Oil/gas partition coefficient.
§Minimum alveolar concentration required to prevent movement of 50% of patients in response to a surgical stimulus. The concentration may vary with age, as noted in the text. (Data from Barash et al., 2001.)

When inhaled continuously for 24 hours or more in concentrations greater than 50%, $O_2$ is toxic to lung tissue. In premature infants, it is also toxic to the retina.

# VOLATILE ANAESTHETICS

## Diethyl Ether

This agent, once the most widely used, is now only of historical interest in the Western world, and it is rarely used anywhere. Diethyl ether is a potent anaesthetic agent that maintains good respiration during light anaesthesia. It maintains a stable blood pressure by releasing endogenous catecholamines. However, this same action may give rise to cardiac arrhythmias. Unfortunately, this agent is explosive, making it a great hazard in modern-day operating rooms.

## Halothane

This volatile agent was introduced into anaesthetic practice in the late 1950s and was for many years the most common agent of its class in use in North America.

Halothane (see Fig. 20-5 and Table 20-1) is a pleasant-smelling, non-irritating, and non-explosive liquid with a boiling point of 50.2°C and a vapour pressure of 243 torr (mmHg) at 20°C. It is soluble in rubber and is therefore taken up by the tubing in anaesthetic equipment.

### Pharmacokinetics
The uptake of halothane from the lung is moderately rapid (see Fig. 20-3), so it can be used for inhalational induction of anaesthesia in concentrations up to about 4% (v/v). It is used for the maintenance of anaesthesia at 0.5 to 2% (v/v). About 20% of the inhaled dose is biotransformed in the liver; the remainder is rapidly eliminated via the respiratory tract after administration is discontinued.

### Pharmacological effects

*CNS.* Halothane is a potent anaesthetic agent, with a MAC of 0.75%. It has only a mild, clinically unsatisfactory analgesic effect, usually requiring the addition of an analgesic agent such as $N_2O$ or an opioid.

*Respiratory.* Halothane vapour does not irritate the respiratory mucosa. It produces a dose-dependent depression of ventilation, with increased rate of respiration but a greater reduction in tidal volume, resulting in a characteristic pattern of short, rapid breaths during anaesthesia. There is a reduced respiratory response to raised $CO_2$ and a greatly depressed response to decreased $O_2$ (hypoxia).

*Cardiovascular.* Halothane causes a dose-dependent depression of the myocardium coupled with a relaxation of vascular smooth muscle, resulting in a *fall in blood pressure. The drug sensitizes the myocardium to catecholamines,* so exogenous administration of these agents can produce arrhythmias.

*Other.* It causes dose-dependent relaxation of uterine contractility that can lead to increased bleeding in obstetrical surgery such as Caesarean sections. It also depresses motility and tone of the gut. Halothane is a poor skeletal muscle relaxant, but it will potentiate neuromuscular blocking agents, allowing for the use of less neuromuscular blocker to achieve the same degree of muscle relaxation.

*Toxicity.* Although halothane has the lowest mortality risk of any general anaesthetic, post-operative hepatitis has been described as a rare complication in about one in 35 000 cases of halothane anaesthesia (see Chapter 43). However, a cause–effect relationship is difficult to establish.

In genetically susceptible subjects, halothane (and other volatile general anaesthetics) may precipitate a malignant hyperthermia crisis (see Chapter 10).

## Methoxyflurane

This volatile anaesthetic agent was specifically designed to have high solubility in blood (see Table 20-1), resulting in a slow induction and emergence. These properties were chosen deliberately because they were thought to provide more safety due to better control during induction, even though they also meant slower recovery from anaesthesia. Methoxyflurane (see Fig. 20-5) gained some popularity in the late 1960s. However, approximately 50% of the inhaled dose is biotransformed, releasing free fluoride, which is toxic to the kidney. Therefore, this agent is rarely used in North America today. It is a good analgesic and has been used for pain relief during labour or short procedures such as wound dressing changes.

## Isoflurane

This drug is the most popular volatile anaesthetic in use today in North America. Isoflurane (see Fig. 20-5 and Table 20-1) is a pleasant-smelling, non-irritating, non-explosive vapour. Its boiling point is 48.5°C, and its vapour pressure is 238 torr at 20°C.

### Pharmacokinetics
The uptake of isoflurane is similar to that of halothane. The concentration in an $O_2$ and $N_2O$ mixture that is used for induction of anaesthesia is usually 2 to 4% (v/v) and for maintenance, 1 to 2% (v/v). Only about 0.2% of the inhaled dose is biotransformed.

### Pharmacological effects

*CNS.* This potent inhalational anaesthetic has mild analgesic properties. It produces CNS depression, reducing cerebral metabolic rate. The MAC for isoflurane is 1.16% (v/v).

*Respiratory.* A concentration-dependent depression of minute ventilation occurs, resulting in increasing arterial $P_{CO_2}$. There is a reduced ventilatory response to $CO_2$ and a greatly depressed response to hypoxia. Isoflurane inhalation results in bronchodilatation.

*Cardiovascular.* Isoflurane produces concentration-dependent depression of the myocardium, with a resulting fall in blood pressure. However, this agent does not sensitize the myocardium to catecholamines, which is one of its advantages over halothane. One of the advantages of isoflurane is that it tends to maintain cardiac output; however, blood pressure and afterload will still be decreased by its vasodilating action on peripheral vascular beds.

*Other.* It produces only a mild degree of muscle relaxation, but it will potentiate neuromuscular blocking agents.

This agent will also precipitate malignant hyperthermia in genetically susceptible individuals.

## Enflurane

This isomer of isoflurane (see Fig. 20-5 and Table 20-1) is a potent inhalational anaesthetic with a MAC of 1.68%. It has physical and pharmacological properties that offer some advantages when compared with isoflurane. However, enflurane produces excitation at higher doses, resulting in seizure-like activity in the electroencephalograph (EEG) that may be manifested as twitching of muscles. Like isoflurane and halothane, it causes bronchodilatation. For surgical cases lasting more than 8 hours, the administration of this agent results in elevated circulating fluoride concentrations, since about 2% of the inhaled dose is biotransformed. Enflurane can precipitate a malignant hyperthermia crisis in susceptible individuals.

## Sevoflurane

This volatile anaesthetic (see Fig. 20-5 and Table 20-1) was first used in humans in 1971. It is a colourless, sweet-smelling, non-flammable liquid at room temperature. Its physical properties also include a boiling point of 58.5°C, blood/gas partition coefficient of 0.69, and saturated vapour pressure of 160 torr (at 20°C).

### Pharmacokinetics

Sevoflurane is eliminated primarily unaltered through the lungs, but up to 5% is metabolized in the liver by CYP2E1, forming the metabolites inorganic fluoride ion and an organic fluoride (hexafluoroisopropanol), which are excreted in the urine.

### Pharmacological effects

*CNS and neuromuscular effects.* Despite being a potent inhalational agent, sevoflurane usually requires concomitant analgesic medication such as opioids and/or nitrous oxide. It produces CNS depression with reduced cerebral metabolic rate, although paradoxical seizure-like activity has been reported in some patients. The MAC of sevoflurane varies with age from 3.3 in neonates to 1.7 to 1.8 in healthy adults to 1.48 in the elderly. The clinical effect of neuromuscular blocking agents is potentiated by sevoflurane.

*Respiratory.* Sevoflurane depresses ventilatory response to carbon dioxide stimulus in the brain stem, resulting in reduced minute ventilation (decreased tidal volume and increased respiratory rate). Sevoflurane is an excellent bronchodilator, second only to halothane.

*Cardiovascular.* Sevoflurane produces a concentration-dependent depression of the myocardium and systemic vascular resistance, but it does not sensitize the myocardium to catecholamines or elicit a positive chronotropic response. Clinically, a slightly decreased or stable heart rate with a fall in blood pressure is observed.

*Other.* Nephrotoxicity may potentially develop after sevoflurane administration, because of (1) production of inorganic fluoride ions and hexafluoroisopropanol as urine metabolites and (2) production of Compounds A to E when sevoflurane is exposed to dry soda lime or Baralyme in the canister, which are used to absorb carbon dioxide. This problem can be prevented by humidifying the canister content and avoiding prolonged sevoflurane exposure at a fresh gas flow of less than 2 L/min.

As with all currently used inhalational anaesthetic agents, sevoflurane can trigger malignant hyperthermia.

*Clinical use.* Due to its physical properties and pharmacological effects, sevoflurane is an excellent agent for inhalational anaesthesia because it allows for quick induction and emergence and rapid change in depth of anaesthesia. This feature makes it desirable for use in ambulatory and pediatric patients.

## Desflurane

This volatile anaesthetic (see Fig. 20-5 and Table 20-1) was first used in humans in 1987. It is a pungent agent with physical properties that include a boiling point of 22.8°C, blood/gas partition coefficient of 0.42, and saturated vapour pressure of 664 torr (at 20°C). Due to these properties, desflurane requires a special heated vaporizer for administration.

### Pharmacokinetics

Desflurane is almost completely eliminated through the lungs. Only 0.02% is metabolized, and no increase of serum or urine fluoride levels has been reported after desflurane exposure. Desflurane is therefore a good anaesthetic agent for ambulatory surgery because of its rapid elimination and minimal metabolism.

## Pharmacological effects

*CNS and neuromuscular effects.* Desflurane has mild analgesic properties. It produces CNS depression with reduction in the cerebral metabolic rate. The MAC of desflurane in healthy adults is 6.6 but varies with age. Desflurane potentiates the effect of neuromuscular blocking agents.

*Respiratory.* Like sevoflurane, desflurane decreases ventilatory response to carbon dioxide stimulus, resulting in clinical reduction of minute ventilation (decreased tidal volume and increased respiratory rate). Among all the inhalational anaesthetics currently available, desflurane is one of the most irritating to the airway; near-MAC concentrations may cause coughing, breath-holding, and laryngospasm. It is not suitable for inhalational induction of anaesthesia.

*Cardiovascular.* Desflurane produces concentration-dependent depression of the myocardium, decreased systemic vascular resistance, and a positive chronotropic response. Clinically, tachycardia and a slight decrease in blood pressure with sustained cardiac output are observed. Desflurane does not sensitize the myocardium to catecholamines.

*Other.* Due to minimal desflurane metabolism, nephrotoxicity and hepatotoxicity are unlikely. However, carbon monoxide may be produced when desflurane is exposed to desiccated Baralyme or soda lime, which are used in the canister to prevent accumulation of carbon dioxide in the closed system. Desflurane can also trigger malignant hyperthermia.

*Clinical use.* Desflurane is a good choice for patients requiring early mobilization following ambulatory surgical procedures because of its minimal metabolism and rapid excretion.

## INTRAVENOUS ANAESTHETICS

Rapidly acting and short-acting intravenous agents are commonly used today for the induction of anaesthesia. The most commonly used drug is propofol, which has replaced thiopental as the primary agent used for this purpose. Other agents include methohexital and ketamine. High doses of opioid analgesics, such as fentanyl, can also be used intravenously for the induction and maintenance of anaesthesia. The disadvantages associated with all of these are the irrevocability of intravenous administration of a potent drug and the consequent dangers of overdosing the patient.

Furthermore, while quite safe in the hands of specialists who are prepared to deal with side effects and anaesthesia accidents, the intravenous anaesthetics are very dangerous when used on an occasional basis by the inexperienced practitioner who falls prey to the temptations of convenience.

## Propofol

Propofol, 2,6-diisopropylphenol, belongs to a new class of anaesthetic agents. It is practically insoluble in water, so that for clinical use, it must be formulated as a 1% aqueous emulsion containing soybean oil, glycerol, and egg phosphatide.

### Pharmacokinetics

Intravenous administration of propofol, like that of thiopental, results in rapid distribution of the drug into the vessel-rich group of tissues, including brain. Unconsciousness is induced in 15 to 30 seconds, depending on the speed of injection. Propofol can be irritating to the blood vessel at the site of injection; this can be minimized by prior administration of intravenous lidocaine or a slower rate of injection (and thus a slower onset of anaesthesia). The termination of action is due to redistribution of the drug out of the brain into less-well-perfused tissues such as muscle and fat, such that the patient will wake up in 5 to 10 minutes. When it is given as a bolus for induction, the redistribution and elimination half-lives are approximately 5 minutes and 3 hours, respectively. When it is given as an infusion or in repeated boluses, the half-lives may vary greatly.

Propofol is rapidly and extensively metabolized in the liver. About 98% is excreted in the urine: 40% is found as propofol glucuronide or sulfate, while approximately 60% is metabolized by the cytochrome P450–dependent mixed-function oxidase system to 2,6-diisopropyl-1,4-quinol, which is then conjugated to glucuronide or sulfate. This elimination process has a half-life of about 2 to 3 hours. Because of rapid biotransformation and elimination, propofol does not accumulate in the body to any great extent, and therefore, unlike thiopental, it can be used to maintain anaesthesia with continuous infusion. At sub-hypnotic doses, propofol can be used for sedation and amnesia.

### Pharmacological effects

*CNS.* Propofol is useful for intravenous sedation and for maintenance of anaesthesia during surgery. It can produce a subjective feeling of well-being and may have abuse potential. It has anticonvulsant properties, but, unlike thiopental, it does not cause hyperalgesia. Propofol reduces brain basal metabolic rate, cerebral blood flow, and intracranial pressure. However, it does not affect cerebrovascular autoregulation and vasomotor response to carbon dioxide. Unconsciousness is induced following an intravenous dose of 1.5 to 2.5 mg/kg. The duration of anaesthesia is about 5 to 10 minutes, depending on the dose used. The infusion dose is between 25 and 75 µg/kg/min for sedation and 100 to 200 µg/kg/min for hypnosis. Recovery from propofol is associated with less residual sedation, fatigue ("hangover"), and cognitive impairment than with other intravenous anaesthetics.

*Respiratory.* Induction of anaesthesia with propofol is frequently accompanied by a period of apnea that may last for more than 1 minute, depending on the dose administered. The maintenance of anaesthesia with propofol results in a dose-dependent decrease in ventilation (decreased tidal volume and increased respiratory rate) and a rise in blood $CO_2$ levels. This respiratory depression is increased when propofol is administered together with other anaesthetic adjuvants such as opioids and benzodiazepines. In contradistinction to inhalation anaesthetics, propofol does not inhibit hypoxia-induced pulmonary vasoconstriction. It may offer some bronchodilatation in patients with chronic obstructive pulmonary disease.

*Cardiovascular.* Propofol administration reduces both systolic and diastolic blood pressure because of its direct myocardial depressant effect with associated reduction in cardiac output and systemic vascular resistance. The baroreflex mechanism is also blunted. These effects are potentiated by prior administration of opioid analgesics. When propofol is used for the maintenance of anaesthesia, the blood pressure is reduced by about 20%, or even more in elderly patients.

*Clinical use.* As with most other induction agents, propofol must be used with great caution in patients with hypovolemia or shock and in the elderly. Propofol does not trigger malignant hyperthermia crises and can be used to induce and maintain anaesthesia in susceptible individuals. Propofol in sub-anaesthetic doses shows antiemetic activity due to its anti-dopaminergic activity. It also relieves pruritus induced by spinal injection of opioids.

## Thiopental Sodium

This thiobarbiturate, which was the prototypical intravenous induction agent in the past, is available as a pale yellow powder. It is a weak acid, $pK_a$ 7.6, and is therefore readily soluble in alkaline medium. It is usually prepared as a 2.5% aqueous solution at pH 10.5.

### Pharmacokinetics

Thiopental is highly lipid-soluble, having a $P_{o/w}$ of 35 in the unionized form. Thus, it can readily cross cell membranes and rapidly enter brain tissue.

With rapid intravenous administration, there is prompt distribution into the vessel-rich group of tissues (brain, heart, lung, kidney, liver, intestine, endocrine glands), which induces unconsciousness in 10 to 15 seconds. The onset of action, therefore, is partly a function of the speed of injection.

The termination of action, however, is due to redistribution of the drug out of the brain and other vessel-rich tissues into less-well-perfused tissues, including skeletal muscle, and then into adipose tissue, where peak levels are not reached until more than 2 hours later (Fig. 20-6).

Thiopental is biotransformed in the liver by the cytochrome P450–dependent mixed-function oxidase system, resulting in side-chain oxidation and demethylation. This process, with a half-life of 6.5 hours, is much slower than the redistribution process. Because of the long half-life, with repeated doses of thiopental, the various body stores begin to fill up and the drug accumulates. As a result, patients with such accumulation may be asleep for a very long period (i.e., days). This is why thiopental is not used as the sole anaesthetic agent except for procedures of very short duration. Renal excretion of the parent compound is negligible.

Thiopental crosses the placenta readily, and peak fetal blood levels occur in about 3 minutes.

## Pharmacological Effects

*CNS.* The rapid injection of 3 to 5 mg/kg will produce loss of consciousness in a single arm–brain circulation time. The duration of anaesthesia is approximately 5 minutes, depending on the dose given. However, thiopental lowers the threshold for pain, resulting in an increased sensitivity to pain (hyperalgesia). It is also a poor muscle relaxant.

It reduces brain metabolic rate and consequently brain blood flow. This will reduce intracranial pressure. Therefore, under controlled conditions, thiopental is very effective for the acute treatment of raised intracranial pressure.

*Respiratory.* It is a potent respiratory depressant, so there is usually a period of apnea during induction of anaesthesia. This effect is enhanced by premedication with other

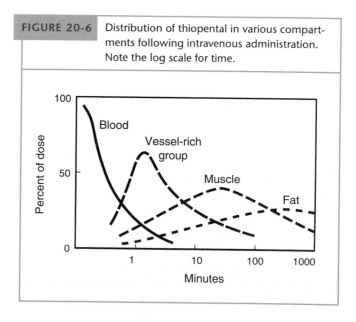

| FIGURE 20-6 | Distribution of thiopental in various compartments following intravenous administration. Note the log scale for time. |

depressant drugs. Thiopental causes a dose-dependent decrease in the response of the respiratory centre to changes in $P_{CO_2}$ and $P_{O_2}$.

*Cardiovascular.* Thiopental is a direct myocardial depressant and vascular smooth muscle relaxant, producing a dose-dependent fall in blood pressure. Accidental intra-arterial injection of concentrations greater than 2.5% causes vascular spasm, primarily due to the alkalinity of thiopental solutions. The vasospasm can result in tissue damage and loss of part of the limb.

*Other.* Clinically, thiopental is used in doses of 3 to 5 mg/kg in a normal patient. This agent would be relatively contraindicated in patients with hypovolemic shock, and the dose must be greatly reduced in the elderly and in patients with myxedema. The use of all barbiturates, including thiopental, is contraindicated in patients with the relatively rare defect in heme synthesis seen in the porphyrias. Barbiturate administration results in a marked increase in the porphyrin synthetic pathway, resulting in an overproduction of intermediate products of heme synthesis, and it can therefore exacerbate the disease process.

## Methohexital

This is an ultrashort-acting oxybarbiturate with pharmacological properties similar to those of thiopental. It is about three times as potent as thiopental, the usual intravenous induction dose being about 1 mg/kg.

## Etomidate

Etomidate is a methylbenzyl-imidazole derivative that is structurally unlike the other intravenous anaesthetics. It is a weak base, $pK_a$ 3.0, that is dissolved in propylene glycol for use as an intravenous anaesthetic. At a dose of 0.3 mg/kg, it produces a rapid induction of anaesthesia much as thiopental does. Consciousness is regained in 5 to 10 minutes, but full recovery may take longer than with thiopental. The drug is biotransformed in the liver with a half-life of 2.9 hours. The major advantage of etomidate is its minimal effect on the cardiovascular system. It produces a dose-related depression of respiration.

The drug depresses adrenal steroidogenesis and therefore cannot be used for long-term administration. Although available in Europe and the United States (Amidate), this drug has not been licensed for use in Canada.

## Midazolam

Midazolam is a water-soluble benzodiazepine that is most commonly used for sedation or as an adjunct to anaesthesia. It can also be used for the induction and maintenance of anaesthesia. In a dose of 0.15 to 0.4 mg/kg administered over 4 to 5 seconds, it induces unconsciousness in about 60 seconds, and patients remain asleep for 7 to 15 minutes, which is longer than with thiopental or propofol. The induction of anaesthesia with midazolam is generally preceded by administration of an opioid such as fentanyl, which will prolong the sleep time. Midazolam provides a smooth induction of anaesthesia with minimal effects on the cardiovascular system.

Midazolam is biotransformed in the liver. It has a half-life of elimination of about 2.7 hours, which is considerably shorter than the 24 to 36 hours for diazepam (see Chapter 23).

## Ketamine

Ketamine is a phenylcyclohexylamine derivative that can be used for rapid induction of anaesthesia by the intravenous (1 to 2 mg/kg) or intramuscular (5 to 10 mg/kg) route. In lower doses, it induces sedation, analgesia, and amnesia. As with other intravenous anaesthetics, it is initially distributed to highly perfused tissues and is then redistributed to less-well-perfused tissues. The redistribution results in termination of its action. The redistribution half-life is about 10 to 15 minutes. Ketamine is biotransformed in the liver into multiple metabolites, including norketamine, which has an anaesthetic potency approximately one-third that of ketamine. Its elimination half-life is 2 to 3 hours.

Ketamine exerts its anaesthetic and analgesic actions by blocking the cation channels that are activated by the *N*-methyl-D-aspartate (NMDA) subtype of receptor for the excitatory neurotransmitter glutamate.

Ketamine produces a unique state that has been described as *dissociative anaesthesia,* which is characterized by profound analgesia, amnesia, and catalepsy. The dissociation component refers to a functional and electrophysiological separation of the normal communications between the sensory cortex and the association areas in the brain. The result resembles catalepsy, in which the eyes may remain open with slow nystagmus and intact corneal reflexes. Patients are generally non-communicative, although they appear to be awake. Varying degrees of skeletal muscle hypertonus may be present, along with non-purposeful skeletal muscle movements that are independent of surgical stimulation.

Ketamine differs from most anaesthetic agents in that it *stimulates the cardiovascular system,* producing increases in heart rate, cardiac output, and blood pressure. Its ability to maintain arterial blood pressure is particularly useful in hypovolemic patients and those in cardiogenic shock. Conversely, ketamine is contraindicated when an elevation of blood pressure should be avoided, as in patients with a history of significant coronary artery disease, hypertension, or cerebrovascular disease. Furthermore, ketamine potentially increases cerebral blood flow and is therefore contraindicated in patients with raised intracranial pressure.

Ketamine can maintain normal lung volumes and can induce bronchodilatation. It is therefore useful in patients with asthma. It is a potent stimulator of salivary and tracheobronchial secretions; therefore, anti-muscarinics such as atropine are often administered concurrently. Emergence phenomena, described as vivid dreams, hallucinations, and delirium, have been reported (see Chapter 26). They appear to be related to the dose and rate of drug administration. The incidence of these phenomena is reduced when benzodiazepines are administered concurrently.

## High-Dose Opioid Anaesthesia

This procedure has proven to be highly effective in cardiovascular surgery. Although morphine was used initially, the commonly preferred drug today is fentanyl (see Chapter 23) at doses of up to 150 µg/kg (the usual analgesic dose is only 1 µg/kg). The high dose of fentanyl is combined with a muscle relaxant, endotracheal intubation, and ventilation with 100% $O_2$. This technique of anaesthesia provides a high degree of stability of blood pressure and cardiac output, but because of the very large dose of fentanyl used, ventilatory support is required post-operatively while the opioid is biotransformed and excreted.

## Neuroleptanalgesia/Intravenous Sedation

Neuroleptanalgesia has been described as a state of drug-induced depression of activity, lack of initiative, and reduced response to external stimuli. The patient has good analgesia and is sedated yet is able to respond to simple commands. Neuroleptanalgesia in a 60- to 70-kg individual is usually produced by means of intravenous injection of a combination of a potent short-acting opioid such as fentanyl (50 to 100 µg) and a short-acting benzodiazepine such as midazolam (0.5 to 1.0 mg). To this may be added a small dose of the butyrophenone droperidol (0.5 to 1.25 mg), or propofol (10 to 20 mg), as required for adequate sedation.

This neuroleptanalgesic state can be readily converted into unconsciousness (neuroleptanaesthesia) by the addition of small doses of an induction agent, such as propofol or thiopental, or by the addition of a mixture of $O_2$ and $N_2O$ or $N_2O$, $O_2$, and sevoflurane.

Intravenous sedation is now commonly used for many minor surgical procedures in conjunction with local infiltration or regional anaesthesia. Agents such as fentanyl, midazolam, and propofol are used to help the patient relax and perhaps experience amnesia for part of the surgical procedure. These patients must be monitored closely because of respiratory depression and the severe consequences of an overdose.

## SUGGESTED READINGS

Barash PG, Cullen BF, Stoelting RK. *Clinical Anesthesia.* 4th ed. Philadelphia, Pa: JB Lippincott; 2001.

Campagna JA, Miller KW, Forman SA. Mechanisms of actions of inhaled anesthetics. *N Engl J Med.* 2003;348:2110-2124.

Dripps RD, Eckenhoff JE, Vandam CD. *Introduction to Anesthesia: The Principles of Safe Practice.* Philadelphia, Pa: WB Saunders; 1982.

Franks NP, Lieb WR. Mechanisms of general anesthesia. *Environ Health Perspect.* 1990;87:199-205.

Miller RD, ed. *Anesthesia.* 5th ed. New York, NY: Churchill Livingstone; 2000.

Tanelian DL, Kosek E, Mody I, MacIver MB. The role of the GABA$_A$ receptor/chloride channel complex in anesthesia. *Anesthesiology.* 1993;78:757-776.

Thompson S-A, Wafford K. Mechanism of action of general anaesthetics—new information from molecular pharmacology. *Curr Opin Pharmacol.* 2001;1:78-83.

Ueda I, Kamaya H. Molecular mechanisms of anesthesia. *Anesth Analg.* 1984;63:929-945.

# 21

# Local Anaesthetics
## DA HAAS AND FJL CARMICHAEL

## CASE HISTORY

A 58-year-old male patient required local anaesthesia for the surgical removal of an abscessed tooth, a procedure that was estimated to require 30 minutes of surgical time. The patient's medical history included mild hypertension, which was well controlled with daily administrations of a diuretic; his blood pressure on examination was 124/80 mmHg. His history also included a pseudocholinesterase deficiency that had been discovered some years earlier in relation to surgery under general anaesthesia and succinylcholine, and he reported that he had had a "bad reaction" to the administration of a local anaesthetic in the past. When questioned on this last point, he recalled that he once fainted following an injection of local anaesthetic for a dental procedure many years ago, but since that time, has had local anaesthetic administered uneventfully.

The presence of infection necessitated administration of local anaesthetic in a site away from the abscess, and a regional nerve block was chosen instead of infiltration directly adjacent to the tooth. The estimated length of time for the surgical procedure indicated that the use of a local anaesthetic with an intermediate duration of action, in combination with a vasoconstrictor, would be appropriate. The history of pseudocholinesterase deficiency ruled out an ester-type anaesthetic. Because of the patient's cardiovascular history, a relatively low concentration of vasoconstrictor was advised as a cautionary measure. The combination of drugs selected for this regional nerve block was therefore 1.5 mL of lidocaine 2% with 5 μg/mL (1:200 000) adrenaline.

Within 2 minutes of injection, the patient felt faint. He was placed in a supine position with his legs elevated, which quickly relieved his symptoms. This reaction was quite likely psychogenic in nature, unrelated to the selection of drugs. Addressing the patient's anxiety might have helped to lessen the likelihood of this reaction.

Once the patient reported feeling well, the signs and symptoms of a successful nerve block were noted, and the surgery was carried out without further incident.

Local anaesthetics are drugs that can reversibly block the generation and propagation of nerve impulses. They are capable of depressing conduction in all excitable cells and therefore potentially interfere with the function of tissues in which impulse transmission occurs. This includes both sensory and motor peripheral nerves, autonomic ganglia, the central nervous system (CNS), neuromuscular junction, cardiac muscle, and smooth muscle. Their primary indications are to temporarily eliminate sensation at a specific site in order to permit surgical treatment or to relieve pain. A number of these agents can also be used as anti-arrhythmics, as discussed in more detail in Chapter 33. Overall, local anaesthetics rank among the most widely used drugs.

The history of local anaesthetics began with cocaine, which was isolated in 1860. It was the active ingredient of the extracts of the leaves of the Andean shrub *Erythroxylon coca*, which were known to confer insensitivity to delicate tissues. In 1884, Koller demonstrated the local anaesthetic effects of cocaine on the conjunctiva of animals, and Hall used cocaine in dentistry. It was used by Halstead in 1885 for nerve blocks and by Bier in 1898 for the first spinal anaesthesia in humans. In 1904, Einhorn synthesized procaine, and in subsequent years, many new local anaesthetic agents have been synthesized and used clinically.

## CHEMISTRY

Local anaesthetics have specific, fundamental structural features in common, as illustrated in Figure 21-1. The first of the three characteristic features is a lipophilic portion composed of an aromatic nucleus derived from para-aminobenzoic acid (PABA), as in procaine, or derived from

**FIGURE 21-1** Structural formulae of local anaesthetics, illustrating common structural features (see text).

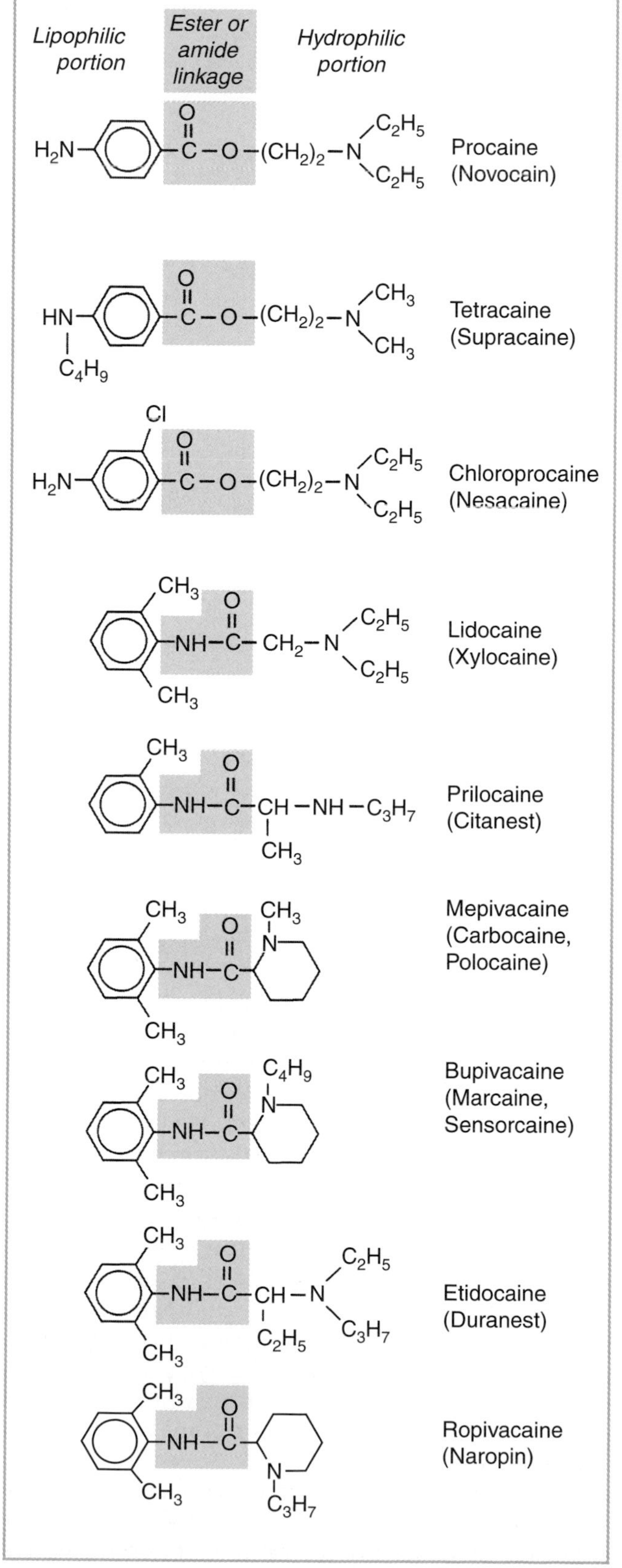

aniline, as in lidocaine. This portion is joined by an amide or ester linkage to an intermediate alkyl chain, the second characteristic feature. The third feature is a hydrophilic secondary or tertiary amino terminus. The lipophilicity of the aromatic group facilitates penetration into the nerve sheath and, subsequently, into the neuronal membrane itself. Both the hydrophilic and lipophilic groups are necessary for drug action. Because of the amino terminus, local anaesthetics are weak bases that can exist as either charged or uncharged molecules. The free base form is only slightly soluble in water, and local anaesthetics are therefore usually formulated as the water-soluble hydrochloride salts. The properties of local anaesthetics are summarized in Table 21-1.

# MECHANISM OF ACTION

## Nerve Membrane and Action Potentials

The function of the nerve cell is to convey information from one part of the body to another. This information is passed along the nerve fibre, or axon, in the form of electrical action potentials, or impulses. Peripheral nerves are generally a mixed population of nerve fibres with different diameters and rates of impulse conduction. These nerve fibres are arranged in a series of bundles, or fascicles, that are surrounded by layers of connective tissue. A single axon is a long cylinder of neural cytoplasm, the axoplasm, surrounded by the neuronal membrane, which is further encased in either a thin sheath, in the case of non-myelinated nerves, or multiple layers of myelin, in the case of myelinated nerves.

The neuronal membrane itself consists of a double layer of phospholipid molecules, with their polar headgroups oriented toward the two surfaces and their non-polar carbon chains oriented toward the middle of the membrane (see Fig. 20-1, Chapter 20). Interspersed among the lipids are protein molecules that constitute the various ion channels, also known as *ionophores,* as well as structural proteins and enzymes. The ionophores are very selective for specific ions, including $Na^+$ and $K^+$, and are regulated, or *gated,* by a membrane potential that is measured in terms of its voltage differential between the inside and outside of the membrane. Therefore, these are known as *voltage-gated channels.* There are also passive ion channels for $Na^+$, $K^+$, and $Cl^-$, which contribute to the resting membrane potential and the leakage of ions into and out of the nerve cell.

The electrophysiological properties of the neuronal membrane are dependent on the concentration of electrolytes on either side of the membrane as well as its permeability to $Na^+$ and $K^+$. The resting neural membrane is relatively impermeable to $Na^+$ and selectively permeable to $K^+$. In the resting state, there is a voltage gradient across the nerve membrane of approximately −70 mV, with the

| TABLE 21-1 | | Properties of Representative Local Anaesthetics | | | | | |
|---|---|---|---|---|---|---|---|
| Drug | pK$_a$ | Ionized to Unionized Ratio at pH 7.4 | Partition Coefficient* | Plasma Protein Binding (%) | Onset of Action | Duration of Action | Relative Toxicity[†] (non-vascular administration) |
| Procaine | 8.9 | 32:1 | 0.02 | 6 | Slow | Short | 0.3 |
| Tetracaine | 8.2 | 6:1 | 4.1 | 85 | Slow | Long | 5 |
| Chloroprocaine | 9.0 | 40:1 | 0.14 | ? | Rapid | Short | 0.3 |
| Lidocaine | 7.9 | 3:1 | 2.9 | 64 | Rapid | Intermediate | 1 |
| Prilocaine | 7.9 | 3:1 | 0.9 | 55 | Rapid | Intermediate | 1 |
| Mepivacaine | 7.6 | 1.6:1 | 0.8 | 8 | Rapid | Intermediate | 1.4 |
| Bupivacaine | 8.1 | 5:1 | 10 | 95 | Slow | Long | 4 |
| Etidocaine | 7.7 | 2:1 | 141 | 94 | Rapid | Long | 2 |
| Ropivacaine | 8.1 | 5:1 | 2.9 | 94 | Rapid | Short-long | 3 |
| Levobupivacaine | 8.1 | 5:1 | 10 | 95 | Rapid | Short-long | 3 |

*Heptane/buffer (pH 7.4).

[†]Toxicity relative to lidocaine (value of 1).

interior negative relative to the exterior. This potential difference is maintained by the Na$^+$/K$^+$-ATPase pump through the constant extrusion of Na$^+$ from inside the cell in exchange for K$^+$, with resultant high intracellular K$^+$ and high extracellular Na$^+$ concentrations.

Action potentials are transient depolarizations of these excitable nerve cells. The reversal of the membrane potential during the generation or conduction of an action potential has been shown to be due to increased membrane permeability to Na$^+$. This leads to the membrane potential becoming less negative, which in turn is followed by a rapid influx of Na$^+$ into the cell, thereby further accelerating depolarization. The Na$^+$ channels then begin to close while an outflow of K$^+$ of a similar magnitude develops more slowly, and these changes result in repolarization of the membrane. Figure 21-2 shows the changes in membrane potential and the corresponding ionic currents during an action potential.

Ionophores can be present in three configurations. In the resting nerve, most Na$^+$ channels are in a *closed* state, such that the neuron is relatively impermeable. Depolarization causes these channels to be in the *open,* or *activated,* conformation, which allows Na$^+$ influx. Rapidly after this, however, the channels change to an impermeable *inactivated* conformation. This latter state is refractory to further stimulation until it returns to the resting, or *closed,* state. The *inactivated* state results in nerve conduction being unidirectional. The impulse is propagated along the axon by a local electrotonic current created by the potential difference between the depolarized section and the adjacent non-depolarized membrane.

## Site and Mode of Action of Local Anaesthetics

Local anaesthetics exert their effect on impulse conduction through a direct action on the sodium channel within the neuronal membrane. They induce a reversible and dose-dependent reduction in the rate of rise and height of the action potential, progressing to the point of total inhibition. There is also an elevation of the firing threshold and a slowing of the spread of conduction down the length of the axon as the concentration of the local anaesthetic increases. In myelinated nerves, these phenomena occur at the nodes of Ranvier.

As shown in Figure 21-3, voltage clamp experiments have demonstrated that local anaesthetics exert their effects by reducing the conductance of Na$^+$ into the cell, thereby preventing the expected transient increase in its permeability. This is accomplished by the binding of the ionized drug to a site directly on the inner surface of the Na$^+$ channel itself. This prevents opening of the channel by inhibiting conformational changes of the protein and preventing the normal cycling process. The effect of local anaesthetics on K$^+$ conduction is less than that on Na$^+$ conduction. Local anaesthetics share this property of blocking Na$^+$ entry with the highly specific channel blockers tetrodotoxin and saxitoxin, which have been used to advance our understanding of the mechanism of action of local anaesthetics.

The charged cationic form of the local anaesthetic molecule blocks neuronal conduction more effectively than the uncharged free base; this can be demonstrated

**FIGURE 21-2** (Top) The course of changes in membrane potential ($E_m$) and membrane conductance of Na$^+$ ($g_{Na}$) and K$^+$ ($g_K$) during propagation of an action potential in squid giant axon. (Bottom) The related Na$^+$ currents ($I_{Na}$), K$^+$ currents ($I_K$), and total membrane ionic current ($I_i$). The early, inward $I_{Na}$ drives the regenerative depolarizing phase of the impulse, whereas the more slowly developing $I_K$ underlies the rapid phase of repolarization. (Adapted from Butterworth and Strichartz, 1990, with permission.)

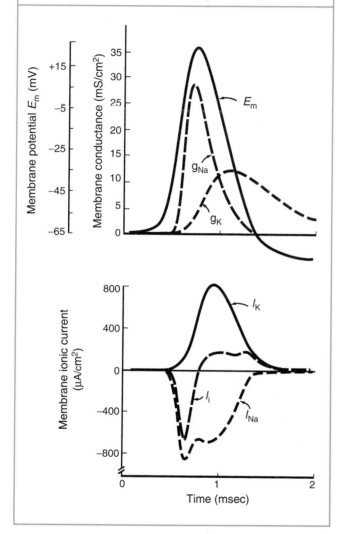

which represents both a small- and large-diameter axon, each having approximately the same density of Na$^+$ channels per unit of surface area. Following generation of the nerve impulse, depolarization spreads electrotonically further and more rapidly down the large axon than down the smaller axon. These local currents trigger the opening of the Na$^+$ channels, drawn as empty circles in Figure 21-5. The spread is unidirectional as the open channels then cycle into the refractory closed state. The large axon will have more excited channels than the small axon. When the anaesthetic is applied in a fixed concentration to a limited area of each axon, the small axon becomes completely blocked because its few excited channels are prevented from opening by the anaesthetic. The larger axon escapes blockade because more Na$^+$ channels are being excited and the limited amount of anaesthetic blocks only a portion of them. This property leads to a differential sensitivity of nerve fibres, such that the smaller fibres are more susceptible to blockade than are larger fibres. As a result, there is a differential blockade of sensory and motor functions. There are no intrinsic differences between sensory and motor nerves; however, there are differences in fibre size and myelination that account for this phenomenon.

Anaesthetic action can be increased by repeated stimulation of the nerve fibre. This is known as a *frequency-dependent* or *phasic block,* and it appears to be due to the local anaesthetic more readily gaining access to the binding site, as well as having a greater affinity for the binding site, when the channel is open. The result is that noxious stimuli, which can cause repeated bursts of depolarization, may be blocked more readily than motor activity, which normally has a lower frequency of discharge.

**FIGURE 21-3** Voltage clamp experiments show that the local anaesthetics primarily block the entry of Na$^+$ without affecting the exit of K$^+$.

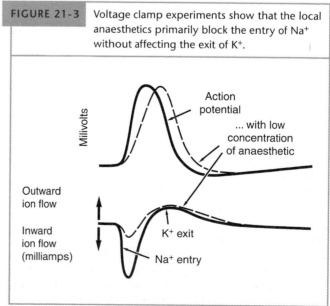

by altering the pH of the bathing solution in an isolated nerve preparation. The effect of pH on the ability of local anaesthetics to block action potentials is illustrated in Figure 21-4. The local anaesthetic is more effective at pH 7.0, when more of it is in the form of the charged cation, than at pH 8.0, when more is present as uncharged free base.

Once the necessary minimum number of channels is blocked over a length of the axon, the action potential cannot be propagated. This is illustrated in Figure 21-5,

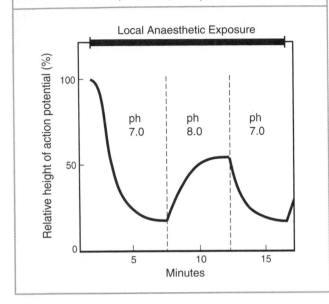

FIGURE 21-4  Effect of changing the pH of the internal bathing solution on the height of the action potential in the isolated giant axon of the squid while exposed to local anaesthetic action. (Adapted from Narahashi T, Frazier DT, Yamada M. The site of action and active form of local anesthetics. I. Theory and pH experiments with tertiary compounds. *J Pharmacol Exp Ther.* 1970;171:32-51, with permission.)

## TYPES OF LOCAL ANAESTHETIC BLOCKS

**Topical.** Local anaesthetic is applied to the surface of the skin, wounds, burns, or mucous membranes.

**Infiltration.** Local anaesthetic is injected directly into or around an area to be treated. This type of block is used for minor surgical procedures.

**Regional nerve block.** To obtain regional anaesthesia, local anaesthetic is injected in close proximity to the nerve supplying the area to be anaesthetized. This block is used for surgical and dental procedures as well as for pain relief.

**Spinal.** Local anaesthetic is injected into the cerebrospinal fluid in the lumbar subarachnoid space to reach the roots of the spinal nerves that supply the surgical site. Spinal block is used in surgery on the lower limbs and pelvis, as well as in obstetrics.

**Epidural, peridural, or extradural.** Local anaesthetic is injected into the extradural space through which the nerve roots pass. Uses are the same as for spinal anaesthesia, but the advantage is that the anaesthetic agent is less likely to rise accidentally to a higher segment of the spinal cord than was intended.

**Intravenous.** Local anaesthetic is injected into the venous system of a limb, distal to the point at which the circulation in that limb is interrupted by a tourniquet. Intravenous block is used for surgery on a limb.

**Sympathetic.** Sympathetic nerve blocks can be used in the treatment of pain caused by reflex sympathetic dystrophies such as causalgia and the shoulder–hand syndrome or for the intractable pain of carcinoma of the pancreas or upper abdomen.

## PHARMACOKINETICS

### Absorption and Onset of Action

The *absorption* of local anaesthetics is dependent upon the site of administration, dose, vasodilating properties, and presence of vasoconstrictor. With the exception of an intravenous block, it is important to understand that local anaesthetic action, unlike that of systemically administered drugs, is not dependent on absorption into the cir-

FIGURE 21-5  Blockade of impulse propagation in small- and large-diameter axons (see text).

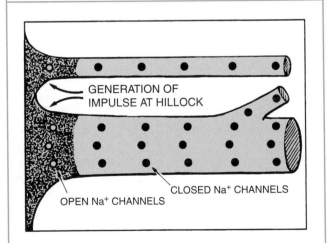

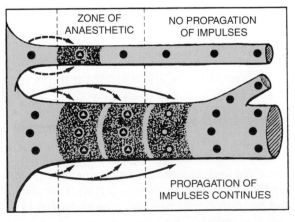

culation. On the contrary, absorption into the systemic circulation is a major factor in terminating the action. The *speed of onset* of the action of local anaesthetics depends on the following factors.

## Dose

To a limited extent, increases in the administered dose will result in a more rapid onset of action due to the greater number of molecules available to reach the site of action.

## Lipid solubility

Uptake by the nerve is facilitated by an increase in lipid solubility of the agents, as this allows more rapid penetration through the nerve sheath. Theoretically, however, increased lipid solubility may lead to sequestration into myelin and other lipid sites, which, on balance, tends to slow the onset of action. As listed in Table 21-1, relative lipid solubility is reflected in the lipid–water partition coefficient, which is related to the potency of the drug.

## Site of injection

Diffusion to the site of action is a factor in the onset of action; the further the drug is deposited from the nerve fibre, the longer it will take to act. Thus, the onset for the infiltration technique is quite rapid, whereas that for brachial plexus block may be prolonged. The speed of diffusion is influenced by tissue binding, removal by the circulation, and, in the case of esters, local hydrolysis.

## Nerve morphology

The morphology of the nerve bundle must be taken into account when considering the onset of action, as each nerve fibre has a differential sensitivity to the conduction-blocking effects of the agent, as stated earlier. The small, slowly conducting A-δ and C fibres, which conduct pain sensation, are blocked with lower concentrations of local anaesthetics than the larger A-α motor fibres. The result of this is a *differential sequence of onset of anaesthesia, with pain sensation being affected earliest, followed by temperature, touch, proprioception, and finally, motor function.*

## pH of the tissue

This will determine the ratio of ionized to unionized drug. Although local anaesthetics are usually formulated as the hydrochloride salt, and therefore are acidic, the strong buffering ability of extracellular fluid rapidly brings the pH of the solution to physiological levels. Carbonation of the local anaesthetic may improve the depth of neuronal blockade because the diffusion of carbon dioxide through the nerve membrane will decrease axoplasmic pH. This, in turn, promotes the formation of the charged form of the anaesthetic molecule. Carbonated local anaesthetics are formulated by the manufacturer by adding $CO_2$ and sealing the vial under pressure. The clinical advantage of carbonation is equivocal with respect to speed of onset, but it does appear to improve depth of blockade when the local anaesthetic is administered epidurally.

## p$K_a$ of the drug

The ratio of ionized to unionized drug is also dependent on the p$K_a$ of the drug. The relative degree of ionization has an important influence on rate of onset, duration, and pharmacodynamics. The uncharged base penetrates the membrane and has some activity of its own; therefore, a higher ratio of uncharged to charged species will increase the speed of onset of action. Some local anaesthetic solutions are prepared in buffered alkaline media with the intention of promoting a faster onset attributable to the higher proportion of uncharged molecules. Again, the strong buffering ability of the tissue minimizes this effect. Furthermore, there is a limit to the amount that the pH can be raised because of the need to avoid causing local tissue irritation or necrosis.

The ionization of local anaesthetics depends on the hydrogen ion concentration of their environment and their p$K_a$, for example,

$$R-N \begin{matrix} CH_3 \\ \\ CH_3 \end{matrix} + H^+ \rightleftharpoons R-\overset{\oplus}{N} \begin{matrix} CH_3 \\ H \\ CH_3 \end{matrix}$$

These effects may be represented in the following:

$$BH^+ \rightleftharpoons H^+ + B \rightleftharpoons \| B \| \rightleftharpoons B + H^+ \rightleftharpoons BH^+$$

| Aqueous phases | Nerve sheath | Membrane phase |

Let $B$ represent the local anaesthetic base (unionized), and $BH^+$ the ionized form. The anaesthetic has been administered by injection in an aqueous solution in which the ionized and unionized forms exist at equilibrium. Only the unionized form, $B$, can effectively penetrate through the nerve sheath into the neuronal membrane, where it once again establishes equilibrium with the ionized molecule. Once inside the neuronal membrane, it is the ionized form that is necessary for effective blockade of $Na^+$ influx. The less ionized, the greater the uptake into the nerve; the more ionized, the greater the effect at the membrane itself.

The relative ratios are determined by the p$K_a$ of the agents. This relationship is described by the Henderson–Hasselbalch equation:

$$pK_a - pH = \log [\text{ionized/unionized}]$$

The p$K_a$ of most anaesthetics ranges from 7.6 to 9.0. At physiological pH 7.4, most of the local anaesthetic will therefore be in the ionized state, as a charged base. An example is lidocaine, which has a p$K_a$ of 7.9. At physiological pH, it exists in a ratio of 3:1 ionized to unionized, based on this formula. Another example is procaine, with a p$K_a$ of 8.9. The higher p$K_a$ value means that, at physiological pH, procaine exists in a ratio of approximately 32:1 ionized to unionized. Since lidocaine has a relatively greater proportion of the unionized form than procaine does, it would be expected to have a more rapid onset of action, which is confirmed clinically. In general, all other factors being equal, the most rapid onset would be expected from agents with the lowest $pK_a$ values (see Table 21-1).

Although the buffering capacity of the body is significant, the pH of the tissue may become more acidic during a localized infection and cause a greater proportion of ionized anaesthetic molecules, thereby delaying or preventing the onset of action. For example, if lidocaine ($pK_a$ 7.9) is administered into a site of infection in which the local pH is 5.9, there would be 100 times as many ionized as unionized forms. Greatly reduced penetration into the nerve tissue would be expected, and this is confirmed clinically. As well, additional factors may be present during an acute infection that may also predispose to local anaesthetic failure.

## Duration of Action

The duration of action of local anaesthetics depends primarily on the redistribution of the drug away from the site of action. These drugs can often be categorized as short-acting, such as procaine and chloroprocaine; intermediate-acting, such as lidocaine, mepivacaine, and prilocaine; and long-acting, such as bupivacaine, etidocaine, ropivacaine, and tetracaine. The duration of action can be altered by the following factors, some of which also influence onset.

### Dose
Increases in the administered dose can increase the duration of action. Doubling the dose prolongs duration by about one half-life.

### Lipid solubility
Within limits, increases in lipid solubility increase the potency and duration of action. This is due to the greater ease with which the drug penetrates the connective tissue layers and nerve sheath into the hydrophobic portion of the neuronal membrane. Since it penetrates more readily, more molecules are now present at the site of action, thus allowing for a longer duration. The relative potencies of local anaesthetics, as well as their protein binding, correlate reasonably well in rank order with their lipid solubilities, as measured by their partition coefficients.

### Diffusion from site of administration
This is the major factor in determining duration of action. It is dependent in part on the vascularity of the tissue surrounding the nerve. Removal from the site is highest with intercostal nerve blocks, followed by lumbar epidural blocks and brachial plexus blocks; slowest removal occurs in poorly vascularized subcutaneous sites. Vasodilating properties differ among the agents, with procaine and lidocaine having strong dilating properties and agents such as bupivacaine having weaker effects. Except for cocaine, all local anaesthetics are inherently vasodilating to an extent such that administration in vascular tissues alone can result in an inappropriately short duration of action.

Diffusion from the site can be reduced by the addition of a vasoconstrictor. This causes a local reduction in blood flow, which, in turn, reduces the rate of uptake of the drug into the circulation, thereby allowing a longer exposure of the nerve to the local anaesthetic. In addition, this reduces the likelihood of systemic toxicity by decreasing the rate of systemic uptake, and it provides localized hemostasis during infiltration for surgery. Adrenaline is most commonly used for this purpose, being supplied as an accompanying agent in a range of concentrations from 5 µg/mL (1:200 000) to 20 µg/mL (1:50 000). Other vasoconstrictors that have been used include phenylephrine, noradrenaline, and levonordefrin.

### Protein binding
Highly protein-bound agents such as bupivacaine, etidocaine, ropivacaine, and tetracaine have an extended duration of action. It is assumed that the degree of plasma protein binding of local anaesthetics correlates with the degree of binding to the neuronal membrane proteins that constitute the ion channels. Greater affinity at this latter site would be expected to prolong action. Binding to tissue proteins may also contribute to the duration of action by reducing the concentration of the free form and thus reducing its rate of diffusion away from the site. Furthermore, increased protein binding of the more lipid-soluble compounds tends to decrease their toxicity and reduce transfer across the placenta.

## Distribution, Biotransformation, and Elimination

The distribution of local anaesthetics when absorbed into the circulation can be described by a two- or three-compartment model. They distribute widely, with highly perfused tissues having greater concentration, as expected. There is rapid extraction by lung tissue.

Biotransformation is dependent on whether the drug is an ester or amide. Esters are hydrolyzed by plasma cholinesterase or by liver esterases, in most cases releasing free PABA, which is known to be allergenic. As discussed in Chapter 10, patients with atypical plasma cholinesterase would be expected to metabolize procaine at a much lower rate. Clinically, however, this is of little consequence unless potentially toxic levels of anaesthetic are employed. Half-lives of elimination of ester-type agents are less than 1 minute.

Amides are biotransformed exclusively by the liver, with the exception of prilocaine, which is also metabolized in the plasma and kidneys. Lidocaine, mepivacaine, bupivacaine, and etidocaine undergo *N*-dealkylation followed by hydrolysis. Ropivacaine undergoes extensive biotransformation by hydrolysis and conjugation. Articaine undergoes hydrolysis by plasma esterases prior to hepatic biotransformation. One of the active metabolites of lidocaine is monoethylglycine xylidide, which is approximately 80% as potent as lidocaine and may be responsible for the toxicity and adverse effects, such as sedation, when excessive doses are used. One of the metabolites of prilocaine is ortho-toluidine, which reduces hemoglobin to methemoglobin and may lead to methemoglobinemia if produced in excess. Half-lives of elimination of amide-type agents range from 90 to 160 minutes.

The pharmacokinetic characteristics may be altered by the health of the patient. If hepatic function or blood flow is significantly altered by disease, changes in the plasma levels of the amide anaesthetics would be expected. Reduced hepatic function would predispose to toxicity (see below) but, unlike its effect on systemically administered drugs, it would not be expected to cause a significant increase in the duration of action of locally administered anaesthetics.

## ADVERSE REACTIONS AND TOXICITY

Adverse reactions may be a result of toxicity, allergy, or an anxiety-induced psychogenic reaction. **Toxic effects** are a function of systemic absorption. High blood levels may be secondary to excessive amounts injected extravascularly, or they could be the result of a single inadvertent intravascular administration into a major vessel. Many factors modify toxicity, such as a raised $CO_2$ or $H^+$ level in the patient, which will increase the amount of the more active ionized form of the anaesthetic. In general, toxicity manifests itself in the CNS and cardiovascular system. The nervous system effects include both excitatory and inhibitory phenomena. With increasing doses, CNS effects are characterized progressively by mild sedation, lightheadedness, dizziness, sensory disturbances, disorientation, tremors, muscle twitching, tonic–clonic seizures, cardiovascular instability, and ultimately by respiratory arrest, cardiovascular collapse, and coma. The ability to cause central excitation is correlated with the intrinsic anaesthetic potency.

Local anaesthetics have significant cardiovascular effects, both on the myocardium and peripheral vascular smooth muscle. The direct effect on the myocardium is also correlated with anaesthetic potency and is reflected in a depression of excitability, rate of conduction, and force of contraction, resulting in decreased cardiac output, hypotension, and eventually cardiovascular system collapse. The effects on myocardial conduction are related to those of some of the anti-arrhythmic agents (see Chapter 33). Bupivacaine is noted to have enhanced cardiotoxicity compared with the others, due to its ability to bind more strongly to resting sodium channels of the myocardium and dissociate more slowly during diastole.

Generally, local anaesthetics are devoid of direct toxicity to nerves when used in therapeutic concentrations, and nerve function recovers completely following a nerve block or spinal anaesthesia. Higher concentrations, however, such as 5% lidocaine, 4% prilocaine, or 4% articaine, have been associated with irreversible conduction block. Local skeletal muscle damage may occur, but this effect is reversible.

In general, the incidence of toxicity of local anaesthetics is very low. This is largely due to the administration of these drugs into a restricted area of the body, from which systemic absorption occurs only gradually. Recommendations for maximum doses are often given, but these must be assessed critically. Toxicity is dependent upon numerous factors, such as site of administration, speed of injection, and presence or absence of vasoconstrictor. Given this caveat, the maximum recommended doses for infiltration or regional nerve block anaesthesia in healthy adults are summarized in Table 21-2.

A true **allergy** to an amide local anaesthetic is rare, whereas esters are somewhat more allergenic because of the PABA metabolite. Allergies to other ingredients in the drug formulation are possible. These include the preservative methylparaben or the antioxidant metabisulfite.

**Anxiety-induced psychogenic events** are relatively common adverse reactions associated with local anaesthetic administration. They may manifest as syncope, hyperventilation, nausea, vomiting, or alterations in heart rate or blood pressure, or they may mimic an allergic reaction. Adverse events may also be the result of inadvertent intravascular administration of a vasoconstrictor, which would produce the expected cardiovascular signs of sympathetic stimulation.

| TABLE 21-2 | Maximum Recommended Doses of Local Anaesthetics* | |
|---|---|---|
| Drug | Plain Solution (mg/kg) | With Vasoconstrictor (mg/kg) |
| Procaine | 5 | 8 |
| Tetracaine | 1.4 | 2.8 |
| Chloroprocaine | 11 | 14 |
| Lidocaine | 4 | 7 |
| Prilocaine | 8 | 8 |
| Mepivacaine | 4 | 6.6 |
| Bupivacaine | 2 | 2 |
| Etidocaine | 4 | 6 |
| Articaine | 7 | 7 |

*Toxicity depends on numerous factors, of which the total administered dose is only one (see text).

# COMMONLY USED LOCAL ANAESTHETICS

Local anaesthetics are usually classified by structure on the basis of intermediate linkage of ester or amide type (see Fig. 21-1).

## Esters

**Cocaine** is primarily of historical interest for regional block techniques; this drug is too toxic for any use other than topical. Cocaine is unique among local anaesthetics in that it induces vasoconstriction and has addiction potential. It may be used for topical application to mucous membranes, including oropharyngeal and nasal cavities, prior to local surgical procedures, bronchoscopy, or nasal intubation.

**Procaine** was the first synthetic local anaesthetic. It has a slow onset, short duration of action, and weak potency. Although procaine has low systemic toxicity, esters in general, as noted above, are more allergenic than the amides. Procaine is most effective when used for infiltration anaesthesia or nerve blocks. Although used widely in the past, it has been superseded by amides.

**Tetracaine** is approximately 10 times as potent as procaine with respect to its anaesthetic action and systemic toxicity. It has a long duration of action but a slow onset, due to its relatively high $pK_a$. Its major clinical application is spinal anaesthesia, where it has a more rapid onset due to the reduction in barriers to diffusion. Tetracaine is effective topically, but this use is limited by its significant toxicity, which may occur following absorption through mucous membranes.

**Chloroprocaine** has a rapid onset of action, short duration, and relatively low systemic toxicity. Its rapid onset of action occurs in spite of its high $pK_a$ because it is formulated in relatively high concentrations, which is feasible because of its low toxicity. It is used for infiltration, nerve block, intravenous, and epidural techniques. Potential local neurotoxicity was shown to be due to the antioxidant metabisulfite, which is no longer contained in the formulation.

**Benzocaine** is poorly soluble and therefore available for topical use only. Excessive absorption may lead to methemoglobinemia.

**Propoxycaine** is formulated in combination with procaine and a vasoconstrictor, which provides a prolonged duration of action.

## Amides

**Lidocaine** is the most commonly used local anaesthetic agent. This xylidine derivative is the prototype for the amide group; it has a rapid onset with an intermediate duration of action. It has prominent vasodilating properties and therefore specific formulations include adrenaline. It is effective for most types of local anaesthetic blocks.

**Prilocaine** is a toluidine derivative similar to lidocaine in properties and uses, except that it is less inherently vasodilating. It provides a similar duration of action and has similar indications to those of lidocaine. It is associated with the risk of methemoglobinemia.

**Mepivacaine** is a xylidine derivative similar to lidocaine; it may be used for infiltration, nerve block, and epidural procedures. It is not effective as a topical agent, and it is not used in obstetric anaesthesia because its biotransformation is prolonged in the fetus.

**Bupivacaine** is a xylidine derivative characterized by a long duration of action. Its onset of action is slower than that of lidocaine, but it is very potent and has good separation of sensory and motor blockade. Bupivacaine has a greater relative toxicity than lidocaine—in particular, a greater potential for cardiotoxicity. Compared with other amides, it has a smaller difference between the doses that lead to cardiovascular collapse and to CNS effects. It can be used for infiltration, nerve block, epidural, and spinal procedures.

**Etidocaine** is a xylidine derivative similar to bupivacaine in that it is characterized by a long duration of action, strong potency, and relatively high cardiotoxicity. However, it differs in that it has a rapid onset of action and little separation of sensory and motor blockade. It is used for infiltration and nerve block.

**Levobupivacaine** is the pure *S*-enantiomer of bupivacaine and was introduced in an attempt to reduce the cardiotoxicity associated with bupivacaine, which is racemic, as are most other local anaesthetics. It may be given by continuous infusion to provide prolonged postoperative analgesia.

**Ropivacaine** is the propyl homologue of bupivacaine and is a pure *S*-enantiomer. It was also introduced in an attempt to reduce the cardiotoxicity associated with bupivacaine. The indications for its use are similar to those for bupivacaine and levobupivacaine.

**Articaine** is a thiophene derivative that appears to be similar to lidocaine. It has wide use in dentistry.

# SUGGESTED READINGS

Berde CB, Strichartz GR. Local anesthetics. In: Miller RD, ed. *Anesthesia*. 5th ed. New York, NY: Churchill Livingstone; 2000.

Butterworth JF, Strichartz GR. Molecular mechanism of local anesthesia: a review. *Anesthesiology*. 1990;72:711-734.

Catteral W, Mackie K. Local anesthetics. In: Hardman JG, Limbird LE, Goodman Gilman A, eds. *Goodman & Gilman's The Pharmacological Basis of Therapeutics*. 10th ed. New York, NY: McGraw-Hill Medical; 2001:367-384.

Liu SS, Hodgson PS. Local anesthetics. In: Barash PG, Cullen BF, Stoelting RK, eds. *Clinical Anesthesia*. 4th ed. Philadelphia, Pa: Lippincott Williams & Wilkins; 2001:449-469.

Thomas JM, Schug SA. Recent advances in the pharmacokinetics of local anaesthetics. *Clin Pharmacokinet*. 1999;36:67-83.

# 22

# The Alcohols

## H KALANT AND JM KHANNA

### CASE HISTORY

J.N., a 56-year-old vice-president of a brokerage firm, was required to undergo a thorough medical examination in connection with a large company-sponsored insurance policy. He denied any current illness, but laboratory test results indicated mildly elevated levels of aspartate transaminase (79 mU/mL), γ-glutamyl transpeptidase (62 mU/mL), and carbohydrate-deficient transferrin (41 mg/L). His physical examination had also revealed a slightly enlarged liver, but of normal consistency and not tender. The physician therefore took a more detailed history and functional inquiry and learned that J.N. had been under gradually but steadily increasing pressure at work for the past 6 or 7 years. He had previously used alcohol socially without apparent problems but had started to increase his intake and now drank an average of five or six drinks a day, and as much as eight drinks on occasion. One uncle on his father's side was said to have had an alcohol problem of long duration.

J.N.'s blood pressure had increased in the last few years and was now 185/100 mmHg, despite the initiation of enalapril therapy by his own family physician. He had also been using diazepam more frequently for relief of tension, and he used flunitrazepam two or three times a week for relief of insomnia. Some years earlier, he had consulted a gastroenterologist because of epigastric pain, which was diagnosed as being due to a duodenal ulcer, and he was started on therapy with ranitidine, which he continued up to the present. However, the gastric discomfort had recurred twice in the past 2 years, during therapy with naproxen, a non-steroidal anti-inflammatory agent that he took during flare-ups of osteoarthritis in his knees.

Finally, J.N. admitted to the physician that, 3 years ago, he had been arrested for impaired driving when coming home from a party. A breath test had indicated a blood alcohol concentration of 154 mg/dL, and he had pleaded guilty. He was fined and his licence was suspended for 1 year. This had been a major inconvenience to him, as well as an emotional jolt, and he claimed that, since his licence had been restored, he never drove after drinking, but his wife hinted that this might not be entirely true.

The use of ethyl alcohol dates from prehistoric times and occurs in almost all parts of the world. Probably this is because the requirements for production of alcohol are extremely simple: some plant material containing starch or sugar, some moisture, yeast (even wild strains from the air), and an ambient temperature high enough to permit fermentation. The earliest technological "improvement" (still used in some technologically undeveloped societies) was to chew the grain or tubers to crush them and mix them with yeasts from the chewer's mouth, then spit them back into a container with water, and leave them to ferment. In ancient times, this crude method gradually evolved into fairly sophisticated methods for producing wines and beers of relatively low alcohol content. Distillation was invented by Arabic chemists, from whom it spread to Europe in the Middle Ages, and it permitted the production of much more potent beverages.

In view of the long association of alcohol with human life and culture, it is not surprising that alcohol has many religious, symbolic, social, economic, and legal roles. These are reviewed in Chapter 70. The present chapter deals primarily with pharmacological, biochemical, and clinical aspects.

## CHEMISTRY, METABOLISM, AND METABOLIC EFFECTS

### Physical Chemistry

The aliphatic alcohols form a homologous series beginning with methanol:

| | |
|---|---|
| CH₃–OH | Methanol (wood alcohol) |
| CH₃–CH₂–OH | Ethanol (grain alcohol) |
| CH₃–CH₂–CH₂–OH | *n*-Propanol |
| CH₃–CH–CH₃ <br>    &#124; <br>    OH | Isopropanol |
| CH₃–CH₂–CH₂–CH₂–OH | *n*-Butanol |

etc.

The first two are completely miscible with water and have very low lipid–water partition coefficients, but water solubility decreases as chain length increases, so octanol is virtually insoluble in water. Within the series of straight-chain alcohols, potency in a variety of biological assays is proportional to the chain length, increasing by a factor of two to three with each additional carbon. However, because of the decrease in water solubility, it is hard to achieve a toxic concentration in the body with longer-chain alcohols than pentanol or hexanol. All of the lower alcohols are used as solvents, but only ethanol is sufficiently non-toxic to be used as a beverage, though trace amounts of other alcohols are found in many alcoholic beverages. The amount of alcohol contained in 1.5 oz. (43 mL) of distilled spirits (40% v/v), 12 oz. of most regular beers (5% v/v), or 5 oz. of an average table wine (12% v/v) is approximately the same (13.6 g). This is referred to as a standard drink in Canada and the United States, but the size of a "standard" drink in other countries varies greatly, from 6 g in Austria to 19.75 g in Japan. There is no relation between the size of a standard drink and the average per capita alcohol consumption in any given country.

### Absorption and Distribution

Ethanol is readily absorbed through any mucosal surface by simple diffusion. This can occur in the stomach but is faster in the intestine, so a delay in gastric emptying, as by food or strenuous physical activity, slows the absorption. The rate of ethanol absorption is highest with 20 to 30% ethanol; it is slower with very dilute solutions because of a lower diffusion gradient. More concentrated alcohol may slow absorption by causing gastric irritation and pylorospasm. Ethanol vapour can also be absorbed readily through the lung, and rats and mice can easily be deeply intoxicated by this route.

After absorption from the gastrointestinal (GI) tract, ethanol is carried to the liver and then to the systemic circulation, diffusing into all tissues and body fluids, including the cerebrospinal fluid (CSF), sweat, urine, and breath. The equilibrium partition coefficient for ethanol between blood and alveolar air in humans is, on average, approximately 2400:1 but varies considerably among individuals; one study of almost 800 drinking drivers in Sweden found that it could range from less than 2100:1 to more than 2700:1. Nevertheless, the ethanol concentration in end-expiratory air can be measured and multiplied by the average partition coefficient (e.g., by Breathalyzer or Intoxilyzer instruments) to provide a fairly accurate estimate of the ethanol concentration in the blood.

Since ethanol is highly water-soluble and its molecular weight is only 46 Da, it moves easily through aqueous channels in cell membranes. *Therefore, it distributes and equilibrates quickly throughout the entire body water,* and its $V_d$ equals the volume of total body water. Alcohol dilution can therefore be used to measure total body water (see "Pharmacokinetics" below and Fig. 22-3). The blood alcohol concentration (BAC) produced by a given number of standard drinks varies from one person to another as a function of individual differences in volume of total body water. This volume is greater in persons with greater height and weight. However, as a percentage of total body weight it is inversely related to the percentage of body fat, so that it tends to decrease with age, to be lower in women than in men, and to be lower in obese individuals than in lean muscular ones of the same body weight.

Though alcohol passes rapidly across capillary walls, differences in blood flow to different tissues result in differences in the rates at which alcohol concentrations in the various tissues and fluids come into equilibrium with the concentration in the blood. This is most marked during the phase of rapid rise of blood alcohol level. During this phase, the rapid diffusion of ethanol from capillary blood into tissue fluid causes the ethanol concentration to be lower in the venous blood leaving the tissue than in the arterial blood entering it. The smaller the volume of blood flow per gram of tissue per minute, the larger is this early arterial–venous (A–V) difference in ethanol concentration. During this time, therefore, the concentration in a sample of blood from a hand or forearm vein is misleadingly low in comparison with the concentration reaching the brain (Fig. 22-1). Once distribution is complete, the A–V difference disappears and may be reversed after the BAC begins to fall. The point at which this happens (i.e., the time of peak BAC) is, on average, about 40 to 60 minutes after the end of drinking, but it varies greatly between individuals, and within the same individual on different occasions, depending on the rate of gastric emptying, the presence or absence of food in the stomach, the type and intensity of physical activity at the time, and the effects of other drugs that may be taken concurrently.

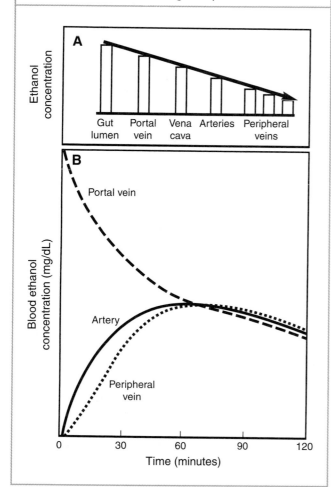

**FIGURE 22-1** (A) Schematic representation of the concentration gradient of ethanol from jejunal lumen to peripheral veins during the early stage of absorption and distribution. (B) Time course of arterial–venous (A–V) differences in ethanol concentration during absorption and distribution.

dizing system **(MEOS)**, which is essentially CYP2E1 and its related coenzymes. All evidence favours the view that, normally, *ADH is by far the most important hepatic enzyme responsible for the in vivo oxidation of ethanol.* Small amounts of ADH are also present in the gastrointestinal mucosa, renal tubular epithelium, lung, and brain and may be responsible for a small amount of extrahepatic oxidation of ethanol.

### Metabolic pathways

ADH is not a single enzyme, but a family of enzymes that are grouped in classes (Class I to Class V). Each enzyme molecule consists of two subunits, which may be identical (homodimer) or different from each other (heterodimer). Seven types of subunit are known, of which six are found in the human. Each subunit is coded for by a different gene. The various subunits differ from each other by only a single amino acid, but the effects on the substrate specificity and kinetics are large. Though ADH is found in virtually all tissues, there is considerable difference in the tissue distribution of the different subunits and enzyme classes. The relationships among the different enzyme classes, genes, subunits, and enzymatic activities are summarized in Table 22-1.

Chronic ingestion of substantial amounts of ethanol leads to induction of the cytochrome P450 system, especially CYP2E1, which has high substrate specificity for ethanol. This induction may be an important factor in the increased rate of alcohol oxidation seen in regular heavy drinkers. It is also related to the ability of chronic heavy drinking to induce the metabolism of a number of other drugs that are substrates of the P450 system.

Since diffusion is a first-order process, the rate at which ethanol is lost from the body in the urine, breath, and sweat is proportional to the plasma concentration of ethanol. Over the range of concentrations produced by light to very heavy drinking, between 2% and 10% of the ingested dose can be lost in this way.

## Biotransformation

Minute amounts of ethanol are conjugated with glucuronic or sulfuric acid (see Chapter 4) and excreted in the urine. By far the most important biotransformation reaction, however, is oxidation to acetaldehyde and then to acetate, primarily in the liver (Fig. 22-2).

The three principal enzymatic mechanisms that can oxidize ethanol to acetaldehyde are **alcohol dehydrogenase (ADH), catalase,** and a **microsomal ethanol-oxi-**

**FIGURE 22-2** The two initial steps of ethanol metabolism in the liver.

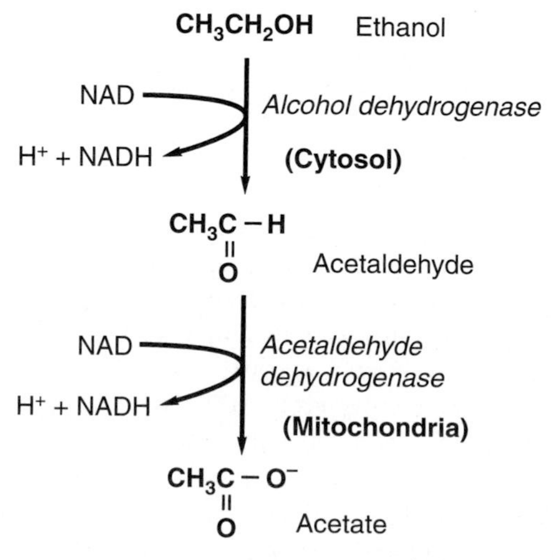

$$CH_3CH_2OH \quad \text{Ethanol}$$

NAD → | Alcohol dehydrogenase
$H^+ + NADH$ ← | **(Cytosol)**

$$CH_3C-H$$
$$\underset{O}{\overset{\|}{}} \quad \text{Acetaldehyde}$$

NAD → | Acetaldehyde dehydrogenase
$H^+ + NADH$ ← | **(Mitochondria)**

$$CH_3C-O^-$$
$$\underset{O}{\overset{\|}{}} \quad \text{Acetate}$$

| TABLE 22-1 | Characteristics of Alcohol Dehydrogenases in the Human | | | | | |
|---|---|---|---|---|---|
| ADH Class | Gene | Subunit | Main Substrate | EtOH $K_m$ (mM) | Tissue Locations |
| I | ADH 1 | $\alpha$ | Short-chain alcohols | 0.05–4 | Liver, adrenals; lower levels in lung, kidney, etc.; absent in brain |
| | ADH 2 | $\beta_{1-3}$ | | | |
| | ADH 3 | $\gamma_{1,2}$ | | | |
| II | ADH 4 | $\pi$ | Ethanol? | 34 | Liver, small intestine |
| III | ADH 5 | $\chi$ | Long-chain alcohols, omega-hydroxy-fatty acids | | All tissues, some tumours |
| IV | ADH 7 | $\sigma$ ($\mu$) | Retinal | 28 | Stomach and upper GI tract |

Most of the acetaldehyde formed from ethanol is oxidized to acetate by the mitochondrial acetaldehyde dehydrogenase in the liver. Small amounts of acetaldehyde that escape into the circulation are oxidized rapidly in other tissues. Acetaldehyde is a highly reactive substance, and even transient elevation of levels in the blood can result in formation of permanent (covalently bonded) complexes with hemoglobin and plasma proteins. These complexes act as antigens, which can be measured by appropriate antibodies. Alcoholics have significantly raised plasma levels of such antigens, and this finding may possibly give rise to a useful diagnostic or screening test for heavy drinking.

Some of the acetate is converted to acetyl–coenzyme A (acetyl–CoA) in the liver and oxidized to $CO_2$ and $H_2O$, or is converted to amino acids, fatty acids, or glycogen in the same way as acetyl–CoA from other sources. However, large amounts of acetate pass into the systemic circulation and are taken up in other tissues, converted to acetyl–CoA, and oxidized in those tissues.

The rate-limiting step in the whole process is the oxidation by ADH. The rate of this reaction in normal, well-nourished individuals is determined by the concentration of the ADH enzyme and by the concentration of NAD, or the NAD:NADH ratio, which, in turn, depends on the rate of reoxidation of NADH. The activity of ADH can be strongly inhibited by pyrazole and 4-methylpyrazole (fomepazole). Fomepazole is now a recommended treatment for poisoning with methyl alcohol or ethylene glycol, to prevent them from being converted by ADH to the highly toxic products formic acid and oxalic acid, respectively. A number of other drugs (e.g., ciprofloxacin, cimetidine, ranitidine, various formamide derivatives, nitric oxide) can also act as inhibitors of different types of ADH and thus prolong the effects of alcohol under some circumstances.

## Pharmacokinetics

There are differences between individuals and within the same person, but *on average, a 70-kg human can oxidize about 10 g of ethanol per hour.* This means that the typical blood alcohol curve, after oral ingestion in the fasting state, rises to a peak level in 30 to 90 minutes, depending on the dose, and then falls at a fairly steady rate of 15 to 20 mg/dL/hr until the concentration reaches about 25 mg/dL; below this point, it falls exponentially (Fig. 22-3). However, ADH actually exhibits Michaelis–Menten kinetics, so the apparently linear portion of the curve is really a very shallow curve, and its slope is affected by the maximum concentration reached before the BAC starts to fall: the higher the maximum concentration attained, the greater is the initial rate of descent.

If the apparently linear ("pseudolinear") portion of the curve is projected back to $t_0$ (see Fig. 22-3), the intercept on the vertical axis is $C_0$, which is the theoretical concentration that would have been found if all the administered dose of ethanol had been instantaneously absorbed and uniformly distributed throughout its $V_d$. Since ethanol is distributed almost entirely in the body water, and blood contains about 80% water, $C_0$ in the blood corresponds to 80% of the $C_0$ in the water phase, or $C_{0\,water} = 1.25 \times C_{0\,blood}$. As well, $C_{0\,water}$ = dose/volume of body water. Therefore, if dose and $C_{0\,water}$ are known, total body water can be estimated; this method has been used clinically for that purpose, and the determined values are in close agreement with those obtained by isotope dilution methods.

It has been suggested that a gender difference in gastric mucosal $\sigma$ADH activity (lower in women than in men) may cause a difference in gastric first-pass metabolism of ethanol and therefore be responsible for higher BACs in women than in men after the same dose of ethanol per unit of body weight. However, it is extremely doubtful that gastric first-pass metabolism of ethanol plays any significant role in humans, because estimates of total body water by the ethanol dilution method are identical whether the ethanol is given by mouth or intravenously. This means that bioavailability of alcohol by mouth must be essentially complete. Moreover, BACs in men and women are identical if they are given the same dose of alcohol per unit of body water rather than per unit of body weight.

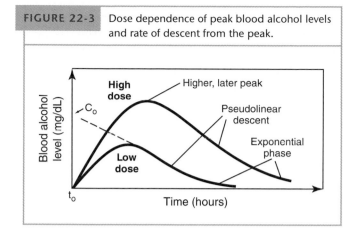

**FIGURE 22-3** Dose dependence of peak blood alcohol levels and rate of descent from the peak.

Since the oxidation of ethanol requires simultaneous reduction of NAD to NADH, anything that makes NAD more available by reoxidizing NADH more rapidly will help to keep the rate of alcohol metabolism at the maximum permitted by the amount of ADH present. Fructose, insulin plus glucose, and other sources of pyruvate may do this. However, it is not possible to speed up the process past its normal maximum by this means. Dinitrophenol can increase the rate of NADH reoxidation (and hence of ethanol oxidation) beyond the normal limit by uncoupling oxidation from phosphorylation, but it is too toxic to use clinically.

## Metabolic Effects of Ethanol

The change of NAD to NADH, resulting from the metabolism of ethanol and acetaldehyde, affects other NAD-linked metabolic processes. Some of the better-studied examples are listed below and in Fig 22-4.

1. Pyruvate is reduced to lactate by lactate dehydrogenase (simultaneously oxidizing NADH to NAD), causing varying degrees of *elevation of serum lactate and metabolic acidosis*. The raised lactate inhibits renal secretion of urate and thus can *precipitate attacks of gout.*
2. Increased hepatic NADH also favours reduction of glyceraldehyde-3-phosphate to glycerol-3-phosphate and inhibits glycerophosphate dehydrogenase, leading to an elevated glycerol-3-phosphate level.
3. At the same time, the excess production of acetate from acetaldehyde, together with the raised NADH level, stimulates the synthesis of fatty acids in the liver, while their oxidation via the tricarboxylic acid cycle is blocked.
4. The excess of glycerol-3-phosphate and fatty acids leads to increased esterification and accumulation of neutral triglycerides in the liver. Ethanol itself can also form ethyl esters with fatty acids, glucuronic and sulfuric acids, and others.

5. The increase in NADH and decrease in pyruvate result in a reduced rate of gluconeogenesis. Therefore, if hepatic glycogen supplies are depleted by lack of adequate food intake, ethanol causes hypoglycemia.
6. The raised NADH level also inhibits the enzyme systems that convert galactose to glucose and that conjugate glycine and benzoate to form hippuric acid (see Chapter 4), so the liver function tests based on these enzymes are disturbed.

All these changes above are reversible when alcohol oxidation is complete.

7. However, chronic heavy ingestion of alcohol increases not only the rate of alcohol oxidation in the liver but also the rate of hepatic $O_2$ consumption. Consequently, the risk of hypoxia in the liver is increased, especially at the hepatic venous end of the sinusoid, where the $PO_2$ is normally lowest anyway (see Chapter 43). This is one suggested explanation why liver cell necrosis in heavy drinkers is found chiefly around the collecting veins ("central veins").
8. In the brain, ethanol can be oxidized to acetaldehyde by the very small amount of Class III alcohol dehydrogenase present there, as well as by catalase and possibly other neuronal or glial enzymes. Even though the amount of acetaldehyde formed is probably quite small, its high reactivity causes it to form condensation products with dopamine, serotonin, and other neuroamines or with the aldehydes produced by the action of monoamine oxidase (MAO) on these amines (Fig. 22-5). The possible roles of such condensation products in the actions of ethanol on the brain are not yet clear.

Numerous other metabolic effects of ethanol are produced in other tissues, but their pharmacological or pathological significance is not yet well established.

# ETHANOL ACTIONS AND INTOXICATION

## Membrane and Cellular Effects of Ethanol

All tissues and cells can be affected by certain concentrations of ethanol, but they differ greatly in sensitivity. At bactericidal concentrations (about 70% or more), protein denaturation and precipitation occurs, as in fixation of tissues for histology. At much lower concentrations (e.g., less than 0.1%), the actions are quite different and involve a reversible modification of various cell membrane functions.

Although ethanol is much more water-soluble than the major anaesthetic agents, its membrane actions are similar in many respects to those of other anaesthetics on excitable cell membranes (see Chapters 20 and 21). In very

**FIGURE 22-4** Evolving concepts of the relationhip between ethanol metabolism and alcohol-related organic damage. The pre-1960 vision of ethanol metabolism is shown in the central shaded area. Discoveries since 1960 have added the rest of the information shown in the figure. The end results, in terms of organ damage or its detection, are circled. (From Kalant, H. Research on alcohol metabolism: a historical perspective. *Keio J Med.* 1991;40(3):113-117. Reproduced by permission of *The Keio Journal of Medicine.*)

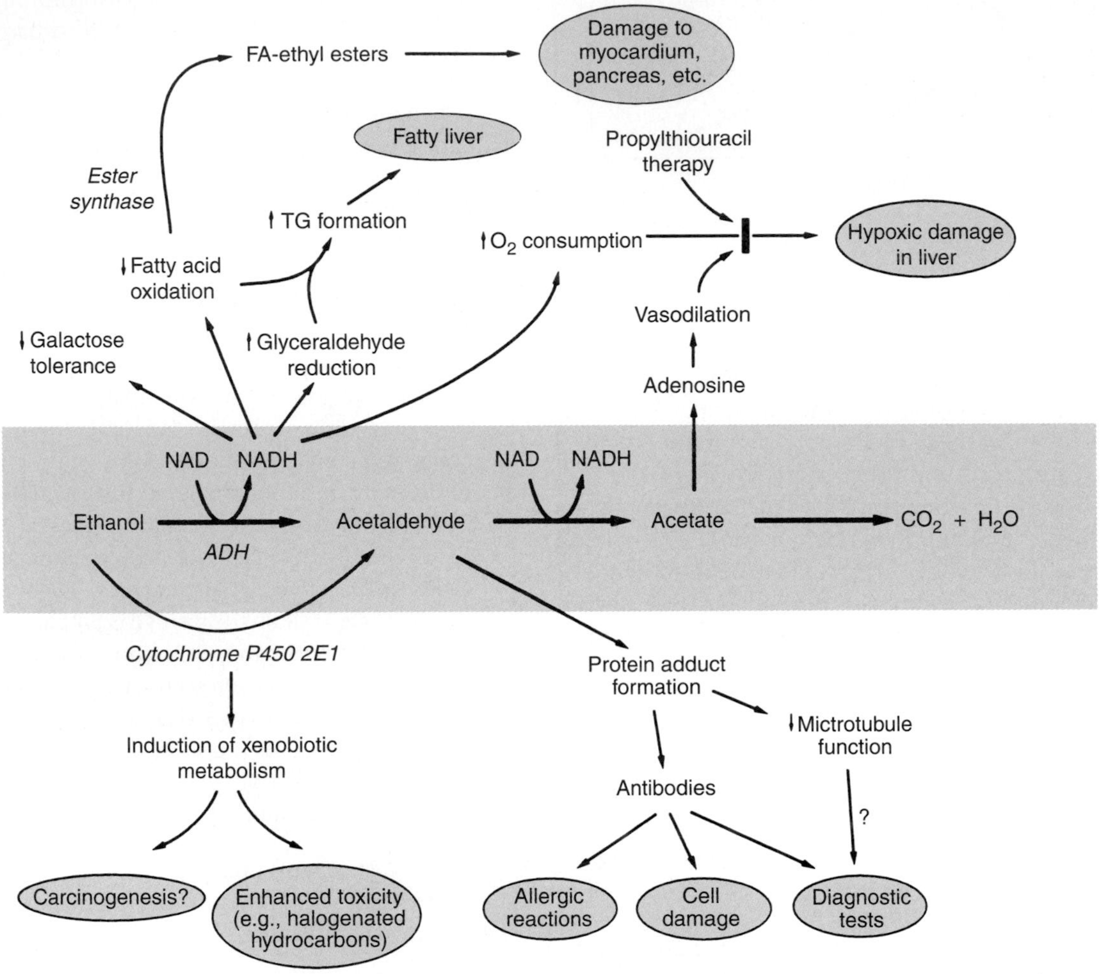

high concentrations that cause profound general anaesthesia or death, ethanol causes expansion and fluidization of the membranes, just as other general anaesthetics do.

At much lower ethanol concentrations, however, such as those resulting from moderate social use of alcohol, the membrane effects are much less diffuse and more selective. This may reflect a more specific interaction of ethanol at the lipid–protein interfaces of particular protein inclusions in the cell membrane, such as receptors, membrane-bound enzymes, and ion channels. As a result, almost every membrane function is altered in ways that produce or reflect altered excitability.

Among these membrane alterations are the following:

1. Acute exposure to relatively low concentrations of ethanol (20 mM or higher) produces a concentration-dependent inhibition of the NMDA subtype of glutamate receptor. Glutamate is the major excitatory neurotransmitter in the brain, and activation of NMDA receptors opens a receptor-linked cation channel, leading to influx of $Ca^{2+}$ and $Na^+$ into the neuron. This influx activates processes involved in learning and memory, but more massive influx can cause epileptic seizures and neuronal death. Inhibition of NMDA receptors may explain the impairment of learning and memory formation (alcoholic amnesia or "blackout") during severe alcohol intoxication, as well as the elevation of stimulus intensity needed to elicit seizures. The other subtypes of glutamate receptor (kainate and AMPA receptors) are also inhibited by ethanol, but the functional consequences are not yet as clear.

FIGURE 22-5    Formation of biogenic aldehyde condensation products through the action of alcohol in the brain. MAO = monoamine oxidase.

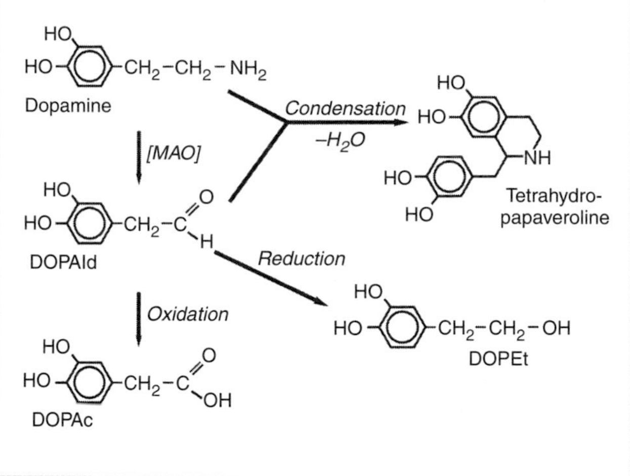

4. Receptor-activated second-messenger systems are also affected by ethanol. Noradrenaline-activated adenylyl cyclase activity is increased by ethanol in some types of neuron, whereas noradrenaline- and acetylcholine-activated phosphoinositol turnover is inhibited. However, the pattern of changes in different parts of the nervous system is complex, and it is not yet clear what role they play in mediating the actions of ethanol.

5. At higher concentrations, ethanol inhibits the active reuptake of adenosine, thus increasing the free adenosine concentration at adenosine receptors.

6. At quite high ethanol concentrations, $Na^+$ channel opening is impaired. Therefore, the rate of rise of action potentials is reduced, so their maximum height is diminished. Nerve conduction and muscle contraction, including myocardial contraction, are thus impaired. At the same time, active transport of $Na^+$, $K^+$, and amino acids by the cell membrane $Na^+/K^+$-ATPase is impaired. This may affect the resting potential of the membrane, on which maintenance of excitability depends.

7. Ethanol increases both the spontaneous and the impulse-triggered release of acetylcholine at cholinergic nerve terminals at the nerve–muscle junction and the recurrent collateral branch of the anterior horn cell axon. In brain slices, however, alcohol inhibits the synaptic release of acetylcholine more than that of other neurotransmitters. In the living organism, the overall effect of alcohol on acetylcholine release is complex, but intoxication generally reduces it, in parallel with the onset of drowsiness.

8. Nicotinic acetylcholine receptors consist of many combinations of eight different types of α subunit and three different types of β subunit, and the predominant subunit combinations in brain neuronal nicotinic receptors are different from those in peripheral ganglia and in nerve–muscle junctions. The different combinations of subunits confer different sensitivities and types of alcohol effect at the different locations. In the brain, the predominant ethanol effect is inhibition of excitatory response to acetylcholine. An analogous dependence on specific subunit composition is seen in the potentiating effect of ethanol on 5-HT$_3$ serotonin receptors in various brain sites.

When the brain is exposed chronically to ethanol, however, the number of NMDA receptors is increased. This up-regulation may result in neuronal hyperexcitability, contributing both to tolerance to the neuronal depressant actions of ethanol and to the major signs of ethanol withdrawal, such as tremor, exaggerated tendon reflexes, and seizures. Overactivity of glutamate receptors, and the consequent increase in $Ca^{2+}$ influx, may also be one factor in the production of alcoholic brain damage.

2. Low concentrations of ethanol have also been reported to enhance the effects of γ-aminobutyric acid (GABA) on the GABA$_A$–benzodiazepine receptor/Cl$^-$-ionophore complex (see Chapters 17 and 23). Under normal conditions, GABA increases Cl$^-$ influx into the cell body and increases Cl$^-$ efflux from axon terminals, in both cases lowering the excitability of the membrane. Enhancement of this action by ethanol varies greatly in different GABA receptors, depending on the respective combinations of subunits of which the receptors are composed. Since the subunit combinations differ in GABA receptors at different locations in the nervous system, there is greater regional selectivity than originally thought with respect to ethanol potentiation of GABA and the consequent inhibition of neurons bearing GABA receptors. Recent evidence suggests that ethanol enhancement of GABAergic transmission in the central amygdala (a part of the brain involved in modulation of tension and anxiety) may be produced via one type of receptor for corticotrophin-releasing factor (CRF).

3. At somewhat higher concentrations, ethanol reduces the excitation-dependent influx of $Ca^{2+}$, thus diminishing $Ca^{2+}$-dependent cell responses such as neurotransmitter release.

While these membrane effects are most prominent in excitable tissues such as brain and muscle, they probably apply to all tissues, but at different alcohol concentrations. Even in the central nervous system (CNS), some cells are more sensitive than others, and complex polysynaptic pathways are generally more sensitive than simple spinal reflex arcs. In general, ethanol causes a dose-dependent reduction of both spontaneous and evoked firing rates of single units in the cerebral cortex, hippocampus, and other parts of the brain. However, depending on differences in sensitivity of small interneurons, large pyramidal or Purkinje cells, myelinated versus unmyelinated fibres, and so forth, some units may show increased activity (disinhibition) at concentrations that decrease activity in others. Death occurs by depression of the respiratory control mechanism at blood alcohol concentrations too low to produce serious *direct* effects on most other tissues.

## Effects of Ethanol on Integrated Functions of the Nervous System

It was formerly thought that there was a hierarchical order of sensitivity to alcohol effects on the CNS, with the cerebral cortex being most sensitive to alcohol at the lowest concentrations, and impairment of thalamic, midbrain, and brainstem functions appearing sequentially at progressively increasing BACs. This concept is outmoded, and it is now generally accepted that sensitivity to alcohol is determined by the degree of complexity of the neural circuitry underlying the various functions that are studied and by the types of neurotransmitters and receptors involved, rather than by anatomical "level."

Relatively low concentrations of ethanol affect the hippocampus, the hypothalamus, and the ascending reticular formation, which is an important arousal mechanism for the forebrain. One of the earliest effects produced by small doses of ethanol (10 to 20 g, equivalent to 1 to 2 oz. of distilled spirits in an adult) is cutaneous vasodilatation of central origin. This appears to be due to disturbed functioning of the thermoregulatory centre in the preoptic area and anterior hypothalamus. The skin is flushed and warm, and there is sweating and increased heat loss from the skin. As a result, in a cool environment, there may be a fall in body temperature. The vasodilatation also contributes to a fall in peripheral arteriolar resistance, tachycardia, and increased amplitude of pulse pressure. Conjunctival vasodilatation, giving rise to reddening of the eyes, is commonly said to be a sign of moderate to severe intoxication, but its cause is not clear.

Hypothalamic actions of ethanol also lead to increased gastric secretion of HCl and increased gastrointestinal motility.

Subjectively, low doses usually produce relaxation and mild sedation in an individual at rest. If alcohol is slowly infused intravenously, the progressive increase in BAC leads to increasing sedation and sleep and, ultimately, to anaesthesia and coma.

In the usual social setting in which alcohol is drunk, the picture is modified. At first, the sedation is accompanied by loss of inhibitory control of emotions, and the *subjects become talkative and emotionally labile.* This is not a unique effect of alcohol; it can be caused by many sedatives in appropriate doses, but these are not normally taken in a social setting. *Small doses* do not impair complex intellectual ability and may even improve it slightly by reducing tension in nervous people. Even after somewhat *higher*

*doses,* the impairment stems principally from slowing of response (increased reaction time) and the inability to concentrate, rather than from loss of actual intellectual ability. However, *high alcohol levels* do produce marked impairment of mental functioning, including impaired judgement, increased risk taking, confusion, and disruption of rational thought. Impaired memory formation may lead to blackouts (i.e., inability to recall, in the sober state, events that occurred during the intoxicated state). The impairment of the reticular activating system results in decreased ability to attend to incoming sensory information from several sources simultaneously, so complex tasks requiring alertness and rapid decision making (e.g., choice reaction time) are more readily disrupted than those in which time is not a critical factor. Visual and other sensory acuity is impaired, and at still higher blood alcohol concentrations, anaesthesia is produced.

**Electroencephalograph (EEG) changes** are not specific for ethanol but are reflections of the state of arousal or depression. At low blood alcohol levels, during the stage of excitation and talkativeness, there is a desynchronized (aroused) EEG with an increase in the mean frequency of $\beta$ activity. At higher levels, with increasing drowsiness, there is a progressive shift toward EEG synchronization with increased amplitude and a steady fall in dominant frequency toward the 1 to 3-Hz range. Cortical and hippocampal evoked responses at first show increased amplitude, but as severe depression develops, the amplitude falls. The latency is also increased, not only in the cortex but also in the afferent paths in the brainstem; this is indicative of a fall in conduction velocity and of a delay in synaptic transmission.

The action of ethanol on the midbrain and medullary reticular formation, and on the input to cerebellar Purkinje cells, also affects descending fibres that modulate the responses of sensory organs and spinal motor synapses. The loss of descending inhibitory control at synapses in the motor pathways, together with impaired proprioceptor sensation, results in *motor ataxia, positive Romberg sign,* and *slurred speech.* Changes in reflexes vary with the complexity of the pathways. Loss of descending inhibitory influences may facilitate simple reflexes, such as tendon jerks, at low or moderate alcohol levels. In contrast, *complex polysynaptic reflexes* are impaired easily. At very high alcohol levels, even monosynaptic reflexes are blocked.

## Endocrine Effects

Numerous endocrine effects, mediated via the hypothalamus, have been shown.

1. Pituitary **antidiuretic hormone secretion is inhibited** by rising blood ethanol levels, causing *diuresis* of low specific gravity and of variable intensity and duration. This can be *abolished by the action of nicotine* on

the hypothalamus. This led to the suggestion that the effect of ethanol might result from decreased excitatory input to the supraoptic and paraventricular nuclei, rather than from direct suppression of secretory cells in the neurohypophysis. However, low concentrations of ethanol have also been shown to inhibit $Ca^{2+}$ channels and enhance $K^+$ currents in the secretory cells, so inhibition of arginine vasopressin release may be due in part to direct action of ethanol on these cells.

2. **Secretion of oxytocin is inhibited,** and intravenous infusion of dilute ethanol was, for a time, used clinically to stop uterine contractions and prevent premature labour. This practice has been abandoned because of the risk of damage to the fetus.

3. **Release of β-endorphin** from the intermediate lobe and probably the anterior lobe of the hypophysis is *increased.* The possible role of increased endorphin release in the effects of ethanol is not yet clear, but there is now considerable evidence that release of β-endorphin within the brain itself, in parts of the limbic system (see Chapters 16 and 70), plays an important role in the neural mechanisms of reinforcement ("reward").

4. **Increased secretion of adrenaline, noradrenaline, and adrenal corticosteroids** occurs during severe intoxication associated with respiratory and circulatory depression. However, small doses of ethanol *diminish* stress responses to a variety of stressors. This anti-stress effect includes reduction or prevention of the elevations in plasma corticosteroid and catecholamine levels. The blood ethanol level at which stress reduction is replaced by ethanol-induced stress probably varies with the person and the circumstances. Some investigators also postulate a role of corticotropin-releasing factor, adrenocorticotrophic hormone, and adrenal corticosteroids in the brain mechanisms of reinforcement.

5. **Secretion of luteinizing hormone is impaired,** and, as a result, serum **testosterone levels tend to fall.** Another factor contributing to the reduction in testosterone output is the inhibition of steroid hydroxylation in the testis as a result of NADH accumulation caused by alcohol dehydrogenase activity in the testis itself.

## Ethanol Intoxication

Signs of intoxication appear at different blood levels depending on individual differences in tolerance and also on the speed of drinking and thus on the rate of rise of the blood ethanol level.

Mild signs appear in most people at levels below 500 mg/L (0.05% or slightly over 10 mmol/L). Frank intoxication with psychomotor impairment is present in many subjects at levels below 1000 mg/L (0.1% or 21 mmol/L), but is present in practically everyone at 1500 mg/L (0.15%,

just under 33 mmol/L). Profound intoxication, with anaesthesia or coma, is likely at 2500 mg/L (0.25%, 54 mmol/L) or higher, although chronic heavy use of ethanol many increase tolerance to such a degree that some individuals are still conscious and active at blood levels of well over 0.35%.

Death occurs, as a result of respiratory depression in most cases, at levels of 5000 mg/L (0.5% or 108 mmol/L) or higher. *Barbiturates and other sedatives, benzodiazepines, phenothiazines (both antipsychotics and antihistamines), opioids, many antidepressants, and many over-the-counter cough and cold medications show additive or potentiating effects when taken together with alcohols.* When such drugs are used to quiet someone who is "roaring drunk," great care must be taken to avoid fatal overdosage.

In many countries, it is illegal to drive a motor vehicle at blood levels specified in the traffic criminal codes. In various European countries, this level is 0.05% (500 mg/L, about 11 mmol/L). In Canada and most states of the United States, it is 0.08% (800 mg/L, 17 mmol/L). In some countries it is 0.1%. These values do not, in most jurisdictions, constitute a legal definition of intoxication, but they form the basis of "per se legislation"; that is, at 0.08%, some individuals with higher than average tolerance might not be demonstrably intoxicated, but enough drivers are likely to be impaired to varying degrees at this designated blood alcohol level to justify making it an offence to drive at this level, whether a given individual is demonstrably impaired or not.

## Treatment of Acute Intoxication

Treatment might theoretically be aimed at either (1) speeding the disappearance of alcohol from the body or (2) counteracting its effects. As already mentioned, metabolic disappearance cannot be speeded up very much. In extreme cases, where death may occur, hemodialysis is undoubtedly rapid and effective in removing the alcohol. Usually, however, such treatment is not needed.

Pharmacological reversal of the effects of ethanol is not usually attempted in mild intoxication. Many compounds have been tested for their claimed **amethystic** (anti-intoxicant) properties; one example is the anti-parkinsonian and antiviral agent amantadine (see Chapters 17 and 55). However, the results are not very convincing. The benzodiazepine receptor inverse agonist Ro 15-4513 can reverse some of the signs of alcohol intoxication, but it does not antagonize the lethal effect of ethanol overdose and has found little or no use in clinical treatment of severe intoxication. The opioid antagonist naloxone has been claimed to reverse alcoholic coma, but there are numerous reports that it has failed to work, and in experimental animals, it works only at doses that have an analeptic effect of their own. Therefore, *supportive therapy (e.g., intravenous fluids, artificial respiration if needed) is the principal approach.* This is continued until metabolism lowers the blood alcohol level to the point where the danger is past.

## ALCOHOLISM AND RELATED PROBLEMS

### Alcoholism ("Chronic Alcoholism," Alcohol Dependence, Alcohol Addiction)

Alcoholism constitutes a very complex medical and social problem. The factors involved include such things as the prevalent social attitudes toward drinking and drunkenness, parental attitudes and habits, drinking practices among certain occupational groups, personal emotional conflicts, and perhaps excessively rewarding pharmacological effects of ethanol. There is considerable evidence of a hereditary (genetic) predisposition in many cases. Much research is currently being directed at a search for biochemical markers for detecting those who have a genetic predisposition (e.g., platelet adenylyl cyclase type VII) and also for biochemical tests for identifying heavy drinkers at an early stage (e.g., plasma carbohydrate-deficient transferrin and gamma-glutamyltransferase). In almost every case, most of these factors are involved to varying degrees, so there is no single cause of alcoholism. This question is examined in more detail in Chapter 70.

The adverse consequences of alcoholism are also seen in many different aspects of the individual's life, including physical and mental health, family relations, work and economic performance, accidents, legal problems, and others. Most of these are beyond the scope of this chapter. Only a few of the pharmacological problems are covered here.

### Nutritional Problems

Oxidation of ethanol yields 7 cal/g. At an average oxidation rate of 10 g/hr or 240 g daily, one could derive nearly 1700 cal/day from ethanol. In many individual cases, especially in regular heavy drinkers, the amount may be much higher. If the average dietary intake of a man with sedentary occupation is 2500 to 3000 cal/day, steady drinking can provide well over half of the total calories. Since alcoholic beverages contain little or no protein, vitamins, or lipotropic factors, a variety of nutritional deficiency diseases can result. **Peripheral neuropathy, Korsakoff's psychosis, Wernicke's disease,** and **pellagra** are examples of *B vitamin deficiencies occurring in alcoholics;* they became much less frequent once vitamin supplementation of bread and other foods began. Since nutrition is frequently insufficient during drinking bouts and hepatic glycogen content is reduced, serious hypoglycemia can occur, as explained above under "Metabolic Effects of Ethanol."

### Organ Damage

Fatty liver is common among alcoholics as a result of the metabolic disturbances described earlier in this chapter. **Alcoholic hepatitis and cirrhosis,** however, appear to result from different processes than fatty liver. The pathophysiological mechanisms responsible for these changes are discussed in Chapter 43, and will not be covered here. Even if the hepatocellular damage is reversible, the cells remain sensitive to ethanol for months after the cessation of heavy drinking; even small doses can produce a prompt rise in serum alanine aminotransferase and gamma-glutamyltransferase levels.

Other parts of the digestive system that are frequently damaged by heavy consumption of ethanol are the stomach and pancreas. Alcoholic gastritis, with inflammatory infiltration of the mucosa, mucosal erosion, ulceration, and bleeding ranging from microscopic to frank hemorrhage, is common among heavy drinkers. Alcoholic pancreatitis has been attributed to accumulation of fatty acid ethyl esters in the pancreas and to formation of oxidative free radicals by cytochrome P450 oxidation of ethanol in the pancreatic acinar cells. It is characterized by inflammatory cell infiltration, foci of necrosis, pseudocyst formation, fibrosis, and impairment of both exocrine and endocrine secretion. The reduction of exocrine secretion gives rise to impaired utilization of dietary protein and fat and to steatorrhea (large fatty stools). Impaired insulin secretion causes a diabetes-like disturbance of carbohydrate metabolism, which may be irreversible even if the person stops using alcohol. The carbohydrate disturbance can also create a diagnostic problem in a comatose patient in that it may be difficult to differentiate between a diabetic coma and an alcoholic coma in a patient with pancreatitis.

The cardiovascular system is subject to alcohol-induced disturbances of several types. Hypertension increases progressively with increasing alcohol intake and may be accentuated during the period of hangover following a drinking bout. This is thought to be a contributory factor to the risk of stroke. Alcoholic cardiomyopathy, with degenerative lesions of the cardiac muscle fibres and impaired contractile function, is a less frequent complication of alcoholism. However, in one minor epidemic of cardiac disease in alcoholics ("beer drinker's heart"), the lesion was found to be due not to the alcohol itself, but to cobalt present as a contaminant in the beer because of a production fault.

Another important type of organ damage in alcoholics is **cerebral cortical atrophy,** with widening of the sulci and enlargement of the ventricles. This can be revealed by computerized tomography (CT) scanning and magnetic resonance imaging (MRI) at a stage before gross neurological or psychological deficits are clinically detectable. This is a different type of lesion from the nutritional deficiency effects previously noted, and it may possibly reflect a direct toxic effect of ethanol itself. Fortunately, it is often reversible if drinking is stopped at an early stage.

Some alcoholics, after years of heavy drinking, show a relatively sudden "break" or loss of tolerance, becoming quite intoxicated by amounts of alcohol that previously produced only mild symptoms. This should be taken as a warning of serious medical problems because it is usually the result of damage to either the liver or the nervous system. Liver damage, resulting in reduced ethanol oxidizing ability, causes the same amount of consumed ethanol to yield higher and more prolonged blood alcohol levels than previously. Brain damage, with cortical and hippocampal neuron loss, may render the nervous system more sensitive to the same blood alcohol level.

The **fetal alcohol syndrome** (FAS) is a complex picture of *irreversible* damage to the fetus and results from ingestion of alcohol by pregnant women. The complete picture includes small head, widely separated eyes with short palpebral fissures and epicanthic folds, a broad upper lip that lacks the normal midline vertical groove (the philtrum), a short nose, mental and physical retardation, cardiac valvular defects (often), and continued postnatal retardation of development. FAS appears to be a toxic effect of ethanol and/or acetaldehyde, perhaps in part by impairment of placental circulation, rather than a consequence of maternal malnutrition. Several different molecular mechanisms have been proposed, but the explanation is not yet fully clear. The severity appears to be dose-dependent, but the minimum dose required to produce it is not known. Therefore, many obstetricians advise total abstinence during pregnancy.

## Public Health Aspects of Alcohol Use

In general, alcoholics have a higher mortality rate than the general population of the same age and gender. The excess mortality is due not only to liver cirrhosis, but to many different causes, including hypertensive heart disease, stroke, cancer of the pharynx and esophagus, and accidents. In contrast, there is considerable epidemiological evidence that a low or moderate alcohol intake, defined as not more than 1 to 2 standard drinks a day, reduces total mortality by reducing certain specific risks such as that of fatal myocardial infarction, type 2 diabetes, and possibly Alzheimer's disease; the mechanisms of these risk reductions are not yet fully known. However, at average daily alcohol intakes in excess of two standard drinks, a progressive increase in total mortality outweighs the cardiac and other protective effects.

## Tolerance and Physical Dependence

With steady intake of alcohol, tolerance develops (i.e., larger amounts of alcohol are required to produce the same degree of effect). This reflects both **metabolic tolerance** produced by faster oxidation in the liver and **functional tolerance** resulting from an actual change in sensitivity in the CNS. Absorption may actually be somewhat faster in tolerant individuals because they show less alcohol-induced delay of gastric emptying. Distribution of the alcohol is not significantly altered.

*Acute tolerance* occurs progressively within the course of a single exposure to ethanol, so there is less intoxication at a given blood alcohol level on the descending limb of the blood alcohol curve than there was at the same level on the rising limb (the Mellanby effect). *Chronic tolerance* is the gradual decrease in degree of intoxication at the same blood alcohol level over the course of repeated alcohol exposures. The relation between acute and chronic tolerance is not yet wholly clear, but there is strong evidence that they share many or most of the same mechanisms. One theory is that acute and chronic tolerance are different aspects of the same process, and that the gradual increase of tolerance during chronic alcohol ingestion is in fact a reflection of faster development of acute tolerance. The maximum degree of tolerance to ethanol is considerably smaller than the maximum tolerance that can develop to opioids or to benzodiazepines.

The mechanism of functional tolerance to ethanol is complex and not yet fully known. Experimental evidence indicates that it is not only the presence of alcohol itself, but also the genetic background of the individual, the environmental and behavioural circumstances under which alcohol is consumed, and the degree of use of drugs with effects that resemble those of alcohol (such as benzodiazepines and other sedatives) that all influence the speed and degree of the development of alcohol tolerance. The neural mechanisms underlying tolerance appear to include serotonin, glutamate (NMDA receptors), acetylcholine, vasopressin, dopamine, and GABA receptors, especially in pathways in the septum and hippocampus that are also involved in learning and memory. Tolerance appears to be related to the development of physical dependence, with which it proceeds more or less in parallel. **Physical dependence** is revealed by the occurrence of physiological disturbances, referred to as **withdrawal symptoms,** when alcohol intake is abruptly reduced or stopped (see also Chapter 70).

## Ethanol Withdrawal Syndrome

Since ethanol depresses neuronal excitability and spontaneous activity in various parts of the brain, adaptation must involve some type of compensatory hyperactivity to offset the alcohol effect. This is seen as tolerance when the alcohol is present. When the alcohol is withdrawn, the hyperactivity gives rise to the withdrawal symptoms. Their severity and duration depend upon the severity and duration of the preceding period of drinking.

Following a single intoxicating dose of alcohol or a single short period of drinking (e.g., one evening), the only consistent physiological change that can be correlated with "hangover" (and is suggestive of withdrawal effect) is some degree of *neuronal hyper-excitability* (Fig. 22-6).

After longer drinking bouts lasting several days or more, the symptoms include marked hyperirritability, exaggerated reflexes, sleeplessness, tremor, muscular tension, cold sweaty skin, nausea, and marked thirst. In severe cases, there may be generalized convulsions. Such symptoms have been attributed to rebound hypersensitivity of excitatory glutamate (and possibly cholinergic) receptors that were inhibited during the drinking phase and to hypoactivity of GABA (inhibitory) receptors.

After chronic drinking for many weeks or months, abrupt cessation or even some reduction of alcohol intake can precipitate a two-stage withdrawal reaction. In addition to the symptoms already described, which begin very soon after withdrawal, there can be a second stage beginning two or more days later. This is characterized by severe hyperactivity with delirium, hallucinations, fever, profuse sweating, intense vasodilatation, and severe tachycardia. This stage (delirium tremens) is still sometimes fatal despite the newer treatments. One hypothesis is that this picture results from rebound hypersensitivity of β-adrenergic receptors that have been suppressed during prolonged intoxication and early withdrawal.

Treatment of the withdrawal syndrome depends on its severity. In many mild cases, rest, quiet, and reassurance are all that are required. In more severe cases, long-acting benzodiazepines such as **diazepam** are usually effective in reducing the irritability, tremor, and sleeplessness and are the drugs of choice. The first dose is sometimes given parenterally for rapid action (see Chapter 23). **Chlormethiazole (clomethiazole)** is widely used in Europe to treat alcohol withdrawal symptoms, but it is not available in North America. Symptoms due to adrenergic overactivity may be relieved by the $\alpha_2$-adrenoceptor agonist clonidine (see Chapter 13).

**Phenothiazines** do not prevent convulsions and may even increase the risk, so they are no longer used in the treatment of alcohol withdrawal reactions. The anticonvulsant benzodiazepine **carbamazepine,** either alone or in combination with **tiapride,** may be helpful in such cases. **Barbiturates, paraldehyde,** and other older-type hypnotic–sedative drugs are less safe and probably somewhat less effective and are now very seldom used clinically. Ethanol itself is effective in treating withdrawal symptoms, and a tapering-off treatment is preferred in some countries. However, such a regimen is hard to adhere to and is psychologically bad for the patient who wishes to stop drinking, unless the alcohol is given by a different route (intravenously) that is not associated with the stimuli and mental associations that ordinarily accompany the ingestion of alcohol. Supportive therapy may include large amounts of fluid, either orally or intravenously, but fluid should be used carefully because some patients are actually over-hydrated when first seen. A high-calorie balanced diet with vitamin supplements, especially thiamine, is usually recommended.

## Pharmacotherapy of Behavioural Dependence

Physical dependence, though commonly found in alcoholic patients, is not the fundamental feature of alcoholism. Rather, it is "psychological," or behavioural, dependence that is believed to be related to the reinforcing effects of ethanol. These topics are discussed in Chapters 69 and 70. Drug therapies aimed at reducing dependence by blocking or decreasing the reinforcing effects are not specific for alcohol but are also used in dependence on other drugs. Therefore, they are covered in Chapter 70.

| **FIGURE 22-6** | Effects of alcohol withdrawal on neuronal excitability by pentylenetetrazol (metrazol) or electric shock. (A) After a single large dose of ethanol at time zero. (B) After prolonged ingestion of ethanol. Note the difference in the time scales in A and B. |
| --- | --- |

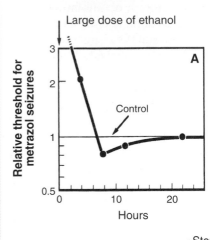

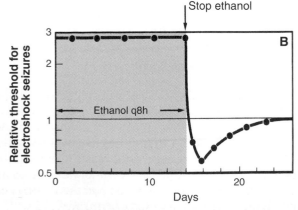

Disulfiram and other drugs described below are specific for alcoholism but do not act directly on the reinforcement system. Instead, they interact with the metabolism of alcohol in such a way as to give rise to highly unpleasant effects. The hope is that the patient's desire to drink alcohol will be offset by the fear of these consequences.

## Disulfiram and Related Drugs

**Tetraethylthiuram disulfide** (disulfiram, or TETD) inhibits the hepatic enzymes that oxidize acetaldehyde to acetate. Consumption of ethanol and disulfiram therefore produces an accumulation of acetaldehyde in the blood and tissues, causing acetaldehyde poisoning. Within minutes, the subject becomes hot, flushed, and cyanotic. The pulse rate, cardiac output, and respiratory rate rise. These effects are thought to result from excessive release of catecholamines from sympathetic nerve endings under the influence of acetaldehyde. However, disulfiram also inhibits dopamine hydroxylase, so the stores of catecholamines in the nerve endings are low to begin with. Therefore, after 30 to 60 minutes, the sympathetic tone falls abruptly and there is a marked drop in blood pressure, with pallor and nausea. This reaction lasts for up to 2 hours and can be very severe and occasionally fatal. Alcoholics are often given disulfiram so that fear of a reaction will deter them from drinking. *It is not a cure for alcoholism,* merely a deterrent (see Chapter 70).

Disulfiram is absorbed rapidly from the GI tract, begins to act within 2 to 4 hours, and reaches its maximum effect in 24 hours. It should not be started until 12 to 24 hours after the last drink of alcohol. The drug is metabolized in the body by splitting the disulfide bond to form diethyldithiocarbamate, which in turn is broken down to form carbon disulfide, which appears in the breath, and sulfate, which is excreted slowly in the urine over the next week. Disulfiram is thought to react with a dithiol site on the acetaldehyde dehydrogenase, oxidizing it to a cyclic disulfide that is inactive as an enzyme.

Disulfiram itself has some toxicity apart from the inhibition of acetaldehyde dehydrogenase and dopamine β-hydroxylase and possibly some other enzymes. Toxic symptoms may include weakness, dizziness, mental disturbances, cardiac arrhythmias, skin reactions, and impotence. It can also inhibit the metabolism of other drugs by liver microsomal enzymes, thus altering the effects of these drugs. Patients using disulfiram must be monitored carefully.

**Tolbutamide, metronidazole, cephalosporins, and calcium carbimide** have similar interactions with alcohol. Patients being treated with these drugs should be warned not to drink alcohol. Conversely, chronic intake of alcohol may result in induction of hepatic cytochrome P450 activity and thus cause faster biotransformation of tolbutamide, warfarin, propranolol, phenytoin, and various other drugs, with corresponding shortening of their duration of action (see Chapter 4). With certain other drugs such as acetaminophen, alcohol induction of cytochrome P450 activity can lead to increased production of toxic metabolites (see Chapter 43).

## METHANOL INTOXICATION

Methanol is a milder intoxicant than ethanol in that larger doses are necessary to produce the same degree of intoxication. Its serious toxicity is not that of methanol itself, but of its metabolic products. It is oxidized by catalase, as well as by alcohol dehydrogenase, to **formaldehyde,** which is oxidized to **formic acid.** These substances are specifically toxic to the retina and optic nerve and may produce partial or complete permanent blindness. In addition, the formic acid gives rise to severe metabolic acidosis, which may be fatal.

Treatment requires vigorous measures to correct the acidosis (caused by the methanol that has already been oxidized) with intravenous sodium bicarbonate solution, and attempts to eliminate the remaining methanol before it can be oxidized. This can be achieved by combining hemodialysis (for removing methanol) with the administration of repeated doses of ethanol, which competitively inhibits oxidation of the methanol. However, precise titration of the ethanol (to avoid excessive intoxication) is difficult, and fomepazole is now the preferred agent for preventing further oxidation of methanol. Folate is also used to enhance oxidation of any formate produced.

## HIGHER ALCOHOLS

**Propyl and isopropyl alcohols** are used as antiseptics and for alcohol rubs. The higher alcohols (e.g., butyl, pentyl) are used mainly as solvents for industrial processes. They are of pharmacological concern for two reasons: (1) distilled beverages contain small amounts of higher alcohols and aldehydes, referred to as "congeners," and there is some slight evidence that they may contribute to the toxicity of the ethanol; and (2) these alcohols are often consumed by "skid row" alcoholics in the form of antifreeze, cleaning fluid, and numerous other toxic mixtures with gasoline, benzene, and so forth. The intoxicating effects are similar to those of ethanol but much more severe for the same dose. Organ toxicity, especially to the liver, kidney, and bone marrow, is also more severe with these mixtures.

Certain other higher alcohols and certain acetaldehyde derivatives (trichloroacetaldehyde hydrate or paraldehyde) were formerly used fairly widely as sedatives and hypnotics. Paraldehyde is still used occasionally by intramuscular injection, but the others have been replaced almost completely by the benzodiazepines.

## SUGGESTED READINGS

Anton RF, Lieber CS, Tabakoff B, et al. Carbohydrate-deficient transferrin and gamma-glutamyltransferase for the detection and monitoring of alcohol use: results from a multisite study. *Alcohol Clin Exp Res.* 2002;26:1215-1222.

Apte MV, Wilson JS. Alcohol-induced pancreatic injury. *Best Pract Res Clin Gastroenterol.* 2003;17:593-612.

Brewer C, Hardt F, Petersen EN, eds. Antabuse—experiences from 40 years of clinical use and the discovery of an active metabolite. *Acta Psychiatr Scand Suppl.* 1992;369:1-72.

Deitrich RA, Dunwiddie TV, Harris RA, Erwin VG. Mechanism of action of ethanol: initial nervous system actions. *Pharmacol Rev.* 1989;41:498-537.

Edenberg HJ. Regulation of the mammalian alcohol dehydrogenase genes. *Prog Nucleic Acid Res Mol Biol.* 2000;64:295-341.

Gorelick DA. Overview of pharmacologic treatment approaches for alcohol and other drug addiction. Intoxication, withdrawal, and relapse prevention. *Psychiatr Clin North Am.* 1993; 16(1):141-156.

Jones AW. Disposition and fate of ethanol in the body. In: Garriott JC, ed. *Medical and Legal Aspects of Alcohol.* 4th ed. Tucson, Ariz: Lawyers & Judges Publishing; 2003:47-112.

Kalant H. Pharmacokinetics of ethanol: absorption, distribution and elimination. In: Begleiter H, Kissin B, eds. *The Pharmacology of Alcohol and Alcohol Dependence.* Vol 2. New York, NY: Oxford University Press; 1996:15-58.

Kalant H, Lê AD. Effects of ethanol on thermoregulation. In: Schönbaum E, Lomax P, eds. *Thermoregulation: Pathology, Pharmacology, and Therapy.* International Encyclopedia of Pharmacology and Therapeutics. Section 132. Oxford, United Kingdom: Pergamon Press; 1991:561-617.

Lê AD, Khanna JM. Dispositional mechanisms in drug tolerance and sensitization. In: Goudie AJ, Emmett-Oglesby MW, eds. *Psychoactive Drugs—Tolerance and Sensitization.* Clifton, NJ: Humana; 1989:281-351.

Lieber CS. Alcohol: its metabolism and interaction with nutrients. *Annu Rev Nutr.* 2000;20:395-430.

Lieber CS. Alcohol and the liver: 1994 update. *Gastroenterology.* 1994;106:1085-1105.

Majchrowicz E, Noble EP, eds. *Biochemistry and Pharmacology of Ethanol.* Vols 1 and 2. New York, NY: Plenum Press; 1979.

Narahashi T, Kuriyama K, Illes P, et al. Neuroreceptors and ion channels as targets of alcohol. *Alcohol Clin Exp Res.* 2001;25 (5 suppl):182S-188S.

Nie Z, Schweitzer P, Roberts AJ, et al. Ethanol augments GABAergic transmission in the central amygdala via CRF1 receptors. *Science.* 2004;303:1512-1514.

Preedy VR, Watson RR, eds. *Comprehensive Handbook of Alcohol-Related Pathology.* Oxford, United Kingdom: Academic Press/ Elsevier Science; 2005.

Suwaki H, Kalant H, Higuchi S, et al. Recent research on alcohol tolerance and dependence. *Alcohol Clin Exp Res.* 2001;25: 189S-196S.

Tabakoff B, Hoffman PL. Alcohol: neurobiology. In: Lowinson JH, Ruiz P, Millman RB, eds. *Substance Abuse: A Comprehensive Textbook.* 2nd ed. Baltimore, Md: Williams & Wilkins; 1992:152-185.

Tabakoff B, Hellevuo K, Hoffman PL. Alcohol. In: Schuster CR, Gust SW, Kuhar MJ, eds. *Pharmacological Aspects of Drug Dependence.* Handbook of Experimental Pharmacology. Vol 118. New York, NY: Springer-Verlag; 1996:373-458.

Treistman SN, Bayley H, Lemos JR, et al. Effects of ethanol on calcium channels, potassium channels, and vasopressin release. *Ann NY Acad Sci.* 1991;625:249-263.

Wallgren H, Barry H III. *Actions of Alcohol.* Vols 1 and 2. Amsterdam, Netherlands: Elsevier; 1970.

Zuo Y, Kuryatov A, Lindstrom JM, et al. Alcohol modulation of neuronal nicotinic acetylcholine receptors is $\alpha$ subunit dependent. *Alcohol Clin Exp Res.* 2002;26:779-784.

# 23

# Drugs Used for Anxiety, Stress Disorders, and Insomnia

## MK ROMACH, KA SCHOEDEL, AND EM SELLERS

### CASE HISTORY

Ms. K., 30 years old, was referred by her family doctor for assessment and management of her pattern and amount of alcohol consumption. Since her early teens, she had experienced anxiety accompanied by heart palpitations, light-headedness, tremulousness, muscle tension, sweating, and difficulty concentrating when she was in any social situation—one-on-one discussions with her teachers, parties, and family gatherings. As a result, she frequently avoided such situations. She then discovered that alcohol facilitated her ability to socialize, and she would drink two to three glasses of wine to relax in these situations.

By the time she entered university, her anxiety had generalized to other situations, and even to the anticipation of them. As a result, she started drinking alcohol before leaving home to attend such events. She found the alcohol to be moderately effective, but she noted that as she drank more, her anxiety became more persistent throughout the day. Her consumption of alcohol had increased over the past 10 years from two to three glasses of wine twice weekly to five or more glasses daily.

Ms. K. was embarrassed by these symptoms and had not discussed them with anybody until 3 months ago, when she confided to her family doctor the difficulties she was having, but she did not reveal how much she was drinking. Following a discussion about ways of managing symptoms of anxiety, her doctor prescribed alprazolam 0.5 mg twice a day. There was little discussion about how long the medication would be prescribed.

Within the first week of medication, Ms. K. found her anxiety significantly but not entirely reduced. Over the next 3 weeks, the dose was titrated to 0.5 mg four times per day. At this dosage, she felt able to conduct her daily activities in a calm and competent manner and became engaged in more social interactions. At times she felt somewhat drowsy, but this abated over time. She also decreased her alcohol consumption significantly. Her intention was to stop drinking entirely, but she wished to reduce her intake gradually.

After 3 months, her physician suggested tapering off the alprazolam because he was concerned that she might become "addicted." However, the patient feared that she might find it impossible to stop taking the drug.

Her ambivalence over the doctor's recommendation to stop the medication and her fear of relapse of her anxiety began to generate an anxiety of its own. She related her concerns about a relapse to the physician, as well as her fear that she would resort once again to heavy drinking. Hearing of her past drinking history, the physician became more insistent that she stop the alprazolam and referred her to a treatment centre for substance abuse. Ms. K. was not currently using any other drugs, licit or illicit, aside from the prescribed alprazolam and four to six glasses of wine per week.

## HISTORICAL BACKGROUND

Anxiety disorders are among the most prevalent psychiatric disorders in the general population. They are associated with significant morbidity and disability and are usually chronic in nature. When alcohol, opioids, and belladonna were the only available therapeutic agents, a wide variety of behavioural disorders were managed by sedating the anxious or disturbed patient. A sedative drug decreases physical activity and agitation. The word "hypnotic," on the other hand, is derived from the Greek word *hypnos* for sleep and is applied to drugs used to promote sleep in any patient, not necessarily an anxious or agitated one.

Older drugs that were used to sedate or induce sleep all shared similar side effects because their mechanism of action was relatively non-selective. Hence, all such drugs tended to cause drowsiness, impaired memory, and often physical dependence (e.g., barbiturates, benzodiazepines). Advances in neuroscience have led to a better understanding of the neurobiology underlying anxiety and stress disorders and hence to new targets for drug treatments that are proving to be as effective as benzodiazepines, which have been the mainstay of anxiety treatment for the past 40 years. Newer drugs have more selective mechanisms of action and are targeted to specific symptoms (anxiety, concurrent depression, particular types of insomnia). This chapter focuses on the medications used to treat the most common forms of anxiety, stress disorders, and insomnia. Chapter 25 reviews the treatment of depression and is particularly important and relevant to the present chapter.

## ANXIETY AND STRESS DISORDERS

## Clinical Definitions and Epidemiology

Anxiety is a normal emotion under conditions of perceived threat and is part of the "fight or flight" reaction that is essential for human evolutionary survival. However, when anxiety symptoms become maladaptive and are associated with distress and impaired daily functioning, they can constitute a psychiatric disorder. The diagnostic criteria and characteristics of the different anxiety disorders are outlined in the *Diagnostic and Statistical Manual of Mental Disorders, Fourth Edition (DSM-IV)* and the *International Classification of Diseases, Tenth Edition (ICD-10)* (see References at end of chapter). Five subtypes of anxiety disorders will be referred to in this chapter: generalized anxiety disorder, panic disorder, social phobia, post-traumatic stress disorder, and obsessive–compulsive disorder.

### Generalized anxiety disorder

The definition of generalized anxiety disorder (GAD) has evolved over the past two decades. GAD is the anxiety disorder that primary care physicians are most likely to have to address in their daily practice. Individuals are diagnosed with GAD if they have experienced a number of physical and psychological symptoms of anxiety and chronic worry for a minimum of 6 months. Most estimates of the lifetime prevalence of GAD are in the range of 2 to 5%. As with most anxiety disorders, females are at greater risk than males, and prevalence increases with age, so in women over the age of 40 years, the lifetime prevalence may be 10% or higher.

Historically, GAD was treated with some of the first psychotropic drugs available, the tricyclic antidepressants and barbiturates, but these were replaced by the benzodiazepines by the 1960s. Concerns about non-therapeutic use, physical dependence, and withdrawal symptoms with benzodiazepines resulted in a gradual shift to the use of antidepressant medications that alter the serotonin and noradrenaline systems: selective serotonin reuptake inhibitors (SSRIs) in the 1980s and serotonin–noradrenaline reuptake inhibitors (SNRIs), including venlafaxine, in the 1990s.

### Panic disorder

Panic disorder (PD) is characterized by (1) recurrent, unexpected anxiety attacks consisting of a number of physical symptoms along with fear and anxiety, (2) anticipatory anxiety, and often (3) phobic avoidance of situations where such attacks may occur. PD is frequently an antecedent to major depressive disorder (MDD) later in life. The lifetime prevalence of PD is estimated to be in the range of 1 to 5%, while up to 10% of the population report experiencing isolated panic attacks at some time in their lives. Women are twice as likely as men to suffer from PD, and one-third to one-half of patients with PD also suffer from *agoraphobia* (anxiety about being in places or situations in which panic attacks may occur, and from which escape might be difficult or embarrassing). The temporal distribution of PD prevalence is bimodal, with a peak in late adolescence and another in the mid-30s.

The preferred current first-line treatments for PD are antidepressants from the SSRI and SNRI classes. Because of their greater efficacy and safety, these antidepressants have displaced benzodiazepines and heterocyclic antidepressants as the mainstay of pharmacological treatment. However, benzodiazepines, in particular the high-potency ones such as alprazolam and clonazepam, continue to be used as adjunctive medications, especially for long-term treatment.

### Social phobia

Social phobia (SP), or social anxiety disorder, is a behavioural disorder consisting of an intense, irrational fear of social or performance situations in which the individual anticipates humiliation or embarrassment. SP can be divided into two further subtypes, discrete and generalized, which vary in the level of disability burdening the patient. In Western nations, the lifetime prevalence of social phobia ranges from 6 to 13%. As with other anxiety disorders, the prevalence is higher in women (about twofold). The onset of SP tends to be relatively early in life, and prevalence does not vary greatly by age category. One of the most common treatments of social phobia is self-medication with alcohol. Therapeutic interventions with SSRIs and SNRIs have become the first line of treatment.

### Post-traumatic stress disorder

Post-traumatic stress disorder (PTSD), a reaction to a traumatic life event, is an anxiety disorder characterized by a constellation of symptoms including chronic mood alterations, anxiety, impaired sleep, and recurring memories of the traumatic event. In a survey of American adults, PTSD was more common in women (10.4% compared with 5% in men), in whom it is frequently associated with sexual abuse. War veterans also frequently suffer from PTSD. In a sample of Vietnam War veterans, the lifetime prevalence was 26.9% in women and 30.9% in men. Current treatments reduce PTSD symptoms, and, of these, the SSRIs are the treatment of choice.

## Obsessive–compulsive disorder

Obsessive–compulsive disorder (OCD) is characterized by the presence of obsessions and/or compulsions that interfere with normal daily functioning, are time-consuming, and cause significant distress to the individual. Obsessions are intrusive inappropriate thoughts, while compulsions refer to repetitive behaviours aimed at preventing distress or a dreaded event. In community studies, the lifetime prevalence of OCD was shown to be approximately 1 to 3%, although it has been estimated that this condition has been clinically recognized in less than 0.1% of the population. This indicates that a large number of patients may not be seeking clinical treatment. This disorder generally has an early age of onset, and 75% of sufferers have comorbid psychiatric conditions, most commonly major depression. SSRIs improve the symptoms of OCD, but responses are less robust than in other anxiety disorders and adjunctive treatments such as benzodiazepines and antipsychotics are frequently required.

## Inter-relationship of Anxiety and Depressive Disorders

Substantial evidence indicates that chronic stress and anxiety symptoms are strongly associated with higher risk of anxiety disorder subtypes and with depression. The fact that all of these disorders appear to result from the interaction of stressful life events and an individual's underlying vulnerability (in part genetic) suggests that a common neuroadaptive pathology underlies the disorders. It is not surprising, therefore, that the same medications are useful for treating all these conditions. The core symptoms of emotional lability, anxiety, depressed mood, and cognitive fears are similar for all; however, the clinical phenotype makes it possible to identify the prominent, yet different, primary disability feature of each (Fig. 23-1).

## Mechanisms of Action

The following section outlines the hypothesized roles of individual neurotransmitter/receptor systems in the neurobiology of anxiety disorders and the pharmacological effects of the relevant psychotropic drugs. However, it is important to remember that the reality is much more complex.

## Serotonergic agents and anxiety

According to earlier hypotheses of etiology, depression was believed to result from decreased brain serotonin (5-HT) levels and anxiety from dysregulation in serotonergic systems. These hypotheses derived from the known pharmacological mechanisms of action of the drugs found to be effective in treating these disorders. Of the 15 known serotonin receptor subtypes regulating central serotonergic activity, at least four have been implicated in mediating

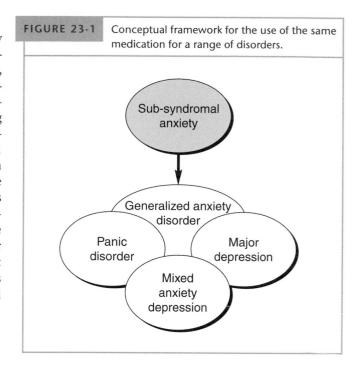

**FIGURE 23-1** Conceptual framework for the use of the same medication for a range of disorders.

anxiety disorders: $5-HT_{1A}$, $5-HT_{2A}$, $5-HT_{2C}$, and $5-HT_3$. As an example, buspirone is a partial agonist that acts on both pre- and postsynaptic $5-HT_{1A}$ receptors to regulate synaptic serotonergic release and actions; it has mild anxiolytic properties but is not effective as an antidepressant. Clinically, antagonists of $5-HT_{2A}$ receptors show anxiolytic properties (e.g., ritanserin), and pre-clinical data suggest that antagonists at $5-HT_{2C}$ and $5-HT_3$ receptors may also be anxiolytic, although clinical studies to date have been negative. SSRIs and SNRIs are thought to increase postsynaptic serotonin levels, and this action is believed to account for both their antidepressant and anxiolytic properties. However, it is now recognized that these are greatly oversimplified hypotheses, and current theories of the etiology of these disorders and mechanisms of action of various medications have evolved to the molecular level. Detailed descriptions of these theories are beyond the scope of this chapter. Interested readers are referred to the Suggested Readings for further information.

## Noradrenergic agents and anxiety

In animal models, overactivity of the central noradrenergic system produced by stimulation of the locus ceruleus can result in behaviour that resembles features of clinical anxiety (e.g., easy startling, increased vigilance, sympathetic arousal, and hyperactivity). Agents that *decrease* noradrenaline release (e.g., presynaptic $\alpha_2$ receptor agonists), deplete noradrenaline stores (e.g., reserpine), or block noradrenergic receptors (e.g., $\beta_1$ receptor blockers) demonstrate some anxiolytic properties in pre-clinical studies. However, clinically, drugs that *increase* noradrenergic neurotransmission by a variety of mechanisms (e.g., mirtazapine, SNRIs, reboxetine) have also shown promise in the treatment of anxiety disorders. These apparently conflicting results underscore the fact that individual receptor/neurotransmitter systems do not operate in isolation, and the interaction of these systems is likely to be as important to the underlying neuropathology of anxiety disorders as any individual receptor system.

## GABA and anxiolytic action

γ-Aminobutyric acid (GABA) is the major inhibitory neurotransmitter in the central nervous system (CNS). There are two main subtypes of GABA receptors: (1) GABA$_A$ receptors are linked with chloride channel conductance and are allosterically modulated by a number of nearby receptors including benzodiazepine and non-benzodiazepine binding sites. Alcohol, barbiturates, and the benzodiazepines all act at this GABA$_A$ receptor macromolecular complex to facilitate chloride channel conductance and hence neurotransmission by GABA. (2) GABA$_B$ receptors are not modulated by benzodiazepines and do not appear to be involved in the mediation of anxiety.

The GABA$_A$ receptor/Cl$^-$-ionophore complex is believed to be composed of combinations of α, β, γ, and a number of other less common subunits, each differing in amino acid composition, and each consisting of a number of variant subunits. While theoretically there could be thousands of GABA$_A$ receptor variants, there are a number of subunit combinations that are more common. More than 30 different GABA$_A$ subunit variants have been identified. These different forms show varying affinity for particular pharmacological agonists and antagonists, and they are differentially distributed in the brain.

Studies of mRNA distribution and receptor binding suggest that the major brain GABA$_A$ subunit combinations consist of $α_1β_2γ_2$ and $α_5β_3γ_2$. In animals, these subunit combinations appear to be associated with differing behavioural effects: sedation, memory, selected aspects of anxiety, sleep, seizure threshold, and self-administration of drugs. For example, studies in transgenic mouse models suggest that anxiolytic functions are mediated partly through the GABA receptor $α_2$ subunit, which is extensively expressed in the limbic system. The $α_1$ subunit, on the other hand, is believed to mediate sedative, amnestic, and anticonvulsant functions.

In 1977, benzodiazepine-specific receptors were discovered in the nervous system. The receptors are most dense in the cerebral cortex, as shown in Table 23-1, but are also present in significant numbers in the cerebellum and parts of the limbic system. Benzodiazepine receptors, although they form a distinct site, are functionally linked to postsynaptic GABA$_A$ receptor/Cl$^-$-ionophore complexes. This entire complex is involved in the mediation and modulation of GABAergic inhibitory neurotransmission.

Figure 23-2 is a schematic model of the GABA$_A$ receptor/Cl$^-$-ionophore complex. This transverse two-dimensional view of the receptor complex represents the centrally located chloride channel surrounded by five subunits that make up the receptor complex and distinct allosteric binding sites: the GABA site, the benzodiazepine site, a neurosteroid site, and a picrotoxin–barbiturate site. Each of these sites has specific GABA subunit compositional requirements for binding, which in turn regulate the nature of the behavioural effects produced by activation of the receptor. Neurotransmitters or drugs such as the benzodiazepines that enhance GABA action and hence open the Cl$^-$ channel are thought to have anti-seizure, sedating, and anxiolytic activity, while those that block GABA transmission and the Cl$^-$ channel (e.g., picrotoxin) are convulsant in nature.

GABA$_A$ receptor subtypes have unique pharmacological properties as a result of the differential subunit composition. This subunit selectivity has led to attempts to synthesize drugs that can target specific symptoms and behaviours. Some success has been found with drugs for insomnia. However, pharmacological selectivity does not necessarily result in effects that are clinically important.

Similarly, the activity of drugs can be controlled by altering their intrinsic activity at the site. The differences in pharmacological profiles of various benzodiazepines are related to differences in their intrinsic activities at the receptor site. Compounds with low intrinsic activity (partial agonists) display anxiolytic activity but are less sedating. These are drugs that increase GABA responses less than 100%. Compounds with high intrinsic activity are anxiolytic and sedating and are often used as sedatives. All the benzodiazepines in current clinical use are full agonists at the benzodiazepine–GABA$_A$ receptor complex.

Both therapeutic and adverse effects result from activation of the benzodiazepine receptor. Hence, undesirable effects such as memory impairment, unsteadiness, and physical dependence can all occur to some degree with full agonists and with partial agonists.

A selective and specific **antagonist**, flumazenil (Ro 15-1788), is available. This drug (see Fig. 23-2) blocks or reverses benzodiazepine effects but has no apparent intrinsic activity of its own. In humans, flumazenil can reverse anaesthesia or benzodiazepine overdose symptoms and could potentially precipitate withdrawal symptoms. Benzodiazepine receptor antagonists have also been discovered among ligands structurally different from flumazenil. Various β-carboline derivatives bind specifically to $^3$H-diazepam receptors but produce effects opposite to those of benzodiazepines (i.e., they show proconvulsant activity and anxiogenic effects). Therefore, they have been called **inverse agonists** rather than antagonists. It has been suggested that β-carbolines produce effects opposite to those of benzodiazepines because these agents reduce the coupling of GABA receptors to the Cl$^-$-ionophore, thereby decreasing the frequency of chloride channel opening. Interestingly, flumazenil also blocks the effect of β-carbolines.

**FIGURE 23-2** Schematic model of the GABA receptor/Cl⁻-ionophore complex with three distinct allosteric sites: the GABA receptor (A), the benzodiazepine receptor (M), and the picrotoxin–barbiturate receptor (B) located within the Cl⁻ ionophore. Although not shown, the neurosteroid site is also located within the Cl⁻ channel. Compounds that bind to these sites are also shown.

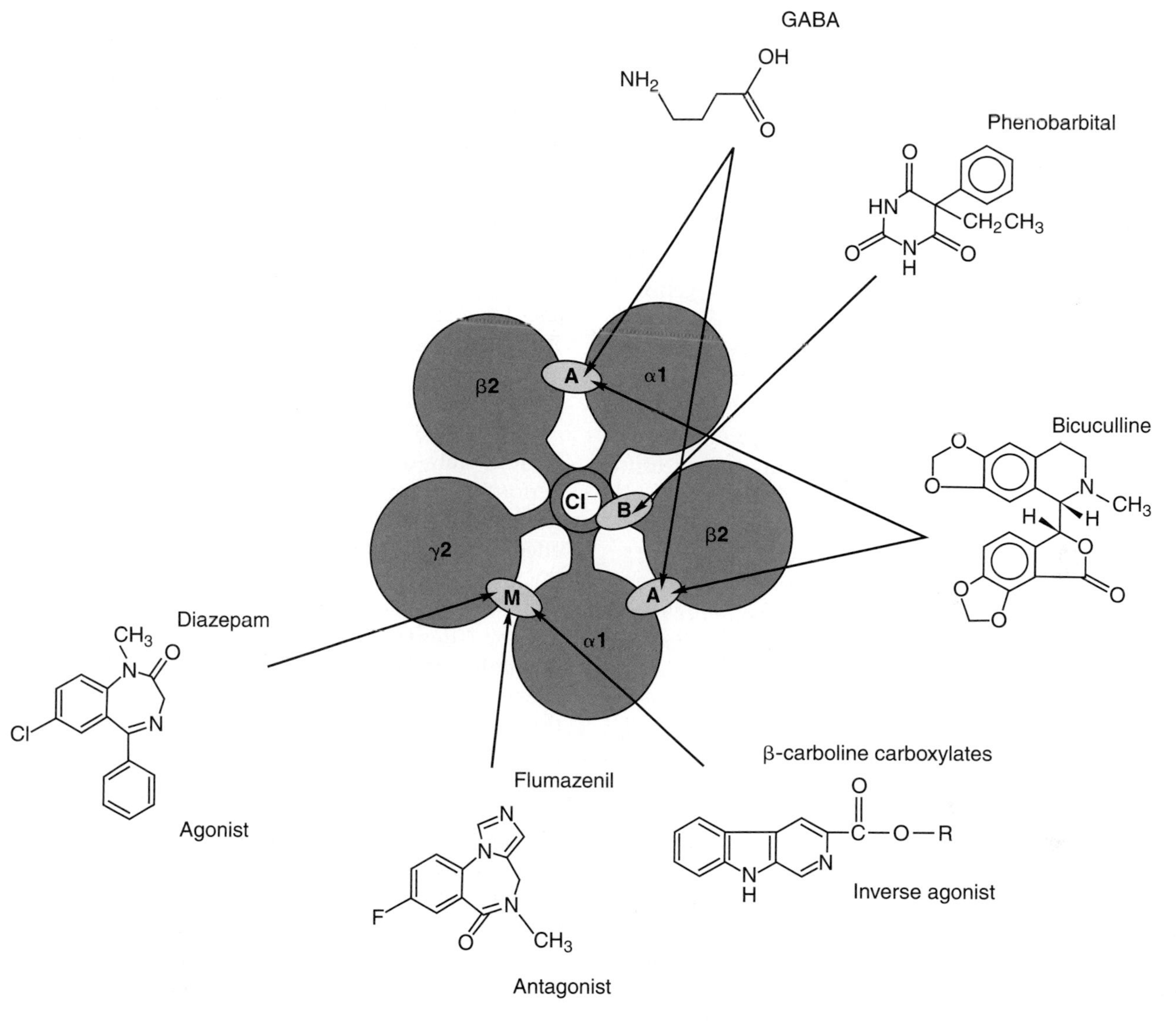

**Barbiturates** are an older class of GABAergic drugs that have fallen out of clinical use in the last two to three decades. Their safety profile is highly unfavourable in overdose situations or when they are co-administered with other psychotropic drugs.

## Other Potential Anxiolytic Mechanisms

### Neurokinin antagonists
Recently, a class of peptide neurotransmitters known as neurokinins has been investigated for a potential role in mood and anxiety disorders. Neurokinin receptors (NK1,

NK2, NK3) are located in areas of the brain implicated in anxiety (e.g., amygdala, hypothalamus, limbic area, locus ceruleus), and it was postulated that antagonists at these sites might have antidepressant and anxiolytic properties. Many NK1 antagonists have been described in the literature. Unfortunately, clinical trials with these compounds have been disappointing, and none are available clinically.

### Glutamate receptor modulators
Glutamate is the major excitatory neurotransmitter in the brain. Glutamate receptors are classified as either iono-

| TABLE 23-1 | Density of Benzodiazepine Binding Sites in Different Regions of the Human Brain |
|---|---|
| Region | $^3$H-Diazepam $B_{max}$ (fmol of $^3$H-ligand per mg protein) |
| Cerebral cortex | 1200 |
| Cerebellar cortex | 730 |
| Amygdala | 720 |
| Hippocampus | 610 |
| Hypothalamus | 520 |

tropic or metabotropic. Ionotropic receptors are coupled to cation-specific ion channels and bind the agonist $N$-methyl-D-aspartate (NMDA). Competitive and non-competitive NMDA antagonists have been evaluated primarily for treatment of stroke, dementia, and brain trauma. Unfortunately, many of these compounds have serious side effects, including psychotic-like symptoms, and their clinical development has been slow. Memantine has recently been approved for use in the treatment of dementia.

### Cholecystokinin (CCK) antagonists

CCK is an anxiogenic neuropeptide present in both the brain and the gastrointestinal tract. CCK is co-localized in neurons with a number of different neurotransmitters, including serotonin, dopamine, GABA, and substance P. There are two types of CCK receptor, A and B, localized in different areas of the brain. A number of selective antagonists to the CCK B receptor have been synthesized, but clinical studies with these agents have not shown significant anxiolytic effects (see Suggested Readings).

### Corticotrophin-releasing hormone (CRH)

CRH is a neuropeptide that plays an important role in mediating the body's physiological and behavioural responses to stress. CRH neurons located in the hypothalamic periventricular nucleus are important modulators of stress-induced activation of the hypothalamic–pituitary–adrenal axis. CRH also plays a neuromodulatory role through neurons and receptors distributed throughout the brain. There is an extensive literature, both pre-clinical and clinical, describing a key role for CRH in anxiety, depressive, and cognitive disorders. CRH acts through two G protein–coupled receptor subtypes, CRH-1 and CRH-2. CRH-1 and CRH-2 receptors have different pharmacology and different localizations in the brain and the periphery. A number of small molecules that show high selectivity for the CRH-1 receptor have been developed for the treatment of depression, anxiety, and stress disorders. Evaluation of several of these CRH-1 antagonists is underway, but none are yet available for clinical use.

## ANXIOLYTIC MEDICATIONS

### Selective Serotonin Reuptake Inhibitors (SSRIs)

The SSRIs, originally developed for the treatment of depression, have also shown efficacy in the treatment of anxiety disorders. Because of their excellent safety profile and low potential for abuse and dependence, SSRIs have become the first-line treatment for most anxiety disorders.

All available SSRIs (including **paroxetine, sertraline, fluvoxamine, fluoxetine, citalopram,** and **escitalopram**) are used clinically for one or more anxiety disorders. These SSRIs are pharmacologically similar in their activity, safety profile (with marginal differences in side effect profiles), and therapeutic efficacy; however, they differ somewhat in their chemical structures, risk for drug interactions, and pharmacokinetic properties (Table 23-2 and Figure 23-3; see Chapter 25 for a complete discussion of SSRIs).

SSRIs have several advantages over benzodiazepines. Most notably, detrimental effects on memory and motor performance seen with benzodiazepines are not as much of a problem with SSRIs. However, with SSRIs, sexual side effects and weight gain can affect patient compliance during treatment. Strategies to address SSRI sexual side effects include the use of adjunctive medication (such as 5-HT$_{2/3}$ and $\alpha_2$-adrenergic receptor antagonists, 5-HT$_{1A}$ and dopamine receptor agonists, and phosphodiesterase enzyme inhibitors) and changes in drug dosage. Additional difficulties include anxiogenic effects at the start of therapy, as well as feelings of restlessness and insomnia that may require control with short-term therapy with benzodiazepines. These difficulties resolve gradually during treatment. Although the abuse potential of SSRIs is low, the abrupt discontinuation of SSRI use after long-term therapy is associated with a discontinuation syndrome. This syndrome (consisting most commonly of dizziness, paresthesias, tremor, nausea, lethargy, and headache) appears within a week of discontinuation and often resolves gradually over 2 to 3 weeks. Although the symptoms are usually mild, discontinuation of SSRI therapy should include a gradual tapering-off period.

Doses used to treat anxiety disorders vary for different SSRIs (from 10 to 20 mg/day for escitalopram up to 100 to 200 mg/day for fluvoxamine) but are generally similar to those used in major depression. Some studies have suggested that doses for OCD may need to be somewhat higher than those used to treat depression.

### Serotonin–Noradrenaline Reuptake Inhibitors (SNRIs)

SNRIs strongly inhibit both serotonin and noradrenaline reuptake, with weak inhibition of dopamine reuptake.

**FIGURE 23-3** Structural formulae of selected anxiolytic and sedative–hypnotic drugs.

**SSRIs:**

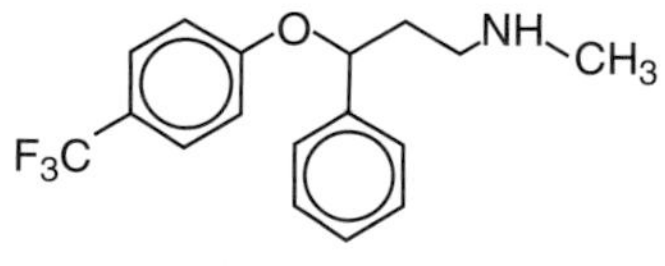

Fluoxetine

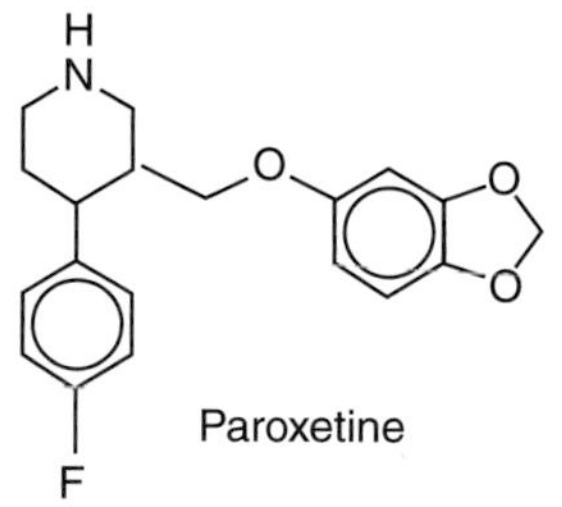

Paroxetine

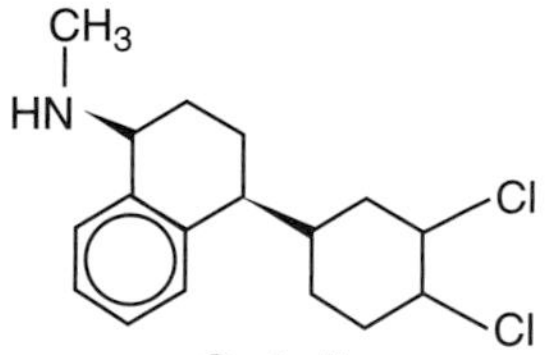

Sertraline

**5-HT$_{1A}$ agonist:**

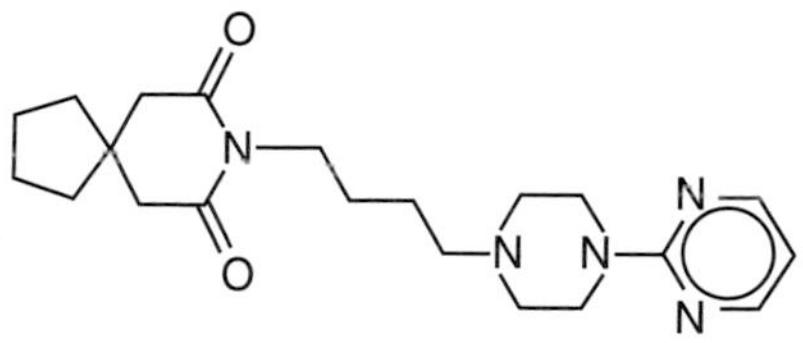

Buspirone

**SNRI:**

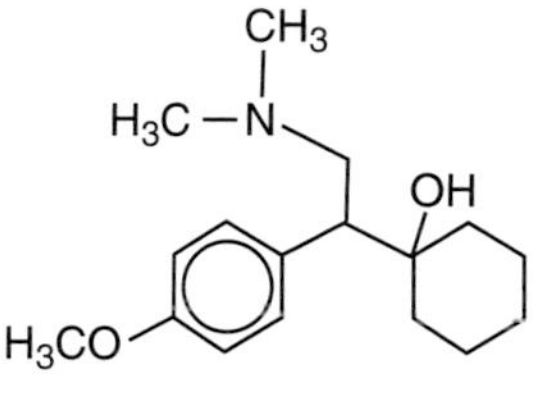

Venlafaxine

**Benzodiazepines:**

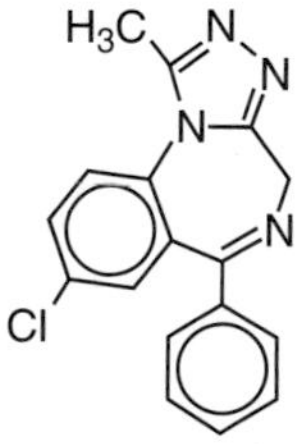

Alprazolam

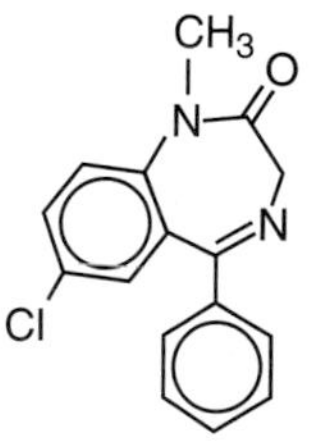

Diazepam

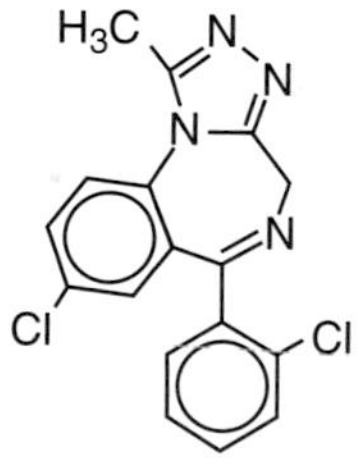

Triazolam

**MAOI:**

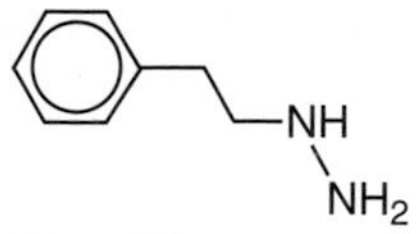

Phenelzine

**TCA:**

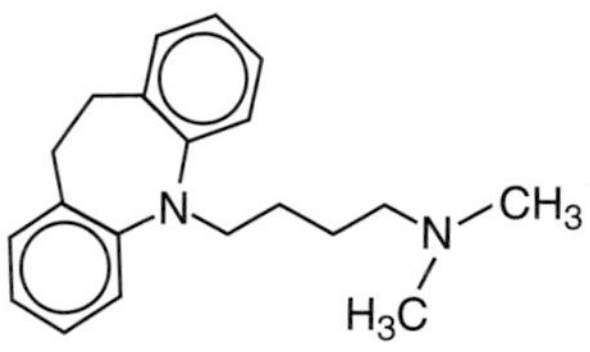

Imipramine

**Non-benzodiazepine sedative–hypnotics:**

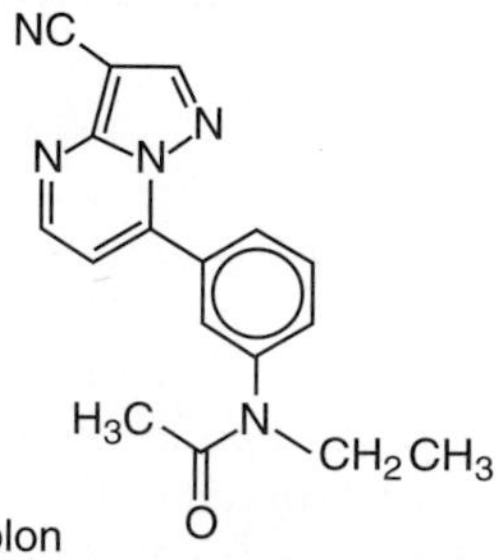

Zaleplon

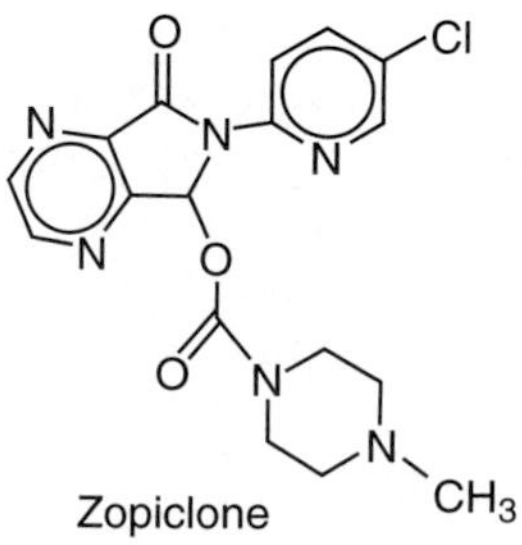

Zopiclone

| TABLE 23-2 | Pharmacokinetic Properties of Selected Anxiolytic Drugs | | | | | |
|---|---|---|---|---|---|---|
| Drug | Representative Trade Name | Therapeutic Indications | Time to Peak Effect (hours) | Half-Life (hours) | Active Metabolites (half-life in hours) |
| **SSRI** | | | | | |
| Paroxetine | Paxil | GAD, PD, PTSD, OCD, SP | 3–7 | 8–43 | |
| Sertraline | Zoloft | OCD, PD | 6–8 | 26 | |
| Fluoxetine | Prozac | OCD | 6–8 | 24–144 | Norfluoxetine (200–225) |
| Fluvoxamine | Luvox | OCD | 1.5–8 | 15–22 | |
| **SNRI** | | | | | |
| Venlafaxine | Effexor | GAD, SP | 2 | 5 | O-DM-venlafaxine (11) |
| **Benzodiazepine** | | | | | |
| Alprazolam | Xanax | GAD, PD | 1–2 | 6–20 | |
| Diazepam | Valium | | 1–2 | 20–100 | DM-diazepam (30–200) |
| Lorazepam | Ativan | Anxiety | 1–6 | 10–20 | |
| **TCA** | | | | | |
| Imipramine | Tofranil | Depression | 2–5 | 9–20 | |
| **MAOI** | | | | | |
| Phenelzine | Nardil | Mixed anxiety/depression | 0.5–1 | 10–12 | |
| **5-HT$_{1A}$ Agonist** | | | | | |
| Buspirone | Buspar | Short-term treatment of GAD | 0.5–1.5 | 2–11 | |

DM = desmethyl; GAD = generalized anxiety disorder; PD = panic disorder; PTSD = post-traumatic stress disorder; OCD = obsessive–compulsive disorder; SP = social phobia.

Side effects and indications are generally similar to those of the SSRIs. **Venlafaxine,** used to treat a variety of anxiety disorders, can ameliorate symptoms in both the short and long term. For GAD (as for MDD) the usual dose is 75 mg/day up to a maximum of 225 mg/day (see Chapter 25 for more details). It is now available in a slow-release formulation. **Duloxetine** is a new SNRI recently approved for the management of major depression and stress urinary incontinence. Its potential therapeutic effect in anxiety disorders has yet to be determined.

## Benzodiazepines

**Chlordiazepoxide** was the first benzodiazepine marketed (in 1960). This was followed by **diazepam** (1963), **oxazepam** (1965), and many others since then. The popularity of these drugs is the result of a combination of their efficacy, their rapid onset of action, and their relative safety. Although SSRIs (and SNRIs) are now the preferred choice by clinicians for long-term treatment of anxiety, benzodiazepines are useful for short-term therapy of intermittent symptoms and for chronic conditions as a bridge treatment before the SSRIs take full effect (e.g., in the first few weeks of therapy). Benzodiazepines can be classified on the basis of their chemical structure, kinetic characteristics, and therapeutic indications.

### Structure

All benzodiazepines are variations upon the 5-aryl-1,4-benzodiazepine nucleus (see Fig. 23-3). 1,5-Benzodiazepines also exist and are similar in pharmacological action. Other than the apparent requirement for the 5-aryl group, the structure–activity relationships are not stringent, and many benzodiazepine metabolites are pharmacologically active.

Chlordiazepoxide and diazepam are the prototypical benzodiazepines. Diazepam and many other benzodiazepines are metabolized to the active metabolite *N*-desmethyldiazepam, also called **nordiazepam** (ND; Table 23-2 and Fig. 23-4). *N*-desmethyldiazepam is marketed as a separate drug in some countries. **Clorazepate** and **prazepam** are quite rapidly converted to ND, one by acid hydrolysis and the other by dealkylation, and owe their clinical effects to this active metabolite.

The 3-OH substituent of oxazepam and lorazepam results in conjugation being the principal metabolic pathway rather than *N*-demethylation. Triazolobenzodiazepines (e.g., **alprazolam, triazolam**) undergo rapid biotransformation without production of active metabolites.

### Pharmacokinetics

*Absorption.* After oral administration, the absorption of diazepam, alprazolam, and triazolam is very rapid. The peak plasma concentrations occur about 1 hour after ingestion. Such rapid absorption accounts for the acute subjective drowsiness, "spaced-out" feeling, and motor impairment after the drugs are ingested. These effects are also dose-related. Diazepam has a systemic bioavailability of 100%. Oxazepam, lorazepam, and prazepam are absorbed more slowly, with the maximum plasma concen-

| FIGURE 23-4 | Patterns of benzodiazepine biotransformation. DM = desmethyl; * = active metabolites. |
|---|---|

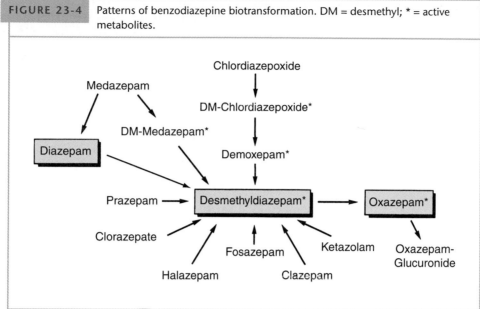

tration occurring 2 to 3 hours after ingestion. The bioavailability of oxazepam taken orally is about 50 to 70%. Since clorazepate is converted by acid hydrolysis in the stomach to its active form, ND, antacids reduce the rate of conversion and decrease the peak effects of the drug.

After intramuscular injection of diazepam or chlordiazepoxide in healthy persons or in alcoholics in withdrawal, absorption is slow (the plasma concentration peaking at 10 to 12 hours) and erratic. As a consequence, clinical effects may be delayed and unpredictable. Therefore, these drugs should generally not be given intramuscularly.

*Biotransformation and disposition of individual benzodiazepines.* All benzodiazepines undergo biotransformation in the liver, mainly by cytochrome P450 activity or by conjugation. Rates and patterns of benzodiazepine biotransformation vary considerably among healthy and ill individuals. The biotransformation of benzodiazepines is impaired in patients with significant chronic liver disease, and the half-life of the drug may increase several-fold. Ethanol can increase both the rate of absorption of benzodiazepines and the associated CNS depression.

Figure 23-4 summarizes the typical pathways of biotransformation for the majority of benzodiazepines. Metabolites indicated with an asterisk are pharmacologically active. Table 23-2 lists pharmacokinetic parameters of selected benzodiazepines.

**Chlordiazepoxide** and **diazepam** each have two major active metabolites that contribute to their clinical effects and toxicity: (1) chlordiazepoxide is converted to desmethylchlordiazepoxide and then to demoxepam; (2) diazepam is converted to ND and then to oxazepam, itself a marketed benzodiazepine. ND has a longer mean half-life than the parent drug (50.9 ± 6.2 hours versus 32.6 ± 11.3 hours). Little diazepam is excreted in the bile, and

enterohepatic recirculation is not responsible for the slow elimination.

These long half-lives and the extent of variation among patients make prediction of the time of maximum clinical effect or toxicity difficult, but during long-term therapy, one can expect cumulative and long-lasting effects of the benzodiazepines with long half-lives. On average, the time for accumulation to peak concentration during long-term oral administration is roughly five times the half-life of the drug (i.e., for chlordiazepoxide it is 3 days, for diazepam 7 days, and for desmethyldiazepam 10 days). The slow accumulation of drug means that the full therapeutic effect or toxicity cannot be determined for a number of days; therefore, the dosage should not be adjusted until accumulation is maximal. Conversely, elimination of the drug is slow, and the offset of drug effect may be delayed.

Because of the long half-lives of chlordiazepoxide and diazepam, multiple daily doses may be unnecessary. However, if the entire 24-hour dosage is given as a single dose, it can cause extreme sedation. It may therefore be best to administer most of the daily dose at bedtime.

**Lorazepam,** a more potent benzodiazepine, is similar to **oxazepam** in structure and in pattern of disposition. Its bioavailability after intramuscular injection is complete. Unlike chlordiazepoxide and diazepam, lorazepam and oxazepam are biotransformed simply by glucuronide conjugation to inactive metabolites. Furthermore, since the mean half-life of oxazepam is 7 hours, accumulation is minor and a full therapeutic response occurs after a few doses. Similarly, sedation diminishes rapidly. However, for the therapeutic effect to be maintained, the drug should be given three times a day. Neither liver disease nor advanced age alters the half-life of oxazepam or lorazepam. These drugs may be preferable for treating acute anxiety symptoms when dose titration is required and daytime sedation is particularly to be avoided.

**Triazolam** is well absorbed, has a rapid onset of action, is rapidly metabolized and excreted, and has no active metabolites. As a result of these properties, it is widely used as a hypnotic agent.

**Flurazepam**, though marketed as a hypnotic, has some disadvantageous properties when used as such. It is rapidly converted to two active metabolites, hydroxyflurazepam and flurazepam aldehyde, which are responsible for its reasonably quick onset of hypnotic action ($T_{max}$ 1 to 2 hours). However, if it is used regularly, accumulation of a third active metabolite, desalkylflurazepam, occurs over 7 to 10 days because this metabolite is slowly eliminated. Its accumulation causes daytime drowsiness as a frequent side effect during long-term use. Older patients are particularly likely to experience adverse effects because they are more sensitive to various psychotropic drugs and may have altered biotransformation of the drug.

**Alprazolam** has been extensively marketed for the treatment of panic disorder and is widely prescribed. It is well absorbed orally and reaches peak plasma concentrations in 1 to 2 hours after a single dose. It has a half-life of about 11 hours, which is increased substantially in the elderly and in patients with liver or kidney disease. One of its primary metabolites, α-hydroxyalprazolam, is further metabolized to desmethylalprazolam, and both of these are active.

**Clonazepam** is a long-acting benzodiazepine; the half-life of the parent compound varies from approximately 18 to 50 hours. Although its pharmacological profile is similar to that of other benzodiazepines, it is used primarily for the treatment of epilepsy.

**Midazolam** is a very short-acting benzodiazepine (half-life 1 to 4 hours) that is available only as an injectable formulation of its water-soluble hydrochloride salt. It is used for both preoperative sedation and induction of anaesthesia. Midazolam itself is highly lipophilic, and the onset of effect is rapid; the offset of effect is also rapid, because of both redistribution and biotransformation. Administration of midazolam is often followed by anterograde amnesia.

### Behavioural effects

*Anti-anxiety action.* The effects of the benzodiazepines can be readily demonstrated in classical animal models of anxiety. In conflict punishment procedures (see Chapter 69), benzodiazepines greatly reduce the behaviour-suppressing effects of punishment, so the animals will continue to seek food or water despite the concurrent presence of electrical shock. Other drugs such as barbiturates may show similar effects, but the benzodiazepines produce these effects at doses that do not cause sedation or alteration of other behaviours.

No benzodiazepine has been shown to be superior in efficacy at equipotent doses to chlordiazepoxide for the treatment of acute anxiety states or chronic anxiety disorders. The majority of the benzodiazepines have been approved for short-term use (6 to 12 weeks) in anxiety disorders. However, many of them end up being prescribed chronically despite some evidence that their anxiolytic effects may diminish over time. The major concern with long-term use is physical dependence, resulting in a withdrawal syndrome on abrupt discontinuation of the medication.

For short-term anxiety-related conditions, such as symptoms following a stressful life event, benzodiazepines can be very helpful if use is limited to several days or weeks. For conditions likely to require longer treatment, such as generalized anxiety disorder, panic disorder, or anxiety related to major depression, other treatment options should be considered in view of the concerns about physical dependence and withdrawal. In these conditions, benzodiazepines are often used as short-term adjuncts to antidepressant medication to provide rapid relief from anxiety and to control the agitation, insomnia, and occasional exacerbation of anxiety seen with the initiation of antidepressant therapy

*Anticonvulsant activity.* All benzodiazepines elevate seizure threshold and are anticonvulsant (see Chapter 18). They have been shown to prevent or abolish seizures in various animal models of epilepsy. Although very effective in the treatment of status epilepticus (e.g., diazepam), absence attacks, and other types of childhood seizures (e.g., clonazepam), oral benzodiazepines have a limited role in the long-term management of seizure disorders because of the development of tolerance to their anticonvulsant effects.

*Alcohol withdrawal.* Most benzodiazepines are effective in the treatment of alcohol withdrawal syndrome (see Chapter 22). The longer-acting benzodiazepines, such as chlordiazepoxide or diazepam, are more useful than the shorter-acting forms because their gradually falling blood levels provide more sustained pharmacological protection against withdrawal symptoms.

*Muscle relaxant effects.* Benzodiazepines reduce elevated skeletal muscle tone and are effective in various neuromuscular disorders including cerebral palsy, tetanus, and "stiff-person syndrome" (a rare autoimmune disease of the CNS, in which auto-antibodies against glutamate decarboxylase interfere with GABA interneuron function in the spinal cord). However, they are frequently used in a variety of situations for which their efficacy is unproven, such as lower back pain and muscle trauma.

*Amnesia with sedation.* The wide margin of safety of the benzodiazepines permits their use in a variety of clinical situations in which the objective is to produce rapid sedation and amnesia (e.g., endoscopy, bronchoscopy, preanaesthetic sedation, anaesthesia induction, cardioversion, childbirth). In these situations, intravenous diazepam is at least as effective as and safer than barbiturates, but it is probably not superior to other parenterally administered benzodiazepines. Midazolam, a benzodiazepine with very rapid elimination, is available for induction of anaesthesia or acute sedation, but it also produces anterograde amnesia in over two-thirds of such cases.

## Responsiveness

Dose requirements for patients vary greatly. For example, the diazepam plasma concentration required to produce sufficient sedation and relaxation to permit passage of a gastroscope varies up to 22-fold among individuals. This implies great variability in receptor sensitivity, and it is not possible to predict clinical response at a particular dose in a particular patient. The sensitivity to benzodiazepines increases with age and liver disease and decreases with smoking and with recent use of benzodiazepines, alcohol, or other CNS drugs that produce cross-tolerance to benzodiazepines. As a rule of thumb, the initial dose of benzodiazepine prescribed should be reduced by 50% in the elderly (over 65 years), patients with liver disease, or those concurrently receiving other CNS depressants.

## Tolerance, dependence, and withdrawal

Acute, subacute, and chronic tolerance to benzodiazepines has been demonstrated in studies with animals and humans (see also Chapter 70). During long-term administration, tolerance commonly manifests itself as a decrease in side effects.

Tolerance to benzodiazepines appears to be primarily functional rather than metabolic in nature. Tolerance to the sedative, anticonvulsant, and muscle relaxant effects of benzodiazepines has been shown. In general, their anxiolytic effects persist during chronic treatment, although there is some disagreement about this. Physical dependence may develop in patients taking both therapeutic and high doses of benzodiazepines (diazepam more than 40 mg/day or chlordiazepoxide more than 200 mg/day), and the consequent signs and symptoms of withdrawal may be seen when use of the drug is stopped abruptly. However, elimination of diazepam and chlordiazepoxide (and their metabolites) is slow enough that the withdrawal reaction is delayed and often mild, because tissue levels of these benzodiazepines decline slowly and neuroadaptation can occur. This is equivalent to clinical tapering of the dose. More rapidly eliminated benzodiazepines may produce a more severe clinical withdrawal syndrome. Abrupt termination of a short-acting benzodiazepine results in a rapid decline in the tissue levels of drug and onset of withdrawal symptoms before any neuroadaptation can occur. If a withdrawal reaction occurs, the typical clinical features include anxiety, tremor, insomnia, disorders of perception, and, rarely, seizures.

Psychological dependence can occur at any dose, and the resultant signs and symptoms may be difficult to distinguish from those of the original anxiety disorder. Patients who have taken therapeutic doses of benzodiazepines for a long time frequently experience severe anxiety when an attempt is made to discontinue the drug. Reassuring the patient that alternate treatments are available if needed and very gradual tapering, or in fact starting them concurrently on a different medication, usually an antidepressant, can aid in successful discontinuation of the benzodiazepines. Before starting therapy with benzodiazepines, the desired therapeutic goals and planned duration of treatment should always be discussed with the patient, as well as the procedure for ending treatment (gradual tapering off).

## Drug interactions

Significant interactions of benzodiazepines with other drugs are infrequent. However, they do produce an additive effect when taken with other CNS depressants. The combination of alcohol and a benzodiazepine can impair driving skills to a degree greater than that caused by the same amount of either drug alone. Physicians should caution patients about the risks of drinking alcohol while they are taking a benzodiazepine. Interactions of benzodiazepines with analgesics, antihistamines, antipsychotics, and tricyclic antidepressants also cause excessive sedation and cognitive and motor impairments.

Benzodiazepines do not induce the synthesis of drug-biotransforming enzymes and are safe to use in combination with anticoagulants, anti-arrhythmics, anti-neoplastic agents, and anti-epileptics.

## Adverse reactions

**Orally administered** benzodiazepines cause non life-threatening side effects in fewer than 10% of patients who receive them. The most common adverse effects are direct extensions of the pharmacological actions of these drugs: drowsiness, ataxia, lethargy, and, rarely, coma.

Benzodiazepines may interfere with memory acquisition, consolidation, and recall, and all can produce anterograde amnesia.

The frequency of side effects of chlordiazepoxide and diazepam increases with age, dose, duration of therapy, and presence of liver disease and hypoalbuminemia.

Hematological, renal, and hepatic toxicities have seldom been reported for benzodiazepines. Various unusual responses have been described, including nightmares, paradoxical delirium and confusion or excitation, depression, aggression, and hostile behaviour. Rarely, patients experience a dry mouth, a metallic taste, or headaches.

Uncommon but important acute adverse effects after **intravenous** administration include respiratory or cardiac arrest or both, hypotension, and phlebitis at the site of injection. Life-threatening adverse reactions occur with a frequency of about 2% after rapid intravenous administration of diazepam. Patients particularly at risk often have coexisting severe pulmonary or cardiac disease or have concurrently received other cardiorespiratory-depressant medications. Whenever possible (and practical), the rate of injection should be less than 12.5 mg/min for chlordiazepoxide and less than 2.5 mg/min for diazepam.

The question of possible teratogenic or other toxic effects on the fetus when benzodiazepines are used during pregnancy is controversial. The risk that has been raised most persistently, but not effectively proven, is a small increase in the potential for midline cleft deformities of the lip or palate, but these remain below the overall risk of birth defects in the general population (2 to 5%).

An **overdose** of benzodiazepines alone is almost never fatal. However, because a large proportion of drug overdoses involve more than one drug, combinations of benzodiazepines and other CNS drugs, such as alcohol, are common and may cause coma and death.

## Other Anxiolytic Agents

**Buspirone** is a partial agonist at the 5-HT$_{1A}$ receptor and may have additional indirect effects on other neurotransmitter systems. It is rapidly absorbed and its half-life is 2 to 3 hours. The recommended daily dosage of buspirone is from 15 mg daily up to a maximum of 60 mg. It has demonstrated efficacy in the treatment of generalized anxiety disorder, with or without concomitant depressive symptoms. Recent prior treatment with a benzodiazepine has been shown to predict poorer response to buspirone, possibly due to benzodiazepine withdrawal and/or exacerbation of withdrawal symptoms by buspirone. Advantages of using this medication rather than a benzodiazepine include the absence of significant interactions with alcohol or sedative–hypnotic drugs and no development of physical dependence and consequent withdrawal reaction after chronic use.

**Monoamine oxidase inhibitors** (MAOIs), **tricyclic antidepressants** (TCAs), and atypical antidepressants (such as **trazodone** and **mirtazapine**) have shown some efficacy in the treatment of anxiety symptoms and disorders. Irreversible MAOIs and the tricyclic antidepressant imipramine are effective treatments for panic disorder. However, MAOIs, because of their relatively narrow margin of safety and their risk of drug interactions (e.g., tyramine-induced hypertensive reactions), are generally considered to be third-line treatments.

## INSOMNIA

Insomnia is a symptom and is not a diagnosis in itself. Except for the occasional patient who may have a primary sleep disorder, insomnia is almost always secondary to a medical or psychiatric illness, medications, or a stressful life event. Insomnia is defined as difficulty initiating or maintaining sleep, which results in psychological distress and impaired daily functioning both at work and socially. Individuals with insomnia not only report drowsiness and fatigue on awakening as well as sleepiness during the day, but they also complain of various physical complaints and visit physicians more often than healthy controls do.

Transient insomnia is short term (less than 2 weeks) and is typically due to factors known to disrupt sleep (e.g., jet lag, situational anxiety, shift work, physical factors such as noise and cold, bereavement, pain). Medications are often not needed, and simple "sleep hygiene" and behavioural changes are sufficient. If a hypnotic is prescribed, the shorter-acting medications (e.g., zaleplon) are preferred in order to minimize morning "hangover."

Chronic insomnia requires a comprehensive medical and psychiatric assessment since it can be associated with a wide range of etiologies (e.g., alcohol or drug abuse, affective and anxiety disorders, dementia, medical illnesses, medication side effects, chronic pain, use of excessive amounts of caffeinated beverages). Treatment of these conditions often alleviates the insomnia, and hence, sedative–hypnotics can be avoided.

The lifetime prevalence of chronic insomnia has been estimated from large population-based surveys to be about 10%; up to 45% of individuals report experiencing insomnia symptoms in the past year. Insomnia is more common in women and the elderly.

## Sleep Architecture

**Normal sleep** consists of at least two phases: (1) slow-wave sleep (SWS, or stages 3 and 4), during which polysomnography shows predominantly high-voltage synchronous activity, but with sustained tonus of skeletal muscles; and (2) rapid-eye-movement (REM) sleep, in which the electroencephalogram (EEG) shows an arousal pattern, the eyes move rapidly and irregularly, skeletal muscles relax completely, and dreaming is thought to take place. These two phases alternate throughout the total sleep period, REM sleep making up about 25% of the total. This cycling appears to depend upon a balance of serotonin and catecholamine influences on the reticular formation.

The **sleep produced by hypnotic**s differs from normal sleep: sleep latency is reduced, SWS patterns are altered and shortened by the appearance of EEG spindles, REM sleep is suppressed, and total sleep time is prolonged. Most of the benzodiazepines produce similar effects on the patterns of sleep. With chronic use, the effects tend to decrease but do not disappear. If, after 3 to 4 weeks, the drug is suddenly stopped, the amount and intensity of REM increase to levels greater than in normal sleep ("REM rebound"). This is considered by some investigators to represent a mild degree of physical dependence and a withdrawal reaction.

## Prescribing Guidelines for Insomnia

Prior to using sedative–hypnotics, it is important to consider the differential diagnosis of insomnia in the patient so that these medications are appropriately prescribed. Sleep experts suggest that these drugs should not be used for longer than several weeks, and product labelling reflects this recommendation. Chronic insomnia should be treated intermittently when possible. However, many patients suffer from insomnia for years, and treatment may need to extend for long periods of time. There is little evidence that sedative–hypnotics lose their efficacy over time, but there is a risk of developing dependence on these drugs. Therefore, the continuing need for these medications should be re-evaluated every few months. The initial use of sedative–hypnotics should be at the lowest effective dose. The elderly are more sensitive to most psychotropic drugs, and lower initial doses should be used in those over 60 years of age.

The most common side effect of sedative–hypnotics is feeling sedated or mentally "fuzzy" in the morning. The longer the drug's half-life, the greater the probability of this complaint. After short-term use, some patients may experience mildly disrupted sleep for a few nights. Sedative–hypnotics should not be combined with alcohol, and patients should be warned of the dangers of this interaction.

## Specific Drugs

The newer non-benzodiazepine sedative–hypnotics are more commonly considered for first-line treatment of insomnia. These include zaleplon, zopiclone, and zolpidem (available only in the United States; see Fig. 23-3). All three drugs have a rapid onset of effect and a short duration of action (Table 23-3).

**Zaleplon** is rapidly absorbed and short-acting (half-life of 1 hour). In common with benzodiazepines, it acts allosterically at the GABA$_A$ receptor but at a different site. The drug is metabolized to inactive metabolites by CYP3A; hence, CYP3A inhibitors (e.g., cimetidine) increase, and CYP3A inducers decrease, zaleplon plasma concentrations. The dose may have to be decreased or increased, respectively, in these situations. Zaleplon is effective in both chronic and transient insomnia in adults and is recommended for individuals having difficulty falling asleep. Doses of 5, 10, and 20 mg have been shown to be more effective than placebo and demonstrate a dose-response relationship. Rebound insomnia may occur after 14 to 28 days of treatment; however, withdrawal emergent phenomena are generally not significantly different than after placebo.

Somnolence is the most common side effect. As expected, the drug interacts with ethanol and with other CNS drugs that cause sedation (pharmacodynamic interaction). The recommended adult dose is 10 mg immediately before bed. There is a risk of abuse in individuals with a past history of alcohol or drug dependence.

**Zolpidem** is similar to zaleplon in pharmacological properties, but it has later peak drug concentrations (2 to 3 hours) and a somewhat longer half-life (1.5 to 3 hours). Late-night administration has been associated with side effects that are absent with zaleplon (e.g., morning sedation, delayed reaction time, and anterograde amnesia). Therefore, it has been approved for bedtime use only.

**Zopiclone** is structurally not a benzodiazepine, but a cyclopyrrolone derivative. Nevertheless, its pharmacological properties are so similar to those of the intermediate-acting benzodiazepines that it is usually grouped with them. It has a rapid onset of action, and the peak plasma concentrations occur within 1.5 hours. Its half-life is 3.5 to 6 hours, longer than that of zaleplon or zolpidem. The usual dose is 7.5 mg at bedtime. Lower doses (3.75 mg) should be given to the elderly. The most common adverse reaction seen with zopiclone is taste alteration (bitter taste).

Benzodiazepines continue to be prescribed for insomnia. Shorter-acting benzodiazepines are preferred because their effects will wear off by morning, but in practice, almost all benzodiazepines are used for treatment of insomnia (**triazolam, nitrazepam, lorazepam,** and **alprazolam**; see Table 23-3 and Fig. 23-3). Treatment can be tailored to the individual's sleep patterns by considering the half-life of the drug.

**Triazolam** is a short-acting benzodiazepine indicated for short-term treatment (7 to 10 days) of transient insomnia. Experience with triazolam is far more extensive than

| TABLE 23-3 | Pharmacokinetic Properties of Selected Sedative–Hypnotic Drugs | | | |
|---|---|---|---|---|
| Drug | Representative Trade Name | Therapeutic Indication(s) | Time to Peak Effect (hours) | Half-Life (hours) |
| Benzodiazepine | | | | |
| Flurazepam | Dalmane | Insomnia | 1–2 | 1.5 |
| Midazolam | Versed | Sedation | 0.25–0.5 | 1.5–5 |
| Nitrazepam | Mogadon | Insomnia | 2 | 15–40 |
| Temazepam | Restoril | Insomnia | 0.8–1.4 | 10–20 |
| Triazolam | Halcion | Insomnia | 1–2 | 1.5–5 |
| Non-benzodiazepine | | | | |
| Zaleplon | Starnoc | Insomnia | 1 | 1 |
| Zolpidem | Ambien | Insomnia | 1.6 | 2.5 |
| Zopiclone | Imovane | Insomnia | <2 | 3.5–6 |

with most of the other hypnotics, but concerns about its safety have been raised. It has received extensive negative publicity because of complaints of confusion, amnesia, bizarre behaviour, agitation, and hallucinations. This drug has been withdrawn from sale in some countries. In North America, the recommended starting dose has been reduced to 0.125 mg from 0.25 mg, and the recommended maximum dose is now 0.25 mg instead of 0.5 mg. Triazolam has been reported to be associated with paradoxical rage reactions, but these are extremely rare, and it is not clear in most cases that the drug was an important etiological factor.

**Temazepam** has a delayed onset of action but an intermediate half-life, and it may be more useful for individuals with middle-of-the-night insomnia.

Disadvantages to using benzodiazepines for insomnia are similar to those encountered in prescribing them for anxiety: daytime sedation, memory impairment, and a withdrawal syndrome after chronic use and sudden discontinuation. Stopping the medications should always be done by gradually tapering off.

## SUGGESTED READINGS

Adams JB, Pyke RE, Costa J, et al. A double-blind, placebo-controlled study of a CCK-B receptor antagonist, CI-988, in patients with generalized anxiety disorder. *J Clin Psychopharmacol.* 1995;15:428-434.

American Psychiatric Association. *Diagnostic and Statistical Manual of Mental Disorder, Fourth Edition, Text Revision (DSM-IV-TR).* Arlington, Va: American Psychiatric Publishing, Inc; 2000.

Blanco C, Raza MS, Schneier FR, Liebowitz MR. The evidence-based pharmacological treatment of social anxiety disorder. *Int J Neuropsychopharmacol.* 2003;6:427-442.

Busto UE, Kaplan HL, Wright CE, et al. A comparative pharmacokinetic and dynamic evaluation of alprazolam sustained-release, bromazepam, and lorazepam. *J Clin Psychopharmacol.* 2000;20:628-635.

Busto U, Sellers EM, Naranjo CA, et al. Withdrawal reaction after long-term therapeutic use of benzodiazepines. *N Engl J Med.* 1986;315:854-859.

Davis KL, Charney D, Coyle JT, Nemeroff C, eds. *Psychopharmacology: The Fifth Generation of Progress.* Philadelphia, Pa: Lippincott Williams & Wilkins; 2002.

Fricchione G. Clinical practice. Generalized anxiety disorder. *N Engl J Med.* 2004;351:675-682.

Kaplan A, Hollander E. A review of pharmacologic treatments for obsessive-compulsive disorder. *Psychiatr Serv.* 2003;54:1111-1118.

Romach MK, Busto U, Somer G, et al. Clinical aspects of chronic alprazolam and lorazepam use. *Am J Psychiatry.* 1995;152:1161-1167.

Rouillon F. Long term therapy of generalized anxiety disorder. *Eur Psychiatry.* 2004;19:96-101.

Sanger DJ. The pharmacology and mechanisms of action of new generation, non-benzodiazepine hypnotic agents. *CNS Drugs.* 2004;18(suppl 1):9-15.

Schoenfeld FB, Marmar CR, Neylan TC. Current concepts in pharmacotherapy for posttraumatic stress disorder. *Psychiatr Serv.* 2004;55:519-531.

Whiting PJ. The $GABA_A$ receptor gene family: new opportunities for drug development. *Curr Opin Drug Discov Devel.* 2003;6:648-657.

# 24

# Antipsychotics

## D MAMO, S KAPUR, AND P SEEMAN

## CASE HISTORY

W.G. was 19 years old when he enrolled in university. His academic record was good, he won a place on the university rowing team, and he enjoyed his share of late nights throughout first year. When he returned to school for his second year, his roommate observed that W.G. was staying by himself, avoiding the company of friends, and skipping school and athletic training, things he had never done before. Some time later, he was heard speaking to himself as he sat isolated in his room, mumbling and smiling. Soon after, he confided to his roommate that he had uncovered a "grand conspiracy" to rob him of his athletic abilities and that he could hear the conspirators' voices as they made plans to destroy him. Finally, he accused his roommate of being part of the conspiracy.

At this point, his friends called his parents and he was taken to see a psychiatrist. The psychiatrist diagnosed him as showing early symptoms of schizophrenia, and he was admitted to the hospital. Blood and urine tests were negative for signs of any general medical condition or the presence of any street drugs. He was therefore treated with risperidone at a starting dose of 6 mg/day. On the second day of his treatment, while a medical student was interviewing him, he seemed to develop a "seizure." His neck was strained backward with his face turned upward toward the ceiling. He was having difficulty speaking but was quite conscious of his surroundings. The attending physician recognized this as an acute dystonic reaction to the medication rather than a seizure. The doctor immediately ordered an injection of benztropine, which resolved the situation in a matter of minutes. The doctor suggested a small decrease in the dose of his current medication, but W.G. refused to have anything more to do with risperidone. However, he agreed to take olanzapine instead after it was explained to him that he was less likely to have the dystonic reaction with this drug.

The dose of olanzapine was gradually increased to 20 mg/day. He experienced sedation, blurred vision, drying of his eyes that made it difficult for him to wear contact lenses, and dry mouth. However, over the next 3 weeks, his delusions and hallucinations disappeared. He developed insight into his problems, and the sedation, dry mouth, and dry eyes became much more bearable. He left the hospital a month later, went back to his dormitory, and resumed his academic life.

Over the next few months, W.G. put on about 5 kg (11 lb.) of weight and started feeling "low" since he had lost his physical prowess and was experiencing difficulties in concentration at school. About 6 months after discharge, his physician noticed a return of some of the previous delusions and hallucinations. On detailed inquiry, it turned out that he had been taking "pep pills," on the recommendation of a fellow athlete, to help him with his problems of weight gain and feeling low. The doctor asked him to bring in one of these pep pills, which were identified as amphetamine in the hospital laboratory. On receiving the report of the analysis, the doctor advised him never to take those pills because they might be responsible for the relapse of his delusions and hallucinations.

Since then, W.G. has continued treatment as an outpatient. Life hasn't been perfect, but he has been able to lose most of his weight gain through diet and exercise. With some accommodations for the time lost, he was able to achieve a passing grade for that year, and while he missed the university rowing squad, he was allowed to train with them on the B team.

As the name suggests, antipsychotic drugs are used to treat psychosis, and while they are most commonly prescribed for schizophrenia, they are also effective in a number of other psychiatric and neuropsychiatric con-ditions presenting with psychotic symptoms. The older term "neuroleptic" is still occasionally used to describe these drugs: this term derives from the profound sedation and abnormal motor posturing noted in animals treated with these drugs, almost as if the nervous system had been "seized" by the drug (*neuro* for nerve, and *lepsis* for seizure). However, with the advent of newer antipsychotic drugs that result in less or even no motor side effects, this term was dropped in favour of the term "antipsychotics."

The primary clinical indication for antipsychotics is the treatment of psychosis, which is the name given to a clinical syndrome characterized by one or more of the following symptoms:

1. **Delusions,** which are fixed false beliefs (e.g., W.G.'s idea of a "grand conspiracy" to rob him of his athletic abilities)
2. **Hallucinations,** which are the experiences of perceptual sensations in the absence of any stimulation (e.g., W.G. hearing the conspirators' voices as they made plans to destroy him)
3. **Grossly disorganized behaviour and speech** (i.e., patients may be unable to take care of themselves, may be mute, mumbling incoherently, or smiling to themselves, and may respond to questions or comments in incomprehensible speech)

The most common indication for antipsychotics is schizophrenia, a psychiatric disorder characterized by delusions, hallucinations, and disorganized behaviour or speech (also known as *positive symptoms*), as well as cognitive disabilities (e.g., impairments of memory, concentration, attention, executive function) and a related cluster of symptoms called *negative symptoms* (e.g., apathy, low mood, restricted range of emotion). Antipsychotics are most helpful in alleviating positive symptoms of schizophrenia, and with the possible exception of clozapine, show little if any effect on cognitive and negative symptoms.

# MECHANISMS OF ACTION OF ANTIPSYCHOTICS

## The Dopaminergic System

While the precise mechanism by which antipsychotics decrease delusions, hallucinations, or disorganized behaviour remains unknown, it is now well established that all antipsychotic drugs used in clinical practice are antagonists of the dopamine $D_2$ receptors. The dopaminergic system arises from groups of cells in the midbrain and the hypothalamus (Fig. 24-1). Of the cells originating in the midbrain, the neurons arising in substantia nigra ascend to the striatum (the nigrostriatal pathway) and are primarily involved in the modulation of motor behaviour. This pathway is implicated in Parkinson's disease and in the parkinsonian side effects induced by antipsychotics, particularly the older (neuroleptic) drugs. The other prominent midbrain projections arise from the ventral tegmental area, projecting to various limbic ("emotional") areas (including the nucleus accumbens

and septum) and cortical regions (cingulate, entorhinal, prefrontal, and pyriform cortices). They are thus referred to as the mesolimbic and mesocortical pathways, respectively, and are involved in cognition, modulation of motivation, reward-linked behaviour, and emotion. In addition, discrete groups of dopaminergic cells originate in the hypothalamus and project to the pituitary and are involved in the neuroendocrine regulation of prolactin secretion (see also Chapter 16, especially Figs. 16-5 and 16-7A, and Chapter 44).

The **receptors for dopamine** consist of two receptor families, namely the $D_1$-like and the $D_2$-like receptors. The *$D_1$-like family* includes the $D_1$ and $D_5$ receptors, which share a similar genetic sequence and activate adenylyl cyclase, thereby increasing the production of the second messenger cyclic AMP (cAMP). The *$D_2$-like family* includes the $D_2$, $D_3$, and $D_4$ receptors, which also share a high degree of genetic sequence similarity and have a similar, though not identical, pharmacological profile. The $D_2$ receptor subtype is predominantly expressed in the caudate–putamen regions, while the $D_3$ and $D_4$ receptors have a higher distribution in the limbic regions of the brain.

Dopamine receptors are localized both pre-synaptically and post-synaptically. The presynaptic receptors located on the cell bodies are termed somatodendritic autoreceptors, while those on the axon terminal are called terminal autoreceptors. The somatodendritic autoreceptors modulate the firing of the dopamine neurons, whereas the autoreceptors on the axon terminal modulate the release of dopamine. The postsynaptic dopamine receptors mediate the effect of dopamine on the non-dopaminergic cell bodies. $D_1$ receptors are primarily postsynaptic, while the $D_2$- and $D_3$ receptors are found both pre- and post-synaptically. To add to this complexity, studies have revealed that both $D_1$ and $D_2$ receptors exist in forms with high affinity and low affinity for dopamine, and it is suggested that the high-affinity conformation may be more relevant to the actual signal transduction and may play a special role in the production of psychotic symptoms.

## Action of Antipsychotics on the Dopaminergic System

The fundamental molecular explanation for the selective blocking of dopamine receptors by antipsychotics is that these drugs adopt a conformation in which certain aspects of the drug molecule are identical to the corresponding features of dopamine. The molecular formulae of **chlorpromazine** (a **phenothiazine**) and **haloperidol** (a **butyrophenone**) and their similarity to dopamine are shown in Figure 24-2. One can readily appreciate that the antipsychotic medications share an affinity for the dopamine system, which is recognized as a crucial aspect of their clinical effectiveness. Several observations buttress the essential connection between the antipsychotic effect of these drugs and their action on the dopamine system:

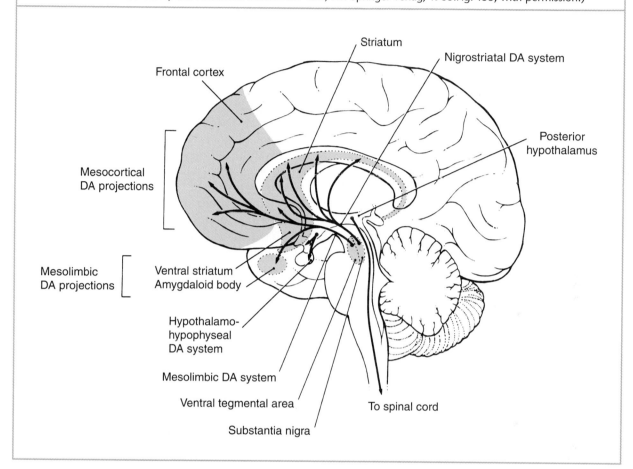

FIGURE 24-1 Dopaminergic pathways. The nigrostriatal dopamine system originates in the substantia nigra and terminates in the main dorsal part of the striatum. The ventral tegmental area gives rise to the mesolimbic dopamine (DA) system, which terminates in the ventral striatum, amygdaloid body, frontal lobe, and some other basal forebrain areas. The hypothalamohypophyseal system innervates the median eminence as well as the posterior and intermediate lobes of the pituitary, and dopamine neurons in the posterior hypothalamus project to the spinal cord. (Adapted from Heimer L. *The Human Brain and Spinal Cord. Functional Neuroanatomy and Dissection Guide*. New York, NY: Springer-Verlag; 1983:Fig. 133, with permission.)

1. Reserpine, one of the first drugs to be studied for its antipsychotic effect, results in depletion of dopamine (as well as of noradrenaline) in the nerve terminals.
2. Amphetamine, a commonly abused stimulant that results in a release of dopamine from the vesicles in dopaminergic nerve terminals, can induce psychosis in humans (an effect that can be blocked by prior administration of antipsychotics).
3. The motor effects (e.g., involuntary movements) of the dopamine agonists L-dopa, apomorphine, and bromocriptine can be blocked by antipsychotic drugs.

The one feature common to all antipsychotics is their ability to bind to dopamine receptors. While most antipsychotics have both $D_1$- and $D_2$-blocking abilities when tested in vitro, in clinical practice they are used at doses that result in substantial central $D_2$ receptor antagonism but little or no $D_1$ receptor antagonism (Fig. 24-3).

Drugs that act exclusively to block the $D_2$ receptors (e.g., raclopride) are effective antipsychotics, but those that act only on the $D_1$ receptors are not effective as antipsychotic agents. Finally, there is a high correlation between the $D_2$ affinity of a drug and the dose at which it is used as an antipsychotic agent (Fig. 24-4 on page 308), whereas no such correlation exists for the $D_1$ receptors.

It is presently held that psychosis is related to a hyperdopaminergic state in the mesolimbic and the mesocortical dopamine tracts. While this theory suggests that it would be ideal to use a drug that blocks the transmission in these circuits and spares transmission in the nigrostriatal (motor) circuits, all current antipsychotics act on both pathways to various degrees, contributing to some of the adverse effects that often accompany treatment with these drugs. Blocking the nigrostriatal pathway (involved in the coordination of movement) results in the parkinsonian side effects, while blocking the hypothalamohy-

FIGURE 24-2 Structural overlap (benzene rings and nitrogen atoms; broken lines) of dopamine and the antipsychotics chlorpromazine (a phenothiazine) and haloperidol (a butyrophenone).

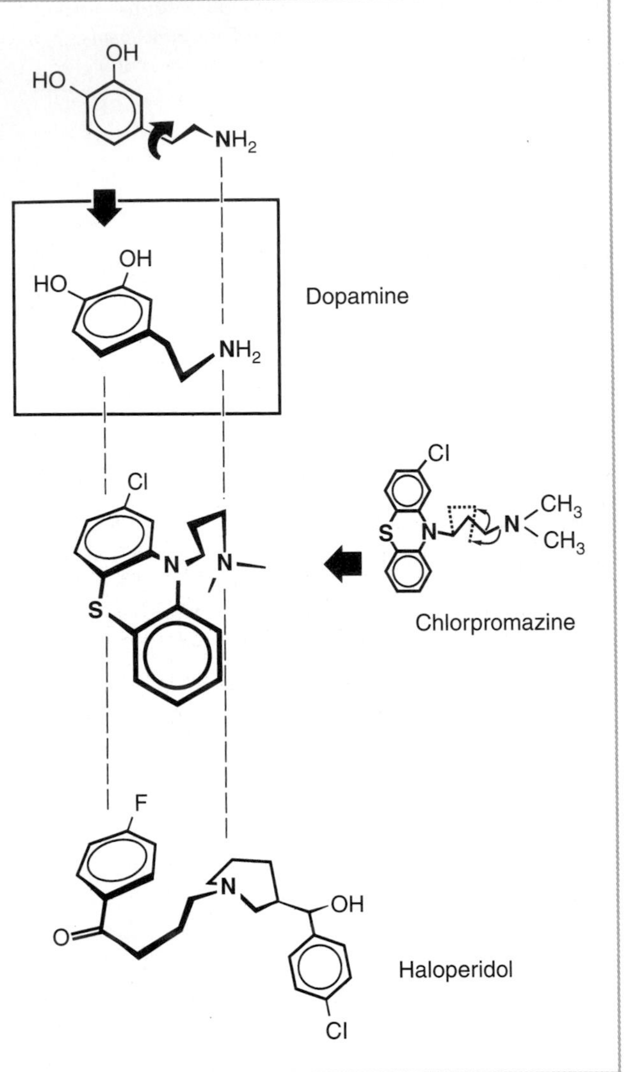

pophyseal pathway (which is involved in the control of prolactin secretion) results in the endocrine side effects (see "Adverse Effects of Antipsychotics"). However, there is some preclinical evidence that clozapine, which is known to be free of parkinsonian side effects and may show some enhanced efficacy for treatment of negative symptoms, may produce functional alterations (as measured by dopamine release and single-cell firing) in the mesocortical tracts while sparing the nigrostriatal system.

## Antipsychotic Action: Beyond Dopamine $D_2$ Receptors

Action at $D_2$ receptors appears to be necessary to produce an antipsychotic response with the currently available antipsychotics, and all currently available antipsychotics were first identified through their ability to block the dopamine system. However, most antipsychotics also act on multiple other neurotransmitter systems, and it is thus fair to ask whether this also contributes to their antipsychotic effects.

Clozapine (Fig. 24-5 on page 309) is the only antipsychotic that, at least in some studies, appears to have greater efficacy than all the other antipsychotic drugs. Clozapine shows affinity not only for dopamine receptors, but also for serotonin, cholinergic, and adrenergic receptors. Most research over the past decade has focused on clozapine's action at serotonin $S_2$ receptors. Clozapine has much higher affinity for the serotonin $S_2$ receptors than for dopamine $D_2$ receptors. However, a number of clinical trials using drugs known to be antagonists of the serotonin $S_2$ receptor (but not of dopamine receptors) have not shown any antipsychotic efficacy. Nevertheless, the possible role of the $S_2$ receptor needs to be tested by determining whether efficacy of treatment is increased if a specific serotonin $S_2$ receptor antagonist (none available at this time) is combined with a specific dopamine $D_2$ receptor antagonist.

Clozapine is also the prototypical "atypical" antipsychotic, in that clinically effective doses do not produce parkinsonian side effects or prolactin elevation. The most commonly cited theory to explain this aspect of clozapine's pattern of effects is based on the drug's high serotonin $S_2$ receptor affinity relative to its dopamine $D_2$ receptor affinity. Since serotonin normally acts on inhibitory somatodendritic autoreceptors in the substantia nigra, it is proposed that when patients take clozapine, its $S_2$-blocking action releases the nigrostriatal circuit from the endogenous serotonin inhibition, thus blocking the manifestation of parkinsonian symptoms that would otherwise result from dopamine $D_2$ receptor blockade. The $S_2/D_2$ hypothesis has been influential in the introduction of four **atypical antipsychotic** medications (**risperidone, olanzapine, quetiapine, and ziprasidone**), all designed to have in common a high ratio of $S_2$ to $D_2$ receptor affinity and a lower incidence of both parkinsonism and hyperprolactinemia. However, at least in the case of risperidone and olanzapine (and possibly also ziprasidone), this atypical nature may be lost at higher doses that produce too high a degree of $D_2$ receptor blockade. Moreover, positron emission tomography (PET) studies have shown that the relationship between clinical effects and drug occupancy of the $D_2$ receptors found with risperidone and olanzapine is very similar to that found with older antipsychotic drugs (i.e., good clinical response is most likely when more than 60% of the $D_2$ receptors are occupied by the drug). On the other hand, clozapine and quetiapine are effective at a lower level of $D_2$ receptor occupancy and do not show sustained hyperprolactinemia at doses used in clinical practice. Thus, it seems that while serotonin receptor binding is a very prominent feature of all the new atypical antipsychotics, the effects at dopamine $D_2$ receptors are still relevant for the antipsychotic effect as well as for side effects.

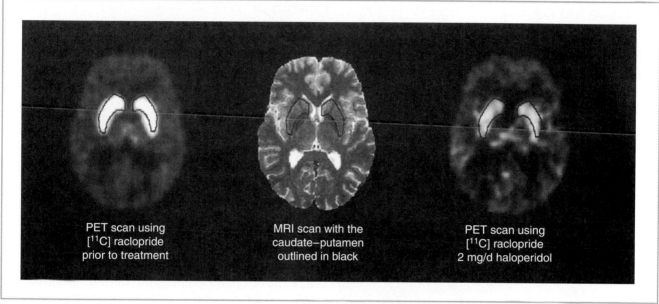

FIGURE 24-3  Positron emission tomography (PET) scans showing the effect of antipsychotics on the dopamine $D_2$ receptors. The figure on the left is a PET scan using $^{11}$C-raclopride, an agent that binds specifically to $D_2$ receptors. The scan shows a high intensity of dopamine receptors localized in the caudate–putamen. The caudate–putamen can be better appreciated on a corresponding magnetic resonance imaging (MRI) scan (middle) from the same subject. The subject then received 10 days of treatment with 2 mg haloperidol. Haloperidol occupies $D_2$ receptors in the caudate–putamen, and as a result, the $^{11}$C-raclopride ligand is unable to bind to them. Therefore, as seen on the scan on the right, the signal from the caudate–putamen is much attenuated. Mathematical modelling of the data revealed that in the second scan the number of receptors measured by $^{11}$C-raclopride was 30% of that found in the first scan, suggesting that 70% of the receptors were occupied by haloperidol. (Scan courtesy of S. Kapur, The PET Centre, Clarke Institute of Psychiatry, University of Toronto. Reprinted with permission of Dr. Shitij Kapur.)

PET scan using [$^{11}$C] raclopride prior to treatment

MRI scan with the caudate–putamen outlined in black

PET scan using [$^{11}$C] raclopride 2 mg/d haloperidol

Research studies are now evaluating whether the mechanism of "atypicality" may be better explained by a preferential binding of atypical antipsychotics to limbic rather than striatal dopamine $D_2$ receptors. Recent studies also suggest that the apparent low occupancy of striatal $D_2$ receptors seen with quetiapine and clozapine may be a result of their loose binding at these receptors (i.e., high $K_{off}$ resulting in low affinity for $D_2$ receptor). Hence, an appreciable amount of bound drug may be displaced by endogenous dopamine or by the trace concentrations of the radioligands used in PET studies, resulting in an underestimation of $D_2$ receptor occupancy.

The most recent antipsychotic to be introduced in the United States, **aripiprazole,** is of particular interest in understanding the mechanism of action of antipsychotic drugs. Aripiprazole is a partial agonist at $D_2$ receptors, with high affinity for the dopamine $D_2$ receptor, but with low intrinsic activity: in conditions of high dopaminergic tone (as in rats treated with apomorphine), aripiprazole has been shown to function as an antagonist (e.g., it blocks apomorphine-induced stereotypy), while in conditions of dopamine depletion (as in rats treated with reserpine), it has properties of an agonist (e.g., it blocks the reserpine-induced dopamine synthesis). For this reason, it has been proposed that aripiprazole functions as a "dopaminergic stabilizer," restoring normal dopaminergic tone when used in the treatment of psychotic symptoms, though the molecular mechanisms whereby these partial agonist properties give rise to clinical antipsychotic effects is not clear. Nevertheless, consistent with its pharmacological profile, aripiprazole has been shown to result in very high striatal dopamine $D_2$ receptor occupancy (>85%) in the absence of extrapyramidal side effects, and it is considered a "second-generation" atypical antipsychotic to distinguish it from the "first-generation" atypicals, all of which result in at least some transient, dose-dependent hyperprolactinemia or extrapyramidal side effects if administered in high enough doses.

Moreover, while the definition of an atypical antipsychotic drug has traditionally included the absence of sustained hyperprolactinemia, risperidone is known to have a particular propensity for causing this side effect at clinical doses. This is related to its relatively high ratio of peripheral to central drug levels, such that to reach a certain level in the CNS, its plasma levels have to be several times higher in the periphery. Since the pituitary lies outside the blood–brain-barrier, doses of risperidone that give rise to appropriate drug levels and receptor occupancy in the brain give rise to in inappropriately high occupancy in the pituitary, leading to elevated prolactin levels.

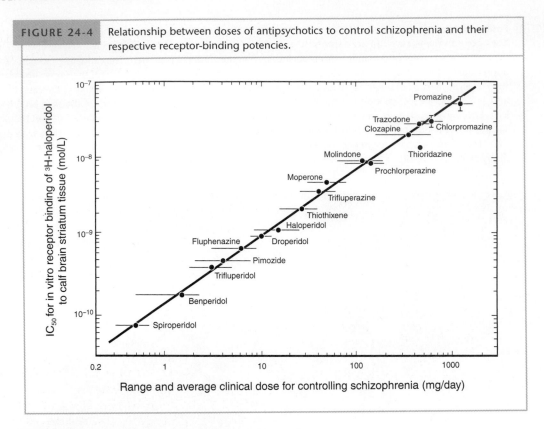

FIGURE 24-4    Relationship between doses of antipsychotics to control schizophrenia and their respective receptor-binding potencies.

## FUNCTIONAL EFFECTS OF ANTIPSYCHOTIC AGENTS

The story of antipsychotics begins in the early 1950s with Laborit, a surgeon in Paris, who was testing various anti-histamine drugs for the prevention of post-operative surgical shock. It was noted that these drugs (including promethazine) resulted in a calming effect that was beyond what would be expected from sedation, described (inappropriately) at the time as a form of "autonomic stabilization." At about the same time, Charpentier synthesized a chemically related compound, chlorpromazine, which was tested by Laborit, who noted that it not only reduced the amount of surgical anaesthetic required but also reduced the patient's anxiety. Subsequently, Laborit urged psychiatrists to use it for treating psychosis, and the first psychotic patients were treated by Delay and Deniker in 1952. Since then, antipsychotic drugs have transformed psychiatric wards and the quality of life of the majority of patients with chronic psychotic disorders, so today we rarely see psychotic patients who are violent, incontinent, catatonic, and require physical restraint. Furthermore, antipsychotics have made it possible for a large number of these patients to leave mental hospitals and live in the community, either free of, or with greatly reduced, symptoms (Figs. 24-6 and 24-7).

When administered to patients suffering from psychotic symptoms, antipsychotic drugs result in a decrease in bizarre or agitated behaviour and an attenuation of delusions and hallucinations. Antipsychotics are also effective in decreasing anxiety (or nervousness) and promoting sleepiness or sedation, and they were also used for these purposes in the past. For this reason, they were referred to as "major tranquillizers," a term still occasionally heard in clinical practice. However, there are now very effective anti-anxiety and sleep-inducing agents that are not effective as antipsychotics (see Chapter 23). Conversely, some of the antipsychotics can achieve antipsychotic effects without prominent sedative effects. In other words, sedative effects of these medications are not a prerequisite for antipsychotic activity. Nonetheless, in clinical practice it may often be desirable in the acute setting to decrease agitation while psychotic symptoms gradually abate.

## PHARMACOKINETICS AND DOSAGE

### Absorption, Biotransformation, and Elimination

Despite their high lipid solubility, the commonly used antipsychotics show quite variable bioavailability. This may indicate a large and variable first-pass effect in the gastrointestinal mucosa or the liver. Bioavailability (see Chapter 5) is increased as much as tenfold by intramuscular injection. Most of these drugs show a high degree of serum protein binding, and they also accumulate in tis-

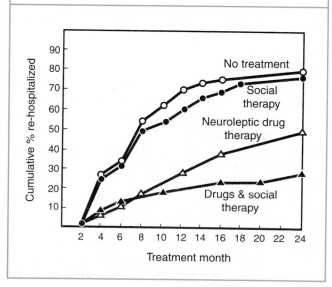

**FIGURE 24-5** Structural formulae of the "atypical" antipsychotics clozapine and risperidone, and their dopamine and serotonin receptor-subtype affinities (see text).

Clozapine
(Affinity for $D_4$ and $S_2$ receptors)

Risperidone
(Affinity for $D_2$ and $S_2$ receptors)

sues with a large blood supply, such as brain, lung, and kidney. They also cross the placenta quite readily into the fetal circulation.

The kinetics of elimination are complex because these drugs follow multiple pathways of biotransformation with different rate and affinity constants. Sulfoxidation, *N*-dealkylation, ring hydroxylation, and glucuronide conjugation are among the more important reactions, and each parent compound may have a large number of different metabolites, most of them inactive. Prolonged administration may cause some induction of hepatic microsomal enzymes, and the plasma concentrations of the drugs may fall despite a constant level of dosage. Excretion occurs in the urine (the more polar metabolites) and the bile.

Most of these agents, with the exception of quetiapine, show plasma elimination half-lives in the range of 10 to 20 hours. However, if body fat has accumulated a large store of drug, traces of the drug and its metabolites may continue to appear in the urine for many weeks or months after the last dose. With the exception of quetiapine (half-life of 5 hours), the long half-life and the lipid accumulation allow for the administration of antipsychotic drugs in once-a-day dosage. These factors may also partly account for the observation that, at least for the older antipsychotic drugs, there may be a considerable delay between discontinuation of chronic treatment and relapse of psychotic symptoms.

Onset of antipsychotic action has often been claimed to occur only after several weeks of treatment. While it is true that the convalescent period for an acute psychotic

episode is often prolonged, a decrease in psychotic symptoms is usually apparent within the first few days of treatment and is not necessarily related to anxiolytic or sedative effects. Most patients treated with antipsychotic drugs show at least some response to treatment, though a sizeable minority of patients with schizophrenia do not respond at all. For some of these treatment-resistant patients, clozapine may result in amelioration of symptoms. Unfortunately, there is no laboratory test available to predict which patients would be expected to respond; nor are we able to predict which patients would be expected to respond to the lower end of the recommended dose range of the respective antipsychotic drugs. While it is now possible to measure the concentration of most antipsychotics in the plasma of patients receiving these medications, this provides minimal predictive power in terms of clinical efficacy, and it is largely used for research purposes only.

## Depot Injections of Antipsychotics

Some antipsychotics, of which **fluphenazine** is perhaps the most common example, have an alcohol substituent (OH) at the end of the molecule, and an ester can be formed by linking the molecule to such fatty acids as decanoic acid (Fig. 24-8). When injected intramuscularly, the fluphenazine esters remain as an oil drop within the

**FIGURE 24-6** Re-hospitalization rates of schizophrenic patients. After being discharged from hospital after a 2-month stay, patients taking antipsychotic medication were much less likely to be re-hospitalized. (Adapted from Hogarty GE, Goldberg SC, Schooler NR, et al. Drug and sociotherapy in the aftercare of schizophrenic patients. II. Two-year relapse rates. *Arch Gen Psychiatry*. 1974;31:603-608, with permission.)

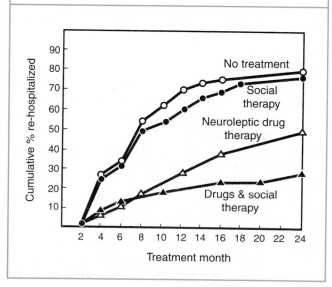

FIGURE 24-7 Effect of antipsychotic medication on relapse rate of schizophrenic patients. (Adapted from Davis JM. Comparative doses and the costs of antipsychotic medications. *Arch Gen Psychiatry.* 1976;33:858-861, with permission.)

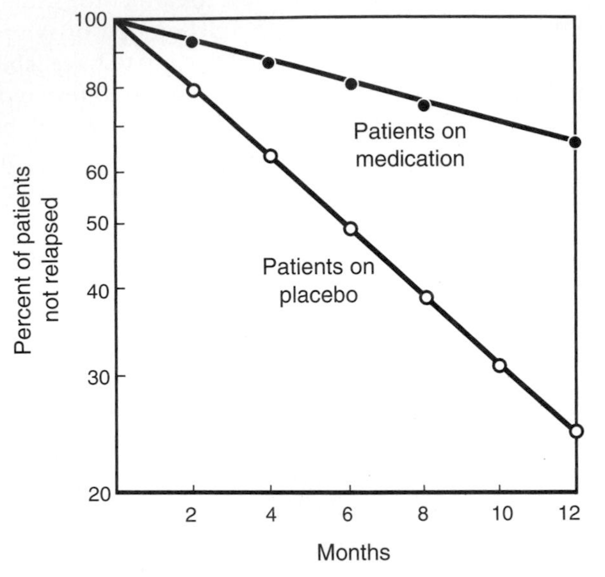

disorders in North America, globally, the older antipsychotics remain the most widely prescribed because of their low cost and widespread availability.

The typical antipsychotics can be functionally divided into different classes, based mainly on their affinity for the dopamine receptors and hence the dose at which they are administered. Most of the side effects of typical antipsychotic drugs originate from their actions on the cholinergic, adrenergic, and histaminergic receptors. Thus, drugs with very high affinity and selectivity for the dopamine receptors (high-potency agents) can be administered at lower doses that result in occupation of a requisite number of dopamine receptors without disturbing the other receptor systems to any appreciable degree. However, since they block the dopamine system with great affinity, high-potency agents such as haloperidol give rise to dopamine-related side effects much more prominently (e.g., parkinsonian and endocrine side effects). On the other hand, the low-potency agents such as chlorpromazine have lower relative affinity for the dopamine system and thus are not very selective. At the doses needed to occupy the requisite number of dopamine receptors, these agents also block the cholinergic, adrenergic, and histaminergic systems to a substantial degree, resulting in a high level of sedation, anticholinergic effects, and hypotension but with minimal motor side effects.

muscle tissue, diffusing out slowly because they are poorly soluble in the tissue and plasma water. When the fluphenazine ester does diffuse into plasma, the plasma esterases immediately split off the fatty acid, freeing the fluphenazine to act directly on the brain. Depot injections are useful in the clinical management of certain patients as they reduce the inconvenience of having to take a pill every day and, more importantly, ensure adherence to the medication regimen.

## FUNCTIONAL CLASSIFICATION OF ANTIPSYCHOTIC AGENTS

All the antipsychotics (with the possible exception of clozapine) are equally efficacious clinically. The choice of medication is thus a highly individualized decision based primarily on the side-effect profile of the respective drug. Over the past decade, the use of older ("typical") antipsychotic drugs in North America has decreased dramatically because of the increased tolerability of the newer (atypical) antipsychotics. Nonetheless, there remains a role for the typical antipsychotics in clinical practice for patients who are unable either to take atypical antipsychotics (e.g., because of the need for a long-acting injectable medication) or to tolerate them (e.g., development of metabolic complications). Finally, while atypical antipsychotics are now the first-line agents for the treatment of psychotic

FIGURE 24-8 Fluphenazine enanthate (Moditen) is slightly less lipid-soluble and is injected intramuscularly at a dose of 25 mg once every 2 weeks. The more lipid-soluble decanoate ester (Modecate) needs to be injected only once every 3 weeks on average.

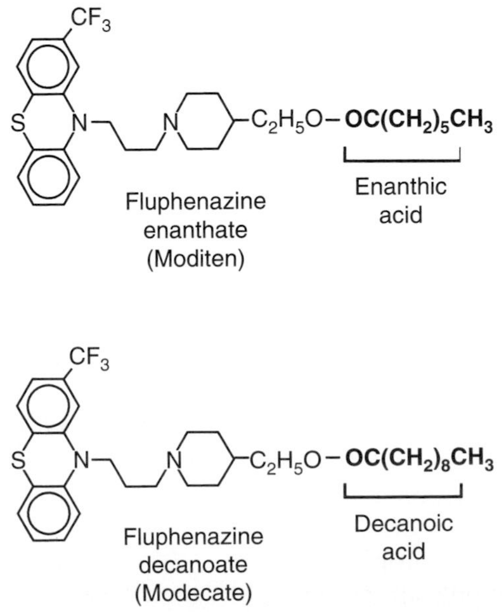

This classification based on potency does not reliably extend to the novel antipsychotic drugs. These include risperidone, olanzapine, quetiapine, ziprasidone, and more recently, aripiprazole. Compared with the typical antipsychotics, clozapine behaves more like a low-potency agent with more cholinergic, adrenergic, and histaminergic side effects, while risperidone resembles high-potency agents. With the advent of the atypicals, the focus has shifted from motor side effects to other equally troubling side effects that will be discussed below.

# ADVERSE EFFECTS OF ANTIPSYCHOTICS

Many side effects of antipsychotic drugs can be easily predicted from the pharmacological properties of the drugs, whereas some side effects (such as the tendency of clozapine to depress the formation of white blood cells and increase salivation) cannot be explained on the basis of our current understanding of their pharmacology. Nonetheless, some basic principles can be applied to all antipsychotics. All antipsychotic drugs have both peripheral effects, all of which are "adverse effects" (e.g., hypotension, constipation, tachycardia), and central effects, which may be either beneficial or adverse, and which result from actions on a variety of receptors other than the dopamine receptors. Some of the adverse effects appear within days or weeks of initiation of therapy (e.g., parkinsonism, dyskinesias, dystonias, and akathisia), whereas others (e.g., tardive dyskinesia, weight gain, and diabetes) may develop months or years after initiation of treatment.

## Antipsychotic-Induced Parkinsonism and Dystonia

Extrapyramidal side effects (EPS) are signs that mimic Parkinson's disease, resulting from the unwanted effects of the antipsychotics on the nigrostriatal pathways, the mechanism of which is shown schematically in Figure 24-9. The signs include the following:

*Akinesia.* The patient has shorter steps that appear as a shuffling gait, reduced arm swing, and cramped handwriting called "micrographia." In addition, the patient may show little spontaneous motion, and there is difficulty in initiating motion, such as getting up from a chair.

*Rigidity.* The patient complains of feeling stiff, and examination reveals a uniform stiffness throughout the range of motion (often superimposed on tremor and felt on physical examination as a "cogwheel" type of rigidity).

*Tremor.* This tremor is similar to the "pill-rolling" tremor seen in Parkinson's disease and may interfere with the patient's ability to carry out fine manual tasks.

*Acute dystonias.* These consist of involuntary twisting motions of the neck, the pelvis, and the eyes (oculogyric crises). Acute dystonias arise early in the course of treatment, and young muscular men are particularly susceptible.

While the incidence and severity of parkinsonism and dystonia have diminished since the use of atypical antipsychotic drugs became widespread, they remain some of the more common short-term adverse effects of antipsychotic drug use. For most patients, an adjustment in dose or change to a drug that is less likely to cause EPS is usually sufficient to control these side effects. Occasionally, a short-term trial of an anticholinergic drug such as benztropine is indicated, restoring the balance between

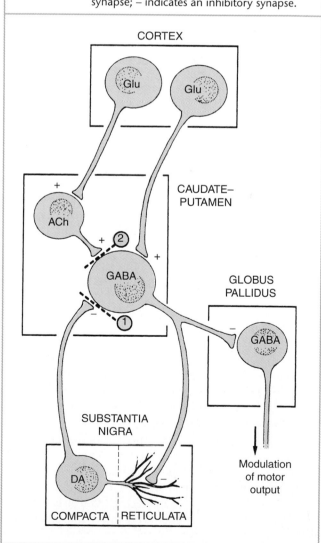

**FIGURE 24-9** (1) Sites of production of extrapyramidal (parkinsonian) signs by antipsychotics. (2) Sites of production of "antiparkinsonian" therapeutic effects by benztropine and other anticholinergic agents. Glu = glutamate; ACh = acetylcholine; GABA = γ-aminobutyric acid; DA = dopamine; + indicates an excitatory synapse; – indicates an inhibitory synapse.

the cholinergic and dopaminergic inputs into the neurons in the striatum (see Fig. 24-9).

It is generally not advisable to routinely prescribe anticholinergic medication together with antipsychotic therapy because of inherent side effects of anticholinergic medication, particularly in the elderly. Titration of an antipsychotic drug from a low starting dose, especially if given to a patient who has never received these drugs before, usually prevents the need for concomitant use of anticholinergic medication. However, it may be considered in certain situations in which dystonia may be more likely to occur or result in non-adherence to the prescribed regimen of medication (e.g., in young male adults with schizophrenia-like symptoms who are particularly susceptible to dystonia). The use of concomitant anticholinergic medication should be reassessed within 3 months because most patients develop tolerance to the motor side effects of the antipsychotic, and the anticholinergic drug may no longer be needed in the majority of patients. However, about 25% of patients will continue to require anticholinergic therapy together with the antipsychotic drug for an indefinite period.

## Neuroleptic Malignant Syndrome

This is a rare but very severe and sometimes fatal side effect that may be seen with all antipsychotic drugs, including the atypicals. It resembles severe parkinsonism in that one of the cardinal features is extreme rigidity. This is accompanied by fever, marked autonomic disturbances, and muscle destruction that results in very high levels of creatine phosphokinase in the blood, as well as myoglobinemia and myoglobinuria. Although the syndrome is related to dopamine $D_2$ receptor blockade, it is unpredictable and is not directly dose-related. Some individuals seem to have a greater susceptibility to it, although there is not yet any prospective method to identify them.

## Antipsychotic-Induced Akathisia

Akathisia, or restlessness, is a common side effect of antipsychotic therapy. Despite the fact that the patient feels rigid or stiff and has difficulty initiating motion, there is a tremendous urge to move, which may be clinically evident in a patient's need to pace about the room intermittently. This is a particularly difficult side effect to diagnose, as restlessness and anxiety usually accompany psychosis itself. In typical cases of akathisia, the onset of the restlessness coincides with the start of the medication, and patients claim that their restlessness has a "physical" component, almost as if the legs themselves were restless. Also, the patients report a marked relief if they move their legs, either on the spot or by pacing. Akathisia is important to recognize since patients are rarely able to verbalize the discomfort spontaneously. Hence, regular screening for this side effect is warranted, especially soon after starting a medication or when assessing a patient who appears "agitated" while on antipsychotic medications. The biological mechanisms involved in akathisia are not understood, but it responds well to lowering of the dose (if possible) or to the addition of low doses of either $\beta_2$-adrenergic blockers such as propranolol or benzodiazepines such as lorazepam.

## Antipsychotic-Induced Dyskinesias

Dyskinesia may set in within 1 to 3 days of antipsychotic therapy (acute dyskinesia) or develop after many months or years (tardive dyskinesia, or TD). Clinically, dyskinesia presents as involuntary oral, buccal, and lingual motion, as if the patient were chewing gum. It may also be accompanied by dystonic motions of the neck, chest, and trunk.

It has generally been thought that TD was caused by an up-regulation of dopamine receptors in response to the prolonged dopamine receptor blockade by the antipsychotic drug. This synthesis of additional receptors was thought to make the cell more sensitive to the small amounts of dopamine still getting through the drug-induced blockade. However, since up-regulation occurs rapidly, whereas the dyskinesia develops very slowly and gradually, other mechanisms are likely to be involved.

Two paradoxical aspects of TD are noteworthy. First, it may seem to improve when the dose of the antipsychotic is increased. This increase of dose may intensify the rigidity side effect and thus mask the involuntary movements of TD. However, anticholinergic drugs, which improve parkinsonian side effects, may worsen TD. This may represent cholinergic effects on dopamine and γ-aminobutyric acid (GABA) systems, although the exact mechanism is unclear.

Treatment of TD by depleting the brain dopamine content by means of reserpine or by giving cholinergic agonists to stimulate the GABA cells, has not been very successful. Some clinicians feel that the most effective measure so far is to discontinue antipsychotic therapy for a time, provided the patient's psychotic symptoms are improved enough to permit this. For patients whose TD is made worse by the antipsychotic, but who cannot do without it, the introduction of the atypical agent **clozapine** provides a useful treatment option. Most of the patients who can be switched to clozapine notice a diminution, or at least no further worsening, of TD. However, clozapine is not used routinely in all patients because it is a low-potency agent that has attendant side effects of sedation, anticholinergic activity, and hypotension. In addition, it causes agranulocytosis (which may be fatal) in about 1% of patients receiving it; therefore, if it is given, the blood must be monitored regularly (initially on a weekly basis).

## Unwanted Sedation

One of the troubling side effects of antipsychotics is sedation, because sedative effects are not essential for the antipsychotic actions and are, in most situations, unwanted. The sedation reflects a complex interaction of the antihistaminergic, antiadrenergic, and anticholinergic actions of these agents. As a general rule, the sedation is greatest for the low-potency agents and least for the high-potency agents. It manifests itself as excessive daytime drowsiness, tiredness, and fatigue and as difficulty with attention and concentration. Thus, it may be an important disabling side effect that can interfere with the rehabilitation and routine functioning of a patient.

## Orthostatic Hypotension

Most antipsychotics depress blood pressure by dilating the arterioles via a direct blocking action on the α-adrenergic receptors responsible for vasoconstriction. The patients thus show orthostatic hypotension. In addition, the drugs may have a direct effect on the vasomotor centre, which may contribute to the hypotension observed with these agents.

## Anticholinergic Side Effects

Some antipsychotics have prominent cholinergic blocking activity, which leads to a series of side effects. Cholinergic blockade in the eye produces blurred vision by causing mydriasis and by weakening the ciliary muscles. It may also lead to dry eyes (xerophthalmia) due to decreased tear secretion. Furthermore, mydriasis may decrease the outflow of aqueous humor and thus may precipitate glaucoma in subjects with a tendency toward narrow-angle glaucoma. Dry mouth and constipation result from anticholinergic action in the gastrointestinal tract, while urinary hesitancy results from such action on the bladder. These adverse effects can be particularly troublesome and even dangerous in the elderly. Low-potency agents tend to be highly anticholinergic, while high-potency agents are less so.

## Weight Gain and Metabolic Side Effects

Recent studies have highlighted concerns of metabolic complications due to treatment with atypical antipsychotics. The risk appears to be highest for clozapine and olanzapine, and least for ziprasidone and aripiprazole. Schizophrenia has been associated with diabetes even in the pre-neuroleptic era; recent publications indicate that diabetes may be up to three times more prevalent in schizophrenics than in the general population. Atypical antipsychotics have recently been associated with a substantial increase in the risk of new-onset diabetes, as well as an increased risk for diabetic ketoacidosis and non-ketotic hyperosmolar coma. The mechanisms involved are poorly understood but may involve dysregulation of insulin secretion and insulin resistance.

Atypical antipsychotics have also been associated with weight gain and increased triglyceride levels (which, in turn, are associated with acute pancreatitis). Diabetes is not necessarily a direct result of increased weight, and between 25 and 50% of patients who develop diabetes while on atypical antipsychotics do not have a history of concomitant increase in weight since starting the medication. Due to the potential for serious cardiovascular morbidity and mortality associated with these metabolic side effects (accentuated by cigarette smoking, which is highly prevalent in patients with chronic mental illness), these complications have highlighted the need for close ongoing monitoring of weight, fasting glucose levels, and lipid profiles in patients treated with atypical antipsychotic agents. Behavioural strategies, including nutritional counselling and increased physical exercise, are recommended in all patients on these medications, and the impact of these strategies on the prevention and amelioration of serious complications is now being studied.

## Pseudopregnancy

The dopamine neurons in the hypothalamus (arcuate cells) release dopamine, which then travels via the hypophyseal portal blood vessels down to the pituitary to inhibit the release of prolactin from the mammotroph cells (Fig. 24-10). Antipsychotics, particularly the older, or typical, drugs, will block the dopamine receptors on these mammotrophs, resulting in a release of prolactin. At the same time, the antipsychotics block the release of follicle-stimulating hormone (FSH) and luteinizing hormone (LH). Thus, a woman does not ovulate, does not menstruate, but has hyperprolactinemia with swollen breasts and possibly galactorrhea; the whole picture simulates pregnancy. Breast swelling and galactorrhea can also occur in men during treatment with atypical antipsychotics.

## Seizures

Since high doses of antipsychotics decrease the seizure threshold, they can produce seizures in susceptible patients who are epileptics or have other predisposing causes. This effect is most prominent with the low-potency agents, including clozapine, and is more often seen at the high end of the dose range.

## Jaundice

Phenothiazine-induced jaundice occurs in a very small number of patients. It is of the obstructive type with elevated plasma bilirubin and alkaline phosphatase, but

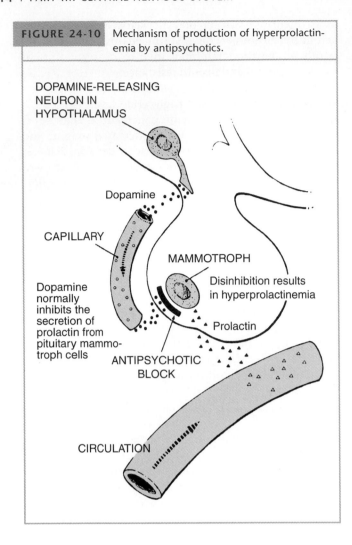

**FIGURE 24-10** Mechanism of production of hyperprolactinemia by antipsychotics.

DOPAMINE-RELEASING NEURON IN HYPOTHALAMUS

Dopamine

CAPILLARY

MAMMOTROPH

Disinhibition results in hyperprolactinemia

Dopamine normally inhibits the secretion of prolactin from pituitary mammotroph cells

Prolactin

ANTIPSYCHOTIC BLOCK

CIRCULATION

without fever, liver tenderness, or pruritus. It is thought to be a hypersensitivity reaction since it is accompanied by eosinophilia, and the severity of the jaundice is not related to the dose of the antipsychotic.

## Dermatitis and Photosensitivity

This occurs in a small number of patients, mostly those who are receiving low-potency older antipsychotics. These patients become excessively sensitive to sunlight, and they develop exaggerated sunburn. Some patients also notice a general hyperpigmentation of the skin, cornea, and the lens.

## ANTINAUSEANT AND ANTIEMETIC ACTION

The chemoreceptor trigger zone (CTZ) in the medulla oblongata lies outside the blood–brain barrier and is therefore readily accessible to noxious chemical stimuli from the periphery that evoke nausea and vomiting. The CTZ is rich in $D_2$ receptors, which are involved in these responses, and $D_2$-blocking agents, including the antipsychotics, can therefore prevent nausea and vomiting induced by other drugs, pregnancy, radiation, cancer, and so forth. However, various other agents, including serotonin-$S_3$ receptor blockers and cannabinoids, are also effective anti-nauseants. Moreover, since the CTZ lies outside the blood–brain barrier, the anti-nauseant action is not directly related to antipsychotic action. Therefore, the topic of anti-nauseant and antiemetic drugs is dealt with in Chapter 42, in relation to the gastrointestinal system.

## FUTURE DIRECTIONS

For historical reasons, currently available antipsychotic medications act primarily on the dopamine system through their actions at dopamine $D_2$ receptors. It is widely accepted that optimal treatment of schizophrenia will require action at other neurotransmitter systems. Indeed, recent studies in schizophrenia have focused on the role of glutamate, an excitatory neurotransmitter, in the pathophysiology of the disorder. Furthermore, it is likely that the current pharmacological approach of using a single "antipsychotic" to treat "psychosis" will give way to specific pharmacotherapeutic approaches targeting different aspects of the disorder (e.g., delusional thinking vs. cognitive manifestations vs. negative symptoms), not unlike the optimization of therapy in other branches of medicine that involve complex physiological dysfunction. This would go a long way from the current focus on positive symptoms of schizophrenia, especially given the marked heterogeneity of clinical presentation of psychotic disorders as well as the significant functional impact of cognitive and negative symptoms. Finally, with the rapid advances in pharmacogenetics, we can look forward to a time when the physician not only can flexibly target different dimensions of psychosis but also have the tools to predict the response of individual patients to antipsychotic treatment.

## SUGGESTED READINGS

Farde L, Nordström AL, Wiesel FA, et al. Positron emission tomographic analysis of central $D_1$ and $D_2$ dopamine receptor occupancy in patients treated with classical neuroleptics and clozapine. Relation to extrapyramidal side effects. *Arch Gen Psychiatry.* 1992;49:538-544.

Healy D. *The Creation of Psychopharmacology.* Cambridge, Mass: Harvard University Press; 2002.

Kapur S, Mamo D. Half a century of antipsychotics and still a central role for dopamine $D_2$ receptors. *Prog Neuropsychopharmacol Biol Psychiatry.* 2003;27:1081-1090.

Kapur S, Seeman P. Does fast dissociation from the dopamine D$_2$ receptor explain the action of atypical antipsychotics? A new hypothesis. *Am J Psychiatry.* 2001;158:360-369.

Lebovitz HE. Metabolic consequences of atypical antipsychotic drugs. *Psychiatr Q.* 2003;74:277-290.

Mamo DC, Sweet RA, Keshavan MS. Managing antipsychotic-induced parkinsonism. *Drug Saf.* 1999;20:269-275.

Meltzer HY. The role of serotonin in schizophrenia and the place of serotonin-dopamine antagonist antipsychotics. *J Clin Psychopharmacol.* 1995;15:S2-S3.

Nordström AL, Farde L, Wiesel FA, et al. Central D$_2$-dopamine receptor occupancy in relation to antipsychotic drug effects: a double-blind PET study of schizophrenic patients. *Biol Psychiatry.* 1993;33:227-235.

Seeman P, Lee T, Chau-Wong M, Wong K. Antipsychotic drug doses and neuroleptic/dopamine receptors. *Nature.* 1976;261: 717-719.

Yokoi F, Grunder G, Biziere K, et al. Dopamine D2 and D3 receptor occupancy in normal humans treated with the antipsychotic drug aripiprazole (OPC 14597): a study using positron emission tomography and [$^{11}$C]raclopride. *Neuropsychopharmacology.* 2002;27:248-259.

# 25

# Antidepressant and Mood-Stabilizing Agents

## JJ WARSH AND PP LI

## CASE HISTORY

A 44-year-old man with a history of bipolar affective disorder had his first medical contact for a manic episode 20 years ago, when he was hospitalized and treated initially with haloperidol in doses of 20 to 40 mg/day. Pre-treatment hematology, serum electrolytes, and renal, hepatic, and thyroid function indices, as well as electrocardiogram (ECG), were normal, showing no contraindications to lithium therapy. The patient was placed on lithium carbonate, beginning with 900 mg/day and increasing to 1500 mg/day, administered as a single daily dose in the evening. On discharge after 22 days in hospital, serum lithium levels were 0.75 mmol/L, and monthly serum lithium levels thereafter were in the range of 0.6 to 0.8 mmol/L. The patient remained symptom-free on a maintenance dose of 1500 mg/day.

Two years later, he was hospitalized for another manic episode during which he received haloperidol, and the lithium dosage was increased to 2100 mg/day during the acute episode, resulting in serum levels of 0.9 to 1.1 mmol/L. His mood stabilized over a 3-week period, haloperidol was slowly discontinued, and he was discharged on lithium carbonate 2100 mg/day. This was then slowly reduced to 1800 mg/day, plasma lithium levels stabilized at 0.8 to 1.0 mmol/L, and over the next 15 years on this maintenance therapy, the patient experienced only two depressive episodes of moderate severity, the second of which responded to the addition of nortriptyline. Hematological, biochemical, thyroid, and cardiac monitoring performed at 6-month intervals remained normal. In recent years, however, the patient reported increased urinary output and increased thirst and consumption of liquids.

About a year ago, the patient's serum lithium levels gradually rose to 1.0 to 1.1 mmol/L, and serum creatinine increased to 110 µmol/L. The lithium carbonate dosage was decreased to 1200 mg/day to maintain plasma lithium concentrations in the range of 0.8 to 1.0 mmol/L. At a routine visit 6 months later, the patient's blood pressure was 160/110 mmHg, serum creatinine was 160 µmol/L, blood urea nitrogen (BUN) was 7.5 mmol/L, and microhematuria was noted on urinalysis. ECG indicated first-degree heart block. Elevated IgA antibodies, elevated serum creatinine, and 24-hour urine output of 4.5 L with reduced urine osmolality were consistent with the diagnosis of IgA nephropathy and lithium-induced nephrogenic diabetes insipidus.

Because of the medical problems and absence of recurrences of mania or hypomania for many years, the patient requested a trial period off lithium before considering an alternative mood stabilizer. The lithium dosage was gradually reduced and stopped at the end of an 8-week interval. The hypertension was controlled with enalapril 20 mg/day. A week after lithium had been stopped, he experienced an abrupt shortening of his usual sleeping time, increased activity, irritability, and expansive mood. He was brought to the hospital in a hypomanic state, which escalated rapidly into a full manic episode within 48 hours. Treatment was instituted with olanzapine 10 to 20 mg/day, clonazepam 2.5 mg/day in three to four divided doses, followed by carbamazepine 400 mg/day in divided doses. After 1 week, serum carbamazepine levels were 20 µmol/L, which rose to 24 µmol/L over the next week and then declined to 17 µmol/L. His mania resolved quickly, and after 16 days in hospital, he was discharged with maintenance doses of carbamazepine 400 mg/day and olanzapine 10 mg/day.

He soon experienced increasing tiredness and lack of interest, felt "a bit slowed down," and complained of difficulty reading, annoying dryness of the mouth, and some constipation. Therefore, the dose of olanzapine was tapered and discontinued, and the carbamazepine dosage was increased to 600 mg/day to bring serum levels to 20 µmol/L. Shortly thereafter he began to have feelings of depression and expressed inappropriate guilt about some past decisions. He lost interest in activities he previously enjoyed and did not want to socialize with friends, staying at home much of the time. He found it difficult to make decisions and to concentrate. His appetite was poor and his weight began to decrease. His sleep became fragmented, and he began to awaken 2 hours earlier than usual, with marked anxiety and agitation in the morning. He felt a failure in his life and expressed thoughts of suicide, but no clear suicidal planning. He still complained of poor visual accommodation and dry mouth. It was decided to treat this depressive episode with sertraline, increasing from a starting dose of 50 mg/day at weekly intervals to 150 mg/day. The concomitant treatment with carbamazepine and sertraline, to which was added clonazepam 2.0 mg/day in divided doses to control anxiety and insomnia, brought this episode under control after 4 weeks. The patient's depression subsided and suicidal thinking ceased. Clonazepam was gradually decreased and discontinued after a dose of 0.25 mg/day was reached. Further symptomatic improvement occurred gradually between 8 and 12 weeks of therapy, and the patient became symptom-free thereafter. He was maintained on the combination of carbamazepine and sertraline for a subsequent 3 months in full remission. Sertraline was then tapered gradually and discontinued over a 4-week period. The patient remained symptom-free for the next 2 years, maintained on carbamazepine.

## MAJOR AFFECTIVE DISORDERS

### Clinical Features

Antidepressants and mood-stabilizing agents such as lithium salts, carbamazepine, and valproate are used to treat the major affective disorders. These disorders include unipolar, or major depressive, disorder (depressive episodes without a history of mania) and bipolar, or manic–depressive, disorder (characterized by episodes of mania and of depression). The cardinal feature of a major depressive episode is sustained (at least 2 weeks) depressed mood and/or pervasive loss of interest or pleasure in activities, accompanied by sleep disturbance, changes in appetite and body weight (usually reductions), loss of energy, altered psychomotor activity (retardation or agitation), feelings of worthlessness or inappropriate guilt, reduced ability to think or concentrate, and recurrent thoughts of death or suicide. In a manic episode, the mood state is marked by abnormal and sustained (at least 1 week) elevation, expansiveness, or irritability, and the patients show at least three of the following symptoms: inflated self-esteem or grandiosity, decreased sleep, hyper-talkativeness, racing thoughts, distractibility, increased goal-directed behaviour, and excessive involvement in pleasurable activities with the potential for painful consequences. Hypomania is distinguished from mania on the basis of duration and severity of the symptoms, which are shorter-lasting and less severe in the former.

### Pathophysiology

While the etiology of the major affective disorders is still unknown, dramatic advances in the understanding of the pathophysiology of these illnesses and the mechanisms of action of antidepressants and mood stabilizers have occurred since the first hypotheses were proposed some 40 years ago, implicating alterations in brain monoamine neurotransmitter function. This "monoamine hypothesis" proposed that manic and depressive symptoms are caused by disturbances in brain neurotransmission mediated by 5-hydroxytryptamine (5-HT) and/or catecholamines (noradrenaline [NA], dopamine [DA]). Genetic, neuroimaging, and psychobiological studies and research on antidepressant/mood-stabilizing drugs have revealed a multi-tiered cascade of disturbances. These extend from the monoamine neurotransmitter systems in cerebral cortical and limbic brain regions at the neuroanatomical level, to signal transduction and gene transcription mechanisms at the intracellular level, and to neuronal plasticity, synaptogenesis, and cell death processes at the cytomorphological level. The multifactorial etiology of these disorders and the differences in clinical picture, course of illness, response to treatments, and clinical outcome all support the view that these disorders are heterogeneous, both diagnostically and pathophysiologically.

### Pharmacotherapy

The antidepressant drugs are the mainstay of treatment for moderate to severe major depression, whereas mood stabilizers are used as first-line treatment for bipolar disorder. Because of the risk of induction of hypomania or mania in bipolar depressed patients, antidepressants are now used for management of bipolar depression adjunctively and only under the cover of a mood stabilizer, if response to the latter alone is incomplete.

The first groups of antidepressants, the tricyclic antidepressants (TCAs) and the monoamine oxidase inhibitors (MAOIs), were identified on the basis of empirical observations and were introduced into clinical practice in the late 1950s. The demand for antidepressant drugs with fewer side effects (especially less anticholinergic and cardiotoxic effects), faster onset of action, and greater efficacy led to the synthesis of a large number of new antidepressant compounds, often referred to as second-, third-, and fourth-generation antidepressants. The observation that TCAs blocked the neuronal reuptake of NA and/or 5-HT, and shared the ability to down-regulate certain neurotransmitter receptors, considerably influenced the focus on the selectivity of action of potential new antidepressants. This led to the development of antidepressants with much greater selectivity of inhibition of reuptake of one or a specific combination of the monoaminergic neurotransmitters: 5-HT (selective serotonin reuptake inhibitor, SSRI), NA/DA (noradrenaline–dopamine reuptake inhibitor, NDRI), and 5-HT/NA (serotonin–noradrenaline reuptake inhibitor, SNRI). Like the SSRIs, potential new antidepressants were identified and developed principally on the basis of screening for specific modes and monoaminergic targets of pharmacological action.

Common to all antidepressants is the delayed onset of therapeutic efficacy, generally over a period of 2 to 6 weeks. This phenomenon is thought to reflect the need for development of biochemical and physiological adaptive changes in monoaminergic function and neural plasticity that underlie the therapeutic response. Regardless of the class, all antidepressants exhibit side effects. These vary, however, with the specific group of agents and have become increasingly important considerations in the choice of drug for management of depression. Because of their favourable side-effect profile, better tolerability, and negligible risk of cardiotoxicity, the SSRIs and SNRIs have largely supplanted the TCAs and MAOIs as the first-line treatment for major depression. However, TCAs are still regarded as having greater efficacy for the treatment of severe depression than a number of the newer antidepressants. This may be attributable to the broader spectrum of action of the TCAs than of the newer antidepressants that were developed to provide greater selectivity of action on brain 5-HT or NA systems. For these reasons, TCAs and MAOIs are still regarded as important treatments in the armamentarium of antidepressants available today, and they represent the standard against which the efficacy and tolerability of newer antidepressants are compared and weighed.

## NEUROADAPTIVE EFFECTS OF ANTIDEPRESSANTS

There is a growing appreciation that neurotransmitter function can be modulated indirectly through the regulation of post-receptor intracellular signalling and gene expression. Recent work seems to implicate adaptive changes in the guanine nucleotide binding (G) protein–coupled cyclic AMP (cAMP) second-messenger and neurotrophin signalling pathways in the mode of action of antidepressants (Fig. 25-1). These adaptive changes occur with a time course that parallels the delayed onset of therapeutic effect.

While chronic treatment with antidepressant drugs is known to reduce the density and/or sensitivity of $\beta_1$-adrenergic receptors ($\beta_1$-Ars), several lines of evidence indicate that antidepressant treatments up-regulate the cAMP signalling cascade at several levels. Thus, there is an increase in the coupling between the stimulatory G protein $\alpha$-subunit and adenylyl cyclase in response to antidepressant treatment. Chronic antidepressant treatment increases cAMP-dependent protein kinase (PKA) activity, activates gene expression mediated by cAMP response element (CRE), and also increases the expression, phosphorylation, and activity of cAMP response element binding protein (CREB) in limbic brain structures, including the cerebral cortex and hippocampus. CREB is a nuclear transcription factor that modulates gene expression and is vital to a variety of cellular processes such as long-term memory and neuronal survival. CREB activity can be stimulated directly following activation of 5-HT$_4$ and 5-HT$_7$ receptors linked to adenylyl cyclase activation; this could explain, in part, how enhanced serotonergic neurotransmission by chronic antidepressant administration could impact a common downstream target, the cAMP signalling pathway.

Among the many potentially relevant target genes regulated by the cAMP signalling pathway, brain-derived neurotrophic factor (BDNF), a member of the nerve growth factor family, which is important in the development, growth, and survival of neurons, has emerged as a common target of antidepressant drugs. Chronic antidepressant treatment increases the expression of BDNF and the autophosphorylation and activation of its receptor, TrkB (tyrosine receptor kinase B). Moreover, long-term antidepressant treatment in rats attenuates the ability of repeated restraint stress to down-regulate BDNF messenger RNA (mRNA) levels. This indicates a relationship between reduced BDNF expression, stress-induced depressive-like behaviour, and antidepressant treatments. In addition, chronic, but not acute, antidepressant treatment increases the proliferation, differentiation, and survival of new neurons derived from progenitor cells in the dentate gyrus of rat hippocampus. These effects may also be linked to the increased expression of CREB and BDNF. The induction of CREB and BDNF by antidepressant treatment assumes particular therapeutic significance in view of recent post-mortem morphometric and brain imaging studies showing reduced grey matter volumes in the prefrontal cortex and hippocampus in patients with major depressive disorder, as well as subtle cell loss and atrophy, both neuronal and glial, in discrete cerebral cortical regions and layers.

These results suggest an interesting model in which CREB and BDNF may represent one of the final common pathways of a complex chain of intracellular events triggered by treatment with different classes of antidepressants that promote neurotrophic effects. Infusion or expression of CREB/BDNF in rat hippocampus produces antidepressant-like effects in two animal behavioural models of depression, the forced swim and learned helplessness paradigms (see Chapter 69). It is conceivable that enhanced cAMP and neurotrophin signalling in response

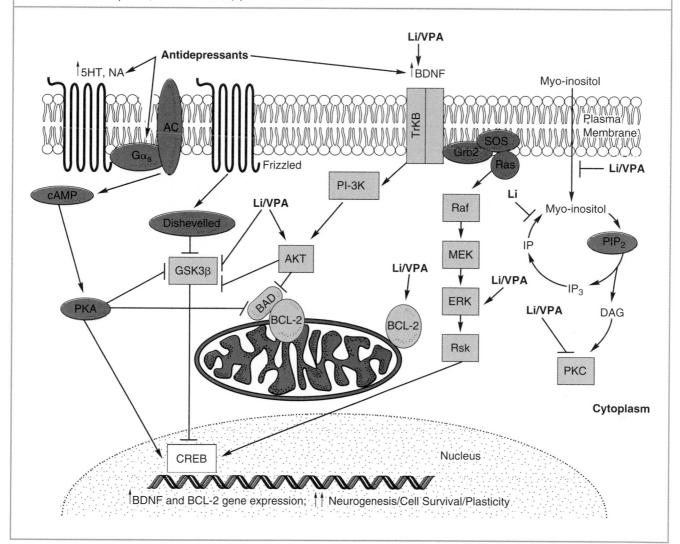

**FIGURE 25-1** Schematic diagram showing several intracellular signalling pathways implicated in the mechanism of action of antidepressants and mood stabilizers. AC = adenylyl cyclase; Akt = protein kinase B; BAD = Bcl-2 associated death agonist; Bcl-2 = B-cell leukemia/lymphoma 2; BDNF = brain-derived neurotrophic factor; CREB = cAMP-response element binding protein; DAG = diacylglycerol; ERK = extracellular signal-regulated kinase; $G\alpha_s$ = stimulatory guanine nucleotide binding protein; Grb2 = growth factor receptor-bound protein 2; GSK3$\beta$ = glycogen synthase kinase 3$\beta$; IP = inositol monophosphate; IP$_3$ = inositol trisphosphate; Li = lithium; MEK = ERK kinase; NA = noradrenaline; PI-3K = phosphatidylinositol 3-OH kinase; PIP$_2$ = phosphatidylinositol-4,5-bisphosphate; PKA = protein kinase A; PKC = protein kinase C; Rsk = ribosomal S6 kinase; Sos = "son of sevenless" (*sevenless* is a gene encoding a tyrosine kinase receptor); VPA = valproate; → = stimulation; |—— = inhibition.

to antidepressant treatment may induce the formation and strengthening of synaptic connectivity (that is thought to be impaired during depression), which gradually results in recovery from the depressive episode.

# TRICYCLIC ANTIDEPRESSANTS

These drugs, of which there are several types, were developed by modification of the central ring of the phenothiazine molecule, as shown in Figure 25-2. The iminodibenzyl type, including imipramine and related drugs, has a C–C bridge in place of the S atom. This is also true of the dibenzocycloheptene derivatives (e.g., amitriptyline), which, in addition, have the N atom of the phenothiazine ring replaced by a doubly bonded carbon. Additional modifications gave rise to the dibenzoxazepine and dibenzoxepine types (see Fig. 25-2). Although many of the original compounds of this class, including imipramine and amitriptyline, were synthesized as potential antipsychotic agents, they were found to be ineffective in quieting agitated psychiatric patients but proved to be effective in treating "endogenous" depression, a depressive subtype now referred to as melancholic.

**FIGURE 25-2** Structural formulae of commonly used tricyclic antidepressants.

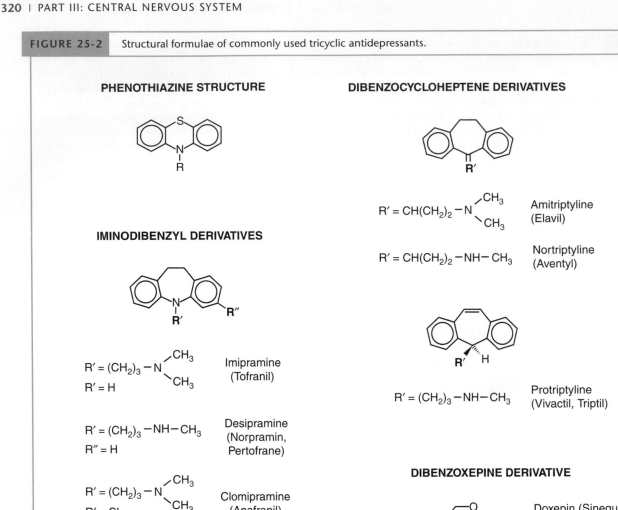

## Pharmacological Properties

### Actions on central nervous system and behaviour

Tricyclic antidepressants do not elevate mood or the level of arousal in normal persons. In fact, they tend to produce drowsiness and fatigue in healthy subjects. In depressed patients, however, they cause a rise of mood, interest level, and pleasure in activities, which develops gradually, generally over a period of 2 to 6 weeks.

In laboratory animals, TCAs prolong hexobarbital-induced sleep and impair both learning and performance of various behaviours, such as conditioned avoidance responses. These sedative-like effects are accompanied by slowing and synchronization of the electroencephalogram (EEG), as seen with barbiturates or other sedatives. Only at high doses do the tricyclics produce EEG signs of stimulation, such as an increase in fast beta wave activity and seizure activity.

### Inhibition of noradrenaline and serotonin reuptake

Tricyclic antidepressants (Table 25-1) are potent inhibitors of the neuronal reuptake of NA and 5-HT. Generally speaking, tricyclic secondary amines (e.g., desipramine, nortriptyline) are more potent than the corresponding tertiary amines in inhibiting NA reuptake. However, tertiary amine tricyclics (e.g., imipramine, amitriptyline, clomipramine) are more potent inhibitors of 5-HT reuptake than the corresponding secondary amines. In humans, tertiary amine tricyclics are biotransformed by demethylation into the secondary amine tricyclics (e.g., imipramine is converted to desipramine, and amitriptyline to nortriptyline).

**TABLE 25-1** Relative Effects of Antidepressants on Neurotransmitter Reuptake and Receptor Blockade, and Other Pharmacological Actions

| Drug | Reuptake Inhibition | | | Receptor Blockade | | | | | | | Side Effects | | |
|---|---|---|---|---|---|---|---|---|---|---|---|---|---|
| | NA | 5-HT | DA | $5\text{-}HT_1$ | $5\text{-}HT_2$ | mACh | $H_1$ | $\alpha_1\text{-}AR$ | $\alpha_2\text{-}AR$ | $D_2$ | Sedation | Anticholinergic | Cardio-toxic |
| **Tricyclics** | | | | | | | | | | | | | |
| Amitriptyline (Elavil) | ++ | ++ | − | ++ | +++ | ++++ | ++++ | ++++ | ++ | + | ++++ | ++++ | +++ |
| Clomipramine (Anafranil) | ++ | ++++ | − | + | +++ | ++++ | +++ | ++++ | + | + | + | ++++ | +++ |
| Desipramine (Norpramin) | ++++ | + | − | + | ++ | ++ | ++ | ++ | + | ± | + | ++ | + |
| Doxepin (Sinequan) | ++ | + | − | ++ | +++ | ++++ | ++++ | ++++ | + | + | ++++ | ++++ | +++ |
| Imipramine (Tofranil) | ++ | +++ | − | + | ++ | +++ | +++ | +++ | + | + | ++ | +++ | +++ |
| Nortriptyline (Aventyl) | +++ | + | − | + | +++ | +++ | +++ | +++ | + | + | ++ | ++ | + |
| Protriptyline (Triptil) | ++++ | + | − | + | ++ | ++++ | +++ | ++ | + | + | − | ++ | +++ |
| Trimipramine (Surmontil) | + | + | − | + | ++ | ++++ | ++++ | ++++ | | ++ | ++++ | ++ | +++ |
| **Other cyclic agents** | | | | | | | | | | | | | |
| Amoxapine (Asendin) | +++ | + | + | ++ | ++++ | ++ | +++ | +++ | + | ++ | ++ | ++++ | ± |
| Maprotiline (Ludiomil) | +++ | + | + | + | + | ++ | ++++ | +++ | + | ++ | ++ | ++++ | ± |
| Trazodone (Desyrel) | + | + | − | +++ | +++ | − | + | ++++ | ++ | + | ++++ | ++ | ± |
| Bupropion (Wellbutrin) | + | − | ++ | − | − | − | ± | + | − | − | + | ++ | ± |
| Mirtazapine (Remeron) | + | + | − | − | ++++ | ++ | ++++ | ++ | +++ | + | +++ | ++++ | ± |
| **SSRIs** | | | | | | | | | | | | | |
| Fluoxetine (Prozac) | + | +++ | ± | ± | + | + | ± | + | ± | ± | ++ | ++ | ± |
| Fluvoxamine (Luvox) | ± | +++ | ± | ± | ± | + | − | + | ± | + | ++ | ++ | − |
| Sertraline (Zoloft) | ± | ++++ | +++ | − | + | + | − | ++ | + | + | ++ | ++ | ± |
| Paroxetine (Paxil) | + | ++++ | ++ | − | ± | ++ | − | + | ± | + | ++ | ++ | ± |
| Citalopram (Celexa) | + | ++++ | − | ± | ± | + | ++ | + | ± | ± | ++ | ++ | ± |
| **SNRI** | | | | | | | | | | | | | |
| Venlafaxine (Effexor) | ++ | ++++ | + | ± | ± | − | − | − | ± | ± | ++ | ++ | ± |

$\alpha_1\text{-}AR$ = $\alpha_1$-adrenergic receptors; $\alpha_2\text{-}AR$ = $\alpha_2$-adrenergic receptors; mACh = muscarinic cholinergic receptors; $D_2$ = dopamine $D_2$ receptors; DA = dopamine; $H_1$ = histamine $H_1$ receptors; 5-HT = serotonin; NA = noradrenaline; −, ±, +, ++, +++, ++++ = absence, or increasing degrees, of reuptake inhibition, receptor blockade, and side effects.

## Receptor effects

Tricyclic antidepressants have potent antagonist effects at a number of central nervous system (CNS) receptors, as listed in Table 25-1. These effects, however, account not for the therapeutic action, but for the profile of adverse effects elicited by these agents, which parallel their respective receptor affinities. In general, all TCAs exhibit significant anticholinergic effects (e.g., blurred vision, dry mouth, constipation, and urinary retention), although the tertiary TCAs are more potent in this regard than the demethylated TCAs such as desipramine and nortriptyline. Various TCAs are also potent blockers of histamine $H_1$ receptors and $\alpha_1$-adrenergic receptors; this action accounts for the sedative and hypotensive effects seen with a number of these agents. The receptor antagonist effects of TCAs also occur rapidly and account for the early onset of side effects seen during treatment. Moreover, these effects occur at lower dosages than those required for therapeutic response.

Two very important receptor changes induced by TCAs may be more directly related to the mechanism of their therapeutic action. These are down-regulation of cerebral cortical $\beta_1$-ARs and sensitization of postsynaptic serotonergic receptors leading to enhanced serotonergic neurotransmission. The former effect is produced not only by different types of antidepressant drugs (TCAs, MAOIs, and some second-generation antidepressants), but also by electroconvulsive therapy (ECT), which is a very effective treatment modality for depression.

Initially, the increased intrasynaptic levels of 5-HT activate somatodendritic $5\text{-HT}_{1A}$ autoreceptors and axon terminal $5\text{-HT}_{1B/D}$ receptors, thus reducing the neuronal firing rate and synaptic release of 5-HT at axon terminals (Fig. 25-3). With time (1 to 2 weeks), however, the somatodendritic and terminal autoreceptors become desensitized, so 5-HT neuronal firing rate progressively recovers, and release of 5-HT from presynaptic terminals is enhanced. These changes, together with the elevated intrasynaptic 5-HT levels at axonal terminals resulting from the continuing blockade of 5-HT reuptake, cause a net increase in serotonergic neurotransmission, an effect hypothesized to be an important component initiating downstream signalling and gene regulatory effects that are essential to the therapeutic action of all antidepressant agents.

## Pharmacokinetics

Absorption of TCAs from the gastrointestinal tract is essentially complete. Patients treated with identical doses show great inter-individual differences in their steady-state plasma concentrations. These differences may be related to inter-individual variation in hepatic blood flow and in the cytochrome P450 hepatic enzyme biotransformation system, resulting in differences in the amount of drug being biotransformed on first pass through the liver. Clinical improvement has been shown to correlate well with plasma drug levels of some TCAs (nortriptyline, imipramine, desipramine).

The slow onset of antidepressant action may also be related, in part, to the time required to achieve adequate steady-state tissue levels for changes in central 5-HT or NA pathways (e.g., receptor desensitization) to take place. The half-life of TCAs in humans ranges from 9 to 20 hours (more than 48 hours has been reported in some studies), and a steady-state plasma concentration is generally not reached until the second week of treatment. The pharmacokinetics of the many active metabolites have not been thoroughly studied, however.

In elderly patients, the steady-state levels of tricyclics tend to be higher than in younger subjects on the same dose because of reduced rates of hepatic clearance. This may explain the increased risk of cardiotoxicity and the need for lower doses in the elderly.

The biotransformation of TCAs involves demethylation, hydroxylation, and conjugation. Many of the metabolites have antidepressant action themselves. In patients receiving the tertiary amine TCAs, the ratio between the plasma concentrations of the tertiary amine and its secondary amine metabolite shows large interindividual differences. Much of the variation appears to be genetically determined (see Chapter 10).

Excretion of TCAs is slow (40% in 24 hours, 70% in 72 hours). The greatest portion is excreted as the N-oxide or as the unconjugated or conjugated 2-OH derivative.

## Adverse Effects

### Pronounced anticholinergic activity (atropinic effects)
In addition to the regularly observed atropine-like side effects of the tricyclics, such as blurred vision, dry mouth, constipation, and urinary retention, there is a danger of acute glaucoma; TCAs must therefore be prescribed with caution to patients with narrow-angle glaucoma or prostatic hypertrophy.

### Cardiovascular system
TCAs have potent and complex effects on the cardiovascular system related to their anticholinergic properties, their inhibition of catecholamine uptake, and their quinidine-like actions. The TCAs also exhibit lidocaine-like effects that can aggravate some pre-existing cardiac disorders, yet, almost paradoxically, may be of therapeutic benefit in preventing certain ventricular arrhythmias. Side effects include postural hypotension, tachycardia, hypertension, ECG changes (T-wave abnormalities, arrhythmias, impaired conduction), and congestive heart failure. These reactions are more likely to occur in the presence of existing cardiovascular disease and with high doses. The risk of cardiotoxic effects of TCAs increases proportionately with plasma concentrations above 1 µg/mL.

### CNS effects
Drowsiness is very common with the tertiary tricyclics. A fine rapid tremor, especially in the upper extremities, occurs in about 10% of elderly patients; it may be treated with propranolol 40 mg twice daily. TCAs lower the seizure threshold, as do phenothiazines, and may produce tonic–clonic seizures in high doses. Psychotoxic side effects vary from impaired memory to delirium. Although best documented for tricyclics, there is a definite risk with

FIGURE 25-3    Mechanisms and sites of action of (1) monoamine oxidase inhibitors (MAOI), (2) selective serotonin reuptake inhibitors (SSRI), and (3) tricyclic antidepressants (TCA) in the regulation of 5-HT-mediated neurotransmission. $\alpha_2$ and $\beta$ = noradrenergic receptors; NA = noradrenaline. *The overall effect of all three classes of drug is increased 5-HT synaptic transmission* (see text).

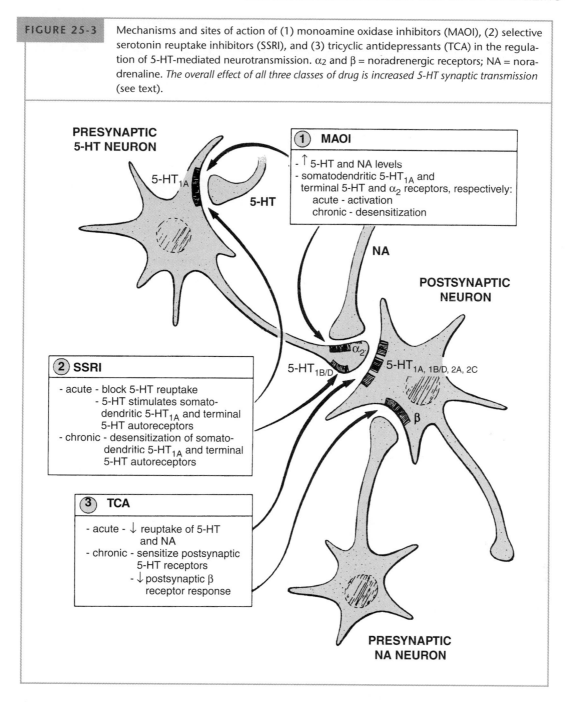

all antidepressants of precipitating a hypomanic or manic episode in depressed patients with a history of bipolar affective disorder.

### Withdrawal symptoms

In patients receiving more than 150 mg of imipramine or its equivalent daily for more than 2 months, withdrawal symptoms may start as early as 4 days, but usually between 1 and 2 weeks, following abrupt discontinuation. Symptoms consist of gastrointestinal disturbances, anxiety, and insomnia. Gradually reducing the dose over a period of several weeks can avoid or substantially reduce such symptoms.

## Drug Interactions

Hypertension and elevated body temperature (hyperpyrexia) may result when TCAs are given in combination with MAOIs, because both groups of drugs tend to increase the amounts of monoamines available to act at postsynaptic receptors. For this reason, practitioners should wait 2 weeks after stopping an MAOI before starting treatment with a TCA to allow regeneration of MAO activity and a return of metabolism of monoamines to normal levels.

Concurrent administration of TCAs and sympathomimetic amines can augment the amine pressor effects to the point of a hypertensive crisis. These antidepressants can also interfere with the therapeutic effects of certain antihypertensive agents (e.g., guanethidine, clonidine; see Chapter 14).

In epileptic patients maintained on anticonvulsant drugs, reduction of the seizure threshold by the tricyclics could be clinically important.

TCAs tend to enhance the effects of all oral hypoglycemic agents.

Because of the extensive hepatic microsomal metabolism of TCAs, co-administration of drugs that induce (e.g., carbamazepine) or inhibit (e.g., SSRIs) these enzymes can cause up to twofold reductions or elevations, respectively, in plasma TCA levels, resulting in prominent adverse effects. Thus, considerable attention must be paid to such potential metabolic interactions whenever TCAs are co-administered with other medications that affect hepatic drug metabolism.

## Overdosage

The clinical picture of overdosage is dominated by marked anticholinergic activity (see "Pronounced anticholinergic activity (atropinic effects)" above). In severe cases, myoclonic seizures, hyperpyrexia, hypotension, impaired cardiac conduction and contractility, ventricular arrhythmias, and coma may occur.

In addition to routine life-support measures and gastric lavage, anticholinergic toxicity marked by confusion, delirium, agitation, or coma may be managed with physostigmine (1 to 2 mg by slow intravenous injection, repeated at 30- to 60-minute intervals as necessary), which counteracts both the central and peripheral anticholinergic effects. Close monitoring of cardiac function is critical in the early stage of TCA overdose treatment. Hemodialysis may be required to prevent or treat cardiotoxic complications.

## Choice among Tricyclic Antidepressants

There is no conclusive evidence that any one TCA or class of antidepressant drugs is superior to another with respect to antidepressant response. The choice in clinical practice depends largely on the individual patient's tolerance of the side effects of a particular antidepressant and the presence of any pre-existing medical illness. Certain TCAs may be chosen for their strong sedating properties (e.g., amitriptyline) when insomnia or excitation is present. Nortriptyline produces less hypotension and therefore may be preferred in the treatment of the elderly, who are at greater risk of injuries from falls brought on by unsteadiness and lightheadedness due to orthostatic hypotension. Several new antidepressants such as the SSRIs (see later in this chapter) are the first choice for treating those patients who are particularly predisposed to the cardiotoxic effects of the tricyclics.

## Other Therapeutic Uses

Tricyclics are also used in other conditions that are not obviously related to depression. In **chronic pain syndromes,** such as trigeminal neuralgia or post-traumatic pain syndrome, amitriptyline and nortriptyline have an analgesic action at low doses (up to 75 mg/day) that are well below the range required for antidepressant action. The mechanism of the analgesic action is unclear.

# MONOAMINE OXIDASE INHIBITORS

Iproniazid (an isopropyl derivative of isoniazid, an antitubercular drug) was synthesized in 1951 in a search for a better chemotherapeutic agent for tuberculosis. When this drug was given to patients, they became cheerful and energetic and showed marked improvement in their outlook, even though there was no change in their lung pathology. In 1952, Zeller and co-workers discovered that iproniazid inhibits the enzyme MAO. Iproniazid was introduced for treatment of depression in 1957 but was abandoned because of its hepatotoxicity. However, its effects on mood spurred pharmaceutical chemists to synthesize other MAOIs in a search for less toxic ones. The structures of some of the MAOIs used clinically are shown in Figure 25-4.

Monoamine oxidase exists in two forms—MAO-A, for which 5-HT and NA are preferred substrates, and MAO-B, for which phenylethylamine is the specific substrate. In the human brain, MAO-B is the predominant form, but its localization is mostly extracellular. The intracellular enzyme is mainly the MAO-A subtype. Inhibition of MAO-A may be more important for antidepressant effects, as the selective MAO-B inhibitor deprenyl (selegiline; see Chapter 17) produces only weak or no response in depressed patients.

## Pharmacological Properties

Because of their potential to produce a serious hypertensive reaction in patients who inadvertently consume foods high in tyramine or medications containing pressor amines, the MAOIs were relegated for many years to a secondary role in the treatment of depression. The results of numerous studies, however, now indicate that these agents have therapeutic efficacy comparable to that of other antidepressants.

Following inhibition of MAO, concentrations of 5-HT, DA, and NA are markedly elevated in the body. It has been hypothesized that it is the increased availability of 5-HT in the brain, producing a net increase in serotonergic neurotransmission, and not the inhibition of MAO-A per se, which is particularly important in the MAOI antidepressant mechanism of action. In addition, the simultaneous effect of MAOIs in increasing NA levels may be instru-

FIGURE 25-4 Structural formulae of representative monoamine oxidase inhibitors.

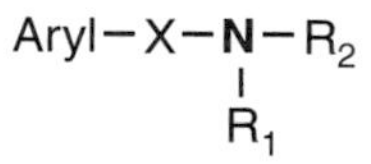

Basic structure of clinically important MAOIs

**IRREVERSIBLE**

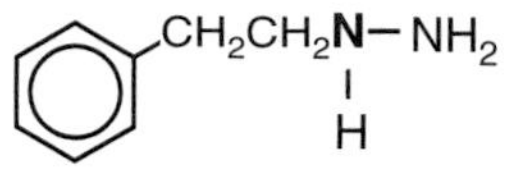

Phenelzine (Nardil)

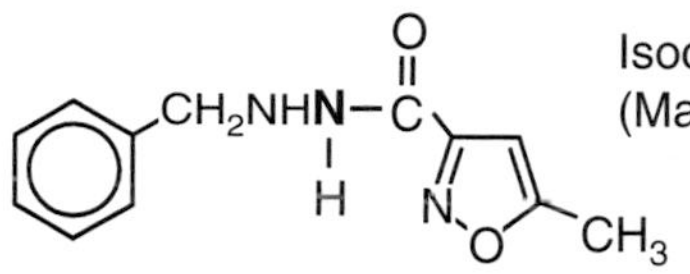

Isocarboxazid (Marplan)

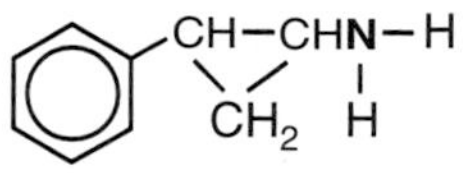

Tranylcypromine (Parnate)

**REVERSIBLE**

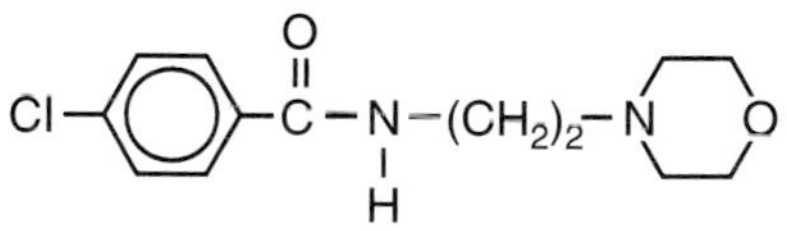

Moclobemide (Aurorix)

mental in actually enhancing net serotonergic neurotransmission. It has been proposed that the increased levels of NA caused by inhibition of MAO desensitize inhibitory $\alpha_2$-adrenoceptors located somatodendritically and pre-synaptically on 5-HT axon terminals. This results in the release of 5-HT neurons from $\alpha_2$ receptor–mediated inhibition and therefore an increased rate of neuronal firing and release of 5-HT. Just as in TCA therapy, the 2- to 3-week latency in producing receptor desensitization, post-receptor signalling, and gene expression effects following the initiation of MAOI treatment mirrors the delayed onset of therapeutic response to these agents.

MAOIs lower blood pressure, but it is uncertain whether this action is related to MAO inhibition. Some MAOIs (e.g., phenelzine, tranylcypromine) also have sympathomimetic activity similar to that of amphetamine due to increased release of stored noradrenaline.

The currently available MAOIs are readily absorbed when given by mouth, but excretion is slow. The onset of antidepressant action is slow, but because the drugs inhibit MAO irreversibly, their effects are long-lasting. Termination of drug effects depends upon synthesis of fresh enzyme, a process taking more than a week to reach normal levels.

## Adverse Effects

Because MAO is widely distributed throughout the body and is present in many different cell types, diverse pharmacological effects can be expected to occur after the administration of MAOIs.

Unlike some tricyclics, of which the whole dose is sometimes administered at night for the beneficial effect on sleep, MAOIs cause insomnia, and therefore evening and night doses should be avoided. Tranylcypromine may produce stimulant effects in some individuals, which is thought to be related to its amphetamine-like structure.

Other side effects are similar to those of the TCAs. They may be grouped as (1) signs of excessive CNS stimulation, including insomnia, irritability, ataxia, and seizures; (2) peripheral vascular effects, including orthostatic hypotension and dizziness; and (3) atropine-like effects such as dry mouth, impotence, urinary retention, constipation, and other gastrointestinal disturbances that probably reflect an imbalance between sympathetic and vagal tone. Orthostatic hypotension is thought to result from the displacement of noradrenaline from vesicular stores and depletion in peripheral sympathetic neurons by the accumulation of the hydroxylated trace amine, octopamine. This acts as a "false neurotransmitter" with little α- or β-adrenergic activity.

As noted, these agents may also precipitate a manic or hypomanic episode in patients with personal or family histories of bipolar disorder.

## Drug Interactions

Because MAOIs inhibit catecholamine breakdown, co-administration of other substances that contain or release catecholamines may result in marked increase in adrenergic activity, with such consequences as hypertension, tachycardia, agitation, occipital headache, and occasionally, intracranial bleeding (secondary to increase in blood pressure, see Chapter 14). Drugs that may interact in this way with MAOIs include TCAs, reserpine, L-dopa, and opioid analgesics. Foods containing large amounts of tyramine, including aged cheeses, bananas, beer, wine, yeast products, yogurt, and meat extracts (e.g., Bovril), can also precipitate a hypertensive reaction. Patients being treated with MAOIs must be warned to consult their physicians before using over-the-counter medications of any kind (especially medicines for coughs and colds, many of which contain sympathomimetic amines), and they must receive detailed instructions about their diet. Hypertensive crisis resulting from such interactions can be treated with short-acting α-adrenergic receptor blockers (e.g., phentolamine) or calcium-channel blockers (e.g., nifedipine).

MAOIs potentiate the effects of numerous other drugs, including alcohol, sedative–hypnotics, general anaesthetics, opioids, and other analgesics. This effect is thought to be due mainly to the inhibition of biotransformation of these other drugs, but direct CNS interactions cannot be ruled out. After the discontinuation of MAOIs, MAO-inhibiting action will continue for at least a week. If TCAs or another MAOI is to be substituted for an MAOI that is being discontinued, it is recommended that an interval of 2 weeks be allowed before the new drug is started. Treatment with MAOIs should also be discontinued at least 10 days prior to elective surgery in order to avoid possible interactions with the anaesthetic or pre-anaesthetic medications. Similarly, a medication-free interval of at least 5 half-lives of any previously administered antidepressant (or that of its active metabolite, if longer than that of the parent drug) should be allowed before initiating MAOI treatment in order to avoid interaction with drugs that may have been used previously.

When co-administered with tryptophan (the precursor of serotonin) or SSRI antidepressants, MAOIs may produce a neurological syndrome characterized by confusion, restlessness, hyperpyrexia, and muscle spasms (myoclonus). This "serotonin syndrome" is now recognized to be due to the marked elevation of 5-HT levels produced under these conditions.

## Overdosage

The clinical picture of MAOI overdosage consists of hyperpyrexia, hypertension, hyper-reflexia, involuntary movements, agitation, hallucinations, and coma. These signs and symptoms closely resemble those of major overdosage with amphetamine or atropine-like drugs (see Chapters 12 and 26), which result in excessive central and peripheral catecholaminergic and anticholinergic activity, respectively. Hypotension may sometimes occur, probably as a result of a different type of pharmacological action.

There is an initial asymptomatic period of up to 12 hours after drug ingestion during which manifestations of overdosage may not be apparent.

Utmost care is recommended in the management of overdosed patients. Many drugs (e.g., sympathomimetics, barbiturates) tend to be potentiated by MAOIs, as noted above, and should be used only under expert guidance.

## Indications for MAO Inhibitors

Although a number of earlier studies suggested that MAOIs are more effective for "atypical depressions" characterized by depression with profound feelings of lethargy, mood reactivity, sensitivity to rejection, increased sleep, and increased food intake with carbohydrate craving, more recent investigations have shown these agents to be effective in the treatment of major depressive episodes in general, as well as in panic disorder (see Chapter 23). Because of their potential to induce serious side effects and the need for dietary restrictions, however, they have been relegated to use as a third line of treatment in individuals who have responded poorly to SSRI, tricyclic, or other antidepressants.

## Dosage

Therapeutic doses for phenelzine (Nardil) and tranylcypromine (Parnate) range from 45 to 90 mg/day and 20 to 60 mg/day, respectively. There is no good evidence supporting the use of a lower dosage during maintenance therapy with these agents. Because insomnia is not uncommon during treatment with MAOIs, they are usually given in divided doses early in the day.

## Reversible MAOIs

Several newer MAOIs have been developed that do not block MAO irreversibly. **Moclobemide,** a benzamide derivative chemically distinct from the irreversible MAOIs, which inhibits MAO-A, is a member of this subclass. It is rapidly absorbed, is subject to a high first-pass effect, and has a short elimination half-life of 1 to 2 hours. Treatment with it is initiated in a dose range of 300 to 450 mg/day in divided doses, and it has a therapeutic range of 300 to 600 mg/day. The adverse effects of this agent are similar to those of the irreversible MAOIs, with the important exception that it shows a much reduced ability to elevate tyramine levels following ingestion of tyramine-containing foods. Thus, there is a greatly reduced possibility of developing a hypertensive reaction with tyramine-containing foods, although moderation in the use of such foods, and avoidance of over-the-counter drugs, should still be observed as with other MAOIs.

The therapeutic indications for moclobemide are similar to those for MAOIs in general, (i.e., for treatment of major depression).

# SECOND- AND THIRD-GENERATION ANTIDEPRESSANTS

The introduction of TCAs and MAOIs in the late 1950s revolutionized the treatment of affective disorders. However, both types of drug produced troublesome or potentially dangerous adverse effects, as noted above. Moreover, only about 70 to 80% of patients responded to treatment with these agents. Therefore, there was a need for new compounds of equal or greater clinical efficacy with fewer and less serious side effects. This led to the development of a number of new antidepressants, the so-called "second- and third-generation antidepressants." Many of these are not tricyclic, and they have structures and pharmacological effects quite distinct from those of the typical TCAs (Fig. 25-5) but are effective in treating depression. A brief description of some of the compounds follows (see also Table 25-1).

# Amoxapine

In addition to being a strong inhibitor of NA reuptake, amoxapine (Asendin) has strong 5-HT receptor blocking activity. It has no significant effect on 5-HT reuptake, and its anticholinergic activity is weak. Although its anti-dopaminergic activity is theoretically useful for some patients, it has many side effects (orthostatic hypotension) similar to those of TCAs and of antipsychotics (see Chapter 24).

# Maprotiline

Maprotiline (Ludiomil) strongly inhibits NA reuptake but only weakly blocks reuptake of 5-HT. It has a strong anti-

**FIGURE 25-5** Structural formulae of second- and third-generation antidepressants.

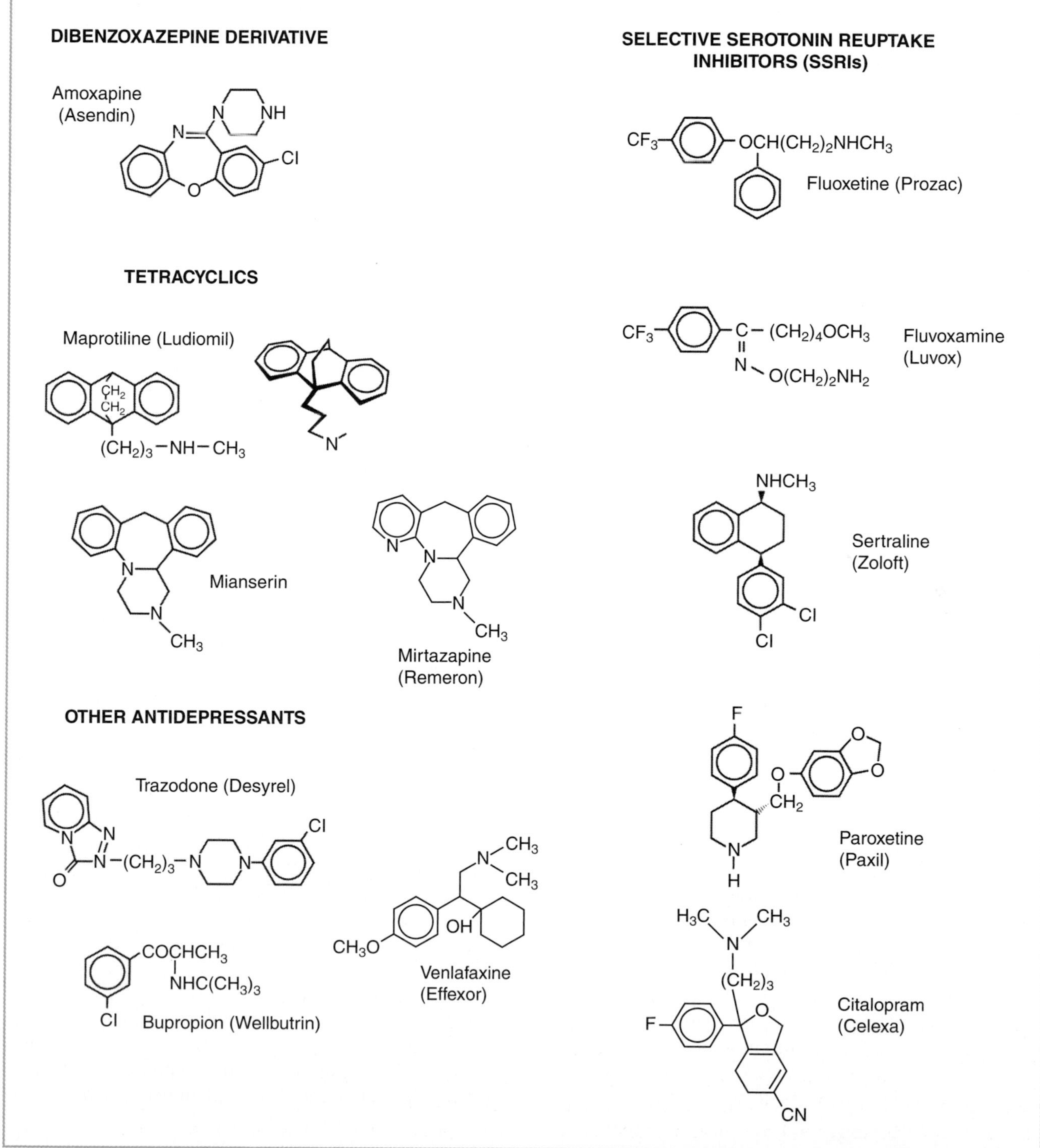

histaminergic and a weak anticholinergic action. There is a lower incidence of cardiovascular complications associated with its use than with that of the TCAs. A higher risk of seizures with this antidepressant has resulted in recommendations for administering lower treatment dosages than originally suggested.

## Mianserin

Mianserin has only weak effects in blocking monoamine reuptake, but it blocks presynaptic $\alpha_2$-adrenergic receptors, thereby increasing NA turnover. In addition, its independent strong sedative and anxiolytic properties are useful for some patients. Mianserin, like maprotiline, has no significant anticholinergic effects and is much less cardiotoxic than TCAs in therapeutic doses. Mianserin is not available in the United States and Canada.

## Trazodone

A relatively selective but weak inhibitor of 5-HT reuptake, trazodone (Desyrel) also has weak anticholinergic and cardiovascular effects. It does, however, produce sedation. Nefazadone, which is related to trazodone, was withdrawn from use because of hepatotoxicity that became evident in adverse reaction reports after its release for treatment of depression.

## Bupropion

Bupropion (Wellbutrin) is an aminoketone structurally related to the phenylethylamines. Unlike most other antidepressants, bupropion has no effect on 5-HT uptake and only exhibits modest DA and weak NA reuptake-blocking actions. Bupropion is rapidly absorbed, reaching peak plasma levels in 1 to 3 hours, and has a mean half-life of about 10 hours. Its three biologically active metabolites, hydroxybupropion, erythrohydrobupropion, and threohydrobupropion, have half-lives of 20 to 27 hours.

Clinically, bupropion has a stimulating effect that may cause agitation, increased motor activity, tremor, and insomnia. Its low anticholinergic potency and lack of effect on cardiac conduction account for its lower potential for cardiotoxicity. It produces a range of gastrointestinal side effects similar to those of the SSRIs, including nausea, vomiting, loss of appetite, insomnia, and headache, and it is more likely to be associated with weight loss. A particularly worrisome side effect of bupropion is its propensity to produce seizures at dosages above 450 mg/day, particularly within the time interval between peak plasma levels. For these reasons, it is recommended that bupropion be administered in divided doses not greater than 150 mg/dose, at least 4 hours apart; the maximum total daily dose should not exceed 450 mg for the immediate-release formulation and 300 mg for the sustained-release formulation.

## Selective Serotonin Reuptake Inhibitors (SSRIs)

Evidence implicating reduced brain serotonergic function in depression led to the search for potential antidepressant compounds that acted selectively on the 5-HT systems. It was reasoned that such agents might have enhanced therapeutic effects with fewer troublesome side effects attributable to non-selective actions on other neurotransmitter systems and receptors. A number of SSRIs (see Fig. 25-5) are now in clinical use throughout the world, the widest experience in North America being with **fluoxetine** (Prozac), **sertraline** (Zoloft), **fluvoxamine** (Luvox), **paroxetine** (Paxil), and **citalopram** (Celexa). Unlike the TCAs, the SSRIs do not share a common chemical structure but are classified on the basis of their common functional effects. All are potent and more selective inhibitors of neuronal 5-HT reuptake, showing little or no inhibition of NA or DA reuptake, with the exception of sertraline and to some extent paroxetine, which exhibit some capacity to inhibit DA reuptake (see Table 25-1). They also cause essentially no or very little blockade of $\alpha_1$-, $\alpha_2$-, or $\beta_1$-adrenergic receptors, dopamine $D_2$ receptors, 5-HT$_{1 \text{ and } 2}$ or histamine $H_1$ receptors (see Table 25-1).

### Pharmacological effects

As with other antidepressants, the clinical response to SSRIs is delayed for several weeks following institution of treatment. Thus, the mechanism of therapeutic action of SSRIs is also thought to be related to adaptive changes in neuronal function resulting in enhanced brain serotonergic neurotransmission and cellular resilience, as already described for TCAs and MAOIs.

### Pharmacokinetics

The SSRIs are generally well absorbed from the gastrointestinal tract, reaching peak plasma levels in 2 to 8 hours. Sertraline tends to be absorbed a little more slowly than the other SSRIs. At therapeutic concentrations, all of these agents show extensive binding to plasma protein (citalopram 80%, fluoxetine 94%, fluvoxamine 77%, paroxetine 95%, and sertraline 99%). Sertraline and citalopram have single-dose plasma half-lives in the range of 24 and 36 hours, respectively; fluvoxamine and paroxetine, about 15 and 12 hours, respectively. In contrast, fluoxetine has a half-life of 3 days.

The SSRIs undergo extensive hepatic biotransformation. The primary metabolite of sertraline, desmethylsertraline, is a weak inhibitor of 5-HT reuptake with only half to one-tenth the potency of sertraline; no active metabolites have been identified for paroxetine or fluvoxamine. Citalopram is primarily metabolized by demethylation, but the demethylated metabolites show much lower potency of 5-HT reuptake inhibition and low CNS penetration. The major metabolite of fluoxetine, norfluoxetine, is also a specific and potent inhibitor of 5-HT reuptake and has a half-life of 7 to 15 days. This prolonged half-life for fluoxetine and its major metabolite merits close consideration when this agent is used to treat depression as it may prolong the duration of intolerable side effects encountered by some patients because of the slow elimination of the drug. However, it may have an advantage in individuals who show poor compliance because occasional missed doses will not result in marked reductions in steady-state plasma levels.

There is little evidence supporting a relationship between plasma levels and response to SSRIs. Fluoxetine and paroxetine show non-linear pharmacokinetics because these agents inhibit their own clearance, leading to an increased half-life at higher doses and a disproportionate elevation in plasma concentrations with subsequent dose increases. Some patients require higher dosage levels of certain SSRIs to produce a clinical response, which may reflect genetic differences in CYP450 drug-metabolizing activity. However, such differences in dose requirements may also rest in part on differential affinities of 5-HT receptor subtypes expressed in prefrontal cortical regions that are thought to be the target of SSRI action in depression and certain anxiety disorders, such as obsessive–compulsive disorder. While these factors can be assessed with genotyping and neuroimaging techniques, cost-effective tests to identify such individuals in advance of instituting therapy are still in development.

### Adverse effects

The lack of effect of SSRIs at various neuroreceptors noted above (see Table 25-1) accounts for the different profile of adverse effects reported for these antidepressants compared with the classical TCAs. For example, they do not cause orthostatic hypotension and cause significantly less frequent anticholinergic symptoms such as dry mouth, constipation, sweating, or blurred vision than TCAs do. The SSRIs have a much greater margin of safety and are less toxic in overdosage than the tricyclics. As they exhibit no significant cardiotoxicity, they are particularly suitable for treatment of depression in individuals with coexisting cardiovascular disease and post-myocardial infarction. However, they can interfere with the metabolism of other drugs that are cleared through the CYP450 system (see "Drug interactions" below) and that may induce cardiac arrhythmias, for example, ketoconazole producing QTc prolongation.

The SSRIs do, however, produce troublesome side effects, including nausea, nervousness, insomnia, and headache. Some of these adverse effects may be related to the increased stimulation of 5-HT receptor subtypes, such as $5-HT_{1A}$, as a result of the 5-HT elevation. This may account for the increased feelings of anxiety and restlessness experienced by as many as 15 to 20% of patients taking these agents. Other common side effects include significant sexual dysfunction, particularly anorgasmia in

women and delayed or absent ejaculation in men, drowsiness, and, in long-term use, weight gain. Extrapyramidal side effects have been reported with some of these agents, possibly mediated by an indirect action on dopaminergic function. Although rare, the possibility of such occurrences should be carefully monitored in long-term maintenance treatment with these agents. Finally, discontinuation of SSRIs taken for longer than a month can be accompanied by a syndrome of dizziness, lightheadedness, vertigo or faint feeling, paresthesias, tremor, visual disturbances, anxiety, nausea, vomiting, insomnia, somnolence, irritability, headache, fatigue, and impaired concentration. This discontinuation syndrome can be avoided or minimized by gradually tapering off the SSRI over several weeks.

### Drug interactions

Most of the SSRIs are competitive inhibitors of specific hepatic CYP450 isozymes, although to varying degrees, and they therefore have the potential for significant drug interactions. Fluoxetine and paroxetine are potent inhibitors of the hepatic CYP2D6 isozyme in vitro and in vivo, whereas sertraline is much less potent. Thus, fluoxetine and paroxetine can produce marked elevations in the plasma levels (and consequently the side effects) of other drugs that are biotransformed by this hepatic isozyme. For example, plasma tricyclic levels can double during co-administration of fluoxetine, a situation that may occur while switching from a TCA to this SSRI. Fluoxetine also inhibits the hepatic CYP3A3/4 and CYP2C isozymes, interfering with the clearance of alprazolam and diazepam, respectively; however, at the usual minimum effective dose of fluoxetine, the effect on CYP2D6-mediated drug metabolism is much greater than on the CYP3A3/4 and CYP2C isozymes. Sertraline at usual therapeutic doses of 50 to 150 mg is much less likely to interfere with the clearance of other drugs. Citalopram shows only weak inhibition of CYP2D6, 1A2, and 2C19 and no inhibition of CYP3A3/4 and, accordingly, has low potential for clinically significant interaction with other drugs cleared through this hepatic drug-clearance pathway.

Because of their high degree of protein binding, SSRIs can increase the plasma-free drug levels and toxicity associated with other drugs (e.g., warfarin, digitoxin) that also show extensive plasma protein binding.

Ample time must be allowed for the washout of these drugs (2 weeks for sertraline, paroxetine, and fluvoxamine; 5 weeks for fluoxetine) when switching from SSRI to MAOI treatment to avoid the production of a hypermetabolic state marked by hyperpyrexia, confusion, agitation, muscular rigidity, myoclonus, and autonomic instability. This reaction has considerable similarity to the serotonin and antipsychotic malignant syndromes and may involve marked augmentation of central serotonergic function.

## Serotonin–Noradrenaline Reuptake Inhibitors (SNRIs)

Among other third-generation antidepressants are those that act on both the noradrenergic and serotonergic neurotransmitter systems. **Venlafaxine** (Effexor; see Fig. 25-5) is a dual action drug. As it is a more potent inhibitor of 5-HT than of NA reuptake, venlafaxine acts like an SSRI at lower therapeutic doses (75 to 225 mg/day) and a dual mode 5-HT and NA reuptake inhibitor at higher doses. Like the SSRIs, it is well absorbed from the gastrointestinal tract and reaches peak plasma levels in 1 to 3 hours. It shows low plasma protein binding, in contrast to the SSRIs. It is metabolized through O-demethylation, forming the active metabolite O-desmethylvenlafaxine (ODV). The half-life is about 6 hours for the parent drug and 15 hours for ODV. Like the SSRIs, venlafaxine is also metabolized through the hepatic P450 system and is a weak inhibitor of CYP2D6, whereas ODV inhibits CYP3A3/4. Venlafaxine has a side-effect profile similar to that of SSRIs: nausea, headache, nervousness, sweating, sexual side effects, and dry mouth are the more common complaints. It can also produce a modest but sustained dose-related elevation in blood pressure, indicating the need for caution when it is used in patients with pre-existing hypertension, but like the SSRIs, it shows very little cardiotoxicity.

## Antidepressants Acting on Specific Adrenergic and Serotonergic Receptors

**Mirtazapine** (Remeron) is a tetracyclic antidepressant that enhances noradrenergic and 5-HT$_{1A}$-mediated neurotransmission. Antagonism of presynaptic α$_2$-adrenergic autoreceptors increases NA release while blockade of α$_2$ heteroreceptors on 5-HT neurons increases 5-HT release. The concomitant blockade of postsynaptic 5-HT$_2$ and 5-HT$_3$ receptors by mirtazapine also contributes to the net increase in 5-HT$_{1A}$-mediated neurotransmission. It has little effect on 5-HT or NA uptake, however. Mirtazapine exhibits low affinity for dopaminergic and muscarinic cholinergic receptors in vitro but high affinity for histamine H$_3$ receptors. It shows high (85%) protein binding but moderate bioavailability (50%), and its pharmacokinetic parameters are independent of dose or drug concentration within the effective dose range of 15 to 45 mg daily. The half-life is relatively long, ranging from 20 to 40 hours.

Mirtazapine undergoes extensive hepatic metabolism through the P450 isozymes: CYP2D6 (8-hydroxylation), P1A2 (N-demethylation), and CYP3A3/4 (N-oxidation). As a weak competitive inhibitor of these isozymes in vitro, it would not be expected to cause clinically significant interactions with other drugs that are substrates for these CYP450 subtypes, but there are few in vivo studies to confirm this. The most prominent side effects encountered with mirtazapine reflect its pharmacodynamic profile and include sedation at the lower dose range, attributable to the H$_1$ receptor blockade, anticholinergic side effects such as dry mouth and blurred vision, and increased appetite and weight gain.

## OTHER PSYCHIATRIC INDICATIONS FOR ANTIDEPRESSANTS

There is substantial evidence that antidepressants are useful in the management of other psychiatric disorders, particularly a number of the anxiety disorders (see Chapter 23). For example, patients with **panic disorder, generalized anxiety disorder, and social phobia** respond to a number of different antidepressants, including the SSRIs, tricyclics, and MAOIs. Although still equivocal in the case of bupropion, all of these antidepressant groups are effective for panic disorder and may show similar efficacy across the groups in treating generalized anxiety disorder. SSRIs, however, are often preferred because of fewer side effects. Patients with panic disorder are likely to be more sensitive to the stimulating side effects (e.g., nervousness, agitation, anxiety) of SSRIs and some tricyclics; therefore, treatment of panic disorder with these antidepressants should be initiated at lower doses and increased much more gradually than when treating depression. The optimal dose range for anti-panic activity of SSRIs is similar to that for the management of depression. Similarly, the SSRIs and **clomipramine**, a tricyclic antidepressant with more potent 5-HT reuptake blocking action, have proved useful in the management of **obsessive–compulsive disorder**. Therapeutic doses for treatment of this anxiety disorder are often higher than for treating major depression and other anxiety disorders.

## MOOD STABILIZERS

Since the introduction of lithium more than 50 years ago, it is still, to this date, the first choice for the acute and prophylactic treatment of bipolar disorder. In general, lithium is most effective in patients who have a classical course of illness; the response rates are lower for bipolar patients with psychotic symptoms, dysphoric mania (coexisting manic and depressive symptoms), rapid cycling, and comorbid substance abuse. The discovery of mood-stabilizing properties of several of the anticonvulsants has expanded the treatment options for bipolar disorder. The recognition of their potential psychotropic effects arose from observations that some patients with seizure disorders and concomitant mood disturbances often showed improved mood while being treated with the anti-seizure agents **carbamazepine** or **valproate** (see Chapter 18). This observation stimulated intensive work in recent years to explore the role of these anticonvulsant drugs in the management of mania and as mood-stabilizing agents.

There is now substantial evidence supporting the anti-manic actions of these agents and growing support for the notion that these agents, valproate in particular, may be more effective in treating manic and hypomanic episodes in certain subtypes of bipolar disorder. These include bipolar disorders with rapid cycling (four or more episodes of mania and depression per year), dysphoric mania, and mania secondary to neurological disorders. However, valproate and carbamazepine show only modest antidepressant efficacy at best, and their effectiveness in preventing the recurrence of manic and depressive episodes still remains to be demonstrated unequivocally in long-term studies. **Lamotrigine** appears to be somewhat different in that it exhibits significant antidepressant efficacy without the risk of inducing hypomania, and it is becoming a favoured first-line agent in treating bipolar depression. While substantial data support the use of valproate as an anti-manic agent, it is not completely clear whether it has similar or better efficacy than lithium for long-term mood-stabilizing effects. For these reasons, valproate, carbamazepine, and lamotrigine are most often introduced adjunctively if there is incomplete or little response to lithium alone. Alternatively, they may be used as monotherapy or, as is more common, in combinations with each other, if lithium is poorly tolerated or medically contraindicated.

Another important pharmacological treatment modality gaining increasing prominence in the management of bipolar disorder is the use of atypical antipsychotics (e.g., olanzapine, quetiapine, risperidone) for the treatment and prevention of recurrence of mania. These agents are particularly useful in bipolar patients who show poor or only partial response to mood stabilizers and more prominent psychotic symptoms over the course of illness. Although some evidence suggests that these agents may exert mood-stabilizing effects as well, this remains to be fully clarified. Consequently, their use in the maintenance phase of bipolar disorder treatment is primarily adjunctive.

## Mechanisms of Action

Lithium differs from other psychotropic drugs in that it does not produce obvious depressant or euphoriant effects in healthy individuals. It has, however, multiple clinical profiles in the treatment of mood disorders, including anti-manic, antidepressant, and long-term prophylactic (i.e., reducing or preventing the relapses and recurrences of subsequent affective episodes) efficacies, antidepressant augmenting effect, and anti-suicidal action. Thus, it is unlikely that the therapeutic actions of lithium are mediated by a single molecular target or "master switch" governing many of the above therapeutic effects. Moreover, the substantial delay between the initi-

ation of mood-stabilizer treatment and the appearance of clinical benefit suggests that the mechanism of action probably involves long-term alterations in cellular signalling pathways and, in most cases, changes in gene expression in critical neuronal circuits. In this context, an intracellular network of parallel and intersecting signal transduction cascades (e.g., cAMP, phosphoinositide [PI], calcium, phosphatidylinositol-3-kinase/protein kinase B [PI-3K/Akt], wingless [Wnt], BDNF, and mitogen-activated protein [MAP] kinase signalling pathways) regulating neuronal and structural plasticity and cellular resilience (see Fig. 25-1) has been implicated in the action of mood-stabilizing drugs, including lithium, valproate, and carbamazepine. The modulatory effects of these agents on the cAMP, PI, and calcium signalling pathways appear to be of therapeutic relevance in view of the growing appreciation that disturbances in these signalling pathways are central to the pathophysiology of bipolar disorder. Thus, it is conceivable that these mood-stabilizing drugs act as a "homeostatic lever" to reset the putative signalling disturbances in bipolar disorder back toward their normal functional range.

Among the actions of lithium that are thought to be of particular relevance to its therapeutic effects (see Fig. 25-1) as they occur at clinically effective tissue drug concentrations are the following:

- Uncompetitive inhibition of inositol monophosphatases (IMPase; $K_i$ = 0.8 mM) that leads to depletion of intracellular *myo*-inositol and, in turn, dampens hyperactive synaptic signalling by receptors that are coupled to PI turnover (i.e., inositol depletion hypothesis)
- Elevation of baseline cAMP levels but decreased stimulation of cAMP formation, leading to the hypothesis that lithium exerts a bimodal effect, adjusting and stabilizing signalling activities within an optimal range and preventing excessive uncontrolled fluctuations
- Attenuation of resting and agonist-stimulated intracellular $Ca^{2+}$ mobilization responses
- Attenuation of cell death in response to cytotoxic insults and promotion of neurogenesis, involving
  - inactivation of NMDA receptors
  - increased expression of BDNF and the anti-apoptotic and cytoprotective protein B-cell lymphoma protein 2 (Bcl-2)
  - reduced expression of the pro-apoptotic proteins p53 and Bax
  - activation of the cell survival kinases PI-3K/Akt and ERK/MAP kinase
  - inhibition of the pro-apoptotic kinase glycogen synthase kinase 3β (GSK-3β)

A problem inherent in researching the mechanism of action of antidepressant and mood-stabilizing medications is the difficulty in deciding which of the multitude of biochemical and cellular findings are relevant to the therapeutic effect and which are merely epiphenomena, or are even responsible for unwanted side effects. It is conceivable that, in the future, pre-clinical and clinical studies of the various intracellular signalling pathways mediating neuroplasticity and cellular resiliency, and their interactions with other genetic or environmental vulnerability factors, will greatly advance our understanding of the molecular mechanisms underlying therapeutic response and of the pathogenesis of major affective disorders.

## Lithium

### Pharmacokinetics and dosage

Lithium absorption from the gastrointestinal tract is rapid, with peak blood levels occurring about 2 to 4 hours after a single dose. The serum half-life is approximately 24 hours. However, it has been reported that the half-life of lithium increases with continuous lithium therapy, and a mean half-life of 57.6 hours has been demonstrated in patients who had been on lithium for more than a year.

Lithium is not protein-bound. The optimal serum lithium concentration for control of manic symptoms is 0.6 to 1.2 mmol/L measured 12 hours after the most recent dose. A daily dose of 900 to 1800 mg, depending on the patient's weight and age, generally provides serum lithium levels within the therapeutic range for mood stabilization (0.5 to 1.0 mmol/L).

There is a competitive interaction between sodium and lithium ions in the renal tubule. An increase in sodium intake decreases renal reabsorption of lithium and thus lowers the serum lithium level slightly, while reduced sodium intake elevates it. Thus, patients on a sodium-restricted diet or taking drugs that impair sodium reabsorption, such as diuretics and non-steroidal anti-inflammatory agents, are at risk of lithium intoxication and must be carefully monitored if treatment with such agents cannot be avoided or lithium cannot be discontinued. As lithium is excreted mainly by the kidneys, patients with impaired renal function are also at great risk of lithium accumulation and intoxication. Where the severity of illness justifies the increased teratogenic risk of continuing lithium during pregnancy, plasma lithium levels also must be monitored carefully in pregnant women because renal lithium clearance increases during pregnancy and decreases after childbirth.

### Side effects and toxicity

Gastrointestinal disturbances, polyuria and polydipsia, fatigue, dizziness, muscle hyper-irritability (fasciculation and twitching), and fine tremor of the hands may occur at serum lithium levels within the therapeutic range.

Severe poisoning (serum lithium above 2 mmol/L) primarily affects the CNS. Disturbances in higher cortical functions, motor incoordination, slurred speech, and coma may develop.

Endocrine and metabolic effects may occur during lithium therapy. These include hypothyroidism and goiter, alterations in carbohydrate and steroid metabolism, and vasopressin-resistant diabetes insipidus–like syndromes. These endocrine effects may be consequent to lithium's effects on various intracellular signalling cascades. For example, by attenuating receptor-activated adenylyl cyclase signalling at the level of both the G proteins that couple receptors to adenylyl cyclases and the adenylyl cyclases themselves, lithium may suppress hormonal responses in peripheral tissues (e.g., thyrotropin activation of thyroid adenylyl cyclase and antidiuretic hormone activation of renal adenylyl cyclase).

Some patients show leukocytosis during long-term lithium therapy, which is reversible when therapy is stopped.

ECG changes (especially T-wave depression), arrhythmias, and peripheral circulatory disturbances have been observed.

The key measure to avoid toxicity is the monitoring of serum lithium levels and the avoidance of tissue accumulation. Lithium therapy is generally not recommended for patients with renal and cardiovascular diseases.

## Mood-Stabilizing Anticonvulsant Agents

The pharmacology of these agents is described in Chapter 18. Their use in the management of bipolar disorder is subject to the same pharmacological and side-effect considerations that apply to their use in seizure disorders. The onset of anticonvulsant effects of these drugs is relatively rapid (24 to 48 hours), in contrast to the delay in anti-manic response. For this reason, it is unlikely that their effects on voltage-sensitive sodium channels, peripheral-type benzodiazepine receptors, and chloride or other membrane ion channels, to which their anticonvulsant effects are ascribed, are responsible for their effects on mood. Rather, it is now thought that their effects on intracellular signalling cascades, neurogenesis, and neuro-adaptation, and their neuroprotective properties, as discussed in "Mechanisms of Action" above, are responsible for their efficacy in bipolar disorder. Side effects encountered with carbamazepine, valproate, and lamotrigine in the treatment of bipolar disorder are the same as those found when these drugs are used for the management of neurological disorders. There is no evidence to support a specific range of doses or plasma concentrations for the anti-manic effects of carbamazepine and valproate. Accordingly, the therapeutic plasma concentration ranges established for anti-seizure activity are also used as a guide in treating mania. Anti-manic response to valproate appears to be optimal at levels in the range of 350 to 700 μmol/L. Antidepressant efficacy of lamotrigine in bipolar disorders is evinced in the dose range of 100 to 200 mg daily; the value of determination of plasma concentrations to monitor lamotrigine therapy in bipolar disorder has not been established, however.

## SUGGESTED READINGS

American Psychiatric Association. Practice guideline for the treatment of patients with bipolar disorder (revision). *Am J Psychiatry.* 2002;159(4 suppl):1-50.

American Psychiatric Association. Practice guideline for the treatment of patients with major depressive disorder (revision). *Am J Psychiatry.* 2000;157(4 suppl):1-45.

Ballenger JC, Davidson JR, Lecrubier Y, et al. Consensus statement on generalized anxiety disorder from the International Consensus Group on Depression and Anxiety. *J Clin Psychiatry.* 2001;62(suppl):1153-1158.

Blier P, de Montigny C. Serotonin and drug-induced therapeutic responses in major depression, obsessive-compulsive and panic disorders. *Neuropsychopharmacology.* 1999;21:91S-98S.

Cookson J. Use of antipsychotic drugs and lithium in mania. *Br J Psychiatry.* 2001;41(suppl):s148-s156.

Coyle JT, Duman RS. Finding the intracellular signaling pathways affected by mood disorder treatments. *Neuron.* 2003;38:157-160.

DeVane CL. Metabolism and pharmacokinetics of selective serotonin reuptake inhibitors. *Cell Mol Neurobiol.* 1999;19:443-466.

Gould TD, Manji HK. Signaling networks in the pathophysiology and treatment of mood disorders. *J Psychosom Res.* 2002;53:687-697.

Manji HK, Drevets WC, Charney DS. The cellular neurobiology of depression. *Nat Med.* 2001;7:541-547.

McElroy SL, Keck PE Jr. Pharmacologic agents for the treatment of acute bipolar mania. *Biol Psychiatry.* 2000;48:539-557.

McDaniel KD. Clinical pharmacology of monoamine oxidase inhibitors. *Clin Neuropharmacol.* 1986;9:207-234.

Pinder RM, Wiering JH. Third-generation antidepressants. *Med Res Rev.* 1993;13:259-325.

Preskorn SH, Magnus RD. Inhibition of hepatic P-450 isoenzymes by 5-HT selective reuptake inhibitors: in vitro and in vivo findings and their implications for patient care. *Psychopharmacol Bull.* 1994;30:251-259.

Rotzinger S, Bourin M, Akimoto Y, et al. Metabolism of some "second"- and "fourth"-generation antidepressants: iprindole, viloxazine, bupropion, mianserin, maprotiline, trazodone, nefazodone, and venlafaxine. *Cell Mol Neurobiol.* 1999;19:427-442.

Rudorfer MV. Monoamine oxidase inhibitors: reversible and irreversible. *Psychopharmacol Bull.* 1992;28:45-57.

Sanchez C, Hyttel J. Comparison of the effects of antidepressants and their metabolites on reuptake of biogenic amines and on receptor binding. *Cell Mol Neurobiol.* 1999;19:467-489.

van Harten J. Clinical pharmacokinetics of selective 5-HT reuptake inhibitors. *Clin Pharmacokinet.* 1993;24:203-220.

# 26

# Hallucinogens and Psychotomimetics

## H KALANT

## CASE HISTORY

R.W., a 19-year-old male, was brought to the physician by his roommate, who found him in a very depressed state, his arms covered with scratches, lacerations, and small abscesses.

The history revealed that R.W. was a chronic drug user who had started using alcohol when he was only 11 years old. His absentee father was alcoholic; his mother had to work full-time to support the children. An older brother had personality problems but was not using drugs and had obtained employment in another city. At age 13, R.W. started using cannabis, often together with alcohol. He had a poor academic record and dropped out of school at age 15. His friends introduced him to "crack" cocaine, and he became both a regular user and a small-scale dealer. When using cocaine, he tended to use alcohol, benzodiazepines, or marijuana to "cool off." He tried LSD several times, and although he enjoyed the visual effects, he did not like the drug in general because it made him feel rather anxious and strange. He also experimented with the amphetamine derivative MDMA (also known as "ecstasy") and with something that was sold to him as mescaline.

A year ago, worsening personal problems led him to escalate his use of cocaine. It made him feel powerful and euphoric but also made him suspicious of his friends and led to frequent fights with them. If he stopped using the drug, his depression returned in a more acute form. Three weeks ago, he markedly raised his daily dosage, taking between 1 and 2 g of cocaine a day, around the clock. He became extremely hyperactive, with fragmented sleep of not more than 2 hours at a time. He became quite paranoid, heard voices talking to him from the ceiling, and thought people in the next room were pounding drums to annoy him. The pattern on the wallpaper began to move, and he thought he was able to make it move at will. He had sexual fantasies that he sustained for hours, but without orgasm. He had no interest in food, and lost 3.2 kg (7 lb) in weight. When he began to feel crawling sensations under his skin, he started to dig into his arms with a needle to extract the imaginary worms. Finally, he ran out of the drug and went into a deep sleep from which he woke feeling severely depressed, tremulous, and still anorexic.

On examination he was thin and malnourished, restless, and slightly short of breath. He had moderate tachycardia, cold clammy skin, some tremor, and a very short attention span. The physician began to treat him with desipramine but referred him immediately to the youth program of a local drug-dependence treatment agency.

A hallucination is defined as the subjective experience of a perception in the absence of a corresponding external reality. Many drugs can produce transient distortions of perception, sometimes giving rise to hallucinations and behaviour such as may be seen in psychotic patients. The drugs that are most potent and selective for this action, and that are sometimes used deliberately to produce it, are called **hallucinogens**, or **psychotomimetics**. They have also been given a variety of other designations reflecting different points of view. Those who advocate their use as a means of self-discovery call them **psychedelics**. In some people, the drug experience may trigger a panic state or a true psychosis, so the drugs are also sometimes called **psychodysleptics** and **psychotogens.**

All these names are inadequate because each emphasizes one effect, rather than the underlying actions and the full spectrum of the effects. Moreover, the drugs are not identical in their mechanisms and consequences of action. Amphetamines and cocaine can produce a true psychotic state that has frequently been mistaken for paranoid schizophrenia; therefore, the term "psychotomimetic" is appropriate. In contrast, the pictures produced by lysergic acid diethylamide (LSD), mescaline, and similar drugs may contain elements reminiscent of true psychoses, but they

334

are seldom mistaken for psychoses, and the user can generally recognize that the symptoms are due to the drug. Therefore, "hallucinogens" is a better term for such drugs, despite the limitations mentioned above.

## DRUGS AND METHODS OF STUDY

The two largest groups of drugs considered in this chapter are indolealkylamine derivatives related chemically to serotonin (5-hydroxytryptamine, 5-HT) and phenylethylamine derivatives related chemically to catecholamines. The chemical structures of a number of drugs in each group are shown in Figures 26-1 and 26-2, respectively.

In addition to these major groups, dissociative anaesthetics such as ketamine, drugs related pharmacologically to atropine, and drugs derived from cannabis can sometimes produce hallucinations when given in high dose or under certain circumstances. Therefore, they are also reviewed here in relation to their perceptual and behavioural effects.

Unfortunately, this division into families does not correspond to any clear-cut separation of pharmacological actions and effects. The mescaline-like drugs shown in the lower half of Figure 26-2 are closely similar in actions and effects to the LSD-like drugs shown in Figure 26-1, even though they are chemically related to amphetamine. Therefore, a meaningful classification must be based on a functional approach, and three complementary techniques have been used to generate such a functional classification.

The first technique is that of **receptor-binding studies.** LSD is extremely potent: a hallucinogenic dose in an adult human can be as little as 2 μg/kg (150 μg total dose). Moreover, it is highly stereospecific; only the *d*-form has activity. These characteristics are consistent with receptor-mediated action, but there has been scientific debate for several decades concerning the identity of the receptors involved in hallucinogen action and the nature of the drug–receptor interaction. The indole nucleus in LSD and related compounds (see Fig. 26-1) is structurally related to 5-HT, and the phenylethylamine structure of the amphetamines and related drugs (see Fig. 26-2) is related to dopamine and noradrenaline). However, the molecular structures of LSD and similar compounds also correspond in part to that of dopamine, and the amphetamine and mescaline families also overlap with essential parts of the 5-HT structure. Therefore, recent investigations have involved systematic comparison of the in vitro binding affinities of all of these compounds at both 5-HT and dopamine receptors, using the techniques described in Chapter 7.

The results demonstrate an extensive overlap of binding patterns. For example, LSD has about equal affinity for 5-HT$_2$ and dopamine D$_2$ receptors and slightly less for the

**FIGURE 26-1** Structural formulae of some representative members of the lysergic acid and psilocybin families of hallucinogenic substances. LSM = lysergic acid monoethylamide; LSD = lysergic acid diethylamide.

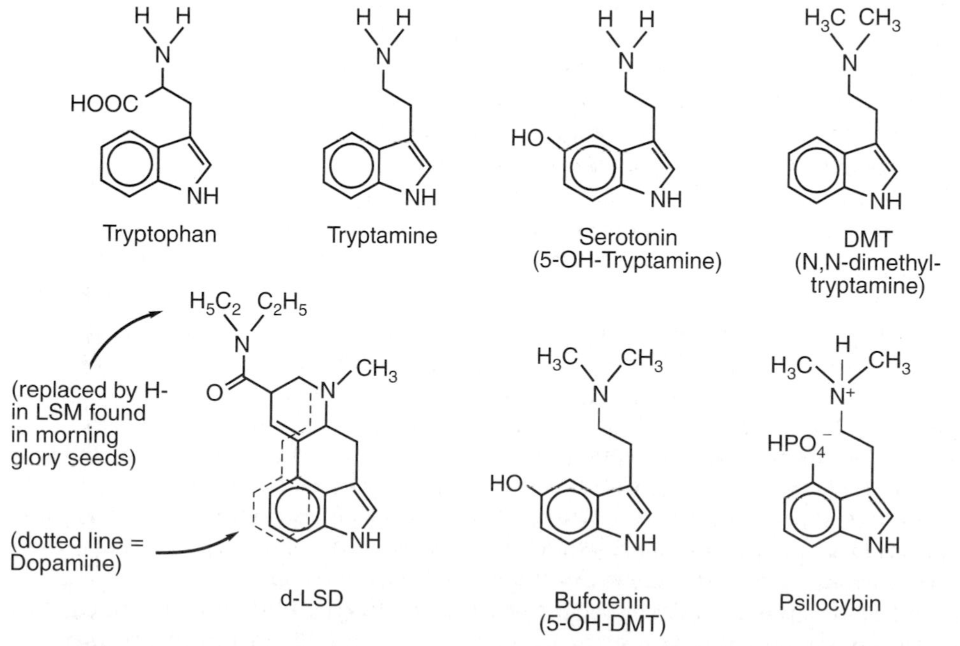

**FIGURE 26-2** Structural formulae of noradrenaline and some representative members of the phenylethylamine group of hallucinogens. (Upper row) Members of the amphetamine family. Superimposed on the amphetamine formula are the main features of the 5-hydroxytryptamine molecule (broken lines). (Lower row) Mescaline and related compounds.

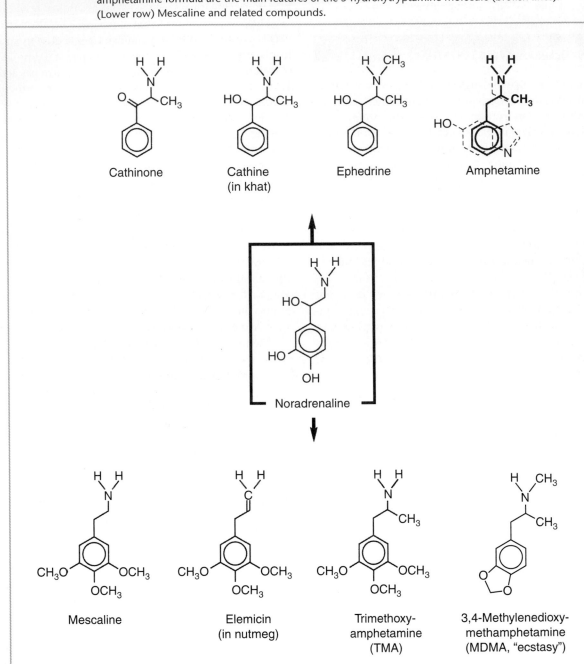

$D_1$ receptors. Its affinity for the dopamine receptors is equal to that of lisuride, a potent dopamine agonist. Conversely, hallucinogenic amphetamine derivatives such as DOM (4-methyl-2,5-dimethoxyamphetamine) bind strongly to $5\text{-HT}_2$ receptors. The strongest evidence at present implicates $5\text{-HT}_{2A/2C}$ and $D_2$ receptors in the hallucinogenic actions of these two major groups of "classical" hallucinogens. For example, ritanserine and spiperone displace LSD from the $5\text{-HT}_{2A}$ receptors and block many of its subjective and behavioural effects and neurophysiological actions. But LSD is also antagonized by clozapine, a blocker of $D_2$, muscarinic, and $5\text{-HT}_2$ receptors, and by sulpiride, which displaces it from $D_2$ receptors.

The second technique is the in vivo observation of the **patterns of behavioural effects** produced by the drugs in experimental animals. The behaviours that are especially useful in this connection are exploratory activity, stereotypy, food-reinforced operant behaviour, and certain motor patterns such as head-twitching and ear-scratching (see Chapter 69). The LSD-like hallucinogens produce decreases in exploratory activity, a tendency for the animal to stay close to the walls and corners of the observation chamber, sudden interruptions in food-rewarded bar-pressing activity, stereotypy, and bizarre behaviours such as prolonged staring or visually following the movement of non-existent objects.

The third technique, also in vivo, is the study of **discriminative stimulus generalization** (see Chapter 69). Rats are trained to press one lever for food reward while under the influence of a drug and a second lever while under placebo. They are then tested under a different drug, and the relative numbers of responses they make on the training drug lever and on the placebo lever indicate whether they perceive the subjective effects of the test drug to be more like those of the training drug or more different from them. Again, the results indicate a considerable overlap of subjective effects. When compared against the training drugs quipazine (predominantly a 5-HT agonist), 5-methoxy-DMT (a pure $5-HT_1$ agonist), and amphetamine (predominantly a catecholamine receptor indirect agonist), most of the drugs of both the indolealkylamine and phenylethylamine groups show varying degrees of cross-generalization.

In general, the results of the receptor-binding studies are in agreement with those of the discriminative stimulus generalization studies and with the behavioural observations. A drug with a very high affinity for $5-HT_1$ receptors is likely to show high generalization to 5-methoxy-DMT training stimuli and little or none to amphetamine stimuli. A drug with lower receptor specificity will show more cross-generalization. There appears to be a continuum of gradation between the two "pure" pictures. Therefore, the spectrum of subjective and objective effects contains similar elements for the two families, but in different proportions. The typical pictures for the various drug groups are described below.

## LSD SYNDROME

## Typical Sequence

The typical sequence of effects of LSD and similarly acting drugs includes three phases: somatic symptoms, perceptual symptoms, and psychic symptoms.

### Somatic symptoms

The first phase, beginning within minutes of the administration of an effective dose, includes a variety of subjective symptoms, such as dizziness, weakness, tremors, nausea, wakefulness, restlessness, and paresthesias, indicative of strong central stimulant action. Muscle tension and hyper-reflexia result in some degree of incoordination. Centrally produced sympathomimetic effects include pupillary dilatation, blurred vision, hyperthermia in some species, tachycardia, hyperglycemia, piloerection, and dry mouth. There is also a direct stimulatory effect on uterine muscle, reflecting the relation between LSD and the ergot alkaloids (see Chapter 44).

### Perceptual symptoms

These begin about an hour after ingestion of the drug and tend to be mainly visual. The first effect is fluctuation in the perceived brightness of illumination. Shapes become distorted and undulating; colours become brilliant, constantly varying in tone and intensity; and objects appear surrounded by coloured halos or rainbows. Distances between objects become confused. The body image becomes distorted, hands and feet may feel enormous, or the whole body may seem to be shrinking away. Sense of hearing is sharpened, and, occasionally, the senses become fused (synesthesia), for example, "the noise of water gushing from the faucet was transformed into optical illusions," or colours appear to have specific smells. With mescaline, there is a tendency to see geometric patterns, even with the eyes closed. The sense of time may become distorted; things seem to hang in suspended animation for a long time that, to an observer, is really only a few seconds. During this stage, there are often rapid mood changes, with the subject being happy, sad, irritable, meditative, or frightened at various times during the same drug experience; some degree of anxiety is almost universal.

### Psychic symptoms

At the peak of the experience, about 2 hours or more after ingestion of the drug, there is marked difficulty in expression of thoughts, a dream-like feeling, and difficulty in concentration on voluntary thought. At the same time, there is a tendency to fixation on specific stimuli and difficulty in moving the attention away from them. The visual illusions may lead into actual hallucinations. Depersonalization is common; the subject feels that the mind has left the body and is looking down on it from a distance. In this state, the users may feel that they are freed from their bodies and are becoming united with the whole universe, much as in a state of religious ecstasy obtained without drugs. In contrast, the same feeling of drifting away from one's concrete self may prove terrifying and give rise to panic or an acute psychosis. *The emotional reaction is strongly influenced by the setting and by other people present,* as well as by the user's personality, previous drug experience, expectations, and emotional state at the time of taking the drug.

## Psychological Effects

As with all hallucinogenic drugs, the content and nature of the experience depend strongly on the individual user.

The neurological and perceptual phenomena are probably the same in all subjects, but the way in which these effects are subjectively perceived differs widely. Aesthetically sensitive people place great emphasis on the beauty of the experience, while insensitive people experience mainly the mood changes. Artists refer to the effect of these drugs on creativity, but their artistic skills actually deteriorate greatly during the drug effect, so it is the memory or insight retained *after* the drug experience that may be relevant. This memory tends to be selective; most subjects remember only pleasant or beneficial aspects of the drug experience, while jitteriness, depression, hostility, auditory hallucinations, and paranoid delusions tend to be forgotten unless they are severe and threatening.

## Pharmacological Mechanisms

Small doses of LSD, mescaline, and related drugs cause increased frequency and desynchronization of the electroencephalogram (EEG), and they reduce the stimulation threshold of the midbrain reticular formation. This hyperarousal state resembles that produced by amphetamines and raises the possibility that sensory overload plays a role in the hallucinogenic effect. With larger doses, the EEG shows intermittent bursts of slow-wave high-voltage activity that appear to coincide with hallucinatory periods. Spontaneous electrical activity of the retina increases and its excitation threshold is lowered, but synaptic transmission in the lateral geniculate nucleus is partially impaired, and the cortical evoked potentials after visual stimuli are markedly altered. These findings suggest that the predominantly visual nature of the hallucinations is due to excessive input from the retina, coupled with incomplete transmission to the optic and association cortex. One functional consequence is that afterimages are prolonged, intensified, and fused ("palinopsia"), possibly contributing to the production of visual hallucinations. Effects on spinal reflexes are variable, but small doses tend to facilitate tendon reflexes and to inhibit polysynaptic reflexes.

Like LSD, MDMA appears to act on serotonergic nerve terminals, but it has a neurotoxic action on these terminals that is preventable by citalopram (a blocker of 5-HT uptake) or by SKF 525A (an inhibitor of cytochrome P450 activity), so the neurotoxicity may be due to a toxic metabolite of MDMA formed after uptake into the nerve terminals. The resulting decrease in 5-HT levels is thought to increase the effects of released dopamine.

## Molecular Mechanisms

As noted earlier, there is considerable evidence that LSD acts primarily at 5-HT receptors but also to some extent at dopamine and other receptors. However, the nature of the actions at these receptors is not entirely clear. Both the phenylethylamine and the indolealkylamine hallucinogens produce the same electrophysiological effects at the 5-HT$_2$ receptors: decreased spontaneous and evoked neuronal activity, prolonged post-activity inhibition, decreased resting K$^+$ conductance, and increased inositol 1,4,5-trisphosphate (IP$_3$) turnover; the net effect is increased excitability. LSD acts as an agonist or partial agonist at both 5-HT and dopamine receptors, but other evidence appears to support an antagonist action. For example, LSD decreases the turnover of both 5-HT and dopamine in some parts of the brain and increases it in others, but the non-hallucinogenic analogue lisuride has the same effects. Another analogue, 2-brom-LSD, inhibits the activity of 5-HT–containing neurons in the midbrain raphe nuclei, and pretreatment with 2-brom-LSD blocks the action of LSD, yet 2-brom-LSD has no hallucinogenic effect of its own. LSD stimulates dopamine receptors in the striatum, and this effect (as well as the hallucinogenic effect) is blocked by chlorpromazine, yet depletion of brain catecholamines does not block the effect of LSD and may even enhance it. These examples illustrate the complexity of interaction of the 5-HT and dopamine systems in the brain and underline the fact that the mechanism of action of LSD is not yet fully understood.

## Absorption, Distribution, and Biotransformation

All the commonly used drugs in this group are readily absorbed by mouth, except DMT, which must be injected, sniffed, or smoked. Effective doses vary widely; for example, for LSD, 2 µg/kg is usually quite potent in humans, while equivalent doses are 150 µg/kg for psilocybin and 5 mg/kg for mescaline. In part, this difference is due to distribution differences: mescaline is tightly bound to plasma proteins, and only a small proportion is free to diffuse into the tissues. In contrast, LSD is also largely protein-bound in the plasma, but the binding is loose and the drug passes rapidly into the tissues. This also affects duration of action; the half-life of LSD in humans is about 3 hours while that of mescaline is about 6 hours. With all of these drugs, the bulk of a given dose is found in the liver, spleen, kidneys, and adrenals, and only a minute fraction in the brain. However, LSD enters the brain rapidly, possibly by active transport. Within the brain, the highest concentrations are found in the pituitary, pineal gland (possibly in relation to 5-HT uptake sites), hypothalamus, limbic system, and visual and auditory relays.

Biotransformation occurs in the liver by routes that differ for each drug. LSD is converted chiefly (almost 90%) to its glucuronide, which is excreted mainly in the bile and a little in the urine; the remainder (10 to 12%) is oxidized to 2-oxy-LSD and a variety of other oxygenated or hydroxylated derivatives. Mescaline undergoes oxidative deamination to 3,4,5-trimethoxyphenylacetic acid. Psilocybin is dephosphorylated to psilocin, which is also active, but is in turn *N*-demethylated and oxidized to a hydroxyindole acetic acid.

## Tolerance and Cross-Tolerance

Tolerance develops rapidly to LSD on repeated use if the drug is taken at too short intervals. This is apparently due to down-regulation of 5-HT$_2$ receptors, which occurs within 2 to 3 days of repeated exposure to LSD; no withdrawal reaction has been reported. Cross-tolerance is then found to the other drugs in this group, but not to cannabis or amphetamine.

## Therapeutic Use

Shortly after the discovery of LSD, numerous attempts were made to facilitate or enhance insight in psychiatric patients by the administration of LSD. It was suggested that under the influence of the drug, repression of unwanted memories could be overcome and the patients would thus gain understanding of the nature and causes of their problems. Despite many early claims of benefit from this approach, a 10-year follow-up of patients treated in this way found no lasting improvement in outcome in comparison with patients not receiving LSD. This method is no longer used.

## LSD Toxicity

LSD has a very large margin of safety; no human fatality due to direct toxicity of the drug has been reported. The few known deaths were the result of accidents (e.g., falls, jumps) occurring during the hallucinated state.

The most common ill effects are psychological: "bad trips," or panic states, arising from the loss of contact with reality, may trigger serious psychotic breakdown in people with chronic emotional problems. The preferred symptomatic treatment for acute adverse reactions to all of these drugs is diazepam. Reserpine enhances the effects of all of them. "Flashbacks" are spontaneous (and usually frightening) sensations of being under the influence of LSD even though the person has taken none. They occur in regular users and can be triggered by cannabis in former LSD users. It is not known whether they are really a form of drug toxicity or are a conditioned behavioural response to subjective stimuli formerly experienced under the effects of the drug.

Chromosome damage, leukemia, and teratogenic effects have been reported in humans and other species exposed to LSD, but there are many contradictory reports, and the question is not settled. Women using LSD appear to have a higher proportion of spontaneous abortions, and their offspring have more chromosome breaks and more congenital anomalies than non-users. But the role of LSD is not clear, since other drugs, viral infections, and other incidental factors may have been important causative or contributing factors.

## SALVINORINS

The salvinorins are a family of closely related compounds derived from the leaves of a Mexican variety of *Salvia* ("magic mint"). They are of interest primarily because they differ from the LSD-like drugs in their mechanism of action, despite having hallucinogenic effects that resemble those of LSD. Of the salvinorins so far isolated, salvinorins A and D-F are hallucinogenic, and salvinorin A is the best studied. It is almost as potent a hallucinogen as LSD itself, and like LSD, it has very little toxicity otherwise.

Salvinorin A can be used by chewing the fresh leaves, squeezing the juice from the leaves and sipping it, or smoking the dried leaf material. When taken by mouth, salvinorin A is absorbed across the buccal mucosa, and the degree of effect is proportional to the length of time it is left in the mouth (when swallowed, it is destroyed in the gastrointestinal tract). An effective human dose by this route is 200 µg or more, compared with 50 to 250 µg for LSD. The first effects appear within 5 to 10 minutes, build up to a plateau lasting about an hour, and fade away over the next hour. In contrast, when it is smoked, or the vapour is inhaled, the onset of action occurs in about 30 seconds, the peak is reached in 5 to 10 minutes, and the effect disappears over the next 20 to 30 minutes.

Unlike the LSD-like drugs, salvinorin A contains no N atom, and it has no affinity for 5-HT$_{2A/2C}$ receptors. It is a diterpene (see Fig. 26-3), and it binds selectively to the κ-opioid receptor (see Chapter 19), at which it is a potent and complete agonist. Like other κ agonists, it has analgesic activity (determined by the tail-flick test), which is blocked by naloxone and which does not occur in κ receptor knockout mice. The pattern of psychoactivity includes visions of people, objects, places, and surface patterns such as films or membranes. The user often experiences sensations of turning into an object, of revisiting the past, or of being in several different places at the same time. At high doses (1 mg or more), there may be the feeling of loss of identity, or depersonalization, and the user may get up and move around aimlessly or laugh hysterically.

Although experienced users find the pattern of effects different from that of LSD, the numerous resemblances despite the completely different mechanism of action indicate that our understanding of the mechanism(s) of hallucinogenic action is still incomplete.

## AMPHETAMINES, COCAINE, AND OTHER CNS STIMULANTS

### Amphetamines

#### Pharmacology

The amphetamines (amphetamine itself, and methamphetamine) and related compounds are strong central

FIGURE 26-3  Structural formula of salvinorin A, a diterpene hallucinogen that binds to the opioid κ receptor and has analgesic action.

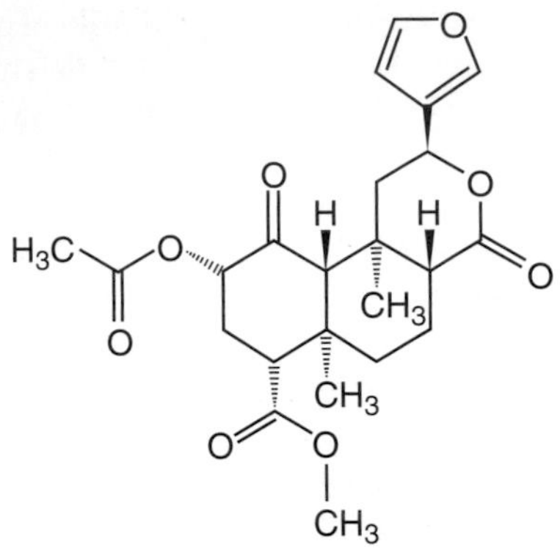

nervous system (CNS) stimulants that are related, both chemically and pharmacologically, to noradrenaline (see Fig. 26-2). Amphetamine has an asymmetric carbon, so optical isomers, *d*- and *l*-forms, exist (Fig. 26-4). While both forms are active peripherally, only the *d*-form (Dexedrine) is a central stimulant. Methamphetamine differs from amphetamine only in the presence of a methyl group on the amino terminus, which makes it somewhat more lipophilic than amphetamine and therefore a little faster in entering the brain. However, it is virtually identical to amphetamine in most respects.

These drugs are sympathomimetics, which act by causing the release of noradrenaline and dopamine from their storage sites in catecholaminergic nerve terminals. Amphetamine also appears to have some direct agonist effect on postsynaptic receptors and a weak inhibitory effect on monoamine oxidase. It has peripheral effects on the heart, gastrointestinal motility, blood vessels, and pupil similar to those of ephedrine and other sympathomimetic drugs (see also Chapter 13). In the CNS, *d*-amphetamine causes a higher turnover rate and a reduced content of catecholamine neurotransmitters. The resulting noradrenergic hyperactivity is probably responsible for the marked increase in wakefulness, alertness, speed of response, hyper-reflexia, and amount of voluntary activity. In normal individuals, this often leads to feelings of well-being or even euphoria and of increased energy and capacity for work. With overdose, however, mental processes are speeded up so much that the subject becomes submerged in a flood of thought associations, and the attention jumps rapidly and ineffectually from one thought to another, as in manic psychosis.

Dopaminergic hyperactivity is believed to be responsible for the reinforcing effect (see Chapter 69) but also for a different set of effects, including stereotypy (continuously repeated, purposeless movements), paranoid ideas, and

hallucinations. All of these effects have been produced experimentally in human volunteers by the administration of large doses of amphetamine, and they were blocked by phenothiazines or butyrophenones. The picture can be mistaken for paranoid schizophrenia.

## Medical and other uses

Amphetamine was originally developed as a substitute for ephedrine to raise the blood pressure if hypotension occurred during surgical anaesthesia. Its vasoconstrictor properties also led to its use as a nasal decongestant. For both of these uses, it has been replaced by newer sympathomimetics with less central effect.

In many activities, amphetamines will delay the onset of mental and physical fatigue, and they are sometimes used to **enhance performance**—for example, by soldiers on forced marches, by truck drivers on long overnight drives, by students "cramming" for examinations, or by athletes striving for peak performance. In rare situations, such as a temporary emergency, this use may be justified, but in the other cases mentioned, it can be very danger-

**FIGURE 26-4**  Structural formulae of amphetamines and related compounds.

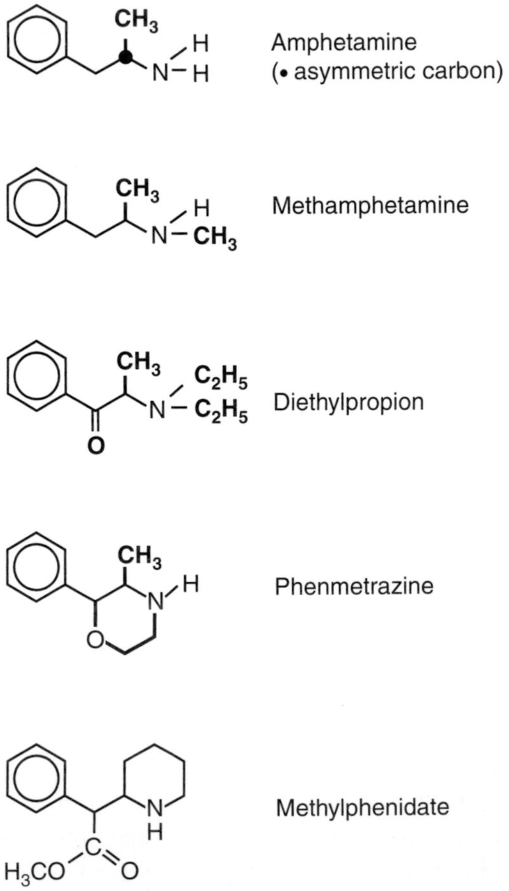

ous. *It maintains performance not only by maintaining wakefulness, but also by diminishing the awareness of fatigue,* which normally warns a person that reserve strength is nearly exhausted. Therefore, the subject may push the exertion to the point of serious damage or even death.

In neurology, the main use of the amphetamines is for treatment of **narcolepsy**, a disease of unknown cause characterized by sudden attacks of sleep occurring in completely inappropriate situations. Large doses of amphetamine, as much as 30 to 200 mg/day, depending on the frequency of attacks, are quite effective. Because of its dopamine-releasing action, which occurs in the striatum as well as in other locations, amphetamine is also useful as a supplementary therapy in some cases of Parkinson's disease (see Chapter 17).

Amphetamine-type drugs, especially methylphenidate (Ritalin), are also widely used in the treatment of behavioural disorders in children. They reduce the restlessness, hyperactivity, and impairment of sustained attention in **hyperkinetic children** (i.e., those with attention deficit hyperactivity disorder, ADHD). There is no adequate explanation for this apparently paradoxical effect of these drugs. However, barbiturates are also known to produce an opposite effect in these children (i.e., hyperactivity rather than sedation) and further aggravate the condition. It has been reported that all children show sedation with amphetamines, but that the effect is more obvious in hyperkinetic children. There is considerable argument about the long-term value of amphetamine-like drugs in the treatment of hyperkinetic children.

In psychiatry, these drugs are sometimes used to **raise the mood and activity** of certain depressed lethargic patients. However, stimulation of the reticular activating system only guarantees an increase in mental activity, not necessarily a change in mood, and cases have been recorded of depressed inert patients who were roused by amphetamines to the point that, instead of remaining inert, they committed suicide. This risk is not confined to the amphetamines. The U.S. Food and Drug Administration issued a warning concerning increased risk of suicidal thoughts and actions in depressed patients treated with the SSRI paroxetine (see Chapter 25). Atypical reactions to the amphetamines are by no means rare: some patients become acutely anxious and irritable; some become relaxed and drowsy. Therefore, these drugs should be used only under close supervision.

By far the most common use was formerly as an aid in losing weight. Amphetamine causes anorexia by some central nervous action that is not fully understood and thus helps people to adhere to a reducing diet. Amphetamine itself is no longer permitted to be used for this purpose. It was replaced by newer drugs such as **diethylpropion** (amfepramone; Tenuate, M-Orexic), **phenmetrazine** (see Fig. 26-4), and **phentermine** (e.g., Ionamin, Fentrol). Although these are merely modifications of amphetamine, they have somewhat less peripheral sympathomimetic action; however, they are basically similar and have correspondingly similar dangers. (For this reason, phenmetrazine was withdrawn from the market, although the closely related phendimetrazine is still sold in the United States.)

## Absorption, distribution, and elimination

Amphetamines are readily absorbed from the gastrointestinal tract, so they can be administered orally as well as parenterally. They are sufficiently lipid-soluble (in the non-ionized form) to cross cell membranes readily, including the blood–brain barrier, so they distribute rapidly to all tissues. Biotransformation occurs almost entirely in the liver, and several different pathways are involved: hydroxylation of the phenyl ring, *N*-demethylation (in the case of methamphetamine and related drugs), deamination, and conjugation reactions. The metabolites, as well as an appreciable fraction of the unchanged drug, are excreted in the urine. Because of the numerous different reactions involved, the half-life of drug in the plasma shows considerable variation between individuals, but it is usually in the range of 12 to 18 hours.

## Side effects and toxicity

When these drugs are given for one purpose, the other usual actions constitute the principal side effects: for example, when they are given as a mental stimulant, anorexia is considered a side effect, and vice versa.

When death occurs from poisoning, it is by excessive sympathomimetic activity, resulting in hypertension, severe tachycardia and collapse, hyperpyrexia, delirium, and convulsions.

The two main non-lethal risks are (1) psychic dependence and tolerance, and (2) psychotic episodes. Dependence was much more common than physicians first realized when the drugs were widely used for treatment of obesity or mild depression. Psychotic episodes usually occur after repeated intake of large amounts and closely resemble paranoid schizophrenia, for which they have been mistaken. Tolerance may be very marked; some addicts take hundreds of milligrams daily. (The normal dose is 5 mg of *d*-amphetamine, two to three times daily.) The drug is largely excreted in the urine for a day to a week or more after the last ingestion, depending on the amount taken. Disappearance from the body is thus gradual, and withdrawal symptoms are relatively mild, consisting of profound sleepiness and depression and a huge rebound in appetite.

## Amphetamine syndrome

In high doses, amphetamines give rise to an acute psychotic picture with hyperactivity, anxiety, paranoid delusions, and auditory and tactile hallucinations, but with clear consciousness and little or no disorientation. This last point differentiates the picture from that of the delirium produced by atropine-like drugs (see "Atropine Syndrome" below). The picture is differentiated from that of the LSD group by the prominence of paranoid ideas and the predominance of auditory and tactile rather than visual hallucinations. Moreover, amphetamine-induced hallucinations are more a matter of misinterpretation than of distorted perception. Stereotyped behaviour is a common finding and is probably related to dopamine release by amphetamine.

Intravenous injection of amphetamine (also known as "speed") greatly increases the rate of onset and intensity of effects. Experiments in human volunteers produced typical amphetamine psychoses in 2 to 3 days, as compared with weeks or months with oral use.

After the drug is stopped, the psychotic picture usually clears rapidly at a rate that depends directly upon the speed of elimination of the drug from the body. The rate can be increased by acidification of the urine, which increases the degree of ionization of the N atom and thus reduces the reabsorption of amphetamine in the renal tubule. However, in some instances, a frank schizophrenic state is precipitated by the drug use in persons already close to clinical breakdown, and in such cases, the symptoms may continue even after the drug is totally eliminated.

In addition to the amphetamine toxicity already mentioned, death also may result from opportunistic complications of intravenous injection, such as viral hepatitis, necrotizing angiitis, acquired immunodeficiency syndrome (AIDS), or septicemia. However, most deaths in amphetamine users are due to violence—accident, suicide, or murder related to aggressiveness and abnormal behaviour while "high."

## MDMA ("Ecstasy") and Related Drugs

Despite the many common features, other drugs in the group of phenylalkylamine and indolealkylamine hallucinogens do show some differences from both amphetamine and LSD. One of the most widely used is MDMA (3,4-methylenedioxy-methamphetamine), an amphetamine derivative that is commonly called ecstasy (see Fig. 26-2). A closely related drug, MDEA, or 3,4-methylene-dioxy-ethamphetamine (also called ecstasy, but more commonly called "Eve"), has an ethyl rather than a methyl substituent on the amino terminus, but it is virtually identical to MDMA in its actions. The methylenedioxy group gives them some resemblance to the properties of mescaline. Like both LSD and amphetamine, these drugs increase the release of catecholamines from dopamine and noradrenaline nerve terminals and block the reuptake of serotonin, so the net release of all three monoamines is increased.

These drugs have become very popular in many countries, mainly among young people attending "raves" or all-night dance parties, because they produce an initial rush of energy and alertness, starting between 20 and 60 minutes after ingestion. The users thus postpone fatigue and are able to dance for hours. This initial stage is later followed by a period of calm, decreased anger and hostility, greater sociability, and increased sensory awareness but without visual distortions; this phase may last for several hours.

### Pharmacokinetics

MDMA is well absorbed by mouth. A typical oral dose of about 100 mg produces a peak plasma concentration of about 150 to 200 ng/mL approximately 2 hours after ingestion. It passes easily into the tissues, including the liver, where CYP2D6 and other enzymes convert it to at least 14 metabolites. One of these, MDA, is also active as a hallucinogen. The elimination half-life of MDMA is about 8 hours, so the drug can be detectable in the plasma and urine for up to 2 days after its ingestion.

### Adverse effects

Like amphetamine, MDMA increases both mental and physical tension and can cause anxiety, jaw clenching, tooth grinding, and muscular pain in the lower back and limbs. This may be partly due to the excessive strenuous muscular activity during raves. MDMA also causes tachycardia and hypertension, which are followed by cardiovascular lability for a day or two after use of the drug. The drug itself, together with the strenuous muscular activity in a hot environment, can raise the body temperature to dangerous levels (hyperthermia) and cause profuse sweating and loss of sodium. If the users drink large amounts of water without salt replacement, the resulting hemodilution can cause cerebral edema and seizures. Hyperthermia can cause acute liver cell damage as well as muscle cell necrosis (rhabdomyolysis) and release of myoglobin into the circulation. Myoglobin is toxic to the renal tubules, so renal failure has also been reported. Another effect of hyperthermia is intravascular clumping of platelets, giving rise to microembolism as well as to reduced clotting ability and thus to risk of hemorrhages. All of these mechanisms have caused numerous deaths among MDMA users.

An additional serious problem attributed to MDMA has been neurotoxicity to serotonergic cells and, to a lesser extent, to dopaminergic cells. The damage, which has been clearly demonstrated in experimental animals, is believed to be due to free radical formation by metabolism of the large amounts of 5-HT and dopamine released by the action of the drug. The resulting neuronal damage has been held responsible for depression, memory deficits, impaired mental functions, and other psychiatric problems in long-term heavy users of MDMA, although the causal role of the drug has not yet been clearly proven in humans.

## Cocaine

Cocaine was isolated from coca leaves in the 1850s, but clinical interest in it did not arise until 1884, when both its central stimulant and local anaesthetic actions were reported. It was at first recommended for the treatment of depression and morphine and alcohol dependence, but within a few years, it was recognized to give rise to dependence itself. It rapidly became popular among drug addicts (see Chapter 70) and eventually came under strict legal controls in most countries.

The pharmacology of cocaine is discussed in Chapter 21. The main points in the present context are that it is absorbed rapidly through the nasal mucosa, enters the CNS rapidly, inhibits the reuptake of noradrenaline and dopamine in catecholaminergic neurons by binding to the transporter in the presynaptic membrane, and thus gives rise to intense central stimulation. Cocaine is *almost identical to amphetamine* in its acute effects and its patterns of toxicity. Double-blind experiments in humans have shown that even experienced cocaine users have great difficulty in distinguishing between the two drugs after intravenous injection. The *main differences* are the following:

- Cocaine has a shorter duration of effect than amphetamine.
- Cocaine users have a lower incidence of the types of complication associated with intravenous use than amphetamine users do, since cocaine is usually sniffed or smoked (as "crack"; see below); instead, rhinitis and perforated nasal septum can occur.

The evidence about tolerance is ambiguous for cocaine, just as it is for amphetamine. With both drugs, tolerance occurs to some effects, such as anorexia, but it is not clear whether there is any tolerance to the hallucinatory and stereotypy effects, and there may even be sensitization.

Cocaine is biotransformed in several ways. The major reaction is hydrolysis of the ester linkage by the non-specific serum esterase, but substantial amounts are also hydroxylated by hepatic cytochrome P450 activity, yielding a reactive metabolite that is thought to be responsible for the small number of cases of serious hepatotoxicity resembling that caused by acetaminophen (see Chapter 43).

In recent years North America has seen a rapid increase in the use of a crudely prepared (and therefore inexpensive) cocaine in the free base form popularly known as "crack." This form, unlike the salts of cocaine, is volatile when heated. It can be volatilized directly by heating it on a piece of aluminum foil, or it can be mixed with tobacco in a cigarette or pipe, and, as the tobacco burns, the free cocaine base volatilizes because of the heat of the combustion zone. The cocaine vapour can be inhaled, and it is absorbed rapidly into the pulmonary circulation so that its central effects are experienced more rapidly. This is entirely analogous to the amphetamine free base that, being volatile, could be used in nasal inhalers and has a very rapid onset of effect, whereas the hydrochloride or sulfate salts are non-volatile, must be taken orally or by injection, and have much slower onset of action when swallowed.

# Modafinil (Provigil)

This drug was introduced as a treatment for the abnormal sleepiness that occurs in narcolepsy, shift work sleep disorder, and obstructive sleep apnea/hypopnea syndrome. It increases wakefulness and locomotor activity, increases speed of ideation and reactions, and produces elevation of mood or euphoria as amphetamine and other sympathomimetic amines do. The subjective sensations experienced by users of the drug (discriminative stimulus properties; see Chapter 69) resemble those produced by amphetamines, and the drug is also reinforcing, as shown by self-administration in monkeys (Chapter 69).

However, the mechanism of action of modafinil differs from that of the sympathomimetic amines and is still unknown. The structural formula of modafinil differs from those of amphetamine and its congeners, especially in the spatial relationship between the aromatic ring and the N atom. Modafinil is neither a direct- nor an indirect-acting agonist at either noradrenaline or dopamine receptors, and it does not produce typical catecholamine effects on the physiological or biochemical responses of circulatory and other systems. It binds to the dopamine reuptake transporter and increases the extracellular concentration of dopamine, but its arousal effect is not blocked by haloperidol, though it is attenuated by the $\alpha_1$-adrenergic receptor blocker prazosin (see Chapter 14). Modafinil also does not bind to the receptors for other neurotransmitters known to modify sleep–wake cycles, including serotonin, GABA, histamine, and melatonin.

## Pharmacokinetics

Modafinil is well absorbed by mouth despite its limited water solubility, and peak plasma concentration after a dose of 200 or 400 mg is reached in 2 to 4 hours. It is about 60% bound to plasma proteins, but does not displace bound warfarin or other drugs. About 90% of a dose is metabolized and excreted in the urine. There are several routes of biotransformation, but the two main metabolites are modafinil acid (produced by hydrolytic deamidation) and modafinil sulfone. Modafinil is a reversible inhibitor of CYP2C19 and therefore can increase the plasma levels of diazepam, phenytoin, and propranolol if given together with those drugs. On the other hand, it is an inducer of CYP3A4 when administered chronically and hence can decrease the circulating levels of other CYP3A4 substrates. The biotransformation of modafinil is slowed in severe liver disease.

## Adverse effects

The most frequent side effects that can lead to discontinuation of therapy are headache, nervousness, anxiety, insomnia, nausea, stomach upset, and diarrhea. In post-marketing surveillance, cases of mania and psychotic reaction have been reported, although the relationship to amphetamine-induced psychosis is not clear. Modafinil also differs from amphetamines in that no reports of drug dependence or of distinctive withdrawal reaction have yet appeared.

## ATROPINE SYNDROME

The pharmacology of anticholinergic drugs is described in Chapter 12. In the present context, the important point is that antimuscarinic agents that can cross the blood–brain barrier induce a toxic delirium that is deliberately sought by some people as another form of drug "high" and that can be mistaken for the effects of LSD-type drugs. The drugs include atropine, scopolamine, benactyzine, piperidyl benzylate esters, and a variety of crude belladonna preparations. The main features of the atropine syndrome are the following:

- Strong peripheral antimuscarinic effects (see Chapter 12)
- Much more severe disruption of thought processes than with LSD-type drugs
- Confusion, disorientation, and memory loss (the basis of the former use of these drugs in the so-called "twilight sleep" analgesia in obstetrics)
- Tactile, auditory, and visual hallucinations, including microhallucinations (vivid and brightly coloured images of tiny humans, animals, scenery, and so forth)
- Somnolence combined with restlessness, incoordination, and hyper-reflexia
- Hyperthermia, with dry, hot skin and flushing

The full-blown drug state may last for well over 24 hours, and residual effects may last for several days. Chlorpromazine does not relieve the symptoms and may even make them worse because phenothiazines and tricyclic antidepressants have some degree of atropine-like effect of their own. Treatment is usually symptomatic, using diazepam or some other sedative.

## PHENYLCYCLOHEXYLAMINE DERIVATIVES

These compounds, of which phencyclidine (PCP) was the first example, produce a mental state similar in some respects to that caused by the atropine group. However, there are some major differences in the clinical picture and a different basic action. They are chemically and pharmacologically related to the dissociative anaesthetic ketamine (Fig. 26-5).

### Pharmacological Effects

The pattern of peripheral autonomic effects of these drugs differs somewhat from that of atropine. Although they are predominantly antimuscarinic, phencyclidine tends to cause hypersalivation rather than the dryness of the mouth typical of atropine action. In addition, phenylcyclohexylamines have direct sympathomimetic action (e.g., they enhance the effect of noradrenaline on isolated gut preparations). They cause tachycardia, hypertension, and hyperthermia, as amphetamine does in high doses, and these effects can be life-threatening. Muscle tone is increased, sometimes to the point of rigidity, and the resulting heat production may contribute to the hyperthermia. At higher doses, the drugs cause hyper-reflexia and seizures. The EEG shows rhythmic spontaneous discharges in the parietal cortex and increased amplitude of sensory evoked responses.

**FIGURE 26-5** Structural formulae of ketamine and its phenylcyclohexylamine analogues. The thienyl ring in TCP is sterically equivalent to a phenyl ring.

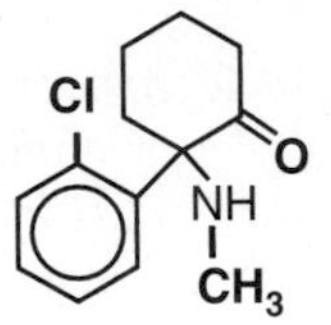

Ketamime

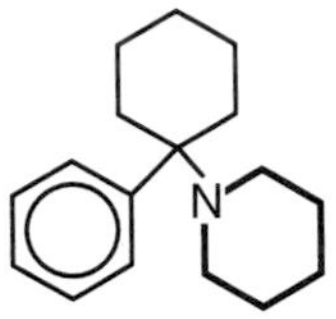

Phenylcyclohexyl-piperidine (PCP) (Phencyclidine)

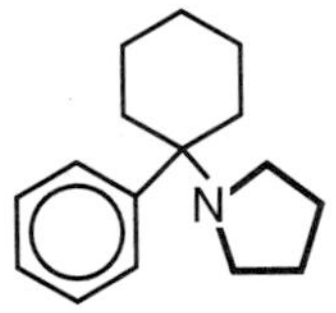

Phenylcyclohexyl-pyrrolidine (PHP)

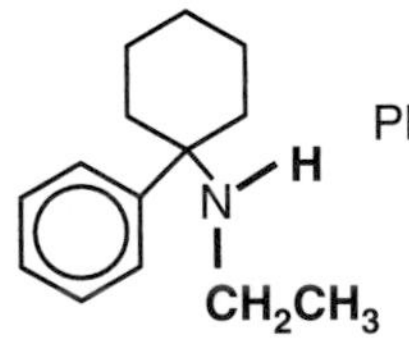

Phenylcyclohexyl-ethylamine (PCE)

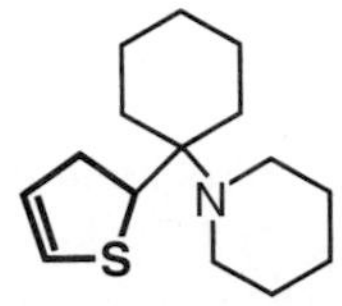

Thienylcyclohexyl-piperidine (TCP)

The behavioural effects of PCP and its congeners are characterized by restless, bizarre, repetitive movements (stereotypy), as well as by the analgesia and anaesthesia for which the drugs were clinically introduced. Ataxia and dysarthria are common, and the person appears drunk. Excitement, agitation, depression, euphoria, and dysphoria may alternate rapidly or even coexist. After a large dose, the person may not return to normal for up to 2 weeks. In addicts, PCP can cause a schizophrenia-like psychosis characterized by flattened affect, dissociative thought disturbances, depersonalization, catatonia, and long-lasting memory deficits; it can also exacerbate true schizophrenia.

## Mechanism of Action

Like the indolealkylamines, the phenylcyclohexylamines interact with multiple neurotransmitters. They are non-competitive blockers of the $Ca^{2+}$ channel associated with the NMDA type of glutamate receptor (see Chapter 16). This action is important in the hippocampus, resulting in marked impairment of memory and learning. These agents indirectly increase the firing rate of midbrain dopamine neurons, transiently increase dopamine output, and inhibit its uptake in the striatum. They also stimulate release and inhibit reuptake of noradrenaline in the nucleus accumbens and hypothalamus; the resulting increase in noradrenaline activity correlates well with the duration of motor hyperactivity. The increased dopamine activity causes a secondary increase in neurotensin levels in the striatum that is prevented by $D_1$ receptor blockers. PCP-like drugs are also much more potent inhibitors of 5-HT uptake. The stereotypy is reversed or prevented by dopamine blockers, but the motor hyperactivity is much more effectively blocked by clonidine, a presynaptic $\alpha_2$ receptor blocker. Many of the other effects are preventable only by administration of metabotropic glutamate receptor agonists combined with blockade of both $D_2$ and $5-HT_2$ receptors (e.g., by risperidone). It was formerly thought that the PCP receptor was identical to the $\sigma$ receptor (see Chapter 19). However, an irreversible blocker for $\sigma$ receptors had no effect on PCP receptor binding, and it is now thought that the $\sigma$ receptor modulates the NMDA receptor independently of the PCP binding site.

## Pharmacokinetics

PCP undergoes hydroxylation of the cyclohexyl ring in humans, and of all three rings in the rat. The 4-hydroxy derivatives are pharmacologically active. However, the hydroxy derivatives undergo subsequent conjugation reactions that inactivate them and allow them to be excreted in the urine. The biotransformation of other drugs may be affected by the fact that PCP itself suppresses the activity of CYP2C11 and CYP2D in the liver. PCP itself is highly lipid-soluble and accumulates in brain and fat,

where it persists for days or weeks. This may account for the slow return to normal after a large dose.

## CANNABIS

The hemp plant (Cannabis sativa) produces a series of related compounds called "cannabinoids," of which $l$-$\Delta^9$-tetrahydrocannabinol (THC) is the main psychoactive one (Fig. 26-6 on page 348). Cannabidiol (CBD) is another cannabinoid that occurs in relatively high concentration. It is not psychoactive, but it has other pharmacological activities that may find medical application in the future. THC and CBD are constituents of the resinous material that coats the immature flowering tops and also occurs at lower concentration in the upper leaves at a certain stage during the life of the plant. The dried leaf material is variously known in different parts of the world as "marijuana," "bhang," "ganja," "maconha," and various other names. The resinous material is known as "hashish," "kif," "charas," and so forth and is five to 10 times as potent as marijuana in terms of the THC content. In the past two decades, the average content of THC in marijuana sold in North America has increased from about 1 to 4% or more, and carefully selected and cloned plants yield as much as 15 to 20%. "Hash oil" is an extract of hashish made with ethanol or a lipid solvent and concentrated by evaporation of the solvent. The THC content varies widely depending on the starting material and the extraction technique; seized samples have ranged from 15 to 70% THC.

## Pharmacological Effects

At doses typically used by humans, cannabis produces a wide range of physiological effects. The most consistent are a dose-dependent increase in heart rate, congestion of the conjunctival blood vessels, and a tendency to orthostatic hypotension due to vascular smooth muscle relaxation. Bronchial and gastrointestinal smooth muscle is also relaxed, but there is as yet no agreement about a claimed anti-spasticity effect on skeletal muscle (see below under "Therapeutic Uses of Cannabinoids") that appears to be produced partly by central and partly by peripheral action. Intraocular pressure is reduced, but the mechanism is not yet clear. High concentrations of THC also decrease immune functions of macrophages, lymphocytes, and natural killer cells (see Chapter 40).

In the CNS, cannabis functions essentially as a sedative. The EEG shows somewhat more persistent alpha rhythm of slightly lower frequency than normal. Cerebral blood flow is decreased by cannabis in inexperienced users; this may be an effect of anxiety rather than a primary pharmacological action. Both THC and CBD have anti-seizure activity resembling that of phenytoin (see Chapter 18). Cannabis and pure THC have significant analgesic activity, especially against neuropathic pain, and a centrally mediated anti-nausea and anti-emetic effect. Sensory acuity may be sharpened slightly. However, thinking is slowed and less accurate. Impairment of short-term memory is one of the most consistent findings; free recall is more impaired than recognition. Emotional reactions are more labile, and there is usually mild euphoria, talkativeness, laughter, and a subjective feeling of relaxation. These changes are very similar to those found with mild alcohol intoxication, but cannabis does not appear to disinhibit aggressive behaviour, as alcohol often does.

In experimental animals, THC displaces the dose–response curves for ethanol and PCP to the left (sensitization) in tests of response rate and accuracy of performance on complex schedules of food-reinforced responding (see Chapter 69). Similarly, in humans, driving skills are impaired (e.g., decreased alertness, shorter attention span, longer response latency, decreased accuracy of motor responses), and the effects are at least additive with those of alcohol. A growing number of studies in various countries have shown increased risk of involvement in motor vehicle accidents and fatalities in drivers under the influence of cannabis. In the early stages of cannabis action there may be synergism with amphetamine, but later there is usually drowsiness and synergism with benzodiazepines and other sedatives. Part of this effect may be due to CBD (rather than THC itself), which can impair the biotransformation of THC and a number of other drugs by microsomal enzymes in the liver.

After very high doses of THC (i.e., 400 µg/kg or more in humans), there are effects similar in some ways to those of mescaline and LSD, including marked distortion of time and space perception, altered body image, depersonalization, auditory and visual hallucinations, transcendental or panic reactions, and even acute psychotic episodes. Visual hallucinations tend to be more of the reverie or daydream type, rather than abstract forms and colours. Ataxia can occur, with selective impairment of polysynaptic reflexes.

The mechanism of action is not yet fully known but has been greatly clarified in recent years. THC binds stereospecifically to a receptor, designated $CB_1$, that is found in high density in the cerebral cortex, hippocampus, and striatum and in moderate density in parts of the hypothalamus, amygdala, central grey, and laminae I to III and X of the spinal cord. A second type of receptor, termed $CB_2$, is found only in the periphery, in vascular smooth muscle, splenic macrophages, and in various cells of the immune system. Both receptors are G protein–linked, decrease adenylyl cyclase activity, inhibit N-type calcium channels, and disinhibit $K^+_A$ channels. The endogenous ligands for the CB receptors are several lipid materials derived from arachidonic acid (compare with prostaglandins, Chapter 27), known as **endocannabinoids.** These include arachidonylethanolamine (anandamide; see Fig. 26-6), 2-arachidonoylglycerol, 2-arachidonoylglyceryl ether, O-arachidonoylethanolamine, and possibly others. They are found in many parts of the CNS, in sites where the CB receptors are located, are formed in situ from constituents of the cell membrane in response to stimulation of the neurons, and are degraded rapidly by local esterases. They appear to function as neurotransmitters or neuromodulators in a wide variety of neuronal pathways. Selective competitive antagonists against THC at the $CB_1$ and $CB_2$ receptors have been synthesized and have helped greatly to elucidate the normal functions of the receptors and the mechanisms of action of THC and the endocannabinoids.

Activation of the $CB_1$ receptor increases the firing rate of dopamine neurons in the ventral tegmental area and the release of dopamine from dopamine terminals in the nucleus accumbens. The increased release of dopamine may be due to disinhibition (i.e., inhibition of an inhibitory neuron that decreases dopamine release). The effect on dopamine release is believed to be linked to the reinforcing effects of cannabis (see Chapter 69). The actions of cannabis are more complex, however, and probably involve interactions with several different neurotransmitters. There is evidence, for example, that modulation of dopamine activity is involved in the effects of cannabis on response latency (see "Pharmacological Effects" above), whereas 5-HT is involved in its effects on stimulus differentiation, and interaction with endogenous opioids is involved in the analgesic action of cannabinoids, even though the cannabinoids do not act directly via opioid receptors.

The effects of cannabis are different from those of other hallucinogens: there is neither discriminative stimulus generalization nor cross-tolerance with either the LSD-like or the amphetamine-like drugs. Some tolerance develops on regular use of high doses of cannabis, but not uniformly to all its effects.

## Pharmacokinetics

THC is highly lipid-soluble and is absorbed rapidly across the alveolar and capillary membranes when cannabis smoke is inhaled, so the onset of drug action is rapid. It is less well absorbed by mouth, and equivalent intensity of effects requires about three times as large an oral dose as an inhaled one. Absorption from the rectum is better than by mouth. THC is converted rapidly to 11-hydroxy-THC in the liver, especially by first-pass metabolism after oral administration, but this metabolite is also pharmacologically active so the drug effect outlasts measurable THC levels in the blood. The principal inactive metabolite is 11-nor-9-carboxy-THC, which is excreted in both the urine and the feces. Because of its lipid solubility, measurable amounts of THC persist in body fat for days after a single dose. This slow phase of elimination has a half-life of about 56 hours in humans, and urine tests for the carboxy metabolite may remain positive for 2 to 3 days after use of cannabis on a single occasion.

## Chronic Toxicity

The best-documented adverse effect of chronic heavy use of cannabis by humans is bronchopulmonary irritation caused by the inhalation of cannabis smoke. Cannabis smoke has a higher tar content than most tobacco smoke, and the tar contains a higher percentage of known irritants and procarcinogens. Chronic heavy smokers of cannabis, therefore, have a high incidence of **chronic bronchitis** with increased airway resistance and impaired gas exchange. Most cannabis users are also tobacco smokers, and the observed effects of cannabis are at least additive with those of tobacco smoke. Precancerous changes have been found in bronchiolar epithelium after only a few years of daily smoking of hashish or marijuana, and a number of cases of bronchopulmonary cancer have been reported in heavy cannabis smokers at a much earlier age than is usual for tobacco-induced cancer. One epidemiological case–control study found that chronic cannabis smokers have a higher risk of developing upper airway cancer than non-smokers do, and the increase in risk is proportional to the total exposure to cannabis smoke.

Chronic heavy users of cannabis often exhibit a condition of mental slowing, loss of memory, difficulty with abstract thinking, loss of drive, and emotional flatness. This picture probably represents a chronic intoxication state, and in most cases, it clears gradually when use of the drug stops. In some cases, however, the symptoms remain long afterward, and they may be indicative of organic brain damage analogous to that seen in severe alcoholics. It is possible that malnutrition, injury, infections, or concurrent use of other drugs may contribute to this picture. However, experimental studies in rats have shown that daily administration of cannabis alone, in moderately heavy doses for 3 months, does not impair general health but does cause long-lasting or permanent impairment of learning of a type resembling that caused by hippocampal damage.

Studies in experimental animals and in humans have shown decreased output of gonadotropic hormones, reduced serum testosterone level, low sperm count in males, and anovulatory cycles in females as a result of daily use of cannabis during a period of several weeks. However, tolerance appears to develop to these effects.

**Chromosomal damage** has been reported in leukocyte cultures from regular cannabis users. As in the case of LSD, the information is so far inconclusive. This also applies to reports of **impaired immune responses** in cannabis users, although experimental studies in animals and in cells in vitro have confirmed that cannabis at high concentrations does indeed depress T-lymphocyte function.

Psychiatric problems consist mainly of short-duration **psychotic episodes** characterized by severe anxiety or panic provoked by high-dose effects on perception. These usually respond rapidly to reassurance and sedation with benzodiazepines, although they occasionally last for several days or weeks. A more serious problem is the precipitation of relapse of true endogenous psychosis (schizophrenia) in patients who were previously compensated or borderline. This has been found repeatedly in well-structured large-scale epidemiological studies. Recent large-scale studies in several countries have also shown increased prevalence of depression and sociopathic behaviour in young heavy users of cannabis, though it is not yet clear whether the cannabis use is a causal factor in these mental problems.

Newborn infants of mothers who smoke cannabis regularly during pregnancy tend to be small for their age and show chronic hyper-irritability and poor feeding for several months after birth. By the time they reach school age, their physical development is normal, but they tend to show mild deficits in verbal learning, memory, problem solving, and impulse control that persist throughout the school years and into young adulthood.

## Therapeutic Uses of Cannabinoids

Cannabis extracts were used extensively in the nineteenth and early twentieth centuries, on medical prescription, as sedatives, hypnotics, and "tonics," but their variability of composition and their limited shelf life made them unreliable, and they were replaced by pure synthetic drugs of known composition and more reliable potency. In recent years, there has been a revival of interest in the possible use of cannabis and of pure cannabinoids for a number of other purposes, including relief of nausea and vomiting, anorexia, pain, epilepsy, glaucoma, spasticity, migraine, and Tourette's syndrome. The first of these applications to find some measure of medical acceptance is the treatment of nausea and vomiting due to anti-AIDS and anti-cancer chemotherapy and to radiation therapy in a small number of cases that do not respond to conventional anti-emetic medications. Oral capsules containing **dronabinol** (Marinol), a synthetic preparation of pure THC, are approved for this purpose in Canada and the United States. THC has also been tested and approved as an agent for improving appetite and promoting weight gain in patients with anorexia and tissue wasting caused by AIDS or advanced malignancy. Conversely, the synthetic $CB_1$ antagonist **rimonabant** (SR 141716A) reduces appetite and helps weight reduction in obesity; it has undergone clinical trials and is at present being reviewed for official approval.

Numerous basic and clinical studies have demonstrated that cannabis extracts or THC have a reproducible analgesic effect that is sufficiently strong to be useful for treatment of pain. THC has also been claimed to relieve muscle spasms in multiple sclerosis, but other studies have failed to confirm significant benefits; it has not been shown to produce significant objective reduction of muscle tension, but it does appear to provide subjective relief, which may be a reflection of its analgesic action. THC is not yet approved for use in treatment of spasticity. Cannabis smoke has not proven useful in the treatment of

**FIGURE 26-6** Structural formulae of anandamide (an endogenous ligand for the cannabinoid receptor), $\Delta^9$-tetrahydrocannabinol (THC), and two synthetic analogues, nabilone and levonantrodol, that have THC-like activity. Dexanabinol (HU-210) is a synthetic analogue that lacks THC-like psychoactivity but has potent analgesic and anti-inflammatory actions.

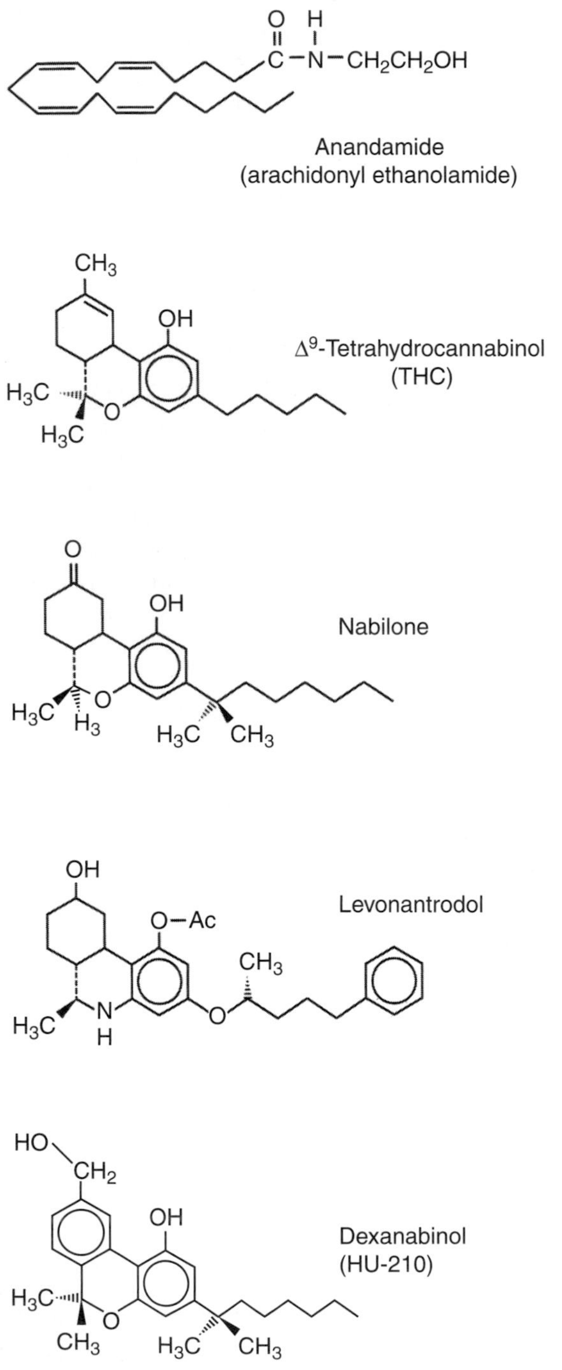

asthma because the chronic inflammatory effect of the smoke quickly overcomes the acute bronchodilatory action of THC. Similarly, the lowering of intraocular pressure by THC has not been clinically useful in treating glaucoma because the action must be maintained throughout the 24-hour period to prevent optic nerve damage, and it has not been possible to separate the ocular activity from the psychoactivity, so the patient would have to be constantly intoxicated in order to gain any benefit to the eye.

When cannabinoids are used for these purposes, most patients find the psychoactive effects undesirable. Therefore, there has been interest in developing modified cannabinoids with greater selectivity of action. **Nabilone** (Cesamet), a 9-keto derivative of THC with a modified side chain (see Fig. 26-6), is about 10 times as potent as THC but very similar in its actions, except that it may have relatively slightly less psychoactive effect. **Levonantrodol,** another synthetic modification of THC (see Fig. 26-6) that can be given parenterally as well as orally, is also under study. None of these agents appears to have any major therapeutic role at present, but the recent advances in the pharmacology of the cannabinoids and cannabinoid receptors may lead to more useful drugs in the future. For example, dexanabinol (see Fig. 26-6) is not a $CB_1$ receptor ligand and lacks psychoactivity but has a potent neuroprotective effect against traumatic and hypoxic brain injury that has been attributed to its ability to inhibit release of tumour necrosis factor $\alpha$. Another synthetic derivative of THC, known as ajulemic acid, has potent anti-inflammatory and analgesic activity with much less psychoactivity than THC. Both of these agents are currently being studied clinically. Other methods of administering cannabinoids that do not involve combustion and the production of smoke are also being explored. Sativex, a **standardized extract of cannabis** containing THC and CBD in 1:1 ratio, has recently been approved in Canada for treatment of neuropathic pain. It is administered from a "puffer" that sprays a metered dose on to the buccal mucosa or under the tongue.

## SUGGESTED READINGS

Adams IB, Martin BR. Cannabis: pharmacology and toxicology in animals and humans. *Addiction.* 1996;91:1585-1614.

Asghar K, De Souza E, eds. *Pharmacology and Toxicology of Amphetamine and Related Designer Drugs.* NIDA Research Monograph 94. Rockville, Md: National Institute on Drug Abuse; 1989.

Bock GR, Whelan J, eds. *Cocaine: Scientific and Social Dimensions.* CIBA Foundation Symposium No. 166. Chichester, United Kingdom: Wiley-Interscience; 1992.

Carrera MR, Meijler MM, Janda KD. Cocaine pharmacology and current pharmacotherapies for its abuse. *Biorgan Med Chem.* 2004;12:5019-5030.

Chavkin C, Sud S, Jin W, et al. Salvinorin A, an active component of the hallucinogenic sage salvia divinorum, is a highly efficacious kappa-opioid receptor agonist: structural and functional considerations. *J Pharmacol Exp Ther.* 2004;308:1197-1203.

Ellison G. The N-methyl-D-aspartate antagonists phencyclidine, ketamine and dizocilpine as both behavioral and anatomical models of the dementias. *Brain Res Rev.* 1995;20:250-267.

Gable RS. Comparison of acute lethal toxicity of commonly abused psychoactive substances. *Addiction.* 2004;99:686-696.

Green AR, Mechan AO, Elliott JM, et al. The pharmacology and clinical pharmacology of 3,4-methylenedioxymethamphetamine (MDMA, "ecstasy"). *Pharmacol Rev.* 2003;55:463-508.

Hall W, Solowij N, Lemon J. *The Health and Psychological Consequences of Cannabis Use.* National Drug Strategy, Monograph Series No 25. Canberra: Australian Government Publishing Service; 1994.

Hammer RP Jr, ed. *The Neurobiology of Cocaine: Cellular and Molecular Mechanisms.* Boca Raton, Fla: CRC Press; 1995.

Heym J, Jacobs BL. Serotonergic mechanisms of hallucinogenic drug effects. In: Marwah J, ed. *Neurobiology of Drug Abuse.* Frontiers of Neurology and Neuroscience. Vol 13. Basel, Switzerland: Karger; 1987:55-81.

Iversen L. Cannabis and the brain. *Brain.* 2003;126(pt 6):1252-1270.

Kalant H. Medicinal use of cannabis: history and current status. *Pain Res Manage.* 2001;6:80-91.

Kalant H. The pharmacology and toxicology of "ecstasy" (MDMA) and related drugs. *Can Med Assoc J.* 2001;165:917-928.

Kalant H, Corrigall WA, Hall W, Smart RG, eds. *The Health Effects of Cannabis.* Toronto, Ontario: ARF Books (CAMH); 1999.

Kalant OJ. *The Amphetamines—Toxicity and Addiction.* 2nd ed. Toronto, Ontario: University of Toronto Press; 1973.

Kalant OJ, trans-ed. *Maier's Cocaine Addiction [Der Kokainismus].* Toronto, Ontario: ARF Books; 1987.

Lin GC, Glennon RA, eds. *Hallucinogens: An Update.* NIDA Research Monograph 146. Rockville, Md: National Institute on Drug Abuse; 1994.

Pletscher A, Ladewig D, eds. *50 Years of LSD: Current Status and Perspectives of Hallucinogens.* New York, NY: Parthenon; 1994.

Schultes RE. Hallucinogens of plant origin. *Science.* 1969;163:245-254.

Siebert DJ. *Salvia divinorum* and salvinorin A: new pharmacologic findings. *J Ethnopharmacol.* 1994;43:53-56.

Swanson CJ, Schoepp DD. A role for noradrenergic transmission in the actions of phencyclidine and the antipsychotic and antistress effects of mGlu2/3 receptor agonists. *Ann NY Acad Sci.* 2003;1003:309-317.

# Part IV

## Mediators and Modifiers
## of Tissue Responses

# 27

# The Eicosanoids

## CR PACE-ASCIAK AND D KADAR

## Case 1

A 26-year-old woman was brought to the emergency department with gross edema of both legs and some cyanosis of the feet. She had started using oral contraceptives at the age of 16, but after using them for 9 months, she developed bilateral deep vein thrombosis and a small pulmonary embolus. At that time, she responded well to anticoagulant therapy and discontinuation of the contraceptive pills. At age 22, she had two spontaneous abortions, one at 9 weeks and one at 8 weeks. A third pregnancy was terminated at 30 weeks because of intrauterine death, and 2 weeks later, she developed left iliofemoral venous thrombosis despite being treated with heparin. Four weeks later, while she was still on heparin, a large thrombus was removed surgically from the lower aorta and both iliac and femoral arteries. She developed renal failure as a result of an extension of the thrombus into the renal arteries. Intravenous epoprostenol (prostacyclin) was therefore combined with the heparin, and her renal function improved progressively. After 6 weeks, both drugs were discontinued. For the past 2 years, she has been maintained on warfarin, aspirin, and dipyridamole and has remained asymptomatic.

## Case 2

A 55-year-old woman was brought to hospital with an 8-year history of Raynaud's phenomenon associated with intractable pain and ischemic skin ulcers of the extremities. She had sclerosis of the systemic arteries and nongangrenous digital ulcers. In addition, she had borderline hypertension (145/85 mmHg) and mild angina on effort. In the past, she had been treated with systemic as well as topical antibiotics to care for the ulcers, and nifedipine as a vasodilator, but the results had not been satisfactory.

On this admission, all other medications were discontinued for 24 hours, and she was then given alprostadil (in a solution of 1 mg/mL in 0.9% saline) by constant infusion pump through a central venous line. The initial rate of infusion was 6 ng/kg/min for 12 hours. As she experienced no adverse effects, the infusion rate was increased to 10 ng/kg/min for 60 hours. The blood pressure, pulse, and respiratory rate were monitored frequently. After 4 weeks, there was a remarkable improvement in the pain and increased warmth of the hands. Attacks of vasospasm were much less severe, and four of the five ulcers that she had on admission were healed. The treatment with alprostadil was repeated with the same dosage, and by 2 weeks later the remaining ulcer was healed. After discharge, she was followed up for a period of 18 months, during which time the Raynaud's symptoms remained much improved, and the cutaneous ulcers did not recur.

The eicosanoids (*eicosa*, Greek for twenty) constitute families of oxygenated products derived from 20-carbon-atom polyunsaturated fatty acids in which successive double bonds are separated by methylene groups. They are formed via three main oxidative pathways that utilize molecular oxygen as a co-substrate (Fig. 27-1). Products in these pathways possess a variety of biological activities and are believed to act as "local hormones," since they are rapidly inactivated in the circulation. The precursors of the eicosanoids are arachidonic, linoleic, linolenic, eicosapentaenoic, and docosahexaenoic acids, which are obtained from dietary sources.

Since arachidonic acid is the most abundant of the polyunsaturated fatty acids and products derived from

**FIGURE 27-1** Three major pathways for the biological oxidation of eicosanoid fatty acids.

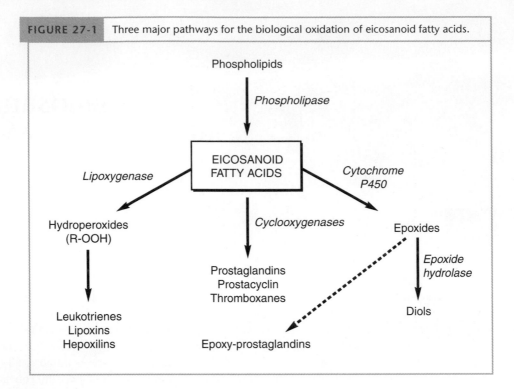

this fatty acid are the most investigated, the pathway of reactions is termed the **arachidonic acid cascade**.

## THE CYCLOOXYGENASE PATHWAY

Since their discovery in the early 1930s and their chemical identification in the early 1960s, considerable effort has been expended on the study of the biological properties and cellular importance of the eicosanoids derived from the cyclooxygenase pathway (Fig. 27-2).

### History

Prostaglandins (PGs; Table 27-1) were once believed to be the most potent pharmacologically active compounds known; however, the thermolabile prostaglandin endoperoxides ($PGG_2$ and $PGH_2$, with a half-life of 5 minutes) were isolated later and shown to be 50 to 200 times more potent than the prostaglandins in certain test systems. Prostaglandins were originally thought to be part of the seminal fluid from the prostate gland but were later shown to be more general; however, the name was retained.

A compound derived from the endoperoxides, isolated from human platelets and termed thromboxane $A_2$ ($TXA_2$), is also unstable (with a half-life of 30 seconds). Thromboxanes are not prostaglandins; they are named after a hypothetical "thrombanoic acid" with a six-member oxane ring. $TXA_2$ possesses 1000 times greater potency than the prostaglandins in inducing platelet aggregation and in contracting the isolated rabbit aorta. Prostacyclin

(prostaglandin $I_2$, or $PGI_2$) was isolated from eluates of the rat stomach fundus and the vascular endothelium along with prostaglandin endoperoxides and was found to oppose the actions of $TXA_2$ on platelets.

### Synthesis

The **prostaglandins** constitute a family of naturally occurring cyclopentane-containing straight-chain 20-carbon carboxylic acids of varying degrees of unsaturation. All "primary" prostaglandins contain the same carbon skeleton, termed **prostanoic acid,** from which stems the systematic numbering and naming of structures of biological origin and those derived through chemical synthesis. There are 10 groups of prostaglandins, designated A through J to indicate the differences in their molecular structures. The E and F classes are named according to whether a keto or a hydroxyl group, respectively, is present in the cyclopentane ring at the C-9 position; the D class is distinguished from the E class by having its keto group at the C-11 position instead of C-9. The number of double bonds in the alkyl side chains distinguishes members within each class and is indicated by subscript 1, 2, or 3 (see Fig. 27-2). Four subclasses, A, B, C, and J, are formed chemically in vitro by dehydration with either mild mineral acid or alkali.

All of the prostaglandins and related substances can be produced from free eicosatrienoic acid (1-series), arachidonic acid (2-series), and eicosapentaenoic acid (3-series), which are released from tissue glycerophospholipids by the enzyme phospholipase $A_2$ or by a combination of

**FIGURE 27-2** General structures of prostaglandins (PGs) and thromboxanes (TXs).

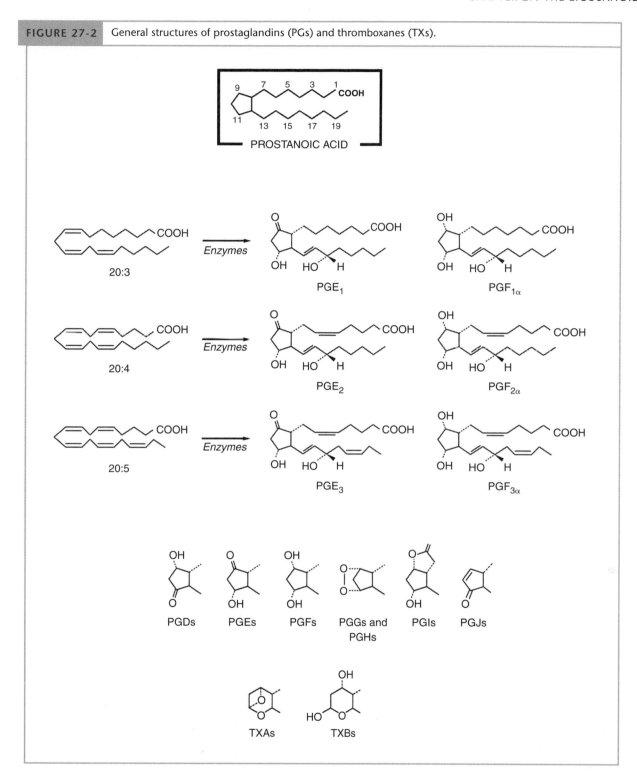

phospholipase C and glyceride lipase. The other essential enzymes in the synthesis of prostaglandins, prostacyclin, and thromboxanes are **cyclooxygenases** (COX). COX-1 (the predominant form) and COX-2 are sensitive to inhibition by steroids and non-steroidal anti-inflammatory drugs such as acetylsalicylic acid (ASA), indomethacin, meloxicam, and others. COX-1 is constitutively expressed in almost all cells. COX-2 is an inducible isoform, but it is also constitutively expressed in the kidney (macula densa, adjacent cortical thick ascending limb of the renal tubule, and glomerular podocytes) and the central nervous system (hypothalamus, thermoregulatory centre, and dorsal root ganglia). A splice variant of COX-1, designated COX-3, plays a significant role in the production of pain and

| TABLE 27-1 | Analogues of the Principal Prostaglandins in Clinical Use or Under Development | | | | |
|---|---|---|---|---|---|
| Prostaglandins | Alprostadil (PGE$_1$) | Dinoprostone (PGE$_2$) | Dinoprost (PGF$_{2\alpha}$) | Epoprostenol (Prostacyclin, PGI$_2$) | Synthetics |
| Analogues | Enisoprost | Arbaprostil | Carboprost | Beraprost | Nocloprost |
| | Gemeprost | Enprostil | Cloprostenol | Ciprostene | Rosaprostol |
| | Limaprost | Meteneprost | Fenprostalene | Iloprost | |
| | Mexiprostil | Sulprostone | Fluprostenol | OP-41833 | |
| | Misoprostol | Trimprostil | Luprostiol | | |
| | Ornoprostil | Viprostol | Prostalene | | |
| | Rioprostil | | Tiaprost | | |
| | | | Xalatan | | |

fever and is quite sensitive to inhibition by acetaminophen. Cyclooxygenases convert arachidonic acid to unstable cyclic **prostaglandin endoperoxides** (PGG$_2$ and PGH$_2$). The enzyme **prostaglandin endoperoxide isomerase** converts the endoperoxides to the prostaglandins PGD$_2$, PGE$_2$, and PGF$_{2\alpha}$. TXA$_2$ and PGI$_2$ are formed by the cytochrome P450 enzymes **thromboxane synthase** and **prostacyclin synthase,** respectively (Fig. 27-3). All these enzymes together are referred to as the **prostaglandin synthase complex** and are bound to the plasma membrane and/or endoplasmic reticulum of many types of cells. The synthesis of eicosanoids is stimulated by the release of arachidonic acid as a result of trauma to the cell membrane, antigen–antibody reactions, oxygen deprivation, changes in ion influxes, proteases such as thrombin, and hormones.

Although the prostaglandin synthase complex is ubiquitous, there is a considerable degree of tissue specificity in the occurrence of each of the pathways. Human platelets convert the endoperoxides into TXA$_2$, important for initiation of the "release reaction" and aggregation of platelets (see Chapter 38). The thromboxane synthase enzyme is also abundant in macrophages, lung, spleen, and brain, yet it is almost undetectable in many other organs, including heart, stomach, and liver. Prostacyclin synthase, a cytochrome P450 enzyme in the stomach wall smooth muscle and endothelial cells of blood vessels, converts endoperoxide to PGI$_2$, which opposes the action of TXA$_2$ (i.e., it inhibits platelet aggregation and potently lowers systemic arterial blood pressure). PGI$_2$ (half-life of 3 minutes) undergoes spontaneous hydration to the inactive 6-keto PGF$_{1\alpha}$ and is excreted in urine.

The kidney appears to contain enzymes that specifically convert the endoperoxides into PGD$_2$, PGE$_2$, and PGI$_2$. It is not yet known what endogenous factors channel the enzymatic activities to favour one pathway or another, but it should be quite possible to manipulate these transformations in the future with drugs that act specifically to block or activate one or several of these related and competing pathways to support adequate renal perfusion.

The whole sequence of prostaglandin synthesis is dependent on the availability of the precursor fatty acids in the free form, since phospholipid-bound fatty acid or the ester derivatives are not converted into prostaglandins. At the opposite end of the sequence, a specific NAD-dependent enzyme, 15-hydroxyprostaglandin dehydrogenase (15-PGDH), which is abundant in all tissues investigated, inactivates PGE$_2$, PGF$_{2\alpha}$, and PGD$_2$. This inactivation is rapid and extensive; for example, a single passage through the lungs inactivates over 90% of PGE$_2$. The metabolic products, mostly inactive, are then excreted into the urine.

## Enzymatic Sites of Drug Action

There are at least four stages at which drugs can influence the fate of products of the arachidonic acid cascade (Fig. 27-3).

1. Phospholipase step: liberation of arachidonic acid from phospholipids
2. Cyclooxygenase and lipoxygenase steps: conversion of arachidonic acid into the prostaglandin endoperoxides or HPETE precursors of leukotrienes, hepoxilins, and lipoxins
3. Prostaglandin endoperoxide catabolic step: channelling of the endoperoxides to TXA$_2$, PGE$_2$, PGF$_{2\alpha}$, PGD$_2$, or PGI$_2$
4. Catabolic step: termination of the biological activity of prostaglandins, prostacyclin, thromboxanes, and leukotrienes

The **corticosteroids** influence the arachidonic acid cascade by moderating the activity of phospholipase A$_2$ by inducing synthesis of the inhibitory protein lipocortin-1 (LC-1, or annexin-1) and by preventing the induction of COX-2 by interleukin-1. However, calcium, calmodulin, and vasoactive peptides such as bradykinin and angiotensin II activate the release of fatty acids, resulting in an enhancement of prostaglandin biosynthesis.

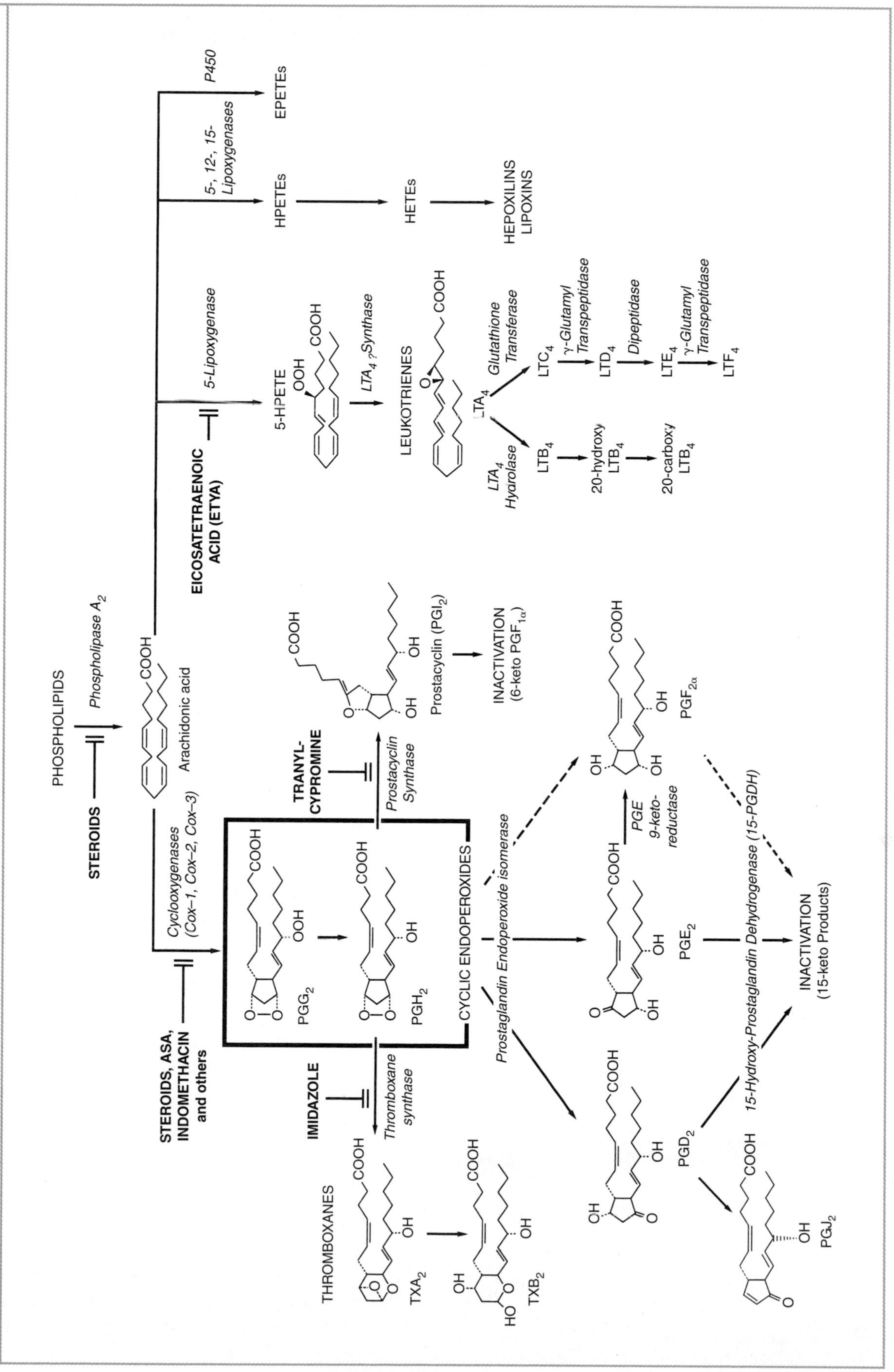

**FIGURE 27-3** Pathways in the eicosanoid fatty acid cascade (simplified). Some sites of inhibition by selected pharmacological agents are indicated by ||. (See text for explanation of abbreviations.)

The activities of COX-1 and COX-2 are inhibited by **non-steroidal anti-inflammatory drugs** (NSAIDs). Acetylsalicylic acid (ASA) and indomethacin inhibit both, but act preferentially on COX-1, whereas diclofenac and celecoxib preferentially inhibit COX-2. ASA inactivates the cyclooxygenase by irreversible acetylation of a serine residue in COX-1 and COX-2, but the other NSAIDs compete with arachidonic acid for the active site of the enzyme. The excess arachidonic acid may enhance the formation of leukotrienes because NSAIDs do not influence lipoxygenase activity. Imidazole and substituted derivatives inhibit thromboxane synthase. While cyclooxygenase is activated by hydroperoxides, prostacyclin synthase is destroyed by hydroperoxides and inhibited by tranylcypromine (a monoamine oxidase inhibitor). Phenylbutazone affects cyclooxygenase and prostaglandin endoperoxide isomerases as well.

It is quite obvious that drugs with a great deal of specificity for the individual pathways would be of immense benefit to the understanding of the functional importance of each pathway. Several such drugs that show selectivity as COX-2 inhibitors have become available for therapeutic use, with specific application to rheumatoid arthritis, osteoarthritis, dysmenorrhea, and acute post-surgical and post-dental extraction pain. They are celecoxib (Celebrex), rofecoxib (Vioxx), meloxicam (Mobicox), valdecoxib (Bextra), and parecoxib sodium (Paracoxib). Another analogue, etoricoxib, which is claimed to have greater selectivity for COX-2, is currently under clinical investigation. Rofecoxib, in 2004, and valdecoxib, in 2005, were removed from the market because large-scale studies revealed that they produce a significant increase in thrombosis, cardiovascular mortality, and other serious complications.

## Inactivation

Intravenously administered prostaglandins are rapidly inactivated, not only by 15-PGDH, but also by numerous other enzymes present in many tissues. The prostaglandin biotransformation products are finally excreted in the urine. Figure 27-4 illustrates some of these pathways. In humans, the major urinary product of $PGE_2$ is the 16-carbon dicarboxylic acid shown. These pathways are tissue- and species-specific, and the activity of several of these enzymes has been shown to change with age.

## THE LIPOXYGENASE PATHWAY

The lipoxygenase pathway involves the addition of molecular oxygen at one or the other of the double bonds of the polyunsaturated fatty acid via different site-specific enzymes (see Fig. 27-3). Different lipoxygenases are designated according to the site at which they insert molecular oxygen into the arachidonic acid molecule, with the formation of the corresponding hydroperoxyeicosatetraenoic

acid (HPETE). The most important products in humans are 5-HPETE, 12-HPETE, and 15-HPETE. These are unstable peroxides that yield their corresponding hydroxy derivatives (HETEs) or are converted to other biologically potent compounds.

Leukotriene (LT) biosynthesis starts with the transformation of 5-HPETE, the precursor, into the unstable triene $LTA_4$, which is converted into $LTB_4$ in polymorphonuclear leukocytes and into $LTC_4$ in mast cells. $LTD_4$, $LTE_4$, and $LTF_4$ are metabolites of $LTC_4$. Slow-reacting substance of anaphylaxis (SRS-A), first described in 1938 and later found to be released from guinea pig lungs upon antigen–antibody reaction, appears to be a mixture of $LTC_4$ and $LTD_4$.

Hepoxilins A and B, with a corresponding hydroxyl group at C-8 or C-10, respectively, and an epoxide at C-11 and C-12, are derived from 12-HPETE by intramolecular rearrangement to hydroxyepoxides. These products are inactivated via specific epoxide hydrolases to the corresponding inactive trihydroxy derivatives.

Metabolites of 15-HPETE with biological activity give rise to the lipoxins (LX), products that possess three hydroxyl groups at positions 5, 6, and 15 for LXA and positions 5, 14, and 15 for LXB.

## THE EPOXYGENASE PATHWAY

A cytochrome P450 monooxygenase system has been described that epoxidizes the double bonds of the precursor acid to form the corresponding mono-epoxide deriva-

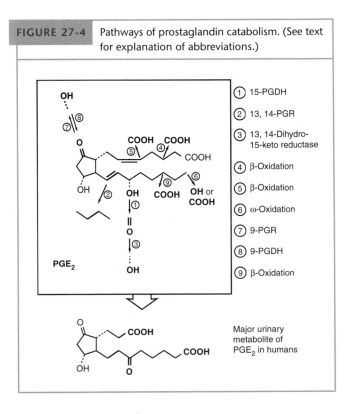

FIGURE 27-4    Pathways of prostaglandin catabolism. (See text for explanation of abbreviations.)

① 15-PGDH

② 13, 14-PGR

③ 13, 14-Dihydro-15-keto reductase

④ β-Oxidation

⑤ β-Oxidation

⑥ ω-Oxidation

⑦ 9-PGR

⑧ 9-PGDH

⑨ β-Oxidation

$PGE_2$

Major urinary metabolite of $PGE_2$ in humans

tives of the fatty acid (epoxy eicosatetraenoic acids, or EPETEs; see Fig. 27-3). These compounds may be involved in the maintenance of vascular tone, ion transport, cellular growth, signal transduction, hemostasis, and hematopoiesis. The epoxide products are transformed into the corresponding dihydroxy derivatives through the action of epoxide hydrolases.

# MECHANISM OF ACTION OF EICOSANOIDS

The eicosanoids act on distinctive cell membrane-bound G protein–coupled receptors that modify adenylyl cyclase activity or that activate phospholipase C and increase the formation of diacylglycerol and inositol trisphosphate, which brings about increased cytosolic calcium concentration and activates some forms of protein kinase C (see Chapter 9). At present, five main types and several subtypes of distinctive eicosanoid receptors are known. They are named after the eicosanoid with the highest affinity for them, the type of tissue they are found in, and the type of response elicited. These receptors are designated as DP ($PGD_2$), FP ($PGF_{2\alpha}$), IP ($PGI_2$), TP ($TXA_2$), and EP ($PGE_2$). The EP receptors have been further subdivided into $EP_1$, $EP_2$, $EP_3$, and $EP_4$, and the TP receptors into $TP_\alpha$ and $TP_\beta$. $PGG_2$, $PGH_2$, and $TXA_2$ initiate platelet aggregation by increasing calcium concentration, but $PGE_1$, $PGD_2$, and $PGI_2$ inhibit platelet aggregation by increasing cyclic-adenosine monophosphate (cAMP) concentration. In general, eicosanoid-induced calcium release causes contraction of smooth muscles (by stimulating myosin light-chain kinase), while increased cAMP generation causes relaxation (by activating protein kinase A, which phosphorylates intracellular $Ca^{2+}$ pumps, resulting in decreased intracellular $Ca^{2+}$). See Table 27-2 for a descrip-

tion of receptors, and Table 27-3 for two antagonists of the leukotriene family.

# BIOLOGICAL EFFECTS

The eicosanoids are formed when the phospholipases or other lipases are activated in a tissue. This activation can result from the action of a physiological stimulus (e.g., angiotensin, bradykinin, noradrenaline) or a pathological stimulus (tissue injury or disease). Once the substrate is released from its esterified stores in the membrane, it is then transformed into the spectrum of products guided by the specific enzymes that it is exposed to. Thus, although the cyclooxygenase and the lipoxygenases in general are ubiquitous, there is considerable tissue specificity in the types of products that are formed. Because prostaglandins and lipoxygenase products are formed in all tissues, and because they exhibit considerable biological potency in test systems, yet are readily inactivated in one or two passes in the lungs and liver, several physiological roles as local hormones have been proposed, some of which are outlined below.

## Prostaglandins, Prostacyclin, and Thromboxane

### Cardiovascular system
In vascular beds of most species studied, **prostaglandins $D_2$, $E_2$, and $I_2$** evoke dilatation of arterioles, pre-capillary sphincters, and post-capillary vessels and thus increase blood flow; cardiac output is increased, and blood pressure generally falls. $PGF_{2\alpha}$ in most species is a vasoconstrictor of pulmonary arteries and veins, albeit a weak one. $TXA_2$, previously termed rabbit aorta contracting substance, is a potent vasoconstrictor. In certain vessels, such as those in

| TABLE 27-2 | Prostaglandin, Thromboxane, and Leukotriene Receptors | | | | |
|---|---|---|---|---|---|
| PG Receptor Type | Platelet Aggregation | Smooth Muscle Tone | Natural Antagonist | G Protein | Second Messenger |
| DP | − | +/− | $PGD_2$ | Gs | cAMP (↑) |
| $EP_1$ | | + | $PGE_2$ | $G_q$ (?) | $IP_3$/DAG/$Ca^{2+}$ (?) |
| $EP_2$ | | − | $PGE_2$ | Gs | cAMP (↑) |
| $EP_3$ | | + | $PGE_2$ | $G_i$, $G_s$, $G_q$ | cAMP (↑↓); $IP_3$/DAG/$Ca^{2+}$ |
| $EP_4$ | | − | $PGE_2$ | $G_s$ | cAMP (↑) |
| FP | | + | $PGF_{2\alpha}$ | $G_q$ | $IP_3$/DAG/$Ca_{2+}$ |
| IP | − | − | $PGI_2$ ($PGE_1$) | $G_s$ | cAMP (↑) |
| TP | + | + | $TXA_2$, $PGH_2$ | $G_q$ | $IP_3$/DAG/$Ca^{2+}$ |
| $CysLT_1$ | | + | $LTC_4$ | | |
| $CysLT_2$ | | + | $LTC_4$ | | |

| TABLE 27-3 | Eicosanoid Receptor Antagonists in Clinical Use | |
|---|---|---|
| Antagonist | Receptor Affected | Use |
| Montelukast | cysLT$_1$ | Asthma |
| Zafirlukast | cysLT$_1$ | Asthma |

the nasal mucosa, prostaglandins evoke a vasoconstrictor effect and have been proposed as nasal decongestants. TXA$_2$ is a powerful initiator of platelet aggregation; conversely, **PGI$_2$** opposes the aggregation through elevation of cyclic AMP levels within the platelet. PGI$_2$ is further capable of deaggregating platelet clumps. It inhibits thrombus formation and is regarded as one of the co-operative factors responsible for the maintenance of hemofluidity (see Chapter 38). The opposing properties of TXA$_2$ and PGI$_2$ on platelet function provide a mechanism of regulation of hemostatic function; thus, an imbalance of the TXA$_2$ to PGI$_2$ ratio might provide an explanation of some pathological states of thrombus formation and inflammation. In experimental models, PGI$_2$ reduces the size of myocardial infarcts, reduces hypoxic damage in the isolated perfused cat liver, and reduces ischemic damage during kidney transplantation in the dog. PGI$_2$, PGE$_2$, and nitric oxide are simultaneously released from endothelial cells. PGE$_2$ inhibits B-lymphocyte differentiation into antibody-secreting plasma cells, the proliferation of T lymphocytes, and the release of lymphokines.

## Smooth muscle

Smooth muscle can be either contracted or relaxed by prostaglandins, depending on the organ studied, the species, and the prostaglandin. **Bronchial muscles** are relaxed in humans and most other species by PGE$_1$, PGE$_2$, and PGI$_2$, although they are contracted by TXA$_2$, LTC$_4$, and LTD$_4$. **Human pregnant uterine muscle** is always contracted in vivo by PGE$_1$, PGE$_2$, and PGF$_{2\alpha}$; hence, these compounds induce abortion. The non-pregnant uterus is contracted by PGI$_2$ and TXA$_2$ but is relaxed by PGEs.

## Gastrointestinal tract

PGEs and PGI$_2$ **inhibit the secretion of gastric acid** (see Chapter 41). Also, the volume of secretion and the pepsin content are reduced, but bicarbonate secretion, mucus production, and blood flow are increased. The secretion of pancreatic enzymes and mucus from the small intestine is increased. Prostaglandins also induce the movement of water and electrolytes into the intestinal lumen; therefore, they can produce **diarrhea.** While prostaglandins and prostacyclin are cytoprotective, TXA$_2$ is pro-ulcerogenic in the dog and can exert cytolytic effects in myocardial and hepatic tissues.

PGEs promote peristalsis by contraction of intestinal longitudinal muscle and relaxation of the circular muscle, but PGFs, PGG$_2$, PGH$_2$, TXA$_2$, PGI$_2$, LTB$_4$, and LTC$_4$ contract both muscle layers.

## Renal system

Prostaglandins increase urine formation, natriuresis, and kaliuresis by altering renal blood flow and renal tubular function. PGD$_2$, PGE$_2$, and PGI$_2$ stimulate renin release. PGEs inhibit the reabsorption of water that is induced by antidiuretic hormone (see also Chapter 44).

## Nervous system

After intracerebroventricular injection, prostaglandins cause catatonia and sedation in experimental animals. More importantly, PGE$_2$ induces a **hyperthermic** response that may be related to pyrogen-induced fever. The antipyretic action of ASA and similar drugs results from their interference with cyclooxygenase (COX-1, COX-2, and COX-3) activity. In humans, prostaglandins cause **pain** when injected intradermally, and PGEs, PGI$_2$, and LTB$_4$ sensitize the nerve endings to the pain caused by histamine, bradykinin, or mechanical stimuli. Inhibition of cyclooxygenase is thus one basis of the analgesic action of salicylates and related drugs (see Chapter 28).

## Endocrine systems

Different prostaglandins can stimulate the release of adrenocorticotrophic hormone, growth hormone, prolactin, and gonadotropins, and in addition, they have thyrotropin-like and luteinizing hormone–like effects. In several mammals, PGF$_{2\alpha}$ can evoke regression of the corpus luteum, which interrupts early pregnancy in these animals; however, this effect has not been observed in humans. 12-HETE increases aldosterone release both directly and indirectly through angiotensin II formation.

## Possible roles in physiology and pathology

Eicosanoids have been implicated in the function of almost all physiological systems, some of which have been mentioned. One of the roles of eicosanoids is the support of renal perfusion in many diseases associated with decreased effective circulation volume, such as heart failure. However, ASA (an inhibitor of COX-1 and COX-2) does not influence most of these physiological systems in low therapeutic doses. Stronger evidence exists for a role of eicosanoids in tissue inflammation and injury. Prostaglandins act synergistically with agents producing pain, possibly by lowering pain thresholds and sensitizing pain receptors (e.g., potentiating the pain induced by histamine or bradykinin). As PGE$_1$, PGE$_2$, and PGI$_2$ are also potent vasodilatory substances, they potentiate the abilities of histamine, bradykinin, and LTD$_4$ and LTB$_4$ to produce edema. The inhibition of cyclooxygenase may be the basis of the analgesic action of NSAIDs (e.g., indomethacin, ibuprofen) and their ability to suppress inflammation-induced edema. Eicosanoids may play a further role in chronic inflammatory joint diseases, which induce destruction of cartilage and resorption of bone (see also Chapters 28 and 30).

## Leukotrienes

Leukotrienes are now believed to be the biologically active constituents of slow-reaching substance of anaphylaxis (SRS-A). They are formed from arachidonic acid by 5-lipoxygenase. The leukotrienes $LTB_4$, $LTC_4$, and $LTD_4$ can be produced in human, rabbit, and rat polymorphonuclear leukocytes, and upon immunological challenge, they are released from human and guinea pig lungs.

$LTC_4$, $LTD_4$, $LTE_4$, and $LTF_4$ possess potent vasoconstrictor activity (e.g., in the coronary arteries) and cause constriction of small airways. Tracheal mucus secretion is also increased.

$LTB_4$ is a powerful chemotactic agent and promotes superoxide generation and transendothelial neutrophil migration. Leukotrienes increase vascular wall permeability, evoking leakage from post-capillary venules and thus causing tissue edema. These actions are potentiated by prostaglandins.

Leukotrienes may play an important role in immediate hypersensitivity responses as mediators of allergic bronchoconstriction and increased vascular permeability. The ability of corticosteroids to reduce the production of leukotrienes, by decreasing the release of arachidonic acid and formation of endoperoxides, might explain the anti-allergic, anti-inflammatory, and anti-asthmatic activity of the corticosteroids. ASA, which does not influence leukotriene production, is devoid of anti-allergic and anti-asthmatic properties. In fact, ASA-induced asthma might be brought on by the redirection of the substrate, arachidonic acid, into the leukotriene synthesis pathway.

$LTB_4$ can be produced by human polymorphonuclear leukocytes and is a potent chemokinetic, chemotactic, and aggregating agent in many types of cells. It may have a role in inflammation and tissue damage. $LTB_4$ has been found to induce accumulation of polymorphonuclear leukocytes in joint diseases such as gout and arthritis, as well as in skin lesions of patients with psoriasis.

## Derivatives of HPETEs and EPETEs

The **HPETE derivatives** have been shown to possess a variety of biological actions in vitro. These actions lead to such diverse effects as relaxation of vascular smooth muscle of the isolated rat and rabbit stomach, in which contraction has previously been induced with noradrenaline; reversal of the effects of $PGI_2$ on the release of insulin from perfused rat islets of Langerhans; and modulation (inhibition) of the effects of $PGI_2$ on the release of renin. The effects could be produced by the HPETEs themselves or, since they are rap-

idly transformed into other products, may be due to conversion into the leukotrienes, lipoxins, or hepoxilins.

Few studies have concentrated on the biological role of the **EPETE derivatives.** These products have been shown to possess marginal activity on the release of calcium from liver microsomes and on the release of pituitary hormones from the hypothalamus.

## THERAPEUTIC USES

### Uterus Stimulation

Prostaglandins induce contractions of the pregnant uterus and, in larger doses, of the non-pregnant uterus. Various preparations are available.

#### Dinoprostone (PGE₂)

Prostin $E_2$ vaginal suppositories contain 20 mg of dinoprostone and are used primarily to induce abortion between the 12th and 20th gestational weeks. They are administered every 3 to 5 hours for not more than 48 hours, until abortion occurs. This product is available only in a limited number of countries.

Prostin $E_2$ oral tablets contain 0.5 mg dinoprostone for elective induction of labour and for induction made necessary by post-maturity, hypertension, toxemia of pregnancy, premature rupture of amniotic membranes, Rh incompatibility, diabetes mellitus, intrauterine death, or fetal growth retardation. It is administered orally every hour until a satisfactory response is obtained. Single doses should never exceed 1.5 mg, and the **duration of treatment should not exceed 18 hours.** If oxytocin is to be used, it should not be administered within 1 hour of the last dose. The most frequently observed adverse reactions are nausea, vomiting, diarrhea, fetal heart rate changes, and uterine hypertonus.

Prostin $E_2$ vaginal gel is a semi-translucent, viscous vaginal gel supplied in a special applicator syringe that contains 1 or 2 mg of dinoprostone per 3 g of gel. It is used for induction of labour at term or near term. The dose is 1 to 2 mg intravaginally and may be repeated 6 hours later depending on the patient's initial response. The adverse effects are very similar to those observed with oxytocin, such as fetal heart rate abnormalities, fetal distress, and uterine hypercontractility.

#### Carboprost (15-methyl PGF₂α)

Carboprost tromethamine salt (Hemabate, Prostin/15M) is used only by intramuscular administration to induce abortion during the 12th to 20th gestational weeks. The dose is 250 µg every 1 to 3 hours depending on the uterine response. It is also used for refractory postpartum bleeding due to uterine atony. Carboprost methyl (U-36384) is carboprost methyl ester.

## Dinoprost (PGF$_{2\alpha}$)

Dinoprost (Leutalyse, Prostin F$_2$ Alpha) injectable is for intra-amniotic administration to induce abortion or labour. It is marketed in 5 mg/mL strength. The initial dose is 5 mg, which is repeated as required up to a total of 40 mg. If response is not satisfactory within 24 hours and the membranes are still intact, an additional dose of 10 to 40 mg can be administered. This product is available in North America but is not advertised or promoted.

## Ductus Arteriosus

In premature infants, the ductus may remain open, probably because of excessive prostaglandin production. In such cases, injectable indomethacin is administered to reduce prostaglandin synthesis and close the ductus.

In neonates with congenital heart defects such as pulmonary atresia or stenosis, tricuspid atresia, coarctation of the aorta, tetralogy of Fallot, interruption of the aortic arch, or transposition of the great vessels, a patent (open) ductus may be essential for survival. In such cases, PGE$_1$ is administered to keep the ductus open until surgical correction can be carried out. The preparation used for this purpose is **alprostadil** (PGE$_1$; Prostin VR), an injectable preparation containing 0.5 mg of PGE$_1$ in anhydrous ethanol. Before administration, it must be properly diluted with sterile sodium chloride or dextrose solution. It is administered with the aid of a pump capable of delivering small volume (constant) infusions. The initial infusion rate is 0.1 µg/kg/min until the desired effect is achieved; it is then reduced to 0.05 to 0.01 µg/kg/min. The drug can be administered into a large vein or through an umbilical artery catheter positioned with its tip at the ductal opening. Numerous precautionary measures must be followed (as listed in the product monograph) before administration is started. The most frequently observed serious side effects are apnea and seizures. The others which are considered to be less serious are flushing, bradycardia, fever, and diarrhea. Long-term use may cause weakening of the walls of the ductus arteriosus and pulmonary arteries; gastric outlet obstruction and cortical proliferation of long bones may occur.

## Gastrointestinal Tract

**Misoprostol** (Cytotec) is a synthetic methyl ester analogue of PGE$_1$ used for the prevention of drug-induced gastric ulceration during NSAID, corticosteroid, or anticoagulant administration. In addition, it can be used alone or in combination with antacids for the treatment of duodenal ulcer (see Chapter 41). It is available in oral tablet formulations of 100 and 200 µg. The dosage for the prevention of drug-induced ulcer is 400 to 800 µg/day and for duodenal ulcer, 800 µg/day in divided doses. Women should be advised not to become pregnant while taking misoprostol. The most frequent side effects are diarrhea, abdominal pain, flatulence, and spotting.

## Platelet Aggregation

**Epoprostenol** (PGI$_2$, prostacyclin; Cyclo-Prostin, Flolan) is used as a replacement for heparin in some hemodialysis patients and for the prevention of platelet aggregation in extracorporeal circulation systems. PGI$_2$ improves the harvest and storage of platelets for therapeutic transfusion. The drug is available in North America on request from the manufacturer.

## Impotence

**Alprostadil** (PGE$_1$; Caverject) was formerly used in the treatment of erectile dysfunction, by injection into the corpora cavernosa, to initiate and maintain complete or partial erection lasting for 1 to 3 hours. However, it has now been replaced by drugs such as sildenafil (Viagra), tadalafil (Cialis), and verdenafil (Levitra), which can be taken by mouth and produce selective inhibition of a phosphodiesterase (PDE5) found in the corpus cavernosum, thus permitting increased blood inflow (see Chapter 34). It has been reported recently that a few users of these medications for erectile dysfunction have suffered permanent blindness due to non-arteritic ischemic anterior optic neuropathy. The nature of the relationship between the drug use and the blindness is currently being investigated.

## SUGGESTED READINGS

Bandeira-Melo C, Bozza PT, Diaz BL, et al. Cutting edge: lipoxin (LX) A$_4$ and aspirin-triggered 15-epi-LXA$_4$ block allergen-induced eosinophil trafficking. *J Immunol*. 2000;164:2267-2271.

Bergström S, Carlson LA, Weeks JR. The prostaglandins: a family of biologically active lipids. *Pharmacol Rev*. 1968;20:1-48.

Coleman RA, Smith WL, Narumiya S. International Union of Pharmacology classification of prostanoid receptors: properties, distribution and structure of the receptors and their subtypes. *Pharmacol Rev*. 1994;46:205-229.

Fiddler GI, Lumley P. Preliminary clinical studies with thromboxane synthase inhibitors and thromboxane receptor blockers: a review. *Circulation*. 1990;81:169-178.

Janssen-Timmen U, Tomic I, Specht E, Beilecke U, Habenicht AJ. The arachidonic acid cascade, eicosanoids, and signal transduction. *Ann NY Acad Sci*. 1994;733:325-334.

Moncada S, ed. Prostacyclin, thromboxane and leukotrienes. *Br Med Bull*. 1983;39(3):209-300.

Narumiya S, Sugimoto Y, Ushikubi F. Prostanoid receptors: structures, properties and functions. *Physiol Rev*. 1999;79:1193-1226.

Pace-Asciak CR, Reynaud D, Demin P, Nigam S. The hepoxilins—a review. In: Pace-Asciak CR, Nigam S, eds. *Lipoxygenases and*

*Their Products: Biological Functions*. Advances in Experimental Medicine and Biology Series. Vol 447. New York, NY: Plenum Press; 1999:123-132.

Reilly M, Fitzgerald GA. Cellular activation by thromboxane $A_2$ and other eicosanoids. *Eur Heart J*. 1993;14(suppl K):88-93.

Samuelsson B, Paoletti R, eds. *Advances in Prostaglandin and Thromboxane Research*. New York, NY: Raven Press; 1987.

Schror K, Hohlfeld T. Inotropic actions of eicosanoids [editorial]. *Basic Res Cardiol*. 1992;87:2-11.

Walt RP. Misoprostol for the treatment of peptic ulcer and anti-inflammatory drug-induced gastroduodenal ulceration. *N Engl J Med*. 1992;327:1575-1580.

# 28

# Anti-inflammatory Analgesics

## D KADAR

**CASE HISTORY**

A 64-year-old man who had been treated for several years with hydrochlorothiazide 25 mg every other day for moderate hypertension began to experience mild pain and discomfort in the hip area. He started self-medication with ibuprofen 600 mg at bedtime. During a routine checkup 2 months later, his blood pressure was found to be moderately elevated, and the dose of diuretic needed to be increased to 50 mg for adequate control. Ibuprofen was replaced with enteric-coated acetylsalicylic acid (ASA) 650 mg to control the discomfort of the patient's arthritis. A few weeks later, the patient complained of epigastric pain and painful swelling of one of his big toes. History revealed that he was a regular moderately heavy drinker. He was found to have hyperuricemia, and ASA was replaced with acetaminophen 500 mg. The diuretic was changed to furosemide 40 mg every other day, and allopurinol 100 mg daily (taken with food) was added to control the hyperuricemia. After 2 months, the antihypertensive medication was changed to the more specific agent fosinopril 10 mg daily, and allopurinol was discontinued because the blood uric acid concentration had normalized and the pain and swelling of the toe had subsided. After 4 months he refused to moderate his alcohol intake. Therefore acetaminophen was replaced with diclofenac sodium 50 mg and misoprostol 200 µg twice daily, supplemented with occasional acetaminophen if needed. Blood uric acid tests and general follow-up examinations were ordered at 3-month intervals.

## HISTORY

The effect of willow bark extract in relieving fever and pain was known to ancient civilizations, but the first reliable description of its antipyretic effect is attributed to Edmund Stone, who was searching for an inexpensive substitute for cinchona bark in the eighteenth century. The active ingredient, salicin, a bitter glycoside, was isolated in 1829, and various derivatives were later found in other plants. Acetylsalicylic acid (ASA) was synthesized by Gerhardt in 1853 and was introduced into medicine by Dreser in 1899 under the Bayer Pharmaceutical Co. trade name of Aspirin. (In Canada, "Aspirin" is still a patented trade name, but in the United States and most other countries, "aspirin" is a non-proprietary name.)

The sharp increase in the number of anti-inflammatory drugs released for medicinal use since 1971 can be attributed to the ease and reliability of modern in vitro and in vivo testing for the desired pharmacological action. All of these drugs inhibit prostaglandin synthesis and prevent the development of carrageenan-induced rat paw edema. With these two rather simple experimental models, hundreds of chemicals can be screened in a relatively short time. Since prostaglandin synthesis is tissue- and species-specific, however, the final evaluation of the beneficial and toxic properties of such drugs requires extensive long-term experience in human subjects.

Other designations for this group of drugs are antipyretic analgesics, anti-inflammatory agents, nonsteroidal anti-inflammatory drugs (NSAIDs), and nonnarcotic analgesics.

## INFLAMMATION AND RELATED PROCESSES

### Pain

Pain is essential for survival. It can serve as a warning of impending or actual tissue or organ injury. Humans usually do not "adapt" to pain. The sensation originates from stimulation of naked nerve endings found in all parts of the body. The pain receptors (nociceptors) can be stimulated by mechanical or chemical means. Pain-producing substances such as histamine or kinins stimulate the naked nerve endings directly, while prostaglandins (PGs) lower the pain threshold by increasing the sensitivity of the receptors to the stimulus. $PGE_2$ and $PGF_{2\alpha}$ are known to cause vascular pain, headache, and local pain at sites of injection.

The sensation of pain is transmitted from the periphery through the spinal cord to higher integrative centres in the central nervous system (CNS) by "fast" myelinated A$\delta$ fibres at 10 to 30 m/sec and by non-myelinated "slow" C fibres at 0.5 to 2 m/sec. When first-order sensory neurons from a diseased organ and from another area of the body synapse on the same second-order neurons in the spinal cord, pain actually originating in the diseased organ may be perceived as coming from the other area; this is known as "referred pain." The intensity of pain sensation can be influenced by distraction (e.g., "white noise"), hypnosis, placebo or suggestion, acupuncture, local anaesthetics, nerve section, or analgesic drugs. Anxiolytics and neuroleptics may diminish the emotional response to pain through action on the limbic system and hypothalamus. Morphine and other opioid analgesics act on opiate receptors in the grey matter around the cerebral aqueduct and adjacent to the third and fourth ventricles, as well as in the spinal cord (see Chapter 19).

## Fever

Fever is the body's response to exogenous or endogenous substances called pyrogens. Bacteria, moulds, yeasts, and viruses elaborate high-molecular-weight lipopolysaccharides capable of stimulating the release of "pyrogens," such as cytokines (interleukin-1$\beta$ [IL-1$\beta$], IL-6, and IL-8) from polymorphonuclear leukocytes and monocytes, and tumour necrosis factor alpha (TNF$\alpha$) from other cells. These pyrogens act on the thermoreceptive region in the preoptic anterior hypothalamus to release arachidonic acid, stimulate $PGE_2$ synthesis (see Chapter 27), and raise the set point of the temperature-regulating centre, which in turn will lead to vasoconstriction in the skin, decreased heat loss, increased heat generation, and increased body temperature. Administration of type E prostaglandin to the cerebral ventricles of experimental animals causes fever. Fever arising from extensive tissue damage, autoimmune disease, neoplasia, or following thromboembolism is thought to be due to the release of a leukocyte-type pyrogen from the affected tissue. Salicylates and other antipyretic drugs appear to act by inhibiting the synthesis or release of prostaglandins in the thermoregulatory centre.

## Inflammatory Process

The inflammatory process can be initiated by invading microorganisms, immunological reactions, tissue decay, and many other less-known phenomena. Mediators of inflammation are thought to cause increased release of the fatty acid precursors of prostaglandins and to increase the rate of prostaglandin synthesis. Prostaglandins may cause inflammation on their own, or they may aggravate a pre-existing inflammatory condition. Endogenous mediators of inflammation may originate from the plasma (such as bradykinin, $C_3$ and $C_5$ fragments, $C_{567}$ complex, fibrinopeptides, fibrin degradation products) and from tissues (such as histamine, serotonin, leukotrienes such as slow-reacting substance of anaphylaxis [SRS-A], prostaglandins, lysosomal proteases, migration inhibitory factor, chemotactic factors, lymphotoxin, skin reactive factors, mitogenic factors, lymph node permeability factor, IL-1, platelet-activating factor [PAF]). Endogenous pyrogens and leukocytosis factors may be liberated, causing local redness, swelling, heat, pain, and disturbed function of the involved organ. Most prostaglandins are known to cause peripheral vasodilatation with local redness and edema formation and to synergistically increase the effect of bradykinin. Practically every part of the body may suffer damage as the result of an inflammatory process. Drugs do not reverse the damage, but they may arrest the process or slow its progress. In addition, the intensity of the pain may be significantly reduced or eliminated.

Anti-inflammatory drugs reduce pain and tissue damage by inhibiting prostaglandin synthesis. In addition, one or more of the following may contribute to the anti-inflammatory effect: (1) inhibition of leukocyte migration and phagocytosis, during which histamine, serotonin, and other substances (autacoids) may often be released; (2) stabilization of lysosomal membranes, thus preventing the escape of lysosomal enzymes into the cytoplasm and hence damage to cell structures; and (3) inhibition of plasmin, a plasma proteolytic enzyme that may activate kinin formation. The composition, biosynthesis, or metabolism of connective tissue mucopolysaccharides can also be affected.

The suppression of antigen–antibody reactions by anti-inflammatory drugs may be due to depressed antibody production, interference with antigen–antibody reactions, reduced histamine release, or cell membrane stabilization.

## SALICYLATES

Acetylsalicylic acid (ASA) is the most frequently used member of this class of anti-inflammatory drugs. The others are salicylic acid, sodium salicylate, choline salicylate, choline magnesium salicylate, salicylamide, methylsalicylate, salsalate (in the United States but not in Canada), and diflunisal. 5-Aminosalicylate is used principally as an intestinal anti-inflammatory agent (see Chapter 42). The chemical structures of salicylic acid, ASA, and diflunisal are shown in Figure 28-1.

## Mechanism and Site of Action

The analgesic and anti-inflammatory actions of salicylates are attributed to their ability to inhibit cyclooxygenases, primarily the COX-1 and COX-2 isoforms (see Chapter 27, Fig. 27-3), the enzymes responsible for the conversion of arachidonic acid to prostaglandin peroxides. This action of the drugs is exerted both in the periphery and at the hypothalamic thermoregulatory centre. ASA acetylates the serine moiety at position 530 of COX-1, and therefore the binding of arachidonic acid to the active site is inhibited. Similarly, acetylation of serine at position 516 in COX-2 blocks the synthesis of prostaglandin, but not of **15R-hydroxyeicosatetraenoic acid** (15R-HETE), which gives rise to the production of epilipoxin, which has anti-inflammatory properties (Table 28-1). The inhibition is irreversible, and restoration of prostaglandin production requires biosynthesis of new enzyme. In addition, salicylates may inhibit formation of plasmin and thereby of bradykinin. They also block the production of pain by kinins acting on chemoreceptors. Recently, it was found that ASA is bound to phospholipase A2, interacting with the release of arachidonic acid.

## Pharmacokinetics

Orally administered ASA is absorbed by passive diffusion, partly in the stomach but to a large extent in the small intestine. The absorption of all acidic drugs including the salicylates is influenced by the pH of the aqueous layer next to the mucous membrane. In the stomach, the low pH enhances absorption because the uncharged molecules of weakly acidic drugs are able to penetrate lipid membranes with relative ease. In the intestines, at almost neutral pH, the effect of reduced absorption due to ionization is offset by the greater solubility in water, which aids in the dispersal of these drugs over the large absorbing sur-face, thereby enhancing absorption. Antacids may reduce the rate of ASA absorption from the stomach by increasing the pH of the gastric juice, but the increased rate of gastric emptying may make more drug available for intestinal dissolution and absorption. The end result on ASA absorption may be negligible. Rectal absorption is slow and unreliable. Salicylates, especially methylsalicylate, are absorbed through the intact skin.

After oral administration of usual therapeutic doses of ASA, absorption is more than 90%. Enteric-coated preparations are designed to release the drug at the pH of the small intestine. Occasionally, the acid-resistant coating fails to dissolve and the intact tablet is found in the feces. The amount of drug available for absorption from delayed-release preparations is greatly influenced by gastrointestinal motility.

Salicylates are unevenly distributed in the body. High levels of ASA are found in organs of the central compartment, such as blood, renal cortex, and liver, and considerably less (one-sixth to one-tenth that of the plasma concentration) is found in other sites, such as brain, spinal fluid, muscle, intestine, aqueous humor, lens, and semen. The ASA concentration in synovial fluid taken from an inflamed joint is about five times as high as the plasma concentration of free ASA, and the half-life of the drug is considerably longer in synovial fluid. Salicylates cross the placenta and also appear in breast milk. Salicylate competes with other drugs and with bilirubin for serum albumin binding sites.

The liver is the principal site of the dose-dependent salicylate biotransformation by the microsomal and mitochondrial enzymes. ASA is first hydrolyzed to salicylic acid and is then converted to salicyluric acid (up to 80%), the acyl and phenolic glucuronides of salicylic acid, gentisic acid, and other minor metabolites.

The metabolites, along with a fraction of the unchanged salicylic acid, are excreted in the urine. Excretion of the unchanged drug is enhanced by sodium bicarbonate administration because, in alkaline urine, the drug is ionized and cannot back-diffuse from the renal tubules. This procedure is especially useful to hasten excretion after an overdose. Salicylates reduce the renal elimination of methotrexate.

The plasma half-life of ASA is about 15 minutes. That of salicylic acid is longer and is dose-dependent—about 2 to 3 hours after a 600-mg dose and 6 to 12 hours after larger doses. At therapeutic doses, the elimination follows first-order kinetics, but after toxic doses, it follows a mixed order because of enzyme saturation, and the plasma half-life may increase to 15 to 30 hours.

**Diflunisal**, a substituted salicylic acid derivative, has powerful analgesic and anti-inflammatory activity but mild and unreliable antipyretic properties. It is completely absorbed after oral administration, is distributed similarly to ASA, and has a plasma half-life of 8 to 12 hours. The

| TABLE 28-1 | Comparison of Prostaglandin Synthase Inhibitory Activity and Anti-inflammatory Potency of Selected Non-opioid Analgesics | |
|---|---|---|
| Drug | Inhibition of Prostaglandin Synthase (IC$_{50}$, µg/mL) | Reduction of Carrageenan-Induced Rat Paw Edema (ED$_{50}$, mg/kg) |
| Piroxicam | 0.06 | 4.0 |
| Indomethacin | 0.06 | 6.5 |
| Mefenamic acid | 0.17 | 55.0 |
| Phenylbutazone | 2.23 | 100.0 |
| ASA | 6.62 | 150.0 |
| Acetaminophen | 100 | Inactive |

pharmacokinetics of diflunisal are dose-dependent, and doubling the dose more than doubles the plasma concentration. Steady state is achieved only after several days of administration. More than 99% is bound to plasma proteins. The drug may appear in human breast milk at a concentration of up to 7% of the total plasma concentration.

## Pharmacological Effects

### Analgesia

Low-intensity pain, such as headache, myalgia, arthralgia, and other pain arising from integumental structures rather than from viscera, is alleviated by salicylates. Part of the analgesia arises from actions on subcortical sites of the CNS, probably the hypothalamus, because at therapeutic concentrations, mental function and alertness are not affected. In contrast to the opioid analgesics (see Chapter 19), these drugs do not produce tolerance or physical dependence during chronic administration. Paradoxically, salicylates cause headache in toxic doses. ASA is frequently combined with codeine or other opioid analgesics and sedatives; such combinations are claimed to give more pain relief with less toxicity than any of the ingredients given alone in effective doses, although this claim has not been clearly proven. The analgesic dose range is between 300 and 1000 mg three or four times a day.

### Antipyresis

Salicylates lower the body temperature in febrile patients by a direct action on the hypothalamic thermoreceptive region and the temperature-regulating centre concerned with heat production and heat loss. Normal body temperature is not affected by therapeutic doses. The increased heat loss produced by salicylates in febrile patients is due to secondary peripheral vasodilatation, especially in cutaneous areas, and to increased sweating. Sweating is important but not essential in this process, because atropine

(which prevents sweating; see Chapter 12) does not prevent salicylates from lowering the elevated temperature. Heat production is not inhibited, and toxic doses of salicylates actually produce fever. The antipyretic dose range is similar to the analgesic range.

### Effects on rheumatic, inflammatory, and immunological processes

Salicylates in large doses (5 to 8 g daily) are used for the treatment of rheumatoid diseases and other inflammatory conditions. The increased capillary permeability during inflammation is reduced by salicylates, which thereby prevents edema formation, cellular exudation, and pain. Their ability to block cellular immune responses appears to contribute to the therapeutic effect.

### Uricosuric effect

Salicylates in doses of 500 mg inhibit both the renal tubular secretion of uric acid and the uricosuric effect of probenecid and sulfinpyrazone by competition for the same proximal tubular transport systems. In large doses of 5 to 10 g daily, however, the tubular reabsorption of uric acid is also inhibited by competition of salicylates with uric acid for more distal active transport sites in the tubule. The net effect of the larger doses is that most of the uric acid filtered by the glomeruli is excreted, and the uric acid concentration in the blood is lowered. When this occurs, the urate crystals already deposited in joints (in cases of gout) are slowly eliminated.

### Additional and adverse effects

*Respiration.* Salicylates in medium or large therapeutic doses directly, or indirectly by increased $CO_2$ production, stimulate the respiratory centre, leading to respiratory alkalosis that is normally compensated by increased urinary elimination of bicarbonate. In toxic doses, salicylates cause central respiratory depression, as well as increased $CO_2$ production by mitochondria in muscle. These effects result in a combination of uncompensated respiratory and metabolic acidosis. Reduction of plasma bicarbonate level by the salicylates, which are acidic, may also contribute to the acidosis.

*Gastrointestinal.* Epigastric distress, nausea, and vomiting are quite common complications of salicylate therapy, and microscopic bleeding is almost universal. Exacerbation of peptic ulcer symptoms, gastrointestinal hemorrhage, and blood loss occurs in sensitive patients on prolonged salicylate therapy. Pain of gastritis from other causes (e.g., alcoholic gastritis) should not be treated with salicylates because of the increased danger of bleeding.

All anti-inflammatory drugs have the potential to cause damage to the gastrointestinal tract. Weakly acidic drugs such as salicylate may be trapped intracellularly in high concentrations because, at intracellular pH, the ionized form of the drug predominates and cannot readily diffuse out of the cell. High intracellular salicylate levels may contribute to the production of gastric mucosal erosion. This is similar to the gastritis following excessive consumption of vinegar or vinegar-containing salad dressing.

Prostaglandins, especially PGI2 and PGE2, act cytoprotectively on the gastrointestinal mucosa by increasing blood flow and the formation of mucus and sodium bicarbonate while reducing the release of HCl and digestive enzymes. Inhibition of prostaglandin synthesis by salicylates therefore may also contribute to damage of the gastrointestinal epithelium.

Corticosteroids, which are powerful anti-inflammatory drugs that are not acidic, also cause gastric ulceration with long-term use because they inhibit the phospholipase A2–induced release of arachidonic acid and suppress the expression of COX-2, thus secondarily reducing prostaglandin synthesis.

*Blood.* Large doses of salicylates administered over a prolonged period of time shorten erythrocyte survival and interfere with iron metabolism. In addition, the plasma prothrombin level is reduced, and anticoagulants may have to be given in reduced dosage. Since ASA acetylates the active site of cyclooxygenase responsible for prostaglandin endoperoxide and subsequent thromboxane A2 (TXA2) synthesis in platelets, platelet aggregation is inhibited and the bleeding time is prolonged. Platelets do not synthesize new enzyme; therefore, this action is irreversible, and the effect lasts until new platelets are formed. The daily administration of 81 mg of ASA in the form of enteric-coated tablets is beneficial for the prophylaxis of thromboembolism of coronary and cerebral blood vessels. ASA might be responsible for the transient hemolysis in patients who have glucose-6-phosphate-dehydrogenase deficiency.

*Metabolic processes.* Oxidative phosphorylation is inhibited by large doses of salicylates, and the energy normally used for ATP production is dissipated as heat. This explains the pyretic effect of toxic overdose. The occasionally observed hyperglycemia may be caused by increased adrenaline release through the activation of central sympathetic centres and the resulting increase of glucose-6-phosphatase activity. Salicylates are also known to cause hypoglycemia, probably by increased utilization of glucose, inhibition of gluconeogenesis, and reduced lipogenesis.

*Endocrine functions.* In addition to stimulating adrenaline release, ASA increases plasma adrenocorticosteroid levels by increasing the release of adrenocorticotropic hormone (ACTH) from the hypothalamus. It also competes with thyroid hormones for binding sites on plasma proteins. This effect leads to higher tissue uptake of thyroxine and triiodothyronine, which may contribute to the higher metabolic rate seen with overdoses of salicylates.

*Pregnancy.* Some data show a slight correlation between consumption of large doses of ASA during the first 16 weeks of pregnancy and the incidence of fetal malformations. If taken regularly during the last trimester, it may contribute to prolonged gestation, prolonged labour, and increased maternal blood loss during delivery. There is no evidence, however, that occasional use of small doses of ASA during pregnancy is harmful. The administration of NSAIDs should be terminated toward the last trimester to avoid premature closure of the ductus arteriosus and postpartum bleeding. ASA is excreted in breast milk, which may sensitize the infant to NSAIDs.

*Hypersensitivity.* The incidence of hypersensitivity reactions to ASA is about 5%, but true allergy is estimated at less than 1% (see Chapter 27, "Leukotrienes"). It is usually manifested as bronchoconstriction, urticaria, or angioneurotic edema; fatal anaphylactic shock is rare. Many patients sensitive to salicylates also may be sensitive to the other anti-inflammatory drugs and to tartrazine, a yellow dye used in numerous pharmaceutical and food preparations. Some foods and beverages containing salicylate, such as curry powder, paprika, licorice, Benedictine liqueur, prunes, raisins, gherkins, and tea, may contribute to allergic reactions.

*Drug interactions.* The combination of salicylates with oral anticoagulants or heparin can lead to hemorrhage for reasons already mentioned above.

Absorbed ASA is hydrolyzed to salicylic acid, and about 80% is bound to serum albumin. Other drugs that are also bound to albumin, such as sulfonamides, can be displaced by salicylates, raising the concentration of free drug in the plasma and therefore increasing the toxicity. For the same reason, infants with incompletely developed bilirubin-conjugating enzyme systems may develop kernicterus after salicylate administration (see Chapter 4).

The risk of toxicity of methotrexate, a cancer chemotherapeutic agent, is increased by salicylates because they inhibit the active renal tubular secretion of methotrexate and displace the anti-neoplastic compound from plasma protein binding sites. This type of interaction may also be a limiting factor when low doses of methotrexate are used in combination with NSAIDs in the treatment of rheumatoid arthritis.

Interaction with the uricosuric effects of probenecid and sulfinpyrazone may effectively cancel urate excretion, as explained above, but this risk is very small with the occasional use of ASA for headache or other minor pain.

Increased gastrointestinal blood loss following simultaneous ingestion of alcohol and ASA is probably due to additive but independent effects of the two agents on the gastric mucosa.

Ammonium chloride, acid sodium phosphate, and ascorbic acid may acidify the urine and thus increase the reabsorption of salicylic acid. The resultant accumulation can be hazardous with large ASA doses.

The interaction of oral hypoglycemic agents and ASA is complex; the plasma concentration of both drugs may increase through competition for plasma protein binding sites and reciprocal interference with urinary elimination.

ASA increases the plasma half-life of penicillin because it competes with penicillin for the active transport (secretory) mechanism in the renal tubules.

## Toxicity

Salicylism, a mild form of intoxication, is characterized by headache, dizziness, mental confusion, tinnitus, nausea, and vomiting. Marked hyperventilation is also present, resulting from the direct stimulatory effect of salicylates on the respiratory centre. Prolonged hyperventilation leads to respiratory alkalosis, but compensatory increases in sodium and potassium bicarbonate excretion may produce a slight improvement in the condition of the patient. The improvement is only temporary if a large dose was ingested. Serum salicylate concentration and pH should be measured to indicate the type of procedure required for further treatment.

If the dose is large enough, and the condition remains untreated, the preceding symptoms are followed by respiratory and metabolic acidosis, restlessness, delirium, hallucinations, convulsions, coma, and death from respiratory failure.

Symptomatic treatment is sufficient in mild cases of poisoning. Alkalinization of the urine (e.g., with sodium bicarbonate) will enhance salicylate elimination. In serious cases, intravenous administration of fluids, frequent measurement and correction of acid–base and electrolyte imbalance, and hemodialysis or peritoneal dialysis are mandatory. Methylsalicylate, the methyl ester of salicylic acid, is non-ionizable and therefore rapidly crosses cell membranes, including those in the CNS. Therefore, it is the most toxic salicylate: one teaspoonful (4 g) may cause death in children.

The occurrence of nephropathy following long-term analgesic therapy is not rare and may lead to a requirement for long-term hemodialysis. The mechanism of development of this toxicity is due partly to the reduction of $PGE_1$, $PGE_2$, and $PGI_2$ production with subsequent reduction of glomerular filtration. The formation of a reactive metabolite that depletes glutathione and binds to cellular macromolecules in the renal tubules may only partly explain the observed cell damage. ASA may cause transient shedding of renal tubular cells, alteration in excretion, and reduced glomerular filtration with consequent retention of water, sodium, and potassium. Patients with active systemic lupus erythematosus, advanced liver cirrhosis, and chronic renal insufficiency appear to be most at risk.

Prostaglandins have an important role in the maintenance of cellular integrity and renal blood circulation. Inhibition of prostaglandin synthesis may cause renal vascular constriction and alteration in vasomotion. In addition, chloride reabsorption in the renal tubules is more complete, and antidiuretic hormone (ADH) activity (via production of cyclic AMP) is unaffected, resulting in increased water reabsorption. This may cause significant water retention, especially in patients with congestive heart failure, and diminished effectiveness of diuretics. Most patients with analgesic nephropathy are middle-aged women with histories of peptic ulcer, anemia, psychiatric disorders, headaches, and arthralgias. If the renal abnormalities are diagnosed early, the condition may stabilize or improve after drug withdrawal.

The recently observed increase in the number of infants, children, and young adults suffering from Reye's syndrome (an often fatal fulminating hepatitis with cerebral edema) following a feverish prodromal viral infection has been attributed to the indiscriminate use of ASA. Although other factors such as dosage have also been implicated, this highlights some of the risks of prescribing antipyretics such as ASA, especially for infants and children.

Finally, it is important to know that salicylate intoxication is a leading cause of accidental poisoning in all age groups, particularly children.

## Therapeutic applications

Sodium salicylate, choline salicylate (available in liquid formulation), choline magnesium salicylate, and ASA are used as antipyretics and analgesics and for the treatment of gout, acute rheumatic fever, and rheumatoid arthritis. Salsalate (salicylsalicylic acid) is a weak inhibitor of prostaglandin synthesis that is used only for the treatment of arthritis. ASA also inhibits platelet aggregation irreversibly. Salicylic acid is used topically as a keratolytic agent (for corns and calluses) and for the treatment of epidermophytosis and hyperhidrosis. Salicylamide is included in a number of over-the-counter analgesic and sedative preparations, but its effect is variable. Methylsalicylate is a colourless or yellowish liquid used in liniments for cutaneous counter-irritation. Recently, adhesive patches containing 15% salicylic acid were made available for transdermal systemic administration.

Several clinical trials involving thousands of patients were carried out to determine the beneficial effect of ASA, administered alone or in combination with dipyridamole, for the prevention or treatment (secondary prevention) of cerebral and coronary thrombosis. In most studies of coronary thrombosis, the mortality rates of the treated and placebo groups were not significantly different, but the rate of re-infarction was significantly reduced by drug treatment.

The inability to precisely define the etiology of the disorders is partly responsible for the equivocal results and interpretation. However, recently, ASA administration in females, but not in males, was found to be moderately beneficial in the prevention of cerebrovascular-induced transient ischemic attacks and visual disturbances (see also Chapter 38). On the other hand, similar treatment for the prevention or recurrence of coronary thrombosis and mortality was significantly more effective only for males. The source of the sex-oriented variability in response is under investigation. Several other inhibitors of thromboxane synthesis are in advanced clinical trials as candidates for the treatment of conditions in which vasoconstriction, platelet aggregation, and bronchoconstriction may endanger the life of the patient.

**Diflunisal** is recommended for the relief of mild to moderate pain accompanied by inflammation in conditions such as musculoskeletal trauma, pain after dental extraction, post-episiotomy pain, and osteoarthritis. It has a slow onset (2 to 4 hours for maximum analgesia) and long duration of action (8 to 12 hours). Only large doses inhibit platelet function, and the inhibition is reversible. Diflunisal in daily doses of 500 mg or more increases uric acid elimination, but on prolonged use, it may cause significant fluid retention. Drug interactions may occur with oral anticoagulants, tolbutamide, diuretics, and other anti-inflammatory drugs. The most often reported side effects are gastrointestinal complaints, headache, drowsiness, cholestatic jaundice, skin eruptions, and confusion. The drug is not recommended during pregnancy or breastfeeding, it should not be administered to patients with ASA hypersensitivity or allergy, and upward dose adjustments should not be made without proper instructions to the patient.

**Misoprostol,** a synthetic prostaglandin $E_1$ analogue (see Chapter 27), increases the secretion of mucus and bicarbonate by secretory cells of the stomach, and it increases capillary blood flow. These properties are utilized for the prophylaxis and treatment of gastric and duodenal ulcers and to prevent the gastrointestinal complications induced by long-term use of anti-inflammatory analgesics and corticosteroids. The usual dosage and frequency of administration of misoprostol is 0.2 mg given alone or simultaneously with the prescribed anti-inflammatory agent for the prevention of gastrointestinal complications, but more frequently for the treatment of established NSAID-associated gastric ulceration.

## PARA-AMINOPHENOLS

The antipyretic analgesic action of **acetanilid** was discovered in 1886 by an accidental mix-up in compounding a prescription. Later, the drug was introduced into medicine but was abandoned several decades later because of its toxicity. **Acetaminophen** and **phenacetin** are congeners of acetanilid, with analgesic and antipyretic effects similar to those of ASA, but they have no therapeutically significant anti-inflammatory or anti-rheumatic proper-

ties. Phenacetin is no longer used in North America because of its toxic side effects.

## Acetaminophen

### Mechanism and site of action
Although its antipyretic and analgesic properties are similar to those of ASA, acetaminophen (Fig. 28-2 and Table 28-1) is a very weak inhibitor of COX-1 and COX-2. In some in vitro systems, the COX-2 inhibitory potency of acetaminophen is comparable to that of fenoprofen, ticlopidine, or sulindac. However, it is possible that the sensitivity of the enzyme is different in various parts of the body and that sufficient inhibition does occur with acetaminophen to produce analgesia and to reduce fever in environments that have low peroxide concentration. An alternative explanation of the analgesic and antipyretic actions of acetaminophen is based on recent evidence that a splice variant of COX-1, designated COX-3, found only in the dog CNS so far, is quite sensitive to inhibition by acetaminophen. If COX-3 plays a significant role in the production of pain and fever, it could be the primary locus of action of acetaminophen.

### Pharmacokinetics
Acetaminophen is rapidly absorbed from the gastrointestinal tract, and peak plasma levels are reached in 30 to 60 minutes. The bioavailability is influenced by the rate of absorption because significant first-pass biotransformation takes place in the luminal cells of the intestine and in the hepatocytes. From ordinary doses of less than 1 g, only 60% of the drug will reach the central compartment in active form. From doses greater than 1 g, up to 90% or more is available for distribution after absorption. The drug diffuses quickly into most tissues and concentrates mainly in the liver. The apparent volume of distribution is 1 L/kg, and less than 10% is bound to plasma proteins. Pharmacokinetic data are summarized in Table 28-2.

Acetaminophen is conjugated in the liver to form inactive metabolites. Following ordinary clinical doses, 54% is conjugated with glucuronic acid, 33% with sulfuric acid, 4% with cysteine, and 5% as a mercapturic acid

| FIGURE 28-2 | Structural formula of acetaminophen. |

(see Chapter 4). A minor amount of acetaminophen is converted in the hepatocytes (and probably in other organs with significant cytochrome P450 activity) to a chemically reactive intermediary metabolite. Under normal circumstances, the active metabolite reacts with glutathione to form a harmless end product; however, following the consumption of large doses, glutathione is depleted and the active metabolite will attach covalently to macromolecules that have an essential role in the normal biochemical processes of the cell. In some individuals, this leads to liver-cell death, which constitutes a serious and life-threatening toxicity (see also Chapters 43 and 72).

The plasma half-life of acetaminophen depends on the dose, rate of absorption, and biotransformation. The average normal half-life is 1 to 2 hours, which may increase to 4 to 5 hours following large doses or in severe hepatic insufficiency. Mild or moderately severe liver disease does not affect the biotransformation. About 2 to 5% of the dose is eliminated unchanged in the urine; the rest is conjugated mainly to the glucuronide or sulfate.

### Pharmacological effects

The antipyretic and analgesic properties of acetaminophen are similar to those of ASA, but the duration of action is slightly shorter. It is an ideal analgesic for patients who suffer from gastric complaints or who cannot tolerate ASA. The analgesic effect appears to be mediated entirely by an action on the CNS.

### Adverse effects and toxicity

At ordinary dosage, acetaminophen is virtually free of significant adverse effects. Its only significant drug interaction is increased risk of hepatotoxicity (see below) in alcoholics or users of other hepatotoxic drugs.

Skin rash or other minor allergic reactions occur infrequently, and minor alterations in the leukocyte count are transient. Renal tubular necrosis and hypoglycemic coma are rare complications of prolonged large-dose therapy. Renal damage is independent of hepatic toxicity. Potentially fatal hepatic necrosis may occur from overdose of 10 g or more in an adult. The reactive metabolite formed in the liver can easily deplete the normal glutathione supply and cause irreversible cell damage. In this case, the administration of *N*-acetylcysteine can be life-saving if administered within 12 to 20 hours (see also Chapters 43 and 72). Currently available *N*-acetylcysteine preparations are administered orally, but they are equally effective when administered intravenously.

Phenacetin is still marketed in a number of countries as a substitute for acetaminophen. Its pharmacological and toxicological properties are similar to those of acetaminophen, but in addition, it may cause hemolytic anemia, methemoglobinemia and, in toxic overdose, cyanosis, respiratory depression, and cardiac arrest.

## NON-STEROIDAL ANTI-INFLAMMATORY DRUGS (NSAIDs)

The drugs in this section are commonly known as NSAIDs. Although they share many properties and applications with the salicylates (notably ASA), they are by convention regarded as a separate group. Personal preference by the physician or the patient and individual tolerance are the main criteria for selecting one or another of these largely similar drugs.

The NSAIDs are chemically diverse (i.e., pyrazolones, indoles, phenylpropionic acids, naphthylpropionic acids, naphthylalkalones, anthranilic acids, pyrroleacetic acids, phenylacetic acids, and oxicams), but they share to a large extent the same mechanisms of action and adverse effects. These are therefore discussed collectively. Pharmacokinetic data are summarized in Table 28-2.

### Mechanisms of Action of NSAIDs

All NSAIDs inhibit the cyclooxygenase required for conversion of arachidonic acid to endoperoxide intermediates (see Chapter 27) $PGG_2$ and $PGH_2$. They act as competitive inhibitors of the binding of arachidonic acid to the active site of the enzyme. Therefore, in contrast to ASA, the inhibition is either readily or slowly reversible, depending on the compound and the tissue source of the microsomal enzyme tested. The antipyretic, analgesic, and platelet-inhibitory effects in most cases are primarily a function of cyclooxygenase inhibition. The actions on rheumatic, inflammatory, and immunological processes, as well as acute gout, depend to varying degrees on inhibition of cyclooxygenase and on many other poorly understood processes, such as inhibition of leukocyte migration and phagocytosis, stabilization of lysosomal membranes, inhibition of plasmin, increased cell-wall integrity, uncoupling of oxidative phosphorylation, inhibition of phosphodiesterase, depression of mucopolysaccharide biosynthesis, and increased release of adrenaline and adrenocorticosteroids. Studies on the reduction in the incidence of colon cancer by ASA and of familial polyposis by sulindac administration are underway. The benefit of COX-2 inhibitors in preventing or arresting the progress of neurological diseases (Alzheimer's or Parkinson's) has not been proven.

### Adverse Effects and Toxicity Attributed to Inhibition of Cyclooxygenase

These are more or less the same as those produced by ASA, but they are probably less frequently encountered and are of reduced intensity. However, NSAIDs may occasionally cause agranulocytosis, which is not observed with salicylates.

**TABLE 28-2**    Recommended Dosages and Known Pharmacokinetic Data for the Anti-inflammatory Analgesics Described in This Chapter

| Generic Name | Trade Name | Recommended Daily Dose (mg) | IC$_{50}$ Ratio (COX-2: COX-1) | Bioavailability (%) | $T_{max}$ (hours) | Serum Half-Life (hours) | Protein Binding (%) |
|---|---|---|---|---|---|---|---|
| **Salicylates** | | | | | | | |
| Acetylsalicylic acid (ASA) | Aspirin,* others | 325–1000 | 32 | 70 | 1–2 | 0.2[†] | 80 |
| Sodium salicylate | | 350–1000 | 2 | – | 1–2 | 2–30 | 80 |
| Choline salicylate | Arthropan, Teejel | 1000–7000 | – | – | 1–2 | 2–30 | 80 |
| Choline magnesium salicylate | Trilisate | 1000–3000 | – | – | 1–2 | 9–18 | 80 |
| Diflunisal | Dolobid | 500–1000 | 1 | 95 | 2–3 | 8–12 | 99 |
| **Para-aminophenol** | | | | | | | |
| Acetaminophen | Tylenol, others | 325–3900 | ? | 60–90 | 0.5–1 | 1–5 | 10 |
| **Pyrazolones** | | | | | | | |
| Sulfinpyrazone | Anturan | 200–800 | | 95 | 1–2 | 3–8 | 98 |
| **Indoles** | | | | | | | |
| Indomethacin | Indocid, Indocin | 50–200 | 46 | 95 | 3 | 4–12 | 90 |
| Sulindac (Indene) | Clinoril | 150–400 | ? | 90 | 1 | 7[†] | 93[†] |
| active metabolite | | | | | 2 | 18 | |
| Etodolac | Ultradol | 400–600 | 0.1 | 80 | 1–2 | 7 | 99 |
| **Phenylpropionic acids** | | | | | | | |
| Fenoprofen | Nalfon | 900–2400 | 7 | 90 | 1.5 | 2.5 | 99 |
| Flurbiprofen | Ansaid | 150–200 | 41 | 95 | 1.5 | 4 | 99 |
| Ibuprofen | Advil, Motrin, Ruefen, others | 600–2400 | 2 | 98 | 1–2 | 2 | 99 |
| Ketoprofen | Orudis | 100–200 | 7 | 98 | 1–2 | 1–35 | 91 |
| Oxaprozin | Daypro | 600–1200 | – | 95 | 1–2 | 26–92 | 99 |
| Tiaprofenic Acid | Surgam | 600–1800 | – | – | 0.5–1.5 | 1.7 | 99 |
| **Naphthylpropionic acids** | | | | | | | |
| Naproxen | Naprosyn | 500–1000 } | 3.5 | 99 | 2–4 | 12–15 | 99 |
| Naproxen sodium | Anaprox | 825–1375 | | | | | |
| **Naphthylalkanones** | | | | | | | |
| Nabumetone | Relafen | 600–1200 | 1 | – | 3–6 | 26–92 | 99 |
| **Anthranilic acids** | | | | | | | |
| Meclofenamate | Meclomen | 300–600 | 2 | 99 | 0.5–2 | 2 | 99 |
| Mefenamic acid | Ponstan | 1000 | 0.1 | 99 | 2–4 | 2–4 | 99 |
| Floctafenine | Idarac | 600–1200 | – | – | 1–2 | 8 | 99 |
| **Pyrroleacetic acid** | | | | | | | |
| Tolmetin | Tolectin | 600–1800 | 3 | 99 | 0.5–1 | 1–6 | 99 |
| Ketorolac tromethamine | Toradol | 30–40 PO | | | | | |
| | | 90–120 IM | 421 | 80 | 0.5–1 | 5 | 99 |
| **Phenylacetic acid** | | | | | | | |
| Diclofenac sodium | Voltaren | 75–150 | 0.4 | 95 | 2.5 | 1–2 | 99 |
| **Oxicams** | | | | | | | |
| Piroxicam | Feldene | 20 | 2 | 99 | 2–4 | 35–90 | 99 |
| Tenoxicam | Mobiflex | 20 | – | 99 | 0.5–6 | 72 | 99 |
| Meloxicam | Mobicox | 15–30 | – | 89 | 9–11 | 22–24 | 99 |
| **Coxibs** | | | | | | | |
| Celecoxib | Celebrex | 100–400 | 0.5 | ? | 2–4 | 11–15 | 97 |
| Rofecoxib | Vioxx | 25–50 | 0.1 | 93 | 1–2 | 17–20 | 87 |
| Valdecoxib | Bextra | 10–40 | – | 83 | 1–3 | 8–11 | 98 |

| Vd (L/kg) | Biotransformation | Excretion | Therapeutic Use | Side Effects |
|---|---|---|---|---|
| 0.1–0.35 | Hyd, Con, Oxi | Ren | AN, AP, RA, OA, AS, JA | GI, tinnitus, hypersensitivity, hyperuricemia, Reye's syndrome, salicylism |
| 0.1–0.35 | Con, Oxi | Ren | AN | GI, salicylism |
| 0.1–0.35 | Con, Oxi | Ren | AN, AP, RA, OA | GI, salicylism |
| 0.1–0.35 | Con, Oxi | Ren | AN | GI, salicylism |
| 0.09 | Con | Ren | AN, RA, OA, JA, AS | GI, headache, rash, jaundice, drowsiness, confusion, hypersensitivity |
| 1.0 | Con, Oxi | Ren | AN, AP | Skin rash, hepatic necrosis, renal tubular necrosis |
| 0.16 | Oxi, Con | Ren | Thrombosis, gout | GI, ↓ renal function, blood dyscrasias |
| 1.0 | Oxi, Con, Dem | Ren, Bil | Gout, AS, RA, OA | GI, headache, dizziness, tinnitus, somnolence, agranulocytosis |
| 2.0 | Oxi, Red | Ren, Bil | Gout, AS, OA, RA | Same as indomethacin but milder |
| 0.41 | Hyd, Con | Ren, Bil | AN, OA | GI, chills, fever, nervousness, depression, blurred vision |
| 0.08 | Oxi, Con, Dem | Ren | AP, AN, RA, OA, D | GI, dizziness, nervousness, palpitations, somnolence |
| 0.1 | Oxi, Con | Ren | RA, OA | GI, headache, edema |
| 0.12 | Oxi, Con | Ren, Bil | AN, AP, OA, D | GI, dizziness, rash, edema, blurred vision, agranulocytosis |
| 0.1 | Oxi, Con | Ren | AP, AN, RA, OA, D | GI, renal, headache |
| 0.25 | Con | Ren | OA, RA | GI, rash, depression, tinnitus |
| 0.1 | Unchanged | Ren | OA, RA | GI, dizziness, drowsiness, headache, rash, edema |
| 0.1–0.35 | Dem | Ren | OA, RA, AS, AN, D, gout | GI, edema, headache, drowsiness, tinnitus |
| 0.25 | Con | Ren | OA, RA | GI, dizziness, headache, rash, edema, tinnitus |
| – | Oxi, Con | Ren, Bil | AN, D, RA, OA | GI, edema, rash, headache, dizziness, tinnitus |
| – | Oxi, Hyx | Ren, Bil | AN, D | GI, dizziness, agranulocytosis |
| – | Oxi, Con | Ren, Bil | AN | GI, dysuria, polyuria, drowsiness, dizziness, headache |
| 0.1 | Con, Hyx | Ren | RA, OA, AS | GI, hypersensitivity, edema, headache, dizziness, ↑ blood pressure |
| 0.25 | Con, Hyd | Ren | AN | GI, headache, dizziness, rash, edema |
| 0.13 | Con | Ren, Bil | RA, OA | GI, dizziness, headache, palpitations, rash, edema |
| 0.12 | Hyx, Con, Hyd | Ren | RA, OA, AS, D | GI, headache, rash, edema, ↓ hemoglobin, ↑ liver enzymes |
| – | Oxi, Con | Ren | RA, OA, AS | GI, rash, headache, dizziness, edema |
| 0.1–0.2 | Oxi, Hyx | Ren, Bil | RA, OA | GI, dyspepsia, nausea, vomiting, pain, bowel perforation |
| 0.1–0.3 | Con Oxi | Ren | AN, AS, OA, RA | GI, pain, edema, hypertension, renal |
| 1–1.5 | Red, Con | Hep, Bil | AN, OA, RA, D | GI, hypertension, edema, thrombosis, renal |
| 1.5–2.0 | Oxi | Ren | RA, OA, AN, D | GI, edema, hypertension, renal |

Bil = biliary; Con = conjugation; Dem = demethylation; Hyd = hydrolysis; Hyx = hydroxylation; Oxi = oxidation; Red = reduction; Ren = renal; AN = analgesic; AP = antipyretic; AS = ankylosing spondylitis; D = dysmenorrhea; JA = juvenile arthritis; OA = osteoarthritis; RA = rheumatoid arthritis; Hep = hepatic.

*In Canada only.

†See text for variations.

## Gastrointestinal

Like ASA, the NSAIDs are weak organic acids and can cause gastric mucosal damage, both by inhibiting prostaglandin synthesis and by accumulating intracellularly because of the low pH in the gastric lumen. The following adverse effects have been reported: occult gastrointestinal bleeding with anemia, gastritis, epigastric pain, hematemesis, dyspepsia, ulcerative esophagitis, acute and reactivated gastric and duodenal ulcer with perforation and hemorrhage, and ulceration and perforation of the large bowel and rectum. These effects are delayed if the drugs are administered rectally, parenterally, or in enteric-coated formulations, and the co-administration of $H_2$ receptor blockers or of prostaglandin analogues (e.g., misoprostol) will increase gastric tolerance during chronic administration of NSAIDs.

## Platelet function

The synthesis of thromboxane $A_2$ (TXA2), derived from cyclic endoperoxides $PGG_2$ and $PGH_2$ (see Chapter 27) that are synthesized from arachidonic acid by cyclooxygenase, is reversibly inhibited by most NSAIDs. Platelets may fail to aggregate. Prostacyclin ($PGI_2$) formation, which opposes platelet aggregation, is also inhibited by NSAIDs, but because of the abundance of cyclooxygenase in endothelial cells and their ability to synthesize new enzyme, the reduction of $PGI_2$ production during long-term NSAID administration is of minor significance. The interaction of NSAIDs with warfarin, however, may have serious consequences.

## Renal

The participation of prostaglandins in normal renal function is complex. COX-2 is constitutively expressed in the macula densa and adjacent cortical thick ascending limb of the renal tubule of the renal cortex. In sodium chloride restriction, COX-2 appears to control renin release. COX-2 is also present in glomerular podocytes and small blood vessels. $PGI_2$ and $PGE_2$ cause direct renal vasodilatation and increased cortical and medullary blood flow, which results in increased glomerular filtration rate, decreased renal vascular resistance, increased natriuresis, and reduced medullary hypertonicity with decreased water reabsorption in the loop of Henle. Also, prostaglandins may indirectly moderate or prevent the action of ADH on tubular epithelium by negative feedback, resulting in increased water elimination. Thus, prostaglandins favour the formation of dilute urine and enhanced water excretion.

NSAIDs, by inhibiting prostaglandin synthesis, remove the negative feedback on ADH (allowing excessive water retention and edema formation), and they permit humoral or neurogenic renal vasoconstriction and sodium and water reabsorption. The administration of NSAIDs to patients with normal renal hemodynamic function may cause temporary water retention and "weight" gain. Patients suffering from marginal or significantly reduced renal function, congestive heart failure, hypertension, or conditions that require the administration of a diuretic, however, are at great risk of serious adverse effects. These adverse effects usually consist of edema, fluid and electrolyte disturbances, sodium and chloride retention, and plasma dilution. NSAID-induced renal failure is usually temporary, and normal renal function returns shortly after the drug is terminated. Of the presently used NSAIDs, sulindac appears to be the least nephrotoxic.

## Respiratory

The administration of NSAIDs to persons suffering from asthma or other respiratory ailments may provoke acute rhinitis, angioneurotic edema, urticaria, bronchial asthma, bronchoconstriction, hypotension, and shock. These reactions do not appear to have an antigenic component, but they may be due to inhibition of cyclooxygenase and a consequent overabundance of leukotriene production (see Chapter 27).

## Pregnancy and labour

NSAID administration during the last trimester of pregnancy may prolong gestation, delay labour, and cause excessive postpartum bleeding and hemorrhage by inhibition of $PGE_2$, PGF2., and TXA2 synthesis.

# Side Effects That Appear to Be Unrelated to the Inhibition of Cyclooxygenase

The rate of occurrence of these side effects is different for each drug. Without regard for rank order or frequency and severity, they can be summarized as follows:

- **Allergic:** Hypersensitivity reactions, bronchospasm, anaphylactic/anaphylactoid reactions, serum sickness, arthralgia, fever
- **Cardiovascular:** Vasodilatation, pallor, elevated blood pressure, palpitation, angina, arrhythmias, pericarditis, perivascular granulomata
- **CNS:** Headache, dizziness, dry mouth, sweating, nervousness, excessive thirst, inability to concentrate, insomnia, stimulation, vertigo, confusion, lightheadedness, convulsions, syncope, paresthesia, peripheral neuropathy, psychic disturbances, tiredness, disorientation, nightmares, hallucinations, migraine, speech disorder, tremor, muscle twitch
- **Dermatological:** Urticaria, rash, erythema, pruritus, angioedema, angiitis, hair loss, photosensitivity, erythroderma, Stevens–Johnson syndrome, toxic epidermal necrolysis
- **Ear:** Tinnitus, vertigo, impaired hearing, hearing loss
- **Endocrine:** Hyperglycemia, hypoglycemia, thyroid hyperplasia, toxic goitre, gynecomastia
- **Eye:** Macular and corneal deposits, corneal opacity, blurred vision, orbital and preorbital pain, diplopia,

optic neuritis, retinal detachment, toxic amblyopia
- **Gastrointestinal:** Flatulence, diarrhea, constipation, gastrointestinal fullness, epigastric distress, stomatitis, glossitis, coated tongue, abnormal taste, salivary gland enlargement, ulcerative stomatitis, colitis
- **Hematological:** Purpura, leukopenia, thrombocytopenia, agranulocytosis, pancytopenia, hemolytic anemia, bone marrow depression, aplastic anemia
- **Liver:** Liver function abnormalities, elevated liver enzymes, reversible hepatitis and jaundice, fulminant hepatitis
- **Musculoskeletal and whole body:** Myalgia, asthenia
- **Renal** (rare in patients with normal renal functions but in the elderly any of the following may occur): interstitial nephritis, glomerulonephritis, acute tubular necrosis, papillary necrosis, proteinuria, oliguria, anuria, nephrotic syndrome, bilateral renal cortical necrosis, renal calculi, renal failure with azotemia
- **Respiratory:** Dyspnea, asthma, respiratory distress, respiratory alkalosis, pharyngitis, rhinitis, sinusitis, voice alteration
- **Urogenital:** Increased urinary frequency, hematuria, glycosuria, vaginal bleeding, impotence
- **Others:** Pancreatitis, metabolic acidosis

## Pyrazolones

**Antipyrine, aminopyrine, phenylbutazone** (Table 28-1), and **oxyphenbutazone** have been used extensively in the past for the treatment of rheumatic fever, ankylosing spondylitis, rheumatoid arthritis, osteoarthritis, and gout. In hypersensitive patients, they cause agranulocytosis; therefore, their use is restricted. However, two chemically related compounds, **sulfinpyrazone** and **apazone**, are used clinically (see below).

### Sulfinpyrazone

Sulfinpyrazone (Fig. 28-3) is a phenylbutazone derivative without anti-rheumatic, antipyretic, analgesic, or sodium-retaining activity. It is a powerful uricosuric agent used for the treatment of chronic gout. The drug is also used to inhibit platelet aggregation in the treatment of transient ischemic attacks, thromboembolism associated with vascular or cardiac prostheses, recurrent venous thrombosis, and arteriovenous shunt thrombosis (see also Chapter 38). The side effects and toxicity of sulfinpyrazone are blood dyscrasias (very rare) and gastrointestinal complaints. Concurrent salicylate therapy is not recommended because salicylates and citrates antagonize the uricosuric effect of sulfinpyrazone, and ASA may prolong bleeding time.

### Apazone

Apazone is one of the recently developed pyrazolone derivatives that is a weak inhibitor of cyclooxygenase and has analgesic, antipyretic, and anti-inflammatory proper-

ties similar to those of phenylbutazone. It is a strong uricosuric agent with various side effects. It is used primarily for acute gout, rheumatoid arthritis, and osteoarthritis. The drug is not yet available in North America.

## Indoles

From the many compounds containing an indole group that have been tested for antipyretic, analgesic, and anti-inflammatory actions, **indomethacin** and **etodolac** were found to be clinically useful. **Sulindac** is an indene, chemically related to indomethacin but lacking the indole nitrogen (Fig. 28-4).

### Indomethacin

The analgesic, antipyretic, and anti-inflammatory actions of indomethacin (see Table 28-1) are similar to those of the salicylates. It is a very potent inhibitor of cyclooxygenase. It also uncouples oxidative phosphorylation, depresses the biosynthesis of mucopolysaccharides, inhibits phosphodiesterase, inhibits the motility of polymorphonuclear leukocytes, and reduces the natriuretic effect of furosemide. The drug is O-demethylated and conjugated with glucuronic acid by hepatic microsomal enzymes.

Indomethacin is a very potent anti-inflammatory agent. Although it has antipyretic and analgesic properties, it also tends to cause serious gastrointestinal and other complications. Therefore, it should be used only for the treatment of rheumatoid arthritis, ankylosing spondylitis, osteoarthritis, and acute gout and for the control of pain in uveitis and post-operative ophthalmic pain.

### Etodolac

Etodolac, a relatively selective and potent inhibitor of COX-1 and COX-2 isoforms involved in inflammatory conditions, is similar to indomethacin but requires higher

**FIGURE 28-3** Structural formulae of pyrazolones.

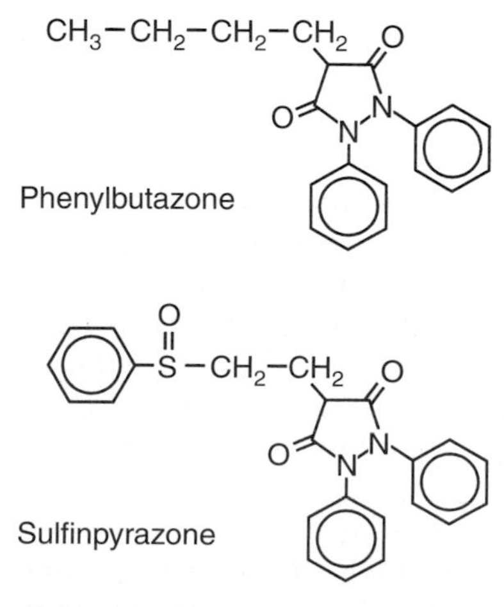

FIGURE 28-4 | Structural formulae of indole compounds.

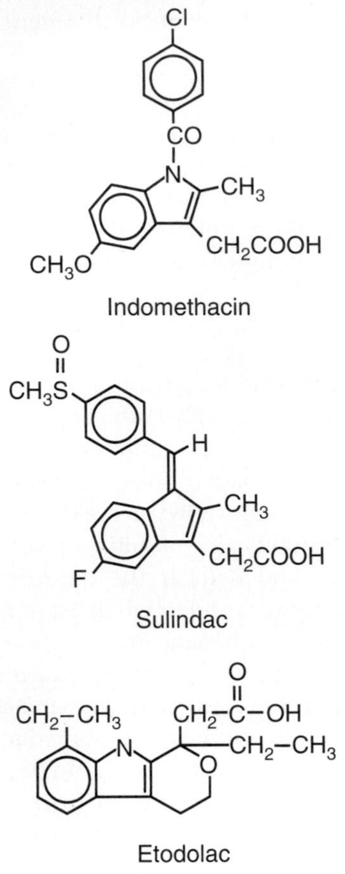

microsomal enzymes oxidize the molecule to a sulfone and reduce it to a sulfide, which is the active form of sulindac. It inhibits prostaglandin synthesis and is about half as potent as indomethacin. The absorption, distribution, and plasma protein binding are also similar to those of indomethacin (see Table 28-2). The plasma half-life of sulindac is about 7 hours, but for the sulfide metabolite, it is about 18 hours. Sulindac spares the kidney because it does not affect renal $PGI_2$ synthesis.

## Phenylpropionic Acid Derivatives and Analogues

The drugs in this group (Fig. 28-5) share many pharmacological and toxicological properties. They are all substi-

FIGURE 28-5 | Structural formulae of propionic acid derivatives.

doses for comparable effects. Gastric prostaglandin synthesis appears less affected.

The drug is well absorbed orally, is unevenly distributed, and is eliminated after conjugation as unchanged drug (20%) and as hydroxylated metabolites (45%) in urine (73%) and feces (14%).

Etodolac is a potent anti-inflammatory, analgesic, and antipyretic drug recommended for the management of rheumatoid arthritis, osteoarthritis, and pain. The dose should not exceed 1200 mg in 24 hours, and it should be reduced if renal function is significantly impaired.

Gastrointestinal disturbances are the most frequent adverse effects, but they are usually less serious than those associated with most other NSAIDs. Drug interactions with other highly protein-bound drugs may occur, but preliminary observations with glyburide, phenytoin, and warfarin were negative. The phenolic metabolites of etodolac may produce a false-positive urinary bilirubin test.

### Sulindac

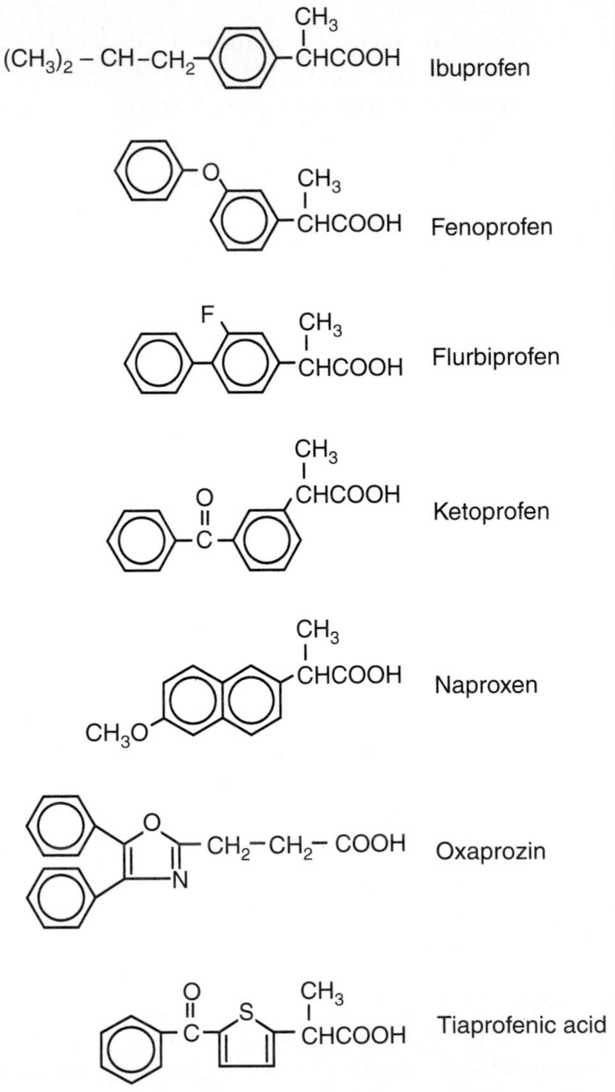

Sulindac, which is closely related to indomethacin, requires biotransformation to become active. Hepatic

tuted phenyl-, naphthyl-, or thienyl-propionic acids, which are chemically and pharmacologically analogous. The drugs inhibit prostaglandin biosynthesis in vitro and in vivo but differ in their potency, which is reflected in the respective doses required to produce analgesia, reduce fever, and inhibit inflammatory processes. Table 28-2 summarizes the pharmacokinetics, the uses, and the most significant side effects.

**Ibuprofen** is probably the best tolerated for long-term use, even by patients who cannot tolerate ASA because of gastric complaints. Oral absorption is complete, but rectal absorption is slow and erratic. A variety of flavoured ibuprofen suspensions and chewable tablets are available for treatment of pain and fever in children, and a preparation of liquid in gelatin capsules is available for the quick relief of prodromal signs and symptoms of migraine headache.

**Fenoprofen** is less popular than the other members of this group, probably because of less intensive commercial promotion. Oral absorption is fast, but it is not complete in the presence of food.

**Ketoprofen** is absorbed rapidly and completely after oral administration, but it is distributed unevenly in body water. The plasma half-life may vary between 1 and 35 hours; the causes of this variability are unknown.

**Flurbiprofen** cannot be tolerated by a small number of patients because of side effects occurring after a few days of administration.

**Naproxen** is well tolerated by most patients. It is completely absorbed after oral or rectal administration. Antacids containing magnesium oxide or aluminum hydroxide reduce the rate of absorption.

**Oxaprozin** is a long-acting NSAID recommended primarily for the symptomatic treatment of rheumatoid arthritis and osteoarthritis. It has analgesic, anti-inflammatory, and antipyretic properties. Care must be taken to avoid overdosage because of the drug's long plasma half-life of 26 to 92 hours. The adverse effects are similar to those of other NSAIDs. Drug interaction with other highly protein-bound drugs is a distinct possibility.

**Tiaprofenic acid** is rapidly absorbed from the stomach, duodenum, and jejunum and is largely (98%) carried in protein-bound form in the plasma. The plasma half-life is only 1.5 to 2 hours, but the drug can be detected in synovial fluid for up to 11 hours. Over 90% of the dose is excreted unchanged in the urine. Therefore, the dose should be reduced for patients with impaired renal function.

## Naphthylalkanones

**Nabumetone** (Fig. 28-6) is a prodrug that requires biotransformation by liver enzymes to form the active metabolite, 6-methoxy-2-naphthylacetic acid (6-MNA), which is a potent inhibitor of COX-1 and COX-2 and has anti-inflammatory, analgesic, and antipyretic effects.

Orally administered nabumetone is absorbed mainly in the duodenum. Maximum concentration of 6-MNA is achieved in serum in 3 to 6 hours and in synovial fluid in 4 to 12 hours. Free and conjugated 6-MNA as well as other active free and conjugated metabolites are excreted in urine (80%) and feces (10%).

Nabumetone is used for its anti-inflammatory and analgesic effect in the symptomatic treatment of rheumatoid arthritis and osteoarthritis. Its value in other conditions, such as ankylosing spondylitis and self-limited soft tissue and musculoskeletal conditions, is unclear.

Adverse effects are similar to those of other NSAIDs. Hepatic or renal impairment and cross-sensitivity with other NSAIDs should be evaluated before commencement of treatment. Drug interactions with other highly protein-bound drugs (e.g., warfarin, tolbutamide, chlorpropamide) or with digoxin, lithium, and methotrexate are possible.

## Anthranilic Acids

**Mefenamic acid** (Fig. 28-7 and Table 28-1), in addition to inhibiting prostaglandin synthesis, appears to inhibit the action of $PGF_2$ on isolated bronchial smooth muscle. It is unevenly distributed in body water, and it has several metabolites that are eliminated in urine along with the unchanged drug. Mefenamic acid has analgesic, antipyretic, and anti-inflammatory properties, but because of gastrointestinal side effects, including occasionally severe diarrhea, the drug is used primarily for short-term analgesia and dysmenorrhea.

**Meclofenamic acid** (see Fig. 28-7) acts similarly to mefenamic acid. It produces significant analgesia in about 30 minutes.

**Floctafenine** (see Fig. 28-7) is a recently introduced anti-inflammatory analgesic. It is completely absorbed after oral administration, attains peak plasma levels in 1 to 2 hours, and has an initial plasma half-life ($\alpha$ phase) of

| FIGURE 28-6 | Structural formulae of nabumetone and its active metabolite 6-methoxy-2-naphthylacetic acid (6-MNA). |

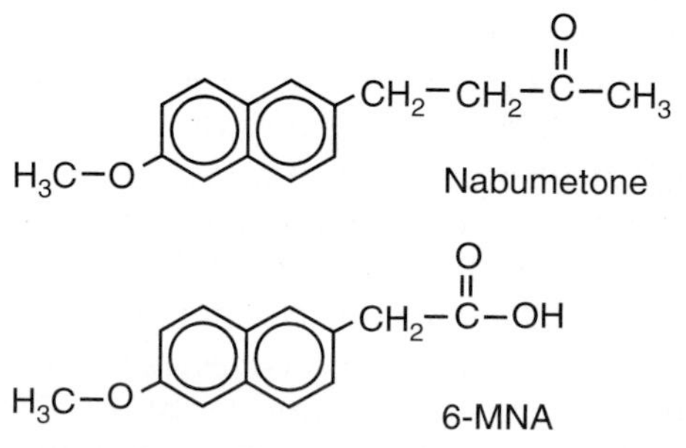

FIGURE 28-7    Structural formulae of anthranilic acids.

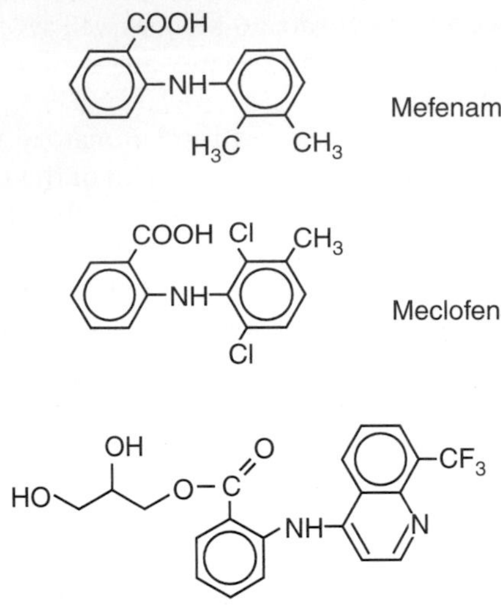

Mefenamic acid

Meclofenamic acid

Floctafenine

1 hour and a β phase of 8 hours. The drug is recommended primarily for the short-term treatment of mild to moderately severe pain.

## Pyrroleacetic Acid and Phenylacetic Acid Derivatives

**Tolmetin,** a substituted pyrroleacetic acid derivative (Fig. 28-8), has analgesic, antipyretic, and anti-inflammatory properties similar to those of ASA. Tolmetin is recommended as an anti-inflammatory drug, but many patients cannot tolerate the side effects (gastric erosion, ulceration, bleeding, nervousness, drowsiness, insomnia).

**Ketorolac tromethamine,** a substituted pyrrolizine-carboxylic acid (see Fig. 28-8), is a potent analgesic with minimal anti-inflammatory and antipyretic activity. It is recommended as an analgesic for mild to moderately severe pain, to be used for up to 3 to 4 weeks. Side effects are mainly gastrointestinal effects and somnolence.

**Diclofenac sodium,** a substituted phenylacetic acid derivative (see Fig. 28-8), has analgesic, antipyretic, and anti-inflammatory properties similar to those of ASA. It is recommended for the treatment of rheumatoid arthritis and severe osteoarthritis, including degenerative joint disease of the hip. It has many of the side effects commonly encountered with this group of drugs, the most serious being gastrointestinal bleeding, cardiac arrhythmias, water retention, and reversible depression of the hematopoietic system. Enteric-coated tablets or a combination product with misoprostol is recommended for oral administration to reduce gastric irritation. Diclofenac sodium 1.5% solution containing dimethyl sulfoxide has been introduced for topical application to relieve pain of

osteoarthritis in the knee. The occurrence of undesirable side effects indicates systemic absorption of diclofenac.

## Oxicams

**Piroxicam** (Fig. 28-9 and Table 28-1) is an amphoteric compound and may behave either as a weak acid or a weak base. It is absorbed slowly after oral administration. Because of its long half-life (in excess of 40 hours), with daily doses of 20 mg, the plasma levels rise for about 5 to 7 days to reach a steady state. Food in the stomach does not influence bioavailability. Because of its potential for cumulation, caution is required when the drug is administered to patients with impaired hepatic or renal function.

**Meloxicam** (Mobicox) is a substituted benzothiazine carboxamide with preferential COX-2 isoform inhibitory properties. It is usually administered orally, but rectal suppositories and intravenous and intramuscular injectable preparations are marketed in some countries. It has antipyretic, anti-inflammatory, and analgesic properties, but it is used primarily for the treatment of rheumatoid arthritis, osteoarthritis, ankylosing spondylitis, and other rheumatological disorders.

Following oral, rectal, or parenteral administration, meloxicam is readily absorbed, with at least 89% bioavailability. Maximum plasma concentrations are achieved in 9 to 11 hours. The plasma half-life is 22 to 24 hours, so it takes 3 to 4 days of oral administration to achieve steady-state concentration. Therefore, intravenous administration is preferred for treating acute flare-ups of osteoarthritis.

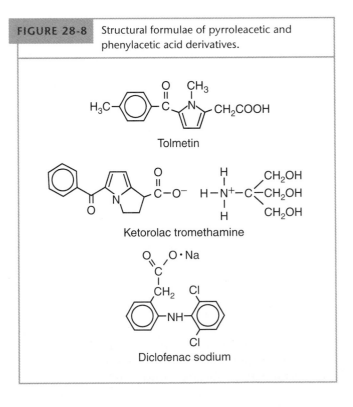

FIGURE 28-8    Structural formulae of pyrroleacetic and phenylacetic acid derivatives.

Tolmetin

Ketorolac tromethamine

Diclofenac sodium

The apparent volume of distribution of meloxicam is 0.1 to 0.2 L/kg, and over 99% is bound to serum albumin. It can be found in perivascular spaces, and the concentration in synovial fluid is about half of the corresponding plasma concentration at steady state.

Meloxicam is metabolized in the liver to four inactive metabolites that are excreted in urine and feces. CYP2C9, 2C8, and 3A4 are the most important P450 isoforms involved in its biotransformation. Related metabolic drug interactions include meloxicam inhibition of tolbutamide oxidation, and sulfaphenazole and ketoconazole inhibition of meloxicam biotransformation. It appears that meloxicam undergoes enterohepatic recirculation because cholestyramine administration increases its clearance by about 50%.

The usual daily dose of meloxicam is 15 to 30 mg. The observable clinical effect (analgesia) is somewhat delayed because of slow absorption following oral administration. Peak plasma concentration may occur only after 10 hours. Intramuscular administration gives relief of pain in 1 hour or less.

In equal therapeutic doses, meloxicam produced less gastrointestinal adverse effects (transient mild gastroduodenal ulceration, dyspepsia, nausea, vomiting, pain, perforation, or hemorrhage) than piroxicam or diclofenac. The usual oxicam precautions and close monitoring are required for patients receiving antihypertensive medications and for patients with renal failure, congestive heart failure, or hepatic insufficiency.

**Tenoxicam** (see Fig. 28-9) is an anti-inflammatory agent with analgesic and antipyretic properties. It inhibits prostaglandin synthesis in vitro and in vivo, and it may act as a scavenger of active oxygen at the site of inflammation. The plasma half-life may vary from 32 to more than 100 hours. Steady-state plasma concentration is reached within 10 to 15 days with daily doses of 20 mg. The main hydroxy metabolite is excreted in urine, but appreciable amounts of the glucuronide conjugates are excreted in bile. The most common adverse reactions are dyspepsia, abdominal discomfort, and epigastric pain.

# SELECTIVE CYCLOOXYGENASE 2 (COX-2) INHIBITORS

As noted in Chapter 27, cyclooxygenase exists in two principal forms. COX-1 is constitutively expressed in most tissues, in which it plays a regulatory role in normal physiological processes, such as protection of the gastric mucosa against attack by gastric HCl. COX-2, on the other hand, is induced by the initiators of the inflammatory process. Drugs that inhibit both forms decrease the inflammatory response by their action on COX-2, but they contribute to adverse effects, such as gastric irritation, by their action on COX-1. Thus, the selective COX-2 inhibitors were introduced with the claim that they have significantly fewer side

effects than NSAIDs that primarily inhibit COX-1. They appeared to have less effect on constitutively expressed COX-2 than on the induced COX-2 isoform. The COX-2 inhibitors were also said to have no anti-thrombotic properties and to not prevent platelet aggregation.

Recently, the claims of greater safety of the COX-2 inhibitors have been withdrawn. The manufacturers removed rofecoxib in 2004 and valdecoxib in 2005 from the market because large-scale population studies revealed that they produced a significant increase in thrombosis and cardiovascular mortality. The final decision concerning their fate will depend on a review of the evidence by the regulatory authorities.

## Celecoxib

Celecoxib (Celebrex) is a diaryl substituted pyrazole that primarily inhibits COX-2 with some minor activity on COX-1. Using recombinant human COX enzyme assays, celecoxib was found to be over 300 times more potent for COX-2 than for COX-1. Following oral administration, it is absorbed in 2 to 4 hours and is extensively bound to plasma proteins. The average plasma half-life is about 11 hours. It is metabolized by CYP2C9, and the carboxylic acid and glucuronic acid conjugated metabolites are excreted in the urine and feces. Celecoxib inhibits CYP2D6 and thus inhibits the metabolism of metoprolol in some patients. In contrast, the related compound rofecoxib does not affect the biotransformation of metoprolol.

### Pharmacological effects

Celecoxib has anti-inflammatory, antipyretic, and analgesic properties. It is used for the symptomatic treatment of osteoarthritis, rheumatoid arthritis, and familial adenomatous polyposis. The recommended usual daily dose

FIGURE 28-9    Structural formulae of oxicams.

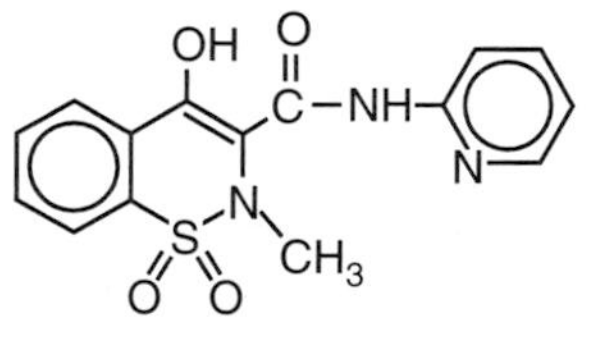

Piroxicam

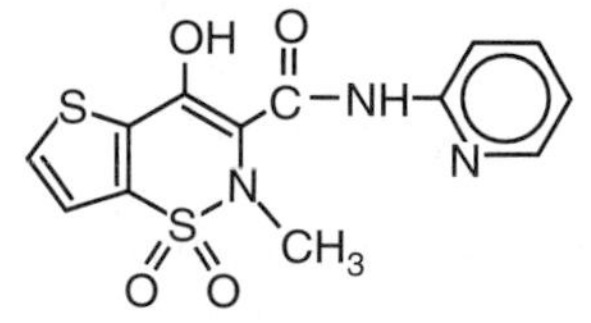

Tenoxicam

is 100 to 400 mg. It should not be administered to patients who are allergic to ASA or sulfonamides. Since the celecoxib molecule contains a sulfonamide grouping, the possibility exists of cross-sensitivity to celecoxib in patients who are allergic to antibacterial or anti-diabetic sulfonamides. Several cases of severe cutaneous allergic reactions to celecoxib have been reported, including erythema multiforme, Stevens-Johnson syndrome, and toxic epidermal necrolysis. It is claimed to have no significant effect on platelet aggregation or bleeding time. Theoretically, increased availability (redirection) of arachidonic acid to platelets may lead to increased TXA2 production, but this can easily be overcome with low doses of ASA. During long-term high-dose celecoxib administration, the patient should be carefully monitored for possible development of upper gastrointestinal ulcers.

### Renal effects

COX-2 is constitutively expressed in the macula densa and adjacent cortical thick ascending limb of the renal tubule in the renal cortex. When sodium chloride intake is restricted, COX-2 appears to control the release of renin and, consequently, of aldosterone. COX-2 in glomerular podocytes and small renal blood vessels has significant influence on glomerular filtration and renal blood circulation (see Chapter 27).

As with other NSAIDs, celecoxib administration may, in some individuals, cause edema, hypertension, interstitial nephritis, and hypophosphatemia. Sodium and potassium retention may occur in normotensive, salt-depleted patients.

## Rofecoxib

Rofecoxib (Vioxx) is a diaryl-substituted furanone with selective strong COX-2 and weak COX-1 inhibition. It has anti-inflammatory, analgesic, and antipyretic properties. Rofecoxib has no effect on platelet aggregation. The recommended oral daily dose of 25 to 50 mg is readily absorbed and provides adequate relief for 24 to 48 hours, respectively. The drug is highly protein-bound. The inactive metabolite dihydrorofecoxib is excreted mostly in urine, and some unchanged drug appears in feces. It has a saturable (zero-order) elimination rate at moderate or high therapeutic plasma concentration, but the average terminal plasma half-life is 17 hours. In metabolic drug interaction studies, it was found that cimetidine increased $C_{max}$ for rofecoxib, and rifampin decreased the rofecoxib plasma concentration. Rofecoxib increased the AUC for theophylline, and the warfarin-induced prothrombin time was increased with reversal of anticoagulation. It reduced the renal elimination of methotrexate. Rofecoxib has moderate inhibitory effect on CYP1A2. Rofecoxib is contraindicated for patients with renal insufficiency because of the powerful inhibitory action on constitutively expressed renal COX-2.

The adverse effects of rofecoxib are similar to those of the other selective COX-2 inhibitors. In sensitive individuals, thrombosis, gastric irritation, gastroduodenal ulceration, and reactivation of pre-existing gastric ulcers may occur. Modest elevation of blood pressure, edema, and altered sodium–potassium elimination is similar to that observed with traditional NSAIDs, especially in patients with hypertension and congestive heart failure. Reduced urinary potassium excretion and reduced glomerular filtration rate may develop in patients with renal insufficiency, congestive heart failure, and in salt-restricted elderly patients. The blood pressure and kidney function of patients on antihypertesive medications or diuretics should be carefully monitored during rofecoxib administration.

Rofecoxib was recommended for symptomatic treatment of rheumatic arthritis, osteoarthritis, and dysmenorrhea and for the control of acute post-operative or post-dental extraction pain. The reaction to rofecoxib of patients who are intolerant or allergic to ASA or other NSAIDs is unpredictable.

## Valdecoxib

Valdecoxib (Bextra) is an isoxazolyl substituted benzenesulfonamide with selective COX-2 isoform inhibitory properties. Its anti-inflammatory, analgesic, and antipyretic activities were evaluated in patients with acute pain, hepatic disease, and renal disease and in healthy young and elderly volunteers.

Valdecoxib is well absorbed following oral administration, and maximum plasma concentration is achieved in 3 hours. The absolute bioavailability is 83%. At dosages exceeding 10 mg twice daily, the increase in plasma concentration is proportionally greater than the increase in dosage; this suggests that some binding sites and/or some routes of biotransformation must be saturable at higher concentrations. Steady-state concentration is achieved by day 4. The volume of distribution is 1.5 to 2 L/kg. The plasma protein binding is about 98%, and the concentration in erythrocytes is 2.5 times higher than that in the plasma. The plasma half-life is 8 hours.

Valdecoxib is biotransformed in the liver by CYP3A4 and 2C9 enzymes to an active metabolite, and it is inactivated by direct enzymatic N-glucuronidation of the sulfonamide moiety. Concomitant administration of fluconazole or ketoconazole may result in increased plasma concentration of valdecoxib. The active metabolite has similar pharmacokinetic properties to those of the parent drug but has considerably less efficacy. Unchanged valdecoxib (5%) and the rest of the dose, as metabolites, are excreted in urine and feces.

Valdecoxib is effective for the control of pain (musculoskeletal, post-surgical, dental, traumatic, and dysmenorrheic) and for symptomatic treatment of rheumatoid arthritis and osteoarthritis when used alone or in combination with corticosteroids, methotrexate, gold compounds, or hydroxychloroquine.

In clinical trials, valdecoxib (10 to 40 mg daily) was found to be superior to placebo and similar in effectiveness to naproxen, diclofenac, and ibuprofen, with significantly less upper gastrointestinal discomfort and gastroduodenal ulcers and bleeding. The adverse effects of valdecoxib related to renal function and blood pressure were similar to those of the comparator NSAIDs, but it had no effect on platelet aggregation or bleeding time.

Valdecoxib should be administered with extreme caution, if at all, to patients with allergic-type (mild or severe) reactions to sulfonamides and NSAIDs or to those who suffer from active peptic ulcer, inflammatory bowel disease, or significant hepatic or renal impairment.

The safety of valdecoxib during pregnancy, labour and delivery, and breastfeeding has not been established.

### Parecoxib sodium

Parecoxib sodium (Parecoxib) is the water-soluble prodrug of valdecoxib. When administered intravenously or intramuscularly, it has analgesic and adverse effects similar to those of intravenous or intramuscular ketorolac for postoperative, dental, gynecological, orthopaedic, or post-traumatic pain. Parecoxib is quickly metabolized in the liver to valdecoxib.

## GOLD COMPOUNDS

Gold compounds, such as **auranofin** (Ridaura), **aurothioglucose** (Solganal), and **sodium aurothiomalate** (Myochrysine), are strictly reserved for the treatment of patients with rapidly progressive rheumatoid arthritis who respond poorly to conventional drug treatment. Reliable results are obtained after intramuscular administration of a solution or oily suspension of the gold compound at weekly or longer intervals. The bioavailability of orally administered preparations is low but sufficient for maintenance therapy. Clinically significant improvements may take months to develop and may last for a year after discontinuation. The distribution of gold in the body is unpredictable; it tends to accumulate in inflamed tissues and joints. After termination of treatment, the concentration in blood will gradually diminish over 2 to 3 months, but significant amounts are excreted in the urine for a year or longer. The mechanism of action is uncertain, the most acceptable theory being that gold compounds suppress immune responsiveness by inhibition of mononuclear phagocyte and T-cell function. There are numerous side effects, including dermatitis, proximal tubular damage, blood dyscrasias, and encephalitis. Gold is contraindicated for patients with heavy-metal hypersensitivity, diabetes mellitus, renal disease, and many other conditions, including pregnancy and breastfeeding.

## DRUGS USED IN THE TREATMENT OF GOUT

A variety of analgesics, uricosuric agents (probenecid and sulfinpyrazone), and corticosteroids are used in the symptomatic or specific treatment of gout. Acute attacks of gout respond well to colchicine, and the chronic form may be controlled by reducing plasma uric acid with allopurinol.

**Probenecid** inhibits the proximal renal tubular secretion *and reabsorption* of uric acid (see Chapter 6). Therefore, the whole filtered load of uric acid is eliminated in the urine. The active tubular secretion of penicillin, indomethacin, cephalosporins, thiazides, and other weakly acidic drugs is also blocked by probenecid. The uricosuric effect of probenecid and of sulfinpyrazone is antagonized by ASA.

**Colchicine** is an alkaloid obtained from the autumn crocus. It is used as an anti-inflammatory drug in the prevention and treatment of acute gouty arthritis. Various plant preparations were used starting in A.D. 600. Colchicine causes the disappearance of the fibrillar microtubules in granulocytes and leukocytes, thereby preventing their mobilization to the site of inflammation. It inhibits the release of histamine and the secretion of insulin, and it arrests cell division in metaphase. It may cause nausea, vomiting, hemorrhagic gastroenteritis, and, following chronic administration, alopecia, agranulocytosis, and aplastic anemia. The usual oral adult dose is about 1 mg initially, but not more than 3 mg in 24 hours. For prophylaxis, a daily dose of 0.5 mg, 2 to 4 days per week, is usually adequate to prevent flare-ups. It is also administered together with allopurinol or uricosuric drugs.

**Allopurinol** and its primary metabolite **alloxanthine** reduce plasma uric acid concentration by inhibiting xanthine oxidase, the enzyme catalyzing the final steps of uric acid synthesis. Thus, hyperuricemia of almost any cause, including that induced by other drugs, is normalized. This facilitates the dissolution of tophi and prevents the development or progression of chronic gouty arthritis. Allopurinol and its metabolites are excreted in dose-dependent fashion by glomerular filtration, but there is significant tubular reabsorption, which is sensitive to probenecid inhibition. The drug is well tolerated, but hypersensitivity reactions may occur even after months or years of continuous medication. The usual daily dose is 100 mg, which may be increased to 300 mg/day.

## SUGGESTED READINGS

Aspirin and acetaminophen [special issue]. *Arch Intern Med.* 1981; 141(3 spec no).

Chaffman M, Brodgen RN, Heel RC, et al. Auranofin. A preliminary review of its pharmacological properties and therapeutic use in rheumatoid arthritis. *Drugs.* 1984;27:378-424.

Davies NM, McLachlan AJ, Day RO, Williams KM. Clinical pharmacokinetics and pharmacodynamics of Celecoxib. *Clin Pharmacokinet.* 2000;38:225-242.

FitzGerald G. COX-2 and beyond: approaches to prostaglandin inhibition in human disease. *Nat Rev Drug Discov.* 2003;2: 879-890.

Fowler PD. Aspirin, paracetamol and nonsteroidal anti-inflammatory drugs. A comparative review of side effects. *Med Toxicol Adverse Drug Exp.* 1987;2:338-366.

Gonzales JP, Todd PA. Tenoxicam. A preliminary review of its pharmacodynamic and pharmacokinetic properties, and therapeutic efficacy. *Drugs.* 1987;34:289-310.

Le Lorier J, Bombardier Cl, Borgess E, et al. Practical considerations for the use of nonsteroidal anti-inflammatory drugs and cyclo-oxygenase inhibitors in hypertension and kidney disease. *Can J Cardiol.* 2002;18:1301-1308.

Petro R, Gray R, Collins R, et al. Randomized trial of prophylactic daily aspirin in British male doctors. *Br Med J.* 1988;296: 313-316.

Rainsford KD. Mechanisms of gastrointestinal damage by NSAIDs. *Agents Actions Suppl.* 1993;44:59-64.

Scott LJ, Lamb HM. Rofecoxib. *Drugs.* 1999;88:499-505.

Singh RK, Ethayathulla AS, Jabeen T, et al. Aspirin induces its anti-inflammatory effects through its specific binding to phospholipase A2: crystal structure of the complex formed between phospholipase A2 and aspirin at 1.9 angstroms resolution. *J Drug Target.* 2005;13(2):113-119.

Sovers JR, White WB, Pitt B, et al. The effects of cyclooxygenase-2 inhibitors and nonsteroidal anti-inflammatory therapy on 24-hour blood pressure in patients with hypertension, osteoarthritis, and type 2 diabetes mellitus. *Arch Intern Med.* 2005;165:161-168.

Valdecoxib [product monograph]. Kirkland, Quebec: Pfizer Canada Inc; 2002.

Van Hecken A, Schwartz JJ, Depre M, et al. Comparative inhibitory activity of rofecoxib, meloxicam, diclofenac, ibuprofen, and naproxen on COX 2 versus COX 1 in healthy volunteers. *J Clin Pharmacol.* 2000;40:1109-1120.

Vane J, Botting R. Inflammation and the mechanism of action of anti-inflammatory drugs. *FASEB J.* 1987;1:89-96.

Vane JR, Botting RM. The mechanism of action of aspirin. *Thromb Res.* 2003;110:255-258.

Warner TD, Giuliano F, Vojnovic I, et al. Nonsteroid drug selectivities for cyclooxygenase-1 rather than cyclooxygenase-2 are associated with human gastrointestinal toxicity: a full in vitro analysis. *Proc Natl Acad Sci USA.* 1999;96:7563-7568.

Weir NU, Demchuk AM, Buchan AM, Hill MD. Stroke prevention. MATCHing therapy to the patient with TIA. *Postgrad Med.* 2005;117(1):26-30.

Werner U, Werner D, Rau T, et al. Celecoxib inhibits metabolism of cytochrome P450 2D6 substrate metoprolol in humans. *Clin Pharmacol Ther.* 2003;74:130-137.

# Autacoids

## D KADAR

### CASE HISTORY

A 57-year-old male high-school teacher with moderate hypertension was adequately treated with atenolol 50 mg daily for several years. In addition, he had suffered from migraine in his youth, but with age it became much less frequent and required no special medication. Recently, he complained that the occasional sexual dysfunction he had experienced since taking atenolol had become more frequent, and he tired easily without any obvious reason. His blood pressure medication was changed to captopril 25 mg twice daily and was increased to three times daily after 2 weeks. His sexual performance and physical endurance improved somewhat after 3 months, but the previously occasional migraine attacks became more frequent and severe, and he experienced frequent coughing. Prophylactic treatment of his migraine with pizotifen, methysergide, or cyproheptadine was not practical because the pain occurred only in the morning and was unpredictable. A trial with sumatriptan succinate produced significant improvement of his headache, but the transient chest pain and sensation of tightness were intolerable side effects. The antihypertensive medication was changed to losartan 50 mg daily to avoid the coughing spells that occurred with captopril. A combination preparation containing acetaminophen 500 mg, caffeine 15 mg, and codeine phosphate 8 mg was prescribed for the headache, two tablets to be taken every 4 hours when required. Blood and urine chemistry were found to be normal after 3 and 9 months of therapy, and the blood pressure was adequately controlled. Routine follow-up 1 year later showed that this treatment plan was satisfactory.

## ANGIOTENSINS, ANGIOTENSIN II–RECEPTOR BLOCKERS, AND ANGIOTENSIN-CONVERTING ENZYME INHIBITORS

### Occurrence and Synthesis of Angiotensins

The angiotensins are peptides of known amino acid composition and structure that are derived from high-molecular-weight angiotensinogen and a plasma $\alpha_2$-globulin. Angiotensinogens are converted to the decapeptide angiotensin I by the enzyme renin, which is released by the kidneys and other organs. Angiotensin-converting enzyme (ACE, peptidyl dipeptidase, kininase II), which is found in high concentration in plasma and tissues (e.g., glands, kidneys, vascular endothelial cells, heart), converts angiotensin I (inactive) to the octapeptide angiotensin II, the biologically most active form, which can then be converted to angiotensin III, a less active heptapeptide, and to inactive fragments by prolyl-carboxypeptidase (Fig. 29-1).

A number of additional "peptidase" enzymes (ACE2) produce angiotensin (1-7) and angiotensin (3-8), which either facilitate or stimulate the release of various hormones and counterbalance the actions of angiotensin II by acting on their specific receptors.

Angiotensin II has a powerful vasoconstrictor action, 40 times more powerful than that of adrenaline. Angiotensin II stimulates the synthesis and release of aldosterone from the adrenal cortex and the release of antidiuretic hormone (ADH, vasopressin) from the pituitary gland, promoting sodium and water retention. Extremely high concentrations of circulating angiotensin II, as seen in terminal liver failure, directly inhibit sodium reabsorption in the distal tubule. This action is only of minor interest, however, because the intense renal artery constriction markedly reduces renal blood flow and reduces glomerular filtration rate almost to the point of complete renal shutdown.

Renin release is initiated by stimulation of $\beta_1$-adrenergic receptors of the juxtaglomerular cells and induced in the macula densa cells by a decrease in blood pressure or blood volume, renal ischemia, or depletion of sodium

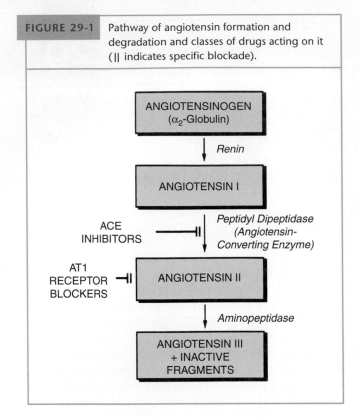

**FIGURE 29-1** Pathway of angiotensin formation and degradation and classes of drugs acting on it (‖ indicates specific blockade).

ions. Adenosine inhibits, and prostaglandins increase, renin release. Non-steroidal anti-inflammatory drugs (NSAIDs) inhibit renin release by inhibition of prostaglandin synthesis. ACE inhibitors, angiotensin II–receptor blockers (ARBs), diuretics, and vasodilators increase renin release, whereas centrally acting sympatholytics and β-adrenergic blockers reduce it. Renin has a short half-life of 15 minutes, so variations in its output provide a mechanism for moderately rapid changes in blood pressure. The induction of renin release by any of these stimuli, and the subsequent production of angiotensin II, increases blood pressure, retention of sodium, cardiac contractility, and heart rate. In addition, angiotensin II causes hypertrophy of vascular and cardiac cells. The elevated blood pressure and angiotensin II concentration act by negative feedback to slow further renin release and bring about a return to homeostasis. Cells in the brain, pituitary, blood vessels, kidney, and adrenal gland can locally produce renin, angiotensinogen, and ACE and, therefore, angiotensins I, II, and III.

Specific oligopeptide inhibitors of renin release and enzymatic activity have been developed. **Ditekiren** is a pseudo-octapeptide, and **enalkiren** is a dipeptide. They are thought to bind to the angiotensinogen binding site of renin and prevent it from forming angiotensin I. These inhibitors have been shown to lower blood pressure in hypertensive subjects, but they are not yet available for clinical use.

The effects of angiotensin II are mediated by AT1 and AT2 G protein–coupled receptors. The effect of stimulating angiotensin receptors is tissue- and species-specific. These effects are mediated by a number of intracellular mechanisms that may involve $Ca^{2+}$ release or influx, Janus kinase, mitogen-activated protein kinase, reactive oxygen species generation, serine/threonine protein kinases, non-receptor tyrosine kinases, small GTP-binding proteins, and inducible transcription factors affecting transcriptional efficiency.

In the kidney, angiotensin II stimulates $Na^+/H^+$ exchange in the proximal tubules and alters renal hemodynamics by acting on the afferent or efferent arterioles.

AT1 receptors are coupled to $G_q$ and $G_i$ proteins, and their activation results in stimulation of phospholipase C activity (thus increasing inositol-1,4,5-trisphosphate and diacylglycerol production) and inhibition of adenylyl cyclase (thus decreasing cAMP formation). The vasoconstrictor action of angiotensin II is mediated both directly through stimulation of AT1 receptors located on pre- and post-capillary vascular smooth muscle cells and indirectly by stimulation of the sympathetic nervous system. The most strongly affected vessels are those of the skin, splanchnic region, and kidney. Vessels of brain and skeletal muscle are less constricted. Elevated circulating levels of angiotensin II and uncontrolled hypertension are responsible for thickening of blood vessel walls, cardiac hypertrophy, fibrosis, and myocardial infarction.

AT2 receptor–mediated effects involve activation of phosphatases, potassium channels, and nitric oxide (NO) production and inhibition of calcium channels. Most of the effects are mediated by AT2 receptor coupling to $G_i$. Selective AT2 receptor blockers are required for more specific elucidation of AT2 receptor–induced mechanism of action. The ratio of tissue- and species-specific distribution of AT2 to AT1 receptors is considerably higher in fetal tissue than in the corresponding adult tissue.

AT2 receptor stimulation upgrades the effectiveness of bradykinin, nitric oxide, cyclic GMP, and prostaglandins to counter-regulate the intensity of AT1 receptor–mediated physiological processes such as protein phosphorylation, cell growth and proliferation, vasoconstriction, and sodium reabsorption. Whether or not the ultimate mechanism of this interaction involves the same biochemical reactions as at AT1 receptor sites, but working in the opposite direction, is not clear.

Angiotensinamide (Hypertensin) is used clinically in some parts of the world to raise blood pressure. It must be given by slow intravenous infusion, with simultaneous monitoring of blood pressure and electrocardiogram (ECG). It may be used to restore blood pressure if the hypotension is due to cardiovascular collapse and not to blood loss.

# Angiotensin II AT1–Receptor Blockers (ARBs)

**Saralasin,** an angiotensin peptide analogue, was the first clinically effective ARB, but it was found to have partial agonist activity that caused transient increases in blood pressure. Additional drawbacks were the short half-life and the lack of effect following oral administration.

Non-peptide, antihypertensive, high-affinity, competitive AT1 receptor blockers with extremely low affinity for AT2 receptors were introduced in the 1980s. Slow dissociation kinetics of ARBs results in a blocking effect that lasts for 24 hours or longer with once-daily drug administration. ARB-induced vasodilation and reduced total peripheral resistance lowers systolic and diastolic blood pressure with minor increases of cardiac output. Aldosterone secretion from zona glomerulosa cells is reduced, with a subsequent increase in serum potassium. ARBs have no effect on the fate of bradykinin, substance P, or ACE. ARBs block the feedback mechanism of angiotensin II; therefore, renin release is increased with subsequent increase of circulating angiotensin II.

ARBs inhibit or reduce the intensity of the following AT1 receptor–mediated biological effects of angiotensin II: vascular smooth muscle contraction, pressor responses, ADH release, aldosterone secretion, adrenal catecholamine release, enhanced noradrenergic neurotransmission, increased sympathetic tone, thirst, renal function changes, and cellular hypertrophy and hyperplasia. The main advantage of ARBs over ACE inhibitors is that they do not reduce angiotensin II generation; therefore, AT2 receptor–induced beneficial physiological functions are retained.

Most of the ARBs are administered as inactive prodrug esters to reduce their ionization in the gastrointestinal tract and improve their bioavailability. Activation takes place during absorption in the intestinal wall or liver. The active drugs are distributed in the extracellular fluid compartment or bound in specific tissues; the extent of this binding can result in an apparent $V_d$ that gives the appearance of distribution throughout the total body water or that greatly exceeds it. The drugs are bound in varying degrees to plasma proteins (especially albumin) and $\alpha_1$- or acid-glycoproteins. The unchanged drugs and their conjugated and oxidized metabolites are excreted in urine and/or bile. The plasma half-life of the prodrug is usually short (minutes or hours) but for the active drug it can be up to 24 hours or longer.

## Therapeutic uses

ARBs are recommended for the treatment of hypertension either alone or in fixed-dose combination with hydrochlorothiazide. ARBs are well tolerated, and the profile and frequency of reported side effects appear to be similar to those of placebo. Exercise tolerance and symptoms of cardiac failure show significant improvement following treat-ment. Extended long-term clinical tests are being carried out to compare ARBs with ACE inhibitors for symptomatic improvement and reduced mortality in cardiac failure, post-myocardial infarction, cirrhosis, and portal hypertension patients. With proper precautions, ARBs can be used in combination with other antihypertensive drugs. The antihypertensive effect appears 5 to 8 hours after the maximum blood concentration is reached and is fully developed after 3 to 4 weeks of continuous drug administration.

## Adverse effects

In comparison with ACE inhibitors, ARBs cause fewer side effects, such as cough or angioneurotic edema, and fewer complications for patients with angiotensin-dependent renal function. Palpitation, hypotension, dizziness, syncope, and back pain occurred at slightly higher rates than in the cross-over placebo controls. Moderate increase of serum potassium concentration is due to reduced aldosterone secretion. There is some genetic variation in ARB biotransformation by CYP2C9 and 3A4.

## Contraindications and warnings

Because they act directly on the renin–angiotensin system, ARBs and ACE inhibitors can cause fetal and neonatal morbidity and death if administered to pregnant women in the second or third trimester. When pregnancy is planned or detected, ARBs should be discontinued as soon as possible. Fetal and neonatal hypotension, skull hypoplasia, anuria, renal failure, death, oligohydramnios, fetal limb contractures, craniofacial deformation, hypoplastic lung, growth retardation, and patent ductus arteriosus have been reported. Repeated ultrasound examinations must be carried out if drug administration is unavoidable during pregnancy (estimated frequency 1:1000). It is not known if ARBs are excreted in breast milk in high enough concentration to harm the infant.

Renal failure and death have been reported in cases of bilateral renal artery stenosis and severe congestive heart failure.

## Pharmacokinetics

Dosages and pharmacokinetic data for candesartan celexetil, eprosartan mesylate, irbesartan, losartan potassium, its E-3174 active metabolite, telmisartan, and valsartan are listed in Table 29-1. Eprosartan is a thienylic acid; the others are biphenylmethyl derivatives. Dozens of other related compounds are in various stages of development. Administration with food delays the absorption of most ARBs and causes clinically insignificant changes in $C_{max}$ and AUC values.

The plasma clearance is affected by both renal and hepatic insufficiency for eprosartan; by only hepatic insufficiency for telmisartan, valsartan, and the active metabolite of losartan; by renal but not by mild or moderate liver insufficiency for candesartan; and by neither for

**TABLE 29-1**  Recommended Dosage and Known Pharmacokinetic Data for the ARBs Described in This Chapter

| Generic Name | Trade Name | Prodrug* | Daily Dose (mg) | Bioavailability (%) | $T_{max}$ (hours) | Half-life (hours) | $V_d$ (L/kg) | Protein Binding (%) | Biotrans-formation | Excretion |
|---|---|---|---|---|---|---|---|---|---|---|
| Candesartan celexetil | Atacand | Y | 80–160 | 15 | 3–4 | 9 | 0.13 | 99 | Con, Oxi | Bil, Ren, U |
| Eprosartan mesylate | Teveten | Y | 300–800 | 13 | 1–2 | 5–9 | 0.18 | 98 | N | Bil, Ren, U |
| Irbesartan | Avapro | N | 75–300 | 60–80 | 1–2 | 11–15 | 0.75–1.3 | 96 | Con, Oxi | Ren, Bil |
| Losartan potassium | Cozaar | N/Y | 50–100 | 33 | 1 | 2 | 0.5 | 98 | Oxi, Con | Bil, Ren |
| E-3174 active metabolite | | | | | 3–4 | 6–9 | 0.17 | 99 | Oxi, Con | Bil, Ren |
| Telmisartan | Micardis | N | 40–80 | 50 | 0.5–1 | 24 | 7 | 99 | Con | Bil, Ren |
| Valsartan | Diovan | N | 80–160 | 23 | 2–4 | 5–9 | 0.24 | 97 | ? | Bil, Ren |

Bil = biliary; Con = conjugation; N = no; Oxi = oxidation; Ren = renal; u = unchanged; Y = yes; ? = unknown.
*Yes indicates that the drug has an active metabolite.

irbesartan. Approximately 14% of the absorbed losartan dose is converted to the significantly more potent carboxylic acid E-3174 metabolite that is responsible for most of the AT1 receptor antagonism. About 1% of patients do not produce this metabolite.

## ACE Inhibitors

ACE inhibitors were developed during a systematic search for inhibitors of the kininases that break down kinins, such as bradykinin and kallidin, and that convert angiotensin I to angiotensin II. ACE inhibitors are classified according to the chemical nature of their ligand, which binds to the zinc ion at the active site of the enzyme. The inhibitors that are used at present, or that are in their final stages of study, are classified as (1) sulfhydryl compounds (alacepril, captopril, fentiapril, moveltipril, pivalapril, zofenopril); (2) carboxyl compounds (benazepril, cilazapril, enalapril, delapril, lisinopril, moexipril, pentopril, perindopril, quinapril, ramipril, spirapril, trandolapril); and (3) phosphoryl compounds (fosinopril and ceronapril). In addition, there are more than 80 compounds in various earlier stages of development.

### Mechanism and site of action

ACE inhibitors act competitively on the enzyme by virtue of their structural resemblance to the dipeptides cleaved by ACE. The inhibition was demonstrated in experimental animals and humans by blocking the conversion of intravenously administered angiotensin I and preventing the resulting pressor effect. This action is specific because the pressor response to exogenously administered angiotensin II or noradrenaline is not influenced by ACE inhibitors.

ACE is also responsible for the breakdown of kinins (e.g., bradykinin). Therefore, enzyme inhibition causes accumulation or synthesis (i.e., prostaglandins) of compounds that are known to produce vasodilatation and lowering of blood pressure. Some of the side effects (e.g., flushing, itching, coughing) can be attributed in part to accumulation of kinins. The direct role of bradykinin in lowering blood pressure is controversial.

Angiotensin II stimulates the synthesis and release of aldosterone to increase sodium–potassium exchange in the distal convoluted tubules of the kidney. The reduced formation of angiotensin II during ACE inhibitor therapy may lead to a significant reduction of plasma aldosterone levels and subsequent increase in serum potassium and depletion of sodium. The reduction of vasopressin release will increase water elimination and contribute to volume depletion by simultaneously administered diuretics.

Proteinuria due to excessive glomerular filtration pressure, often observed in chronic hypertension, is reduced or eliminated after blood pressure reduction.

Plasma renin activity increases during ACE inhibitor administration because the angiotensin II–regulated feedback mechanism is impaired.

### Therapeutic uses

In hypertensive patients, 2 to 3 hours after oral administration of ACE inhibitors, blood pressure is reduced by a decrease in total peripheral arterial resistance and an increase in compliance of large arteries, while there is no change or a slight increase in cardiac output. The renal blood flow is increased, but the glomerular filtration rate remains the same because of compensatory dilatation of both afferent and efferent arterioles. The blood pressure–lowering effects of ACE inhibitors are additive to those of thiazide diuretics. ACE inhibitors can also be combined with α blockers, β blockers, or calcium-channel blockers. The natriuretic effect is the result of reduced aldosterone secretion and improved renal hemodynamics. In congestive heart failure, and post-myocardial infarction, the effects of venodilatation and reductions in pulmonary artery pressure, pulmonary capillary wedge pressure, and left atrial and left ventricular filling pressure lead to increases in stroke volume, cardiac output, and exercise tolerance. After several months of ACE inhibitor administration, in addition to the improvement in overall hemodynamics, the hypertension-induced left ventricular hypertrophy is considerably reduced. Diminished AT2 receptor–mediated function as the consequence of inhibited angiotensin II production is not known. All ACE inhibitors have similar therapeutic indications, adverse effects, and contraindication profiles.

## Additional and adverse effects

In the presence of renal artery stenosis, ACE inhibitors, by lowering the blood pressure, may cause additional reduction of renal perfusion, thus increasing blood urea nitrogen (BUN) and serum creatinine. A significant increase in serum potassium may occur in patients with renal impairment or in those receiving the ACE inhibitor together with potassium-sparing diuretics. The angiotensin II–stimulated renal prostaglandin synthesis may be reduced, causing changes in intrarenal blood distribution. Self-limiting cough and throat irritation due to kinin accumulation is very common, even in patients with low plasma renin activity. Serious hypotension following first dose administration can be avoided by starting therapy with one-quarter or less of the usual dose and then gradually increasing the dose to the therapeutically effective level.

The most frequently observed adverse reactions are dizziness, upper abdominal pain, headache, mental confusion, urticaria, uremia, acute renal failure (in patients with renal artery stenosis), and impotence.

## Toxicity

ACE inhibitors cross the human placenta. Therefore, they are contraindicated in pregnancy for similar reasons as ARBs. Although adverse effects resulting from first-trimester exposure have not been documented, ACE inhibitor administration should be discontinued if pregnancy is planned or suspected. Repeated ultrasound examinations should be carried out if drug administration is unavoidable during pregnancy.

Toxicity associated with ACE inhibitor administration includes transient angioedema of the face, lips, and tongue, with possible fatal outcome if the larynx is involved. In rare cases, neutropenia and agranulocytosis have been reported. Therefore, patients who unexpectedly develop systemic or oral cavity infections during therapy should be closely followed. White cell and differential blood counts should be performed, especially during the early stages of therapy. Transient or long-lasting dermatological reactions such as rash or pruritus (with fever), arthralgia, and eosinophilia may occur any time during ACE inhibitor administration; this requires termination of therapy.

Proteinuria and increased BUN and creatinine levels occur primarily in patients with pre-existing renal disease or in those who receive high doses of ACE inhibitors. Anaphylactoid reactions have been reported in dialysis patients and during desensitization treatment with *Hymenoptera* venom. Patients with liver disease may develop hepatitis and elevated liver enzymes. Temporary dysgeusia (perverted taste sensation) occurs often, accompanied by moderate weight loss.

## Therapeutic application

ACE inhibitors alone, or in combination with thiazide diuretics or other antihypertensive agents, are used for the treatment of hypertension. They are also useful for the treatment of heart failure in patients who do not respond adequately to digitalis and diuretics. Consideration should always be given to the risk of neutropenia, agranulocytosis, and laryngeal edema. In general, patients with chronic renal failure (creatinine clearance <40 mL/min) may require only 25 to 50% of the normal dose, except for fosinopril, which usually requires no dose adjustment. Dosage and pharmacokinetic properties of ACE ihibitors are listed in Table 29-2. The main difference between the them is their potency, pharmacokinetics, and whether they act directly or are prodrugs.

**Alacepril** is rapidly converted first to desacetyl alacepril, which is not detected in plasma, and then to the active metabolite captopril. Maximum drop in systolic blood pressure occurs after 3 to 3.5 hours, and a significant blood pressure–lowering effect is noticeable for up to 24 hours. Because 50 to 70% of the dose is excreted in urine as captopril, it may cause a false-positive urine test for acetone.

**Benazepril** is converted to the active metabolite benazeprilat by liver and plasma esterases. After oral administration, 37% is absorbed in 0.5 to 1 hour; the presence of food in the stomach does not affect bioavailability. Maximum blood concentration of benazepril occurs in 1 to 2 hours.

**Captopril** (Fig. 29-2) was the first clinically useful, orally administered ACE inhibitor. The drug should be administered 1 hour before meals because the presence of food in the stomach reduces its bioavailability. It is unevenly distributed in total body water. A minor amount crosses the blood–brain barrier in experimental animals, but it freely crosses the human placenta. The antihypertensive effect is much longer than the demonstrable inhibition of the circulating ACE, perhaps because the ACE

FIGURE 29-2    Structural formulae of representative ACE inhibitors and the ARB losartan potassium.

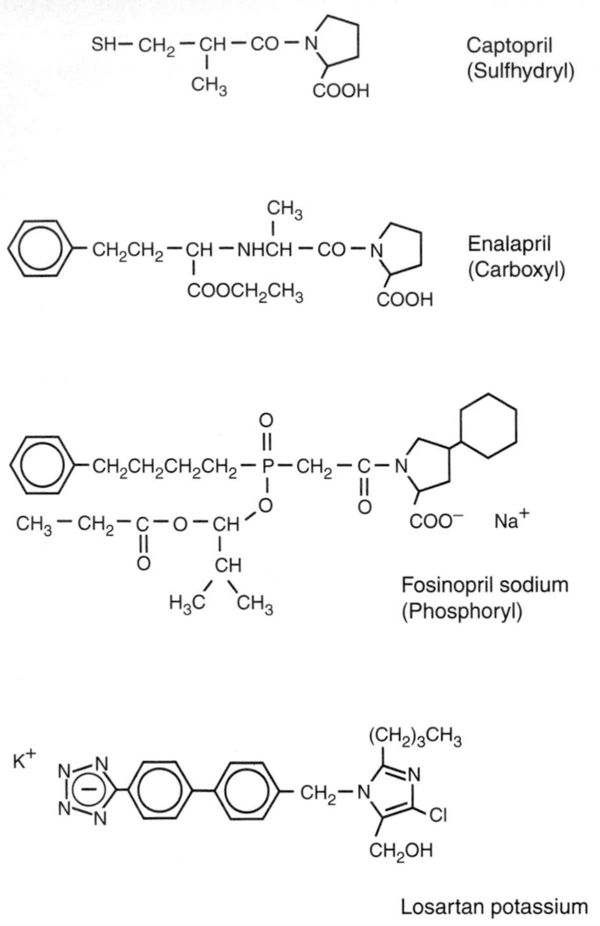

present in vascular endothelium is inhibited by extremely low tissue concentrations of the drug. About half the absorbed dose is excreted in the urine unchanged; the rest is eliminated as the disulfide dimer of captopril and captopril-cysteine disulfide. Captopril may cause a false-positive urine test for acetone.

Cilazapril is rapidly de-esterified in liver and blood after oral administration to form the active metabolite cilazaprilat. Peak effects occur in 2 to 3 hours, but significant lowering of blood pressure persists for 30 to 50 hours.

Enalapril maleate (see Fig. 29-2) is the maleic acid salt of enalaprilic acid ethyl ester, which is the ethyl ester of enalaprilic acid. It is hydrolyzed to enalaprilat, which is much more potent than the parent drug. The drug is not biotransformed further, and 94% of the dose is excreted in urine and feces as enalapril and enalaprilat. There is a prolonged terminal phase in the serum concentration profile of enalaprilat that represents the slow elimination of the ACE-bound drug. The drug and metabolite freely cross the placenta. Enalaprilat is available only in injectable preparation.

Fosinopril (see Fig. 29-2) is a prodrug that is hydrolyzed to the active metabolite fosinoprilat by gut-wall and hepatic esterases. It is present in plasma as fosinoprilat (75%), its glucuronide conjugate, and as a p-hydroxy metabolite. In oliguria, dose reduction is not essential because extensive biliary excretion compensates for reduced renal elimination.

Lisinopril is an analogue of enalaprilat, with lysine replacing alanine. Bioavailability is not affected by food, age, or co-administration of hydrochlorothiazide, propranolol, digoxin, or glyburide. Lisinopril is not a prodrug, it is not bound to serum proteins, and it is excreted unchanged in the urine. Steady-state plasma concentration is achieved after 3 days of administration, and accumulation occurs in patients with severe renal impairment. The effective serum half-life is about 13 hours, but significant blood pressure reduction continues for more than 24 hours.

Pentopril is a prodrug ester that undergoes hydrolysis to form the active metabolite pentoprilat. Following oral administration, 20 to 25% of pentoprilat is excreted in urine unchanged by filtration and active tubular secretion because the renal clearance is 400 mL/min. The plasma half-life of pentoprilat is 2 to 2.5 hours but is significantly prolonged to 15 hours in patients with severe chronic renal failure.

Perindopril is a long-acting prodrug, 17 to 28% of which is hydrolyzed to the active metabolite, perindoprilat.

Quinapril, a prodrug, is well absorbed after oral administration and rapidly hydrolyzed to the active metabolite quinaprilat. Quinaprilat (50 to 60%), a small amount of quinapril, and two diketopiperazine metabolites are excreted in urine. The magnesium content of quinapril tablets may reduce the bioavailability of tetracyclines.

Ramipril is a prodrug that is rapidly hydrolyzed by liver esterases to the long-acting active metabolite ramiprilat.

Zofenopril is a prodrug that is hydrolyzed to the active metabolite zofenoprilat during and after absorption. Almost complete ACE activity is blocked for 6 to 8 hours, but still relevant inhibition is detectable after 24 hours. In addition to the antihypertensive effect, it has significant cardioprotective properties. The magnesium content of the preparation may reduce the absorption of concurrently administered tetracycline.

# KININS

Kinins are a separate class of peptides that are formed from kininogen precursors (which, like angiotensinogen, are $\alpha_2$-globulins) by the proteolytic enzymes kallikreins and some non-specific enzymes such as trypsin. In plasma, the nonapeptide bradykinin (named for its action in producing slow contraction of the gut) is formed. In tissues, the initial

CHAPTER 29: AUTACOIDS | 389

**TABLE 29-2**  Recommended Dosage and Known Pharmacokinetic Data for ACE (Kininase II) Inhibitors Described in This Chapter

| Generic Name | Trade Name | Prodrug* | Daily Dose (mg) | Bioavailability (%) | $T_{max}$ (hours) | Half-life (hours) | $V_d$ (L/kg) | Protein Binding (%) | Biotrans-formation | Excretion |
|---|---|---|---|---|---|---|---|---|---|---|
| Alacepril | Cetapril | Y | | 70 | 1–2 | 2–5 | | | Hyd | Ren |
| Benazepril | Lotensin | Y | 10–20 | 37 | 1 met 1–4 | 11 met 21 | 0.34 | 97 met 95 | Con, Hyd | Ren |
| Captopril | Capoten | N | 25–300 | 75 | 1 | 2 | 0.14 | 30 | Con | Ren |
| Cilazapril | Inhibace | Y | 2.5–10 | 57 | 1 met 2 | 2 met 40 | 0.2–1 | | Hyd | Ren |
| Delapril | Adecist Cupressin | Y | 30–60 | | 1 met 1.2 | 0.3 met 1.2 | | | Hyd, Oxi | Ren |
| Enalapril | Vasotec | Y | 2.5–40 | 60 | 1 met 4–5 | 1.3 met 11 | 0.25–0.70 | | Hyd (some) Met N | Ren, Fec |
| Fosinopril | Monopril | Y | 10–20 | 36 | met 3 | met 11 | 0.34 | 95 | Hyd, Oxi, Con | Ren, Bil |
| Lisinopril | Zestril Privinil | N | 5–40 | 25–30 | 6–8 | 13 | 0.34–0.70 | 0 | N | Ren |
| Pentopril | | Y | 125 | 60–70 | | 2–3 | | | | Ren |
| Perindopril | Coversyl Electan Procaptan | Y | 4–8 | 65–90 | 1 met 3–4 | 1.5–3 met 25–30 | 0.2 | 20 | Hyd | Ren |
| Quinapril | Accupril | Y | 5–80 | 60 | 1 met 2 | 1 met 3–4 | 0.34 | met 97 | Hyd Oxi | Ren, Bil |
| Ramipril | Altace Cardace | Y | 5–20 | 50–60 met 44 | 1 met 2–4 | 2–4 met 9–18 | 1–1.3 | 56 met 73 | Hyd, Oxi | Ren, Bil, Fec |
| Spirapril | Sandopril Renpress | Y | 12.5–50 | | 2 | 1–2 | | 56 | Hyd | Bil |
| Trandolapril | Mavik | Y | 1–8 | 7.5 | 1 met 6 | 15 met 24 | | 80 met 94 | Hyd | Bil, Ren |
| Zofenopril | Zoprace | Y | 30–60 | 96 | 1–1.5 | 2–5 | 0.34 | 88 | Hyd | Bil, Ren |

Bil = biliary; Con = conjugation; Fec = fecal; Hyd = hydrolysis; met = metabolite; Oxi = oxidation; Ren = renal; N = no; Y = yes.

*Yes indicates that the drug has an active metabolite.

product is kallidin, a decapeptide that can be converted to bradykinin by an aminopeptidase that removes a lysine residue. Bradykinin has a very short half-life (15 seconds) and is inactivated by kininases. Kininase II is identical with peptidyl dipeptidase (or, angiotensin-converting enzyme, the enzyme that converts angiotensin I to angiotensin II) and can thus be blocked by ACE inhibitors (Fig. 29-3).

Kinins act on specific receptors ($B_1$, $B_2$, and $B_3$) to activate phospholipase C or $A_2$, causing powerful vasodilatation in most vascular beds.

In addition to vasodilatation, kinins also cause increased vascular permeability and edema. Bronchoconstriction induced by kinins is selectively antagonized by ASA and similar analgesics. In asthmatics, kinins may

cause respiratory distress. In addition, kinins are potent pain-inducing agents. The hyperalgesia, edema formation, and vasodilatation associated with the kinins are at least partially due to increased synthesis and release of certain prostaglandins.

At present, the kinins have no therapeutic use. However, the inhibition of kinin breakdown by ACE inhibitors may contribute to the antihypertensive effects of these agents (see "ACE Inhibitors" above). Currently, several bradykinin analogues are being tested for their kinin-receptor-blocking properties.

**Aprotinin** (Trasylol) is an inhibitor of the enzyme kallikrein, probably identical with the pancreatic trypsin inhibitor of Kunitz, and is used in treating acute pancre-

FIGURE 29-3    Pathways of formation and inactivation of bradykinin (|| indicates blockade at the points shown).

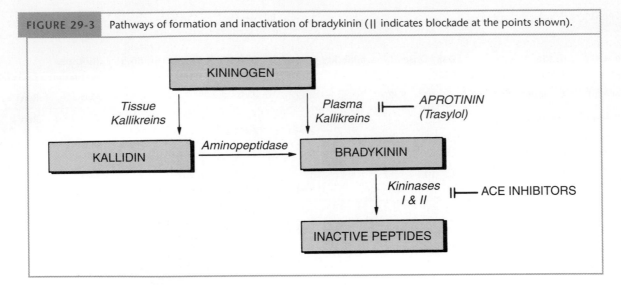

atitis, the carcinoid syndrome, and states of hyperfibrinolysis because of its action as an inhibitor of trypsin, kallikrein, and plasmin.

## NON-OPIOID PEPTIDES OF BRAIN AND GASTROINTESTINAL TRACT

### Substance P

Substance P is an undecapeptide that was first extracted from intestine. It is also found in the brain, in primary afferent neurons, dorsal root ganglia, and dorsal horn of the spinal cord, and in small arterioles of the human heart. It is proposed to be a sensory neurotransmitter associated with pain transmission. Substance P binds to G protein–coupled substance P receptors and causes release of endothelium-derived hyperpolarizing factor (EDHF), resulting in vasodilatation. It contracts smooth muscles of the gut. The functions of substance P in the brain are not yet fully identified, although a co-transmitter role in some serotonin neurons has been postulated (see Chapter 16). Participation of substance P neurons in extrapyramidal motor control has also been proposed. MK-869, a substance P receptor antagonist, is being tested as a possible treatment for chemotherapy-induced emesis.

### Endothelins

Endothelins are peptides released from mammalian vascular endothelial cells. Endothelin-1 (ET-1) acts on $ET_A$-receptors to produce intense and long-lasting vasoconstriction, but it also acts on $ET_{B1}$ receptors to cause vasodilatation by release of nitric oxide. Selective antagonists of the $ET_A$ receptors are being explored for possible use in the treatment of vasospasm.

### Cholecystokinin (CCK)

This is a peptide composed of 33 amino acids; however, a shorter eight-amino-acid fragment of CCK also has full biological activity. CCK is localized in the brain and gastrointestinal tract. When injected into the brain, CCK causes anorectic reactions and may be a factor that triggers peripheral satiety mechanisms (see also Chapter 16).

### Neurotensin

This tridecapeptide was found originally in the brain and subsequently in the intestinal mucosa. Systemic administration of neurotensin causes vasodilatation, hypotension, and increased vascular permeability. These actions may be due at least in part to histamine release.

### Vasoactive Intestinal Polypeptide (VIP)

VIP consists of 28 amino acids. It is present in intestinal neurons and is also found in the brain (including coexistence in some dopamine neurons). The neurons containing VIP in the intestine may be involved in reflexes facilitating intestinal transport. VIP also causes relaxation of tracheal smooth muscles.

The central roles of the five peptides mentioned above are largely unknown at present. They coexist in neurons together with classical CNS neurotransmitters. They seem to act through specific individual receptors and play either a neuroregulator or a neurotransmitter role.

In the intestine, these neuropeptides likely are important in regulating intestinal motility, blood flow, and mucosal transport. If specific antagonists for the individual peptides are discovered, they may greatly assist in clarifying their physiological or pathological roles.

## Somatostatin

The function of somatostatin is primarily to control the activity of growth hormone–releasing hormone (GHRH), but it is also found outside the CNS in D cells of the pancreatic islets and in gastric and duodenal mucosa. It inhibits the secretion of growth hormone, insulin, glucagon, gastrin, VIP, and possibly others.

**Octreotide** (Sandostatin) is a synthetic octapeptide analogue of naturally occurring somatostatin. It inhibits the secretion of peptides of the gastroenteropancreatic endocrine system (insulin, glucagon, gastrin) and of growth hormone. It also inhibits the release of thyroid-stimulating hormone induced by thyrotropin-releasing hormone.

Octreotide is indicated for symptomatic treatment of carcinoid and vasoactive peptide-secreting tumours, and it is most beneficial for the control of diarrhea and flushing episodes associated with these conditions. It is administered intravenously in daily doses of 100 to 600 mg. Adverse effects are local irritation, gastrointestinal disturbances, impaired glucose tolerance, and hepatic dysfunctions.

# 5-HYDROXYTRYPTAMINE (5-HT, SEROTONIN)

The synthesis and degradation of serotonin are described in Chapter 16 and are outlined in Figure 29-4. About 90% of body serotonin is found in enterochromaffin cells of the gastrointestinal tract. The remainder is localized in platelets and in specific neurons in the CNS.

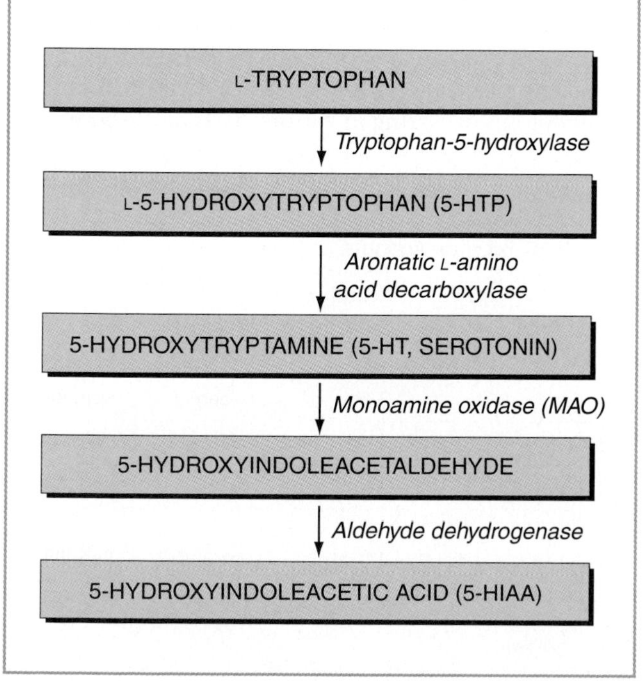

## Physiology and Pharmacology

In the CNS, 5-HT acts as a neurotransmitter localized in neurons originating in the raphe nuclei and distributed throughout the brain. Stimulation of 5-HT$_{1A-D}$ receptors may increase or decrease adenylyl cyclase activity, resulting in increased or decreased (inhibited) K$^+$ conductance and thus, indirectly, in increases or decreases in the release of noradrenaline or acetylcholine.

Stimulation of 5-HT$_2$ receptors causes excitation by activation of phospholipase C and increased synthesis of inositol trisphosphate and diacylglycerol. The central functions of 5-HT relate to regulation of mood, food intake, and sleep. It may also participate in regulating adenohypophysial secretions, in stimulating the release of adrenocorticotropic hormone (ACTH), growth hormone, and prolactin, and in inhibiting the release of luteinizing hormone (LH), follicle-stimulating hormone (FSH), and thyroid-stimulating hormone (TSH). In the pineal gland, 5-HT serves as the precursor of the hormone melatonin.

In the periphery, 5-HT$_3$ receptors found in autonomic ganglia may cause increased noradrenaline or acetylcholine release, and those of the sensory nerves may produce itch or pain.

The cardiovascular system may be affected directly by stimulation of 5-HT receptors or indirectly by influencing noradrenaline release. 5-HT receptors designated as 5-HT$_{1A}$, 5-HT$_{1B}$, 5-HT$_{1C}$, and 5-HT$_{1D}$ are located in various blood vessels in the body and may cause vasodilatation in skeletal muscles and coronary arteries by inhibition of adenylyl cyclase and release of nitric oxide or prostaglandins. 5-HT$_2$ receptor stimulation activates phospholipase C, increases intracellular calcium ion concentration, and produces vasoconstriction in the splanchnic area, lungs, and kidneys.

Stimulation of 5-HT$_1$ receptors in the heart increases the heart rate and force of contraction, but stimulation of 5-HT$_3$ receptors in the coronary arteries and baroreceptors causes significant reflex slowing of the heart rate, hypotension, and vasovagal syncope.

5-HT synthesized in enterochromaffin cells is released into the blood and is actively taken up by platelets. 5-HT and thromboxane A$_2$ are released from platelets during aggregation or after exposure to air (in vitro). Hemostasis is promoted by further platelet aggregation (5-HT$_2$ receptors) and constriction of cutaneous blood vessels.

5-HT receptors located in the gastrointestinal tract, uterus, and bronchial smooth muscle may have some physiological function, but they are also stimulated by 5-HT released from enterochromaffin cell tumours (carcinoid tumours) and are responsible for most of the cardio-

| FIGURE 29-4 | Biosynthetic pathway and metabolism of serotonin. |

L-TRYPTOPHAN

↓ *Tryptophan-5-hydroxylase*

L-5-HYDROXYTRYPTOPHAN (5-HTP)

↓ *Aromatic L-amino acid decarboxylase*

5-HYDROXYTRYPTAMINE (5-HT, SEROTONIN)

↓ *Monoamine oxidase (MAO)*

5-HYDROXYINDOLEACETALDEHYDE

↓ *Aldehyde dehydrogenase*

5-HYDROXYINDOLEACETIC ACID (5-HIAA)

vascular, intestinal, bronchial, and other symptoms associated with these tumours.

5-HT is also involved in the prodromal vasoconstriction stage (aura) of classical migraine, which is followed by pain due to intense vasodilatation caused by liberation of other vasoactive substances such as prostaglandins, kinins, and nitric oxide.

When administered systemically, 5-HT affects the cardiovascular, respiratory, gastrointestinal, and other organ systems in the periphery, but it does not cross the blood–brain barrier. However, its precursors tryptophan and 5-hydroxytryptophan enter the brain fairly readily by facilitated transport.

## 5-HT Receptor Agonists

Drugs with selective 5-HT receptor stimulating properties are of great interest for the investigation and treatment of conditions in which the function of 5-HT neurotransmission or receptors is implicated. Drugs with beneficial effects on mood, mentality, or certain behaviours such as excessive alcohol consumption, and without serious toxic effects, would have an enormous impact on society.

During the late 1980s, several 5-HT receptor agonists (5-HT RAs) were tested for their effects on the extensive vasodilatory phase (pain) of migraine and the trigeminal pathway pain. They are 5-HT analogues that primarily stimulate 5-HT$_1$ receptor subtypes B and D.

There is some evidence that symptoms of migraine headache arise from activation of the trigeminovascular system, which results in vasodilation and neurogenic inflammation involving antidromic release of VIP, substance P, and calcitonin gene-related peptide. The pain relief is attributable to the agonist effect of 5-HT RAs on 5-HT receptors located in the intracranial blood vessels, including meningeal (mainly dural) blood vessels, the arteriovenous anastomoses, and sensory nerves of the trigeminal system, resulting in cranial vessel constriction

and inhibition of the release of pro-inflammatory peptides (kinins) and neuropeptides.

The 5-HT RAs have similar pharmacodynamics and side effects, but they differ in dosage and in certain pharmacokinetic properties listed in Table 29-3. Total plasma clearance and biotransformation is influenced by the severity of renal and/or liver function impairment. In extreme cases, the $C_{max}$, AUC, and half-life are increased to more than twice their normal values, requiring reduction of the dose and frequency of administration. Most patients experience significant pain relief within 4 hours after oral administration.

### Therapeutic uses
5-HT RAs are recommended for the acute treatment of migraine attacks with or without aura. They should not be used in hemiplegic, basilar, or ophthalmogenic migraine. They should not be administered in combination with ergotamine-containing drugs or their derivatives (e.g., dihydroergotamine, methysergide) or with serotonin reuptake inhibitors.

5-HT RAs are contraindicated for patients with coronary artery disease, valvular and congenital heart disease, cardiac arrhythmias, atherosclerosis, uncontrolled or severe hypertension, or seizures.

The age limit for 5-HT RA administration is 18 years or over (for zolmitriptan, 12 years or older), with reduced dosage for patients aged over 70 years. The safety in pregnancy and lactation has not been established. The "triptans" are **not** for prophylactic use.

### Adverse effects
Angina pectoris–like syndromes, arrhythmias, coronary artery vasospasm, myocardial infarction and resulting deaths, cerebral and subarachnoid hemorrhage, stroke, increased blood pressure, and reduced coronary vasodilatory reserve can arise in susceptible individuals.

During placebo-controlled clinical trials, the following symptoms occurring in various parts of the body were

**TABLE 29-3** Recommended Dosage and Known Pharmacokinetic Data for 5-HT Receptor Agonists

| Generic Name | Trade Name | Daily Dose (mg) | Bioavailability (%) | $T_{max}$ (hours) | Half-life (hours) | $V_d$ (L/kg) | Protein Binding (%) | Biotrans-formation | Excretion |
|---|---|---|---|---|---|---|---|---|---|
| Eletriptan | Relpax | 20–40 | 50 | 1.5 | 4 | ? | ? | N-demet | Ren, Bil |
| Naratriptan | Amerge | 1–5 | 74 | 2–5 | 5–8 | 3.7 | 29 | Oxi | Ren |
| Rizatriptan | Maxalt | 5–20 | 45 | 1–2 | 1.7 | 14 | 14 | Oxi | Ren, Fec |
| Sumatriptan succinate | Imitrex | 25–100 | 14 | 0.5–5 | 2–3 | 2.4 | 14–21 | Oxi | Ren, Bil |
| Zolmitriptan | Zomig | 1–5 | 25 | 2–3 | 2.5–3 | 7 | 25 | Oxi | Ren, Bil |

Bil = biliary; Fec = fecal; Ren = renal; N-demet = N-demethylation; Oxi = oxidation; ? = unknown.

recorded: pain, discomfort, pressure, heaviness, constriction, tightness, heat or burning sensation, paresthesia, numbness, tingling, strange sensations, dizziness, nausea, vomiting, and fatigue.

## Preparations

**Eletriptan** (Relpax) is the latest addition to the group of 5-HT RAs. It binds to 5-HT$_{1B}$, 5-HT$_D$, and 5-HT$_F$ receptors. It is recommended for the acute treatment of migraine, with or without aura, in adults. It is *N*-demethylated by CYP3A4 to a less active metabolite. The non-renal clearance accounts for 90% of the total clearance. Ketaconazole, erythromycin, fluconazole, and verapamil inhibit the metabolism of eletriptan. Adverse effects are similar to those of the other 5-HT$_1$ agonists.

**Naratriptan** (Amerge) is one of the most potent 5-HT RAs, with predictable oral bioavailability and long-lasting effect. If creatinine clearance is <40 mL/min or there is moderate liver failure, the $C_{max}$ and AUC are increased, and the half-life is 20 hours or longer. The active metabolite, *N*-desmethyl rizatriptan (accounting for 14% of the dose), has activity and an elimination rate similar to those of the parent drug. Naratriptan and its metabolites are eliminated by glomerular filtration and tubular secretion.

**Rizatriptan** (Maxalt) absorption and elimination are rapid, and the half-life is short. Monoamine oxidase-A (MAO-A) is an important enzyme for the drug's biotransformation to inactive metabolites. Rizatriptan is a competitive inhibitor of CYP2D6.

**Sumatriptan succinate** (Imitrex) is available in tablet and subcutaneous injectable formulations. It was the first "triptan" drug for migraine. MAO inhibitors reduce its clearance and increase systemic exposure. The total plasma clearance is 1160 mL/min. The safety of more than four treatments in 30 days or its use in cluster headache has not been established. The nasal spray containing sumatriptan hemisulfate (5 mg/spray) has identical pharmacodynamic and similar kinetic parameters to those of other preparations. The onset of action is 10 to 15 minutes for subcutaneous injection, 15 minutes for intranasal spray, and 30 minutes for oral administration. Non-renal clearance accounts for about 80% of total body clearance.

**Zolmitriptan** (Zomig, Zomig Rapimelt) is rapidly absorbed by mouth, but its pharmacokinetics are markedly affected during migraine attacks. When it is administered during a moderate or severe attack, $C_{max}$ is reduced by up to 40%, AUC is reduced by 25%, and $T_{max}$ is increased compared with the same subjects in the absence of migraine. The drug is eliminated largely by hepatic biotransformation, followed by urinary excretion of the metabolites. Total body clearance is rapid because of a combination of glomerular filtration and active tubular secretion. About 4% of the dose is converted to the *N*-desmethyl metabolite, which is two- to sixfold more potent than the parent drug. The dose should be reduced in moderate to severe renal or liver failure. About 70% of the patients experience significant pain relief within 4 hours. Zomig Rapimelt, containing 2.5 mg zolmitriptan, is an oral tablet formulated to disintegrate rapidly.

**Ergotamine** and **dihydroergotamine** have been used for many decades for the treatment of migraine headache. Some of their properties, such as stimulation of 5-HT receptors, are similar to those of sumatriptan, but they may have significant additional effects by blocking adrenergic receptors and causing vasoconstriction by a direct action on blood vessels.

## Selective Serotonin Reuptake Inhibitors (SSRIs)

The use and side effects, including the serotonin syndrome, of the SSRIs **citalopram, escitalopram, fluoxetine, fluvoxamine, paroxetine, sertraline,** and **trazodone** in the treatment of major depressions are described in Chapter 25. A recent addition to the group is **dapoxentine**, which has been shown in clinical trials to prolong the latency of ejaculation and is currently awaiting approval for the treatment of premature ejaculation. The mechanism of this action appears to be distinct from that of the antidepressant effect of SSRIs, because it is of rapid onset and short duration.

## Drugs Influencing Endogenous Serotonin

Since tryptophan hydroxylase, the rate-limiting enzyme in 5-HT formation, is not saturated with its substrate, the administration of tryptophan can increase the levels of serotonin. In this manner, tryptophan may be of value in phenylketonuria.

The compounds that lower brain serotonin levels, such as parachlorophenylalanine (an inhibitor of tryptophan hydroxylase) and 5,7-dihydroxytryptamine (which destroys serotoninergic neurons), have no clinical use at present. Reserpine, a drug that depletes serotonin storage sites (but also those of other monoamines), has been used in the treatment of hypertension and psychosis. The effects of reserpine are presumably exerted not only via the serotoninergic system, but also via the analogous effects of reserpine on noradrenergic and/or dopaminergic neurons (see Chapter 25).

Lysergic acid (LSD) and other hallucinogens selectively antagonize many peripheral actions of 5-HT. A similar antagonism of 5-HT actions in the brain has been suggested as the basis of the hallucinogenic effects of LSD, but this is not proven (see Chapter 26). Morphine partially blocks 5-HT action on the intestine.

Compounds that were designed and synthesized specifically to block the peripheral actions of 5-HT include methysergide, pizotifen, and cyproheptadine, as well as several newer agents described below.

**Methysergide** (Sansert), a congener of LSD, is recommended for the prophylactic treatment of migraine. It takes 1 to 2 days to develop its full effect, and therapy should not be initiated during an acute attack. Continuous administration should not exceed 6 months without a drug-free interval of 3 to 4 weeks. Patients should be carefully monitored for side effects, such as retroperitoneal or pleuropulmonary fibrosis, fibrotic changes in aortic and mitral valves, gastrointestinal disturbances, insomnia or mild euphoria, weight gain, dermatological and hematological manifestations, peripheral edema, and alopecia. The dose should be decreased gradually over 2 to 3 weeks before complete discontinuation in order to avoid "headache rebound."

**Pizotifen** (Sandomigran) was introduced for the prophylactic treatment of migraine headache. It is effective in reducing the frequency and severity of attacks. Since it is a potent serotonin and histamine antagonist and also has anticholinergic and sedative effects, the drug should be administered with caution, and drug-free intervals of 3 to 4 weeks should follow every 6 months of continuous therapy. The initial dose is 0.5 mg at bedtime; this is usually increased to 0.5 mg or more, three times a day, but the total dose should not exceed 6 mg in 24 hours. Unpleasant side effects are drowsiness, potentiation of CNS depressants (e.g., alcohol, antihistamines), headache, edema, dry mouth, and impotence. Hepatotoxic effects might occur after prolonged use.

**Cyproheptadine** (Periactin) is a potent 5-HT and histamine antagonist with mild anticholinergic and CNS-depressant properties. It is used primarily as an anti-pruritic agent when itching is caused by the release of 5-HT or histamine. It may cause weight gain and increased rate of growth in children. The CNS-depressant effects of other drugs may be potentiated if taken concomitantly with cyproheptadine. The usual adult dose is 4 mg, three to four times a day.

**Ketanserin** (Ket, Serefrex), a 5-HT$_2$ receptor blocker, relaxes vascular and tracheal smooth muscle and has been studied as a possible antihypertensive agent. It also blocks $\alpha_1$-adrenoreceptors, histamine H$_1$ receptors, and dopamine receptors. It has not yet had wide clinical use.

**Risperidone** (Risperdal), similar to ketanserin, blocks 5-HT$_2$ receptors in low doses and dopamine D$_2$ receptors and $\alpha_1$-adrenergic receptors in high doses. It is used primarily for the treatment of acute and chronic schizophrenic psychoses (see Chapter 24). Adverse effects include insomnia, agitation, extrapyramidal side effects, and headache. The recommended daily dose is 6 mg.

**Ondansetron** (Zofran), dolasetron mesylate (Anzemet), and granisetron (Kytril) are 5-HT$_3$ receptor antagonists used for the prevention and control of nausea and vomiting accompanying radiotherapy or anti-neoplastic chemotherapy. They have no extrapyramidal side effects. The most common adverse effects are headache, constipation or transient diarrhea, asthenia, and cardiac rhythm changes. The drugs are available in oral and parenteral formulation. They have also been tested as an aid for reducing nicotine (tobacco) and excessive alcohol use, but their value for this purpose has not been clearly demonstrated.

## SUGGESTED READINGS

Crackower MA, Sarao R, Oudit G, at al. Angiotensin-converting enzyme 2 is an essential regulator of heart function. *Nature.* 2002;417:822-828.

Deleu D, Hanssens Y, Worthing EA. Symptomatic and prophylactic treatment of migraine: a critical appraisal. *Clin Neuropharmacol.* 1998;21:267-279.

Fitchett D. Have angiotensin receptor blockers lived up to expectations? *Can J Cardiol.* 2005;21:569-575.

Harrington MA, Zhong P, Garow SJ, et al. Molecular biology of serotonin receptors. *J Clin Psychiatry.* 1992;53(suppl 10):8-27.

Horiuchi M, Akishita M, Dzau VJ. Recent progress in angiotensin II type 2 receptor research in the cardiovascular system. *Hypertension.* 1999;33:613-621.

McConnaughey MM, McConnaughey JS, Ingenito AJ. Practical considerations of the pharmacology of angiotensin receptor blockers. *J Clin Pharmacol.* 1999;39:547-559.

Timmermans PB, Wong PC, Chiu AT, et al. Angiotensin II receptors and angiotensin II receptor antagonists. *Pharmacol Rev.* 1993;45:206-251.

Uchida S, Watanabe H, Nishio S, et al. Altered pharmacokinetics and excessive hypotensive effect of candesartan in a patient with the CYP2C9*1/*3 genotype. *Clin Pharmacol Ther.* 2003; 74:505-508.

Vane JR. The history of inhibitors of angiotensin converting enzyme. *J Physiol Pharmacol.* 1999;50:489-498.

Wada A, Ueda S, Masumori-Maemoto S, et al. Angiotensin II attenuates the vasodilating effect of a nitric oxide donor, glyceryl trinitrate: roles of superoxide and angiotensin II type receptors. *Clin Pharmacol Ther.* 2002;71:440-447.

Wagenaar LJ, Voors AA, Buikema H, et al. Angiotensin receptors in the cardiovascular system. *Can J Cardiol.* 2002;18:1331-1339.

# 30

# Histamine and Antihistamines

## D KADAR

**CASE HISTORY**

A 48-year-old female in early menopause had suffered from seasonal hay fever in late summer and early autumn for several years. Self-medication with diphenhydramine or related antihistamines gave sufficient relief of symptoms for many years but was accompanied by a moderate though tolerable degree of sedation. Recent newspaper and TV advertising convinced her that newer antihistamines would cause significantly less or no daytime sedation, whereupon she changed to terfenadine 60 mg three times a day. Because this drug is sold over the counter, she did not bother to inform her physician. She was happy with her choice because she experienced no sedation or any other side effects with this drug. Toward the end of the hay fever season, she came down with an acute bacterial upper respiratory tract infection, for which her physician prescribed clarithromycin 250 mg twice daily. After 3 days of taking both terfenadine and clarithromycin, she complained of fatigue, headache, palpitation, and unusual weakness. An ECG showed a significantly prolonged QT interval with ventricular dysrhythmia (torsades de pointes). On questioning, she told her physician about the terfenadine, and it was replaced by diphenhydramine for the duration of the antibiotic therapy. She was cautioned not to mix the so-called low-sedating antihistamines with any other medication without prior consultation with her physician.

## HISTAMINE AND ALLERGIC PHENOMENA

### Histamine

Histamine is widely distributed in nature. It occurs in plants and in practically all mammalian tissues and body fluids in varying concentrations.

Histamine is an amine formed by decarboxylation of the amino acid histidine (Fig. 30-1). Decarboxylation occurs in the same tissues in which histamine is stored, chiefly the lungs, skin, and gastrointestinal mucosa. In these tissues, histamine is stored in the mast cells as small, dense granules of an inactive histamine–anionic polymer (heparin) complex along with other biologically active chemicals and enzymes. It is also present in blood platelets and basophilic leukocytes (as a chondroitin sulfate complex in the secretory granules), as well as in the central nervous system (CNS) and fetal liver. Histamine is present in lower concentration in tissues not containing mast cells, and it has a rapid turnover because of lack of a storage mechanism.

Histamine is released from tissues in free active form through the following:

1. Destruction of cells (e.g., from bee sting venom, bacterial toxins, cold, injury)
2. Dissolution of cytoplasmic granules (e.g., by surfactants, radiation)
3. Histamine liberators (e.g., drugs, such as $d$-tubocurarine, morphine, and vancomycin, foreign proteins, dextran, X-ray contrast media)

Despite its wide distribution and potent pharmacological actions, the physiological role of histamine is not yet clear. Its effects are mediated through special G protein–coupled histamine receptors that are designated as $H_1$, $H_2$, and $H_3$ types. A number of structural analogues of histamine have been synthesized, and more or less specific agonists have been identified for each of the $H_1$ (2-methylhistamine), $H_2$ (4-methylhistamine), and $H_3$ (N-$\alpha$-methylhistamine) receptors.

FIGURE 30-1 Formation of histamine from histidine.

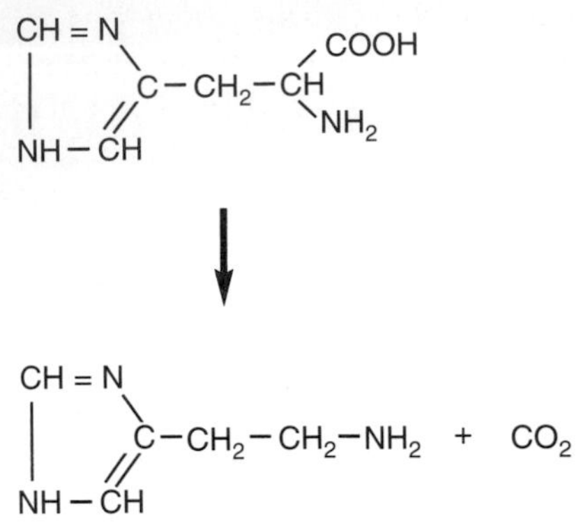

## Mechanism of Action

Histamine $H_1$, $H_2$, and $H_3$ receptors are located on the cell surface, and the stimulus–response coupling is mediated through altered $Ca^{2+}$ flow into the cell or increased utilization of intracellular calcium. $H_1$ and $H_2$ receptors are distributed in resistance vessels, capillaries, venules, gastrointestinal and bronchial smooth muscle, exocrine glands, sensory nerve endings, and the CNS.

Vasodilation is mediated by $H_1$ receptors on endothelial cells and $H_2$ receptors on smooth muscle cells. $H_1$ receptor stimulation leads to increased intracellular calcium ion concentration, activation of phospholipase $A_2$, and production of prostacyclin ($PGI_2$) and NO (nitric oxide). NO diffuses into the smooth muscle cells, activates guanylyl cyclase to increase cyclic GMP, and stimulates protein kinase to decrease intracellular calcium, which results in smooth muscle relaxation. $PGI_2$ is a smooth muscle relaxant vasodilator that activates adenylyl cyclase to increase cyclic AMP (cAMP) generation; cAMP activates protein kinase A, which phosphorylates the intracellular calcium ion pump to decrease intracellular calcium concentration.

Phospholipase C–coupled $H_1$ receptor stimulation leads to inositol-1,4,5-trisphosphate ($IP_3$) and diacylglycerol formation from the cell membrane to release calcium ions from the endoplasmic reticulum. Diacylglycerol activates protein kinase C, and calcium activates $Ca^{2+}$/calmodulin-dependent protein kinases and phospholipase $A_2$ to produce the required response, which is organ and species specific.

Stimulation of $H_1$ receptors mediates contraction of bronchi, intestines, and large blood vessels as a result of $IP_3$-mediated release of intracellular calcium, which activates $Ca^{2+}$/calmodulin-dependent light-chain kinase, phosphorylation of myosin light chain, cross-bridge cycling, and contraction.

$H_2$ receptors located on parietal cells of the stomach are stimulated by histamine released from enterochromaf-fin-like cells to activate cAMP and the phosphorylation of parietal cell effector proteins, which leads to activation of the $H^+/K^+$-ATPase (a proton pump).

$H_2$ receptors appear to have an autoregulatory role since their stimulation by histamine prevents further histamine release in some experimental preparations. Histamine may stimulate $H_2$ receptors of T cells, resulting in elevated cAMP concentration and reduced T-cell-mediated cytotoxicity. Lymphocyte proliferation may also be reduced or suppressed. The suppressor T cell function is inhibited by $H_1$ receptor stimulation.

$H_3$ receptors are located in the CNS and in the periphery and act both as inhibitory autoreceptors on histamine-containing terminals and as inhibitors of the release of various other neurotransmitters. The mechanisms of signal transduction underlying these actions are not yet fully known but appear to involve a G protein ($G_i/G_o$) and reduction of $Ca^{2+}$ influx through an N-type calcium channel.

## Effects of Histamine

Stimulation of $H_1$ and $H_2$ receptors by histamine leads to capillary dilatation and greatly increased permeability of post-capillary venules, with leakage of plasma proteins and fluid and their accumulation in extracellular spaces. In the skin, this gives rise to the classical "triple response" to local injury: reddening, wheal formation, and flare ("halo"). Urticaria is the cutaneous reaction to systemic and local intradermal histamine release or to allergens. Histamine action on $H_2$ receptors blocks the degranulation of basophils by IgE.

The heart responds to medium-high systemic doses of histamine with increased heart rate ($H_2$ receptors) and increased strength of contraction ($H_1$ and $H_2$ receptors).

Histamine stimulates exocrine secretions through action on both $H_1$ receptors (e.g., nasal and bronchial mucus) and $H_2$ receptors (stimulation of gastric HCl secretion; see Chapter 41).

Histamine stimulation of $H_1$ receptors on chromaffin cells causes the release of adrenaline from the adrenal medulla.

Stimulation of sensory nerve endings by histamine produces itch and pain (mainly $H_1$ receptors).

Histamine appears to play an important role in the production of certain types of migraine (vascular) headaches.

It also seems to have some as yet poorly understood neurotransmitter and neuroendocrine function in the CNS; $H_1$, $H_2$, and $H_3$ receptors appear to be involved (see Chapter 16).

## Biotransformation

The inactivation of histamine occurs in many tissues by *N*-methylation or oxidative deamination (Fig. 30-2). The respective products, methylhistamine and imidazole acetic acid, are converted further to a number of other derivatives.

## Allergy and Anaphylaxis

There is a marked similarity between the symptoms elicited by intravenous injection of histamine and those of allergic reactions and anaphylactic shock triggered by consumption of foods by sensitive individuals. In both conditions, contraction of smooth muscle, vasodilatation and increased permeability of capillaries (decreased total peripheral resistance), stimulation of secretions, and stimulation of sensory nerve endings occur. It is generally felt, although without complete agreement, that allergic and anaphylactic reactions are due to the release, from storage sites, of mediators of anaphylaxis, such as histamine, 5-hydroxytryptamine, leukotrienes, eosinophil chemotactic factor of anaphylaxis (ECFA), prostaglandins, thromboxane $A_2$, neutrophil chemotactic factor, platelet activating factor (PAF), kinins, and protease enzymes. Anaphylaxis is an emergency and can be fatal if not immediately managed.

The differences between localized allergic reactions (e.g., cutaneous, respiratory) and generalized anaphylactic reactions depend upon the sites and rates of mediator release. If localized release of histamine is slow enough to permit inactivation of any that gets into the bloodstream, only a local allergic reaction will occur. However, if the release is too rapid for inactivation to keep pace, the reaction will be of the anaphylactic or anaphylactoid type.

Drug-induced histamine release can be triggered by antigen–antibody reactions, but most often, the presence of circulating (IgG) or cell-bound (IgE) antibodies cannot be detected. X-ray contrast media in the absence of antibodies may liberate massive amounts of histamine, causing anaphylactoid reactions, often with fatal outcome.

Measures for the control of allergy and anaphylaxis may be either prophylactic or therapeutic and either specific or symptomatic, depending on their locus of action.

**Prophylactic treatment** of asthma and certain allergic conditions with nedocromil sodium or cromolyn sodium (sodium cromoglycate) hinders the release of histamine and other autacoids from mast cells and other cell types (see Chapter 36). Ketotifen fumarate (Zaditen), a prophylactic anti-allergic agent against pediatric asthma, blocks $H_1$ receptors but, in addition, has an apparently separate anti-inflammatory effect in the lungs. It inhibits release of leukotrienes, prevents bronchoconstriction induced by leukotrienes and by PAF, and decreases PAF-induced platelet and eosinophil accumulation in the airways.

**Specific therapy** would be the avoidance or elimination of offending antigens or foods and the desensitization of the sensitive individual.

**Symptomatic therapy** with $H_1$ receptor blockers ("antihistamines") will relieve the effects of histamine release, as in hay fever. If $H_1$ receptor blockade is not effective or not practical, leukotriene receptor blockers or physiological antagonists such as adrenaline, specific $\beta_2$-adrenoceptor stimulants (that inhibit histamine release), or theophylline can be used. In serious cases, beclomethasone administration by inhalation or nasal spray for localized effects can be as effective as systemic glucocorticoid therapy.

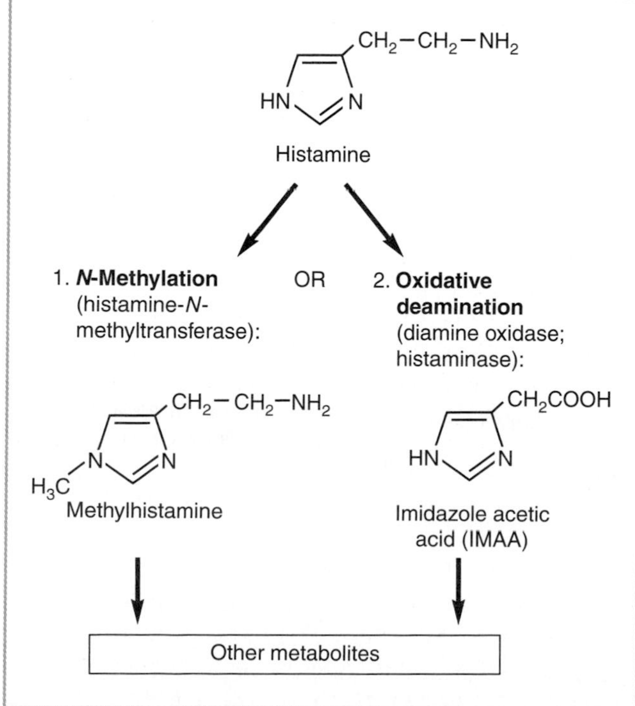

## Clinical Uses

Histamine is occasionally used to assess the ability of the stomach to secrete acid and to test bronchial reactivity. Pentagastrin, a synthetic analogue of gastrin, is now preferred for stimulation of gastric HCl secretion; it has fewer unwanted effects than either histamine or other histamine analogues.

Histamine can be used to test the integrity of sensory nerves and as a provocative agent for the diagnosis of pheochromocytoma, a tumour of the adrenal gland (histamine stimulates the release of catecholamines from the tumour).

## HISTAMINE H₁ RECEPTOR BLOCKERS

In 1937, Bovet and Staub detected histamine-blocking activity in one of a series of amines. This substance (2-isopropyl-5-methylphenoxyethyldiethylamine) protected sensitized guinea pigs against lethal doses of histamine, antagonized histamine-induced spasms of smooth muscle, and lessened the symptoms of anaphylactic shock (these are now known to be $H_1$ receptor–mediated reac-

---

**FIGURE 30-2** Biotransformation of histamine.

Histamine

1. **N-Methylation** (histamine-N-methyltransferase): OR 2. **Oxidative deamination** (diamine oxidase; histaminase):

Methylhistamine

Imidazole acetic acid (IMAA)

Other metabolites

tions). It was too weak and too toxic for therapeutic use, but the synthesis of related substances resulted, in 1942, in the first clinically employed antihistamine, phenbenzamine (Antergan). Other highly effective histamine antagonists followed rapidly. Several decades later, the "non-sedating" $H_1$ receptor blockers were developed and used for symptomatic therapy. Table 30-1 lists the most often used histamine $H_1$ receptor blockers.

## Structure

All antihistamines have the same basic structure, consisting of two aryl rings attached to either a N, O, C, or S atom at one end of a three-atom chain, or its steric equivalent, with a dimethylamine group at the other end, as shown in Figure 30-3. In addition, the terminal dimethylamine group may be incorporated into a ring structure (see Fig. 30-3). Chlorcyclizine is such an example and is illustrated in Figure 30-4, along with some other common antihistamines.

From all these possible constituents, a tremendous number of combinations can be made. There have been more than 4000 such compounds synthesized and tested, and several dozen are in clinical use. However, none of these will inhibit the histamine-induced stimulation of gastric acid secretion, which is an $H_2$ receptor–mediated reaction.

| TABLE 30-1 | Commonly Used Antihistamines |
|---|---|
| **Antihistamine** | **Routes of Administration** |
| Ethanolamines | |
| Diphenhydramine (Benadryl) | oral, parenteral |
| Dimenhydrinate (Dramamine, Gravol)* | oral, rectal, parenteral |
| Ethylenediamines | |
| Tripelennamine (Pyribenzamine) | oral, topical |
| Antazoline (Antistine) | oral |
| Naphazoline (Privine) | nasal |
| Alkylamines | |
| Chlorpheniramine (Chlor-Tripolon) | oral, parenteral |
| Brompheniramine (Dimetane) | oral |
| Piperazines | |
| Cyclizine (Marzine)* | oral, rectal, parenteral |
| Meclizine (Antivert, Bonamine)* | oral |
| Cetirizine (Reactine) | oral |
| Phenothiazine | |
| Promethazine (Phenergan) | oral, rectal, parenteral |
| Piperidines | |
| Loratadine (Claritin) | oral |
| Desloratidine (Aerius) | oral |
| Fexofenadine (Allegra) | oral |
| *Used primarily for prevention of nausea, vomiting, and motion sickness. | |

## Mechanism and Site of Action

The mechanism and site of action are virtually identical for all $H_1$ receptor blockers. The basic structure of conventional antihistamines contains a portion that is similar to the essential structure of histamine itself. This similarity is sufficient to permit the antihistamines to compete for the histamine receptor sites on target cells, while the differences are such as to render them inactive as histamine substitutes (i.e., they are competitive blockers of histamine). This can be demonstrated with isolated tissues in vitro.

In vivo, conventional antihistamines (i.e., $H_1$ receptor blockers) antagonize all the actions of histamine, except the stimulation of HCl secretion in the stomach and that part of the vasodilatation that is mediated by $H_2$ receptors.

## Pharmacokinetics

All $H_1$ receptor blockers are well absorbed following oral administration, and maximum serum levels are achieved within 1 to 2 hours. The bioavailability is high, except that of rectally administered preparations, which are affected by too many variables to be predictably absorbed. The older antihistamines, such as **diphenhydramine** and **chlorpheniramine**, are distributed in all tissues including the CNS, but the newer agents (e.g., **loratidine, desloratidine, fexofenadine**) do not appear to enter the CNS as readily (which explains the relative absence of the sedative effect for these compounds). Plasma protein binding is

| FIGURE 30-3 | Basic structure of antihistamines ($H_1$ receptor blockers). |
|---|---|

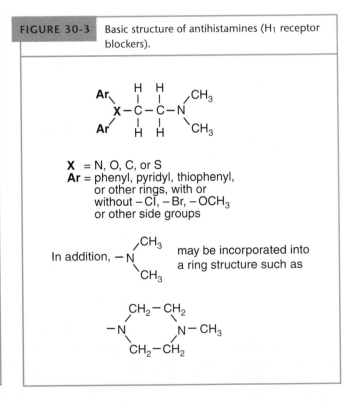

**FIGURE 30-4** Structural formulae of some antihistamines (H$_1$ receptor blockers).

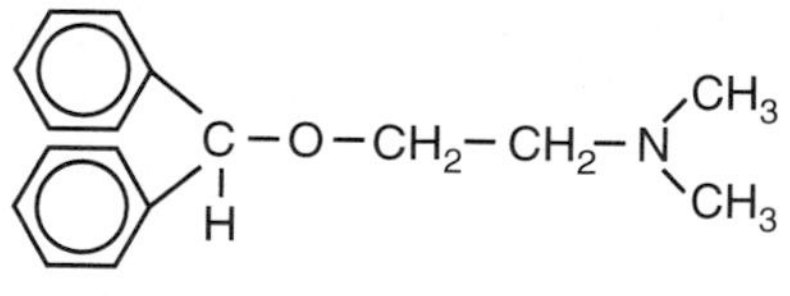

Diphenhydramine (an ethanolamine)

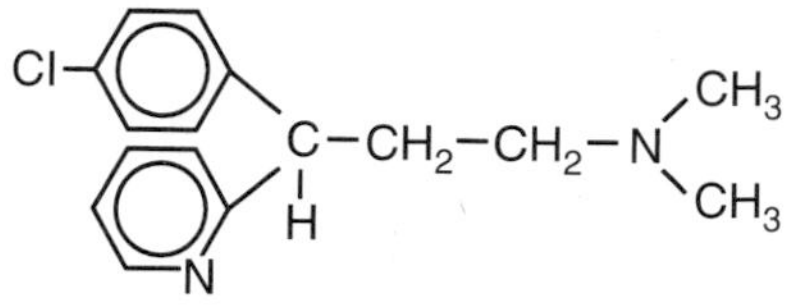

Chlorpheniramine (an alkylamine)

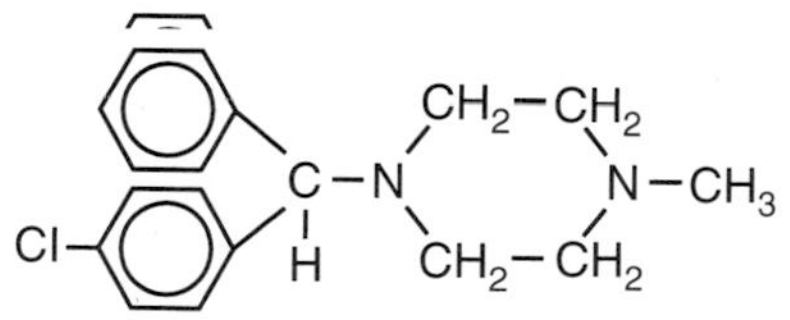

Chlorcyclizine (a piperazine)

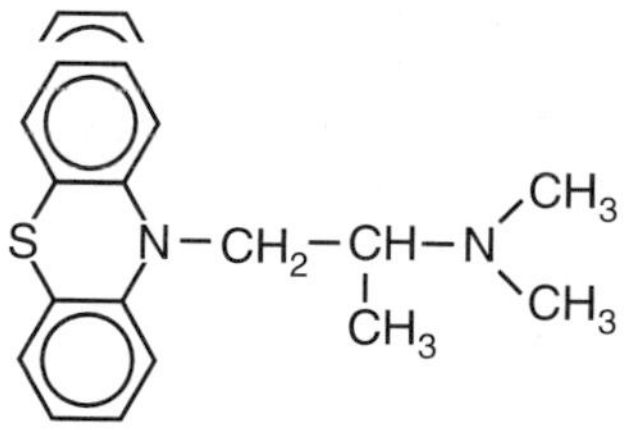

Promethazine (a phenothiazine)

The histamine-induced contraction of gastrointestinal or respiratory smooth muscle is diminished or abolished both in vivo and in vitro. The H$_1$ receptor-mediated component of increased capillary permeability and vasodilatation is inhibited, especially if the antihistamine is administered before liberation of, or exposure to, histamine. Salivary, lacrimal, and bronchial secretions are reduced or arrested if the activity of the glands was due solely to excessive histamine stimulation.

The older H$_1$ receptor blockers have limited effectiveness in severe allergic or anaphylactic reactions. In serious cases, or in the presence of laryngeal edema, adrenaline remains the drug of choice (see Chapter 13). However, a number of the newer non-sedating H$_1$ receptor blockers, including **cetirizine** (Reactine), **mizolastine** (Mizollen), **ebastine** (Kestine), and others, also inhibit the release of leukotrienes and cytokines, and thus have anti-allergy activity. They are useful in the treatment of both acute and chronic urticaria.

The effects of H$_1$ receptor blockers on the CNS are unpredictable. Most often they cause CNS depression, but in some patients agitation or restlessness may occur. The pharmacological effect involved in the prevention of motion sickness is partly due to cholinergic muscarinic receptor blockade, but not all H$_1$ blockers are equally effective against motion sickness.

## Additional and Adverse Effects

All antihistamines have some **CNS-depressant** effects, but these are much less marked with loratadine, desloratidine, and fexofenadine, presumably because of their reduced entry into the CNS. Some antihistamines (e.g., promethazine, diphenhydramine) are good sedatives or hypnotics and are used as the active agents in over-the-counter sleeping pills. Others have antitussive properties (e.g., diphenhydramine). The relative prominence of these effects varies from one antihistamine to another.

All antihistamines have **local anaesthetic** activity, and some are quite potent in this respect. The dimethylaminoethanol group, either in ester or ether linkage, is common to the local anaesthetics and to many antihistamines (see Chapter 21). Like the local anaesthetics, the antihistamines in high doses cause central stimulation and may cause convulsions, as can sometimes be observed in attempted suicide with antihistamines. Also like the local anaesthetics, and like procainamide and amiodarone (which also share the dialkylaminoethyl group), the antihistamines are cardiac depressants when given in high dosage.

Some of the antihistamines, and especially those in which the X atom is oxygen, are potent **anticholinergics** (see Fig. 30-3). If progressively larger groups replace the acetyl group in acetylcholine, the acetylcholine-like action decreases, and it is finally converted into an anticholinergic

variable. The major site of biotransformation of all antihistaminic drugs is the liver, and minute amounts of the unchanged drugs and most of the metabolites are excreted in the urine. Some of the metabolites are active and contribute to the total duration of action of the parent compound. **Cetirizine** is itself a metabolite of the anxiolytic agent **hydroxyzine,** which also has powerful H$_1$ receptor-blocking activity (see Chapter 23). The plasma half-life varies widely: for many of the older compounds it is in the range of 4 to 6 hours, but for the piperazine and piperidine derivatives it tends to be closer to 24 hours or even longer.

## Pharmacological Effects

Antihistamines offer almost complete protection against the effects of injected histamine, but their effectiveness is less complete against endogenously liberated histamine.

effect. Benzilic acid esters of choline (e.g., oxyphenonium) are good examples. Oxygen-containing antihistamines have a chemical resemblance to these choline esters, which suggests a basis for their anticholinergic activity (CNS depression and sedation).

Some antihistamines, especially the phenothiazine derivatives, are adrenergic blockers, while others have a weak ganglioplegic effect.

Thus, all antihistaminic drugs have adverse effects to some degree. It is obvious that the side effects differ for different drugs, because they derive from chemical features other than those responsible for the antihistaminic action. The incidence and severity of side effects also vary greatly between individual subjects. Therefore, in prescribing a given antihistamine, it is essential to know the particular constellation of side effects for that drug and to anticipate that about one person in four will experience some bothersome reaction during antihistamine therapy.

The most frequently observed side effect common to most histamine antagonists is **sedation**. Other untoward reactions, including dizziness, tinnitus, lassitude, incoordination, fatigue, blurred vision, and tremors, are referable to central actions of the antihistamines. Some side effects involve the digestive tract (loss of appetite, nausea), and these drugs may cause dryness of the mouth (atropine-like effect). All of these troublesome symptoms may or may not disappear with continued therapy.

The most recently introduced antihistaminic drugs, cetirizine, loratadine, desloratidine, fexofenadine, ebastine, mizolastine, acrivastine, and others, are claimed to be generally free of CNS-related side effects and to have a lower incidence of other side effects. In addition, they do not appear to intensify the CNS-depressant effects of other drugs or alcohol. Side effects recorded in some clinical trials have been not much greater in frequency than those of placebo. Nevertheless, patients with heart disease should be watched for any changes in cardiac performance.

The simultaneous administration of metronidazole, systemic antifungals (e.g., ketoconazole, fluconazole), macrolide antibiotics (e.g., erythromycin), or any other drug that inhibits the cytochrome P450 isozyme responsible for the biotransformation of terfenadine and astemizole was contraindicated because of serious toxicity due to these two first-generation "non-sedating" antihistamines, which have since been withdrawn from the market in most countries. Severe interference with cardiac rhythm (torsades de pointes) was reported in susceptible individuals taking these medications concurrently.

The antihistamines can themselves evoke allergic reactions, presumably by acting as haptens that combine with some tissue protein to form antigen complexes. These drugs, especially if used topically or intermittently as against the common cold (in which they have relatively little beneficial effect), occasionally produce the usual drug allergies, including agranulocytosis and chronic dermatoses.

**Interactions** of antihistamines with other drugs can have serious consequences. The older antihistaminics potentiate the central effects of all other CNS-depressant drugs, including alcohol. Patients taking antihistamines, even if only one dose, should be warned not to drink alcohol, to drive, or to operate dangerous machinery while under the influence of the drug. In many countries, including the United States and Canada, the use of antihistamines, as in cough and cold preparations, is generally not a mitigating factor in impaired-driving charges. Almost all cough and cold preparations contain substances that are banned by Olympic and other sports organizations.

## Acute Poisoning

Although the margin of safety of antihistamines is relatively high, and chronic toxicity is rare, acute poisoning with these drugs is not uncommon, especially in young children.

In acute poisoning, central effects predominate and are the greatest danger. The syndrome includes hallucinations, excitement, ataxia, and convulsions. The latter are difficult to control. In the child, the picture includes fixed dilated pupils, flushed face, and fever and is remarkably similar to that of atropine poisoning. If untreated, deepening coma and cardiorespiratory collapse may lead to death within a few hours. In the adult, fever and flushing are less severe, and drowsiness and coma often precede the excitatory (convulsive) phase. Since there is no specific therapy for antihistamine poisoning, treatment is generally symptomatic and supportive.

## Therapeutic Applications

### Suppression of allergic phenomena

Antihistamines are beneficial in nasal allergies (hay fever), acute skin reactions (urticaria, drug rashes), and systemic allergic reactions (e.g., serum sickness, transfusion reaction), but they are almost without effect against asthma and chronic skin allergies. Probably it is a matter of differential ability of these drugs to penetrate to the sites of endogenous release of histamine and other autacoids (e.g., 5-HT, prostaglandins; see Chapters 27 and 29). It is also conceivable that different and as yet unrecognized receptor variants are involved. **Levocabastine** (Livostin) eye drops and nasal spray are used for the treatment of seasonal allergic conjunctivitis and allergic rhinitis (itchy or running nose), respectively. The beneficial effect is due exclusively to $H_1$ receptor blocking properties.

### Anti-parkinsonian use

Atropine and various synthetic atropine-like drugs have an anti-parkinsonian effect that generally parallels their anticholinergic activity (see Chapter 17). The oxygen-containing antihistamines, which have anticholinergic side effects as already noted, also have useful activity against acute skeletal muscle spasticity. Orphenadrine is used almost exclusively for this purpose. It is possibly useful in the short-term treatment of parkinsonian symptoms that may occur as a side effect of phenothiazine neuroleptic therapy, but not in the long-term treatment of post-encephalitic parkinsonism because the drug tends to lose its effectiveness after a few months.

## Motion sickness

Nausea and vomiting can result from several different types of stimuli. The phenothiazine neuroleptics are effective suppressants of the chemoreceptor trigger zone, but they do not block the effects of vestibular stimuli. Some, but not all, antihistamines do prevent or diminish nausea and vomiting mediated by both the vestibular and the chemoreceptor pathways. Among the most effective ones are **promethazine, cyclizine, meclizine, and dimenhydrinate.** These are of different chemical types, with different side effects, so the antiemetic action appears to be independent of the antihistaminic and other actions mentioned before.

Recent approaches to the control of hyperemesis of multifactorial origin also employ other antiemetic agents. Nabilone (Cesamet) and dronabinol (Marinol) are cannabinoid antiemetics used in cancer chemotherapy to control nausea and vomiting (see Chapter 26). However, they also have sedative and psychotropic properties, which limit their usefulness in many patients. Transderm-V, a thin, multilayered, circular film containing 1.5 mg scopolamine, is applied to the skin behind the ear approximately 12 hours before an antiemetic effect is required. There is a sustained absorption of scopolamine for about 3 days while the tape is in contact with the skin. Scopolamine produces all the side effects of atropine (see Chapter 12).

## HISTAMINE H2 RECEPTOR BLOCKERS

The H2 receptor–blocking agents constitute a clinically important group having very little if any affinity for H1 receptors. They are clinically effective in blocking the stimulatory effects of histamine and pentagastrin on gastric HCl secretion, and a number of new H2 receptor blockers are now in use. Their molecular structure (Fig. 30-5) contains a portion that resembles the histamine molecule, but the five-member ring varies: cimetidine retains the imidazole ring of histamine, but in newer drugs of this class, it is replaced by furan, thiazol, or other rings.

## Cimetidine

### Mechanism of action

This drug acts on H2 receptors located in stomach, blood vessels, and other sites in the body. It is a competitive antagonist of histamine, and its effect is fully reversible. It has no affinity for H1 or other known neurotransmitter receptors.

Cimetidine (Tagamet, Peptol; see Fig. 30-5) completely inhibits gastric acid secretion induced by histamine, gastrin, or pentagastrin; that induced by acetylcholine or bethanechol is only partly inhibited. In therapeutic concentrations, it inhibits gastric HCl secretion in all phases following solid or liquid food feeding or after insulin and caffeine administration. Extremely high doses paradoxically facilitate histamine release by blocking the H2 receptor–mediated negative-feedback mechanism.

### Pharmacokinetics

Close to 80% of an orally administered dose is absorbed, and maximum blood concentrations are reached in 1 to 1.5 hours. The therapeutic plasma concentration is about 2 μmol/L. It is unevenly distributed in the various organs of the body; it crosses the placental barrier, but it does not cross the blood–brain barrier easily because of its high water solubility. It can be found in the cerebrospinal fluid in concentrations about 30% of those in plasma. Less than 25% is bound to plasma proteins. Cimetidine has two major metabolites, which are excreted in urine together with about 50% of unchanged drug. The serum half-life is short, about 1 to 1.5 hours, but is longer in renal failure.

### Adverse effects

The adverse effects of cimetidine are usually minor and are mainly associated with the reduced gastric juice produc-

FIGURE 30-5 Structural formulae of the H2 receptor blockers cimetidine, ranitidine, and famotidine.

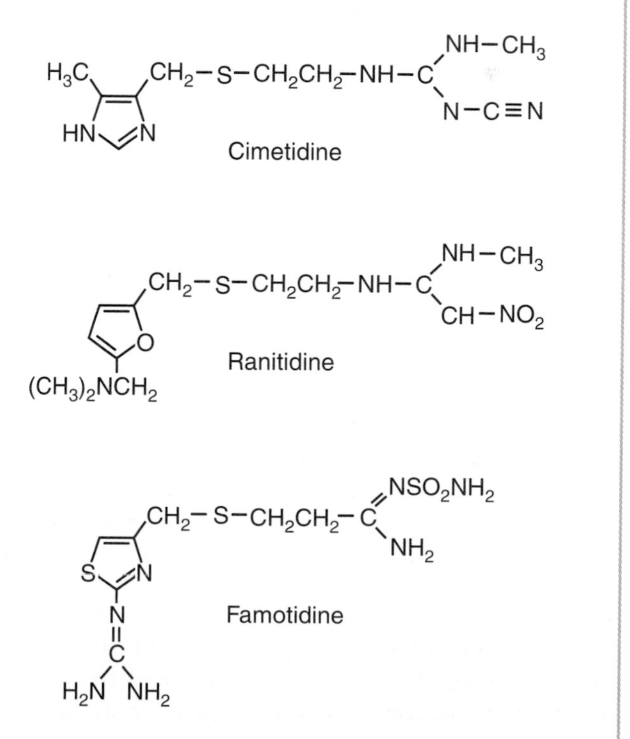

tion. Headache, confusion, hallucinations, dizziness, or other CNS-related side effects may occur primarily in the elderly or following prolonged administration, as for treatment of Zollinger-Ellison syndrome, a chronic gastric hypersecretory state. A few cases of mild gynecomastia have been reported, but no endocrine basis for it has been found. Cimetidine can bind to androgen receptors, and at very high doses it can reduce the sperm count. It is practically non-toxic, even following accidental overdose of 10 g or so. The heart rate may be increased, probably as a reflex response to mild reduction in blood pressure. Cimetidine reduces the rate of hepatic cytochrome P450–dependent biotransformation of a number of drugs. It also may competitively inhibit the renal tubular secretion of other organic bases (e.g., procainamide). The circulating gastrin concentration is elevated during cimetidine administration. The effects of cimetidine on gastric alcohol dehydrogenase are discussed in Chapter 22.

## Ranitidine

### Mechanism of action and pharmacokinetics
Ranitidine (Zantac; see Fig. 30-5) is a very potent $H_2$ receptor blocker. Its mechanism and site of action, as well as its pharmacological effects, are similar to those of cimetidine, but ranitidine is five to 10 times more potent. Only 50% of an orally administered dose is absorbed, and maximum plasma concentration occurs 1 to 2 hours later. The plasma half-life is 3 hours. The distribution and plasma protein binding are similar to those of cimetidine. Ranitidine has two minor metabolites, which are excreted in urine, but most of the drug is eliminated unchanged.

### Adverse effects
Adverse effects of ranitidine include mild and infrequent gastrointestinal complaints and rare CNS side effects (intermittent confusional states). Drug interactions at the renal or hepatic level are less frequent than with cimetidine, because ranitidine does not inhibit cytochrome P450. Endocrine-related symptoms have not been reported, and ranitidine does not block androgen receptors. Ranitidine is considered to be practically non-toxic, although elevation of serum transaminase levels and possible hepatocellular injury have been reported in a few cases.

## Famotidine

Famotidine (Pepcid), another member of the group of very potent $H_2$ receptor blockers, has a thiazole ring in place of the imidazole (see Fig. 30-5).

### Mechanism of action and pharmacokinetics
The mechanism of action, pharmacological effects, site of action, indications, and clinical use are the same as for the other $H_2$ receptor antagonists. Famotidine is three to 20 times as potent as ranitidine. Less than 45% of an oral dose is absorbed; maximum plasma concentration occurs 1 to 3 hours after ingestion. The plasma half-life is 2.5 to 3.5 hours in patients with normal kidney function, but with creatinine clearance of less than 10 mL/min, the elimination half-life can be 12 hours or longer, and 20 hours or more in anuric patients. About 30% of an oral dose and 65 to 70% of an intravenous dose are eliminated in the urine unchanged, and the rest is eliminated as a sulfoxide metabolite. The recommended single daily dose of 20 to 40 mg at bedtime inhibits up to 94% of nocturnal gastric acid secretion, and 25 to 30% for another 8 to 10 hours later. The nocturnal intragastric pH is between 5.0 and 6.4.

### Adverse effects
Adverse effects of famotidine observed during controlled clinical trials were few and of minor importance. They are similar to those of ranitidine. The frequency of these reactions was comparable to those recorded in the placebo group, and a causal relationship could not be established. Most often observed were headache, dizziness, constipation, and diarrhea. Treatment of accidental or intentional overdosage should be symptomatic and supportive. Daily doses of up to 640 mg, administered to patients with pathological hypersecretory conditions, had no serious adverse effects. With chronic treatment, gastric emptying and exocrine pancreatic functions are not affected, but an increase in gastric bacterial flora may occur. Because adverse effects can emerge after years of extensive clinical use, periodic observation of patients treated with famotidine is advised. In healthy volunteers, famotidine in clinical doses caused significant increases in cardiac pre-ejection period and decreases in stroke volume and cardiac output, without significant change in heart rate or blood pressure.

## Nizatidine

Nizatidine (Axid) is an $H_2$ receptor blocker approved for the treatment of acute duodenal and benign gastric ulcers. Its potency is similar to ranitidine. It is absorbed rapidly after oral administration, reaching peak serum concentrations in 0.5 to 3 hours. Food has no significant effect on bioavailability. About 35% is protein-bound, mainly to $\alpha_1$-glycoprotein. The apparent volume of distribution is between 0.8 and 1.5 L/kg, plasma half-life is 1 to 2 hours, and 60% of the dose is excreted in the urine as unchanged drug. The average plasma clearance is about 50 L/hr, which can be reduced to 7 to 14 L/hr in patients with creatinine clearance of 10 mL/min or less, giving rise to a plasma half-life of 4 to 11 hours. An oral dose of 300 mg at bedtime can suppress gastric acid secretion for 10 to 12 hours.

FIGURE 30-6 Structural formulae of two H₃ receptor agonists and the H₃ receptor blocker thioperamide.

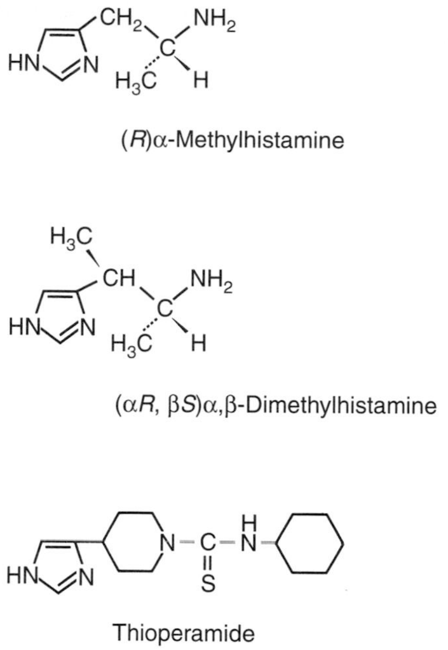

(R)α-Methylhistamine

(αR, βS)α,β-Dimethylhistamine

Thioperamide

In short-term trials, nizatidine was found to be free of hormonal interference and had no effect on the drug metabolizing P450 enzymes. In clinical trials, the frequency of observed side effects such as headache, somnolence, and pruritus was somewhat higher than in the placebo group, but a causal relationship to nizatidine administration could not be established. Serum cholesterol, serum uric acid, serum creatinine, and platelet and white cell counts showed statistically non-significant differences from the placebo group. Serum transaminases have been elevated in a few cases, but the clinical importance of these changes is not clear. In healthy volunteers, nizatidine was shown to have a negative chronotropic influence with increased cardiac pre-ejection period and decreased heart rate and cardiac output, without change in stroke volume.

## Clinical Uses of H₂ Receptor Blockers

Therapeutic applications of these agents are identical. H₂ receptor blockers are useful in the prophylactic treatment of conditions that require a reduction of gastric acid secretion, such as treatment of duodenal ulcer, non-malignant gastric ulcer, gastroesophageal reflux disease, pathological hypersecretion states associated with Zollinger-Ellison syndrome, systemic mastocytosis, and multiple endocrine adenomas. They are also described in this specific context in Chapter 41.

# HISTAMINE H₃ RECEPTOR AGONISTS AND BLOCKERS

Histamine H₃ receptors found in the CNS are located on presynaptic histaminergic, cholinergic, dopaminergic, adrenergic, and serotonergic neurons and produce feedback modulation of the synthesis of histamine and other neurotransmitters and their release into the synaptic cleft. The H₃ receptor agonists, (R)α-methylhistamine and (αR, βS)α,β-dimethylhistamine (Fig. 30-6), are not used clinically, only to study the distribution of H₃ receptors in the brain and peripheral tissues and to determine their physiological and pathological roles.

Thioperamide (see Fig. 30-6) is the most often used histamine H₃ receptor blocker. It appears that most, but not all, histamine-induced actions in vitro and in animal models are blocked by H₁, H₂, and H₃ receptor blockers. In the periphery, additional distinct histamine receptors are likely to be discovered shortly.

# SUGGESTED READINGS

Casale TB, Blaiss MS, Gelfand E, et al. First do no harm: managing antihistamine impairment in patients with allergic rhinitis. *J Allergy Clin Immunol.* 2003;111:S835-S842.

DuBuske LM. Second-generation antihistamines: the risk of ventricular arrhythmias. *Clin Ther.* 1999;21:281-295.

Hill SJ. Distribution, properties, and functional characteristics of three classes of histamine receptor. *Pharmacol Rev.* 1990;42:45-83.

Lebrun-Vignes B, Diquet B, Chosidow O. Clinical pharmacokinetics of mizolastine. *Clin Pharmacokinet.* 2001;40:501-507.

Leurs R, Blandina P, Tedford C, Timmerman H. Therapeutic potential of histamine H₃ receptor agonists and antagonists. *Trends Pharmacol Sci.* 1998;19:177-183.

Magee LA, Mazzotta P, Koren G. Evidence-based view of safety and effectiveness of pharmacologic therapy for nausea and vomiting of pregnancy (NVP). *Am J Obstet Gynecol.* 2002;186(5 suppl):S256-S261.

O'Connor BJ, Lecomte JM, Barnes PJ. Effect of an inhaled histamine H₃-receptor agonist on airway responses to sodium metabisulphite in asthma. *Br J Clin Pharmacol.* 1993;35:55-57.

Pounder R, ed. *Histamine H₂-Receptor Antagonists.* London, United Kingdom: Science Press; 1990.

Raud J, Thorlacius J, Xie X, Lindbom L, Hedqvist P. Interactions between histamine and leukotrienes in the microcirculation. Aspects of relevance to acute allergic inflammation. *Ann NY Acad Sci.* 1994;744:191-198.

Rimmer SJ, Church MK. The pharmacology and mechanisms of action of histamine H₁-antagonists. *Clin Exp Allergy.* 1990;20(suppl 2):3-17.

Russell T, Stolc M, Weir S. Pharmacokinetics, pharmacodynamics, and tolerance of single- and multiple-dose fexofenadine hydrochloride in healthy male volunteers. *Clin Pharmacol Ther.* 1998;64:612-621.

Simons FE, Simons KJ. Pharmacokinetic optimisation of histamine H1-receptor antagonist therapy. *Clin Pharmacokinet.* 1991;21:372-393.

Ten Eick AP, Blumer JL, Reed MD. Safety of antihistamines in children. *Drug Saf.* 2001;24:119-147.

Timmerman H, van der Goot H, eds. *New Perspectives in Histamine Research.* Basel, Switzerland: Birkhauser Verlag; 1990.

Verster JC, Volkerts ER. Antihistamines and driving ability: evidence from on-the-road driving studies during normal traffic. *Ann Allergy Asthma Immunol.* 2004;92:294-303.

Wilson AM, O'Byrne PM, Parameswaran K. Leukotriene receptor antagonists for allergic rhinitis: a systematic review and meta-analysis. *Am J Med.* 2004;116:338-344.

# Part V

## Cardiovascular System

# 31

# Cardiovascular System Overview and Organization

## U ACKERMANN

Pharmacological treatment of cardiovascular dysfunction is directed at pathologies affecting rhythm, cardiac contractile performance, blood vessel function, or blood pressure regulation. This chapter will summarize inter-relationships among cardiac, blood vessel, and nervous functional components of cardiovascular performance.

## OVERVIEW

The cardiovascular system consists of a four-chambered pump, the heart, and a flow-distributing network of blood vessels. Its two primary functions are (1) to provide to all tissues at all times the supply of nutrients required to sustain the metabolic activity of the tissue, and (2) to remove from all tissues the products of their metabolic activity.

Cardiac function is initiated by electrical events in the heart. In each heartbeat, the processes of excitation–activation–contraction coupling convert electrical activity into pulsatile mechanical actions that propel a bolus of blood from the right ventricle into the pulmonary artery and another bolus from the left ventricle into the aorta. Viscoelastic properties of the arterial network convert the pulsatile output of the heart into a smooth, uninterrupted capillary flow within each tissue. The viscoelastic properties of the venous network function mainly to modulate, on a time scale of seconds to minutes, the flow that returns to the heart from the capillary beds. The venous system and the pattern of cardiac relaxation after each contraction are the two major influences on the filling of the ventricles with blood in preparation for the next ejection. Relaxation, like contraction, is initiated by electrophysiological and biochemical events in cardiac cells.

## CARDIAC ELECTROPHYSIOLOGY

The electrical activity of each excitable cardiac cell can be measured as periodic changes in the electrical potential difference between the inside and outside of the cell. The polarity, amplitude, and pattern of change of this potential difference are determined by the transport of ions through highly regulated membrane proteins that form a variety of transporters and channels. Both passive and active transport mechanisms are involved. Passive transport through ion-selective channels and down electrochemical gradients determines cell behaviour on a time scale of milliseconds; active transport mechanisms operate on a slower time scale and are dominant in restoring and maintaining the electrochemical gradients that drive passive transport.

### Ion Channels

Ion-selective channels are members of a closely related family of intrinsic cell membrane proteins. They typically consist of a principal plus one or more satellite subunits each made up of several transmembrane segments. The segments and domains are serially linked in the extracellular space and in the cytosol by polypeptide chains. Channels are formed by monomeric or multimeric arrangements of polypeptides around a central, selective "pore" of variable conductance.

Cardiac electrophysiological behaviour can be adequately described by focusing on **open** and **closed** states of channels that are selective for $Na^+$, $Ca^{2+}$, or $K^+$. Their total numbers, individual conductances, or sensitivity to activation can be modulated by a variety of chemical ligands. However, the ordered and sequential openings of channels that result in the electrical impulses initiating each heartbeat occur almost exclusively in voltage-gated channels. This class of ion channels is controlled by changes in cell membrane potential. They include voltage-sensing elements among their transmembrane domains. Activation of such elements opens each channel, and only milliseconds later, spontaneous or voltage-dependent inactivation processes will close the channel. Such opening and closing sequences result in the action potential that is described below.

## Sodium channels

*Channel activation.* The main functional component of the $Na^+$ channel is a large (269 kDa) transmembrane protein known as the α subunit. It contains the binding site for tetrodotoxin and saxitoxin, both of which will inhibit channel conductance. In different excitable tissues, the α subunit can occur in association with a variable number of smaller subunits, termed $β_1$ and $β_2$, that may modulate channel structure or function but are not essential for ion transport.

*Channel inactivation.* Inactivation probably involves further conformational change in portions of the channel and can result in either a closed refractory state or a closed activatable state. Closed $Na^+$ channels in either state conduct a small leakage current, called the slow $Na^+$ current.

*Transition from refractory to activatable state.* Channels that have gone through an activation–inactivation cycle following membrane depolarization are refractory at first, but they can be made available for future activation. This requires complete membrane repolarization. The time required for this restoration of availability is on the order of 100 ms at –80 to –100 mV.

*Long-term modulation.* Modulation on a time scale that is longer than a few milliseconds occurs by phosphorylation of the channel protein by means of protein kinase C and cAMP-dependent protein kinase A. Their greatest effects are on channel inactivation.

## Calcium channels

Most excitable cells have many types of $Ca^{2+}$ channels, but the L type is prominent in cardiac muscle. T-type channels are often also present. The L channel mediates long-lasting $Ca^{2+}$ currents. Membrane depolarization causes the L channel to admit an influx of $Ca^{2+}$ ($I_{Ca,L}$) that is capable of triggering intracellular responses. $I_{Ca,L}$ is inhibited by $H^+$, by external multivalent cations like $Mn^{2+}$, $Mg^{2+}$, or $Ni^{2+}$, and by at least three structurally different classes of antagonists. These antagonists are the dihydropyridines (e.g., nifedipine and nisoldipine), the phenylalkylamines (e.g., verapamil), and the benzothiazepines (e.g., diltiazem). T channels differ from L channels in that they have (1) a more negative activation threshold voltage; (2) more rapid, voltage-dependent inactivation; (3) an insensitivity to the common L-channel blockers, but a high sensitivity to blockade by $Ni^{2+}$, and (4) a high resistance to β-adrenergic stimulation.

*Channel activation.* Both L- and T-type channels have a distinct threshold voltage: at membrane potentials more positive than threshold, channels are activated quickly, permitting $Ca^{2+}$ current to flow. The L-type channel threshold is near –40 mV (at 2 mM $[Ca^{2+}]_o$) and the T-type threshold is –50 to –65 mV. Both thresholds are influenced by the extracellular concentration of divalent cations such as $Ca^{2+}$; higher extracellular concentrations act to shield surface charges and move the threshold voltage toward more positive values. T-channel activation, where it occurs, is brief. L-channel activation, on the other hand, quickly reaches a peak and then diminishes slowly during an inactivation phase that lasts up to 300 ms in non-pacemaker myocardial cells.

*Channel inactivation.* Inactivation is slow in myocyte L channels, lasting a few hundred milliseconds, and is influenced by both membrane voltage and $Ca^{2+}$ entry into the cell. In T channels, the inactivation process is much more rapid, lasting a little less than 50 ms, and it appears to be primarily voltage-dependent.

*Modulation of $Ca^{2+}$ channel behaviour.* Apart from the pharmacological antagonism that was mentioned above, $Ca^{2+}$ channel function can be altered by a variety of neurohumoral influences.

- β-**Adrenergic receptor** stimulation enhances $I_{Ca,L}$ by a protein kinase A–dependent mechanism.
- Modulation by **muscarinic receptor** stimulation is a controversial matter because muscarinic activation stimulates a transient outward $K^+$ current that overlaps $I_{Ca,L}$. Basal $I_{Ca,L}$ appears to be unaffected by acetylcholine, but catecholamine-stimulated $I_{Ca,L}$ is inhibited by it.
- Modulation by **$G_s$ proteins** may stimulate $I_{Ca,L}$ by a cytoplasmic pathway identical to the one that follows β-adrenergic receptor stimulation.
- Elevation of cytosolic $Ca^{2+}$ concentration inhibits L-type calcium channels.

## Sodium–calcium exchange

Cardiac T-tubule membranes contain a protein that is driven by the extracellular/intracellular $Na^+$ gradient to exchange 3 $Na^+$ inward for each $Ca^{2+}$ outward. This sodium-in/calcium-out direction of the exchanger prevails throughout all phases of the normal human cardiac action potential. However, the direction can be reversed by appropriate changes in membrane potential or the reversal potential of the exchanger.

## Potassium channels

Although the structure of the $K^+$ channel is simpler than that of the $Na^+$ or $Ca^{2+}$ channels, less is known about the details of its function, and it continues to be a target of vigorous investigation. Several **functional subtypes** are known to be important for cardiac function:

- Channels that are sensitive to extracellular acetylcholine
- Acetylcholine-insensitive channels that appear to be the major carrier of basal potassium current ($I_{K1}$) in human heart cells: Their "open" times are longer than those of the acetylcholine-sensitive channels.

- Channels carrying the delayed rectifier currents, $I_{Kq}$, $I_{Kr}$, and $I_{Ks}$, which provide outward current for repolarization of the membrane towards its diastolic potential: As described later for the action potential, $I_{Kq}$, $I_{Kr}$, and $I_{Ks}$, respectively, carry the ultrarapid, rapid, and slow components of what was formerly called THE delayed rectifier current. Their thresholds for activation can be as low as –50 mV ($I_{Kq}$ and $I_{Kr}$), and they show rising strength as membrane potentials increase to +50 mV. These currents are not affected by acetylcholine, but β-adrenergic receptor agonists (1) move minimum threshold 5 to 10 mV more negative, (2) increase the magnitude of the fully activated current, and (3) slow the kinetics of channel deactivation.
- Channels that are inactivated by ATP ($I_{K(ATP)}$): These channels contribute negligibly to the basal potassium current but may become important during ischemia when cellular ATP levels are low.

## Membrane Potentials

Cardiac muscle cells are excitable cells and are, therefore, capable of generating action potentials. Most muscle cells in the atria and ventricles tend to have stable resting membrane potentials in the intervals between action potentials. Some cardiac cells, called **pacemaker cells**, never rest; they have unstable membrane potentials that allow them to reach threshold and generate action potentials spontaneously.

### Resting membrane potential

When they are not excited, most cardiac cells maintain a stable resting membrane potential between –80 and –95 mV. It arises from passive ion fluxes and electrogenic transport (Fig. 31-1) and is largely determined by the ratio of intracellular to extracellular K+, because the resting membrane is far more permeable to K+ than to the other ions in the resting state. An approximation of the steady-state resting membrane potential ($E_m$) can be calculated from the Goldman–Hodgkin–Katz equation:

$$E_m = \frac{RT}{F} \ln \frac{P_K [K^+]_o + P_{Na} [Na^+]_o + P_{Cl} [Cl^-]_i}{P_K [K^+]_i + P_{Na} [Na^+]_i + P_{Cl} [Cl^-]_o}$$

Here, $R$ is the universal gas constant, $T$ is absolute temperature, $F$ is Faraday's constant, $P_X$ is the membrane permeability for ion "X," $[X]_o$ is the extracellular concentration of ion "X," and $[X]_i$ is the intracellular concentration of ion "X."

This equation, based on a simplified model of ion transport through membranes, has guided much experimental design and interpretation and has led to the realization that the resting membrane potential is determined by the behaviour of ion channels and ion transporters. It is, therefore, influenced by changes in the ionic milieu and by any neurohumoral factors or drugs that affect ion transport across cell membranes.

## Action potentials

Cardiac muscle cells respond to an appropriate stimulus with a sequence of electrophysiological changes that constitute the phases of the action potential. They are labelled "0" to "4," as shown in Figure 31-2. Most cardiac muscle cells are quiescent non-pacemaker cells that can be triggered by a stimulus from pacemaker cells. Pacemaker cells generate the initiating stimulus intrinsically and spontaneously. A network of conductive tissue and gap junctions facilitate the distribution of electrical activity throughout the muscle walls.

## Pacemaker potentials

Pacemaker cells give the heart the property of **automaticity.** They differ from other cardiac cells in their phase 4 electrical behaviour, which shows gradual depolarization in pacemaker cells, but not in other cardiac muscle cells. This spontaneous, gradual phase 4 depolarization arises from the presence of an inward current ($I_f$) as well as the absence of the outward current, $I_{K1}$ (see Fig. 31-2). A pacemaker action potential is generated when the gating voltage for L-type $Ca^{2+}$ channels is reached at about –40 mV. Action potential generation by $I_{Ca,L}$ rather than $I_{Na}$ marks another difference between cardiac pacemaker and non-pacemaker cells.

There are two main populations of pacemaker cells. They are found in the region of the sinoatrial (SA) node and in the atrioventricular (AV) node and Purkinje fibres. SA node cells normally show the steeper diastolic rise in potential because they have the lowest density of channels carrying $I_{K1}$, which is the major stabilizing current in non-pacemaker cells. Hence, SA nodal cells are the earliest to depolarize, have the highest discharge rate, and are, therefore, the dominant pacemaker. They normally determine the heart rate. When, for any reason, the AV node takes over the pacemaker role, the heart rate is lower.

## Non-pacemaker action potentials

Most cardiac muscle cells are not spontaneously active. They require an adequate stimulus in order to be depolarized and generate the five phases of an action potential (see Fig. 31-2).

- *Phase 0,* the action potential upstroke: Application of an effective stimulus causes activation of enough Na+ channels to produce rapid depolarization, shown by a steep upstroke in the membrane potential recording that moves rapidly toward the Na+ equilibrium potential. The increase in Na+ flux lasts only 1 to 2 ms because the channels carrying it undergo voltage-dependent inactivation. Channels carrying $Ca^{2+}$ currents ($I_{Ca,T}$ and $I_{Ca,L}$) are activated when the membrane potential reaches their gating thresholds: about

Ion currents contributing to cardiac cell resting membrane potentials. The resting membrane potential in cardiac cells results from a balance among ion fluxes that result from passive diffusion down electrochemical gradients, active transport, or coupled transport. (A) *Passive diffusion mechanisms*. Four currents contribute significantly: an inwardly directed sodium current ($I_{Na}$); a relatively large outwardly directed potassium current ($I_{K1}$); an ATP-sensitive potassium current ($I_{K(ATP)}$) that is small when ATP levels are normal or high; and a small chloride current ($I_{Cl}$) that is directed outward, against the concentration gradient, because the chloride equilibrium potential is positive with respect to the resting membrane potential. (B) *Active transport mechanisms*. The $Na^+/K^+$ pump transports two $K^+$ into the cell while extruding three $Na^+$ ions for each molecule of ATP hydrolyzed. The coupling ratio of 3:2 prevails over a wide range of conditions. There also is an ATP-consuming $Ca^{2+}$ pump that helps to maintain low resting intracellular calcium concentration. (C) *Coupled transport*. The $Na^+/Ca^{2+}$ exchanger operates through a sarcolemmal protein and is driven by the $Na^+$ electrochemical gradient. Reversal to a $Na^+$-out/$Ca^{2+}$-in state can occur under some circumstances but is rare in healthy human myocytes.

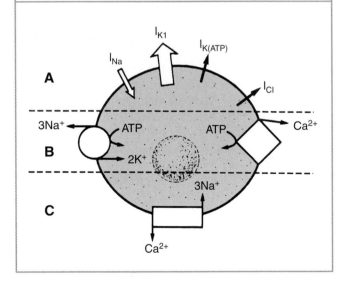

$-50$ mV for $I_{Ca,T}$ and about $-40$ mV for $I_{Ca,L}$. $I_{Ca,L}$ remains activated well into the next two phases. It is a vital controller of excitation–activation–contraction coupling because it triggers and modulates the release of $Ca^{2+}$ from intracellular sarcoplasmic stores.

- *Phase 1,* early rapid repolarization: At the peak of the upstroke, the membrane potential reaches about $+30$ to $+40$ mV and then undergoes rapid repolarization by transient outward currents, $I_{to1}$ and $I_{to2}$.

Their importance lies in determining the magnitude of the plateau (phase 2) voltage.

- *Phase 2,* the action potential plateau: The plateau occurs because the depolarizing and repolarizing currents are nearly in balance during this phase. The major depolarizing influence is the inward $Ca^{2+}$ current, $I_{Ca,L}$, but $I_{NaCaX}$ also contributes net inward flow of positive charge. These two depolarizing influences are opposed by the repolarizing influence of an outward flow of $K^+$ currents carried by several types of channels. While the plateau is maintained, the cell cannot be re-excited. Because of this prolonged period of refractoriness, cardiac muscle cannot be tetanized. This is a major difference from skeletal muscle.

- *Phase 3,* late rapid repolarization: The plateau terminates because the L-type channels are inactivated by processes dependent on time, voltage, and $[Ca^{2+}]_i$. Repolarization then occurs rapidly because the influence of outward $K^+$ currents dominates. As the membrane potential approaches its resting value and the electrochemical gradient for $K^+$ decreases, the $K^+$ current diminishes and the cell enters phase 4.

- *Phase 4:* The inward flow of positive ions ($I_{Na}$ [leak] and $I_{NaCaX}$) is balanced by outward flows $I_{3Na/2K}$ and $I_{K1}$. As the $Na^+$ and other channels that were inactivated by membrane depolarization return to the activatable state, membrane excitability is restored in preparation for the next action potential. The end result of the cycle is a net gain of $Na^+$ and a net loss of $K^+$ during the entire action potential. This imbalance is corrected by the sarcolemmal $Na^+/K^+$-ATPase, which uses the energy from the hydrolysis of ATP to transport $Na^+$ back out of the cell and $K^+$ back in.

## Functional Significance of Cardiac Electrophysiological Phenomena

At the coarsest level, it must be appreciated that there can be no heartbeat and no circulation of blood without cardiac action potentials. At more subtle levels, the frequency and regularity of cardiac contraction are primarily determined by ion currents in pacemaker cells, and the long-term and short-term availability of $Ca^{2+}$ and, therefore, the strength of cardiac contraction, are determined by ion transport phenomena in cardiac muscle cells.

### Current modulation in pacemaker cells

Physiological modulation of pacemaker activity is achieved by extremely subtle changes in transmembrane ion currents. Catecholamines released from the adrenal medulla or from adrenergic nerve terminals increase the frequency of pacemaker action potentials and thus cause an increase in heart rate (**positive chronotropic effect**). The catecholamines increase the levels of cAMP, activat-

**FIGURE 31-2** Cardiac action potentials and the major ion currents influencing them.

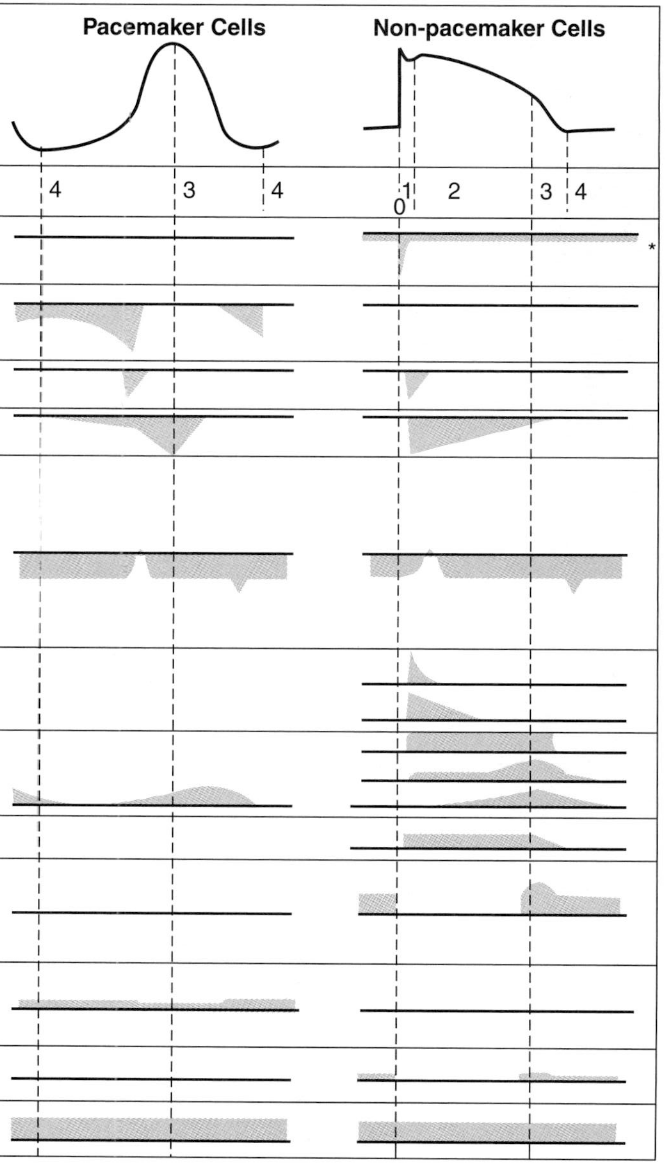

| Current | Action Potential Phase | Pacemaker Cells | Non-pacemaker Cells |
|---|---|---|---|
| | **Membrane Potential vs. Time** | | |
| $I_{Na}$ | Carried by rapidly activating and inactivating, voltage-gated $Na^+$ channels; contains a small non-inactivating component (the slow $Na^+$ current). | | |
| $I_f$ | A non-selective cation current, composed mostly of $Na^+$. The channel carrying $I_f$ opens upon hyperpolarization and this "funny" behaviour has given it the designation "f". $I_f$ is directly modulated by cAMP. | | |
| $I_{Ca-T}$ | A $Ca^{2+}$ current that is carried by voltage-gated T-type $Ca^{2+}$ channels (blocked by nickel). | | |
| $I_{Ca-L}$ | This $Ca^{2+}$ current is carried by voltage-gated L-type $Ca^{2+}$ channels (blocked by dihydropyridine). | | |
| $I_{NaCaX}$ | Carried by the $3Na^+/Ca^{2+}$ exchanger, which is driven by the $Na^+$ electrochemical gradient. Its reversal potential, $E_{NaCaX}$, is calculated from the equilibrium potentials of $Na^+$ and $Ca^{2+}$ as $3E_{Na}-2E_{Ca}$. Fluctuations in intracellular $Ca^{2+}$ concentrations during each cardiac cycle cause the reversal potential to fluctuate between $-15$ mV in diastole when $[Ca^{2+}]_i$ is 50 to 100 nM and $+65$ mV in systole when $[Ca^{2+}]_i$ increases to about 1,200 nM during the action potential. At either extreme $E_{NaCaX}$ is more positive than the prevailing membrane potential and, therefore, operates to transfer positive charge into the cell ($Ca^{2+}$-out mode) throughout the cardiac cycle. Reversal to a $Na^+$-out/$Ca^{2+}$-in state depends critically on the systolic level of $[Ca^{2+}]_i$. It can occur under some normal circumstances and may be of importance in disease states. | | |
| $I_{to1}$ $I_{to2}$ | Two components have been identified in this "transient outward" current: $I_{to1}$ is a rapidly inactivating voltage-gated $K^+$ channel that is blocked by 4-aminopyridine (4-AP); $I_{to2}$ is activated by $Ca^{2+}$ and is inactivated more slowly than $I_{to1}$. It is not yet certain whether $I_{to2}$ is carried by $K^+$ or by $Cl^-$. | | |
| $I_{Kq}$ $I_{Kr}$ $I_{Ks}$ | $I_{Kq}$, $I_{Kr}$ and $I_{Ks}$ form, respectively, the ultrarapid, rapid, and slow components of the delayed rectifier $K^+$ current; $I_{Kq}$ is blocked by quinidine; $I_{Kr}$ is blocked by $La^{3+}$ and the methane-sulfonilide antiarrhythmic drugs; mutations in $I_{Ks}$ are responsible for the long QT syndrome. Pacemaker cells lack $I_{Kq}$ and $I_{Kr}$. They have $I_{Ks}$ only. | | |
| $I_{Kp}$ | This is usually a small $K^+$ current. Its importance is that is highly sensitive to $[H^+]$ changes and might, therefore, provide an important coupling to metabolic states. | | |
| $I_{K1}$ | Although $I_{K1}$ is only one of several inward rectifier $K^+$ currents, it is the most important. Like all inwardly rectifying channels it is highly conductive in the inward direction when the membrane potential is more negative than the $K^+$ equilibrium potential. It is poorly conductive in the outward direction when the membrane potential is more positive than the $K^+$ equilibrium potential. The channel is not voltage-gated. | | |
| $I_{K(Ach)}$ | This $K^+$ current that is carried through an inwardly rectifying channel in pacemaking tissue and atrial myocytes. The channel is directly coupled to a G protein and this makes it susceptible to neuro-humoral regulation. It is responsible for at least half of the negative chronotropic effect of vagal stimulation. | | |
| $I_{K(ATP)}$ | K(ATP) channels are an important link between membrane potential and cellular metabolic status. They are inhibited by physiological levels of ATP and open when cytosolic [ATP] decreases. | | |
| $I_{3Na/2K}$ | This designates the outward current arising from the ubiquitous $3Na^+$ - $2K^+$ membrane $Na^+/K^+$ pump. | | |

*Downward deflection indicates positive ions flowing INTO the cell; upward deflection indicates positive ions flowing OUT OF the cell; distances from the zero line (→) are not drawn to scale.

ing protein kinase A and leading to changes in several transmembrane currents:

- Increase in $I_{Ca,L}$ leads to an accelerated upstroke in the pacemaker potential.
- Increase in $I_{Ks}$ shortens the action potential and begins the diastolic rise of the membrane potential earlier.
- Steeper rise of the diastolic potential towards threshold occurs.

Parasympathetic stimulation of **muscarinic receptors** causes a reduced level of cAMP and increases the activity of cytosolic phospholipase C, which activates the acetylcholine-sensitive $K^+$ channel ($I_{K(Ach)}$; see Fig. 31-2) and increases its outward $K^+$ current. The resultant hyperpolarization and slower rise of diastolic potential both contribute to a decrease in pacemaker frequency.

### Current modulation in non-pacemaker cells

The amplitude and duration of the plateau potential (phase 2; see Fig. 31-2) determine both how much $Ca^{2+}$ enters the cell by way of $I_{Ca,L}$ and how much $Ca^{2+}$ leaves the cell by way of $I_{NaCaX}$, the $3Na^+/Ca^{2+}$ exchanger. Therefore, $I_{Na}$, $I_{to1}$, $I_{to2}$, $I_{Ca,L}$, $I_{NaCaX}$, $I_{Kq}$, $I_{Kr}$, and $I_{Ks}$ can each have profound influences on short-term $Ca^{2+}$ dynamics.

The amplitude of both the resting membrane potential (phase 4; see Fig. 31-2) and the reversal potential for $I_{NaCaX}$ determine how much $Ca^{2+}$ is lost from the cell, mainly in each diastolic interval. As a result, the factors influencing resting membrane potential or $Na^+Ca^{2+}X$ reversal potential can each influence the $Ca^{2+}$ economy of cardiac muscle cells and, with that, the strength of cardiac muscle contraction.

## CALCIUM HANDLING IN CARDIAC MUSCLE

### Sources of Calcium

Most of the calcium that enters the myocyte at the start of an action potential is carried by $I_{Ca,L}$. It contributes no more than 10% of the total $Ca^{2+}$ needed for a maximal contraction, but it provides the trigger for releasing calcium from intracellular stores (sarcoplasmic reticulum) during systole and also acts as a source for topping up the intracellular stores during diastole.

Although the **sodium–calcium exchanger** in human myocytes normally operates in the $Ca^{2+}$-out mode throughout the cardiac cycle, small changes in membrane potentials or electrochemical gradients of $Na^+$, $K^+$, or $Ca^{2+}$ can reduce the rate of $Ca^{2+}$ loss or even flip the exchanger to the $Ca^{2+}$-in mode for part of the cycle. This is one of the beneficial effects of cardiac glycosides.

The **sarcoplasmic reticulum (SR)** functions as the major intracellular source and storage site for ionized cal-

cium. A small influx of $Ca^{2+}$ from the extracellular space through L-type (dihydropyridine) $Ca^{2+}$ channels operates to release $Ca^{2+}$ from the SR through ryanodine channels. In a single contraction, the SR is the major source of $Ca^{2+}$. However, it is the $Ca^{2+}$ transport mechanisms across the sarcolemma and SR membrane that create the intracellular stores and make repeated contraction–relaxation cycles possible.

### Uptake of Calcium

When the action potential has passed and the myocyte has repolarized, calcium is removed from the cytosol. Both the $Na^+/Ca^{2+}$ exchanger and $Ca^{2+}$-ATPases are significant contributors to $Ca^{2+}$ removal from the cytosol.

Two molecularly different **$Ca^{2+}$-ATPases**, present in the sarcolemma and the membrane of the SR, each transfer two $Ca^{2+}$ per molecule of ATP. The SR $Ca^{2+}$-ATPase is intimately associated with the polypeptide **phospholamban**. Phospholamban phosphorylation and dephosphorylation modulates SR $Ca^{2+}$-ATPase: dephosphorylation inhibits $Ca^{2+}$ uptake by the SR, whereas phospholamban phosphorylation promotes $Ca^{2+}$ transport into the SR. Phosphorylation of phospholamban is promoted by several kinases, each of which is activated by different agents, including cAMP, cGMP, and $Ca^{2+}$/calmodulin.

## CARDIAC MUSCLE FUNCTION

### Cardiac Metabolism, Oxygen Consumption, and Work

Although cardiac myocytes are capable of utilizing a variety of metabolic substrates, under normal conditions, fatty acids supply two-thirds of myocardial ATP in the adult human heart. They are, therefore, the key source of energy required for the performance of cardiac work. Fatty acids are actively taken up by the myocardial cell and are converted to fatty acyl-CoA, which is transported into the mitochondria, is converted to acetyl-CoA, and subsequently—in the Krebs (tricarboxylic acid) cycle and the electron transport chain—is metabolized to yield mostly $CO_2$, water, and ATP.

Sustained increase in cardiac work requires an increase in the rate of oxygen-dependent ATP production and utilization. Therefore, anything that impairs coronary blood flow, or reduces pulmonary blood flow or oxygenation, will quickly decrease myocardial performance.

### The Contraction Process

In each cardiac cycle, the processes of **excitation–activation–contraction coupling** link electrical events of the myocyte action potential to the mechanical events of tension development and subsequent diastolic relaxation.

Ionized calcium plays a crucial role because interaction of free intracellular $Ca^{2+}$ with protein constituents of cardiac muscle cells removes steric hindrance and initiates the processes that lead to the development of tension in the power stroke. The crucial protein constituents are myosin, actin, tropomyosin, and troponin. Their organized arrangement in a cardiac muscle cell is shown in Figure 31-3.

## Protein constituents

**Myosin** forms the thick filament. It is a long molecule that consists of two intertwined, immunologically distinct heavy chains, two myosin essential light chains, and two myosin regulatory light chains. Each heavy chain includes a globular "head" ($S_1$) that is attached to the long tail of the molecule by a myosin fragment called $S_2$. Inherent properties of the long-tail portion encourage myosin polymerization in parallel and antiparallel manner around the M-line of the sarcomere. As shown in detail in Figure 31-3, the $S_1$ region includes the actin binding site, the binding and catalytic sites for ATP, the hinge region for cross-bridge rotation, and attachment points for the two light chains. The chemical functions of $S_1$ are (1) to bind to actin and (2) to promote ATP binding and hydrolysis; its mechanical function is internal and involves rotation of its two domains about the hinge region. A single thick filament consists of about 400 myosin molecules, arranged in parallel and distributed symmetrically with half of the molecules on each side of the M-line. The head groups of the myosin are at the end of the molecule that is furthest from the M-line (see Fig. 31-3).

Thin filament **actin** is F-actin. It is formed by two intertwined strands of G-actin, the intertwining being formed by coupling subdomains of the G-actin molecules (see Fig. 31-3, detail). Purified actin functions chemically to bind myosin and release the products of ATP hydrolysis from the $S_1$ region. By way of this product release, actin functions as a promoter of myosin ATP-ase activity.

Controlled muscle function can occur only if the spontaneous coupling of actin to myosin, as well as the associated ATP hydrolysis, can be intermittently inhibited. The regulatory proteins tropomyosin and troponin perform this intermittent inhibitory function.

**Tropomyosin** consists of two chains and its molecules are joined end to end, forming a strand that lies near the groove of the intertwined actin strands (Fig. 31-4). Each molecule interacts with seven actin molecules and is associated with one troponin complex.

**Troponin** exists in muscle as a complex of three dissimilar subunits (see Fig. 31-4), designated troponin-C (Tn-C), troponin-T (Tn-T), and troponin-I (Tn-I). Tn-C is shaped like a dumbbell. It is attached to Tn-I and contains a regulatory $Ca^{2+}$ binding site at its N-terminal. Tn-I exists in one of two binding states: it is tightly bound either to actin (when the sarcomere is relaxed) or to the $Ca^{2+}$-activated Tn-C molecule (when the sarcomere is contracted). The Tn-I domain that binds to actin inhibits myosin ATPase, and this pre-vents formation of strong, cycling cross-bridges in the relaxed state. In addition, tight binding of the Tn-C/Tn-I complex to Tn-T keeps the entire troponin complex in place relative to tropomyosin (see Fig. 31-4).

*Removal of steric hindrance (transition from blocked to cocked actomyosin state.)* When $[Ca^{2+}]_i$ increases after membrane depolarization, $Ca^{2+}$ binds to Tn-C and changes the conformation of the troponin–tropomyosin complex in a way that moves tropomyosin closer to the actin groove (see Fig. 31-3, detail, and Fig. 31-4) and permits formation of a force-generating actomyosin cross-bridge.

## Tension development: the power stroke

Once a strong cross-bridge has been formed between myosin and actin, the myosin head moves rapidly from the cocked to the on state. This is characterized by strong actomyosin binding, high myosin ATPase activity, and high force generation. In this state, there is cyclic myosin–actin interaction during which the $S_1$–$S_2$ portion of the myosin molecule (see Fig. 31-3) tilts relative to the tail of the molecule. This is called the swinging lever model of muscle function, and its sequence is shown in Figure 31-5. It depends on a slight rotation around the hinge region of the myosin head and results in incremental sliding of the thin filament relative to the thick filament. The parallel and antiparallel arrangement of myosin molecules around the M-line (see Fig. 31-3) translates such sliding into shortening of the distance between neighbouring Z-lines. Each rotation causes a displacement of only 5 to 10 nm. A sarcomere shortens by 100 to 300 nm during contraction. To achieve this degree of shortening, repeated release and reattachment of cross-bridges is necessary. This requires both continued availability of $Ca^{2+}$ to give freedom from steric hindrance and a supply of ATP to take each cross-bridge out of the rigor state (see Fig. 31-5B). Lack of ATP arrests the heart in a contracted state ("stone heart").

## Cardiac Performance

All tissues receive their blood flow from a common source, the cardiac output (CO), which is the amount of blood pumped from each side of the heart each minute. CO is determined by the heart rate (HR) and the volume ejected from each ventricle with each contraction (the stroke volume, SV):

$$CO = HR \times SV$$

HR is set by the activity of the pacemaker cells. SV is determined by the effectiveness of ventricular emptying in systole. That effectiveness is termed cardiac performance and is determined by four factors:

- The degree of sarcomere stretch prior to actomyosin cross-linkage (preload)
- The efficacy of actomyosin interaction (contractility)

- The ventricular wall tension required to achieve ejection (afterload)
- The interval between contraction–relaxation cycles (heart rate)

These factors apply equally to the left and right ventricles, but in the following descriptions, the focus is placed on the left ventricle because it is the ultimate source of blood flow to the periphery.

### Preload

Cardiac performance is normally proportional to the degree of diastolic stretch in the ventricles, as described by the Frank–Starling law of the heart. At rest, the Starling

---

**FIGURE 31-3** Contractile and regulatory proteins in cardiac muscle. Cardiac muscle consists of two contractile proteins, myosin and actin, as well as the regulatory proteins, tropomyosin and troponin. Myosin and actin are arranged in an interdigitating pattern of thick and thin filaments and are stabilized by the very large protein, titin. Local magnifications show details of the thick and thin filaments as well as an actomyosin cross-bridge in end-on view.

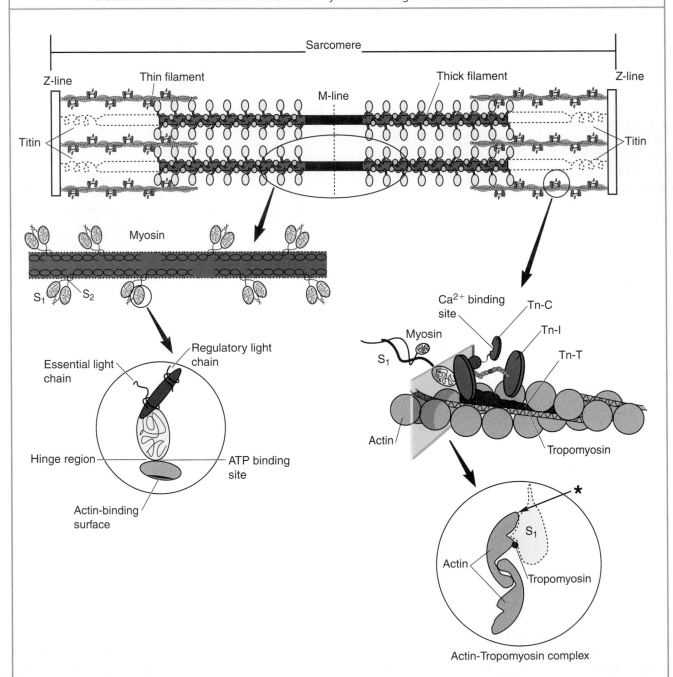

**FIGURE 31-4** Actomyosin cross-bridge formation. When Tn-C interacts with $Ca^{2+}$, strong, force-generating actomyosin cross-bridges are formed after tropomyosin has moved from a blocking position (shown in A) towards the groove formed by the intertwined actin strands. (A) Troponin-C (Tn-C) is attached by its C-terminal to the N-terminal of troponin-I (Tn-I). Tn-I attaches to Tn-C, troponin-T (Tn-T), and to actin by an ATPase-inhibitory domain (shown in darker colour) residing in the central spiral of Tn-I. Tn-T is attached to Tn-I as well as the adjoining and neighbouring tropomyosin molecules. The dotted line indicates the position of tropomyosin when it has been moved away from the blocking position. (B) $Ca^{2+}$ binding to Tn-C initiates changes of conformation and state. Four key changes are involved: (1) high affinity binding between Tn-C and Tn-I; (2) release of the attachment between actin and Tn-I, which then permits (3) physical movement of Tn-I and an associated movement of Tn-T, and (4) physical movement of tropomyosin towards the actin–actin groove so that strongly attached, force-generating actomyosin cross-bridges can form.

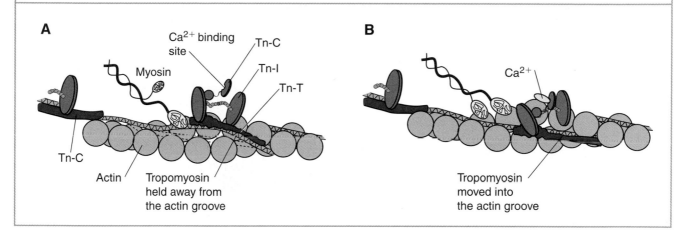

mechanism helps to adapt cardiac performance to postural changes and to match left heart output to right heart output during respiratory changes in venous return. During exercise, responses to changes in preload contribute to the increase in cardiac output, although reflex mechanisms that operate via catecholamines can, during exercise, overshadow the effect of sarcomere stretch in altering cardiac performance. With advancing age, as the effectiveness of catecholaminergic modulation of cardiac performance diminishes in humans, the preload mechanism becomes increasingly important in matching cardiac output to the oxygen demands of the body.

***Cellular basis of the preload mechanism.*** The force developed during muscle contraction is directly related to four general factors: (1) change in the number of actomyosin cross-bridges; (2) modulation of the transient increase in $[Ca^{2+}]_i$ that occurs after excitation; (3) modulation of $Ca^{2+}$–troponin interactions at a given $[Ca^{2+}]_i$; and (4) modulation of the degree of synchronization among individual contractile units.

It was formerly thought that the most important mechanism of the Starling effect was the increase in the number of cross-linkages between actin and myosin that is made possible by stretching the sarcomere. However, this seems unlikely, and more importance is now attributed to (1) increased $Ca^{2+}$ release from the sarcoplasmic reticulum because of stretch-activated ion channels; (2) increased calcium sensitivity of Tn-C, resulting in a greater force generated at a given $[Ca^{2+}]_i$; and (3) a stretch-

associated decrease in lateral distance between neighbouring thin and thick filaments, which allows a higher rate of cross-bridge cycling.

***Functional determinants of preload.*** The degree of ventricular filling in diastole is a function of filling pressure, ventricular compliance, and time available for filling.

- **Filling pressure** is the difference between atrial pressure and ventricular pressure. Left ventricular filling pressure depends greatly on pulmonary vascular pressure. This, in turn, is influenced by right ventricular output as well as intrathoracic pressure.
- **Ventricular compliance** is a measure of the ease with which the ventricle expands while it accepts diastolic inflow. It can be altered by factors that alter the properties of cardiac muscle itself or by factors that alter conditions in the pericardial space. Both occur on a time scale that affects only long-term regulation.
- **Time available for ventricular filling** is inversely related to heart rate. At heart rates in excess of 180 beats/min, the time available for rapid diastolic flow from the atria into the ventricles is significantly reduced.

### Contractility

An increase in contractility, most easily brought about by $\beta_1$-**adrenergic receptor stimulation,** is associated with increased velocity of wall shortening, reduced time to

| FIGURE 31-5 | The sliding-filament, swinging lever hypothesis. At rest, only momentary weak binding of myosin to actin can occur, and ATPase activity is low. However, when $Ca^{2+}$ binds to Tn-C, protein-to-protein interactions are triggered, removing steric hindrance and leading to a cycling, force-generating physical coupling between actin and myosin. (A) Steric hindrance has been removed, a strong actomyosin cross-bridge has formed, and the nearness of actin allows ADP and $P_i$, which were both formed in a preceding cycle, to escape from the $S_1$ head. (B) Escape of $P_i$ allows previously stored energy to move the lower portion of the myosin head around the hinge region of $S_1$. This moves actin to the right by about 10 nm. This conformation is called the rigor complex. Escape from it requires a supply of ATP. (C) Previous release of ADP and $P_i$ allows new ATP to be bound if it is available. Binding of fresh ATP leads to myosin detachment because the triad of actin, myosin, and ATP is unstable. (D) ATP is hydrolyzed by the inherent myosin ATPase activity. The energy that is liberated during ATP hydrolysis rotates the $S_1$ lever about the hinge and returns it to the starting position. The lever is held there as long as $P_i$ stays close to the myosin head. Absence of locally bound ATP allows a new cross-bridge to be formed and the cycle to be repeated provided that sufficient $Ca^{2+}$ is present to remove steric hindrance. |
| --- | --- |

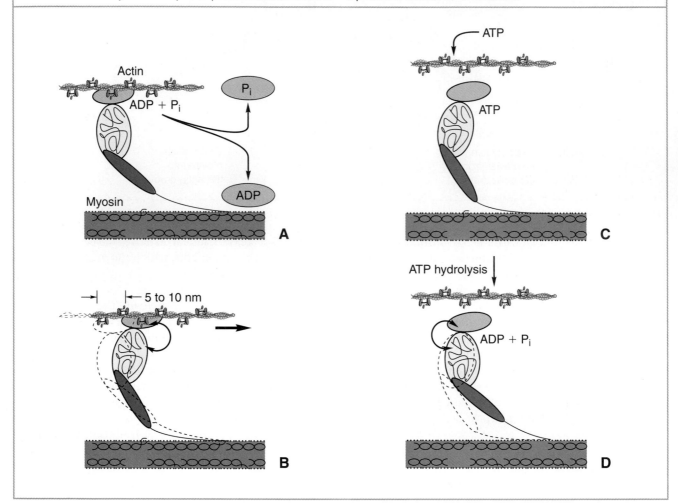

peak tension, more rapid relaxation, shorter duration of systole, greater extent of fibre shortening, greater stroke volume, higher ejection fraction, and decreased end-systolic volume. If the ventricle is made to contract isovolumetrically (without a change in volume) rather than isotonically (at constant tension), there is, in addition to many of the above changes, an increase in peak tension.

Since all myocytes participate in a normal cardiac contraction, the measurable whole-organ changes that accompany changes in contractility cannot be due to changes in the number of active myocytes but must arise from properties associated with $Ca^{2+}$ dynamics, the effectiveness of actin–myosin interactions, and the nature of the contractile proteins themselves. Stimulation of $\beta_1$-adrenergic receptors leads to increased $[Ca^{2+}]_i$ by both direct and indirect mechanisms, as described earlier. In addition, the increase in cAMP resulting from $\beta_1$-adrenergic receptor stimulation promotes the phosphorylation of troponin and hence the tension development, but it also leads to more rapid release of $Ca^{2+}$ from the phosphorylated troponin, so that diastolic relaxation and ventricular filling are facilitated.

## Afterload

The term "afterload" was coined in isolated muscle experiments, where it refers to the load the muscle is required to lift during contraction. In the cardiovascular system, afterload is the load against which the left ventricle ejects its stroke volume, designated the aortic input impedance. This load determines left ventricular wall tension during ejection, which is the major determinant of myocardial oxygen consumption. Wall tension is related to distending pressure, chamber radius, and wall thickness by Laplace's law, and it can be approximately calculated for the ventricle as the product of transmural pressure and chamber radius divided by two times the wall thickness.

An increase in afterload decreases cardiac performance. However, a healthy heart can respond to increased afterload with an increase in contractility. This is called the **Anrep effect**. It is caused by a secondary increase in coronary blood flow that is brought on by an initial buildup of vasodilator metabolites when increased wall stress compresses coronary blood vessels.

## Rate

Over most of the physiological range of heart rates, peak tension increases as the rate increases (the Bowditch effect). This observation is explained by the inability of active pumping to maintain intracellular concentrations of $Na^+$ and $K^+$ at the high frequencies of action potentials. The consequent changes in resting membrane potential and reversal potential of the $3Na^+/Ca^{2+}$ exchanger lead to gradually increasing $[Ca^{2+}]_i$ and result in stronger contraction.

# BLOOD VESSEL FUNCTION

## Vascular Smooth Muscle

### Structure of vascular smooth muscle

Vascular smooth muscle is found in varying proportions in all blood vessels except capillaries. Its cells are spindle-shaped or branched and make extensive electrical and metabolic contact with adjacent cells by means of gap junctions (see Chapter 2). In addition to the gap junction region, the plasma membrane shows histologically (and, presumably, functionally) different portions. One portion has surface invaginations (caveolae), another has closely apposed SR, and a third has attachments for the intermediate filaments that are part of the cytoskeletal structure.

**Caveolae** greatly increase the surface area of smooth muscle cells, but they appear to have no other function. The plasma **membrane apposed to SR** is probably a major site of signal transduction by way of voltage-gated or receptor-mediated mechanisms. Within this region are electron-dense structures that appear to couple the plasma membrane to the SR. Smooth muscle SR, like cardiac muscle SR, is the major intracellular depot for $Ca^{2+}$, and it plays a corresponding role with respect to $Ca^{2+}$ movements in relation to contraction and relaxation.

The contractile machinery of smooth muscle is not organized in spatially repetitive patterns as it is in striated muscle. However, the two muscle types resemble each other in most of the important features, including the thick and thin filaments, their involvement in a sliding-filament mechanism, the presence of both voltage-gated and ligand-gated ion channels, and the role of ion movements in the contraction–relaxation cycle.

### Function of vascular smooth muscle

The trigger for activating smooth muscle contraction is a rise in cytosolic $[Ca^{2+}]$, as is the case in myocytes. However, smooth muscle activation does not necessarily require an action potential because $[Ca^{2+}]_i$ can be increased by either electrical (action potential) or chemical means.

*Electrical triggering.* Electrical triggering of the activation–contraction processes in smooth muscle is by way of membrane depolarization that allows a sufficient increase in cytosolic $[Ca^{2+}]$, but may or may not be sufficient to generate action potentials. When an action potential does occur, most vascular smooth muscle cells differ from myocytes in that the action potential upstroke is caused primarily by $Ca^{2+}$ influx rather than $Na^+$ influx. This action potential–supplied $Ca^{2+}$ is used chiefly to mediate further $Ca^{2+}$ release from intracellular depots. Three electrically distinct types of vascular smooth muscle have been identified: (1) smooth muscle that generates action potentials spontaneously, (2) smooth muscle that generates action potentials in response to an appropriate stimulus, and (3) smooth muscle that responds to excitatory stimuli with a sustained, non-regenerating electrical response that resembles a skeletal muscle end-plate potential. Types 1 and 2 exhibit phasic contractions, whereas type 3 shows more sustained contractions.

*Chemical triggering.* Physiological ligands or drugs can induce contractions of vascular smooth muscle. The two major components of chemical triggering are stimulation of intracellular $Ca^{2+}$ release (predominantly by inositol trisphosphate [$IP_3$]) and modulation of the $Ca^{2+}$ sensitivity of the actin–myosin interaction. Of these two, the $IP_3$ mechanism is by far the more important.

In addition to differences between myocardium and smooth muscle with respect to calcium dynamics, they also show several differences in the details of the contractile processes and their modulation.

*Differences in excitation–activation–contraction coupling.* The processes of cross-link formation, ATP hydrolysis, sliding filaments, and cross-bridge detachment are thought to be identical in smooth and striated muscle. However, in smooth muscle, there is a cascade of many more biochemical steps intervening between $Ca^{2+}$ entry and eventual force generation. In smooth muscle, these steps can be regulated to allow various degrees of tension to be developed for varying durations.

The first step involves a small (15 000 Da) calcium-binding protein, **calmodulin.** Smooth muscle does not use troponin for $Ca^{2+}$ binding. Instead, when $[Ca^{2+}]_i$ reaches approximately $10^{-6}$ M, $Ca^{2+}$ binds to calmodulin and the $Ca^{2+}$/calmodulin complex activates the enzyme myosin light-chain kinase. This, in turn, promotes phosphorylation of the myosin regulatory light chain, which is a necessary and sufficient antecedent to increased myosin ATPase activity and actomyosin force generation.

*Differences in relaxation mechanisms.* Smooth muscle resembles myocardium in that relaxation occurs when $Ca^{2+}$ is removed from the cytosol. However, greater control over the relaxation process is possible in smooth muscle because myosin phosphatases can be used in a controlled manner to dephosphorylate the myosin regulatory light chains.

*Differences in force duration.* Prolonged maintenance of contractile force with low energy consumption is a characteristic feature of smooth muscle. This is known as the **latch state.** It is dependent on the ability of smooth muscle to reduce phosphorylation of myosin regulatory light chain without necessarily disconnecting the associated myosin head from actin.

# Vascular Endothelium

The endothelial lining of blood vessels forms autocrine and paracrine substances that serve two main functions: they prevent intravascular thrombus formation, and they modulate the tone of the underlying smooth muscle. Both relaxing and constricting factors are synthesized by the endothelium and participate in the local regulation of tissue blood flow. They can also influence the effectiveness of neurotransmitters released by autonomic nerve endings on the vascular smooth muscle and thus modulate the effect of the central nervous system on vascular tone.

## Endothelium-dependent relaxation

Four important dilating factors are derived from the endothelium (Fig. 31-6). They are nitric oxide (NO), C-type natriuretic peptide (CNP), endothelium-derived hyperpolarizing factor (EDHF), and prostacyclin (PGI₂). Of these four, NO makes by far the greatest contribution. Its role appears to be the continuous regulation of resistance vessels and, hence, of arterial blood pressure.

*Nitric oxide (NO).* NO is synthesized in vascular endothelial cells from the amino acid L-arginine by endothelial nitric oxide synthase (eNOS; see Fig. 31-6).

*C-type natriuretic peptide (CNP).* This peptide resembles other natriuretic peptides like atrial or brain natriuretic peptide, but it has no natriuretic action. The endothelium is one of its production sites. It has two mechanisms of vasodilator action. One operates through a guanylyl cyclase type of membrane receptor (see Chapter 8) and the other through activation of a K⁺-specific ion channel.

*Endothelium-derived hyperpolarizing factor (EDHF).* Two substances are currently under consideration as the hyperpolarizing vasodilator agents that are produced by acetylcholine action on the muscarinic M₁ receptor. One is an intermediate in the cyclooxygenase pathway of arachidonic acid metabolism, and the other is an acetylcholine-sensitive membrane K⁺ channel.

*Prostacyclin (PGI₂).* PGI₂ is a major intermediary product in the metabolism of arachidonic acid by cyclooxygenase in vascular smooth muscle (see Chapter 27). It is rapidly converted to prostaglandin F₁α, which has no biological activity. PGI₂, however, causes vasodilatation. This action results from elevation of cytosolic cAMP in smooth muscle cells.

## Endothelium-dependent constriction

The vascular endothelium also produces smooth muscle constricting factors. Such production varies greatly among species and also among different vascular beds within a given species. The major contracting factors are the endothelins, locally produced angiotensin II, prostaglandin H₂, thromboxane A2, and an as-yet-unidentified contracting factor, endothelium-derived contracting factor (EDCF), that is produced and released in response to hypoxia. Figure 31-7 summarizes the control of endothelial constrictor release.

*Endothelin.* Endothelin is a 21-amino-acid peptide cleaved from a 203-amino-acid precursor called preproendothelin. Four forms of endothelin have been identified, of which only one, endothelin-1, is produced by endothelial cells. When this agent interacts with the ET_A receptor in vascular smooth muscle, it activates phospholipase C and leads to elevated $[Ca^{2+}]_i$ via the IP₃ pathway, causing powerful, long-lasting vasoconstriction. Endothelin-1 also potentiates the vasoconstrictor effects of hormones and neurotransmitters such as serotonin or noradrenaline.

*Angiotensin II.* Angiotensin II is produced locally because endothelial cells contain angiotensin-converting enzyme and many contain local stores of renin. As a result, both extracellular and locally produced angiotensin I are converted to angiotensin II, a powerful vasoconstrictor agent.

*Thromboxane A2.* Thromboxane A2 (TXA2) and prostaglandin H₂ (PGH₂) are produced in small amounts when arachidonic acid is metabolized in the cyclooxygenase pathway (see Chapter 27). Both mechanical and chemical stimuli promote their formation. Both bind to the throm-

**FIGURE 31-6**  Relaxing factors derived from vascular endothelium. Four notable dilator agents are synthesized by the endothelial cells that line blood vessels. *Nitric oxide (NO)* is the most significant. Its synthesis is promoted by elevated cytosolic calcium concentration. Agonists promoting its release are shear stress and a variety of receptor-mediated activators of phospholipase C. NO interacts with soluble guanylyl cyclase and causes smooth muscle relaxation by way of an increase in cGMP. *C-type natriuretic peptide (CNP)* is synthesized constitutively and can be further increased by agents that elevate phospholipase C. It, too, relaxes muscle in part by way of cGMP. However, membrane (receptor) associated guanylyl cyclase, not soluble guanylyl cyclase, is involved. In addition, CNP hyperpolarizes the membrane by way of $Ca^{2+}$-activated $K^+$ channels. *Endothelium-derived hyperpolarizing factor (EDHF)* is a short-lived product of muscarinic $M_1$ receptor activation. Both epoxyeicosatrienoic acid (EET) and the acetylcholine-sensitive $K^+$ current ($I_{K(Ach)}$) are candidates for the identity of EDHF. It desensitizes smooth muscle by hyperpolarizing its membrane potential ($E_m$). *Prostacyclin (PGI_2)* is an intermediate product of short half-life in the cyclooxygenase metabolic pathway of arachidonic acid. It operates via cAMP to relax vascular smooth muscle. cAMP = cyclic adenosine monophosphate; cGMP = cyclic guanosine monophosphate; COX = cyclooxygenase; eNOS = endothelial nitric oxide synthase; $EP_2$ = prostaglandin $E_2$ receptor; $R_{GC(B)}$ = B-type guanylyl cyclase–linked receptor.

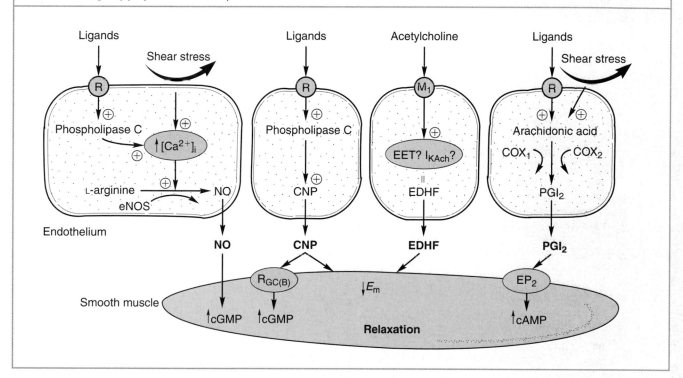

boxane receptor, activate phospholipase C, and promote vasoconstriction because of $IP_3$-mediated elevation of $[Ca^{2+}]_i$ (see Fig. 31-7).

***Endothelium-derived contracting factor (EDCF).*** EDCF is an unidentified constrictor agent that is released from endothelial cells in response to hypoxia. Its release requires activation of voltage-gated $Ca^{2+}$ channels.

## Functional Integration of Endothelium-Derived Factors

A suggested model of functional integration of control of blood flow in microvascular units, by the endothelial factors described above, is as follows:

- The smallest arterioles are controlled mainly by metabolic factors like $CO_2$, $K^+$, adenosine, and oth-

ers; the importance of metabolic control diminishes in larger upstream vessels.
- Mid-sized arterioles are influenced most strongly by pressure-dependent myogenic responses. They may operate through stretch-sensitive ion channels.
- Large arterioles are most responsive to blood flow, which exerts its endothelial effects by way of shear stress.

Receptor-mediated release of endothelial factors has not yet been incorporated into an integrated scheme.

## Cardiovascular Regulation

Regulation of **vascular** function in individual tissues results from a complex interplay among locally produced vasoactive factors and remote influences exerted by nerves and blood-borne agents (hormones and autacoids). The effect of such influences is to alter the hydraulic resistance of the tissue vasculature by altering the effective diameter of the vascular bed. The objective of such local regulation is to ensure an adequate supply of blood to support metabolic activities of that individual tissue.

Regulation of **cardiovascular** function, on the other hand, is a whole-body phenomenon. Its purpose varies with conditions.

- When conditions are normal, the processes of cardiovascular regulation ensure that all tissues receive a flow of blood that is adequate for their metabolic needs under a variety of demands that range from sleep to intense exercise.
- When conditions are critical, cardiovascular regulation ensures survival of the organism by diverting all available flow to the two crucial vascular beds, brain and heart.

The two major aspects of cardiovascular regulation are the regulation of cardiac output (CO) and the maintenance of normal mean perfusion pressure (ABP). Pressure regulation can be accomplished independently of cardiac output regulation by the modulation of total peripheral resistance (TPR). The following equation summarizes the essential features:

$$[HR \times SV = CO] \times TPR = ABP$$

Short-term regulation is based on regulation of arterial blood pressure and is accomplished, in part, through intrinsic mechanisms such as the cardiac responses to varying preload or afterload, and, in part, through the

---

**FIGURE 31-7** Contracting factors derived from vascular endothelium. *Endothelin-1* is generated from the precursor preproendothelin. It is a powerful vasoconstrictor that is preferentially released toward the luminal side of endothelial cells. It is a regulator of local function as opposed to one of general systemic cardiovascular function. *Angiotensin II (AII)* is produced in endothelial cells because they are the locus for angiotensin-converting enzyme (ACE). *Prostaglandin H₂ and thromboxane A2 (TXA2)* both bind to the TXA2 receptor ($R_{TXA2}$). They are produced when cyclooxygenase is activated by mechanical or various chemical stimuli. Preference for production of one or the other is determined by local concentrations of promoters and inhibitors. $PGH_2$ has an extremely short half-life. *Endothelium-derived contracting factor (EDCF)* is responsible for hypoxic vasoconstriction. Its chemical nature has not yet been identified. AI = angiotensin I; AII = angiotensin II; ACE = angiotensin-converting enzyme; $AT_1$ = type 1 angiotensin II receptor; COX = cyclooxygenase; $ET_A$ = A-type endothelin receptor; $PGI_2$ = prostaglandin I₂ (prostacyclin); $PGH_2$ = prostaglandin H₂; TXA2 = thromboxane A2.

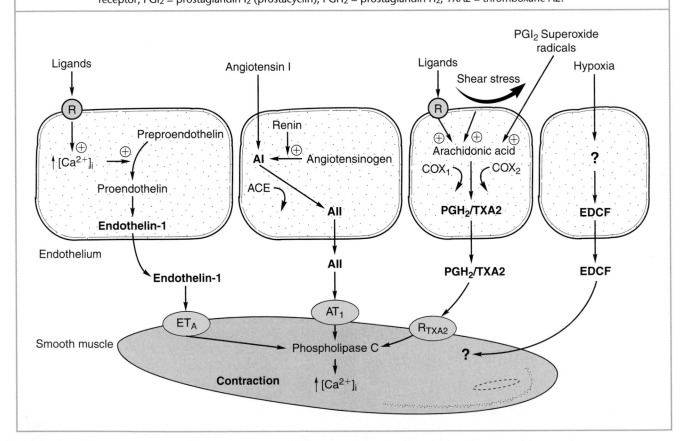

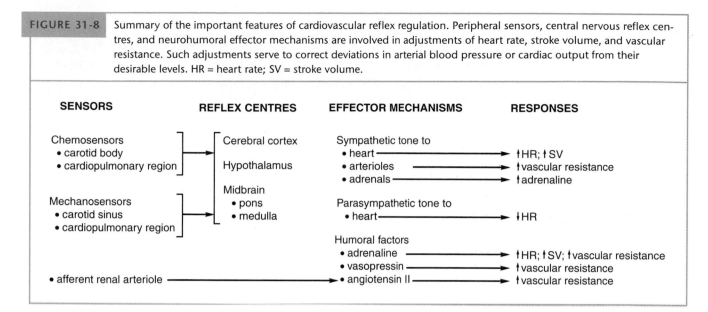

**FIGURE 31-8** Summary of the important features of cardiovascular reflex regulation. Peripheral sensors, central nervous reflex centres, and neurohumoral effector mechanisms are involved in adjustments of heart rate, stroke volume, and vascular resistance. Such adjustments serve to correct deviations in arterial blood pressure or cardiac output from their desirable levels. HR = heart rate; SV = stroke volume.

reflex regulation of autonomic nervous outflow and circulating hormones like the catecholamines, vasopressin, or angiotensin II. Reflex regulation is based on (1) the existence of a *set point for arterial blood pressure*, (2) sensory mechanisms that detect deviations of the pressure from the desired set point, and (3) effector mechanisms that operate to return arterial blood pressure towards the set point. These mechanisms are summarized in Figure 31-8. Long-term regulation involves both the cardiovascular system and systems that regulate body fluid volumes. Three aspects are of particular importance: mechanisms controlling cardiac hypertrophy, the renin–angiotensin–aldosterone system, and a frequently direct relationship between arterial blood pressure and renal $Na^+$ excretion (pressure natriuresis).

## SUGGESTED READINGS

Fuster V, Alexander RW, O'Rourke RA, Wellens HJJ, eds. *Hurst's the Heart.* New York, NY: McGraw-Hill; 2000.

Gordon AM, Homsher E, Regnier M. Regulation of contraction in striated muscle. *Physiol Rev.* 2000;80:853-924.

Katz AM. *Physiology of the Heart.* New York, NY: Lippincott Williams & Wilkins; 2001.

Mifflin SW. What does the brain know about blood pressure? *NIPS.* 2001;16:266-271.

Opie LH. *Heart Physiology: From Cell to Circulation.* 4th ed. Philadelphia, Pa: Lippincott Williams & Wilkins; 2003.

Rowell LB. *Human Cardiovascular Control.* New York, NY: Oxford University Press; 1993.

# Digitalis Glycosides and Other Positive Inotropic Agents

## G MOE

### CASE HISTORY

A 69-year-old male with a long-standing history of congestive heart failure secondary to previous myocardial infarctions was seen in the Heart Function Clinic because of palpitations and increasing shortness of breath. His medical regimen included an angiotensin-converting enzyme inhibitor, lisinopril 10 mg once daily; a β-adrenergic receptor blocker, carvedilol 25 mg twice daily; digoxin 0.25 mg once daily; and furosemide 20 mg once daily. He had undergone several cardiac revascularization procedures, and his left ventricular ejection fraction had been known to be depressed at 25%. On this occasion, he was found to be in atrial fibrillation, which had not been present previously, with a ventricular response of about 110 beats/min. Physical examination revealed pitting edema of both legs and fine crackles at the bases of both lungs. The patient was maintained on digoxin in a dose of 0.25 mg/day, and the furosemide was increased to 40 mg twice daily.

Approximately 1 week after the original visit, the patient returned to the clinic with a complaint of "palpitations," by which he meant periods of irregular heartbeat. An electrocardiogram showed multiple ventricular premature beats with occasional runs of non-sustained ventricular tachycardia. Physical examination no longer revealed signs of congestion, but the serum creatinine was found to be twice the upper limit of normal. Serum digoxin level was 3.8 nmol/L (therapeutic range is 1.0 to 2.6 nmol/L) and serum potassium was 3.0 mmol/L. The patient was admitted to hospital, and the digoxin was discontinued, the dose of furosemide was reduced, and potassium supplement was given. After 6 days, the ventricular arrhythmias were no longer present, renal function had improved, and the serum digoxin level declined to 1.8 nmol/L. The patient was discharged on 0.125 mg of digoxin daily, along with his other cardiac medications.

The therapeutic role of digitalis glycosides in heart failure has diminished over the years. Although digitalis is very useful in controlling ventricular response in patients with atrial fibrillation, its therapeutic benefit in patients with heart failure and in sinus rhythm remains controversial. The case history also highlights the relatively narrow therapeutic window of these agents.

## HEART FAILURE

Heart failure has been recognized as a clinical syndrome since the ancient Egyptian and early Greek civilizations. The continued evolution of the understanding of the pathophysiology of heart failure has resulted in a succession of paradigms to describe this syndrome (Fig. 32-1). A useful contemporary clinical definition of the condition is that heart failure is a clinical syndrome caused by an abnormality in the heart and recognized by a characteris-

tic pattern of hemodynamic, renal, neural, and hormonal responses. This definition incorporates many aspects of the cardiorenal, hemodynamic, and neurohormonal paradigms depicted in Figure 32-1, and it can be further expanded by stating that, in heart failure, the heart is unable to provide an adequate amount of oxygenated blood to meet the needs of the peripheral tissues. This additional statement incorporates many of the signs and symptoms seen in patients with heart failure.

Heart failure can be caused by a variety of conditions that induce damage to the myocardium. These include myocardial ischemia and infarction, long-standing pressure and volume overload, and damage from viral infections and toxins, including alcohol. While the etiologies of heart failure may be diverse, a critical process in the progression of most forms of heart failure is left ventricular (LV) remodelling. The morphological components of cardiac remodelling include a progressive increase in chamber volume, eccentric hypertrophy, and the assump-

**FIGURE 32-1** Heart failure paradigms.

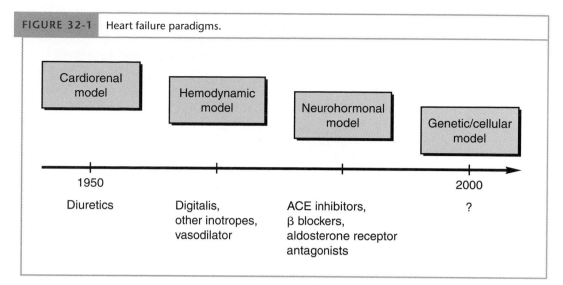

tion of a more globular shape. The process of LV remodelling involves changes in both the myocytes and the extracellular matrix, including activation of proteolytic enzymes and alteration in the myocardial collagen organization. It is important to note that LV remodelling often continues even if the initiating event has resolved, and it tends to progress over time. These changes contribute to alterations in LV chamber geometry and function. The complex relationships between the etiologic factors and the various pathophysiological paradigms and how their interplay ultimately results in adverse clinical outcomes are illustrated in Figure 32-2.

One of the traditional hallmarks of heart failure is impaired LV systolic function, often measured by ejection fraction. However, it is now appreciated that a large proportion of patients who present with symptoms of heart failure have LV ejection fractions within the normal range. Although some have postulated that ventricular systolic function is still impaired, most investigators have concluded that the fundamental abnormality in these patients is a disorder of diastolic (rather than systolic) function, and these patients are frequently referred to as having diastolic heart failure. The use of such terminology is problematic because it presumes that one completely understands the mechanisms leading to this disorder and therefore can justify the substitution of a mechanistic term for a descriptive phrase. A less presumptuous approach is to refer to these patients as having heart failure with preserved ejection fraction, a descriptive approach that makes no assumptions about our knowledge about the pathophysiology of this disorder. It is useful to distinguish patients with heart failure with preserved systolic function from those with impaired systolic function. First, heart failure with preserved systolic function may be more difficult to diagnose. Second, patients with heart failure with preserved systolic function, on balance, have a better prognosis than those with impaired systolic function. Third,

while there exists plenty of evidence to support the use of certain classes of agents to improve clinical outcomes in patients with impaired systolic function, there are as yet no effective evidence-based therapies for patients with heart failure and preserved systolic function.

The treatment of heart failure accompanied by impaired systolic LV function is strongly evidence-based. The goal of treatment is to improve clinical outcomes and alleviate symptoms. As highlighted at the beginning of the case presentation, currently, the angiotensin-converting enzyme (ACE) inhibitors and β-adrenergic receptor blockers, both of which have been shown to improve clinical outcomes in patients with heart failure, constitute the standard therapy in these patients. Adjunctive therapies for relief of symptoms include digitalis, vasodilators such as the nitrates, and diuretics. This chapter will review the use of digitalis and other inotropic agents.

## DIGITALIS GLYCOSIDES

### Structure

All the digitalis glycosides have three structural components: a steroid nucleus, a series of sugar residues in the C-3 position, and a five- or six-member lactone ring in the C-17 position (Fig. 32-3). The steroid nucleus and the lactone ring together are called a genin or aglycone. This aglycone moiety elicits the cardiotonic effects, which are qualitatively similar for all the aglycones. However, absorption, onset, and duration of action vary among different glycosides in relation to the sugar portion of the molecule.

### Preparations

Several formulations of digitalis glycosides are commercially available. However, only a few are in common clini-

FIGURE 32-2    Mechanisms of progression of heart failure. CAD = coronary artery disease; RAAS = renin–angiotensin–aldosterone system; SNS = sympathetic nervous system; ET-1 = endothelin; AVP = arginine vasopressin; TNFα = tumour necrosis factor alpha; IL-1β = interleukin-1 beta; IL-6 = interleukin-6.

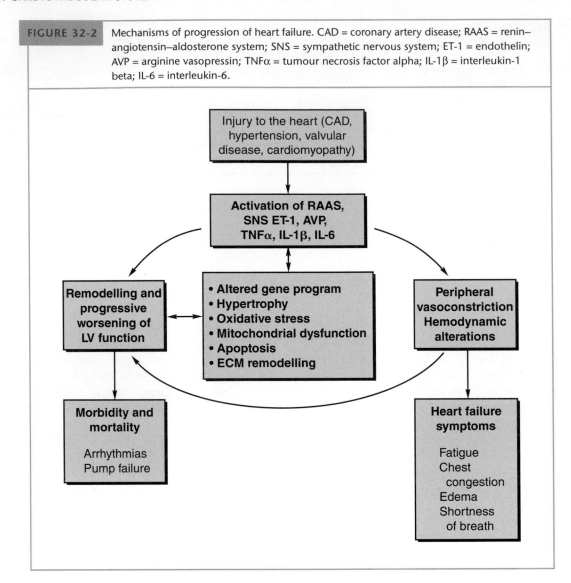

cal use. At least 90% of digitalis therapy in North America is carried out with digoxin, but two other digitalis preparations are occasionally prescribed. Table 32-1 summarizes the pharmacokinetic data for three digitalis preparations, deslanoside (Cedilanid), digoxin (Lanoxin), and digitoxin (Crystodigin). These values are averages, and variations in measurements such as half-life are substantial even in normal subjects.

## Mechanism of Action

### Positive inotropic effect

The fundamental mechanisms by which digitalis glycosides stimulate the contractile forces within the cardiac cell have been widely debated. Present evidence suggests that this action is mediated through potentiation of the process of coupling the electrical excitation and the mechanical contraction (excitation–contraction coupling). The consensus of opinion is that digoxin inhibits the $Na^+/K^+$-ATPase membrane pump. $Na^+/K^+$-ATPase regulates intracellular sodium and potassium concentrations by using the energy from splitting ATP to carry sodium outward and potassium inward against their respective concentration gradients. Inhibition of this enzyme leads to an increase in intracellular sodium concentration (i.e., decreased outward transport) and, ultimately, to an increase in intracellular calcium as sodium–calcium exchange is stimulated by high intracellular sodium concentrations (Fig. 32-4).

Increased intracellular concentrations of calcium allow for greater activation of contractile proteins (e.g., actin, myosin; see Chapter 31). While the contractile proteins and the troponin–tropomyosin system are directly involved in muscular contraction, it is not clear how digoxin augments their action. Digoxin does not directly affect these proteins or the cellular mechanisms that provide energy for contraction, nor does it affect contraction in skeletal muscle. Digoxin also increases sympathetic tone, but this does not

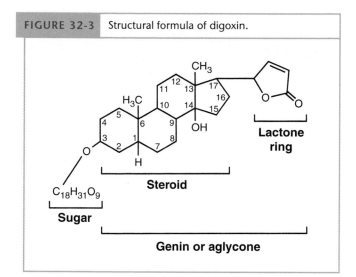

FIGURE 32-3    Structural formula of digoxin.

possesses direct vasoconstrictive properties, as well as enhancing peripheral vasoconstriction reflexes mediated by the central nervous system (CNS). Although this increases vascular resistance, in patients with failing hearts, the effect of increased myocardial contractility predominates and total peripheral resistance drops. In patients with heart failure, an increased cardiac output will decrease sympathetic tone, thereby reducing the heart rate and causing diuresis in edematous patients, and improving coronary blood flow.

## Electrophysiological effects

Some of the therapeutic and also potentially serious toxic effects of digitalis can be related to its action on the electro-physiological properties of the heart. The drug acts directly and indirectly on automaticity, conduction velocity, and the effective refractory period of cardiac tissues. Also, digitalis indirectly increases vagal tone in normal persons and decreases adrenergic nerve action on the failing heart. As mentioned above, digitalis inhibits the $Na^+/K^+$-ATPase, with a resultant decrease in intracellular potassium. This effect is dose-related. An increasing body concentration of digitalis ultimately leads to toxicity manifested by cardiac arrhythmias. The decrease in intracellular potassium leads to an increase in the slope of phase 4 depolarization and a decrease in maximal diastolic membrane potential (i.e., it becomes closer to zero membrane potential). This phenomenon leads to increased automaticity and development of ectopic rhythm. Not only are many of the electro-physiological and arrhythmic effects of digitalis related to intracellular potassium depletion, but it also appears that potassium and digitalis compete for binding sites on myocardial $Na^+/K^+$-ATPase. Potassium is relatively loosely bound to the enzyme, but it delays subsequent binding of digitalis. Once digitalis is bound, however, its rate of dissociation is not increased by potassium.

account for the positive inotropic effect, which persists even in the presence of β-adrenergic receptor blockade.

Administration of digitalis improves cardiac performance, shifting the cardiac function curve to the left so that it approximates the normal curve (Fig. 32-5). By increasing the force of myocardial contraction, digitalis reduces end-diastolic pressure, and consequently the end-diastolic volume. This decrease in ventricular volume increases the efficiency of contraction. Digitalis thus reduces the ratio of myocardial oxygen consumption to contractile force. The effect is largely due to decreased myocardial fibre length and diastolic wall tension. Digoxin directly increases the force and velocity of myocardial contraction in both healthy and failing hearts. In the failing heart, an increased force of contraction raises cardiac output, resulting in greater systolic emptying and smaller diastolic heart size. End-diastolic pressures decrease, leading to a reduction in pulmonary venous pressures. Digoxin also

| TABLE 32-1 | Cardiac Glycoside Preparations | | |
|---|---|---|---|
| | Deslanoside | Digoxin | Digitoxin |
| Gastrointestinal absorption (%) | Unreliable | 60–85 | 90–100 |
| Onset of action (minutes) | 10–30 | 15–30 | 25–120 |
| Peak effect (hours) | 1–2 | 1.5–5 | 4–12 |
| Average half-life | 33 hours | 36 hours | 4–6 days |
| Principal metabolic and/or excretory pathway | Renal excretion | Renal; some gastrointestinal excretion | Hepatic biotransformation; renal excretion of metabolites |
| Protein binding at therapeutic concentration (%) | – | 25 | 90 |
| Average digitalizing dose, oral (mg) | – | 1.25–1.5 | 0.7–1.2 |
| Average digitalizing dose, intravenous (mg) | 0.8 | 0.75–1.0 | 1.0 |
| Usual daily oral maintenance dose (mg) | – | 0.25–0.5 | 0.1 |

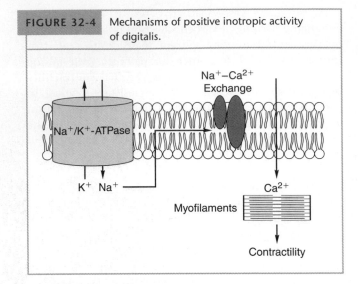

**FIGURE 32-4** Mechanisms of positive inotropic activity of digitalis.

The action of digitalis on **automaticity** (i.e., the property that allows a single cell to spontaneously depolarize without outside influences) is dose-dependent. In therapeutic concentrations, digitalis has little effect on automaticity; however, in toxic concentrations, the slope of phase 4 diastolic depolarization is increased in all cardiac tissues, and ectopic foci of impulse formation may develop. Indirectly, via vagal stimulation, digitalis causes decreased impulse formation in the sinoatrial (SA) node, so ectopic foci can take over control of the cardiac rhythm.

**Conduction velocity** (i.e., the rate at which an impulse is conducted through cardiac tissue) is a function of the amplitude of the action potential and its rate of rise (phase 0). Both of these variables are related to the resting membrane potential present at the onset of the action potential; the more negative the membrane potential, the steeper the slope of phase 0. All concentrations of digitalis diminish conduction velocity, but different parts of the heart respond to different degrees. The atrioventricular (AV) node is most sensitive, followed in descending order by atrial muscle, the Purkinje system, and ventricular muscle. The effect on the AV node is partly direct and partly indirect. It is most prominent when the initial vagal tone is low and adrenergic tone is high, as in heart failure. It should be noted that the direct effect of digitalis on atrial muscle (i.e., decreased conduction velocity) predominates over its indirect vagotonic effect (i.e., increased conduction).

The **refractory period**, consisting of phases 1, 2, and 3 in the transmembrane potential recording, includes the periods in which a cell is unexcitable (effective refractory period, ERP) and poorly excitable (relative refractory period, RRP). The digitalis-induced increase in vagal activity causes a marked decrease in the duration of the ERP in the atria, producing greater discharge frequency of fibrillating atria (or it may convert atrial flutter to fibrillation). However, an increase in vagal activity reduces conduction velocity and prolongs the ERP. As a result, the ventricular

rate is lowered. This prolongation of the ERP of the AV node is the main beneficial effect of cardiac glycosides when used for the treatment of atrial flutter or fibrillation.

The effects of digitalis on the electrophysiology of the heart are summarized in Table 32-2. These form the electrophysiological basis for slowing the ventricular response to atrial arrhythmias and converting supraventricular arrhythmias to normal sinus rhythm.

### Neural effects

The three most important neural effects of digitalis glycosides are increased vagal activity (which can be blocked by atropine), sensitization of carotid sinus baroreceptors, and increased sympathetic outflow from the CNS at high doses. The first two mechanisms likely contribute to the beneficial effects of digitalis. Indeed, some investigators propose that these mechanisms may be more important than the positive inotropic effect of digitalis. Digitalis thus ameliorates heart failure–related autonomic dysfunction by enhancing parasympathetic tone and reducing peripheral muscle sympathetic nerve activity. Baroreceptor responsiveness, which is decreased in heart failure, is increased by digoxin. Reduced baroreflex sensitivity contributes to increased plasma catecholamine, vasopressin, and renin. Digoxin may therefore act as a neurohormonal modulator in patients with heart failure.

## Pharmacokinetics

Digoxin is commercially available as tablets, capsules, oral elixir, and solution for injection. In general, digoxin is rapidly absorbed from the gastrointestinal tract following an oral dose. The major site of absorption appears to be the small intestine. Bioavailability from capsules is essentially complete but is approximately 75 to 85% from oral elixir and 70 to 80% from tablets. However, the bioavailability of digoxin in tablet form varies widely between

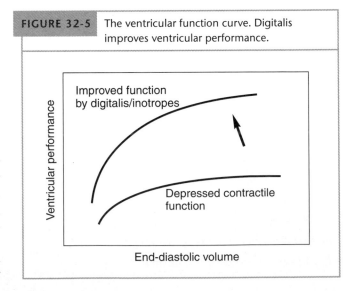

**FIGURE 32-5** The ventricular function curve. Digitalis improves ventricular performance.

| TABLE 32-2 | Electrophysiological Effects of Digitalis | | | | | |
|---|---|---|---|---|---|---|
| | Automaticity | | Conduction Velocity | | Effective Refractory Period | |
| | Direct | Indirect | Direct | Indirect | Direct | Indirect |
| SA node | ↑* | ↓ | | | | |
| Atrium | ↑* | | ↓* | ↑ | ↑ | |
| AV node | | | ↓↓ | ↓↓ | ↑↑ | ↑↑ |
| Purkinje system | ↑* | | ↓* | | ↓ | ↑ |
| Ventricles | ↑* | | ↑↓* | | ↓↓ | |

*At high or toxic doses; ↑ = increase; ↓ = decrease; ↑↑ or ↓↓ denotes therapeutically important effects.

commercial preparations. Even well-standardized preparations show variable absorption within and between patients. Diarrhea, malabsorption syndromes, or food in the stomach may also influence absorption significantly.

Digoxin distributes throughout the body tissues, with the highest concentrations found in the heart, kidneys, intestine, liver, stomach, and skeletal muscle. Small amounts can be found in the brain. The presence of congestion in heart failure slows the rate at which steady-state distribution is achieved. Only 20 to 30% of the drug is protein-bound. Digoxin crosses the placenta, and maternal and fetal plasma concentrations of the drug are equal. Onset of therapeutic effects generally occurs within 30 minutes to 2 hours after oral administration and within 5 to 30 minutes following intravenous administration. The peak effect generally occurs between 2 to 6 hours after oral administration of a dose.

A small amount of digoxin is metabolized in the liver to inactive metabolites. There is some enterohepatic circulation of digoxin. In approximately 10% of patients, however, significant amounts of orally ingested digoxin are metabolized in the gut by intestinal bacteria. Thirty to 50% of a dose is excreted unchanged in the urine. The elimination half-life of digoxin in adults is normally 30 to 40 hours, but heart failure or renal impairment can prolong elimination. Thus, in patients with renal impairment, the half-life is extended to as long as 4 to 6 days.

## Drug Interactions

The action of digitalis may be *enhanced* by substances that (1) slow gastrointestinal motility (e.g., antispasmodics, such as atropine-like agents) and thereby increase gastrointestinal absorption of slowly absorbed digitalis preparations; (2) disturb body electrolytes by lowering plasma potassium levels, eliciting hypomagnesemia and hypercalcemia (e.g., diuretics, amphotericin B, oral or parenteral glucose); (3) change renal clearance and/or alter plasma protein binding (e.g., quinidine, verapamil, amiodarone and other anti-arrhythmics); (4) stimulate β-adrenergic receptors and cause cardiac arrhythmias (e.g.,

adrenaline, ephedrine); and (5) elicit cardiac arrhythmias by unknown mechanisms (e.g., succinylcholine, anticholinesterases). These interactions may predispose to digitalis toxicity. On the other hand, the action of digitalis may be *reduced* by substances that (1) reduce gastrointestinal absorption (e.g., kaolin–pectin, anti-hyperlipidemic agents, and antacids); (2) increase gastrointestinal motility (e.g., metoclopramide); and (3) stimulate hepatic microsomal enzymes and thus enhance the biotransformation of digitoxin (e.g., spironolactone, phenytoin, acetylsalicylic acid, phenylbutazone, and barbiturates).

## Side Effects and Toxicity

The toxic manifestations of digitalis may be classified into cardiac and extra-cardiac. The key manifestation of cardiac toxicity is dose-related arrhythmias, which may terminate in ventricular fibrillation. The common predisposing factor is a decrease in intracellular potassium. Potassium depletion may be hastened by concurrent treatment with certain diuretics or by conditions such as severe vomiting and diarrhea. Irregularities in cardiac rhythm, such as coupled beats (bigeminy), are signals calling for a reduction in digitalis dosage. Other cardiac manifestations of digitalis toxicity are premature ventricular contractions, premature atrial contractions, AV block, paroxysmal atrial tachycardia with or without block, and ventricular tachycardia.

The principal extra-cardiac manifestations of digitalis toxicity are mostly gastrointestinal. Vomiting is caused by stimulation of the chemoreceptor trigger zone. Diarrhea results from the activation of the dorsal motor nucleus of the vagal nerve, increasing gastrointestinal motility. A variety of CNS side effects occur, including anorexia, weakness, lethargy and fatigue, and visual complaints. The visual disturbances include hazy vision, difficulty in reading, various types of scotoma, altered or disturbed colour perception, and photophobia. Other neurological symptoms of digitalis toxicity include dizziness, headache, paresthesias, and, with massive overdose, convulsions, delusions, stupor, and coma.

### Treatment of digitalis toxicity

Digitalis must be discontinued immediately if toxic manifestations occur. Often these symptoms may persist for some time because of slow elimination of the drug. Since there is usually a loss of potassium from the myocardium during treatment with digitalis glycosides, and since the loss of potassium is the probable cause of arrhythmias, immediate relief may be obtained by the intravenous administration of potassium salts. This measure raises the extracellular potassium concentration and thus decreases the slope of phase 4 depolarization so that problems due to excessive automaticity are diminished. There are, however, hazards associated with potassium administration when there is depressed automaticity or decreased conduction, because this may lead to complete AV block. Digitalis-induced, second- or third-degree heart block is the type of arrhythmia in which potassium is contraindicated. In addition to potassium, digitalis-induced cardiac arrhythmias also respond to drugs such as lidocaine or phenytoin (see Chapter 33).

Life-threatening arrhythmias and heart block produced by digoxin or digitoxin can be safely treated with digoxin-specific Fab fragments that have been purified from antibodies raised in sheep by immunization against digoxin. The crude antiserum from sheep is fractionated to separate the IgG fraction, which is cleaved into Fab and Fc fragments by papain digestion. The Fab fragments are not antigenic or complement-binding. They are excreted fairly rapidly by the kidney as a digoxin-bound complex. In patients with life-threatening arrhythmias, treatment with digoxin-specific Fab fragments brings about rapid resolution of the arrhythmias.

## Therapeutic Indications Based on Evidence from Clinical Trials

Historically, the drugs included under the generic term digitalis, also known as cardiac glycosides, have been used primarily to treat heart failure. Digitalis, which is extracted from the foxglove plant, was used before 1785 in folk medicine. In that year, William Withering published his celebrated book *An Account of the Foxglove and Some of Its Medical Uses: With Practical Remarks on Dropsy, and Other Diseases.* Withering initially thought that foxglove was a diuretic, but he later recognized that the heart was affected and that the drug produced cardiac slowing in patients with generalized edema (dropsy). Digitalis is extracted from the dried leaf of the foxglove plant, *Digitalis purpurea.* Seeds and leaves of *Digitalis lanata,* a number of other digitalis species, and a variety of other plants also contain cardiac glycosides.

Despite more than two centuries of use and contemporary outcome data, the use of digitalis in chronic heart failure remains controversial. In certain parts of the world, such as the United Kingdom and some European countries,

digoxin is rarely prescribed for heart failure. Digoxin has also been used to control ventricular rate in patients with chronic atrial fibrillation; however, this use of digoxin has also declined in recent years, being replaced by more effective rate-controlling agents such as calcium-channel blockers. There are sufficient data to support the use of digoxin for *symptomatic* improvement, including quality of life and exercise duration. These data resulted in the United States Food and Drug Administration's approval for its use in mild to moderate heart failure. Furthermore, the American College of Cardiology/American Heart Association, the Heart Failure Society of America, as well as the Canadian Cardiovascular Society heart failure management guidelines recommend digoxin use as adjunctive therapy for *symptomatic* patients in the absence of contraindication.

The data used for these decisions and recommendations included the Digitalis Investigator Group (DIG) survival study sponsored by the National Institutes of Health, along with retrospective analyses from the Prospective Randomized Study of Ventricular Failure and the Efficacy of Digoxin (PROVED) and the Randomized Assessment of the Effect of Digoxin on Inhibitors of the Angiotensin-Converting Enzyme (RADIANCE) efficacy trials. Overall, results of these trials have demonstrated that digoxin increases LV ejection fraction, improves symptoms, and reduces the need for hospitalization for heart failure, but overall mortality is not altered.

Although the beneficial clinical effects of these agents have been known empirically for over two centuries, their mechanisms of action have not been well understood until recently. It is now generally acknowledged that their most clinically significant direct action is augmentation of contraction of the atrial and ventricular myocardium. A thorough understanding of the pharmacology of these agents is particularly important because they are used widely, and as highlighted in the case presentation, they have a narrow margin of safety (i.e., there is a very small difference between the therapeutically effective dose and the toxic or fatal dose). Several studies have indicated that up to 20% of patients taking digitalis show some form of drug-induced toxicity. These toxic manifestations are more pronounced in elderly patients: the incidence is 24% for those over 60 years of age compared with 14% for those under 60 years.

## Clinical Prescription and Therapeutic Monitoring

For the treatment of chronic heart failure in the presence of sinus rhythm, a loading dose is often unnecessary. The recommended dose ranges from 0.125 to 0.25 mg/day, based on body weight, age, and renal function. Most practitioners obtain a serum digoxin concentration as a trough level drawn at least 6 hours after oral dosing, once a steady state is achieved. Serum digoxin concentration need not be measured frequently unless there is suspicion about the patient's compliance, worsening renal function, or digitalis toxicity. Most heart failure specialists recommend a trough digoxin level between 1.0 and 1.5 nmol/L, drug levels that were achieved in the DIG and RADIANCE trials. As illustrated in the case history, the therapeutic index for digitalis is low, and consequently, the dosage must be carefully controlled for each individual. It may be difficult to estimate the initial and maintenance doses because they depend very much on the clinical condition of the patient.

## NON-DIGITALIS INOTROPIC AGENTS

The use of sympathomimetic agents, such as **dopamine** and **dobutamine**, is currently limited to short-term intravenous administration in acute heart failure and other clinical conditions characterized by shock. Phosphodiesterase inhibitors, such as **amrinone, milrinone,** and **enoximone,** increase contractile function by preventing the breakdown of intracellular cyclic AMP. Oral milrinone has been shown to increase mortality in patients with chronic heart failure, so this approach is therefore abandoned. Currently, among the phosphodiesterase inhibitors, only intravenous milrinone is used for short-term administration in the same clinical settings as dobutamine. The most promising class of non-digitalis inotropic agents is the calcium sensitizers. Preliminary data suggest an agent such as **levosimendan,** a calcium sensitizer, improves short-term outcome in patients with acute heart failure.

## CONCLUSION

For decades, cardiac glycosides have been used in the treatment of heart failure and for heart rate control in atrial tachyarrhythmias. Their narrow therapeutic index and the compelling benefits of ACE inhibitors and β-adrenergic blockers have limited the use of cardiac glycosides in the setting of chronic heart failure. Unless further data become available, it is anticipated that the therapeutic role of the cardiac glycosides will continue to decline.

## SUGGESTED READINGS

Falk RH, Leavitt JI. Digoxin for atrial fibrillation: a drug whose time has gone? *Ann Intern Med.* 1991;114:573-575.

Kim RSS, Labella FS. Endogenous ligands and modulators of the digitalis receptor: some candidates. *Pharmacol Ther.* 1981;14:391-409.

Kjeldsen K, Bundgaard H. Myocardial Na,K-ATPase and digoxin therapy in human heart failure. *Ann N Y Acad Sci.* 2003;986:702-707.

Klein L, O'Connor CM, Gattis WA, et al. Pharmacologic therapy for patients with chronic heart failure and reduced systolic function: review of trials and practical considerations. *Am J Cardiol.* 2003;91:18F-40F.

Kulick DL, Rahimtoola SH. Current role of digitalis therapy in patients with congestive heart failure. *JAMA.* 1991;265:2995-2997.

Langer GA. Effects of digitalis on myocardial ionic exchange. *Circulation.* 1972;46:180-187.

Mason DT. Regulation of cardiac performance in clinical heart disease: interactions between contractile state mechanical abnormalities and ventricular compensatory mechanisms. *Am J Cardiol.* 1973;32:437-448.

Packer M, Carver JR, Rodeheffer RJ, et al. Effect of oral milrinone on mortality in severe chronic heart failure. *N Engl J Med.* 1991;325:1468-1475.

Schlant RC, Sonnenblick EH. Pathophysiology of heart failure. In: Hirst JW, ed. *The Heart, Arteries and Veins.* New York, NY: McGraw-Hill; 1990:387-418.

Sidwell A, Barclay M, Begg G, Moore G. Digoxin therapeutic drug monitoring: an audit and review. *N Z Med J.* 2003;116:U704.

Smith TW. Digitalis: mechanisms of action and clinical use. *N Engl J Med.* 1987;318:358-365.

The effect of digoxin on mortality and morbidity in patients with heart failure. The Digitalis Investigation Group. *N Engl J Med.* 1997;336:525-533.

# 33

# Anti-arrhythmic Drugs

## A SARKOZY AND P DORIAN

### CASE HISTORY

A 55-year-old man developed a spontaneous sustained ventricular tachycardia with presyncope, for which he was admitted to hospital. He had had an anterior wall myocardial infarction 5 years previously, which was asymptomatic during treatment with acetylsalicylic acid 325 mg once a day and metoprolol 50 mg twice a day.

Investigation revealed moderate left ventricular dysfunction with an ejection fraction of 42%. There was no inducible myocardial ischemia, but Holter monitoring showed frequent short runs of non-sustained ventricular tachycardia. Soon after, he developed sustained atrial fibrillation with a resting ventricular rate of 110 bpm. Oral digoxin, 0.25 mg/day, was begun, as well as anticoagulation with warfarin to maintain an international normalized ratio (INR) of 2.0 to 3.0 (see Chapter 38). In order to prevent the risk of recurrence of sustained ventricular tachycardia and to attempt to restore and maintain sinus rhythm, amiodarone 1200 mg/day was administered orally in divided doses for 7 days in hospital with no untoward effects. The patient was then discharged with the instruction to take 400 mg/day of amiodarone for 4 weeks and to reduce the dose to 200 mg/day thereafter. Medication with digoxin and warfarin was continued. At the time of discharge, the rhythm was atrial fibrillation with a resting ventricular rate of 70 bpm. The INR was 2.9.

Three weeks later, the patient came to the emergency department with bleeding from the gums, very easy bruising, intermittent epistaxis, as well as extreme fatigue, nausea, and visual disturbances. Physical examination and ECG showed sinus bradycardia, 30 bpm, regular, with no evidence of heart failure. The INR was 6.5, and trough serum dixogin level was 4.5 nmol/L (therapeutic range 0.5 to 2.0 nmol/L). Thus, the patient had clear-cut clinical evidence of excess warfarin and digitalis effects.

The doses of digoxin and warfarin were titrated downward and adjusted to the minimum required to restore a therapeutic INR of 2.0 to 3.0 and to correct overdigitalization in the presence of amiodarone. Once these adjustments had taken effect, the patient was discharged with exact ambulatory dosing instructions and a closely spaced follow-up schedule.

**Comment:** The patient's recovery demonstrated that amiodarone was effective at restoring sinus rhythm in atrial fibrillation and preventing recurrence of ventricular tachycardia. However, the clearance of both digoxin and warfarin was markedly reduced during co-administration of amiodarone. In addition, some of the pharmacodynamic effects of digoxin, such as bradycardia or atrioventricular block, were likely additive with those of amiodarone. Because of these known interactions of amiodarone with drugs that are eliminated by the hepatic microsomal enzyme system, such as warfarin and digoxin, the doses of these drugs should have been reduced by one-half soon after amiodarone was started, and clinical effects and plasma concentrations should have been monitored more carefully.

The management of cardiac arrhythmias is primarily concerned with reducing symptoms from arrhythmias, restoring and maintaining sinus rhythm, and preventing the occurrence or recurrence of symptomatic and/or life-threatening arrhythmias.

## MECHANISMS OF ARRHYTHMOGENESIS AND THE EFFECTS OF ANTI-ARRHYTHMIC INTERVENTION

The normal physiology of the cardiac action potential, including the ionic currents underlying it (Table 33-1) and the differences between myocardial cells and pacemaker cells, was described in detail in Chapter 31. This chapter deals with abnormal automaticity and re-entry and the drugs used to correct it.

## Basic Mechanisms of Arrhythmogenesis

Once depolarization of the cell membrane begins and the action potential has started, the cell becomes refractory to subsequent stimuli. Initially, it will be totally refractory irrespective of the strength of the stimulus (**absolute refractory period**), but during the latter part of the action potential, depolarization can be induced in response to a stronger-than-normal stimulus (**relative refractory period**; Fig. 33-1). Because excitation and recovery do not occur simultaneously in all cardiac cells, asynchrony of repolarization may occur. This results in a vulnerable period during which the heart is susceptible to the induction of arrhythmias since some cells will be able to conduct impulses whereas others will not, thus allowing for the possible occurrence of re-entry phenomena, as described in the following section. The application of a single strong stimulus at this time may elicit an abnormal response such as ventricular fibrillation. This vulnerable period corresponds approximately to the peak of the T wave on the electrocardiogram (ECG; see Fig. 33-6A). Anti-arrhythmic drugs may alter the duration of the vulnerable period or its magnitude, thus altering the likelihood of an arrhythmia developing in response to a given stimulus.

There are two putative causes of arrhythmias: abnormalities in impulse formation leading to **enhanced or abnormal automaticity**, and abnormalities in impulse conduction resulting in **re-entry phenomena**. Although most common arrhythmias, such as sustained ventricular tachycardia in patients with coronary disease, atrial and ventricular fibrillation, and paroxysmal supraventricular tachycardias, are caused by re-entry, the specific mechanism by which many clinical anti-arrhythmic agents act on the factors initiating and maintaining re-entry for a particular arrhythmia episode is not known.

## Effect of Anti-arrhythmic Agents on Automaticity

Spontaneous phase 4 depolarization is a property of the sinus node, atrioventricular (AV) node, His–Purkinje system, and certain specialized atrial fibres. The ability of these cells to depolarize spontaneously is called **normal automaticity.** Arrhythmias caused by alterations in automaticity are thought to arise from **enhanced normal automaticity** at any one of these sites other than the sinus node. Normal myocardial cells do not depolarize spontaneously, and, therefore, arrhythmias due to enhanced normal automaticity cannot originate in these cells.

Damaged myocardial cells often remain partially depolarized, and this failure to reach maximum negative diastolic potential (about −85 mV) may induce abnormal automatic discharges. Unlike enhanced normal automaticity, arrhythmias due to **abnormal automaticity** can occur in myocardial cells as well as in specialized conduction tissue. In the presence of myocardial cell necrosis, hypoxia, or potassium imbalance, the cell fails to repolarize fully and the resting potential only reaches −30 to −40 mV.

Most anti-arrhythmic agents suppress automaticity by decreasing the slope of phase 4 spontaneous depolarization and/or shifting the voltage threshold to a less negative level. In both cases, the threshold potential for initiating an action potential is reached later, leading to less frequent discharges of full action potentials in a given time by the pacemaker cell (see Fig. 33-1). Although this effect also decreases the frequency of discharge of normal pacemaker cells (e.g., the sinus node), it has a more pronounced action on ectopic pacemaker activity. The rela-

| TABLE 33-1 | | Major Ion Fluxes during the Cardiac Action Potential | | |
|---|---|---|---|---|
| **Name** | **Ion** | **Current** | **Phase of Action Potential** | |
| $I_{Na}$ | $Na^+$ | Inward | 0 | (depolarization) |
| $I_{to}$ | $K^+$ | Outward | 1 | (rapid repolarization) |
| $I_{Ca}$ | $Ca^{2+}$ | Inward | 2 | (plateau) |
| $I_{Kr}$ | $K^+$ | Outward | 2, 3 | (repolarization) |
| $I_{Ks}$ | $K^+$ | Outward | 2, 3 | (repolarization) |
| $I_{Kur}$* | $K^+$ | Outward | 2 | (repolarization) |
| $I_{K1}$† | $K^+$ | Outward | 3, 4 | (repolarization, diastole) |
| $I_f$ | $Na^+$ | Inward | 4 | (spontaneous depolarization) |

*$I_{Kur}$ is only identified in atrial tissue.

†$I_{K1}$ during the resting phase (diastole in cells without spontaneous depolarization) maintains the equilibrium responsible for the resting potential at or near the Nernst potential.

**FIGURE 33-1** Diagram of the ventricular action potential. Phase 0 = depolarization; phase 1 = rapid repolarization; phase 2 = plateau; phase 3 = final repolarization; phase 4 = spontaneous depolarization in pacemaker cells. ARP = absolute refractory period; RRP = relative refractory period; TP = threshold potential; RMP = resting membrane potential.

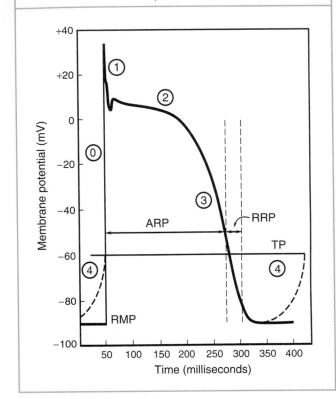

calcium-channel antagonists, magnesium, and by restoring physical or electrolyte balance to the cell milieu.

## Effect of Anti-arrhythmic Agents on Re-entry

Re-entry depends on the existence of two anatomically or physiologically distinct pathways, as shown in Figure 33-3. For example, the normal AV node and an accessory atrioventricular bypass tract (Kent bundle) are anatomically distinct. In other situations, in the presence of myocardial scarring (e.g., from a previous myocardial infarct), scarred tissue can exhibit slowed conduction or prolonged refractoriness (physiological distinction). Normally, impulses will be conducted in the same direction down both pathways, bifurcating to cover the entire ventricular surface. However, should there be a unidirectional block (e.g., from conduction failure or functional refractoriness) in pathway 2, the impulse may only be conducted down pathway 1. If the block in pathway 2 is in the forward direction only (as would be caused by functional as opposed to "anatomical" block), it may be possible for the impulse to return in a retrograde fashion through this pathway, reaching the initial point of bifurcation, provided that the transit time through the circuit exceeds the refractory period in the circuit. Under these circumstances, re-excitation of the myocardium may occur via this "short-circuiting" of the conducting tissue, thus causing a single re-entrant beat. If this re-entry mechanism becomes repetitive, a sustained ventricular arrhythmia such as ventricular tachycardia occurs. Similar re-entry mechanisms have been proposed in the atria as a common cause of atrial flutter and near the AV node as a cause of AV nodal re-entry tachycardia. Arrhythmias in patients with accessory atrioventricular connections (Wolff–Parkinson–White [WPW] syndrome) usually arise from re-entry with anterograde conduction through the AV node and retrograde conduction through the atrioventricular bypass tract.

Anti-arrhythmic agents most likely abolish re-entry by depressing membrane responsiveness, slowing conduction so that propagation around the re-entrant circuit cannot occur, or increasing refractoriness so that the re-entrant wavefront impinges on refractory tissue, halting its further progress. Most anti-arrhythmic drugs appear to act by slowing conduction and/or increasing refractoriness, converting unidirectional into bidirectional block.

## ANTI-ARRHYTHMIC DRUGS

The most widely accepted classification of anti-arrhythmic drug action was initially proposed by Vaughan Williams (and later modified), who separated the action of various agents according to their predominant electrophysiological effects on the action potential. It is impor-

tively selective suppression of ectopic pacemaker foci may abolish an arrhythmia due to abnormal automaticity at doses of a drug that have little effect on normal sinus node function. However, in states where the sinus node or conducting tissue exhibits impaired function (e.g., sick sinus syndrome), suppression of phase 4 depolarization may result in a reduction of the heart rate or possible asystole.

Another form of abnormal automaticity is called **triggered activity.** Under certain pathological conditions, a transient depolarization may occur before a cell is fully repolarized, causing early or delayed afterdepolarizations (EADs or DADs, respectively; Fig. 33-2). These low-amplitude oscillatory depolarizations may give rise to or "trigger" propagated action potentials. Arrhythmias caused by digitalis toxicity, and possibly catecholamine excess, or arrhythmias induced by anti-arrhythmic drugs that prolong repolarization may be examples of this mechanism. Arrhythmias caused by triggered automaticity cannot, in general, be induced by premature extra stimuli, but they can be induced by continuous rapid stimulation. These oscillations in membrane potential can be suppressed by

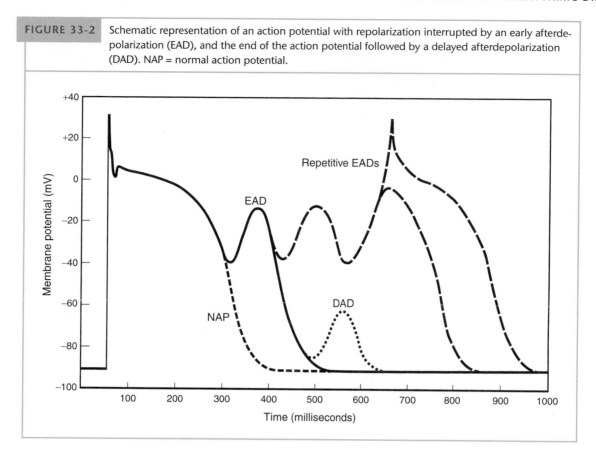

**FIGURE 33-2** Schematic representation of an action potential with repolarization interrupted by an early afterdepolarization (EAD), and the end of the action potential followed by a delayed afterdepolarization (DAD). NAP = normal action potential.

tant to understand that this classification is descriptive, and its clinical relevance has not yet been clarified. Importantly, the classification distinguishes between drug actions and not the drugs themselves. Many of the anti-arrhythmic drugs shown in Figure 33-4 have actions relating to more than one class or subclass in the classification. Moreover, many anti-arrhythmic drugs have active metabolites with a different class of action than that of the parent drug. The classification in Table 33-2 is used in the following paragraphs.

**Drugs with class I anti-arrhythmic properties**, of which quinidine is the prototype, slow the rate of rise of phase 0 ($\dot{V}_{max}$) of the action potential by blocking membrane sodium channels and thus decreasing the rate of entry of $Na^+$. These drugs have little or no effect on the resting membrane potential in doses used in clinical practice. They cause a decrease in excitability and conduction velocity; some also prolong the effective refractory period (and may block $K^+$ channels—this is a "class III" effect) and may decrease the slope of phase 4 spontaneous depolarization in pacemaker cells. Quinidine, procainamide, and lidocaine also exhibit local anaesthetic activity on the myocardial membrane.

**Drugs with class II mechanism of action** include the β-adrenergic receptor antagonists. They depress phase 4 depolarization and exert their anti-arrhythmic effects through competitive inhibition of the β-adrenergic-receptor-mediated stimulation by catecholamines. In high concentrations, many of these agents also show local anaesthetic properties, but this action is not usually seen in clinical practice.

**Drugs with class III mechanism of action** prolong the duration of the action potential with a consequent increase in the absolute and effective refractory period. Some of these agents (e.g., bretylium) have no significant effect on phase 4 depolarization, whereas others (e.g., amiodarone) may depress it.

**Drugs with class IV properties** decrease the inward current carried by calcium across the cell membrane. In the sinus node, this results in less net inward (depolarizing) current during the latter part of spontaneous diastolic depolarization, leading to a decrease in the rate of rise (slope) of phase 4 spontaneous depolarization and a slowing of the heart rate. In addition, these drugs slow conduction in tissues dependent on calcium currents (e.g., AV node), thus prolonging the PR interval in the ECG and prolonging the refractory period of the AV node.

Subclassification of the class I mechanism of action is shown in Table 33-2. It is important to emphasize that many drugs (e.g., amiodarone) possess actions pertaining to more than one class of anti-arrhythmic drug action and that drugs with a similar mechanism of action are not necessarily interchangeable with respect to clinical efficacy.

The pharmacokinetics of the main anti-arrhythmic drugs are summarized in Table 33-3. Table 33-4 lists the

**FIGURE 33-3** Mechanism of re-entry and effect of anti-arrhythmic intervention. The impulse is conducted unimpeded down pathway 1 but encounters an area of anatomical or functional block in pathway 2. The impulse can then be conducted retrogradely through pathway 2, and re-entry into pathway 1 may be established. Drugs can abolish the arrhythmia by improving forward conduction (A) or by preventing retrograde conduction (B).

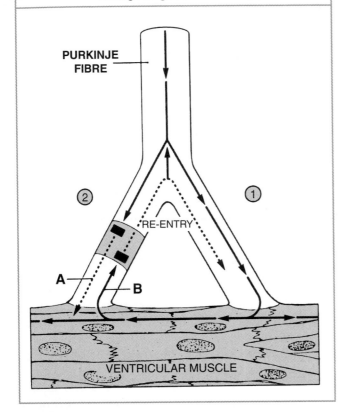

important pharmacodynamic mechanisms, properties, and toxicities of the agents discussed in the following paragraphs. For simplicity, drugs are listed under the "class" pertaining to their predominant mechanism of action.

Given the difficulty with the commonly used modified Vaughan Williams classification of anti-arrhythmic drug action, a new approach to classifying drugs with potential anti-arrhythmic activity has been proposed. Termed the "Sicilian gambit," it proposes to identify a number of potential targets for drug action, to include various ion-conducting channels ($Na^+$, $K^+$, $Ca^{2+}$, $Cl^-$), receptors ($\alpha$-, $\beta$-adrenergic, muscarinic, purinergic), and pumps ($Na^+/K^+$-ATPase). All anti-arrhythmic drugs or substances that affect cardiac electrophysiology would then be characterized by their actions on each of these channels, receptors, or pumps. (These actions may be activation or inhibition with varying kinetics and intensity.) If the most appropriate "target" for drug action for a given

arrhythmia or a given patient were known, therapy could be tailored for that specific situation. Unfortunately, the precise mechanisms of arrhythmias and the specific consequences of actions on particular channels or receptors are poorly understood. Nevertheless, the "Sicilian gambit" is a useful conceptual framework for classifying anti-arrhythmic drugs and helps clinicians to understand the multiplicity of drug actions; it may ultimately allow a "dissection" of the components of drug activity and definition of the best targets for specific arrhythmias and specific situations. A summary of drugs and their effects is illustrated in Figure 33-5.

## Class Ia Drugs

### Quinidine

*Pharmacokinetics.* Quinidine sulfate is rapidly and nearly completely absorbed after oral administration; the gluconate salt is absorbed more slowly and less completely. An intravenous preparation is available but can cause severe hypotension and must be administered with caution. Approximately 80% of a quinidine dose is hydroxylated in the liver, and the metabolites are cardioactive. The remainder of the drug is excreted unchanged by the kidney.

*Anti-arrhythmic effects.* As already described, quinidine slows the rapid sodium current, thereby decreasing the rate of rise of phase 0 of the action potential ($\dot{V}_{max}$). It also decreases the slope of phase 4 spontaneous depolarization, thus tending to inhibit ectopic rhythms due to automaticity. Although quinidine suppresses ventricular arrhythmias caused by increased normal automaticity, it has little effect on abnormal automaticity. Quinidine may also abolish re-entrant arrhythmias: it produces bidirectional block (see Fig. 33-3, example B) by depressing membrane responsiveness and prolonging the effective refractory period.

In the presence of an intact autonomic nervous system, quinidine may cause an increase in heart rate either by a reflex increase in sympathetic activity or by a decrease in vagal tone. In patients with sick sinus syndrome, quinidine may produce severe sinus node depression, causing an aggravation of the bradycardia.

In clinical practice, quinidine is effective in the treatment of a wide variety of arrhythmias including atrial, AV junctional, and ventricular tachyarrhythmias. However, evidence from clinical trials suggests that *quinidine could increase mortality due to proarrhythmic sudden death, especially in individuals with structural heart disease.* Due to the safety concerns and the availability of more effective class Ic drugs, quinidine is now rarely used for the treatment of supraventricular tachycardias. Infrequently, it is still used in combination with class III anti-arrhythmic

**FIGURE 33-4** Structural formulae of anti-arrhythmic drugs in current clinical use.

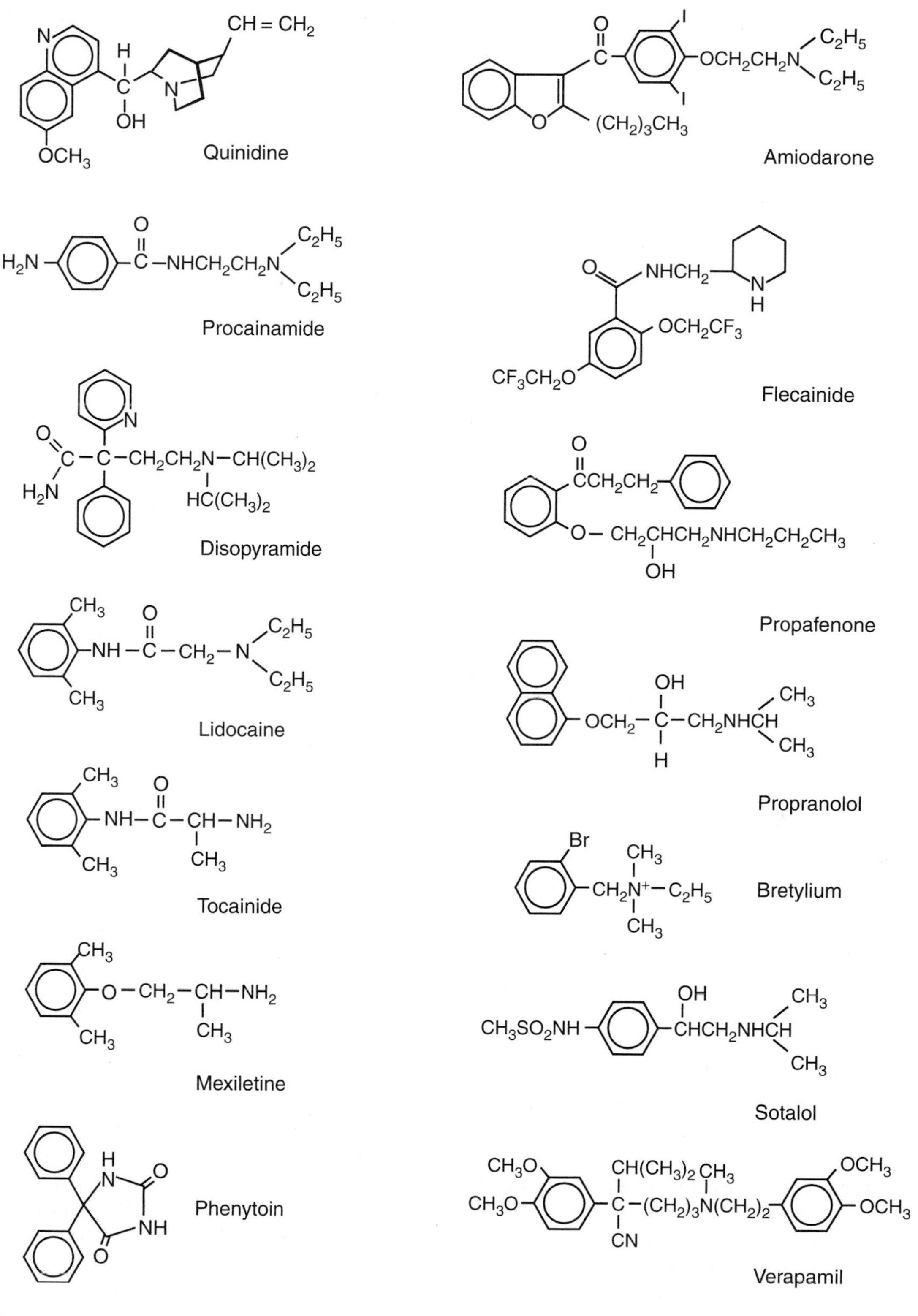

| TABLE 33-2 | Classification of Anti-arrhythmic Drug Action | |
|---|---|---|
| **Class** | **Predominant Action** | **Drugs** |
| Ia | Slowing of rate of rise of phase 0, slowing of conduction, prolongation of refractoriness | Quinidine, procainamide, disopyramide |
| Ib | Slight slowing of conduction, no change in refractoriness | Lidocaine, mexiletine, tocainide, phenytoin |
| Ic | Marked slowing of conduction, little or modest prolongation of refractoriness | Flecainide, propafenone |
| II | β-Adrenergic receptor antagonism | β Blockers (e.g., propranolol) |
| III | Prolongation of action potential duration and of refractoriness | Bretylium, amiodarone, sotalol, ibutilide, dofetilide |
| IV | Blockade of calcium entry, decrease of slope of phase 4 | Verapamil, diltiazem |

(Modified from Vaughan Williams EM. Classification of anti-dysrhythmic drugs. *Pharmacol Ther.* 1975;1:115-138, with permission.)

drugs for the treatment of recurrent, therapy-refractory ventricular tachycardia in patients with an implantable cardioverter defibrillator.

*Effects on the ECG.* Quinidine may increase the heart rate. In therapeutic concentrations, it has little effect on the PR interval, but prolongation of the QRS complex and QTc (QT interval corrected for heart rate) occurs. These effects become more pronounced with increasing plasma concentrations. (Examples of normal and abnormal ECGs are given in Figure 33-6.)

*Cardiovascular and hemodynamic effects.* Quinidine decreases myocardial contractility (negative inotropic effect). However, therapeutic concentrations of quinidine do not usually impair myocardial performance since the negative inotropism is minimal. If administered intravenously, quinidine may produce vasodilatation and marked hypotension.

*Cautions and toxicity.* With increasing plasma levels of the drug, the risk of AV block or asystole increases. Toxic concentrations may induce abnormal automaticity and ventricular tachycardia. Another type of ventricular arrhythmia may be observed in patients who exhibit excessive QT prolongation; this is known as torsades de pointes polymorphic ventricular tachycardia (see Fig. 33-6D) and may occur at therapeutic plasma concentrations of quinidine.

When administered to patients in atrial fibrillation or flutter, quinidine may occasionally cause a paradoxical increase in the ventricular rate. This is because the drug may decrease the number of atrial impulses reaching the AV node to such an extent that 1:1 conduction through the AV node becomes possible and because quinidine may shorten AV nodal refractoriness through its anticholinergic effect. In clinical practice, most patients receive digitalis preparations or β blockers before quinidine is administered in order to avoid this phenomenon.

It is important to note that quinidine can interact with other drugs. In particular, it will cause a twofold increase in serum digoxin concentration in patients at steady state as a result of decreased renal and non-renal clearance of digoxin and the displacement of digoxin from tissue binding sites by the quinidine molecule.

Gastrointestinal intolerance (nausea and diarrhea) is common, and large doses of the drug may produce cinchonism, which is characterized by a spectrum of symptoms including blurred vision, tinnitus, headache, and gastrointestinal upset. Drug fever and rare idiosyncratic reactions, such as thrombocytopenia secondary to antiplatelet antibodies, have also been reported.

## Procainamide

*Pharmacokinetics.* Procainamide is more than 75% bioavailable after oral administration. The intravenous preparation is relatively frequently used but can cause hypotension if rapidly administered. Procainamide has a relatively short half-life of 2 to 3 hours. Like quinidine, procainamide blocks $Na^+$ entry and slows conduction in myocardial tissue.

A variable proportion of the drug is acetylated in the liver to N-acetylprocainamide (NAPA). NAPA, unlike the parent drug, has little effect on $\dot{V}_{max}$ of Purkinje fibres but prolongs the duration of the action potential, thus having the properties of class III drug action. The concentration–response relationship for NAPA is different from that for procainamide; it is therefore not useful to add the concentrations of the parent drug and its metabolite when using plasma level monitoring to estimate drug effect.

The NAPA metabolite is eliminated primarily via the kidneys. Hence, the patient's acetylation status (see Chapter 10) and renal function will be important in determining the plasma concentration at steady state, and dosages will need to be adjusted in renal failure.

*Anti-arrhythmic effects.* The anti-arrhythmic properties of procainamide are similar to those of quinidine; it has comparable effects on automaticity, excitability, responsiveness, and conduction. This results in **electrocardiographic features** *similar to those of quinidine,* at both therapeutic and toxic plasma concentrations.

In clinical practice, intravenous procainamide is still relatively frequently used for the termination of hemodynamically stable ventricular tachycardia. It can also be used for the acute conversion of atrial fibrillation with WPW syndrome or for the conversion of other forms of atrial fibrillation. Oral procainamide is used only in combination with class III anti-arrhythmic drugs for the treatment of recurrent, therapy-refractory ventricular tachycardia in patients with an implantable cardioverter defibrillator.

*Hemodynamic properties.* Procainamide is comparable to quinidine in its minimal negative inotropic effects at usual oral clinical doses. Intravenous administration may produce vasodilatation and hypotension in addition to more marked negative inotropism.

*Cautions and toxicity.* Excessive concentrations of procainamide markedly impair conduction, which may result in asystole or the induction of ventricular arrhythmias. Hypersensitivity reactions include occasional drug fever and, rarely, agranulocytosis. A more common and troublesome reaction is the development of a syndrome resembling systemic lupus erythematosus (SLE), which presents with arthralgia, fever, and pleural–pericardial inflammation. The drug-induced SLE may be accompanied by LE cells in the blood smear. An anti-nuclear factor is often present in the blood of patients receiving procainamide and is not by itself diagnostic of the SLE syndrome. This syndrome usually disappears on withdrawal of the drug, although cases of persistent SLE have been reported following procainamide therapy. The SLE phenomenon is dose- and time-related and is more likely to occur in patients who exhibit slow hepatic acetylation resulting in higher plasma drug concentrations of the parent compound.

Rare CNS side effects include depression, hallucinations, and psychosis, but gastrointestinal intolerance is less frequent than with quinidine.

## Disopyramide

*Pharmacokinetics.* As 50% or more of orally ingested disopyramide is excreted unchanged by the kidneys, the dosage will require downward adjustment in renal insufficiency. Approximately 30% of the drug is converted by the liver to the less active mono-*N*-dealkylated metabolite.

*Anti-arrhythmic effects.* Disopyramide has properties similar to those of quinidine in that it slows the rate of rise of phase 0 ($\dot{V}_{max}$) of the action potential and causes a concentration-dependent decrease in the slope of phase 4 depolarization. Disopyramide also slows the rate of discharge of the sinus node and may cause serious bradyarrhythmias in patients with pre-existing sinus node dysfunction.

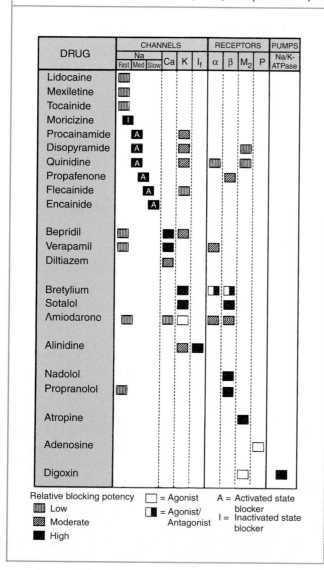

**FIGURE 33-5** Summary of the most important actions of drugs on cardiac electrical activity. Sodium-channel block is divided into fast, medium, and slow according to the kinetics of its development and dissipation and results in little, modest, or marked QRS prolongation at ordinary sinus rates, respectively. Agonists are shown as open squares and antagonists as filled squares. Bretylium has initial agonist action (noradrenaline release) followed by antagonism of α and β receptors. Note that, for simplicity, α and β receptor subtypes are not separated out in this scheme. α = α-adrenergic receptor; β = β-adrenergic receptor; M₂ = muscarinic receptor; P = purinergic receptor. (Adapted from Rosen and Schwartz, 1991, with permission.)

| TABLE 33-3 | Pharmacokinetics of Anti-arrhythmic Drugs | | | | | | |
|---|---|---|---|---|---|---|---|
| Drug | Bio-availability (%) | $V_d$ (L/kg) | Protein Binding (%) | Half-Life (hours) | Therapeutic Range | Biotransformation and Excretion | Metabolites |
| Quinidine | 75 | 2–3 | 75–90 | 4–8 | 2–6 µg/mL (7.3–21.9 µmol/L) | Liver: 80% Kidney: 10–20% unchanged | Hydroxyquinidine, slight activity |
| Procainamide | 75–95 | 1.5–2.5 | 15–25 | 2–4 | 4–10 µg/mL (17–42.5 µmol/L) | Liver: acetylation Kidney: 60% unchanged | N-acetylprocainamide (NAPA): class III activity |
| Disopyramide | 90 | 0.5–1.5 | 35–95 | 6–9 | 2–5 µg/mL | Liver: 25–35% inactive compound Kidney: 50% unchanged | N-dealkyl disopyramide, less active than parent compound |
| Lidocaine | — | 1–2 | 65–75 | 0.3–2 | 1.5–5 µg/mL (5.7–21.3 µmol/L) | Liver: 90% dealkylated | Monoethylglycylxylidine (MEGX), glycine xylidine (GX): relatively inactive |
| Mexiletine | 90 | 5–9 | 75 | 9–12 | 0.5–2 µg/mL | Liver: 90% Kidney: 10% unchanged (↑ with acid urine) | Inactive |
| Tocainide | 100 | 2–3 | 2–22 | 11–15 | 4–10 µg/mL | Liver: 60% Kidney: 40% unchanged | Inactive |
| Phenytoin | Variable | 0.5–1 | 90 | 18–36 | 10–20 µg/mL (39.6–79.2 µmol/L) | Liver: 95% hydroxylated to inactive compound | Inactive |
| Flecainide | 95 | 9 | 50 | 14–50 | 200–1000 ng/mL (0.42–2.11 µmol/L) | Liver: >95% | Inactive |
| Propafenone | 5–12 dose-dependent | 3 | >95 | 3–5 | 500–1000 ng/mL | Liver: >99% genetic variation in biotransformation | 5-OH propafenone: active |
| Propranolol | 25–50 | 3–4 | 85–95 | 3–6 | 50–100 ng/mL (0.19–0.39 µmol/L) | Liver: high first-pass extraction | 4-OH propranolol: slight activity |
| Bretylium | 15–30 | 5–6 | <10 | 6–10 | 0.5–1.5 µg/mL | Kidney: 80% unchanged | None |
| Amiodarone | 20–50 | Very large | Probably high | 20–50 days | 0.5–3 µg/mL | Liver: de-ethylation | Desethyl amiodarone (DEA): active |
| Sotalol | >95 | 1.5 | Negligible | 13 | 1–2 µg/mL (3.7–7.4 µmol/L) | Kidney: 100% unchanged | None |
| Ibutilide | — | 9–13 | 40 | 6 | NA | Liver: 75% | α-Hydroxy: active Other 8 metabolites: inactive |
| Dofetilide | >90% | 3–4 | 60–70 | 7–10 | 0.5–6 ng/mL | Kidney: 70% unchanged Liver: 30% | None |
| Verapamil | 15–30 | 4–5 | 90 | 3–7 | ≈ 100 ng/mL | Liver: high first-pass extraction | Norverapamil: moderately active |

In clinical practice, disopyramide is now only very rarely used; its main use is for the treatment of supraventricular tachycardias in patients without structural heart disease. The **electrocardiographic features** are similar to those of quinidine and procainamide.

*Hemodynamic effects.* In comparison with quinidine and procainamide, disopyramide exerts a marked *negative inotropic effect* and may produce clinically important decreases in myocardial contractility and cardiac output in patients with pre-existing impairment of left ventricular

| TABLE 33-4 | Pharmacological Mechanisms, Effects, and Toxicity of Anti-arrhythmic Agents | | | |
|---|---|---|---|---|
| **Drug** | **Anti-arrhythmic Effects** | **ECG** | **Hemodynamic Properties** | **Toxicity** |
| Quinidine (class Ia) | ↓ Rate of rise, phase 0 ($\dot{V}_{max}$); ↓ slope, phase 4; prolongs ERP, but modest effect on APD | → or ↑ HR ↑ PR ↑ QRS ↑ QT | Minimal negative inotropism; vasodilatation; decreased blood pressure (IV) | Impaired conduction/ bradycardia; ventricular arrhythmias; gastro-intestinal intolerance; cinchonism; thrombocytopenia; drug fever |
| Procainamide (class Ia) | (Similar to quinidine) Decreased normal automaticity; abolishes re-entry by producing bidirectional block | → or ↑ HR ↑ PR ↑ QRS ↑ QT | Minimal negative inotropism; vasodilatation (IV) | Impaired conduction and ventricular arrhythmias; gastrointestinal intolerance; agranulocytosis; drug-induced systemic lupus erythematosus |
| Disopyramide (class Ia) | (Similar to quinidine) | ↑ HR ↑ PR ↑ QRS ↑ QT | Marked negative inotropism; vasoconstriction | Anticholinergic effects: dry mouth, constipation, urinary retention, blurred vision; ventricular arrhythmias |
| Lidocaine (class Ib) | ↓ Rate of rise, phase 0; ↓ slope, phase 4 depolarization; shortens APD and ERP | ± ↓ QT | No impairment of normal contractility | Drowsiness, confusion, irritability; respiratory arrest; convulsions |
| Mexiletine (class Ib) | Abolishes abnormal automaticity | → or ↓ QT | Minimal or no impairment of contractility | Gastrointestinal disturbance; dizziness; ataxia; tremor |
| Tocainide (class Ib) | Abolishes re-entry by producing bidirectional block | | | |
| Phenytoin (class Ib) | | ↓ QT | Decreased blood pressure (IV) | Nystagmus; ataxia; lethargy; gastrointestinal intolerance |
| Flecainide (class Ic) | Marked ↓ $\dot{V}_{max}$ | ↑ PR ↑ QRS | Moderate depression of contractility | Weakness; dizziness; proarrhythmia (due to marked conduction slowing) |
| Propafenone (class Ic) | Marked ↓ $\dot{V}_{max}$ slight ↑ ERP | ↑ PR ↑ QRS → or ↑ QT | Moderate depression of contractility | Dizziness; altered taste; proarrhythmia |
| Propranolol (and other β blockers) (class II) | ↓ Slope, phase 4; competitive β-adrenergic receptor blockade; abolishes catecholamine-dependent arrhythmias | ↓ HR | Negative inotropism; decreased blood pressure | Impaired AV conduction/bradycardia; bronchospasm; fatigue; insomnia |
| Amiodarone (class III, with class I, II, and IV properties) | Prolongs APD and ERP; ↓ $\dot{V}_{max}$ (slowed conduction); Ca²⁺ channel block; prolongs refractoriness of the AV node; non-competitive β-adrenergic receptor blockade; diminishes normal automaticity; abolishes re-entry by producing bidirectional blockade | ↓ HR ↑ QT | No impairment of normal contractility; decreased blood pressure and increased coronary blood flow (IV) | Photosensitivity; skin pigmentation changes; neurologic abnormalities; gastrointestinal symptoms; thyroid and liver function abnormalities; corneal microdeposits; infrequent pulmonary toxicity |
| Sotalol (class III) | ↓ Slope, phase 4; β-adrenoceptor blockade; ↑ APD; ↑ ERP | ↓ HR ↑ QT | Negative inotropism Decreased blood pressure | Fatigue, lethargy; proarrhythmia (torsades de pointes) |
| Ibutilide (class III) | Prolongs APD and ERP | ↑ QT → or ↓ HR | None | Proarrhythmia (torsades de pointes) |
| Dofetilide (class III) | Prolongs APD and ERP | ↑ QT | None | Proarrhythmia (torsades de pointes) |
| Verapamil, diltiazem (class IV) | ↓ Slope, phase 4; ↑ refractoriness of AV node; diminishes normal automaticity; abolishes re-entry by producing bidirectional blockade | ↑ PR | Negative inotropism; vasodilatation; decreased blood pressure | Impaired conduction/bradycardia; gastrointestinal intolerance; constipation (verapamil) |

APD = action potential duration; ERP = effective refractory period; HR = heart rate; PR, QRS, QT = respective ECG intervals; → = remains the same; ↑/↓ = increase/decrease.

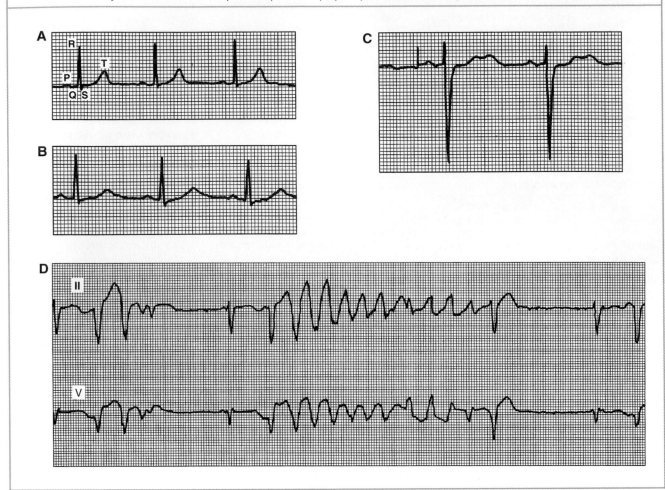

FIGURE 33-6    Illustrative electrocardiogram (ECG) tracings. (A) Normal ECG, showing the P–QRS–T complex (PR interval = 150 ms; QRS duration = 80 ms; QT interval = 410 ms). (B) Prolonged QT interval of 600 ms as seen following a drug with class III anti-arrhythmic action. (C) First-degree AV block (PR interval = 210 ms), QRS prolongation (QRS duration = 135 ms), and QT prolongation (QT interval = 650 ms). These are typical ECG features of amiodarone therapy, which has class I (QRS-prolonging), class III (QT-prolonging), and class IV (calcium-channel blocking, PR-prolonging) activity. Note also the sinus bradycardia (50 bpm) typical of a drug with antiadrenergic activity (class II). (D) Polymorphic ventricular tachycardia with QT prolongation. Note the underlying bradycardia with wide complex escape after a pause. The QT intervals after pauses are greater than 700 ms, and the coupling interval from the QRS to the first beat of ventricular tachycardia is 700 ms. This "pause-dependent" polymorphic ventricular tachycardia is termed "torsades de pointes."

function. This property limits the usefulness of the agent in patients with a history of congestive heart failure.

*Cautions and toxicity.* Most of the side effects seen with disopyramide relate to its anticholinergic activity (e.g., dry mouth, urinary hesitancy or retention, blurred vision, and constipation). *As with quinidine, patients who demonstrate an excessively prolonged QT interval with disopyramide are at risk of developing ventricular arrhythmias related to the therapy itself.* In addition, when disopyramide is used as the sole agent in the management of atrial fibrillation, it may produce an increase in the ventricular rate by a mechanism similar to that described for quinidine.

## Class Ib Drugs

### Lidocaine

*Pharmacokinetics.* Lidocaine is given intravenously because extensive first-pass transformation by the liver prevents the attainment of clinically effective plasma concentrations by the oral route. The drug is dealkylated and eliminated almost entirely by the liver, so dosage adjustments are necessary in the presence of hepatic disease or dysfunction.

*Anti-arrhythmic effects.* Lidocaine causes a reduction in $(\dot{V}_{max})$ (phase 0) of the action potential. It also shortens the duration of the action potential and the effective refractory period of normal Purkinje fibres and ventricular myocardial cells. The shortening effect on the action potential is greater than that on the effective refractory period, and thus the effective refractory period is lengthened relative to the action potential duration. Lidocaine has little activity on the action potential duration in atrial tissue.

Sinus node function is not altered in normal subjects but may occasionally be depressed in patients with pre-existing dysfunction. Unlike quinidine, lidocaine is capable of suppressing abnormal automaticity in conditions such as digitalis excess. Lidocaine abolishes ventricular re-entry by a mechanism similar to that for quinidine (see Fig. 33-3, example B). The drug slows conduction most in diseased (hypoxic or ischemic) tissues and at high rates of stimulation ("use-" or frequency-dependent effect). Lidocaine, in theory, would be especially useful in treating ventricular arrhythmias arising during myocardial ischemia, such as during myocardial infarction, and it has been used extensively in this setting. However, *although lidocaine is of proven benefit in preventing ventricular fibrillation early after myocardial infarction, there is no evidence that it reduces (and it may even increase) mortality in this setting.*

In current clinical practice, lidocaine is no longer used for the prevention of ventricular fibrillation in acute myocardial infarction. It is still occasionally used as an alternative treatment to amiodarone in therapy-refractory, recurrent ventricular fibrillation, especially in the setting of acute myocardial infarction. Although evidence does not support its efficacy, it is also used for the termination of hemodynamically stable ventricular tachycardia. It has little effect on atrial or AV junctional arrhythmias.

*Effects on the ECG.* Lidocaine has minimal effects on the ECG, although shortening of the QT interval is occasionally seen.

*Hemodynamic effects.* In clinical practice, lidocaine does not impair left ventricular function and has little or no negative inotropic effect. Unlike class Ia drugs, lidocaine does not alter autonomic function.

*Toxicity.* CNS side effects predominate; drowsiness, slurred speech, paresthesias, agitation, and confusion are most common. These symptoms may progress to convulsions and respiratory arrest (compare with cocaine, Chapter 26) if higher plasma concentrations of the drug develop.

## Mexiletine

*Pharmacokinetics.* Mexiletine is an orally effective structural analogue of lidocaine. It is well absorbed and biotransformed by the liver to inactive metabolites; the half-life is relatively long (about 12 hours).

*Anti-arrhythmic effects.* The drug has electrophysiological effects similar to those of lidocaine, shortening the action potential duration in normal tissues but slowing conduction, especially in diseased tissues. Mexiletine also suppresses abnormal automaticity in Purkinje fibres. Like lidocaine, it is effective in the treatment of ventricular arrhythmias and relatively ineffective for atrial or AV junctional arrhythmias.

In current clinical practice, mexiletine is only used in combination with class III anti-arrhythmic drugs for the treatment of recurrent, therapy-refractory ventricular tachycardia in patients with implantable cardioverter defibrillator.

*Effects on the ECG.* Mexiletine has minimal effects on the ECG.

*Hemodynamics.* Very little negative inotropic effect is seen, and the drug can be given to patients with significant left ventricular dysfunction.

*Toxicity.* Gastrointestinal (nausea, anorexia) and CNS side effects (tremor, ataxia, dizziness, diplopia, insomnia, confusion) are common and respond to a decrease in dose. As with lidocaine, drug-induced arrhythmias are uncommon.

## Tocainide

Tocainide is another oral analogue of lidocaine with a very similar profile of electrophysiological effects and clinical efficacy to that of lidocaine.

It is well absorbed and has high systemic bioavailability, with a half-life of approximately 12 hours.

Side effects are similar to those of lidocaine and mexiletine, but the drug can, on rare occasions, cause agranulocytosis.

In clinical practice, although it is still available, it is no longer recommended.

## Phenytoin

This drug is described in greater detail as an anti-epileptic agent in Chapter 18 (see also Table 33-3).

*Anti-arrhythmic effects and ECG.* The anti-arrhythmic properties of phenytoin generally resemble those of lidocaine. Phenytoin shortens the QT interval in the ECG.

In clinical practice, this drug is rarely used as an anti-arrhythmic agent in adults, with the possible exception of the treatment of rhythm disturbances secondary to digitalis overdose. It is more often used in children with ventricular arrhythmias.

*Hemodynamic effects.* As with lidocaine, clinically useful doses of phenytoin produce little or no alteration in left ventricular function.

## Class Ic Drugs

### Flecainide

*Pharmacokinetics.* Flecainide has a long half-life of 16 to 20 hours after oral administration; it undergoes partial biotransformation to inactive metabolites. Both the unchanged parent drug and the metabolites are eliminated renally.

*Anti-arrhythmic effects.* The drug is a potent suppressant of $\dot{V}_{max}$ in Purkinje and myocardial fibres, causing marked slowing of conduction in all cardiac tissues with relatively small and variable effects on action potential duration and refractoriness. Automaticity is reduced by an elevation in threshold potential rather than a decrease in the slope of phase 4 depolarization. Like other class Ic agents, the drug is effective in a wide variety of atrial, AV nodal, and ventricular arrhythmias. It is a particularly potent suppressant of premature ventricular contractions ("PVC killer") and is highly effective in slowing conduction over accessory atrioventricular bypass tracts in the WPW syndrome. It is also effective in restoring and maintaining sinus rhythm in cases of atrial fibrillation. In atrial tissues, there is a more marked prolongation of refractoriness.

In current clinical practice, it is only used in patients without structural heart disease. It is widely used for the acute conversion of atrial fibrillation and for the chronic maintenance of sinus rhythm. It is also frequently used for the chronic treatment of paroxysmal supraventricular tachycardia. With rare exceptions, it is no longer used for the treatment of ventricular arrhythmias.

*Effects on the ECG.* Flecainide causes a dose-dependent increase in PR and QRS intervals; QTc intervals are little changed. QRS intervals may increase by up to 50%, and excessive increases appear to be associated with drug toxicity.

*Hemodynamic effects.* Flecainide has negative inotropic effects and can cause worsening of congestive heart failure, especially in patients with severe pre-existing left ventricular dysfunction.

*Toxicity.* The most common side effects include dizziness, blurred vision, headache, and nausea. Like other drugs with class Ic action, *flecainide can cause a severe worsening of pre-existing arrhythmias or de novo appearance of life-threatening ventricular tachycardia resistant to treatment. In patients with frequent PVCs following myocardial infarction, although flecainide is effective in suppressing PVCs, it increases mortality compared with placebo.* For this reason, flecainide is contraindicated in patients with coronary artery disease or other structural heart disease.

### Propafenone

*Pharmacokinetics.* Propafenone undergoes extensive first-pass transformation to a hydroxylated metabolite with reduced electrophysiological effects. The clearance is dose-dependent, and higher doses exhibit lower clearance and prolonged half-life; clearance is impaired in patients with liver disease.

*Anti-arrhythmic effects.* Propafenone, like flecainide, markedly slows conduction in all cardiac tissues. It also prolongs action potential duration in atrial and ventricular tissues, thus also prolonging refractoriness. It decreases the slope of phase 4 in Purkinje fibres but has little effect on sinus node automaticity. Like flecainide, propafenone is a "broad-spectrum" anti-arrhythmic that is effective in a wide variety of arrhythmias.

In current clinical practice, propafenone, similar to flecainide, is used widely for the treatment of supraventricular tachyarrhythmias in patients without structural heart disease.

*Effects on the ECG.* The drug causes an increase in all ECG intervals, including PR, QRS, QT, and QTc duration.

*Hemodynamic effects.* Negative inotropism with worsening of congestive failure is occasionally seen.

*Toxicity.* Propafenone is usually well tolerated but can cause nausea, weakness, and a metallic taste. *It may also have severe proarrhythmic effects similar to those of the other agents with class Ic properties.*

Many anti-arrhythmic drugs, of which those with primarily class I action have been the best studied, are biotransformed by the hepatic microsomal enzyme system (CYP2D6). The activity of this enzyme system is genetically determined (see Chapter 10); there may be wide differences between individuals in the rate of biotransformation and therefore in the concentration of parent drug and metabolites. The electrophysiological effect of a given dose of drug may therefore be very different between individuals due to differences in drug disposition as well as differing concentration–effect relationships at the site of drug action.

## Class II Drugs

### Propranolol (and other β-adrenergic receptor blockers, e.g., bisoprolol, metoprolol, atenolol, timolol, nadolol, acebutolol)

Although propranolol is not a potent suppressant of premature ventricular contractions, it has been shown to *reduce the incidence of sudden, presumably arrhythmic, death following myocardial infarction.* As with metoprolol and timolol, this effect may be a direct anti-arrhythmic and/or an indirect anti-ischemic effect of chronic β-adrenergic receptor blockade. β *Blockers have also been shown to reduce mortality in patients with congestive heart failure.*

This drug and other β-adrenergic receptor antagonists like it are described in greater detail in Chapter 14 (see also Table 33-3).

*Anti-arrhythmic effects.* Propranolol exerts its major anti-arrhythmic effect through competitive inhibition of β-adrenergic receptors, which also results in a relative prominence of vagal effects on the heart. Although the drug also possesses a local anaesthetic action, this property does not contribute to its role as an anti-arrhythmic agent in therapeutic doses. Propranolol decreases the slope of phase 4 depolarization of the sinus node. This action characteristically results in sinus bradycardia. In conditions where catecholamine excess is responsible for generating autonomous ectopic rhythm disturbances (e.g., pheochromocytoma and exercise-induced ventricular tachycardia), propranolol is useful in abolishing the arrhythmia.

*Hemodynamic and adverse effects.* Other properties of propranolol, its hemodynamic effects, and its toxicity are discussed in Chapter 14. In brief, the adverse cardiac effects of propranolol are generally predictable, the most important being left ventricular failure, hypotension, bradycardia, and, rarely, AV block.

## Class III Drugs

### Bretylium

*Pharmacokinetics.* Bretylium tosylate is poorly absorbed from the gastrointestinal tract and is therefore generally administered parenterally. The drug is excreted unchanged in the urine, and dosage adjustment is required in the presence of renal failure.

*Anti-arrhythmic effects.* Bretylium differs from class I anti-arrhythmic agents in that it does not slow the rise of phase 0 ($\dot{V}_{max}$) of the cardiac action potential and does not reduce the slope of phase 4 depolarization. Furthermore, therapeutic serum concentrations do not appreciably alter membrane responsiveness. The drug does, however, prolong both the duration of the action potential and the effective refractory period in Purkinje fibres.

Bretylium is generally reserved for use in life-threatening ventricular arrhythmias, especially recurrent ventricular fibrillation. However, in current clinical practice, amiodarone, being at least as efficacious with fewer side effects, has replaced bretylium for this indication.

*Effects on the ECG.* The drug reduces the sinus rate and prolongs the QT interval.

*Hemodynamic effects.* Bretylium initially displaces catecholamines from sympathetic terminals but then usually causes hypotension as a result of its adrenergic neuron-blocking action (see Chapter 14). Severe postural hypotension can be seen after prolonged administration, most commonly in patients with pre-existing impairment of left ventricular function, and it may cause or worsen congestive heart failure.

*Toxicity.* Nausea and vomiting may occur after rapid intravenous administration, and long-term oral therapy has been reported to produce painful parotid gland enlargement.

### Amiodarone

Amiodarone is a very complex and incompletely understood drug originally introduced as an anti-anginal agent. In the last decade, it became evident that the acute intravenous administration of amiodarone results in a different electrophysiological, anti-arrhythmic, and side-effect profile than chronic oral administration. For this reason, intravenous and chronic administration will be discussed separately.

*Pharmacokinetics.* Amiodarone is incompletely absorbed after oral administration. It is extensively taken up by tissues, especially fatty tissues, and has a half-life of up to 60 days after long-term administration. A large loading dose of total 15 g is generally required to maximize tissue loading. The drug is extensively de-ethylated in the liver to *N*-desethyl amiodarone, which has significant electrophysiological effects. Serum concentration of the active metabolite increases progressively for more than a year after drug initiation, if the maintenance dose is held constant. Full clinical effects may not be achieved for up to 6 weeks after initiation of chronic oral treatment, with a slower onset for some effects (increases in refractoriness) than others (slowing of AV nodal conduction).

The onset of action of intravenous amiodarone is within several hours, possibly within minutes. Elimination half-life after a single intravenous dose is 18 to 36 hours. It takes several days of continous infusion to accumulate even low levels of its active metabolite, desethyl amiodarone.

*Anti-arrhythmic effects.* The drug has complex effects and possesses class I, II, III, and IV actions. During chronic oral administration, its dominant effect is probably through prolongation of action potential duration and refractoriness, which is rate independent. It also slows cardiac conduction, acts as a calcium-channel blocker and as a weak β-adrenergic receptor blocker, and may have central antiadrenergic effects. The high iodine content of amiodarone exerts an anti-thyroid action, which may in itself have anti-arrhythmic effects.

Recent evidence suggests that intravenous amiodarone may acutely exert its effect, in part, through a profound antiadrenergic action. It reduces cardiac presynaptic noradrenaline release and increases noradrenaline metabolism, effects not seen during oral administration. It also increases AV nodal refractoriness, slowing conduction over the AV node, and it reduces conduction velocity in the atrium and ventricle.

In clinical practice, amiodarone, in spite of its unfavourable extracardiac side-effect profile, is *the most widely used anti-arrhythmic drug.* It can be used in the treatment of virtually any clinical tachyarrhythmia. Its oral administration is especially effective in the prevention of atrial fibrillation and ventricular tachycardia. Its intravenous form is widely used for the treatment of recurrent ventricular tachycardia and, recently, shock-resistant ventricular fibrillation.

*Effects on the ECG.* Amiodarone causes an increase in the QT interval and smaller increases in PR and QRS intervals. Sinus bradycardia can occur (see Fig. 33-6C).

*Hemodynamic effects.* The drug is a vasodilator and an effective anti-anginal agent. Its intravenous administration can lead to hypotension. Although it has modest negative inotropic properties, it rarely causes clinically evident hemodynamic impairment, even in patients with severe left ventricular dysfunction.

*Toxicity.* Amiodarone has a very wide spectrum of toxic effects. After use of several years' duration, more than 25% of patients will suffer limiting side effects, often requiring drug discontinuation. Some of the more common side effects include gastrointestinal intolerance, tremor, ataxia, dizziness, hyper- or hypothyroidism, corneal microdeposits (invariable) with disturbance of night vision (occasional), liver toxicity, photosensitivity, slate-grey facial discoloration, neuropathy, muscle weakness, weight loss, symptomatic bradycardia, and proarrhythmia (rare). The most dangerous side effect is pulmonary fibrosis, which occurs in 1 to 3% of patients.

## Sotalol

Sotalol is a β-adrenergic receptor blocker that also prolongs action potential duration and refractoriness in all cardiac tissues.

*Pharmacokinetics.* Sotalol has a half-life of about 12 hours after oral administration. It is eliminated largely by the kidneys, and doses need to be lowered substantially in patients with renal dysfunction.

*Effects on the ECG.* Sotalol prolongs the QT interval and causes sinus bradycardia.

*Anti-arrhythmic effects.* The drug suppresses phase 4 spontaneous depolarization and may produce severe sinus bradycardia. It also slows AV nodal conduction.

Action potential duration and refractoriness are prolonged in atrial and ventricular myocardium. The combination of β-adrenergic receptor blockade and prolongation of action potential duration may be especially effective in the prevention of sustained ventricular tachycardia.

In current clinical pratice, *sotalol is frequently used for the prevention of atrial fibrillation, even in patients with structural heart disease, especially coronary artery disease.* It is also effective in the *prevention of ventricular tachycardia,* therefore reducing the number of discharges in patients with recurrent ventricular tachycardia and implantable cardioverter defibrillator. This indication is also supported by sotalol's ability to lower the defibrillation threshold.

*Hemodynamic effects.* Significant left ventricular dysfunction can occur when sotalol is administered, especially in patients with previous left ventricular enlargement and congestive heart failure.

*Toxicity.* Fatigue, dizziness, and insomnia can occur. *Drug-induced polymorphic ventricular tachycardia can develop in patients with excessive QT prolongation,* especially if hypokalemia is present. This form of proarrhythmia is dose-dependent and is more common in women.

## Dofetilide

Dofetilide is a recently approved new anti-arrhythmic drug (in the United States) with pure class III anti-arrhythmic properties. Although initial investigations were performed with both the intravenous and oral form, only the latter is available for clinical use.

*Pharmacokinetics.* Dofetilide is well absorbed after oral administration, with an absolute bioavailability exceeding 90%. Approximately 70 to 80% of absorbed dofetilide is excreted unchanged by the kidney by an active transport mechanism. In individuals with normal renal function, the remaining 20 to 30% is metabolized by the liver to inactive metabolites, which are then excreted by the kidney. The terminal elimination half-life is 7 to 10 hours. On the basis of data from clinical trials, the dofetilide dosage must be adjusted according to the estimated creatinine clearance in order to avoid toxicity.

*Anti-arrhythmic effects.* Dofetilide is a potent selective blocker of the rapid component of the outward delayed rectifier potassium channel ($I_{Kr}$). This results in prolongation of repolarization, action potential duration, and the effective refractory period in both atrial and ventricular myocardium. This effect shows reverse use dependency; it diminishes as heart rate increases and is augmented at slow heart rates. This results in increased risk of proarrhythmia in the form of torsades de pointes ventricular tachycardia at slow heart rates and in decreased efficacy at fast heart rates.

In clinical practice, dofetilide is relatively effective in the conversion of persistent atrial flutter and fibrillation and in the maintenance of sinus rhythm. Although it does not prevent sudden death in high-risk patients with congestive heart failure or recent myocardial infarction, it proved to be safe and did not increase mortality, as opposed to class I drugs. For this reason, it is used in individuals with severe left ventricular systolic dysfunction when amiodarone has failed or has been ineffective for the treatment of atrial tachyarrhythmias.

*Effects on the ECG.* Dofetilide prolongs QT interval in a dose-dependent manner, which allows safety monitoring. It does not effect the PR and QRS intervals.

*Hemodynamic effects.* Dofetilide has a favourable hemodynamic profile. It does not significantly alter the left ventricular systolic function, even in patients with severe dysfunction. It has been shown to have a very mild negative chronotropic effect.

*Cautions and toxicity.* The main side effect of dofetilide is proarrhythmia, with an incidence of torsades de pointes polymorphic ventricular tachycardia associated with QT prolongation of 0.9 to 3.3%. To minimize this risk, dofetilide should be initiated in hospital, the dose should be adjusted according to the renal function, and it should be discontinued in the case of marked QTc prolongation. Dofetilide does not have any other significant cardiac or extracardiac side effects.

### Ibutilide
Ibutilide is a new class III anti-arrhythmic drug.

*Pharmacokinetics.* Ibutilide is available only in an intravenous formulation, as its first-pass hepatic metabolism is extensive after oral administration. It is rapidly distributed into a large volume, and its electrophysiological effects dissipate rapidly after initial intravenous administration. As a result, the onset of its effects is fast, around 30 minutes, and the risk of a ventricular proarrhythmia event is greatest within the first hour of administration. Interestingly, plasma concentrations of ibutilide have not correlated with anti-arrhythmic efficacy, only with the prolongation of the QTc interval. The half-life of ibutilide and its metabolites is 4 to 8 hours, with an average of 6 hours. It is primarily hepatically eliminated to eight metabolites. One of these metabolites is active but does not appear to contribute significantly to clinical effects.

*Anti-arrhythmic effects.* Ibutilide has the unique effect of activating a slow inward sodium channel during the plateau phase of action potentials. It also blocks the rapid component of the delayed rectifier potassium channel, leading to a class III action. These two effects lead to the prolongation of repolarization and action potential duration both in the atrium and ventricle. This effect may not exhibit significant reverse use dependence.

Clinically, it is used *to terminate acutely persistent (3 hours to 90 days' duration) atrial flutter and fibrillation.* It has higher efficacy in converting atrial flutter. It also lowers the atrial defibrillation threshold.

*Effects on the ECG.* Ibutilide prolongs the QT and QTc intervals in a dose-related manner. It does not influence the PR and QRS intervals.

*Hemodynamic effects.* Ibutilide slightly decreases the sinus rate but otherwise does not have any hemodynamical effect, even in patients with left ventricular systolic dysfunction.

*Cautions and toxicity.* The most significant adverse effect of ibutilide is proarrhythmia, in the form of torsades de pointes ventricular tachycardia. The risk of torsades is 3 to 8%, with the higher incidence in flutter. About 2% of these arrhythmias are sustained and require electrical cardioversion. Bradycardia, hypokalemia, hypomagnesemia, a history of congestive heart failure, and female gender increase the risk of torsades ventricular tachycardia. To minimize the risk, ibutilide should not be given to patients with resting QT prolongation (QTc >440 ms) or concomitantly with class Ia or class III anti-arrhythmic drugs, with the exception of amiodarone. Patients are monitored for a minimum of 4 hours following its administration. Nausea and headache are rare side effects.

## Class IV Drugs

### Verapamil, diltiazem
These drugs are described in greater detail in Chapter 34 (see also Table 33-3).

*Anti-arrhythmic effects.* Verapamil and diltiazem block the inward current carried by $Ca^{2+}$ and exert their main anti-arrhythmic action by slowing AV node conduction and prolonging its effective refractory period; therefore, they slow the ventricular response to atrial fibrillation. Phase 0 of the action potential is not altered and neither is the duration of the action potential. The slope of phase 4 depolarization is decreased, and heart rate is slightly reduced.

In clinical practice, verapamil, when given intravenously, abolishes re-entry rhythms involving the AV node, such as AV nodal re-entrant tachycardia. *Oral diltiazem and verapamil are both widely used for the prevention of paroxysmal supraventricular tachycardias. Oral and intravenous diltiazem is used for rate control in atrial fibrillation.*

*Effects on the ECG.* The PR interval may increase, but QRS duration and the QT interval are not altered.

*Hemodynamic effects.* Verapamil, and to a lesser extent diltiazem, has negative inotropic properties and may impair left ventricular performance in patients with pre-existing myocardial dysfunction. The drugs also cause peripheral vasodilatation with a resultant fall in blood pressure.

*Cautions and toxicity.* Both verapamil and diltiazem may cause bradycardia, and asystole has been reported, particularly if the drugs are used in combination with a β blocker. Side effects include gastrointestinal intolerance and constipation. Diltiazem on rare occasions may cause headache, flushing, and ankle swelling.

## Digoxin

Although extensively described in Chapter 32, some aspects of digoxin are worthy of consideration in the management of arrhythmias. Digoxin prolongs the effective refractory period and diminishes conduction velocity in Purkinje fibres while conversely shortening the refractory period in atrial and ventricular myocardial cells. Prolongation of the effective refractory period of the AV node causes PR interval prolongation in the presence of sinus rhythm and permits digoxin to control the ventricular response rate in atrial fibrillation and flutter, its most important anti-arrhythmic action. Digoxin also increases vagal activity and thus reduces the rate of discharge of the SA node. If present in toxic serum concentrations, digoxin causes increased abnormal automaticity with resulting ventricular rhythm disturbance, which may be potentiated by hypokalemia. This arrhythmia has traditionally been treated with lidocaine or phenytoin.

## Adenosine

Adenosine is a naturally occurring substance that attaches to receptors in the AV and sinus nodes. Intravenously administered adenosine is inactivated in the blood within seconds and thus has a very short duration of action. At therapeutic doses, AV nodal conduction is markedly slowed or interrupted, producing transient AV block. This makes adenosine almost universally effective for re-entrant arrhythmias that use the AV node as a portion of the circuit. Transient bradycardia, flushing, and slight hypotension may also occur, although serious side effects are rare. *This drug can be considered first-choice therapy for AV nodal and atrioventricular re-entrant arrhythmias.*

## Magnesium

Although not directly anti-arrhythmic in most models of arrhythmia, magnesium *effectively abolishes polymorphic ventricular arrhythmias that occur in the context of QT prolongation (i.e., torsades de pointes ventricular tachycardia)* such as is caused by quinidine, procainamide, sotalol, or other drugs that prolong the QT interval (e.g., disopyramide, tricyclic antidepressants, intravenous erythromycin, ter-

fenadine, or astemizole in overdose). It interferes with calcium transfer across the cell membrane and within the cell, and at high doses, it reduces heart rate, slows AV nodal conduction, and may slow intraventricular conduction.

# CLINICAL MANAGEMENT OF ARRHYTHMIAS

It is important to emphasize that no anti-arrhythmic drug, in any patient population, has been definitively shown to prolong life for any arrhythmia. Drug therapy is therefore used to treat ongoing symptoms and prevent symptomatic recurrences of arrhythmias. In the case of class I anti-arrhythmic drugs, the risk of causing proarrhythmia is frequently greater than the benefit, especially in the presence of structural heart disease, except in exceptional circumstances.

## Atrial Premature Beats

These generally do not require treatment. However, if they cause severe symptoms or are responsible for initiating paroxysmal atrial arrhythmias, they can be suppressed with β blockers or class Ia or class Ic agents (Table 33-5).

## Atrial Fibrillation and Flutter

In the acute state, sinus rhythm may be restored by means of electrical cardioversion. Alternatively, drugs with class Ic, Ia, and III action may terminate the arrhythmia. Drugs that slow conduction through the AV node, such as digoxin, verapamil, propranolol, and amiodarone, will tend to control the ventricular response and thus reduce the heart rate (see Table 33-5). Digoxin and verapamil are not useful in restoring or maintaining sinus rhythm.

## Paroxysmal Supraventricular Tachycardia

This often arises via a re-entry phenomenon using the AV node. Accordingly, drugs with AV nodal blocking properties (e.g., adenosine, verapamil) will often terminate this arrhythmia. Propafenone, flecainide, sotalol, and occasionally amiodarone have been used on a chronic basis for prophylaxis of such arrhythmias (see Table 33-5).

## Ventricular Premature Beats

Ventricular premature beats do not usually cause symptoms. There is no specific indication for treating ventricular premature beats per se in any situation. Following acute myocardial infarction, β blockers reduce mortality irrespective of the presence or frequency of ventricular premature beats. Although there is evidence that frequent ventricular premature beats late after myocardial infarc-

| TABLE 33-5 | Therapeutic Choices for the Management of Common Arrhythmias | | | |
|---|---|---|---|---|
| | Acute | | Chronic | |
| Arrhythmia | First-Line | Alternatives | First-Line | Alternatives |
| Atrial premature beats | Usually do not require treatment | | | β Blockers |
| Atrial flutter/fibrillation | DC-cardioversion β Blocker (to control ventricular response) | Ibutilide Flecainide Propafenone Verapamil or digoxin (to control ventricular response) | Flecainide Propafenone + diltiazem or β blockers | Sotalol Amiodarone Dofetilide |
| Paroxysmal supraventricular tachycardia | Adenosine | Verapamil β Blocker | RF catheter ablation Diltiazem Verapamil β Blocker | Flecainide Propafenone Sotalol Amiodarone |
| Ventricular premature beats | Usually do not require treatment | | β Blockers | |
| Ventricular tachycardia | DC-cardioversion | Lidocaine Procainamide Amiodarone Bretylium | Implantable cardioverter defibrillator | Amiodarone Sotalol |

DC = direct current; RF = radiofrequency (catheter ablation).

tion are associated with an increased risk of subsequent sudden death from ventricular tachycardia or fibrillation, suppressing these premature beats does not reduce the risk of death.

## Ventricular Tachycardia

If this arrhythmia occurs acutely with circulatory collapse, it is treated by direct current cardioversion. In less severe cases, reversion to sinus rhythm may be accomplished by means of intravenous procainamide, lidocaine, or amiodarone. In conjunction with the implantable cardioverter defibrillator, amiodarone and sotalol are recommended for long-term control and suppression of ventricular tachycardia in patients with structural heart disease (see Table 33-5).

The treatment of ventricular tachycardia and prevention of ventricular tachycardia or fibrillation are undergoing rapid evolution. It is advisable to refer to an up-to-date textbook of cardiology or recent periodicals for further discussion.

## SUGGESTED READINGS

Gillis AM, Kates RE. Clinical pharmacokinetics of the newer antiarrhythmic agents. *Clin Pharmacokinet.* 1984;9:375-403.

Kavanagh KM, Wyse DG. Recent advances in pharmacotherapy: ventricular arrhythmias. *Can Med Assoc J.* 1988;138:903-913.

Nattel S. Antiarrhythmic drug classifications: a critical appraisal of their history, present status, and clinical relevance. *Drugs.* 1991;41:672-701.

Nattel S, Talajic M, Fermini B, Roy D. Amiodarone: pharmacology, clinical actions, and relationships between them. *J Cardiovasc Electrophysiol.* 1992;3:266-280.

Rosen MR, Schwartz PT, eds. The Sicilian Gambit. A new approach to the classification of antiarrhythmic drugs based on their actions on arrhythmogenic mechanisms. *Circulation.* 1991; 84:1831-1851.

Singh BN. Current antiarrhythmic drugs: an overview of mechanism of action and potential clinical utility. *J Cardiovasc Electrophysiol.* 1999;10:283-301.

# 34

# Vasodilators and the Pharmacological Treatment of Hypertension

## RI OGILVIE

## CASE HISTORY

A 48-year-old man who was overweight, weighing 90 kg (198 lb.) with a BMI of 29, decided to begin an exercise program. In an initial exercise test at the gym, his systolic blood pressure rose from 148 mmHg to 210 mmHg after 10 minutes on the treadmill, and he was told to see his family physician for medical clearance. He was symptom-free, except for nocturia once a night for several years. On physical examination, his fundi showed only slight arteriolar narrowing, without arteriolar-venous crossing changes, hemorrhages, or exudates. His chest and heart sounds were normal. His abdomen was obese, with a waist circumference of 109 cm (ideally <96 cm), but without enlargement of the liver or spleen. His peripheral pulses were full and equal, and there were no bruits over major vessels. His ECG was normal. A random urinalysis was normal, with a microalbumin/creatinine ratio of 1:8. His serum electrolytes, creatinine, uric acid, and sTSH were normal. His fasting blood sugar was 6.3 mmol/L (normal 4 to 6.5 mmol/L), and a two-hour post-lunch value of 8.4 mmol/L (normal <8.5 mmol/L) was found. His fasting LDL cholesterol was 3.5 mmol/L, with an HDL cholesterol of 0.9 mmol/L (ideally >1.2 mmol/L), and triglycerides of 2.5 mmol/L (ideally <2 mmol/L). His office blood pressure was 148/90 mmHg at the first visit and varied between 138 to 150 mmHg systolic and 85 to 92 mmHg diastolic in the subsequent four visits over a 2-month period.

The physician confirmed the need for a regular physical activity program, including a gradual increase in activity and time at the gym, as well as brisk walks for 20 to 30 minutes each day, in addition to caloric restriction and weight loss. The aim was to overcome the cardiovascular risks associated with the "metabolic syndrome" of abdominal obesity, borderline increased blood sugars, low HDL cholesterol, and hypertriglyceridemia combined with an elevated blood pressure. Six months later, the patient had reduced his weight to 82 kg, but his office blood pressure was consistently at 144/92 mmHg. He was started on hydrochlorothiazide 12.5 mg/day, but this was increased to 25 mg/day 3 months later as his pressure was still above 135/85 mmHg. He developed a red painful swollen joint in his foot and an elevated serum uric acid. Acute gout was diagnosed and treated with a short course of a non-steroidal anti-inflammatory drug. The hydrochlorothiazide was stopped and perindopril was started at 4 mg/day. The gout did not recur, and the serum uric acid returned to normal. An increase in the dose of perindopril to 8 mg was required to reduce both the office and self-determined blood pressures to less than 135/85 mmHg.

A few years later, in his mid-fifties, he was given increased work responsibilities, and his time commitment increased. He had gradually abandoned his physical activity program and had regained some of his lost weight. He admitted to drinking a half-bottle of wine plus a cocktail each evening. His blood pressure was more often high, with an average of 145/95 mmHg in the doctor's office. However, he was reluctant to add more medication since his self-determined blood pressures at home were often around 132/85 mmHg. A 24-hour ambulatory blood pressure monitor record confirmed poor control, averaging 138/89 mmHg during the day and 125/85 mmHg at night. The target would be less than 135/85 mmHg during the day (<130/80 mmHg for a diabetic) and less than 120/80 mmHg during the night. A dihydropyridine calcium blocker, amlodipine, was added to the perindopril. The dose of amlodipine was gradually raised from 2.5 to 10 mg/day before the target blood pressure was achieved. The patient was able to increase his physical activity and reduce his alcohol intake to less than 1/3 bottle of wine a day. As part of an educational program, his physician emphasized the increased risk for an adverse cardiac or cerebral vascular event associated with the patient's profile. He reiterated the need for dietary modification and annual monitoring of fasting blood sugar and lipid profile. He predicted that unless weight control and adherence to antihypertensive medications were maintained, the patient would develop type 2 diabetes mellitus and/or worsened dyslipidemia requiring pharmacological management.

# INTRODUCTION

Systemic hypertension accounts for a large proportion of visits to a practitioner's office. In Canada, the overall prevalence of hypertension is 10 to 15%, but by 60 years of age, the prevalence rises to 30 to 40%. Non-drug treatments such as weight control, salt restriction, reduced alcohol use, smoking cessation, and avoidance of drugs that increase blood pressure (such as oral contraceptive agents, non-steroidal anti-inflammatory agents, or nasal vasoconstrictors) are used as preventive measures and as adjuncts to drug treatment. However, the majority of hypertensive patients require antihypertensive medication to achieve blood pressure control. Over the past decade, threshold blood pressure values for initiating treatment and the target blood pressure values for control have decreased for some conditions. For example, it is recommended that diabetic patients have blood pressures below 130/80 mmHg to reduce endpoints such as renal failure, myocardial infarction, and cerebrovascular infarction or hemorrhage. Such patients often require more than one antihypertensive drug to achieve the target blood pressure. Hypertension can be considered a model disease state for application of clinical pharmacological principles of therapy. The treating physician must understand the pathophysiological process underlying the hypertensive state in an individual patient, assess the presence of associated conditions and target organ damage in that patient, then initiate, monitor, and continuously modify appropriate therapy using knowledge of drug effects, both beneficial and adverse.

Hypertension does not cause symptoms unless there are associated conditions or target organ damage involving the eyes, brain, heart, or kidneys. In most individuals, a diagnosis is made by documenting blood pressures above a threshold value that is usually established as a pressure above which treatment would benefit the individual by preventing premature target organ damage or death. However, the benefit of treatment must outweigh the risk of treatment. The risks of a treatment include all of the possible adverse drug effects in the patient being treated. When considering a population of hypertensive patients, the economic costs of the treatment versus the costs of not treating the condition may also be involved in treatment decisions.

The cause of hypertension is unknown for most hypertensive individuals and involves a complex interplay of genetic and environmental factors. Perhaps less than 5% have hypertension secondary to other disorders such as renal parenchymal disease, including chronic glomerulonephritis or pyelonephritis; renal failure associated with diabetes; renal artery stenosis with augmented renin–angiotensin–aldosterone production; or endocrine causes, including adrenal medullary pheochromocytoma with excess catecholamine release and adrenal cortical hyperplasia or adenomas with excess corticosteroid or aldosterone production. Hypertension may be modified by interventions such as dialysis and control of circulating volume in chronic renal disease, but antihypertensive drugs are usually also required. Drug therapy is also required before other interventions, such as angioplasty for renal artery stenosis or surgical removal of an adrenal adenoma or pheochromocytoma.

Blood pressure is a product of cardiac output and systemic vascular resistance. Increased blood pressure can result from a persistent increase in cardiac output (due to increases in heart rate or myocardial contractility), reduced peripheral venous capacitance, or increased circulating blood volume. Normally, homeostatic mechanisms such as baroreflex-induced bradycardia and renal diuresis operate to reduce circulating volume and blood pressure towards normal values. Most individuals with increased blood pressure have elevated peripheral vascular resistance. In younger individuals, hypertension is associated with a greater increase in diastolic than systolic pressure, and the term *diastolic hypertension* is applied. Diastolic blood pressure reflects the state of arteriolar constriction. The cause for excess arteriolar constriction in the absence of other conditions, such as hormonal excess, renal parenchymal disease, or renal artery stenosis outlined previously, is unknown at present. Arteriolar vasodilators have been developed to counter mechanisms involved in arteriolar smooth muscle constriction. Examples include drugs that block the effects of angiotensin, the sympathetic nervous system, or the calcium channel of the smooth muscle contractile system, or that donate nitric oxide to that system, or drugs that cause vasodilatation by some direct effect on vascular smooth muscle. Some classes of drugs such as diuretics or β-adrenergic receptor blocking agents are used as antihypertensive agents without complete knowledge of the mechanism involved in their effect.

With increasing age, hypertension is associated with larger increases in systolic blood pressure. If both the systolic and diastolic pressures are elevated, the term *combined systolic and diastolic hypertension* is applied. In many individuals, the diastolic pressure gradually decreases with age so that the difference between systolic and diastolic blood pressure, termed the *pulse pressure,* is increased to more than about 45 to 50 mmHg. When the systolic pressure is elevated and the diastolic pressure is below 90 mmHg, the term *isolated systolic hypertension* is used. The mechanisms involved in systolic hypertension are a complex interaction of increased aortic and other large conduit blood vessel stiffness, increased velocity of the forward pressure wave with each cardiac contraction, and an early return of the pressure wave reflected back from the smaller peripheral muscular arteries and arterioles. This reflected wave augments systolic blood pressure being developed by cardiac contraction, particularly if it arrives at the heart before closure of the aortic valve. In systolic hypertension, an increase in circulating volume or a reduction in heart rate can increase the cardiac stroke volume. The larger stroke volume ejected into the stiff large blood vessels can further augment systolic blood pressure.

## DRUG TREATMENT OF ESSENTIAL HYPERTENSION

The goal of antihypertensive drug therapy is to prevent or reduce target organ damage such as myocardial infarction, stroke, or renal failure and to reduce mortality from vascular events. Clinical trials have shown that the drug groups commonly used at present (diuretics, β-adrenergic blockers, angiotensin-converting enzyme (ACE) inhibitors, angiotensin receptor blockers (ARBs), and dihydropyridine calcium-channel blockers) improved outcomes compared to placebo. A drug from any one of these classes can be used to initiate antihypertensive therapy for patients without target organ damage or associated clinical conditions such as diabetes, gout, or asthma. However, in the presence of these conditions or of chronic renal disease, proteinuria, angina pectoris, myocardial infarction, congestive heart failure, or stroke, including transient ischemic attacks (TIA), treatment may begin with certain specific agents that have been proven to reduce morbidity and mortality in those situations.

Only 70% of individual patients may respond to a single drug from any of the drug classes, with an average reduction in systolic/diastolic blood pressures of 15/10 mmHg from baseline untreated values. Most patients will require combined therapy with two or more agents to achieve target blood pressure reductions. The clinician must have complete knowledge of the patient's blood pressure, associated target organ damage, other health problems, and the pharmacology of the drugs in order to choose effective combinations of drugs and develop a therapeutic plan to achieve a target blood pressure without adverse effects.

In contrast to the drug classes listed above, there is little or no evidence for long-term benefit from several classes of oral antihypertensive drugs used in the past, including direct vasodilators (hydralazine and minoxidil), centrally acting agents (reserpine, α-methyldopa, and clonidine), or peripherally acting agents inhibiting noradrenaline release from sympathetic nerve endings (guanethidine and guanadrel). Although these drugs can reduce blood pressure, their clinical use has been abandoned or limited to special situations described later in this chapter.

## DIURETICS

Diuretics (see Chapter 37) increase renal elimination of water and sodium. The mechanisms underlying their antihypertensive effect are varied and not quite clear. **Loop diuretics** such as ethacrynic acid and furosemide cause a rapid but brief diuresis and natriuresis, with a limited and brief reduction in blood pressure. They are used to control excess circulating volume in hypertensive states associated with chronic renal failure but not as antihypertensive therapy in the absence of increased plasma volume. They have a small direct vasodilator effect on arterioles, resulting from an unknown mechanism. After 8 weeks of therapy with the low doses of **benzothiadiazides ("thiazides")** and related diuretics recommended for treating hypertension, circulating plasma volume is unchanged even when maximal antihypertensive effect has been established. Perhaps a reduction in total body sodium or its distribution is partly responsible for the antihypertensive effect. Chronic administration of thiazides also reduces sympathetic nerve impulse traffic to vascular smooth muscle. No direct vasodilator effect of thiazides has been demonstrated. **Diazoxide**, a benzothiadiazine derivative resembling the thiazide diuretics but lacking a sulphonamide group, does not cause a diuresis but is a direct arteriolar vasodilator. It activates ATP-sensitive $K^+$ channels, thus causing hyperpolarization and relaxation of arteriolar smooth muscle. Its use was limited to hypertensive emergencies since oral administration causes severe hyperglycemia and water retention. Most clinicians consider diazoxide to be obsolete. **Indapamide** is an indolene with a sulphonamide group but without a thiazide ring. It has both diuretic and antihypertensive effects, but in patients with renal failure, it also lowers blood pressure without producing diuresis. Indapamide may have some calcium-channel blocking activity that causes arteriolar smooth muscle relaxation.

Thiazide diuretics, being both effective and inexpensive, are the preferred drugs of choice in the initial treatment of hypertension. They are useful in combination with other classes of drug, particularly with β blockers, angiotensin-converting enzyme (ACE) inhibitors, or angiotensin receptor blockers (ARBs). Gout is a contraindication unless the serum uric acid concentration has been reduced by allopurinol. Thiazides are not effective in patients with a serum creatinine greater than 150 mmol/L. For these patients, indapamide may be substituted for the antihypertensive effect, or loop diuretics may be used to control excess circulating plasma volume.

Although hydrochlorothiazide has a relatively short plasma half-life of 6 hours, once-a-day dosing in the morning is recommended at a dose of 25 mg or less. Indapamide (plasma half-life 25 hours) or chlorthalidone (plasma half-life 48 to 72 hours) is also used in low doses for the treatment of hypertension.

**Adverse effects** can be limited by using low doses. The dose–response curve for antihypertensive effect is relatively flat at higher doses, so higher doses produce little or no therapeutic gain but can cause electrolyte disturbances such as hypokalemia, hypomagnesemia, or hyponatremia with associated arrhythmias or cerebral disturbances. Dehydration, orthostatic hypotension, hyperuricemia, gout, hyperglycemia or frank diabetes, as well as allergic rashes, are other adverse effects. Lithium toxicity can occur in patients receiving diuretic therapy.

**Potassium-sparing diuretics** are often used to prevent the hypokalemia associated with thiazides. **Amiloride** can be used in combination tablets. Used alone, amiloride has limited diuretic or antihypertensive effect. **Triamterene** has been used to prevent the hypokalemia of thiazide therapy. Triamterene is considered obsolete as it can reduce the bioavailabilty of thiazides and can cause interstitial nephritis and tubular obstruction. **Spironolactone** and **eplerenone** are competitive antagonists of the aldosterone receptor that can be used alone or in combination with thiazides in the treatment of hypertension or congestive heart failure. Eplerenone causes gynecomastia in men and menstrual disorders in women less frequently than spironolactone does. It has far lower affinity for progesterone and androgen receptors than spironolactone. There is considerable interest in both agents in the treatment of congestive heart failure or hypertension since aldosterone antagonism favours beneficial remodelling of the left ventricle. The dose–response curve for reductions in systolic pressure is steeper than for diastolic pressure. The patient must be monitored for dose-related hyperkalemia with all of these agents. Patients with diabetes or renal failure are at increased risk.

# β-ADRENERGIC RECEPTOR BLOCKERS

**Propranolol**, a non-selective $β_{1,2}$-adrenergic receptor blocker, was initially developed for the prevention of angina. Its antihypertensive effect was discovered by serendipity, but the mechanism for this effect is unknown. Acute $β_{1,2}$-adrenergic receptor blockade in normal individuals *increases* blood pressure, as peripheral arterial resistance is increased. α-Adrenergic constrictor influence on arteriolar smooth muscle is unopposed by $β_2$-adrenergic vasodilator effects after β blockade. However, chronic oral therapy with either non-selective or cardioselective β-adrenergic receptor blockers lowers the blood pressure of hypertensive individuals. Resting cardiac output and heart rate are slightly reduced. There is a greater reduction in exercise-induced heart rate and cardiac output. Total peripheral resistance is lowered by some unknown mechanism. β Blockade does reduce renin release and may also have an undetermined effect on the central nervous system (CNS) that reduces sympathetic influence on the vasculature. However, neither of these mechanisms is likely a sufficient explanation for the antihypertensive effect. For a detailed discussion of β-adrenergic blockers, see Chapter 14.

Inter-patient variability in blood pressure response to β blockade may be explained by genetic polymorphism in $β_1$-adrenergic receptors. Polymorphism of these receptors occurs in Caucasians, Blacks, and Oriental Chinese subjects. In addition, some β blockers such as **propranolol, metoprolol,** and **timolol** are biotransformed by hepatic cytochrome P450 2D6, which is also genetically polymorphic. Some 10 to 15% of Caucasians and approximately 1% of Oriental Chinese are poor metabolizers. In general, Blacks may be less clinically responsive, while Oriental Chinese subjects may be more responsive to β blockers than Caucasians are.

## Use in Hypertension

β-Adrenergic receptor blockade is indicated for the initial therapy of hypertension and is useful in combination with other classes of drugs, particularly with diuretics, dihydropyridine calcium blockers, or $α_1$-adrenergic receptor antagonists. β Blockade is the preferred therapy for patients with hypertension and angina or with a recent myocardial infarction. It is contraindicated for patients with asthma. Elderly patients with systolic or combined systolic–diastolic hypertension may not respond with adequate reduction in systolic pressure, and long-term benefits in vascular morbidity and mortality have not been demonstrated. β-Adrenergic blockers, by reducing heart rate and diastolic filling time, may increase systolic pressure as a consequence of the resultant increased stroke volume. In systolic hypertension, use of β-adrenergic blockers is usually restricted to patients with concomitant angina or a recent myocardial infarction, for their symptomatic and cardioprotective properties. As propranolol has a short plasma half-life requiring multiple doses each day, other agents (e.g., **atenolol, bisoprolol**) have largely replaced its use in the clinic. **Metoprolol**, which is biotransformed in the liver, is used for patients with renal failure since dosing of water-soluble drugs such as atenolol or **nadolol** that are eliminated unchanged by the kidney becomes difficult to predict with renal insufficiency. Bisoprolol is about 50% eliminated unchanged by the kidney.

## Use in Angina, Post-myocardial Infarction, and Congestive Heart Failure

β-Adrenergic blockers prevent angina, reduce mortality post–myocardial infarction, and in low doses modify the symptoms and outcome of patients with congestive heart failure. Low-dose β blockade has become a major therapy of chronic congestive heart failure. **Carvedilol** (Coreg) is a non-selective β blocker that also has $α_1$-blocking activity at equal potency, so it lowers peripheral arteriolar resistance while preventing a reflex increase in heart rate. Oral carvedilol is used in congestive heart failure.

**Adverse effects** include asthma, fatigue, reduced exercise tolerance, bradycardia, heart block, congestive heart failure, cold digits, increased claudication, erectile dysfunction, and delayed recognition of hypoglycemia in diabetics.

Mental disturbances and nightmares can occur with lipid-soluble agents such as propranolol or metoprolol but less commonly with water-soluble agents such as atenolol or nadolol. A withdrawal syndrome of increased heart rate and blood pressure or precipitation of angina has occurred with abrupt discontinuation of β blockers. A tapered withdrawal is preferred for discontinuation of therapy.

# CALCIUM-CHANNEL BLOCKERS

Muscle contraction is initiated by an influx of $Ca^{2+}$, which in turn triggers the intracellular events leading to muscle contraction. Inorganic cations, such as manganese, cobalt, and lanthanum, can function as general calcium antagonists. They probably do so by substituting for calcium at a variety of binding sites, where they either block $Ca^{2+}$ channels or enter the cell and substitute for $Ca^{2+}$ at intracellular $Ca^{2+}$ receptors. Several organic calcium-channel blockers have been developed for clinical use (Fig. 34-1). These agents exert their actions at low (nanomolar) concentrations and exhibit stereospecificity; it appears likely that they are recognized by specific structures in the $Ca^{2+}$ channel. The diversity of molecular structure of the organic calcium-channel blockers is consistent with different mechanisms and sites of action. Although the therapeutic effect of dihydropyridine calcium-channel blockers such as **nifedipine, felodipine, nisoldipine,** and **amlodipine** and non-dihydropyridine blockers such as **diltiazem** and **verapamil** is the same, it appears likely that dihydropyridine-type blockers act at a different site within the $Ca^{2+}$ channel than verapamil and diltiazem do.

There is evidence of three different types of voltage-dependent $Ca^{2+}$ channels designated as L, T, and N types (see Chapter 31). The L type is large in conductance, T is transient in duration of opening, and N is exclusively neuronal in distribution. The L type is the most frequent in cardiac and smooth muscle. It is known to contain binding sites that differ for different calcium-channel blockers and has thus been interpreted as containing several different drug receptors. L-type channels are found in neurons, glandular cells, and muscle cells and are involved in excitation–contraction coupling. N-type channels appear to be limited to neuronal membranes, especially at axon terminals, where they mediate the $Ca^{2+}$ influx that triggers neurotransmitter release. This process is not sensitive to dihydropyridine-type blockers. **Mibefradil,** an agent that selectively blocks the T-type channel, was withdrawn from clinical use because of induction of serious and fatal cardiac arrhythmias, serious drug interactions, and liver toxicity.

## Effects on Smooth Muscle

Transmembrane $Ca^{2+}$ influx is responsible for normal resting tone and contractile responses in most types of smooth muscle. The calcium-channel blockers relax these cells. Although relaxation can be demonstrated in bronchial, gastrointestinal, and uterine smooth muscle, smooth muscle in vascular tissues appears to be the most sensitive. Blood pressure is thus reduced, particularly with dihydropyridine-type blockers. Reduction of coronary arterial tone has been demonstrated in patients who have coronary artery spasm.

## Effects on Cardiac Muscle

Calcium influx is particularly important for normal cardiac function. The $Ca^{2+}$-dependent action potentials occurring in the SA and AV nodes may be reduced or blocked by most of the calcium-channel blockers. Similarly, there is a reduction in excitation–contraction coupling in cardiac cells exposed to calcium-channel blockers. Cardiac contraction velocity and cardiac output may be reduced in a dose-dependent fashion by calcium-channel blockers. Thus, patients with angina may benefit by at least two mechanisms: (1) the reduction in peripheral vascular resistance, and (2) the reduction in cardiac output with an accompanying reduction in oxygen requirement.

The different calcium-channel blockers differ in the results of their interaction with $Ca^{2+}$ and $Na^+$ channels.

FIGURE 34-1 Structural formulae of drugs having calcium-channel blocking properties. Only nifedipine, diltiazem, and verapamil are used clinically for their vasodilating action based on calcium-channel blockade.

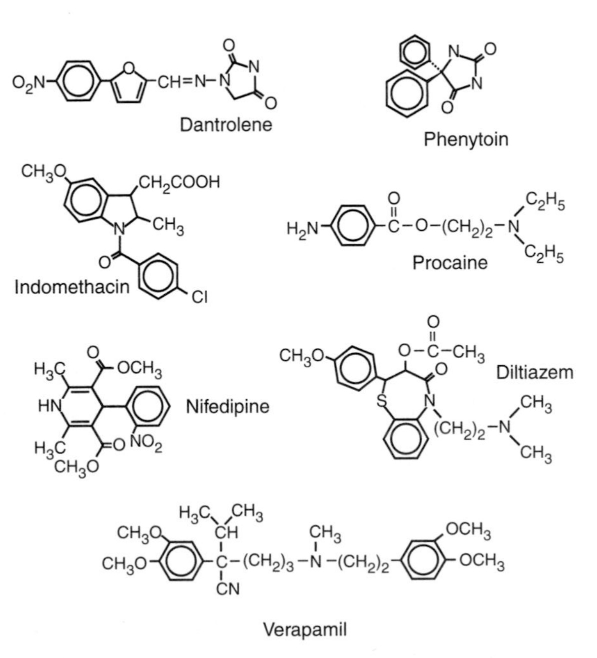

For example, $Na^+$ channels are blocked by verapamil, but less so than $Ca^{2+}$ channels; $Na^+$-channel block is much less marked with diltiazem and nifedipine. Dihydropyridines such as nifedipine block vascular smooth muscle $Ca^{2+}$ channels at concentrations below those required for cardiac $Ca^{2+}$-channel blockade. Other dihydropyridines are even more effective in their smooth muscle action than their cardiac action.

## Hemodynamic Effects

Calcium-channel blockers act preferentially on the arterial side (large conduit vessels to arterioles) rather than the venous side (venules to large veins). As a consequence, both systolic and diastolic blood pressures are reduced without an orthostatic effect. Although dihydropyridine-type blockers such as nifedipine and amlodipine reduce cardiac output in a dose-dependent manner, their effect on cardiac impedance and total peripheral resistance overrides any negative inotropic effect on the heart unless cardiac function is already impaired. Heart rate is usually slightly increased by a baroreceptor-induced reflex response to the lowered blood pressure. The increased heart rate and lowered arterial afterload result in an increased cardiac output, with venous return maintained by a lack of effect on the venous side of the circulation. In contrast, the blood pressure reduction caused by the non-dihydropyridine-type blockers results in little change or reduction in heart rate, in part by impairment of SA and AV nodal transmission and in part due to a weaker effect on blood pressure and cardiac afterload. Both diltiazem and verapamil cause a reduction in cardiac output and can induce congestive heart failure in patients with impaired left ventricular cardiac function.

## Pharmacokinetics

**Oral** or **sublingual nifedipine** has a rapid onset of action, with a large reduction in blood pressure and increase in heart rate. The magnitude is unpredictable, and there may be severe hypotension, precipitating angina pectoris, myocardial infarction, or stroke. Nifedipine has a short plasma half-life of 2.5 hours. However, **sustained-release preparations** have been developed and are preferred for clinical use in both angina and hypertension. Use of immediate-release sublingual or oral nifedipine in the treatment of hypertensive emergencies and urgencies is now considered dangerous and contraindicated. **Felodipine** is also used as a sustained-release preparation that provides a gradual onset and offset of hemodynamic effect. Regular-release preparations are used for **amlodipine**, which has a long plasma half-life of 40 hours. Dihydropyridines are substrates for hepatic CYP3A4. Felodipine therefore undergoes an extensive first-pass effect after oral administration. Bioavailabilty of felodipine, but not usually of nifedipine or amlodipine, can be increased three-to tenfold by concomitant ingestion of CYP3A4 inhibitors such as grapefruit juice.

Although non-dihydropyridine-type blockers have a more gradual onset of hemodynamic effects, the relatively short plasma half-life of 4 hours for both **diltiazem** and **verapamil** has also prompted the development of sustained-release preparations for once-per-day dosing. Metabolites produced by hepatic biotransformation are weaker vasodilators with longer half-lives.

## Coronary Blood Flow and Angina Pectoris

$Ca^{2+}$-channel blockers increase coronary blood flow by inducing coronary vasodilatation. Diltiazem and verapamil reduce myocardial oxygen requirements by their negative effect on heart rate and myocardial contractility. Dihydropyridines can decrease cardiac work by reducing cardiac afterload. β-Adrenergic blockade can enhance the anti-anginal effect of the dihydropyridine-type $Ca^{2+}$-channel blockers by reducing heart rate and contractility. However, β-adrenergic blockade is contraindicated during treatment with diltiazem or verapamil because of additive negative effects on heart rate and contractility. The non-dihydropyridine-type blockers can substitute for β-adrenergic blockade for the treatment of angina in patients who cannot tolerate β-blockade. $Ca^{2+}$-channel blockers are used in the prevention of chronic stable angina and the treatment of unstable and variant (Prinzmetal's) angina.

## Hypertension

Oral $Ca^{2+}$-channel blockers are used for the treatment of chronic systemic hypertension. Clinical trials have provided evidence that dihydropyridine-type (but not the non-dihydropyridine-type) blockers improve treatment outcome, reducing vascular morbidity and mortality. They are indicated as initial treatment of both systolic and diastolic hypertension. Combination with β blockers for added antihypertensive effect also reduces the stimulating effect of dihydropyridines on heart rate and renin release that could limit their antihypertensive effect. Combination therapy with ACE inhibitors or ARBs is also effective. Combination with a diuretic is not as effective for additional antihypertensive effect.

Adverse effects are related to vasodilatation and include dizziness, flushing, nausea, hypotension, headache, and peripheral edema, particularly with dihydropyridines. Arteriolar vasodilatation without venular dilatation causes increased capillary pressure and transudation of fluid. This is enhanced by standing and by physical inactivity and is resistant to diuretic treatment. Dihydropyridines can also cause tachycardia, arrhythmias, angina, myocardial infarction, and heart failure. Non-dihydropyridine-types can also cause heart block and congestive heart failure, as well as constipation.

## ANGIOTENSIN-CONVERTING ENZYME (ACE) INHIBITORS

The renin–angiotensin system has an important role in the regulation of blood pressure and extracellular volume (Chapter 29). Plasma and tissue ACE converts angiotensin I to angiotensin II, an octapeptide that has potent vasoconstrictor activity and stimulates release of aldosterone from the adrenal glands. In addition, angiotensin II can facilitate noradrenaline release from sympathetic nerve endings. By reducing angiotensin II formation, ACE inhibitors can lower blood pressure. ACE is also responsible for the degradation of bradykinin and related vasodilator peptides. Accumulation of these vasodilator peptides after ACE inhibition may contribute to the beneficial effects. Angiotensin II is also a potent stimulator of smooth muscle cell growth. ACE inhibition can reverse or prevent hypertrophy of the heart and arterioles that occurs with long-standing hypertension.

### Hemodynamic Effects

ACE inhibitors act primarily on the arterial side (from large conduit vessels to arterioles) of the circulation and reduce both systolic and diastolic blood pressure. Peripheral resistance and cardiac afterload are decreased with little change in cardiac output. Baroreflexes are modified so that increases in heart rate do not occur. ACE inhibition does have vasodilating effects on the venous side, but orthostatic hypotension is rare unless the patient's blood volume is depleted. Antagonism of aldosterone effect on the cerebral circulation by either ACE inhibition or angiotensin receptor blockade raises the lower limit of cerebral blood flow autoregulation so that cerebral blood flow is preserved at low blood pressures. In congestive heart failure, ACE inhibition increases peripheral venous capacitance, thus reducing venous return, central blood volume, and ventricular filling pressures and decreasing myocardial workload. ACE inhibition may have an anti-anginal effect, either through blockade of the effect of aldosterone on the coronary circulation or by a reduction in ventricular wall stress through decreased cardiac afterload and end-diastolic volumes. In individuals with or without heart failure, arteriolar dilatation and reduction in pre-capillary resistance does not cause peripheral swelling as calcium-channel blockers do. Capillary pressure does not increase since ACE inhibition lowers both pre- (arteriolar) and post-capillary (venular) resistance. In the kidney, angiotensin acts preferentially on efferent rather than afferent glomerular arterioles. As a consequence, ACE inhibition lowers intraglomerular pressure. The reduced intra-glomerular pressure initially lowers glomerular filtration rate (GFR), but it also decreases proteinuria and, in the long term, preserves renal function and may later result in increased GFR. This underlies the use of ACE inhibitors in chronic renal disease, including diabetic nephropathy.

## Pharmacokinetics

The prototype ACE inhibitor, **captopril** (Fig. 34-2), has an onset of antihypertensive effect within 20 to 30 minutes after oral or sublingual administration. The reduction in blood pressure is usually proportional to the baseline (pre-drug) pressure but can be unpredictable and augmented by volume depletion, diuretic use, or other causes of increased renin and angiotensin. The short plasma half-life of 2.5 hours requires the use of multiple doses each day. Other ACE inhibitors with a longer half-life, allowing use of a single dose each day, have replaced captopril for clinical use. Many are prodrugs (e.g., **enalapril, ramipril, perindopril, trandolapril, quinapril**) that undergo conversion in the liver to a more active metabolite (enalaprilat, ramiprilat, perindoprilat, trandolaprilat, quinaprilat, respectively). Most have a hypotensive effect that begins within 2 hours and evolves over many hours to days with daily dosing. Six to 8 weeks of therapy may be required for the maximal effect to be established. The kidney eliminates most ACE inhibitors and their active metabolites. Renal insufficiency can cause accumulation. **Fosinopril sodium** is an exception, as both the liver and kidney eliminate it. The ACE inhibitors differ widely in tissue distribution, but the clinical significance of this difference has not been established. Although there are wide differences in potency, all have a relatively steep dose–response curve at low doses but a flatter dose–response curve at higher doses.

## Clinical Uses

### Hypertension

ACE inhibitors are indicated for the initial treatment of both systolic and diastolic hypertension. There is clinical trial evidence that they reduce vascular morbidity and mortality. Their renal protective effects are beneficial for patients with diabetes or chronic renal disease, particularly in the presence of microalbuminuria or proteinuria. They can be combined with a diuretic or calcium-channel blockers for added antihypertensive effect. Combination of perindopril with indapamide has been effective in reducing the incidence of recurrent stroke.

### Post–myocardial infarction and congestive heart failure

ACE inhibition reduces morbidity and mortality after myocardial infarction and in patients with congestive heart failure, whether the patient has normal blood pressure or hypertension.

## Adverse Effects

The most common **adverse effect** of ACE inhibitors is a dry, irritating cough that can be continuous, intermittent, or nocturnal. It is probably related to the accumulation of bradykinin and related peptide mediators since

| FIGURE 34-2 | Structural formulae of drugs used to reduce peripheral vascular resistance. Calcium-channel blockers also used for this purpose are shown in Figure 34-1. |

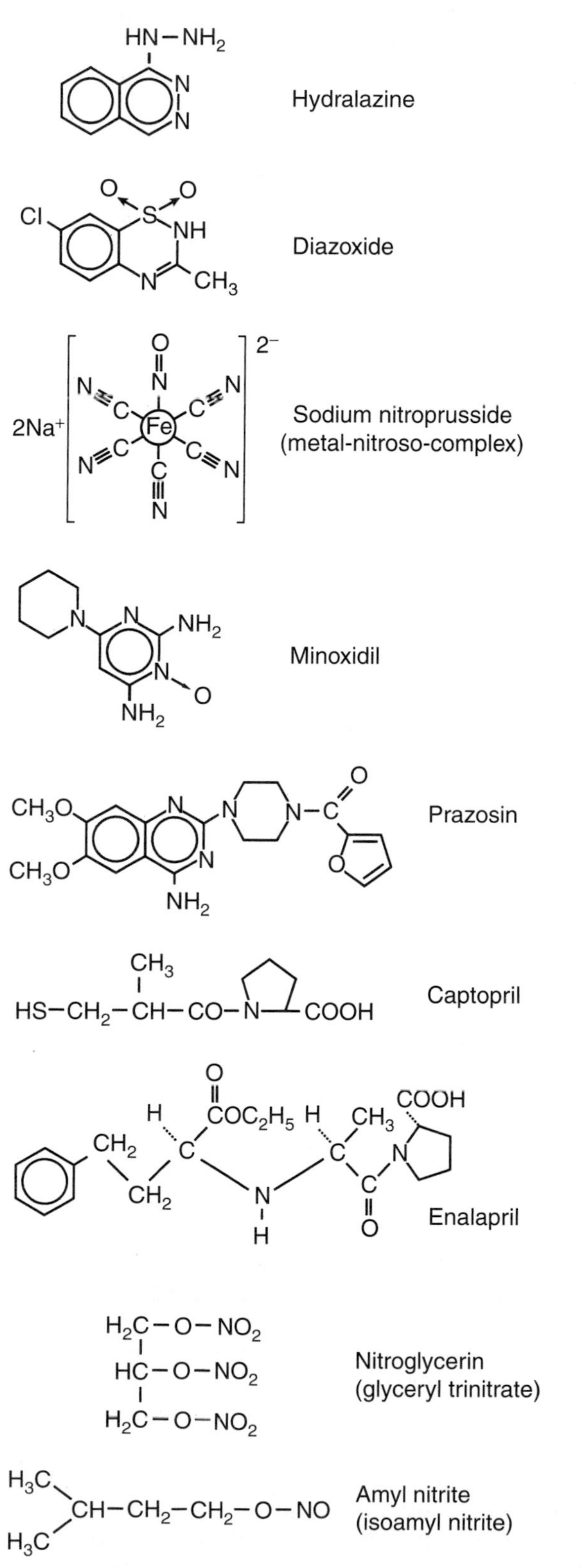

Hydralazine

Diazoxide

Sodium nitroprusside (metal-nitroso-complex)

Minoxidil

Prazosin

Captopril

Enalapril

Nitroglycerin (glyceryl trinitrate)

Amyl nitrite (isoamyl nitrite)

ARBs are not associated with a cough. There must be a genetic influence since the incidence in Caucasians is about 10%, whereas the incidence in Blacks or Oriental Chinese approaches 20 to 30%. There is no evidence that one ACE inhibitor causes less cough than another. A less common but potentially more serious adverse effect when it affects the upper airway is angioedema, with an incidence of about 0.1 to 0.7%. Blacks, but not Oriental Chinese patients, have a fivefold higher incidence than Caucasians. Again, the incidence of angioedema is far lower with ARBs but is not negligible, and cross-sensitivity may exist.

Since ACE inhibitors increase plasma renin but reduce serum aldosterone, hyperkalemia can ensue, particularly in patients with renal impairment or diabetic patients. Renal artery stenosis is accompanied by renin release and augmented angiotensin II effect on the efferent glomerular arterioles, causing increased intra-glomerular pressure and filtration. ACE inhibition can block this compensatory mechanism and reduce glomerular filtration in the under-perfused kidney. When there is bilateral renal stenosis or a solitary kidney with renal artery stenosis, ACE inhibitors can cause acute renal failure with a reversible rise in serum creatinine.

ACE inhibitors are contraindicated in the first trimester of pregnancy since they interfere with the development of the kidneys in the fetus. Like other antihypertensive agents, they can cause hypotension or skin rashes.

## ANGIOTENSIN RECEPTOR BLOCKERS (ARBs)

### Drug Action and Pharmacokinetics

**Losartan potassium** was the first of several non-peptide angiotensin II receptor blockers in clinical use. It acts as a selective competitive antagonist at AT1 receptors. However, its active metabolite EXP-3174 is a non-competitive rather than competitive antagonist at the AT1 receptor and is 10 to 40 times more active than the parent compound. Losartan itself has a short plasma half-life of 2 hours, but its metabolite has a longer half-life of 6 to 9 hours. Other ARBs (e.g., **irbesartan, candesartan cilexate, telmisartan**) have a longer plasma half-life than losartan and its metabolite. Candesartan and irbesartan, like the active metabolite of losartan, are non-competitive antagonists of the AT1 receptor. The clinical significance of these differences is unknown. The half-life of antagonism to exogenous angiotensin II in humans is about 8 hours for losartan and valsartan, about 12 hours for candesartan, and about 15 to 18 hours for irbesartan after single or repetitive doses of these drugs. As selective antagonists of the AT1 receptor, these drugs do not alter the effect of angiotensin II on AT2 receptors that are involved in tissue growth, repair, and remodelling.

Losartan and irbesartan have marked affinity for CYP2C9, CYP3A4, and CYP1A2. CYP2C9 transforms losartan to its more active metabolite. Although there are possible drug interactions with inhibitors and substrates, the clinical significance has not been established. The enzyme responsible for the metabolism of valsartan has not been identified. Candesartan cilexate is completely transformed to candesartan during absorption through the gastrointestinal tract. Candesartan is eliminated in the urine and feces. **Eprosartan** has a plasma half-life of 5 to 9 hours, and it is eliminated unchanged via urinary and biliary routes. **Telmisartan,** the most lipophilic of currently available ARBs, has a plasma half-life of 24 hours and is largely eliminated unchanged via the biliary route.

As ARBs have the same hemodynamic effects as ACE inhibitors, they are often substituted for ACE inhibitors in patients with hypertension or congestive heart failure who develop cough. Recent clinical trial evidence demonstrates a reduction in vascular morbidity and mortality in hypertensive patients treated with AT1 receptor blockers. Overall, reduction in cerebrovascular events has been greater than the reduction in cardiovascular events. Like ACE inhibitors, these drugs delay deterioration in renal function in diabetic patients with microalbuminuria or nephropathy, but they can also cause hypotension, hyperkalemia, acute renal failure in the presence of bilateral renal artery stenosis, and skin rashes. They are contraindicated during pregnancy. Lithium toxicity can occur when it is co-administered with either valsartan or diuretics. Telmisartan and digoxin are substrates for P-glycoprotein, an ATP-dependent pump that transports drugs across renal tubular cells, intestinal walls, and bile canalicular membranes. Telmisartan can increase the $C_{max}$ of digoxin, but this has not been reported to result in digoxin toxicity.

## OTHER ANTIADRENERGIC AGENTS

Several of the earliest drugs developed for the treatment of hypertension either reduce the release of noradrenaline and adrenaline from adrenergic terminals or the adrenal medulla, or they block the effect of these catecholamines on α-adrenergic receptors. Their clinical utility and use have diminished as evidence for improved morbidity and mortality has been acquired for other classes of drugs.

## CENTRALLY ACTING ANTIHYPERTENSIVE AGENTS

α-**Methyldopa** enters the CNS by an active transport process and is biotransformed to an active metabolite, α-methylnoradrenaline, that displaces noradrenaline and acts as an α2-adrenergic agonist in the brainstem, reducing sympathetic nervous discharge. Blood pressure is reduced by peripheral arteriolar dilatation without associated tachycardia. In fact, heart rate and cardiac output are reduced. Although the plasma half-life is quite short (~2 hours), its maximal blood pressure–lowering effect is not seen for 6 to 8 hours. Usually, two or three doses each day are required. **Adverse effects** include a dry mouth, fatigue, reduced mental acuity, sedation that may disappear with continued use, sodium and water retention, hepatic dysfunction, autoimmune disorders, and positive Coombs' test or anti-nuclear antibody titres. Formerly, it was used intravenously in hypertensive emergencies. However, as altered CNS function precludes assessment of intracranial events and the hypotensive effect is not predictable, other agents have replaced it for use in emergencies. Oral α-methyldopa remains the drug of choice for hypertension associated with pregnancy.

**Clonidine, guanabenz**, and **guanfacine** are agonists that stimulate α2-adrenergic receptors in the brainstem, reducing sympathetic nerve discharge and plasma noradrenaline levels. They lower blood pressure by reducing arteriolar resistance while lowering cardiac sympathetic tone and thus reducing heart rate, contractility, and output. Orthostatic hypotension can occur as a consequence of peripheral venodilatation.

**Adverse effects** include a dry mouth, fatigue, reduced mental acuity that may disappear with continued use, sodium retention, and dizziness. Sodium retention can cause loss of the blood pressure–lowering effect of these drugs ("pseudotolerance"), so concomitant use of diuretics may be required. Guanabenz may cause less sodium retention. Abrupt discontinuation can cause a withdrawal syndrome with headache, anxiety, restlessness, sweating, tachycardia, and increased blood pressure. Administration of more clonidine relieves these symptoms, and it also relieves similar symptoms produced by opioid withdrawal in opioid-dependent individuals (see Chapter 19). Large doses can cause hypertension by stimulation of α2-adrenergic receptors on peripheral arterioles, causing vasoconstriction. Clonidine is occasionally used for patients with hypertension resistant to combinations of other classes of drug or as a substitute for β blockers when vasodilators cause tachycardia.

## PERIPHERAL ADRENERGIC BLOCKERS

**Reserpine,** an alkaloid extracted from the root of the Indian shrub *Rauwolfia serpentina,* inhibits the release of noradrenaline from storage vesicles in peripheral as well as central adrenergic neurons. Decreased peripheral sympathetic activity lowers heart rate, cardiac output, vascular resistance, and blood pressure. Although cheap and effective, reserpine has many **adverse effects,** including dry mouth, nasal stuffiness, sedation, difficulty concentrating, psychotic depression, peptic ulcers, salt retention, and other effects that limit its utility.

**Guanethidine** inhibits the release of noradrenaline from peripheral sympathetic nerve endings. Its predominant effect on blood pressure is in the upright position. Increasing doses in an attempt to lower the recumbent blood pressure, or coincidental occurrence of dehydration, can cause severe orthostatic hypotension, due in part to venodilatation and reduced cardiac output. Retrograde ejaculation and diarrhea are other adverse effects of this drug.

## α-Adrenergic Receptor Antagonists

**Prazosin** (see Fig. 34-2), **terazosin,** and **doxazosin** are selective antagonists of the $\alpha_1$-adrenergic receptors on arterioles and veins. Antagonism of the effect of noradrenaline lowers blood pressure by reducing peripheral resistance. Venodilatation can increase peripheral venous capacitance and reduce venous return to the central circulation. Severe orthostatic hypotension can occur, particularly after the first dose and before tolerance to the venodilator effect develops. It is recommended that the initial doses be small and administered at bedtime for a few days. Reduced efficacy can follow chronic administration ("pseudotolerance") due to sodium and water retention, but tachyphylaxis does not occur. In a comparison of doxazosin and chlorthalidone in treatment of hypertension, ALLHAT (the Antihypertensive and Lipid-Lowering Treatment to Prevent Heart Attack Trial) doxazosin was terminated prematurely because of an increased incidence of heart failure. Fatigue, dizziness, and nasal stuffiness are other adverse effects. Prazosin has a shorter duration of antihypertensive effect that requires dosing twice a day in contrast to once-a-day dosing for terazosin and doxazosin. These drugs are used to reduce nocturia, bladder hesitancy, and bladder-neck spasm associated with prostatism and as add-on agents when multiple other antihypertensive agents fail to control hypertension. **Tamulosin HCl,** which selectively blocks $\alpha_{1A}$- adrenergic receptors on the prostate, has little antihypertensive action.

**Phenoxybenzamine** and **phentolamine** are nonselective α-adrenergic blockers used in hypertensive emergencies.

## DIRECTLY ACTING VASODILATORS

**Minoxidil** (see Fig. 34-2) is a "direct" arteriolar dilator without an effect on veins. Its primary metabolite probably acts as an ATP-dependent potassium channel opener, causing potassium loss from smooth muscle cells. As a consequence, the hyperpolarized smooth muscle cells lose intracellular calcium, resulting in relaxation. The reduction in peripheral resistance lowers blood pressure

and stimulates baroreflex-induced tachycardia, peripheral venous constriction, and increased venous return and cardiac output. The renin system is stimulated, and salt and water retention is prominent. Often, β blockers are required to control the tachycardia and increased cardiac output, and diuretics are needed to control the excess circulating volume. Chronic administration has been associated with a failure to reverse, or even an enhancement of, left ventricular hypertrophy. Although minoxidil is very effective in lowering blood pressure in patients resistant to combinations of other agents, there is no evidence that the benefit of such reduction results in reduced vascular events. Most clinicians are reluctant to use minoxidil because of the frequency and intensity of adverse effects.

**Hydralazine** (see Fig. 34-2) is currently limited to use in eclampsia (see "Eclampsia and pre-eclampsia" below).

## HYPERTENSIVE URGENCIES AND EMERGENCIES

A very high blood pressure does not always require immediate reduction. In the absence of other conditions, such as unstable angina pectoris, acute myocardial infarction, pulmonary edema, dissecting aortic aneurysm, eclampsia, hypertensive encephalopathy, seizures, or an intracerebral hemorrhage, gradual reduction is appropriate so as to preserve autoregulated blood flow to the brain, heart, and kidneys. It is the manifestations and consequences of the associated conditions plus a very high blood pressure that defines the need for either immediate or urgent reduction of the pressure. When rapid reduction is required, the choice of the drug will depend on the associated condition and the properties of the drug. Immediate blood pressure reduction, but controlled to prevent reductions below the autoregulatory limits for blood flow to the brain, eye, heart, and kidneys, requires parenteral administration of an agent that has a rapid onset of action, a predictable dose–response, and reasonably limited duration of action in order to allow rapid dose titration to achieve and maintain a target blood pressure. In many clinical situations, an initial 25% reduction in systolic, diastolic, or mean blood pressure will arrest the adverse clinical manifestations of the associated condition (e.g., acute pulmonary edema associated with heart failure, or seizures associated with eclampsia) and prevent their recurrence. Subsequent gradual additional reduction will prevent adverse effects on cerebral, cardiac, and renal function associated with interference with blood flow autoregulation. The choice of drug and the target blood pressure reduction must include consideration for clinical surveillance of ongoing concomitant conditions. A drug that adversely alters cerebral function directly (such as clonidine or α-methyldopa) or indirectly by abolishing cerebral blood flow autoregulation (such as hydralazine)

| TABLE 34-1 | Some Properties and Adverse Effects of Clinically Used Vasodilators | | | | |
|---|---|---|---|---|---|
| Drug | Route of Administration | Main Indication | Venodilatation | Cardiac Output | Adverse Effects |
| Nitrates | Sublingual, oral, cutaneous, intravenous | Angina pectoris, refractory heart failure, hypertensive emergency | Yes | ↑↓ | Headache |
| Sodium nitroprusside | Intravenous | Hypertensive emergency | Yes | (↑)* | Cyanide poisoning (potential danger) |
| Minoxidil | Oral | Severe hypertension | No | ↑ | Hypertrichosis, fluid retention, cardiac hypertrophy |
| Calcium-channel blockers | Oral (verapamil, also intravenous) | Angina pectoris, hypertension, arrhythmia[†] | No | ↑↓ | Headache, constipation, peripheral edema, heart block[†] |
| ACE inhibitors | Oral | Hypertension, congestive heart failure | Yes | ↑↓ | Cough, hyperkalemia, angioedema |
| Angiotensin II–receptor blockers | Oral | Hypertension, congestive heart failure | Yes | ↑↓ | Hyperkalemia, angioedema |

*Only in congestive heart failure.

†Non-dihydropyridine-types verapamil and diltiazem.

↑ = increase; ↑↓ = varies with drug, dose, and method of administration.

would not be a suitable choice for patients with a cerebrovascular event. As outlined previously, oral or sublingual nifedipine has a rapid (within minutes) but unpredictable hypotensive effect. Oral or sublingual captopril also has a relatively rapid onset (within 20 to 30 minutes) but an unpredictable hypotensive effect that cannot be titrated to a target blood pressure. Therefore, neither agent is suitable for hypertensive emergencies or urgencies.

## Hypertensive Emergencies Requiring Drug Therapy in Minutes

Patients with coronary artery disease and acute myocardial infarction plus hypertension often develop **acute pulmonary edema.** Pulmonary congestion will not resolve without reduction of blood pressure. This must be initiated rapidly without interfering with coronary blood flow, which is best preserved by maintaining diastolic blood pressure above 60 to 70 mmHg while reducing systolic pressure. The drug of choice to reduce both cardiac pre- and afterload while preserving coronary flow is **nitroglycerin (glyceryl trinitrate),** an organic nitrate.

### Organic nitrates and nitrites

Nitrates and nitrites are simple nitric and nitrous acid esters of mono- or polyalcohols. They vary from extremely volatile liquids (amyl nitrite) to moderately volatile liquids. Nitroglycerin is considered the prototype of the group (see Fig. 34-2). The formulations of nitroglycerin used in medicine are not explosive. The sublingual tablet form of nitro-

glycerin may lose potency during storage as a result of volatilization and adsorption to plastic surfaces, and it has been largely replaced by a pump-spray applicator. Structure–activity studies indicate that all therapeutically active agents in this group are capable of releasing nitrite ion in vascular smooth muscle target tissues. Unfortunately, they are all also capable of inducing cross-tolerance.

*Pharmacokinetics.* Organic nitrate esters are quite lipid-soluble and therefore are readily absorbed through the well-vascularized sublingual mucosa. The organic nitrate esters are hydrolyzed by hepatic enzymes that convert them into water-soluble, partially denitrated metabolites and inorganic nitrite. The products are considerably less potent vasodilators; they circulate in the plasma for several hours after a dose of nitroglycerin and eventually are excreted in the urine.

The effectiveness of organic nitrates is strongly influenced by extensive first-pass metabolism by hepatic P450 and glutathione-S-transferases. Therefore, bioavailabilty of all orally administered organic nitrates is very low (typically less than 10%). Consequently, the sublingual route (spray or tablet) is preferred for rapidly achieving a therapeutic blood level. Nitroglycerin and isosorbide dinitrate are absorbed efficiently by this route and reach therapeutic blood levels within a few minutes. However, the total dose administered by this route must be limited to avoid excessive effects, and the duration of effect is brief, typically 15 to 30 minutes. When much longer duration of action is needed, oral preparations are available that contain an amount of drug sufficient to result in sustained systemic blood levels of drug or active metabolites despite the high first-pass effect in the liver. Other routes of nitroglycerin administration include transdermal absorption when it is applied to the skin as an ointment or patch and buccal absorption from slow-release buccal preparations. Intravenous administration of nitroglycerin has an onset of action within 0.5 to 2 minutes, slightly faster than with the sublingual spray application, and has a brief duration of effect (~3 to 5 minutes). Continuous intravenous administration is required for a maintained effect, but tolerance develops over time (12 to 24 hours).

*Pharmacological effects.* Low concentrations of nitroglycerin cause greater smooth muscle relaxation in large (veins > arteries) than in small (arterioles > venules) blood vessels. As a consequence, systolic blood pressure is reduced more than diastolic. Higher concentrations can relax arteriolar smooth muscle and reduce diastolic blood pressure. Venodilatation increases peripheral capacitance and reduces venous return and central blood volume, as well as ventricular end-diastolic volumes and pressure. The orthostatic effect of standing upright can further reduce cardiac preload. Cardiac output is reduced by nitroglycerin. Pulmonary vascular resistance is also reduced. Increased arterial capacitance resulting from relaxation of the large conduit arteries, combined with a change in the velocity of forward and reflected arterial pressure waves, reduces systolic blood pressure and cardiac afterload. The reduction in systolic blood pressure triggers a baroreceptor-induced increase in heart rate.

*Adverse effects.* Facial flushing and headache are common manifestations of the arteriolar dilatation associated with nitroglycerin. High doses can further decrease systolic and diastolic blood pressure and cardiac output, causing tachycardia, dizziness, nausea, vomiting, profound weakness and fatigue, and disorientation, all worsened in the upright position. Fatal hypotension can occur with nitroglycerin administration to patients who have used sildenafil for erectile dysfunction in the previous 24 hours.

*Tolerance to nitrates.* Organic nitrates are thought to induce smooth muscle relaxation by the release or formation of nitric oxide (NO) or an NO-like compound, activation of the cytosolic form of guanyl cyclase, and subsequent increases in smooth muscle cGMP content. However, although a number of proteins and enzymes are known to mediate the denitration of organic nitrates to produce inorganic nitrite anion, identification of the enzyme that mediates the three-electron reduction of organic nitrates to NO has remained elusive. Increased cGMP accumulation results in the activation of cGMP-dependent protein kinase (PKG) and subsequent phosphorylation of cell proteins leading to decreased intracel-

lular $Ca^{2+}$ and/or decreased $Ca^{2+}$ sensitivity followed by vascular smooth muscle relaxation. An alternate or additional mechanism by which increases in cGMP may mediate relaxation is inhibition of the cGMP-inhibited cAMP-specific phosphodiesterase (PDE), resulting in increased cAMP levels and activation of cAMP-dependent protein kinase (PKA) or PKG. There is also some evidence that NO may elicit vasodilatation, at least in part, by cGMP-independent mechanisms.

Stimulation of guanylyl cyclase activity and elevation of cGMP by organic nitrates is markedly inhibited in nitroglycerin-tolerant vascular tissue. In the clinical setting, tolerance to the anti-anginal and hemodynamic effects of nitrates is associated with continuous exposure and has led to the use of elliptical dosage regimens to provide a nitrate-free interval during which recovery of sensitivity to the vasodilator effects of the nitrate can occur. This strategy has the disadvantage of leaving patients without the benefits of therapy during the nitrate-free period, and it can result in a rebound phenomenon characterized by an increased frequency of anginal attacks or a deterioration in exercise performance. Tolerance to organic nitrates is multifactorial in nature, and a number of proposed mechanisms of tolerance development have been advanced, both at the cellular level and involving cardiovascular homeostatic mechanisms. These include intravascular volume expansion, neurohumoral counter-regulation, increased vascular superoxide ($O_2^{·}$) production secondary to angiotensin II–induced up-regulation of a vascular NADH/NADPH oxidase, increased vascular endothelin-1 production, depletion of critical sulfhydryl groups, and a reduced cGMP response due to reduced biotransformation of the organic nitrate to NO, desensitization of guanylyl cyclase to activation by NO, or increased cyclic GMP phosphodiesterase activity. Exposure to nitroglycerin causes an endothelium-dependent increase in the bioavailability of superoxide ion due to abnormalities in nitric oxide synthase (NOS) function. Superoxide anion and other oxygen free radicals can directly impair NO bioavailabilty. Folic acid has been used to prevent nitrate tolerance by increasing the bioavailability of tetrahydrobiopterin, which is a cofactor for NOS function.

*Clinical uses.* A major use for nitrate therapy is the treatment and prevention of **angina pectoris**. Anginal pain is the result of an imbalance between myocardial oxygen demand and supply. Since myocardial oxygen extraction is almost complete, demand for increased oxygen delivery to the heart is normally met by increasing the blood flow rather than by more complete extraction of oxygen. Ischemia is the major stimulus for coronary vasodilatation, and it is believed that myocardial regional blood flow is adjusted by autoregulatory mechanisms.

The effects of nitrates on cardiac pre- and afterload are important determinants of myocardial oxygen requirements and relief from anginal pain. Nitrates only transiently increase coronary blood flow by direct vasodilatation of the coronary vascular bed. In patients with organic stenosis of the coronary arteries, nitrates may not increase total coronary blood flow but may alter distribution in favour of more hypoxic regions. Selective vasodilatation of large epicardial vessels redistributes coronary blood flow to the ischemic subendocardial areas. Thus, by a combination of mechanisms, nitrates rapidly relieve angina. When nitrates are used for the prevention of angina, a 12-hour nitrate-free period must be used each day to ensure continued effectiveness.

The patient with **hypertension and acute pulmonary edema** requires immediate treatment with nitroglycerin. While intravenous administration is being prepared, the drug can be sprayed sublingually to begin its effects within a minute or two. The intravenous dose can be titrated to reduce systolic blood pressure without an excessive fall in diastolic pressure that might lower coronary perfusion. The resultant reduction in cardiac pre- and afterload, preservation of coronary blood flow or increase in coronary blood flow to ischemic regions, and reduction in pulmonary vascular resistance can lead to rapid improvement in left ventricular function and resolution of pulmonary congestion. The development of tolerance with continued administration can be partially overcome by using higher doses. However, other ongoing treatment measures should be instituted. Oral or topical nitrates can be used as adjunctive therapy for chronic congestive heart failure but there is no evidence for a reduction in mortality . In contrast, there is clinical trial evidence that ACE inhibitors or ARBs reduce mortality and prolong life in congestive heart failure. Low-dose β-adrenergic blockade can be considered when the patient is stable; there is evidence that it reduces mortality.

Nitrates are not commonly used for the treatment of chronic hypertension. Occasionally, patients with systolic hypertension refractory to multiple drugs in combination can benefit from a 12-hour period each day in which oral or skin patch nitrate is used for additional effect on systolic blood pressure.

**Pre-eclampsia** is a multi-system disorder of pregnancy associated with increased blood pressure and proteinuria. **Eclampsia** is defined by the occurrence of one or more convulsions superimposed on pre-eclampsia. Delivery of the fetus is paramount. The prevention of seizures or their termination is better achieved with intravenous administration of **magnesium sulfate** than with phenytoin or diazepam. A loading dose of magnesium sulfate is given intravenously over 15 minutes, and the effect is monitored by changes in deep tendon reflexes. Loss of deep tendon reflexes precedes respiratory depression. A maintenance dose should follow either intravenously or intramuscularly. Magnesium is a mild direct vasodilator and induces modest reductions in blood pressure, probably by blocking influx of extracellular calcium and promoting intracellular uptake of calcium by the sarcoplasmic reticulum. Nifedip-

ine, a calcium-channel blocker, is increasingly being used for hypertension and pre-eclampsia in the third trimester of pregnancy. However, calcium-channel blockers may interact with magnesium and result in paralysis. In eclampsia, parenteral **hydralazine** or **labetalol** can be used in addition to magnesium sulfate to achieve blood pressure control.

### Hydralazine (Apresoline)
Hydralazine (see Fig. 34-2) is a direct arteriolar smooth muscle relaxant with an unknown mechanism of action. It has little effect on veins, so orthostatic hypotension is not among its adverse effects. Its use is associated with a baroreflex-induced tachycardia. Following intravenous or intramuscular administration, its hypotensive effect is apparent in 10 to 30 minutes and has a variable 3- to 6-hour duration. The hypotensive effect is not predictable or easily titrated to a specific blood pressure goal. The sympathetic nervous system is activated with increased heart rate and contractility and stimulation of the renin system. Intracardiac noradrenaline may be released by a direct action of hydralazine, resulting in increased cardiac contractility. Myocardial ischemia and angina can result. Hydralazine abolishes cerebral autoregulation; increased cerebral blood flow can ensue if blood pressure is not decreased, causing increased intracranial pressure and headache. Hypotension below the lower limit of cerebral autoregulation can severely reduce cerebral blood flow.

**Eclampsia** is the only clinical indication for intravenous hydralazine. Although it is readily absorbed after oral administration, its systemic bioavailability is low and is controlled by acetylator phenotype. *N*-acetylation to an inactive molecule occurs in the bowel wall and liver. Systemic bioavailability is lower in fast than in slow acetylators. Other agents have replaced its oral use in chronic hypertension. Multiple daily doses are required because of its short plasma half-life of about 1 hour. The associated tachycardia limits its hypotensive effect, and concomitant β-adrenergic blockade is required. Occasionally, hydralazine is used with nitrates, diuretics, and low-dose β blockers for patients with chronic congestive heart failure who cannot tolerate ACE inhibitors or ARBs.

**Adverse effects** include headache, gastrointestinal complaints, palpitations, arrhythmia, precipitation of angina, salt and water retention ("pseudotolerance"), and other consequences of arteriolar vasodilatation. Doses at or above 200 mg/day can cause the lupus syndrome, particularly in individuals with a slow acetylator phenotype.

### Labetalol (Trandate)
Labetalol has both $\alpha_1$- and $\beta_{1,2}$-adrenergic receptor blocking properties in a ratio of 1:7, plus intrinsic sympathomimetic activity on $\beta_2$ receptors. Given intravenously as a loading dose, it has an onset of hypotensive action within 5 minutes and a duration of effect from 4 to 8 hours. It

undergoes hepatic biotransformation, and its elimination half-life averages 4 hours. The hypotensive effect is not as readily titratable as with nitroprusside but is more predictable than with nitroglycerin or hydralazine.

Labetalol is useful for urgent treatment of eclampsia and most other hypertensive emergencies except acute heart failure, where the negative inotropic effect of its much stronger β-adrenergic blocking action would counter the hypotensive effect of $α_1$-adrenergic blockade, and pheochromocytoma, where β blockade could allow unopposed α-adrenergic vasoconstriction since the α to β blockade ratio is 1:7. $α_1$-Adrenergic receptor blockade induces vascular smooth muscle relaxation by interfering with sympathetic nervous and catecholamine influences on contraction. There is an initial venodilator effect with increased peripheral capacitance, but tachyphylaxis follows within several hours. The effect on arteriolar resistance persists. The usual baroreflex induced tachycardia associated with a lowered blood pressure after isolated $α_1$-adrenergic receptor blockade is prevented by the $β_{1,2}$-adrenergic receptor blocking properties of labetalol. The mechanism of hypotensive effect of β-adrenergic blockade in the absence of $α_1$-adrenergic receptor blockade is unknown. In normal individuals, $β_{1,2}$-adrenergic receptor blockade *increases* blood pressure as α-adrenergic constrictor influence on arteriolar smooth muscle is left unopposed by normal $β_2$-adrenergic vasodilator effects. Possibly the intrinsic sympathomimetic activity of labetalol on $β_2$ receptors enhances arteriolar relaxation.

Labetalol is not commonly used orally for the treatment of chronic hypertension. An extensive first-pass hepatic clearance reduces its bioavailabilty. Food and changes in hepatic blood flow also alter bioavailabilty.

**Adverse effects** include tingling of the scalp, gastrointestinal upset, fluid retention, and bradycardia as well as impaired cardiac contractility. Excessive intravenous loading doses can cause severe hypotension.

## Pheochromocytoma

Pheochromocytoma is an endocrine tumour of chromaffin cells arising in the adrenal medulla or sympathetic ganglion chain that intermittently or continuously releases catecholamines (noradrenaline > adrenaline) and causes hypertension. Severe increases in blood pressure can occur after sudden large increases in noradrenaline. α-Adrenergic blockade with intravenous **phentolamine** is a rational treatment choice. Alternatively, intravenous **nitroprusside** can be used. As noted above, **labetalol** is not a rational choice. Oral **phenoxybenzamine** is often used preoperatively to control blood pressure before removal of a pheochromocytoma.

### Phentolamine (Rogitine)
Phentolamine is an imidazoline compound that competitively antagonizes $α_1$- and $α_2$-adrenergic receptors, decreasing peripheral arteriolar constriction. However, the $α_2$-blockade results in increased circulating levels of noradrenaline, which causes tachycardia. The reduction in blood pressure also causes a baroreflex-induced tachycardia and increased cardiac output. Phentolamine can block receptors for 5-HT and cause mast cells to release histamine. Part of its vasodilator effect may arise from $K^+$-channel blockade. Intravenously, it has an onset of action within 1 to 2 minutes and a short duration of 3 to 10 minutes. The hypotensive effect is unpredictable and difficult to titrate. **Adverse effects** include hypotension (particularly with dehydration or in the upright position), gastrointestinal upset, headache, flushing, arrhythmia, angina, and myocardial infarction.

### Phenoxybenzamine
Phenoxybenzamine is a haloalkylamine that covalently conjugates with $α_1$- and $α_2$-adrenergic receptors. The blockade is irreversible; therefore, regeneration of new receptors is required for recovery after the drug is discontinued. This may take several days, even though the plasma half-life for the drug itself is less than 24 hours. Just as in the case of phentolamine, the arteriolar dilatation and the fall in blood pressure produced by phenoxybenzamine cause a baroreflex-induced tachycardia that may be enhanced by noradrenaline release. Phenoxybenzamine also inhibits neuronal and extraneuronal uptake mechanisms that usually limit the effects of noradrenaline on vascular smooth muscle and the heart. Control of the tachycardia with β-adrenergic blockade is not indicated and may be dangerous, as the hypertensive effect of excess circulating noradrenaline may be accentuated. Occasionally, β blockade is required to control associated cardiac arrhythmias. Concern over development of malignant tumours in rodents given phenoxybenzamine has led drug regulatory agencies to impose restrictions on its use. In Canada, special permission is required for each patient. After five decades of use, the clinical significance of these animal experiments is still unknown. As a consequence, the intravenous form is rarely available for hypertensive emergencies.

Oral phenoxybenzamine can be used over a 2- to 3-week period to prepare the patient for surgical removal of a pheochromocytoma. While limiting large increases in blood pressure and preventing myocardial damage, its administration in the preoperative period allows the circulating volume to gradually expand, thus preventing severe hypotension that might otherwise occur with surgical removal of the source of excess catecholamines. Long-term oral therapy can be considered for patients with an inoperable or malignant pheochromocytoma.

The **adverse effects** of phenoxybenzamine are similar to those of phentolamine, including hypotension, particularly with dehydration or in the upright position, gastrointestinal upset, headache, flushing, arrhythmia, angina, and myocardial infarction.

### Sodium nitroprusside (Nipride)

Given intravenously, nitroprusside (see Fig. 34-2) undergoes enzymatic or non-enzymatic one-electron reduction in vascular smooth muscle, resulting in the formation of NO, which activates guanylyl cyclase, leading to cGMP formation and rapid vascular smooth muscle relaxation and vasodilatation. The bioactivation system involved is likely different from the one for nitroglycerin, since nitroprusside has a different pattern of vascular effects and tolerance does not develop.

*Pharmacological effects.* Like nitroglycerin, nitroprusside has effects on both arterial and venous sides of the circulation. In contrast to nitroglycerin, at lower concentrations, it has effects on arterioles and venules as well as large conduit vessels. In subjects with normal cardiac function, the increased peripheral venous capacitance and reduced cardiac preload is countered by reduced cardiac afterload; cardiac output is only slightly reduced. Like nitroglycerin, the hypotensive effect of nitroprusside is enhanced in the upright position because of its effect on venous capacitance and venous return to the heart. Nitroprusside causes an immediate reduction in both systolic and diastolic blood pressure. Regional distribution of blood flow is not altered. Stimulation of the renin–angiotensin system aids maintenance of glomerular filtration. For an unknown reason, heart rate is only slightly increased.

*Pharmacokinetics.* Sodium nitroprusside is unstable and readily decomposed by alkaline conditions or light. It must be administered intravenously, preferably using a calibrated pump-delivery system while covering the intravenous reservoir and lines with aluminum foil. It has an onset of action within 30 seconds and a peak hypotensive effect at 2 minutes, lasting less than 3 minutes. This rapid onset and offset of hypotensive effect allows titration of the dose to a given blood pressure target, but it also requires continuous blood pressure monitoring that can only be provided by an intra-arterial pressure line. This usually requires an intensive patient-care environment. The formation of NO in the vascular smooth muscle is accompanied by the formation of cyanide, which is further transformed by the liver to thiocyanate, which is eliminated by the kidney with a half-life of 3 days.

Hypotension is the major **adverse effect**. Higher doses of nitroprusside can promote arteriolar-venous shunting of blood flow in all vascular beds. This "washout" phenomenon can cause myocardial, cerebral, and renal ischemia and reduced organ function, particularly in patients with vascular disease of these organs. It can worsen arterial hypoxemia in patients with chronic obstructive pulmonary disease. Nitroprusside can abolish cerebral blood flow autoregulation, causing headaches and increased intracranial pressure. Arterial blood gases must be monitored for lactic acidosis as a result of cyanide accumulation. When nitroprusside is infused for periods greater than 24 hours, particularly in patients with renal impairment, thiocyanate toxicity can ensue with nausea, vomiting, muscle twitching, weakness, disorientation, toxic psychosis, or seizures. Plasma thiocyanate concentrations should be monitored.

*Hypertensive emergencies.* Nitroprusside is used to lower blood pressure in hypertensive emergencies when an immediate but controlled hypotensive effect is required. With intra-arterial blood pressure monitoring, the dose can be titrated to achieve and maintain a target blood pressure. In patients with left ventricular cardiac failure, nitroprusside can effectively lower cardiac pre- and afterload while increasing cardiac output, as the greater effect is on afterload. However, myocardial oxygen demand may increase, and distribution of coronary blood flow may be adversely altered, in contrast to the beneficial effect of nitroglycerin. On the other hand, tolerance does not occur with nitroprusside, and dose-titration is easier than with nitroglycerin. A rebound increase in blood pressure after termination of dosing is greater with nitroprusside than with nitroglycerin. In patients with an aortic or carotid dissection (see "Dissecting aortic aneurysm" below), β-adrenergic blockade is required to reduce enhanced myocardial contractility and left ventricular ejection consequent to the effect of nitroprusside on arterial impedance, in order to prevent continued arterial wall dissection.

## Hypertensive Emergencies Requiring Drug Therapy within an Hour

There are several situations in which an immediate blood pressure reduction within minutes may not be required, but a controlled reduction to a specific target level within an hour is indicated to reduce morbidity and mortality.

### Dissecting aortic aneurysm

High blood pressure can extend a dissection within the wall of the aorta, leading to rupture or occlusion. Intravenous **nitroprusside** (see Fig. 34-2) can be used for rapid reduction and titration to a systolic and diastolic pressure that prevents propagation of the wall dissection while preserving coronary blood flow. However, **concomitant β-adrenergic blockade** is required to reduce the increase in velocity of left ventricular ejection and forward pressure wave that could easily extend the dissection. Alternatively, intravenous **labetalol** can be administered, since it combines α- and β-adrenergic blocking properties in one drug. Labetalol has a slower onset and less predictable but longer duration of hypotensive effect than nitroprusside, with less rebound hypertension upon discontinuation of the drug. Conversion to chronic oral therapy with other antihypertensive agents is easier following labetalol than nitroprusside. Many patients with an aortic dissection do not require emergency surgery but will need long-term reduction in systolic blood pressure to about 100 mmHg.

## The hypertensive patient requiring emergency surgery

Hypertension by itself is not a contraindication to surgery. In the absence of compelling associated conditions, patients with a systolic blood pressure less than or equal to 220 mmHg or diastolic pressure less than or equal to 120 mmHg are often left untreated. However, a patient with unstable angina pectoris, recent myocardial infarction, or left ventricular failure is at increased risk for additional vascular events or death. If surgery is required, the anaesthetist may consider intravenous **nitroglycerin.** For some associated clinical conditions, **nitroprusside** would be a better choice since it can be more readily and rapidly titrated to a target blood pressure. For example, endotracheal intubation of the patient can cause a large increase in blood pressure, whereas induction of anaesthesia can cause a large reduction in blood pressure. The pump-administration rate of nitroprusside can be rapidly adjusted accordingly. **Labetalol** would *not* be a rational choice. **Esmolol,** a cardioselective β-adrenergic blocker, is occasionally used for rapid reduction of blood pressure. An intravenous bolus has an onset of action within 2 minutes. It is rapidly hydrolyzed by red blood cell esterases and has a plasma half-life of 9 minutes; a continuous infusion is required for maintained effect. Indications include hypertension associated with endotracheal intubation, postoperative angina, or supraventricular tachycardia. Expense and a somewhat unpredictable hypotensive effect have limited the use of esmolol; however, rapid termination of its effect on blood pressure, heart rate, and myocardial contractility provides some advantages over other intravenous β-blocking agents.

### Hypertension and acute intracranial hemorrhage
Hypertension can increase the morbidity and mortality associated with intracerebral or subarachnoid hemorrhage by such processes as expansion of an intracerebral hematoma, resumption of bleeding from a ruptured aneurysm, secondary cerebral vasospasm, impaired cerebral blood flow autoregulation, and an increased lower limit for maintenance of cerebral blood flow. Attempts to lower blood pressure may worsen outcome. Ideal treatment has not been established. If the systolic blood pressure is greater than 200 mmHg or diastolic is greater than 110 mmHg, some clinicians initially lower the pressure about 25% so as to prevent loss of cerebral blood flow that would occur at pressures below the autoregulatory limit. Modest blood pressure reduction may limit renewed bleeding and vasogenic cerebral edema.

Intravenous **labetalol** may be a better choice than intravenous nitroprusside or hydralazine, which interfere with cerebral autoregulation, or nitroglycerin, which is not as predictable in achieving a target blood pressure. Intravenous **enalaprilat,** the active form of the ACE inhibitor enalapril, could be considered as ACE inhibitors do not interfere with cerebral blood flow autoregulation. Unfortunately, its hypotensive effect is very abrupt and unpredictable, particularly in high renin states. Intravenous α-**methyldopa,** a centrally acting $\alpha_2$-adrenergic agonist, is contraindicated as its neurological effects could interfere with clinical monitoring of CNS function.

## Hypertensive Urgencies Requiring Blood Pressure Reduction within Several Hours

Hypertension associated with **encephalopathy, head injury, acute burns,** or **quadriplegia** can be gradually reduced over several hours to prevent falling below the lower limit of cerebral blood flow autoregulation. The patient with hypertensive encephalopathy and marked diastolic or systolic–diastolic hypertension may complain of a severe headache, nausea, vomiting, and visual disturbances. Mental obtundation, stupor, coma, and convulsions may occur. Papilledema and retinal hemorrhages and exudates are found on fundoscopy. Initially, a target reduction of about 25% is used with a subsequent further reduction over 8 to 24 hours. Intravenous **labetalol** is commonly used, although nitroprusside can be given with all of the considerations provided in previous sections of this chapter.

## Hypertensive Urgencies Requiring Blood Pressure Reduction within Several Days

Oral antihypertensive therapy can be used for patients with severe hypertension without target organ damage or associated conditions outlined previously. Patients with **acute glomerulonephritis** or **unilateral renal artery stenosis** can also be treated with oral agents. A single agent such as an ACE inhibitor is started, and the dose is rapidly titrated upward over a few days while observing for clinical and laboratory evidence of reduced perfusion of the brain, eye, heart, and kidneys. A dihydropyridine calcium-channel blocker and, occasionally, a β-adrenergic receptor blocker are required in addition and are added sequentially over the subsequent days to a week or two. Most hypertensive emergencies and urgencies are associated with stimulation of the renin–angiotensin system, which can be countered by aldosterone antagonism with ACE inhibition or angiotensin receptor blockade or by renin inhibition with β blockade. Diuretics can further augment the renin–angiotensin system: their use in combination therapy should be delayed for several days.

### Acute ischemic stroke and hypertension
It has been recommended that treatment of acute hypertension in patients suffering an acute ischemic stroke be

deferred, since hypotension may interfere with cerebral autoregulation, particularly in tissues surrounding the area of cerebral necrosis. Exceptions include patients requiring thrombolytic therapy, severe hypertension with systolic values of 220 mmHg or greater or diastolic values of 120 mmHg or greater, or concomitant conditions such as acute myocardial infarction, unstable angina, left ventricular failure, or aortic dissection. Treatments recommended in such cases include intravenous nitrates, nitroprusside, or labetalol, depending on the clinical situation. Intravenous **nimodipine**, a calcium-channel blocker, has caused neurological deterioration as a consequence of acute hypotension in acute ischemic stroke. In a recent clinical trial, oral **candesartan cilexate**, an ARB, started within 24 to 38 hours of the stroke, reduced recurrent strokes and cardiac events without adverse consequences from hypotension. In another clinical trial, the combination of the ACE inhibitor **perindopril** and the diuretic **indapamide**, started from 1 week to several months after a stroke when the cerebral circulation was stable, was more effective than placebo in preventing recurrent stroke and myocardial infarctions.

### Malignant hypertension

Malignant hypertension is a clinical phase of essential and secondary hypertension characterized by severe diastolic hypertension and accelerated and progressive renal damage often accompanied by papilledema and retinal hemorrhages and exudates. If unrecognized, it has a poor prognosis with early death from renal failure or an abrupt vascular event. The mechanisms underlying widespread arteriolar spasm and dilatation, endarteritis, and necrotizing arteriolitis have not been clarified but involve the renin–angiotensin system, endothelin, and other constrictor substances. Aggressive oral antihypertensive drug treatment is indicated, using combinations of several classes including β blockers, dihydropyridine calcium-channel blockers, and ACE inhibitors. Diuretics are not indicated initially, but loop diuretics may be required for control of excess circulatory volumes after treatment with other agents has been established.

## DRUG TREATMENT OF PULMONARY HYPERTENSION

Compared with systemic hypertension, idiopathic and secondary pulmonary hypertension are uncommon but very difficult to treat and have a high mortality. Primary pulmonary hypertension, characterized by progressive intimal proliferation and pulmonary artery occlusion, often affects young women. Secondary causes include scleroderma and other connective tissue diseases or immunological disorders, HIV, thromboembolic disease, hepatic cirrhosis, and severe congestive heart failure. Attempts to use older and current antihypertensive vasodilator drugs have failed to modify the dismal prognosis, although dihydropyridine calcium-channel blockers have some effect. Increased pulmonary arteriolar vasoconstriction due to excess endothelin (ET) and thromboxane, with deficient vasodilatation due to insufficient prostacyclin, has led to the assessment of recently developed drugs modifying these systems. Suspected deficiencies in the pulmonary NOS system have prompted use of inhaled **nitric oxide**. **Prostacyclin** is a potent arteriolar vasodilator with anti-thrombotic and anti-proliferative properties. Prostacyclin is synthesized in endothelial cells and acts on prostacyclin receptors on the surface of vascular smooth muscle cells, augmenting cAMP and causing vascular relaxation. Treatment with prostacyclin by continuous intravenous administration (**epoprostenol**), continuous subcutaneous administration (**treprostinol**), or inhaled (**iloprost**) or oral (**beraprost**) agents is costly but has had some success, perhaps by limiting intimal proliferation. Headache, flushing, nausea, diarrhea, and jaw and leg pain have been reported. **Bosentan,** a non-selective antagonist of the effects of endothelin-1 on $ET_A$ and $ET_B$ receptors, has improved symptoms and exercise tolerance. Teratogenicity, hepatic dysfunction, and cost are concerns with its use. **Sildenafil**, a selective inhibitor of phosphodiesterase (PDE) 5, enhances erectile function by vascular relaxation in penile arteries, arterioles, and sinusoids. Normally, relaxation of vascular smooth muscle occurs after stimulation of guanylyl cyclase by NO released from non-adrenergic, non-cholinergic nerves and endothelial cells, stimulating the formation of cGMP and ultimately causing reduced cytosolic $Ca^{2+}$ concentration. The hydrolysis of cGMP by PDE5 is limited by sildenafil. The antihypertensive and coronary vasodilator properties of sildenafil are dependent on the degree of activation of the NO–guanylyl cyclase pathway. Combination with an NO donor such as nitroglycerin can cause fatal hypotension. Several PDE isoforms, including PDE5, are involved in regulating pulmonary resistance. Sildenafil is under investigation as a pulmonary vasodilator, either alone or in combination with other oral or inhaled agents, in patients with pulmonary hypertension.

## SUGGESTED READINGS

ALLHAT Officers and Coordinators for the ALLHAT Collaborative Research Group. Major outcomes in high-risk hypertensive patients randomized to angiotensin-converting enzyme inhibitor or calcium channel blocker vs diuretic: The Antihypertensive and Lipid-Lowering Treatment to Prevent Heart Attack Trial (ALLHAT). *JAMA.* 2002;288:2981-2997.

Belfort MA, Anthony J, Saade GR, et al. A comparison of magnesium sulfate and nimodipine for the prevention of eclampsia. *N Engl J Med.* 2003;348:304-311.

Belz GG. Angiotensin II dose-effect curves and Schild regression plots for characterization of different angiotensin AT$_1$ receptor anagonists in clinical pharmacology. *Brit J Clin Pharmacol.* 2003;56:3-10.

Brown NJ. Eplerenone: cardiovascular protection. *Circulation.* 2003;107:2512-2518.

Canadian Hypertension Society. *Recommendations for the Diagnosis and Treatment of Hypertension.* Available at: http://www.hypertension.ca. Accessed October 12, 2005.

Carter BL, Ernst ME, Cohen JD. Hydrochlorothiazide versus chlorthalidone. Evidence supporting their interchangeability. *Hypertension.* 2004;43:4-9.

Dahlof B, Devereux RB, Kjeldsen SE, et al. Cardiovascular morbidity and mortality in the losartan intervention for endpoint reduction in hypertension study (LIFE): a randomized trial against atenolol. *Lancet.* 2002;359:995-1003.

Fox KM, EUROPA Investigators. Efficacy of perindopril in reduction of cardiovascular events among patients with stable coronary artery disease: randomised, double-blind, placebo-controlled, multicentre trial (the EUROPA study). *Lancet.* 2003;362:782-788.

Gori T, Burstein JM, Ahmed S, et al. Folic acid prevents nitroglycerin-induced nitric oxide synthase dysfunction and nitrate tolerance. A human in-vivo study. *Circulation.* 2001;104:1119-1123.

Humbert M, Sitbon O, Simonneau G. Treatment of pulmonary hypertension. *N Engl J Med.* 2004;351:1425-1436.

Johnson JA, Zineh I, Puckett BJ, et al. Beta$_1$-adrenergic receptor polymorphisms and antihypertensive response to metoprolol. *Clin Pharmacol Ther.* 2003;74:44-52.

Julius S, Kjeldsen SE, Weber M, et al. Outcomes in hypertensive patients at high cardiovascular risk treated with regimens based on valsartan or amlodipine: the VALUE randomised trial. *Lancet.* 2004;363:2022-2031.

Lewis EJ, Hunsicker LG, Clarke WR, et al. Renoprotective effect of the angiotensin-receptor antagonist irbesartan in patients with nephropathy due to type 2 diabetes. *N Engl J Med.* 2001; 345:851-860.

Magee LA, Cham C, Waterman EJ, Ohlsson A, von Dadelszen P. Hydralazine for treatment of severe hypertension in pregnancy: meta-analysis. *BMJ.* 2003;327:955-960.

Magpie Collaborative Group. Do women with pre-eclampsia and their babies benefit from magnesium sulphate? The Magpie Trial: a randomized placebo controlled trial. *The Lancet.* 2002;359:1877-1890.

PROGRESS Collaborative Group. Randomized trial of a perindopril-based blood-pressure-lowering regimen among 6,105 individuals with prior stroke or transient ischaemic attack. *Lancet.* 2001;358:1033-1041.

Reffelmann T, Klonor RA. Therapeutic potential of phosphodiesterase inhibition for cardiovascular disease. *Circulation.* 2003;108:239-244.

Rubin LJ, Badesch DB, Barst RJ, et al. Bosentan therapy for pulmonary artery hypertension. *N Engl J Med.* 2002;346:896-903.

Schrader J, Luders S, Kulshewski A, et al. The ACCESS study. Evaluation of acute candesartan cilexil therapy in stroke survivors. *Stroke.* 2003;34:1699-1703.

Staessen JA, Wang J-G, Thijs L. Cardiovascular prevention and blood pressure reduction: a quantitative overview updated until March 2003. *J Hypertens.* 2003;21:1055-1076.

Unger T, Kaschina E. Drug interactions with angiotensin receptor blockers: a comparison with other antihypertensives. *Drug Saf.* 2003;26:707-720.

# 35

# Dyslipidemias and Antihyperlipidemic Drugs

## AYY CHENG AND LA LEITER

**CASE HISTORY**

A 56-year-old post-menopausal woman came to her family physician's office for a routine health examination. Her medical history included type 2 diabetes mellitus and hypertension, both of which were diagnosed 4 years ago. She had no known vascular complications arising from the diabetes. She did not use alcohol, but smoked 20 cigarettes a day. There was a family history of diabetes mellitus, but not of premature coronary disease. Her current medications were a biguanide and a sulfonylurea for her diabetes mellitus; a diuretic, an ACE inhibitor, and a calcium-channel blocker for her hypertension; and low-dose aspirin.

On examination she was found to be overweight, with a body mass index of 27 kg/m$^2$. Her blood pressure was well controlled, at 125/75 mmHg. She did not have xanthelasma, corneal arcus, or xanthoma. Cardiovascular examination revealed no evidence of heart failure and no audible bruits. Peripheral pulses were all palpable. There were no abnormalities of her feet, and protective sensation was normal. Her most recent laboratory results were as follows:

| | | | |
|---|---|---|---|
| Total cholesterol | 5.7 mmol/L | Creatinine | 60 µmol/L |
| Triglycerides | 2.4 mmol/L | Liver enzymes | normal |
| LDL-C | 3.6 mmol/L | | |
| HDL-C | 1.0 mmol/L | | |

Evaluation of her lipoprotein profile indicated a mild elevation in LDL-C, for which there were no obvious secondary causes. It likely represented a primary form (e.g., polygenic) of high LDL-C. The decision to treat was based on an appropriate risk assessment for this patient. Despite the lack of evident vascular disease, the presence of diabetes mellitus placed her in the high-risk category for cardiovascular disease, and the guidelines suggested aggressive treatment to decrease LDL-C and a few other parameters. To achieve this decrease, the patient was assessed and counselled by a registered dietitian regarding potential dietary modifications to improve the lipid profile. In view of her high-risk status, treatment with a "statin" was also initiated.

Three months later, she has followed all the lifestyle advice given at the last meeting. She has lost 3.5 kg in weight and has had no side effects from the statin. Her repeat lipid profile shows the LDL-C to be reduced to 2.2 mmol/L, and the total cholesterol is improved. Since she has achieved her target, she is encouraged to continue the lifestyle modifications and use of the statin.

## INTRODUCTION

Cardiovascular disease remains the leading cause of death in developed countries and is projected to account for more than 40% of all deaths around the world by the year 2020. Many risk factors, both modifiable and non-modifiable, contribute to an individual's risk for cardiovascular disease. Among these risk factors are age, smoking, diabetes, hypertension, and family history of premature coronary artery disease. Another important modifiable risk factor is dyslipidemia, defined as an abnormality in lipoprotein concentrations. In this chapter, normal lipoprotein metabolism and the classification and treatment of dyslipidemia are discussed.

## CLASSIFICATION OF LIPOPROTEINS

Hydrophobic insoluble lipids (cholesterol and triglycerides) need to be transported within the aqueous phase of plasma to provide various tissues with the substrates for energy, lipid deposition, steroid hormone production, and bile acid formation. To achieve this, the lipids are transported in the form of lipoproteins, of which there are five major classes. The lipoprotein complex consists of a core of hydrophobic lipid (cholesteryl esters and triglycerides) surrounded by a surface of hydrophilic phospholipids, free unesterified cholesterol, and apolipoproteins (Fig. 35-1). Apolipoproteins serve as structural proteins, as cofactors for enzymes, and as ligands for binding to certain receptors. Abnormalities of any of these functions can lead to dyslipidemia. All lipoproteins have the same basic structure of core and surface, but they differ in size, density, electrophoretic mobility, lipid composition, and apolipoprotein constituents.

The five major classes of lipoproteins are chylomicron, very-low-density lipoprotein (VLDL), intermediate-density lipoprotein (IDL), low-density lipoprotein (LDL) and high-density lipoprotein (HDL). Each class has specific physiological and anatomical significance (Table 35-1).

**Chylomicrons** are very large low-density particles that are rich in dietary triglyceride and are synthesized in the intestine. A number of apolipoproteins are present in chylomicrons, most notably Apo B48 and Apo CII. The half-life of chylomicrons is only 5 to 30 minutes, and therefore wide fluctuations in plasma triglyceride levels are seen. **VLDLs** are large particles synthesized in the liver, containing endogenous triglyceride and a small amount of cholesteryl ester. Their major apolipoproteins are Apo B100, Apo CII, Apo CIII, and Apo E. The half-life of VLDLs is approximately 12 hours. **IDLs** are smaller particles that are an intermediary step in the conversion from VLDL to LDL. They carry cholesteryl esters and triglycerides and

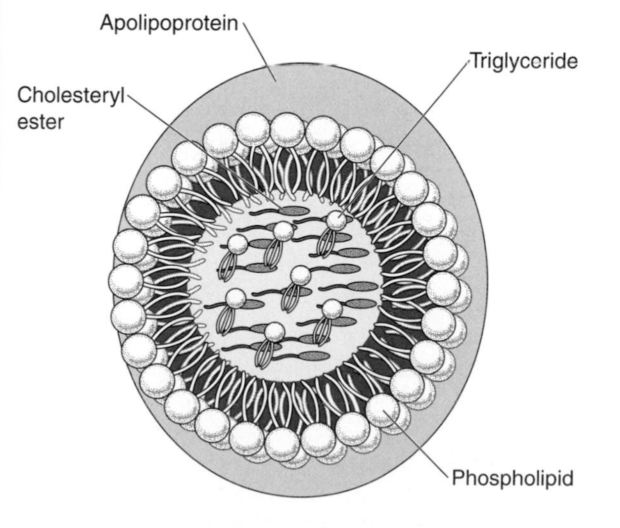

are associated with are even smaller ch from the successive and IDL particles. Th Apo B100. The half-li VLDL, IDL, and LDL pa and are believed to be t The measurement of Apo of the number of atherog LDL). **HDL** particles are sized in the liver and intesti their lipid, predominantly apolipoprotein constituents with the other lipoproteins. number of apolipoproteins, most notably Apo A, and are believed to be "protective" against atherosclerosis.

All five classes of lipoproteins are closely linked through metabolic pathways resulting in the necessary synthesis and delivery of vital lipid components to various tissues of the body. The major metabolic pathways of lipoprotein metabolism are the exogenous, endogenous, and HDL pathways.

## LIPOPROTEIN METABOLISM

### Exogenous Pathway

This pathway is responsible for the absorption of dietary lipids and their transport to the various tissues of the body for utilization or storage (Fig. 35-2). Dietary triglyceride is hydrolyzed in the lumen of the intestine. The free fatty acids are then taken up by the intestinal mucosal cell and combined with glycerol and monoglycerides to form triglyceride again. To a lesser extent, free cholesterol is esterified to cholesteryl ester. The triglycerides and cholesteryl ester are packaged with certain apolipoproteins, including Apo B48, and released into the lymphatic system. These "incomplete" chylomicrons are then released via the thoracic duct into the systemic circulation, where they interact with HDL particles, which provide them with Apo CII and Apo E, thereby rendering the chylomicrons "complete." Thus, a complete chylomicron particle contains a large amount of triglyceride, minimal cholesteryl ester, Apo B48, CII, and E, and a few other apolipoprotein species.

Within the circulation, lipoprotein lipase is an enzyme attached to the endothelial surface. With Apo CII as a cofactor, it hydrolyzes the triglyceride within the chylomicrons, thereby releasing free fatty acids into the circulation to be used for energy or stored within adipocytes. The size of the chylomicron particle becomes progressively smaller. The resulting chylomicron remnant is cleared from the circulation by the liver via a receptor with affinity for Apo E. The cholesterol within the remnant is incorporated into the hepatic cholesterol pool.

FIGURE 35-1 The lipoprotein complex consists of a core of hydrophobic lipid surrounded by a surface of hydrophilic phospholipids and apolipoproteins.

chemical Characteristics of the Major Lipoprotein Classes

| ein | Density (g/dL) | Molecular Weight (Da) | Diameter (nm) | Lipid (%)* | | |
|---|---|---|---|---|---|---|
| | | | | TG | Chol | PL |
| omicrons | 0.95 | $400 \times 10^6$ | 75–1200 | 80–95 | 2–7 | 3–9 |
| VLDL | 0.95–1.006 | $10$–$80 \times 10^6$ | 30–80 | 55–80 | 5–15 | 10–20 |
| IDL | 1.006–1.019 | $5$–$10 \times 10^6$ | 25–35 | 20–50 | 20–40 | 15–25 |
| LDL | 1.019–1.063 | $2.3 \times 10^6$ | 18–25 | 5–15 | 40–50 | 20–25 |
| HDL | 1.063–1.21 | $1.7$–$3.6 \times 10^6$ | 5–12 | 5–10 | 15–25 | 20–30 |

*Percentage of composition.

TG = triglycerides; Chol = cholesterol; PL = phospholipids.

(From Ginsberg et al., 1990. Reprinted with permission.)

## Endogenous Pathway

This pathway begins with the synthesis of VLDL particles by the liver (Fig. 35-3). Free fatty acids (FFAs) released into the circulation are taken up by the liver, where they are either used for energy or combined with glycerol to reform triglycerides. The triglycerides can then either be stored in hepatocytes or packaged into VLDL particles to be released into the circulation. The endothelial surface lipoprotein lipase, with Apo CII as a cofactor, hydrolyzes the triglyceride-rich core, releasing free fatty acids into the circula- tion. The VLDL particle becomes progressively smaller, and some of the excess surface components (Apo C, phospholipids) are transferred to HDL particles. As the VLDL particle size decreases, it is transformed into IDLs, which are triglyceride-depleted. About half of the IDL particles are taken up by the liver via interaction with Apo E. The other half are converted to smaller, cholesteryl-ester-rich LDL particles by hepatic lipase, which is located in the vascular endothelium of the liver. The only apolipoprotein associated with LDL is the same B100 molecule that was secreted with the VLDL particle from the liver.

**FIGURE 35-2**  Exogenous pathway of lipid metabolism. Dietary fat taken up by intestinal mucosal cells is used to produce chylomicrons, which are released into the circulation via the thoracic duct. The major apolipoprotein of chylomicrons is Apo B48. In the circulation, chylomicrons are hydrolyzed by lipoprotein lipase (LPL), releasing some free fatty acids (FFAs) into the circulation. The resulting chylomicron remnant is smaller and is taken up by the liver via a receptor with an affinity for Apo E.

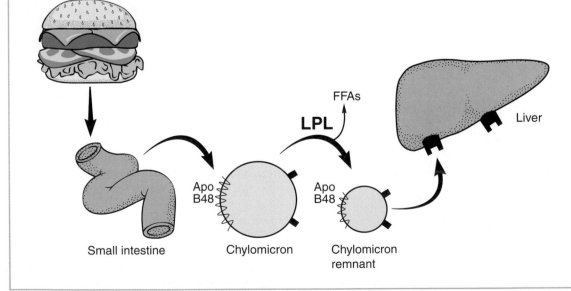

Endogenous pathway of lipid metabolism. Triglyceride-rich VLDL is secreted by the liver. In the circulation, lipoprotein lipase (LPL) hydrolyzes part of the triglyceride component of VLDL, thereby releasing free fatty acids (FFAs) into the circulation and making the VLDL particle smaller. The resulting VLDL remnant, also known as intermediate-density lipoprotein (IDL), either can be taken up by the liver via a receptor that recognizes Apo E or can undergo further hydrolysis via hepatic lipase (HL). The resulting particle is smaller and filled primarily with cholesteryl ester (LDL). The LDL particle can travel to other parts of the body to deliver necessary cholesterol. Alternatively, the liver can uptake LDL due to receptor-recognition of Apo B100.

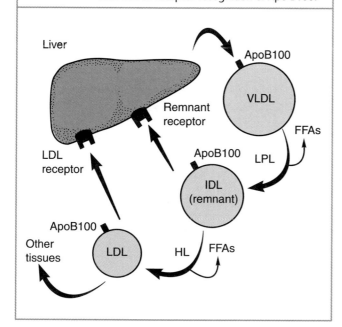

LDL particles can be taken up by the LDL receptors, either in the liver or in non-hepatic tissues, and are used in the synthesis of bile acids or cell membrane constituents or are stored. In the liver, the internalized LDL particle is disassembled by lysosomal hydrolysis, and the free cholesterol is incorporated into the intracellular pool. The intracellular level of free cholesterol in the liver determines the rate of endogenous synthesis of cholesterol and expression of the LDL receptor by the hepatocyte. When the amount of intracellular free cholesterol is high, LDL receptor expression is suppressed. Synthesis of cholesterol is also decreased through inhibition of 3-hydroxy-3-methylglutaryl-coenzyme A (HMG-CoA) reductase, the rate-limiting step in endogenous cholesterol synthesis. Alternatively, low amounts of intracellular free cholesterol will stimulate LDL receptor expression and HMG-CoA reductase activity, thus increasing both uptake of LDL from plasma and synthesis of cholesterol. However, not all LDL particles are cleared via the LDL receptor. Some LDL particles can be taken up by other cells, such as macrophages, via an unregulated scavenger receptor, resulting in intracellular lipid accumulation and formation of foam cells, leading to atherosclerosis.

## HDL Metabolism

The liver and intestine synthesize nascent discoidal HDL particles containing apolipoproteins, phospholipids, and minimal lipid content (Fig. 35-4). These small particles acquire more phospholipid and apolipoproteins through the conversion of triglyceride-rich chylomicrons and VLDL to chylomicron remnants and IDL. The major apolipoproteins of HDL are Apo AI and Apo AII, with some Apo C and Apo E. The discoidal HDL particles then acquire unesterified cholesterol from peripheral tissues, which is esterified to cholesteryl ester by the enzyme lecithin cholesteryl acyl transferase (LCAT), which requires Apo AI as a cofactor. This is the first step in the reverse cholesterol pathway whereby HDL removes cholesterol from peripheral tissues, including macrophages in atherosclerotic lesions, and carries it back to the liver for excretion in bile. After the esterified cholesterol has been incorporated into the discoidal HDL, the particle becomes larger and spherical and can transfer its cholesteryl ester to Apo B–containing particles (VLDL, IDL, and LDL) via the enzyme cholesteryl ester transfer protein (CETP). This transfer is also accompanied by the reciprocal transfer of triglycerides from Apo B–containing particles to HDL, a process that is felt to play a role in the clearance of HDL from the circulation. Hepatic lipase then acts on the triglyceride-enriched HDL particle and converts it back to the discoidal HDL, ready to accept more free cholesterol from peripheral tissues, and the cycle begins again. The net effect of this pathway is the delivery of free cholesterol from peripheral tissues to the liver, where it can either be excreted in bile or re-used in another way.

## Lipoprotein (a)

Lipoprotein (a), or Lp(a), is composed of one LDL particle with an apolipoprotein (a) moiety attached to the Apo B100 molecule. The lipid composition is similar to LDL, but its presence appears to be associated with an increased risk of cardiovascular disease, particularly in patients with other lipid risk factors for cardiovascular disease. The Lp(a) particle is assembled extracellularly. The Apo(a) protein is structurally similar to plasminogen and may compete with tissue plasminogen activator and thus interfere with fibrinolysis. Lp(a) crosses the endothelium by a non-receptor-mediated process and is found within the arterial intima, particularly in association with atherosclerotic plaque.

**FIGURE 35-4** HDL metabolism. The liver and intestine synthesize nascent discoidal HDL particles. The major apolipoproteins of HDL are Apo AI and Apo AII, with some Apo C and Apo E. The discoidal HDL particles then acquire free cholesterol (FC) from peripheral tissues, which is esterified to cholesteryl ester (CE) by the enzyme lecithin cholesteryl acyl transferase (LCAT). The discoidal HDL then becomes larger and spherical and can transfer its cholesteryl ester to Apo B–containing particles (VLDL, IDL, and LDL) via the enzyme cholesteryl ester transfer protein (CETP). This transfer is accompanied by the reciprocal transfer of triglycerides (TG) from Apo B–containing particles to HDL. The Apo B–containing particles can transfer the cholesteryl ester to the liver via the endogenous pathway, allowing the cholesterol to be excreted in the bile.

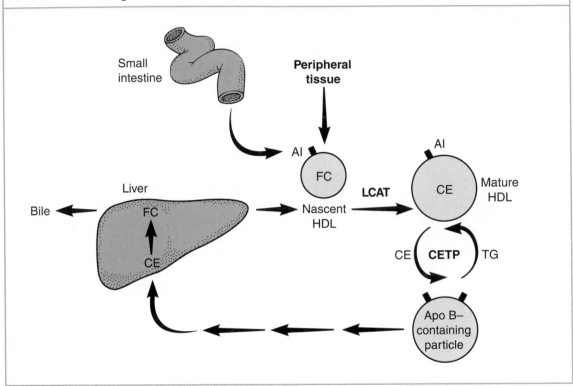

# CLASSIFICATION AND CAUSES OF DYSLIPIDEMIAS

Dyslipidemia is defined as an abnormality in lipoprotein concentrations. Traditionally, the Fredrickson classification (Table 35-2) was used to describe dyslipidemia on the basis of the biochemical phenotype of the lipoprotein that was increased. However, this classification has been replaced in common use by a more clinically relevant description of the lipid abnormality. Most clinical laboratories will report a concentration of total cholesterol (TC), triglycerides (TG), LDL-cholesterol (LDL-C; either calculated or directly measured), and HDL-cholesterol (HDL-C). Typically, lipid abnormalities are now classified as one of the following:

- Isolated elevation of LDL-C
- Hypertriglyceridemia (usually associated with low HDL-C levels)
- Combined elevation of LDL-C and TG
- Isolated low HDL-C
- Isolated high HDL-C

In all of the above dyslipidemias, the characteristic lipid profiles can result from either primary or secondary disturbances, or both (Table 35-3). Not all the primary genetic disturbances have been characterized. For example, by far the most common genetic lipid disorder is polygenic hypercholesterolemia, which does not have a single specific genetic cause and includes all primary causes of an elevated LDL-C that do not fit any of the identified primary disorders.

## Isolated Elevation of LDL Cholesterol

The accumulation of LDL particles resulting in the elevation in LDL cholesterol can occur from a primary defect or from secondary causes. Primary defects include familial hypercholesterolemia, familial defective Apo B, and auto-

| TABLE 35-2 | Frederickson Classification of Dyslipidemia | | |
|---|---|---|---|
| Type | Clinical Designation | Plasma Lipid Changes | Primary Defect |
| I | Familial hyperchylomicronemia | ↑↑ chylomicrons (↑↑ TG, ↑ cholesterol) | Lipoprotein lipase deficiency, Apo CII deficiency |
| IIa | Familial hypercholesterolemia | ↑ LDL cholesterol | LDL receptor deficiency, defective Apo B |
| IIb | Combined hyperlipoproteinemia | ↑ VLDL, ↑ LDL (HDL may be ↓) | LDL receptor deficiency, ↑ production of VLDL |
| III | Dysbetalipoproteinemia | ↑ IDL (↑ cholesterol, ↑ TG) | Atypical form of Apo E, causing poor uptake of IDL by the liver |
| IV | Familial hypertriglyceridemia | ↑ VLDL, ↓ HDL (↑ TG, ↑/normal cholesterol) | ? |
| V | Mixed hypertriglyceridemia | ↑↑ chylomicrons, ↑↑ VLDL | ? |
| VI | Familial hyperalphalipoproteinemia | ↑ HDL | ? |

somal recessive hypercholesterolemia and sitosterolemia. Familial hypercholesterolemia (FH) is by far the most common of the identified primary disorders resulting in isolated elevated LDL-C. It is an autosomal co-dominant disorder causing either defective or absent LDL receptors, so LDL particles accumulate in the plasma and can lead to extremely premature atherosclerotic disease with coronary artery disease occurring in childhood in homozygous individuals and in the third or fourth decade in heterozygous individuals. The heterozygous form has a prevalence of 1:500 in most Caucasian populations but is more common in certain populations such as French Canadians, Afrikaners from South Africa, and Lebanese. Familial defective Apo B is much less common than FH but shares the same phenotype. Defective Apo B is associated with an altered ability of LDL to bind to the LDL receptor for clearance. Hence, similar to FH, there is an accumulation of LDL particles in the plasma. Autosomal recessive hypercholesterolemia and sitosterolemia are

very rare genetic disorders also resulting in isolated elevations in cholesterol. Sitosterolemia results from a genetic defect leading to abnormal retention of sterols in the body, contributing to increased atherosclerotic disease.

There are several secondary causes of isolated elevated LDL cholesterol. Hypothyroidism can be associated with an elevation in LDL-C resulting from decreased clearance of LDL from the plasma. Nephrotic syndrome has also been implicated, likely because of increased loss of lipoproteins in the urine resulting in over-compensated production of all proteins (including lipoproteins) by the liver. Cholestatic liver disease has also been associated with elevated LDL-C, as well as the use of certain medications such as cyclosporine and sirolimus.

## Hypertriglyceridemia

An elevation in triglycerides can result from an accumulation of chylomicrons or VLDL particles. Elevations of triglycerides are often associated with a reduction in HDL-C, perhaps related to increased clearance of triglyceride-rich HDL particles. There are several primary defects and many secondary disturbances that can result in hypertriglyceridemia. Some of the primary genetic defects resulting in hypertriglyceridemia include familial hypertriglyceridemia, as well as the less common lipoprotein lipase deficiency and Apo CII deficiency. No single genetic defect has been identified for familial hypertriglyceridemia, and it is likely that this disorder represents an assortment of genetic defects resulting in the same phenotype. Since lipoprotein lipase is necessary for the hydrolysis of the triglyceride components of both chylomicrons and VLDL particles, deficiency of this enzyme would result in an accumulation of these particles. Apo CII is a necessary cofactor of this interaction, so its deficiency would result in the same phenotype. These disorders are uncommon and result in severe hypertriglyceridemia.

| TABLE 35-3 | Secondary Causes of Dyslipidemia | |
|---|---|---|
| **High LDL** | | **High TG** |

**High LDL**
- Hypothyroidism
- Nephrotic syndrome
- Cholestatic liver disease
- Medications: cyclosporine, sirolimus, tacrolimus

**Low HDL (isolated)**
- Most commonly associated with the insulin resistance or metabolic syndrome
- Smoking
- Lack of physical activity

**High TG**
- Insulin resistance or metabolic syndrome
- Diabetes mellitus
- Alcohol consumption
- Chronic kidney disease
- Hepatocellular disease
- Pregnancy
- Abdominal obesity
- Medications: OCP, estrogen, retinoids, steroids, protease inhibitors, β blockers, thiazides, cyclosporine, sirolimus

There are a number of secondary causes of elevated triglycerides. The most common are likely abdominal obesity, insulin resistance, and the metabolic syndrome. Diabetes, alcohol consumption, chronic kidney disease, hepatocellular disease, and pregnancy are also associated with hypertriglyceridemia. A number of medications can cause high triglycerides. These include estrogens, oral contraceptive pills, retinoids, corticosteroids, protease inhibitors, β-adrenergic receptor blockers, and others.

## Combined Elevation of LDL-C and Triglycerides

Combined elevation of LDL-C and TG can be caused by familial combined hyperlipidemia, which is a genetic disorder of unknown etiology. Patients with this disorder typically have a history of both elevated LDL-C and TG, often not simultaneously. They also frequently have a family history of dyslipidemia and/or premature coronary artery disease, typically in the late fifth or sixth decade. Depending on when the disorder is detected, the patient may be considered to have isolated elevations of LDL-C or TG, when in fact, with time, it will become evident that the patient has a propensity for both abnormalities. Another much less common cause of elevated laboratory values of both LDL-C and TG is classically referred to as "type III hyperlipoproteinemia" or dysbetalipoproteinemia. Individuals with this disorder are generally homozygous for a form of Apo E (Apo E2) that is less efficient at binding to receptors in the liver. Therefore, there is an accumulation of chylomicron remnants and IDL particles, leading to a stereotypical pattern on lipoprotein electrophoresis. These patients are genetically predisposed to the phenotype, but typically however, another factor, such as lifestyle, poorly controlled diabetes, or excessive alcohol intake, is required to exceed the ability of the poorly functioning Apo E to clear IDL and chylomicron remnants, thus leading to expression of the full phenotype with its associated increased cardiovascular risk.

There are no secondary causes that lead to a combined elevation of LDL-C and TG. Rather, there is a combination of individual factors that result in the lipoprotein abnormalities seen.

## Isolated Low HDL Cholesterol

Isolated low HDL cholesterol is uncommon. Typically, low HDL-C is seen in association with elevated TG, even mild elevations. There are a few rare primary causes of isolated low HDL-C. These include ABC transporter deficiency, Apo AI deficiency, and perhaps some LCAT abnormalities. The ABC transporter is primarily responsible for the transport of free cholesterol from peripheral tissues to discoidal HDL particles, allowing them to form mature HDL particles. A deficiency of such a transporter would result in low HDL concentrations. Genetic defects resulting in a deficiency of Apo AI and abnormalities of LCAT are associated with a marked reduction in HDL concentrations. There are a few secondary causes of low HDL-C, independent of hypertriglyceridemia. These include a diet very low in saturated fat, as well as smoking.

## Isolated High HDL Cholesterol

Isolated high HDL-C is uncommon. Some rare primary disorders that result in elevated HDL-C levels include CETP deficiency and abnormalities of hepatic lipase. Some secondary factors that can raise HDL-C are alcohol consumption, estrogens, and exercise. It is believed that, in most situations, elevated HDL-C is protective against cardiovascular disease.

## DYSLIPIDEMIA AND CARDIOVASCULAR RISK

Abnormalities in concentrations of lipoproteins can contribute to atherosclerotic disease. Over 60% of men with premature coronary artery disease have dyslipidemia, defined as total cholesterol, triglycerides, LDL-C, Apo B, or Lp(a) over the 90th percentile or an HDL below the tenth percentile.

High LDL-C concentration is associated with increased cardiovascular risk. LDL particles can be modified by oxidation or glycosylation or both. These modified LDL particles promote atherosclerosis through a number of mechanisms. Macrophages take up these modified LDL particles more readily to form foam cells, a critical component of plaque formation. There is a reduction in nitric oxide release and activity, leading to endothelial dysfunction. There is also increased platelet aggregation, increasing the risk of thrombosis. Together, these mechanisms account for the increased cardiovascular risk associated with elevated LDL levels. Not only is the concentration of LDL important, but also the quality of the LDL particles. For example, an increase in small dense LDL particles is seen in association with hypertriglyceridemia. These small dense LDL particles bind less avidly to the LDL receptor, remain in the circulation longer, and are thus more prone to modification by oxidation or glycosylation. As mentioned previously, Lp(a), which is an LDL particle with the Apo(a) protein attached to it, is also associated with increased cardiovascular risk, particularly in association with other abnormalities of lipoprotein concentration.

HDL particles generally protect against atherosclerosis. The exact mechanisms by which this occurs are not clear. The protective effects of HDL are likely secondary to increased reverse cholesterol transport, the antioxidant and anti-inflammatory properties of HDL, the maintenance of endothelial function, and/or the protection against thrombosis. Therefore, low levels of HDL have been associated with increased cardiovascular risk, and much attention has been paid to the total cholesterol to HDL ratio as a reliable marker of an individual's cardiovascular risk.

The relationship between hypertriglyceridemia and cardiovascular risk remains debatable. Since hypertriglyceridemia is typically associated with low HDL and small dense LDL, both risk factors for cardiovascular disease, it is difficult to determine if hypertriglyceridemia per se is related to increased cardiovascular risk or whether the increased risk is simply a result of the company it keeps.

## PRINCIPLES OF TREATMENT

### Prior to Treatment

Before deciding whether an individual patient requires treatment for dyslipidemia, one must follow a number of steps. First, the type of lipid abnormality must be identified and the cause elucidated. The type of lipid abnormality can be identified easily through measurement of plasma total cholesterol, triglycerides, HDL, and LDL. After identifying the type of lipid abnormality, one must determine if the cause is primary, secondary, or both. A thorough history, physical examination, and routine blood tests are usually sufficient to determine the cause(s) of the dyslipidemia. Once the type and cause have been determined, one can decide whether or not treatment is warranted. Nearly all individuals with dyslipidemia will require advice on lifestyle modifications to improve their lipid status through dietary changes, exercise, weight loss, and/or smoking cessation. However, the decision to begin pharmacological treatment in addition to the lifestyle advice will depend on the severity of the dyslipidemia, the presence or absence of other cardiovascular risk factors (which will allow one to calculate the individual's estimated cardiovascular risk category), and the target lipid levels.

### Assessing Cardiovascular Risk

Many professional organizations from around the world have developed guidelines for the treatment of dyslipidemia based on expert consensus panels and available evidence. Although the details differ somewhat from organization to organization, several principles are common to all. The concept of basing the intensity of treatment on an assessment of the individual's estimate of cardiovascular risk is central to all the guidelines. Many "risk calculators" have been developed from data from large epidemiological studies of dyslipidemia and cardiovascular disease. Based on the number and severity of risk factors, each individual can be assigned a "risk category" based on his or her estimated long-term risk for cardiovascular disease. For example, the National Cholesterol Education Panel

(Adult Treatment Panel III, NCEP-ATPIII) in the United States (Table 35-4) and the Canadian Working Group on Hypercholesterolemia and Other Dyslipidemias (Table 35-5) recommend that risk calculations be based on data from the Framingham epidemiological study of individuals in the United States. If the 10-year risk estimate of hard cardiac endpoints (death and non-fatal myocardial infarction) is less than 10%, the individual is placed in the low-risk category. If their 10-year risk is 10 to 20%, then the individual is in the moderate-risk category, and if their 10-year risk is greater than 20%, they are placed in the high-risk category. Individuals with known atherosclerosis (coronary or non-coronary) or diabetes are automatically considered high risk. Based on newer clinical trial data, the NCEP-ATPIII has modified its recommendations to include a very-high-risk category with even lower lipid targets for patients with established vascular disease plus other high-risk factors. These changes were considered "optional." In contrast, the Joint Task Force of the European and other Societies on Cardiovascular Disease Prevention in Clinical Practice (Table 35-6) recommends the use of the Systematic Coronary Risk Evaluation (SCORE) Model and Risk Charts derived from the SCORE study, a large dataset of prospective European studies. Depending on whether the country of residence is deemed high or low risk, the corresponding risk chart would be used to determine a risk estimate for the individual. In the European guidelines, a 10-year risk of a fatal cardiovascular event greater than or equal to 5% is considered high risk.

### Treatment Decisions Based on Risk Category

Depending on the severity of the risk category assigned, treatment decisions can be made. The higher the risk, the greater the intensity of treatment required. The lipid targets also become lower as risk increases because studies have shown a greater absolute risk reduction with treatment for those at higher baseline risk of a cardiac event. Again, the specific targets differ from organization to organization but the concept remains the same—more aggressive treatment and targets for those at higher risk. The target lipid levels from the NCEP-ATPIII, the Canadian Working Group, and the European Task Force are shown in Tables 35-4 to 35-6.

### Severe Hypertriglyceridemia

Reduction of cardiovascular risk is the main reason for choosing to treat almost all lipid abnormalities, with the exception of severe hypertriglyceridemia (TG >6.0 mmol/L). In the case of severe hypertriglyceridemia, treatment is necessary to prevent some of the associated acute complications of very high triglyceride levels. Acute pancreatitis can be caused by severe hypertriglyceridemia and is

**TABLE 35-4** National Cholesterol Education Program—Adult Treatment Panel III Cholesterol Targets, 2001

| Risk Category | LDL-C Goal (mg/dL) | LDL-C Level at Which to Initiate TLC (mg/dL) | LDL-C Level at Which to Consider Drug Therapy (mg/dL) | Non-HDL-C Goal (mg/dL) |
|---|---|---|---|---|
| Very high risk* | <70 (<1.8 mmol/L) | ≥70 (≥1.8 mmol/L) | ≥70 (≥1.8 mmol/L) | <130 (<3.4 mmol/L) |
| CHD or CHD risk equivalents† (10-year risk >20%) | <100 (<2.6 mmol/L) | ≥100 (≥2.6 mmol/L) | ≥130 (≥3.4 mmol/L) | <130 (<3.4 mmol/L) |
| 2+ Risk factors (10-year risk ≤20%) | <130 (<3.4 mmol/L) | ≥130 (≥3.4 mmol/L) | 10-year risk 10–20% ≥130 (≥3.4 mmol/L) 10-year risk <10% ≥160 (≥4.1 mmol/L) | <160 (<4.1 mmol/L) |
| 0 or 1 Risk factor | <160 (<4.1 mmol/L) | ≥160 (≥4.1 mmol/L) | ≥190 (≥4.9 mmol/L) | <190 (<4.9 mmol/L) |

CHD = coronary heart disease.

*Very high risk = established cardiovascular disease **plus** (1) multiple major risk factors (especially diabetes), or (2) severe and poorly controlled risk factors (especially smoking), or (3) multiple risk factors of the metabolic syndrome, or (4) acute coronary syndrome. Note that these recommendations are considered "optional."

†CHD equivalents = any atherosclerotic disease or diabetes mellitus.

(Adapted from Grundy et al., 2001 and Grundy et al., 2004.)

potentially life-threatening. Eruptive xanthoma is another acute complication, which manifests as an eruptive skin rash of pruritic papules that can cause the patient much discomfort. Although these patients are also at risk for cardiovascular disease, the major rationale to treat is the prevention of these more immediate complications.

## NON-PHARMACOLOGICAL TREATMENT OF DYSLIPIDEMIA

All patients with dyslipidemia should be given advice about appropriate lifestyle interventions. These may include dietary modifications, increased physical activity, weight reduction, and smoking cessation. The specific dietary recommendations will differ depending on the pre-

dominant lipid abnormality. To lower LDL cholesterol, a reduction in saturated fat, hydrogenated fat, dietary cholesterol, and total fat are helpful measures. Increases in soluble fibre, soy protein, and plant sterols are also helpful. Most of these measures will individually reduce LDL cholesterol by approximately 5 to 10%. The "portfolio diet," which is a combination of multiple dietary interventions, has been shown to reduce LDL by as much as 28%; however, long-term palatability of the diet remains questionable. To lower triglycerides, the following lifestyle interventions are helpful: reduction of total fat and alcohol consumption, weight reduction, increased physical activity, substitution of low for high glycemic index foods, and increased ingestion of omega-3 fatty acids. HDL cholesterol levels may also increase with these measures, perhaps due to the reduction in triglycerides as opposed to any direct

**TABLE 35-5** Canadian Working Group Cholesterol Targets, 2003

| Risk Category | 10-Year Risk Estimate of CVD | LDL-C (mmol/L) | | TC to HDL-C Ratio |
|---|---|---|---|---|
| High | • 20% • Diabetes • Any atherosclerotic disease • Chronic kidney disease (including dialysis-dependent and renal transplant recipients) | <2.5 | and | <4.0 |
| Moderate | 10–20% | <3.5 | and | <5.0 |
| Low | <10% | <4.5 | or | <6.0 |

(Adapted from Genest et al., 2003, with permission.)

| TABLE 35-6 | European Task Force Cholesterol Targets, 2003 | |
| --- | --- | --- |
| Risk Category | Total Cholesterol (mmol/L) | LDL-C Level (mmol/L) |
| CHD or CHD equivalent | <4.5 | <2.5 |
| 10-year CV risk ≥5% | <4.5 | <2.5 |
| 10-year CV risk <5% | <5.0 | <3.0 |

CHD = coronary heart disease; CV = cardiovascular.
(Adapted from De Backer et al., 2003.)

effects on HDL metabolism. Smoking cessation is obviously a critical component of reducing cardiovascular risk, irrespective of baseline lipid levels. In addition, it has also been shown that smoking cessation can raise HDL levels.

# PHARMACOLOGICAL THERAPY

Depending on the individual's estimated risk and severity of dyslipidemia, some individuals will be started on pharmacological therapy, along with lifestyle modifications, from initial diagnosis. Others will require pharmacological therapy only after a trial of lifestyle changes has not achieved target lipid levels. The choice of drug is dependent on the desired lipoprotein change. The lipid effects and side effects of the major classes of lipid-lowering agents are outlined in Tables 35-7 and 35-8, respectively, and are discussed below. The classes can be divided into those with primarily LDL-lowering effects (statins, resins, cholesterol absorption inhibitors, stanols/sterols), triglyceride-lowering effects (fibrates, fish oil capsules), or combined effects (niacin). It is important to note that each agent may have effects on all the lipoproteins; however, the degree of effect differs.

## LDL-Lowering Agents

### HMG-CoA reductase inhibitors (statins)

There are currently six agents of this class (Fig. 35-5) that are used clinically—namely, atorvastatin (Lipitor), fluvas-

tatin (Lescol), lovastatin (Mevacor), pravastatin (Pravachol), rosuvastatin (Crestor), and simvastatin (Zocor).

*Mechanism of action and efficacy.* Statins are competitive inhibitors of 3-hydroxy-3-methylglutaryl-coenzyme A (HMG-CoA) reductase and therefore block the synthesis of cholesterol in the liver. This results in lowered intracellular levels of cholesterol, which results in an increase in the number of LDL receptors on the hepatocyte cell surface. The increase in LDL receptors increases the receptor-mediated uptake of LDL by the liver, thus reducing plasma LDL levels. In addition, the statins also decrease VLDL secretion by the liver, which in turn also decreases LDL-C levels. Depending on the statin being used, these drugs typically produce a 24 to 55% reduction in LDL. There are also minor effects on the other lipoproteins. Triglycerides may be reduced by 5 to 20%, and HDL may rise by 5 to 10%. The statins differ in efficacy, with atorvastatin and rosuvastatin producing the largest LDL reduction, apparently as a result of their longer serum half-lives. There may also be benefits beyond their lipid-lowering abilities (so-called "pleiotropic effects"). For example, statins have also been shown to improve endothelial function and provide anti-inflammatory properties, thus perhaps contributing to their protective effects on the cardiovascular system, although it is not clear whether these non-lipid lowering effects are secondary to the lower LDL, to reductions in mevalonic acid (as a result of inhibition of HMG-CoA reductase), or to the drugs themselves.

*Pharmacokinetics.* Lovastatin, simvastatin, and pravastatin are derived from the fungus *Aspergillus terreus*. The other statins are synthetic compounds and are structurally different from the fungal-derived statins. Some of the pharmacokinetic differences between the statins are shown in Table 35-9. With the exception of lovastatin and simvastatin, all the statins are administered as active compounds that inhibit HMG-CoA reductase and are biotransformed to inactive or weakly active metabolites. In contrast, lovastatin and simvastatin are inactive prodrugs that require hydrolysis by the liver to form one or more active metabolites that are then further biotransformed to inactive products.

| TABLE 35-7 | Lipid Effects of Lipid-Lowering Agents | | | |
| --- | --- | --- | --- | --- |
| Medication | Total Cholesterol | Triglycerides | LDL-C | HDL-C |
| Statins | ↓ (15–30%) | ↓ (5–20%) | ↓↓ (25–55%) | ↑ (5–10%) |
| Bile acid binding resins | ↓ (15–20%) | ↑ | ↓↓ (20–30%) | ↑ (2–5%) |
| Cholesterol absorption inhibitors | ↓ (10–15%) | ↓ (5–6%) | ↓ (15–20%) | ↑ (1–4%) |
| Fibrates | ↓ | ↓↓ (40–50%) | ↓ or ↑ | ↑↑ (10–20%) |
| Niacin | ↓ (20–40%) | ↓↓ (20–50%) | ↓ (5–25%) | ↑↑ (15–35%) |

| TABLE 35-8 | Side Effects and Contraindications to Lipid-Lowering Agents | | |
|---|---|---|---|
| Medication | Recommended Dose Range | Side Effects | Contraindications/Cautions |
| **Statins** | | • Myositis | • Active liver disease |
| Atorvastatin (Lipitor) | 10–80 mg | • Hepatitis | • Pregnancy/lactation |
| Fluvastatin (Lescol) | 20–80 mg | | • Renal dose adjustment (for most) |
| Lovastatin (Mevacor) | 20–80 mg | | • Beware of drug interactions |
| Pravastatin (Pravachol) | 10–40 mg | | |
| Rosuvastatin (Crestor) | 10–40 mg | | |
| Simvastatin (Zocor) | 10–80 mg | | |
| **Bile acid binding resins** | | • Constipation | • Biliary obstruction |
| Cholestyramine (Questran) | 2–24 g | • Upper GI discomfort | • Can alter absorption of other drugs |
| Colestipol (Colestid) | | | • Inconvenient |
| **Cholesterol absorption inhibitor** | | • Allergy | • Pregnancy/lactation |
| Ezetimibe (Ezetrol) | 10 mg | | • Moderate to severe hepatic dysfunction |
| **Fibrates** | | • Upper GI discomfort | • Severe kidney dysfunction |
| Bezafibrate | 400 mg | • Cholelithiasis (?) | • Hepatic dysfunction |
| Fenofibrate | 67–200 mg | • Myositis | • Gallbladder disease |
| Gemfibrozil | 600–1200 mg | • Kidney impairment | • Primary biliary cirrhosis |
| | | | • Pregnancy/lactation |
| **Niacin** | 1–3 g | • Flushing | • Active peptic ulcer disease |
| | | • Hepatotoxicity | • Hepatic dysfunction |
| | | • GI discomfort | • Recent active gout |
| | | • Diarrhea | |
| | | • Hyperglycemia | |

GI = gastrointestinal.

All six drugs are well absorbed by mouth but undergo first-pass metabolism by the liver. Lovastatin, simvastatin, and atorvastatin are primarily metabolized by the CYP3A4 isoenzyme. Fluvastatin is primarily metabolized by the CYP2C9 isoenzyme. In contrast, pravastatin and rosuvastatin exhibit minimal, if any, metabolism by the cytochrome P450 system. Pravastatin and rosuvastatin also differ in that these two statins are relatively hydrophilic, unlike the others, which are lipophilic. The elimination half-lives of the drugs range from 2 to 20 hours; atorvastatin and rosuvastatin have the longest half-lives of 15 and 20 hours, respectively. The urinary excretion of statins is relatively minor. It is important to note that fluvastatin, lovastatin, pravastatin, and simvastatin require administration in the evening to maximize efficacy. However, atorvastatin and rosuvastatin can be taken at any time of day with equal efficacy, presumably as a result of their longer half-lives.

*Side effects, drug interactions, and contraindications.* These agents have been widely used, and overall they have an excellent safety profile and are well tolerated. There are a few potential toxicities, however, that may occur. Elevations in liver transaminases can occur in 1 to 2% of patients. These are generally transient, but it is recommended that patients on statins have their liver function tests checked at 3 months and periodically thereafter. Myalgias, with or without elevations in creatine kinase (CK) levels, may also occur. Rarely, severe elevations in CK can result in rhabdomyolysis. Typically, these adverse effects resolve when the medication is discontinued. The risk of toxicity is generally dose-dependent and increases in the context of reduced kidney function and/or drug interactions. There have been several case reports of an association between chronic statin use and peripheral neuropathy. This has not been observed in any of the large cardiovascular outcome trials. Thus, even if this association is true, it should be noted that the increase in risk is very small relative to the large cardiovascular benefit.

Drug interactions are important considerations when using statins as they can increase the risk of toxicities associated with statin use. Given that the majority of the statins are metabolized through the cytochrome P450 system, agents that affect the system can cause changes in the

**FIGURE 35-5** Structural formulae of HMG-CoA-reductase inhibitors.

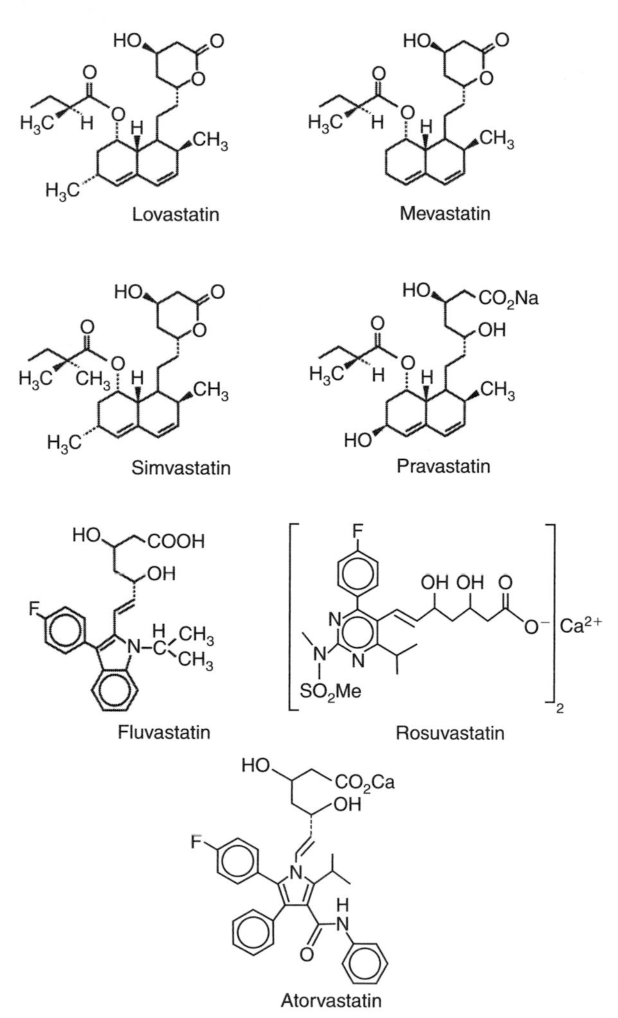

Lovastatin

Mevastatin

Simvastatin

Pravastatin

Fluvastatin

Rosuvastatin

Atorvastatin

is unknown. Rosuvastatin is minimally metabolized by the cytochrome P450 system. However, co-administration with cyclosporine has been shown to increase plasma levels of rosuvastatin tenfold. All the statins have subtle effects on warfarin concentrations; thus, prothrombin time should be monitored carefully when a statin is initiated. All the statins also interact with fibrates, particularly gemfibrozil, although to different degrees. Generally, combination use of statins and fibrates increases the risk of muscle toxicity and therefore should be used cautiously. In addition to the drug interactions resulting from alterations of the P450 system, statins are also substrates for P-glycoprotein, which is a transporter of drugs across cell membranes that can alter the absorption and bioavailability of drugs that compete with statins as a substrate for P-glycoprotein. Antacids, dietary fibre, and bile acid binding resins can decrease the absorption of statins and should be administered at different times.

Given the extensive hepatic metabolism of statins, active liver disease is one of the contraindications to their use. Other contraindications include pregnancy or lactation. Kidney disease is not an absolute contraindication. Although renal excretion is fairly minor, severe kidney dysfunction can lead to increases in plasma levels of statins. Therefore, the dose of statin should be decreased in patients with severe kidney impairment.

*Evidence.* There is an abundance of evidence for the use of statins for both primary and secondary prevention of cardiovascular disease (Table 35-10). Most studies report an approximate relative risk reduction of 30 to 35% for cardiovascular events in primary prevention and 25% in secondary prevention. However, it is important to note that although the relative risk reduction appears to be greater for primary prevention, the *absolute* risk reduction is far greater for secondary prevention. The reduction in cardiovascular risk appears to continue as the LDL is lowered, with no apparent lower limit. The Heart Protection Study, a large, randomized, controlled secondary prevention study comparing simvastatin 40 mg once daily to placebo, demonstrated significant reduction in cardiovascular events, irrespective of baseline lipid levels.

## Bile acid binding resins

The resins (also called bile acid sequestrants) currently in clinical use are cholestyramine (Questran) and colestipol (Colestid).

*Mechanism of action and efficacy.* Bile acid binding resins are insoluble in water, are unaffected by digestive enzymes, and are not absorbed from the intestinal tract. They are cationic resins that bind the bile acids and thus prevent their absorption from the intestine. The net result is increased fecal excretion of bile acids and a compensatory increase in *de novo* production of bile acids from the

plasma levels of the statin. Medications can either be substrates, inducers, or inhibitors of specific isoenzymes in the cytochrome P450 system. Therefore, co-administration of lovastatin, simvastatin, or atorvastatin with a macrolide, an anti-fungal, a protease inhibitor, or cyclosporine, all of which are known inhibitors of CYP3A4, can result in elevated plasma levels of the statin and increased risk of toxicity. Similarly, large amounts (greater than 1 L/day) of grapefruit juice, a potent inhibitor of CYP3A family, can result in similar effects on lovastatin, simvastatin, and atorvastatin. Fluvastatin is metabolized via CYP2C9. Co-administration with cimetidine and omeprazole appears to increase plasma levels of fluvastatin, but the clinical significance is unclear. Pravastatin does not appear to interact with the known inhibitors of the cytochrome P450 system, with the exception of cyclosporine, which can cause an increase in pravastatin levels; however, the clinical significance of this

**TABLE 35-9**    Pharmacokinetic Properties of the Statins

| Drug | Mechanism of Hepatic Metabolism | Protein Binding (%) | Renal Excretion (%) | Lipophilicity | Elimination Half-Life (hours) |
|---|---|---|---|---|---|
| Atorvastatin | CYP 3A4 | >98 | <2 | Yes | 15 |
| Fluvastatin | CYP 2C9 | >99 | 5 | Yes | 3 |
| Lovastatin | CYP 3A4 | >95 | 10 | Yes | 2 |
| Pravastatin | Sulfation | 50 | 20 | No | 2 |
| Rosuvastatin | CYP 2C9 (minor) | 88 | 10 | Slight | 20 |
| Simvastatin | CYP 3A4 | >95 | 13 | Yes | 3 |

cholesterol in the liver. As a consequence of reduction in intracellular cholesterol, there is an increase in LDL receptors, resulting in more receptor-mediated uptake of LDL and a reduction in plasma LDL levels. There is no systemic absorption of the resin.

The amount of LDL lowering is dose dependent. A 20 to 30% reduction can be seen with maximal doses of resin. There is an unpredictable minimal rise in HDL of 2 to 5%. The effect on triglycerides is less favourable. In patients whose triglyceride levels are increased prior to treatment, triglycerides will increase further with resins.

*Side effects.* Nausea, abdominal bloating, indigestion, and constipation are common side effects of resin use. Since the resins bind bile acids, they also impair the absorption of

dietary fat; therefore, they may interfere with the absorption of fat-soluble vitamins and can cause steatorrhea in high doses. These cationic resins have high affinity for acidic compounds and thus bind to and impair the intestinal absorption of certain drugs, such as warfarin, thiazides, phenylbutazone, barbiturates, thyroxine, and cardiac glycosides. Therefore, orally administered drugs should be ingested either 2 hours before or 4 hours after the resin. Finally, the resins are generally taken in the form of powders that have poor palatability. For all the above reasons, their use is often associated with poor compliance.

*Evidence.* Although bile acid binding resins have been available for the treatment of hypercholesterolemia for many years, there is only one trial (the Lipid Research

**TABLE 35-10**    Outcome Trials of Statin Therapy for the Primary and Secondary Prevention of Cardiovascular Disease

| Trial Name | Patient Population | Intervention | Relative Risk Reduction | Number Needed to Treat |
|---|---|---|---|---|
| **Primary prevention** | | | | |
| WOSCOPS | High LDL (men) | Pravastatin | 31% | 45 |
| AFCAPS/TexCAPS | Moderate LDL | Lovastatin | 37% | 50 |
| ASCOT-LLA | Moderate LDL, multiple risk factors, hypertensive | Atorvastatin | 36% | 90 |
| **Secondary prevention** | | | | |
| 4S | High LDL | Simvastatin | 29% | 30 |
| CARE | Moderate LDL | Pravastatin | 23% | 33 |
| LIPID | Moderate LDL | Pravastatin | 23% | 53 |
| HPS | Low to high LDL | Simvastatin | 24% | 18 |
| PROSPER | TC 4.0–9.0 mmol/L Mean LDL 3.8 mmol/L Age >70 years | Pravastatin | 15% | 48 |
| PROVE-IT | TC <6.21 mmol/L Median LDL 2.74 mmol/L ACS within 10 days | Pravastatin 40 mg versus atorvastatin 80 mg | 16% (favour atorvastatin 80 mg) | 26 |
| TNT | LDL <3.4 mmol/L Stable CHD | Atorvastatin 10 mg versus 80 mg | 22% (favour 80 mg) | 45 |

TC = total cholesterol; ACS = acute coronary syndrome; CHD = coronary heart disease.

Clinics-Coronary Primary Prevention Trial (LRC-CPPT) demonstrating a modest reduction in cardiovascular events associated with their use.

## Cholesterol absorption inhibitors

*Mechanism of action and efficacy.* Ezetimibe is the first member of a class of selective cholesterol absorption inhibitors that selectively inhibit dietary and biliary cholesterol absorption at the brush border of the intestinal mucosa. The absorption of triglycerides and fat-soluble vitamins is not affected. The drug is well absorbed following oral administration. Both ezetimibe and its main metabolite, ezetimibe glucuronide, are active cholesterol absorption inhibitors. The parent compound is partially glucuronidated into its main metabolite by the intestinal enterocyte. The compound is further metabolized by the liver, and the active glucuronide metabolite is excreted back into the intestine via the bile duct. Thus, the action of the glucuronide metabolite is prolonged because it is reabsorbed and recirculated through enterohepatic circulation. The half-life of ezetimibe and its main metabolite is approximately 20 to 30 hours.

When used as monotherapy, ezetimibe can reduce LDL levels by approximately 15 to 20%. Studies of combination therapy with statins demonstrate a further 15 to 20% reduction in LDL, beyond that of statin alone. The effect on HDL and triglyceride levels is minimal. Given that ezetimibe exerts its primary effect on LDL-C, it can be used either alone or in combination with a statin in patients with primary hypercholesterolemia who have not achieved their LDL-C target level. Monotherapy should be considered in those patients who are unable to tolerate statins or for whom statins are contraindicated, assuming that they are no more than 15 to 20% above their target LDL-C level. Addition of ezetimibe to statin therapy should be considered if the LDL-C target has not yet been achieved despite the maximum tolerated statin dose. In patients with homozygous familial hypercholesterolemia, ezetimibe can be added to statin therapy to lower cholesterol levels. Sitosterolemia is a rare, inherited recessive disorder characterized by hyperabsorption of plant sterols and decreased biliary excretion, leading to increased circulating levels of plant sterols and increased risk of atherosclerosis. Ezetimibe has also been shown to be a useful adjunct to dietary therapy for patients with sitosterolemia.

*Side effects.* Clinical studies of ezetimibe as monotherapy or in combination with statins have demonstrated adverse event profiles similar to placebo. However, there have been some post-marketing reports of allergy with ezetimibe. Liver enzymes and CK levels are not significantly altered with ezetimibe alone. Unlike the experience with resins, the occurrence of gastrointestinal symptoms is similar to placebo. Fat-soluble vitamin status is not affected. Pharmacokinetic studies demonstrate no significant effect on the cytochrome P450 isoenzymes. No significant interaction has been observed with concomitant warfarin, oral contraceptive, digoxin, or cimetidine use. However, cyclosporine may increase ezetimibe levels, and patients who take both should be carefully monitored. Cholestyramine decreases the bioavailability of ezetimibe; thus ezetimibe should be dosed at least 2 hours before or 4 hours after administration of cholestyramine.

*Evidence.* Studies of ezetimibe have demonstrated its efficacy in lowering LDL-C levels. However, there are no vascular disease outcome data at this time.

## Sterols and stanols

Plant sterols and stanols, which are mainly present in nuts, seeds, beans, cereals, and vegetable oils, are structurally similar to cholesterol. Sitosterol, campesterol, and stigmasterol are the most common sterols in nature. Humans can not synthesize sterols, so they must originate from the diet. Sitostanol and campestanol are saturated plant sterols. Plant sterols and stanols, which are poorly esterified, are poorly absorbed from the intestine because only esterified sterols are incorporated into chylomicrons for absorption. However, these compounds have been shown to decrease intestinal cholesterol absorption, perhaps through replacement of cholesterol in the micelles. Also, there is an increase in the expression of ABC transporters, increasing the excretion of cholesterol from the enterocyte back into the lumen. This reduction in cholesterol absorption results in an increase in endogenous cholesterol synthesis and LDL receptor expression. This results in increased receptor-mediated uptake of LDL from the plasma, leading to decreased plasma LDL-C levels. Animal studies suggest that these compounds also decrease atherosclerotic plaque formation. Studies of the use of sterols and stanols have demonstrated a reduction in LDL-C levels of 10 to 20%, and the effects are additive with other diet and drug interventions. No significant adverse effects of stanol and sterol use have been reported. Some countries have begun to fortify food products, such as margarine and beverages, with sterols and stanols. Although the efficacy data are positive and no adverse effects have been reported, there are still no human vascular outcome data to support the use of sterols and stanols.

# Triglyceride-Lowering Agents

## Fibrates (fibric acid derivatives)

*Mechanism of action and efficacy.* The currently available fibrates are gemfibrozil, fenofibrate, and bezafibrate. The fibrates lower VLDL levels and increase HDL levels in plasma. The fibrates act on the nuclear receptor peroxisome proliferator–activated receptor α (PPARα), which is the primary subtype of PPAR in the liver. PPARα plays a major role in regulating the hepatic metabolism of fat and the synthesis and catabolism of lipoproteins. Activation of PPARα by fibrates leads to the trancription of a number of genes, resulting in increased hepatic fatty acid oxidation, thereby decreasing the substrate for formation of triglycerides and VLDL and decreasing hepatic VLDL synthesis. Activation of PPARα also results in increased lipoprotein lipase activity via inhibition of expression of Apo CIII, an inhibitor of lipoprotein lipase. This results in decreased hepatic synthesis of VLDL and increased plasma clearance of VLDL. In addition, there is an increase in HDL formation through increased expression of Apo AI and AII, the two major proteins in HDL, and there is increased transfer of cholesterol from peripheral tissues to HDL.

The fibrates have been shown to decrease triglyceride levels by up to 40 to 50% and raise HDL levels by up to 10 to 20%. The effect on LDL cholesterol is less predictable. Although there is usually a small decrease in LDL levels, 10 to 15% of fibrate-treated patients may exhibit a paradoxical increase in their LDL levels. Although there is little comparative data, it would appear that bezafibrate and fenofibrate are associated with somewhat greater LDL lowering than gemfibrozil. They also have the advantage of generally once-daily dosing versus the twice-a-day dosing of gemfibrozil.

*Pharmacokinetics.* Following oral administration, the drugs are rapidly hydrolyzed to their active metabolites, which are further glucuronidated. The elimination half-life ranges from 2 hours for gemfibrozil to 20 hours for fenofibrate. All the fibrates are excreted primarily through urine and a small amount through feces.

*Side effects, drug interactions, and contraindications.* Potential side effects of fibrate therapy include epigastric and abdominal discomfort, nausea, and diarrhea. The incidence of gallstones appeared to increase in some studies of gemfibrozil and clofibrate, but this has not been a consistent finding. There is a small risk of myositis with the use of fibrates alone, and this risk is increased further when they are used in combination with statins. Gemfibrozil, in particular, has been shown to increase the risk of myositis when combined with a statin. The incidence of myositis does not appear to be as high when statins are combined with fenofibrate or bezafibrate, although no direct comparisons have been made. A reversible increase in serum creatinine has also been reported with use of fibrates. In the context of reduced kidney function, fibrates should be used cautiously, and renal dose adjustment may be required with fenofibrate and bezafibrate. Other potential laboratory abnormalities include elevation of liver enzymes, anemia, and leucopenia. Fibrates are contraindicated in patients with severe hepatic dys-

function and in pregnant and lactating women, and they should be used cautiously (with dose adjustments) in patients with kidney disease. With respect to drug interactions, as previously mentioned, the combination of fibrate and statin can be used cautiously with appropriate monitoring for myositis. Gemfibrozil has been shown to significantly increase blood levels of repaglinide, a non-sulfonylurea insulin secretagogue, which results in hypoglycemia. Therefore, the combination use is contraindicated. It is not clear if similar interactions occur with the other fibrates. Also, fibrates interact with warfarin; thus the coagulation profile needs to be monitored closely when therapy is initiated.

*Evidence.* There is evidence demonstrating that fibrates can reduce the cardiovascular risk in both primary and secondary prevention in the context of an individual with high triglycerides and low HDL-C (Helsinki Heart Study) or with normal LDL-C and low HDL-C (VA-HIT). There are also angiographic data showing benefit with the use of fibrates in patients with low HDL-C levels.

### Fish oil capsules

The discovery that mortality from myocardial infarction was significantly lower among Greenland Eskimos than among Danes led to the notion that omega-3 fatty acids may be protective against cardiovascular disease. A number of epidemiological studies have demonstrated that fish intake is inversely related to the incidence of cardiovascular disease. The GISSI-Prevenzione trial randomized 11 323 post-myocardial infarction patients to supplements of omega-3 fatty acids (1 g daily), vitamin E, both, or placebo, in addition to optimal pharmacological and lifestyle advice. Treatment with omega-3 fatty acids produced a significant reduction in the cumulative rate of all-cause mortality and non-fatal myocardial infarction. Some of the proposed mechanisms for the cardioprotective effects of omega-3 fatty acids are discussed below.

Omega-3 fatty acids are known to reduce circulating levels of triglycerides by 20 to 50%, perhaps through a reduction in hepatic VLDL synthesis and an increase in lipoprotein lipase activity. Long-chain omega-3 fatty acids appear to decrease platelet aggregation and improve endothelial function. In addition, some researchers have suggested that omega-3 fatty acids have anti-arrhythmic properties, thereby reducing the incidence of arrhythmia and sudden death.

One of the best sources of omega-3 fatty acids is through consumption of a variety of fish species, including halibut, mackerel, herring, and salmon. Omega-3 fatty acid supplements are also available, as are salmon fish oil capsules, which may contain variable amounts of omega-3 fatty acids. To achieve reduction in triglyceride levels, approximately 3 to 4 g/day of omega-3 fatty acids are required. To achieve some of the cardiovascular benefit, smaller amounts are probably sufficient. Only very high doses (>20 g/day) can produce adverse effects, including increased bleeding times, gastrointestinal discomfort, and nausea.

# Combined LDL-Lowering, Triglyceride-Lowering, and HDL-Raising Agent

## Niacin (nicotinic acid)

Niacin is currently available over the counter as an immediate-release formulation or a sustained-release formulation. It is also available in some countries in an extended-release form.

*Mechanism of action and efficacy.* The antihyperlipidemic action of nicotinic acid (niacin), discovered in 1955, is unrelated to its role as a vitamin. Although the mechanism of action is not fully understood, there is some evidence that it involves inhibition of the release of free fatty acids from adipose tissue and their esterification to triglycerides in the liver. Production of VLDL in the liver is reduced, and this in turn decreases IDL and LDL levels in the plasma. HDL-C levels are increased possibly due to inhibition of hepatic uptake of Apo AI, a major component of HDL. Niacin decreases levels of LDL-C by 5 to 25%, raises HDL-C by 15 to 35%, and decreases TG levels by 20 to 50%. There is also a reduction in Lp(a) by 34%, which is currently a unique property of niacin.

*Pharmacokinetics.* Niacin is metabolized by two processes: (1) a low-affinity, high-capacity pathway whereby the drug is conjugated with glycine to form nicotinuric acid, and (2) a high-affinity, low-capacity pathway in which the drug undergoes oxidation–reduction reactions to yield nicotinamide and pyrimidines. The first pathway is associated with flushing, whereas the second pathway is associated with hepatotoxicity. Immediate-release products quickly saturate the second (non-conjugative) pathway, resulting in a large fraction being metabolized by the conjugative pathway; the opposite is true for the sustained-release formulation. The immediate-release formulation needs to be taken three times a day. The sustained-release formulation can be taken once daily. The extended-release formulation is an intermediate-release preparation given once daily at bedtime and is available as a prescription medication in some countries. Drug absorption is distributed over 8 to 12 hours to balance the amounts metabolized by the two metabolic pathways.

*Side effects, drug interactions, and contraindications.* Despite niacin's positive effects on lipid profiles, its use has been limited by side effects, particularly cutaneous flushing, which has led to discontinuation of niacin in up to 25% of patients in some studies. Tolerance can develop over time, but some patients do not continue the niacin long enough to develop it. The use of aspirin prior to the first niacin dose of the day may decrease the severity of flushing. Also, niacin should be started at a low dose and then slowly titrated upwards. Taking the niacin with food and avoiding spicy foods, hot beverages, and/or hot showers close to the time of taking niacin are other measures that may be beneficial. The sustained-release formulation has a lower incidence of cutaneous flushing; however, the lipid-modifying effects may be less, and the risk of hepatotoxicity appears to be increased with some sustained-release niacin preparations, perhaps due to increased metabolism via the non-conjugative pathway. In addition, alternating immediate-release and sustained-release formulations may further increase the risk of hepatotoxicity. Since these preparations are available over the counter, patients need to be instructed to use one type of niacin and to not change it without physician supervision. Extended-release niacin, which is a prescription medication, has a lower incidence of flushing compared with immediate-release formulation and a lower incidence of hepatotoxicity compared with sustained-release formulation. The lipid effects are similar to the immediate-release preparations. In addition to flushing and hepatotoxicity, niacin has also been associated with some gastrointestinal symptoms, including nausea, vomiting, diarrhea, and abdominal pain. Drug interactions are not a major concern with niacin. Bile acid sequestrants may interfere with the absorption of niacin and should be taken at different times. The combination of niacin and a statin may increase the risk of myositis slightly, although this remains controversial.

Niacin should be avoided in patients with active peptic ulcer disease, hepatic insufficiency, or recent history of gout. The presence of diabetes or impaired glucose tolerance should not be an absolute contraindication to the use of niacin. The potential for hyperglycemia should be anticipated and monitored, and appropriate changes to diabetes management should be instituted to maintain optimal glycemic control.

*Evidence.* Data from the 1970s and 1980s show that the use of niacin alone or in combination with a fibrate results in a reduction in cardiovascular adverse events. Niacin has also been studied in combination with bile acid sequestrants for secondary prevention. These studies demonstrated a significant improvement in lipid parameters with angiographic evidence of regression in atherosclerotic disease. These studies did not have sufficient power to detect significant differences in the frequency of clinical events. The combination of niacin and a statin has also been well studied. HATS (HDL-Atherosclerosis Treatment Study) studied patients with established coronary heart disease, normal LDL-C levels, and low HDL-C levels. The combination niacin–statin group experienced a 90% relative risk reduction in the primary composite endpoint of cardiac death, non-fatal myocardial infarction, stroke, or revascularization. In addition, there were marked improvements in all lipid parameters. Clearly, there are data to support the use of niacin, particularly in combination with a statin, to lower cardiovascular risk. The availability of the extended-release niacin formulation with less flushing and hepatotoxicity will improve the tolerability and perhaps increase the use of this medication.

## CONCLUSIONS

Cardiovascular disease remains a leading cause of death around the world, and it is predicted that the burden of disease will continue to grow as the population ages. Treatment of dyslipidemia has been shown to decrease the risk of cardiovascular disease and is an effective means of lowering the burden of disease. At-risk patients should be screened for lipid abnormalities, primary and secondary, and treatment, both lifestyle and pharmacological, should be initiated as appropriate. An understanding of the mechanisms of disease and the available pharmacological treatments will allow the practitioner to make appropriate treatment decisions and avoid potential drug interactions or side effects. Despite all the advances in pharmacological therapy, many patients remain untreated or undertreated. Novel and effective treatment strategies need to be implemented to bridge that treatment gap.

## SUGGESTED READINGS

Ballantyne CM, Corsini A, Davidson MH, et al. Risk for myopathy with statin therapy for high risk patients. *Arch Intern Med.* 2003;163:553-564.

Cheng AY, Leiter LA. Clinical use of ezetimibe. *Can J Clin Pharmacol.* 2003;10(suppl A):21A-25A.

De Backer G, Ambrosioni E, Borch-Johnsen K, et al, for the Third Joint Task Force of European and Other Societies on Cardiovascular Prevention in Clinical Practice. Executive summary: European guidelines on cardiovascular prevention in clinical practice. *Eur Heart J.* 2003;24:1601-1610.

Genest J, Frohlich J, Fodor G, McPherson R, for the Working Group on Hypercholesterolemia and Other Dyslipidemias. Guidelines for the management and treatment of dyslipidemia and prevention of cardiovascular disease. *CMAJ.* 2003;169(9):921-924.

Ginsberg HN, Arad Y, Goldberg IJ. Pathophysiology and therapy of hyperlipidemia. In: Antonaccio M, ed. *Cardiovascular Pharmacology.* 3rd ed. New York, NY: Raven Press; 1990:485-513.

Gotto A, Pownall H, eds. *Manual of Lipid Disorders.* 3rd ed. Philadelphia, Pa: Lippincott Williams & Wilkins; 2002.

Grundy SM, Becker D, Clark LT, on behalf of the National Cholesterol Education Program Expert Panel. Executive summary of the third summary of the third report of the National Cholesterol Education Program (NCEP) expert panel on detection, evaluation and treatment of high blood cholesterol in adults (adult treatment panel III). *JAMA.* 2001;285:2486-2497.

Grundy SM, Cleeman JI, Merz NB, et al., for the Coordinating Committee of the National Cholesterol Education Program. Implications of recent clinical trials for the National Cholesterol Education Program adult treatment panel III guidelines. *J Am Coll Cardiol.* 2004;44:720-732.

Lipsy RJ. Overview of pharmacologic therapy for the treatment of dyslipidemia. *J Manag Care Pharm.* 2003;9:9-12.

Miller M. Niacin as a component of combination therapy for dyslipidemia. *Mayo Clin Proc.* 2003;78:735-742.

National Cholesterol Education Program. *Third Report of the National Cholesterol Education Program (NCEP) Expert Panel on Detection, Evaluation, and Treatment of High Blood Cholesterol in Adults (Adult Treatment Panel III). Final Report.* NIH Publication No 02-5215. Bethesda, Md: National Institutes of Health; 2002. Available at: http://www.nhlbi.nih.gov/guidelines/cholesterol/index.htm. Accessed October 12, 2005.

Pasternak RC, Smith SC Jr, Bairey-Merz CN, et al. ACC/AHA/NHLBI clinical advisory on the use and safety of statins. *J Am Coll Cardiol.* 2002;40:567-572.

Williams D, Feeley J. Pharmacokinetic-pharmacodynamic drug interactions with HMG-CoA reductase inhibitors. *Clin Pharmacokinet.* 2002;41:343-470.

# Part VI

## Respiratory, Renal, Blood, and Immune Systems

# 36

# Drugs and the Respiratory System

## KR CHAPMAN

### CASE HISTORY

A 45-year-old woman was referred to the outpatient asthma clinic after receiving outpatient therapy with oral steroids for her third exacerbation of disease that winter. She reported having had asthma since childhood, with a period of frequent childhood hospitalization followed by a symptom-free period in adolescence. Typical asthma symptoms had reappeared when she was in her late twenties and persisted. The patient had been using inhaled salbutamol (albuterol) on an as-needed basis for many years and for 8 years had used inhaled fluticasone 250 µg twice daily. When stable, she resorted to salbutamol once or twice daily and awoke with asthma symptoms once or twice a week. She avoided aerobic exercise because it typically triggered episodes of wheezing. Exacerbations characterized by increased cough, wheeze, and breathlessness occurred at the rate of one to three episodes a year and typically responded to therapy with a short course of oral prednisone at a dosage of 40 mg daily for 7 days. She was a non-smoker and kept no pets.

On assessment in the clinic, her physical examination was unremarkable, with no findings in the chest. However, spirometry showed moderate airflow obstruction with a brisk but incomplete response to inhaled bronchodilator. Her metered-dose inhaler technique was found to be suboptimal. She was advised to replace inhaled corticosteroid monotherapy with a combination of inhaled fluticasone 500 µg and salmeterol 50 µg to be inhaled via dry powder device twice daily. At a follow-up visit 3 months later, her nocturnal asthma symptoms had disappeared and her need for quick relief bronchodilator had decreased to one administration every 2 or 3 weeks, but her spirometry test showed that mild airflow limitation was still present. No exacerbations had occurred in this interval.

Drugs affect the respiratory system in a number of ways: some by direct local action in the airways, some by influence on circulating cytokine and cellular traffic, and some by remote actions in the central nervous system (CNS) affecting respiratory control mechanisms. The most important local drug effects on the airways are those that influence the inflammatory changes in diseased airways and the degree of constriction or relaxation of bronchial smooth muscle. The most important CNS effects are those that diminish the sensitivity of the cough reflex and those that alter the chemosensitivity of the respiratory control centres in the medulla and thus alter the rate and depth of respiration. These various categories of drug action are reviewed separately in the following sections.

## DRUGS AFFECTING RESPIRATORY TRACT FLUID

The tracheobronchial tree is bathed in a mucus-containing fluid, a complex gel composed of mucoproteins, muco- polysaccharides, proteins, and fats. The fluid functions to protect the lung tissues by warming and moistening inspired air and by trapping foreign airborne particles. Normal human respiratory secretion is 95% water; adequate hydration and high relative humidity of inspired air are necessary for the production of normal mucus. In health the nasal humidification system maintains constancy of humidity and normal mucus movement as long as nasal breathing prevails. Oral breathing, in a dyspneic or unconscious patient, quickly leads to thickening of the bronchial fluid.

The rate of fluid production averages about 100 mL/day but varies with the rate of ventilation and the quantity of airborne material inspired. Infected or stagnant respiratory secretions contain DNA fibres from bacterial and phagocytic cells, which give purulent sputum its yellow or green colour.

The respiratory tract fluid is produced from three sources: goblet cells of the epithelium, bronchial glands in the mucosa, and serous transudate from the mucosal vasculature. In bronchitis, goblet cells are greatly increased in number and produce extremely viscous sputum. Therefore, it has been traditional practice to administer drugs to stimulate secretion of an increased volume of more watery fluid. However, any agent that increases respiratory tract secretions or decreases their viscosity may act to the detriment of the patient unless the material is propelled upward by normal ciliary activity and either expectorated by coughing or removed by mechanical suction. Otherwise, mobilized mucus will gravitate into the most dependent areas of the lungs, where it may impair respiratory function.

## Anti-mucokinetic Agents

The reduction of respiratory tract fluid production may be accomplished by parasympatholytic drugs such as **atropine** (see Chapter 12). This is clinically useful in some situations, such as preparation for general anaesthesia (see Chapter 20).

## Mucokinetic Agents (Expectorants)

Agents that increase the production of respiratory tract fluid are often used in order to prevent the drying out of secretions and the plugging of the airways with mucus and to increase the productiveness of coughing. The most important of these agents are water and saline given as aerosols. The traditional expectorants, whether given by mouth (e.g., **glyceryl guaiacolate**) or by vapour inhalation (e.g., **menthol, camphor,** and **lemon oils**), are of dubious value. However, **potassium iodide** solution may be effective, and **ipecacuanha** (ipecac) apparently initiates a gastric reflex that results in vagal stimulation of the bronchial glands.

## Mucolytic Agents

Mucolytic inhalants are mucokinetic substances that liquefy mucus and that are usually given by aerosol to aid the elimination of excess solidified mucus in patients with respiratory disease. Excess mucus may be liquefied by proteolytic agents and disulfide bond–cleaving agents. **Acetylcysteine** is the *N*-acetyl derivative of the amino acid L-cysteine. It possesses a reactive sulfhydryl group that splits the disulfide bonds of the mucin molecule and thereby reduces the viscosity of mucus. This drug is an extremely effective mucokinetic agent, but it is little used because it causes many side effects, such as stomatitis, nausea, vomiting, rhinorrhea, and especially bronchospasm. Given orally on a regular basis to patients with chronic bronchitis, *N*-acetylcysteine may reduce the frequency of exacerbations, an effect that may reflect an antioxidant mode of action rather than any direct effect on airway secretions. **Pancreatic dornase** is a hydrolytic enzyme (deoxyribonuclease) that is of value in the treatment of purulent secretions in which viscosity is due to the presence of DNA.

## DRUGS AFFECTING CONTRACTION OF BRONCHIAL SMOOTH MUSCLE (BRONCHODILATORS)

### Asthma

Bronchial asthma is a condition characterized by eosinophilic inflammation of the airways and airway hyperresponsiveness manifested by repeated attacks of cough, wheeze, and breathlessness. It is now recognized that the characteristic inflammatory changes are present in the airways of patients even when the disease is asymptomatic. Bronchial hyper-responsiveness, or an exaggerated bronchoconstrictor response to many different stimuli, is characteristic of asthma. Although mast cells have been viewed historically as being important in the response to allergens and exercise, their role in persistent asthma remains less certain. Drugs that stabilize mast cells are not potent in controlling chronic symptoms in asthma. Corticosteroids, which have no direct action on mast cells, inhibit the late response to allergens and thus may prevent or reduce bronchial hyper-responsiveness. Other inflammatory cells such as macrophages, eosinophils, neutrophils, and lymphocytes are also present in the mucosa of patients with asthma, and any of these cells may liberate inflammatory mediators. The most characteristic asthmatic cell is the eosinophil. Lymphokines may be important mediators in the inflammatory response, and interleukin-5 release by lymphocytes also may be important in acting to prime the eosinophils in the mucosa. (See also Chapters 28, 29, and 40.)

### Bronchodilators

The pharmacology of β-adrenergic receptor agonists is described in Chapter 13. Activation of $\beta_2$ receptors on the smooth muscle of the airways causes activation of adenylyl cyclase, resulting in increased intracellular concentrations of cyclic adenosine monophosphate (AMP). In turn, this leads to activation of protein kinase A, which lowers intracellular calcium concentration and thus results in relaxation of the bronchial smooth muscle. $\beta_2$ Receptor agonists relax the bronchial smooth muscle from the trachea down to the terminal bronchioles, irrespective of the stimulus that has caused the bronchial smooth muscle to constrict.

#### Sympathomimetic agents

Stimulation of $\beta_2$ receptors relaxes airway smooth muscle but does not produce the cardiac stimulation that results from $\beta_1$ receptor activation. Therefore, $\beta_2$-selective drugs are the most important group of adrenergic receptor agonists for the treatment of asthma.

Although adrenergic agonists (see Chapter 13) may be administered by any route, delivery by inhalation results in the greatest local effect on bronchial smooth muscle with the least systemic toxicity. Aerosol deposition depends on the particle size, the pattern of breathing (tidal volume and rate of airflow), and the geometry of the airways. Even with particles in the optimal size range of 2 to 5 μm, 80 to 90% of the total dose of chlorofluorocarbon (CFC)-driven aerosol is deposited in the mouth or pharynx. Particles under 1 to 2 μm in size remain suspended in the air within the respiratory tract and may be exhaled. Deposition can be increased by using a spacing chamber. (This is a tube with a mouthpiece or nasal mask at one end and a one-way valve allowing airflow only towards that end. The aerosol is introduced into the other end and can move only toward the mouthpiece or mask.) CFCs used as aerosol propellants are being replaced gradually by newer and safer aerosol propellants, such as hydrofluoroalkanes (HFAs), or by dry-powder inhalers. Many HFA aerosols deliver a dissolved (rather than suspended) medication via fine particles, so a greater percentage of medication is deposited in the lower airways.

Use of sympathomimetic agents by inhalation at first raised fears about possible tachyphylaxis or tolerance to β agonists, cardiac arrhythmias due to β1 receptor stimulation and hypoxemia, and arrhythmias caused by fluorinated hydrocarbons in CFC propellants. However, the concept that β agonist drugs cause worsening of clinical asthma by inducing tachyphylaxis to their own action has not been clearly demonstrated as an important clinical phenomenon. There is speculation that β receptor phenotypic variability may account for a subset of the population with suboptimal or harmful effects from frequent or regular β agonist use.

**Adrenaline** stimulates β2 receptors and produces bronchodilatation in asthma. It also stimulates β1 and α receptors and thus produces hypertension, tachycardia, and cardiac arrhythmias. It is used for treating the acute asthmatic attack and can be given subcutaneously in a dose of 0.5 to 1.0 mg. The drug has also been used by inhalation, but for this route, it has been replaced by more selective β2 receptor agents.

**Salbutamol (albuterol;** Ventolin) is a selective β2 agonist. It is used as an aerosol, an intravenous infusion, and as an oral tablet. The aerosol administration minimizes side effects by delivering the drug directly to its site of action (thus permitting a lower dose), and this is the method of choice for the use of this drug in the relief of bronchoconstriction in chronic asthma or chronic obstructive pulmonary disease. The usual single dose delivered by an appropriate metered inhaler device is 200 μg (two puffs). The onset of action of the inhaled drug is almost immediate. When the drug is given by mouth as 5-mg tablets, the action begins within 30 minutes, rises to a peak between 2 and 4 hours, and gradually declines over a period of 6 hours. The drug causes an increase in heart rate and skeletal muscle tremor when given by mouth. Other selective β2 sympathomimetic agents with similar properties are **terbutaline** (Bricanyl), **orciprenaline**

(**metaproterenol;** Alupent), **fenoterol** (Berotec), and **isoetharine** (Bronkosol). These drugs are not inactivated by catechol-O-methyltransferase and so have a long duration of action compared with adrenaline.

**Formoterol** (Oxeze, Oxis, Foradil) and **salmeterol** (Serevent) are β2 agonist bronchodilators that have a long duration of action, allowing their twice-daily use by inhalation to produce sustained bronchodilator effect. Developed initially as maintenance agents for asthma, they are best used in combination with inhaled glucocorticoids rather than as maintenance monotherapy. Both of these agents produce bronchodilatation lasting about 12 hours and differ only in their speed of onset. Formoterol provides a rapid bronchodilating effect comparable to that of salbutamol. Thus, formoterol can be used in a dosage of 6 to 12 μg on an as-needed basis in replacement of salbutamol. In contrast, salmeterol bronchodilates more gradually, producing its peak effect in 20 to 30 minutes. When these agents are given in combination with inhaled glucocorticoids, they improve asthma control, are more effective than increased doses of glucocorticoids alone, and reduce the rate of asthma exacerbation. Thus, asthma is controlled at lower doses of inhaled glucocorticoids.

Their long duration of action makes formoterol and salmeterol useful in the symptomatic management of chronic obstructive pulmonary disease (COPD). Like most effective bronchodilators used in COPD, these agents not only reduce day-to-day symptoms and as-needed bronchodilator use, but they also appear to reduce the frequency and severity of exacerbations.

## Anticholinergic drugs

**Atropine** is a competitive blocker of acetylcholine at muscarinic cholinergic receptors and thus can cause a variety of effects due to loss of parasympathetic activity, including blurring of vision, increases in heart rate, and drying of secretions in the salivary glands and respiratory tract (see Chapter 12). This limits its usefulness as a bronchodilator.

**Ipratropium bromide** (Atrovent) is a quaternary isopropyl-substituted derivative of atropine that does not cross the blood–brain barrier and therefore has no central effect; it causes no significant cardiovascular effects at usual therapeutic dosages and appears to have no effect on sputum volume or viscosity. The actions of ipratropium bromide are otherwise similar to those of atropine, and its therapeutic use is confined to inhalation. The drug is administered by aerosol metered-dose inhaler delivering 20 μg per puff or by jet nebulizer at doses of 250 to 500 μg.

Ipratropium bromide has found little routine use in the treatment of asthma except as an adjunctive bronchodilator used together with salbutamol in the treatment of acute severe episodes. Its primary use has been in the treatment of COPD, where it appears to be as or more effective than β2-selective agonists. Ipratropium, and perhaps other anticholinergic bronchodilators, appears to act on more central airways than adrenergic agents and to maintain its effect better with chronic administration, as might be expected of an antagonist rather than an agonist. Patients with COPD using ipratropium chronically show small shifts in baseline lung function, particularly improvements in lung volume, that are not seen with chronically administered adrenergic agents.

**Tiotropium (Spiriva)** is the most recently developed anticholinergic bronchodilator with properties that make it particularly useful in the treatment of COPD. Tiotropium is the first clinically useful anticholinergic bronchodilator that is muscarinic receptor subtype–specific. Of the several muscarinic receptor subtypes (see Chapters 11 and 12), the $M_2$ and $M_3$ are the most pertinent to understanding the effectiveness of anticholinergic bronchodilators. $M_2$ receptors are inhibitory autoreceptors found on nerve endings, while $M_3$ receptors are found on the surface of bronchial smooth muscle. Under physiological conditions, acetylcholine (ACh) is released from nerve endings and stimulates the $M_3$ receptor to maintain normal airway tone. However, ACh also diffuses back to stimulate $M_2$ receptors, diminishing the release of additional ACh. Previously available anticholinergic bronchodilators were non-selective, blocking both $M_2$ and $M_3$ receptors and potentially reducing anticholinergic effectiveness by allowing the release of additional ACh from nerve endings.

Although tiotropium binds initially to both $M_2$ and $M_3$ receptors, it diffuses away from the $M_2$ receptor in minutes while remaining bound to the $M_3$ receptor for many hours. In clinical use, tiotropium is inhaled once daily from a dry-powder device in a dosage of 18 μg. Its sustained bronchodilator effect is greater than that seen with ipratropium and similar to or slightly greater than that seen with long-acting $\beta_2$ agonists such as salmeterol. As with other long-acting bronchodilators, its regular long-term use in COPD is associated not only with reduced symptoms but also with reduced frequency of exacerbations. While its side effects are minimal and seldom limit therapy, dry mouth, constipation, and urinary symptoms are consistent with its atropinic heritage.

## Methylxanthines

The three important methylxanthines are theophylline, theobromine, and caffeine. Their major source of intake by humans is beverages such as tea, cocoa, and coffee, respectively. Their effects on the various organ systems are as follows.

In low to moderate doses, the methylxanthines, especially caffeine, cause mild cortical arousal with increased alertness and deferral of fatigue. In unusually sensitive individuals, the caffeine contained in beverages (e.g., 100 mg in a cup of coffee) is sufficient to cause nervousness and insomnia. The methylxanthines have direct positive chronotropic and inotropic effects on the heart. At low concentrations, these effects appear to result from increased calcium influx, probably mediated by increased cyclic AMP. At higher concentrations, sequestration of calcium by the sarcoplasmic reticulum is impaired, so that intracellular calcium concentration is increased and myocardial contraction is strengthened (see Chapter 31) These agents also relax vascular smooth muscle, except in cerebral blood vessels, where they cause contraction. They stimulate secretion of both gastric acid and digestive enzymes. The methylxanthines, especially theophylline, are weak diuretics. This effect may involve both increased glomerular filtration and reduced tubular sodium reabsorption.

The *bronchodilatation* produced by the methylxanthines is their major therapeutic action. Tolerance does not develop, but side effects, especially in the CNS, may limit the dose. In addition to this direct effect on the airway smooth muscle, these agents inhibit antigen-induced release of histamine from lung tissue; their effect on mucociliary transport is unknown.

The therapeutic actions of the methylxanthines may not be confined to the airways, for they also strengthen the contractions of isolated skeletal muscle in vitro (see Chapter 15) and have potent effects in improving contractility and in reversing fatigue of the diaphragm in patients with COPD. This *effect on diaphragmatic performance*, rather than an effect on the respiratory centre, may account for the ability of theophylline to improve the ventilatory response to hypoxia and to relieve dyspnea even in patients with irreversible airflow obstruction.

## Theophylline (Pulmophylline and others)

This 1,3-dimethylxanthine is a plant alkaloid. It is poorly soluble and must be chemically complexed with other drugs to increase the solubility enough for clinical use (e.g., **aminophylline** = diethyl*amine* + the*ophylline*).

*Mechanism of action.* The action of theophylline as a bronchodilator is commonly attributed to its inhibition of phosphodiesterase and the consequent increase in cyclic AMP concentration in smooth muscle. However, inhibition of phosphodiesterase is not prominent at usual therapeutic doses of theophylline (only 10 to 20% inhibition occurs at blood concentrations regarded as therapeutic). It has been suggested that theophylline produces blockage of adenosine receptors, although this effect is probably not important for bronchodilatation. Theophylline may also influence smooth muscle $Ca^{2+}$ concentration to produce bronchial smooth muscle relaxation. It has also been shown to inhibit the effects of prostaglandins on smooth muscle and to inhibit the release of histamine and leukotrienes from mast cells (see Chapters 27, 29, and 30). It is controversial whether or not theophylline offers any clinically relevant anti-inflammatory effect.

*Pharmacokinetics.* Theophylline is rapidly and completely absorbed when given by mouth, and it is distributed into all body compartments. There is marked inter-individual variation in the hepatic transformation of theophylline, and the clearance rate is influenced by many different factors so that the dose necessary to maintain optimal serum concentrations (27 to 82 µmol/L, or 5 to 15 mg/L) varies widely. The clearance of theophylline in men is 20 to 30% higher than that in women. The major routes of biotransformation are 3-demethylation by CYP1A2 and 8-hydroxylation by CYP3A3. Cigarette smoking increases theophylline elimination by inducing these hepatic enzymes (see Chapter 4), and there is decreased biotransformation of theophylline in hepatic cirrhosis and congestive heart failure. The administration of various drugs, including hepatically metabolized antibiotics, may interfere with theophylline metabolism and thus produce accidental toxicity.

*Theophylline toxicity.* Toxicity is related to dose and plasma concentration. Serious toxic effects are uncommon at concentrations below 110 µmol/L (20 mg/L), although a significant percentage of patients have unacceptable side effects even when the plasma concentration does not exceed the usual therapeutic range. The most serious toxicities are cardiac arrhythmias, seizures, and respiratory or cardiac arrest. Minor adverse effects occur frequently; the most common are headache, anorexia, nausea, vomiting, and anxiety.

## Selective phosphodiesterase inhibitors

Although theophylline has been described as a phosphodiesterase inhibitor, it is unclear that it achieves its effects by this mechanism at usual therapeutic doses. However, newer agents have been developed as selective inhibitors of phosphodiesterase isoenzymes and show promise in the treatment of respiratory disease. By selectively inhibiting phosphodiesterase-4, agents such as **roflumilast** and **cilomilast** may find roles in the management of asthma and COPD. These agents are weak bronchodilators but are likely to find a use as oral anti-inflammatory agents. In asthma, the agents block both early and late components of the asthmatic response to allergen challenge. In COPD, the release of neutrophil chemoattractant factors is reduced. Side effects appear to be primarily gastrointestinal.

## Asthma Prophylaxis

### Anti-inflammatory steroids

Glucocorticoid drugs such as **prednisone, prednisolone,** and **dexamethasone** (described in Chapter 48) are known empirically to relieve airway obstruction in bronchial asthma, but the mechanism of their action is complex and not fully understood. The long-term administration of systemic glucocorticoids can produce serious side effects such as Cushing's syndrome, peptic ulcer, osteoporosis, steroid myopathy, diabetes mellitus, sodium retention, hypertension, increased susceptibility to infection, and decreased responsiveness to stress (see Chapter 48). Therefore, the chronic use of systemic glucocorticoids must be avoided if

at all possible. If it is necessary to use these drugs, minimum effective doses should be employed, and therapy should be given on alternate days in order to minimize adrenal suppression. Chronic oral corticosteroid therapy is rarely necessary in the management of typical asthma since the introduction of topically effective inhaled corticosteroids. Oral corticosteroids continue to be used in 7- to 10-day "bursts" for the treatment of acute asthma or COPD exacerbations. Short-term therapy is rarely harmful except in patients with concurrent disease exacerbated by glucocorticoids (e.g., diabetes mellitus).

Topical glucocorticoid drugs such as **beclomethasone dipropionate** and **beclomethasone valerate** were developed for administration by inhalation, providing useful anti-inflammatory effect to the lower airway but with minimal systemic absorption. In addition to these early agents, there are now several other topical steroids with similar properties available for inhalational use. These include **budesonide, triamcinolone, flunisolide, fluticasone,** and **mometasone.** The inhaled corticosteroids are remarkably effective in suppressing the inflammatory process occurring with asthma. In single doses, they block the late asthmatic response to allergen exposure and diminish bronchial hyper-responsiveness. Inhaled corticosteroids reduce the number of mast cells, eosinophils, and lymphocytes in the airway and also reduce the microvascular leakage caused by inflammatory mediators.

Although these agents have far less systemic impact for a given degree of airway treatment effect than oral glucocorticoids, considerable attention must be paid to any potential for systemic side effects given the current practice of using inhaled glucocorticoids as first-line controllers in asthma. It has long been known that high doses of inhaled glucocorticoids can produce biochemical changes that reveal systemic absorption and metabolic effect. More recently, there has been evidence that the long-term use of high-dose inhaled glucocorticoids is associated with measurable decreases in bone mineral density and perhaps an increased risk of fractures in the elderly. These changes in bone and an increased risk of cataract formation appear to be related to dose and duration of use. Of lesser consequence is the dermal thinning that sometimes accompanies use in the elderly. In children, doses of beclomethasone (or equivalent) below 400 µg/day appear to be without risk, although at higher doses there may be some slowing of vertical growth. Adult height seems to be unaffected. Local side effects include hoarseness and oral candidiasis, which are reduced by delivery systems or adjuncts (such as spacing chambers) that reduce upper airway deposition of the medication.

Several approaches have been used to reduce the potential for inhaled corticosteroids to produce systemic effects. Given that some of the corticosteroid intended for deposition in the lower airway will be swallowed, agents with limited oral bioavailability (e.g., fluticasone) or high first-pass hepatic metabolism will have less systemic impact than compounds without these properties. Delivery systems that minimize deposition of drug in the oropharynx (e.g., spacing devices) can reduce systemic absorption. **Ciclesonide** (Alvesco) is a new inhaled corticosteroid that works as a prodrug. That is, ciclesonide is inactive until it is acted upon by lung esterases that convert the molecule to its active metabolite, desisobutyryl-ciclesonide. Upper airway and systemic side effects appear to be reduced.

## Mast Cell Stabilizers

These drugs, including **cromolyn sodium** (Intal and others) and **nedocromil sodium** (Tilade), are used solely for the prevention, rather than the treatment, of asthmatic attacks. They are thought to inhibit the release of mediators such as histamine and leukotrienes from the secretory granules of mast cells following the challenge of antigen interacting with specific IgE antibodies. Although the exact mechanism of action of cromolyn sodium is not clear, the drug is mildly effective in persistent asthma when given chronically, and it may also reduce asthmatic wheezing triggered by exercise and by exposure to cold, dry air. Both exercise and cold air are associated with rapid respiratory loss of heat, which may be a physical stimulus to mast cell degranulation. It has been suggested that cromolyn sodium acts as a non-specific stabilizer of the mast cell membrane and/or granules.

Cromolyn sodium is absorbed poorly from the gastrointestinal tract and therefore is effective in the treatment of asthma only when deposited directly into the airways. Two methods of administration are currently used for asthma. In adults, the drug can be given by a "Spinhaler" apparatus that causes a capsule to be punctured so that its powdered contents are entrained into inspired air and deposited in the airways. The usual dose is 20 mg inhaled four times daily. In children, who may have difficulty in using this device, the drug may be given by aerosol. Other formulations, for topical use in the eye or nose, are intended for the prophylaxis of allergic rhinitis and conjunctivitis (hay fever).

About 10% of the inhaled dose is gradually absorbed from the lungs into the blood, from which it is cleared, unchanged, by urinary and biliary excretion, with a plasma half-life of about 1.5 hours. There are very few toxic effects of cromolyn sodium because very little is absorbed systemically. Local side effects such as throat irritation and cough may follow inhalation of the dry powder. Rashes have been reported, as well as rare cases of anaphylactic reaction.

The use of cromolyn in asthma is diminishing. Although safe, the long-term inhalation of cromolyn is only modestly effective, particularly when compared with currently available inhaled corticosteroids.

Nedocromil sodium is considered to be a mast cell stabilizer similar to cromolyn. It is inhaled as an aerosol via a metered-dose inhaler, in puffs of 1.75 mg each. The usual starting dose is a cumbersome two puffs, four times per day. This inconvenient dosing regimen may be reduced to two puffs twice daily at times of stability. It is not clear that nedocromil offers advantages over cromolyn, and it is similarly less effective than available inhaled corticosteroids. Nedocromil appears equally free of significant side effects, but its taste is often regarded as unpleasant by patients. Neither mast cell stabilizer is recognized to have a role in the management of COPD.

## Anti-Leukotriene Therapy

Early in the process of unravelling the allergic asthmatic diathesis, it was recognized that many transient attacks of wheezing and breathlessness triggered by allergen were followed by more gradual but sustained late responses that perpetuated the episode and allowed asthmatic symptoms to persist or recur. One of the many mediators identified as contributing to this late and sustained process was "slow reacting substance of anaphylaxis," or SRSA. SRSA has since been identified as the leukotriene cascade (see Chapter 27). It is now well established that the sputum of patients with symptomatic asthma contains excess amounts of leukotrienes and that elevated levels of leukotriene breakdown products are present in their urine. Leukotrienes given by inhalation are among the most potent bronchoconstrictor agents known. The cysteinyl leukotrienes $C_4$, $D_4$, and $E_4$ stimulate cysteinyl leukotriene receptors and appear to play a key role in asthma, while the non-cysteinyl leukotriene $B_4$ may be of greater relevance in COPD.

The leukotriene pathway may be blocked either by inhibition of leukotriene synthesis or by blockade of leukotriene receptors. **Zileuton,** an oral therapy given four times daily, inhibits the enzyme 5-lipoxygenase and reduces the production of leukotriene molecules. Its cumbersome dosing schedule limits its usefulness. In laboratory settings, several oral agents including **montelukast, zafirlukast,** and **pranlukast** can block cysteinyl leukotriene receptors and prevent leukotriene-induced bronchoconstriction when given orally. Unfortunately, the orally administered anti-leukotriene agents have been found less potent in clinical use than inhaled corticosteroids. When given to patients with mild to moderate persistent asthma, agents such as montelukast reduce the need for quick-relief bronchodilators, reduce the frequency of daytime and nighttime symptoms, and reduce the frequency of exacerbations. However, the effect is less than that seen with a low dose of inhaled corticosteroids (e.g., beclomethasone 400 µg per day), so montelukast and similar agents are used as second-line maintenance therapy for patients unwilling or unable to use inhaled corticosteroids. By virtue of their systemic administration, these agents can treat the entire airway and can be of value in reducing upper airway allergy symptoms. This effect is modest and is usually adjunctive to first-line therapy such as intranasal corticosteroids in the treatment of allergic rhinitis.

## BIOLOGICAL AGENTS

### Replacement Therapy

Alpha-1 antitrypsin (AAT) deficiency is among the most common of inherited deficiencies and is thought to be present in one in 1500 to 4000 Caucasians. The homozygous deficiency state is associated with abnormally low serum and alveolar levels of the 52 kDa anti-protease protein and thereby predisposes such individuals to accelerated injury from neutrophil elastases. Smokers with homozygous deficiency develop accelerated declines in lung function manifesting as diffuse panlobular emphysema, which occurs most typically at an early age. Homozygous AAT deficiency is thought to account for approximately 2% of COPD cases. Weekly intravenous infusions of replacement protein (Prolastin) made from pooled blood product can restore serum and alveolar levels of AAT protein to what are considered protective thresholds. Although no randomized controlled trials have used spirometry to confirm that replacement therapy prevents further loss of lung function, non-randomized observational spirometric data and sensitive computed tomography (CT) scan lung density measurements provide strong supportive evidence that this form of therapy is effective. Recombinant DNA technology has been used successfully to produce AAT protein, but this has not yet been used clinically in replacement therapy.

### Monoclonal Therapy

Immunoglobulin E is recognized as pivotal in the allergic diathesis. Allergen-specific IgE antibodies produced by B cells bind very tightly to specific high-affinity receptors (FceRI) on the surfaces of inflammatory cells, particularly mast cells in the respiratory mucosa and nasal or conjunctival epithelium. Allergen binding causes the cross-linking of receptor-bound IgE and triggers mast cell degranulation. There is a rough correlation between circulating levels of IgE and asthma severity, a relationship that suggests a pivotal role for the IgE pathway in asthma (and upper airway allergies). **Omalizumab** (Xolair) is a humanized mouse-derived monoclonal antibody available for once or twice monthly subcutaneous injection in the treatment of asthma and upper airway allergy. Omalizumab binds to circulating IgE to form an inert complex that does not activate complement. Levels of free IgE drop precipitously with this therapy, and trials demonstrate improvement in asthma symptoms and reduced need for bronchodilators. Exacerbation rates are reduced

and steroid tapering is possible. Side effects are generally limited to minor local reactions at the injection site, but rare episodes of anaphylaxis have been reported. The expense and cumbersome nature of the therapy will generally limit its use to severe disease inadequately controlled by less expensive conventional inhaled therapy.

## DRUGS AFFECTING THE COUGH REFLEX

The cough reflex is mediated by receptors located in the mucosa or deeper structures of the larynx, trachea, and major bronchi and by mechanoreceptors that detect changes in bronchial intramural tension. Stimuli are transmitted via the vagus to the cough centre in the medulla. Efferent impulses originating from the cough centre are transmitted through cholinergic pathways to the abdominal and intercostal muscles and to the diaphragm, producing sudden, explosive expiratory movements. The effect of coughing is to expel foreign particles that have entered the bronchial tree and to expectorate sputum from the bronchial lumen. This may be beneficial to the patient, protecting against damage by foreign bodies or bacteria and helping to clear the airways. However, repeated non-productive coughing (i.e., coughing that fails to clear mucus from the lower respiratory tract) exhausts the patient and disturbs sleep. Long-term coughing also may lead to the breakdown of elastic tissue in the lung or to damage to the tracheobronchial epithelium. It is therefore often helpful to give drugs to suppress the cough reflex.

### Antitussive Drugs

#### Opioid antitussive agents

Opioid analgesics (see Chapter 19) are most effective in depressing the cough centre. Although the precise mechanism by which they exert their effects is uncertain, they appear to react with a variety of receptors identified at numerous sites in the central and peripheral nervous systems. There is some selectivity among opioids with respect to their antitussive potency. For example, the ratio of $ED_{50}$ for analgesia to $ED_{50}$ for cough suppression is 6.62 for codeine, 4.60 for hydrocodone, and 2.87 for morphine. **Codeine** thus appears to be a more effective cough suppressant relative to its analgesic activity. The antitussive dose of codeine is relatively low, and 10 mg may produce a 62% elevation of threshold to ammonia-induced cough for 60 minutes. The usual antitussive dose is 15 to 20 mg as required. Codeine also has significantly less respiratory depressant effect than morphine.

The development of tolerance and physical dependence is a major drawback to morphine-like drugs, and for this reason their long-term use as antitussive agents is discouraged. They can, however, be used for short-term cough suppression. Because of the low dose of codeine required, and its relatively low addiction liability, it may be more suitable than other opioid drugs for long-term antitussive use.

## Non-opioid antitussive agents

**Dextromethorphan** is a synthetic opioid derivative that is an effective antitussive agent, suppressing the response of the cough centre but lacking analgesic or habituating properties. It is the D-isomer of levomethorphan, which is a potent opioid analgesic. This demonstrates that the analgesic activity as well as the addictive properties are exerted through receptors with stereospecificity, while the antitussive receptor sites lack the opioid stereospecificity (see Chapter 19). **Levopropoxyphene** is an antitussive that similarly lacks the analgesic activity of its isomer, dextropropoxyphene. Other non-opioid drugs that have some antitussive activity in addition to their other pharmacological actions include **phenothiazines, antihistamines,** and **benzononatate.**

## SUGGESTED READINGS

Abboud RT, Ford GT, Chapman KR. Alpha₁ antitrypsin deficiency: a position statement of the Canadian Thoracic Society. *Can Respir J.* 2001;8:81-88.

Barnes PJ. A new approach to the treatment of asthma. *N Engl J Med.* 1989;321:1517-1527.

Drazen JM, Israel E, O'Byrne PM. Treatment of asthma with drugs modifying the leukotriene pathway. *N Engl J Med.* 1999;340: 197-206.

Easthope S, Jarvis B. Omalizumab. *Drugs.* 2001;61:253-260.

Pauwels RA, Buist AS, Ma P, et al. Global strategy for the diagnosis, management, and prevention of chronic obstructive pulmonary disease: National Heart, Lung, and Blood Institute and World Health Organization Global Initiative for Chronic Obstructive Lung Disease (GOLD): executive summary. *Respir Care.* 2001;46:798-825.

# 37

# Diuretics

## RMA RICHARDSON

### CASE HISTORY

A 50-year-old man presented to his family doctor for an annual physical examination. As part of this assessment, his fasting blood glucose was found to be markedly and repeatedly elevated at between 8 and 10 mmol/L. A diagnosis of type 2 diabetes mellitus was made. He was also found to be hypertensive with a blood pressure of 160/100 mmHg. As he was overweight and sedentary, he was instructed on a diabetic, calorie-reduced diet and advised to start a regular exercise program. He was also given a prescription for an angiotensin-converting enzyme (ACE) inhibitor. After 1 month, his blood pressure was still elevated at 140/90 mmHg. Hydrochlorothiazide 12.5 mg once daily was added, and after a further month of therapy, his blood pressure was 130/80 mmHg, which is considered acceptable for a diabetic.

Three years later, he had a myocardial infarction. While in the coronary care unit, he went into cardiogenic shock with hypotension and pulmonary edema. He was given furosemide 80 mg intravenously and drugs to increase blood pressure, resulting in a rapid diuresis and resolution of his pulmonary edema. He underwent coronary artery angioplasty, but his left ventricular function was found to be severely impaired as a result of his myocardial infarction. Because of this, he was continued on an ACE inhibitor and hydrochlorothiazide, and a β blocker and spironolactone 25 mg daily were added.

Two years later, he was noted to have progressive edema of his ankles and lower legs, and his hypertension was more difficult to control. At this time, he was found to have an elevated serum creatinine of 250 μmol/L (normal value 60 to 110 μmol/L), with 2.5 g of protein in a 24-hour urine collection. He was seen by a nephrologist, who diagnosed advanced diabetic nephropathy. As he was already on maximum doses of an ACE inhibitor and a β blocker, a calcium-channel blocker was added for blood pressure control, and his hydrochlorothiazide was changed to oral furosemide 80 mg daily. Over the next few months, his hypertension and edema persisted, and the dose of furosemide was gradually increased to 120 mg twice a day. Since he remained hypertensive and edematous, metolazone 2.5 mg twice daily was added, and he had a brisk diuresis with resolution of his edema. Blood pressure dropped from 145/90 to 135/75 mmHg. However, his serum creatinine increased from 250 to 325 μmol/L. The dose of furosemide was reduced to 80 mg twice a day, and he remained stable on this regimen for more than 1 year.

**Comment:** This case demonstrates some of the important roles played by diuretic drugs in the management of one of the most common and most serious medical conditions occurring in our society today—diabetes mellitus. Thiazide diuretics play an integral role in the management of hypertension, including essential hypertension and, especially, complicated hypertension. Given intravenously, the loop diuretic furosemide is effective therapy for the acute medical emergency of pulmonary edema, which is a manifestation of congestive heart failure. The aldosterone antagonist spironolactone, although a relatively weak diuretic, reduces mortality in patients with advanced congestive heart failure. In diabetics and other patients with advanced renal failure, treatment of sodium retention with high doses of potent loop diuretics is frequently necessary to adequately control blood pressure and edema. Finally, some patients exhibit "resistance" to loop diuretics alone; in these patients, the combination of a loop diuretic with a thiazide-type diuretic such as metolazone may be extremely effective. In this chapter, the physiology, pharmacology, and clinical use of diuretics will be discussed.

## REVIEW OF RENAL PHYSIOLOGY

### Sodium and ECF Volume

Sodium, with its anions chloride and bicarbonate, is by far the most abundant osmotically active molecule in the extracellular fluid (ECF), so that the total amount of sodium determines the amount of water and, hence, the volume of the ECF. Sodium is largely confined to the ECF by the action of the enzyme $Na^+/K^+$-ATPase, which pumps sodium out of cells and potassium into cells across cell membranes. Blood volume is a component of the total ECF volume and is critically important for the perfusion of the brain and other organs; therefore, it is not surprising that mammalian physiology defends the blood volume and the ECF volume aggressively. Although humans probably evolved in a relatively salt-poor environment, we are now exposed to far more salt than is necessary through ready access to high-salt foods. Furthermore, some very common illnesses are characterized by stimulation of the same sodium-retaining systems that were designed to prevent ECF volume depletion. The result is that clinicians commonly see patients whose major disease manifestation is excessive sodium retention and increased ECF volume. The manifestations of sodium retention can include edema (swelling detectable by physical examination, and representing increased volume of the interstitial component of the ECF), ascites (free fluid in the peritoneal cavity), pulmonary edema (fluid in the lung alveoli, causing severe shortness of breath), and hypertension. Diuretics play an important role in the treatment of these conditions because they act on the kidney to increase sodium and water excretion in the urine.

### Sodium Handling by the Kidney

The excretion of sodium in the urine occurs through two processes: filtration of sodium across the glomerular capillary wall into the tubular system and reabsorption of most of the filtered sodium by the tubules. Urinary sodium excretion equals the amount filtered less the amount reabsorbed by the tubules and is usually much less than 1% of the filtered load. In order to maintain a stable sodium content in the ECF, the amount of sodium excreted daily must equal the amount of sodium ingested in the diet less any sodium lost by other routes, such as skin (sweating) or the gastrointestinal tract. Typically, this amounts to between 10 and 300 mmol daily.

Human nephrons have at least 13 segments that can be identified, but for the purposes of simplification, we will discuss only the four segments that are most important for sodium handling and diuretic action. They are the proximal tubule, the thick ascending limb of the loop of Henle, the distal convoluted tubule, and the cortical col-lecting duct. Table 37-1 indicates the relative amounts of sodium reabsorbed by nephron segments and the major sodium transporters.

Figure 37-1 shows the basic mechanism whereby the tubular cells reabsorb sodium from the lumen back into the blood capillaries that surround the tubules. Sodium transport is active, requiring energy and a pump, $Na^+/K^+$-ATPase, which is located at the basolateral side of the cell (i.e., on the cell surface adjacent to the blood vessels and opposite to the luminal cell membrane). The action of

| FIGURE 37-1 | Mechanism of sodium transport across renal tubular cells. Sodium is transported from the lumen (left) to the peritubular space (right). $Na^+/K^+$-ATPase, located on the basolateral membrane, lowers intracellular sodium and creates a negative intracellular potential difference (PD). Luminal sodium enters the cell down an electrochemical gradient through specific luminal membrane transport proteins. There are three general types (shown top to bottom along the luminal membrane): selective sodium channels (e.g., the epithelial sodium channel of the cortical collecting duct); sodium antiporters (e.g., the sodium–hydrogen exchanger in the proximal tubule); and sodium co-transporters (e.g., the sodium–chloride co-transporter of the distal convoluted tubule). Sodium entering the cell is pumped across the basolateral membrane by $Na^+/K^+$-ATPase and can diffuse into peritubular capillaries. Most diuretics act by blocking sodium entry through the luminal transport proteins. |

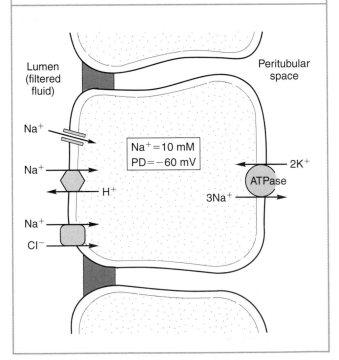

Na$^+$/K$^+$-ATPase lowers intracellular sodium concentration to about 10 mmol/L and renders the interior of the cell electrically negative compared with the lumen of the tubule. This creates a very large electrochemical gradient favouring movement of positively charged sodium ions from the lumen into the tubule cell. Once sodium enters the cell, it is pumped by the Na$^+$/K$^+$-ATPase into the interstitial fluid adjacent to the basolateral membrane, from which it can diffuse into the peritubular capillaries.

However, ions like sodium cannot easily cross cell membranes unless there are specific cell membrane proteins to facilitate sodium transport. There are different sodium transport proteins in each segment of the nephron (see Table 37-1). Diuretics act mainly by inhibiting the activity of these transport proteins, preventing sodium entry from the lumen of the tubule into the cells. Water movement across the tubular cells is entirely passive and follows the osmotic gradients created by sodium transport; thus, when diuretics are taken, both sodium and water reabsorption are inhibited, and urinary sodium and water excretion both increase.

## Regulation of Sodium Excretion

Since maintenance of circulating volume is so critical, it is not surprising that there are multiple mechanisms for regulating sodium excretion. Glomerular filtration rate (GFR) plays a minor role. Regulation of sodium excretion requires sensors and effectors. Changes in circulating volume are sensed by low-pressure volume receptors in the cardiac atria and great veins of the thorax, by pressure receptors or baroreceptors in the carotid sinus, and by specialized cells of the afferent arterioles of the kidney, which form part of what is called the juxtaglomerular apparatus (JGA). Low blood volume and blood pressure stimulate the sympathetic nervous system, which indirectly can stimulate renin secretion by the JGA; low arterial pressure and low GFR directly stimulate renin secretion by the JGA. Renin acts on angiotensinogen to ultimately produce circulating angiotensin II, which, in turn, stimulates the secretion of aldosterone by the adrenal gland.

The effectors of this regulatory system—the sympathetic nervous system, angiotensin II, and aldosterone—all promote sodium reabsorption by the kidney. Angiotensin II stimulates the activity of the sodium–hydrogen exchanger in the proximal tubule. Aldosterone stimulates the activity of the epithelial sodium channel of the cortical collecting duct. These sodium-retaining factors are stimulated by sodium depletion that might occur with severe diarrhea or hemorrhage, but they are also stimulated when cardiac output is impaired (as in congestive heart failure) or when the peripheral arterial resistance vessels are excessively dilated (as in cirrhosis of the liver with ascites). In these latter conditions, prolonged periods of sodium retention lead to edema, pulmonary edema, ascites, or pleural effusions, which are common reasons for using diuretics.

Another regulator of sodium excretion is atrial natriuretic peptide (ANP), which is secreted by cardiac atria in response to increased blood volume. It inhibits sodium reabsorption by the medullary collecting duct. There is as yet no proven pharmacological role for this natriuretic hormone.

# DIURETICS

Diuretic agents have been classified according to their chemical structure and/or site of action (Fig. 37-2). A more clinically useful approach is to consider them also according to efficacy, as listed in Table 37-2.

## Loop Diuretics

### Mechanism and site of action
The loop diuretics (Table 37-3; Fig. 37-3) inhibit the sodium–potassium–2–chloride co-transporter at the luminal membrane of the thick ascending limb of the loop of Henle.

### Pharmacokinetics
**Furosemide** (Lasix, Furoside) is rapidly but incompletely absorbed from the gastrointestinal tract. In the circula-

| TABLE 37-1 | Sodium Reabsorption along the Nephron | | |
|---|---|---|---|
| Nephron Segment | Filtered Sodium Reabsorbed (%) | Sodium Transport Protein | Hormonal Regulation |
| Proximal tubule | 60–70% | Sodium–hydrogen exchanger | Angiotensin II |
| Loop of Henle | 20–30% | Sodium–potassium–2–chloride co-transporter | |
| Distal convoluted tubule | 5–10% | Sodium–chloride co-transporter | |
| Cortical collecting duct | 1–3% | Epithelial sodium channel | Aldosterone |
| Medullary collecting duct | 1–3% | Epithelial sodium channel | Atrial natriuretic peptide |

FIGURE 37-2    Sites of action of diuretic agents in the nephron. (1) carbonic anhydrase inhibitors, osmotic diuretics; (2) "loop" diuretics; (3) thiazide diuretics; (4) aldosterone antagonists; (5) other potassium-sparing diuretics. (→) = specific membrane transport mechanisms; (---→) = passive transfer; ADH = antidiuretic hormone; ANP = atrial natriuretic peptide.

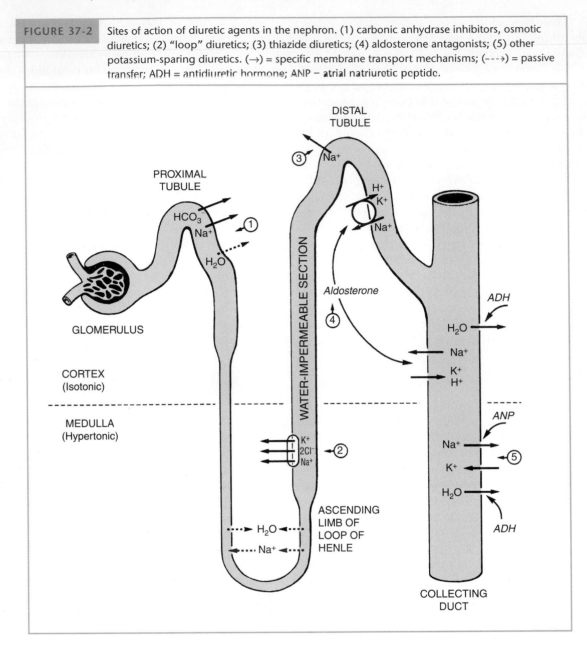

tion, it is 98% protein-bound. Excretion is primarily via proximal renal tubular secretion, at the organic-acid secretory site. As with most diuretics, renal tubular secretion of furosemide is necessary for pharmacological effect of the drug at the luminal membrane.

**Bumetanide** (Bumex) is a sulfamoyl benzoic acid derivative like furosemide. It is almost completely absorbed from the gastrointestinal tract, reaching peak blood concentrations within 30 minutes after an oral dose. In plasma, it is 90% protein-bound. The drug is partially metabolized by the liver, but more than 50% is excreted unchanged in the urine within 6 hours of administration.

**Ethacrynic acid** (Edecrin) is well absorbed from the gastrointestinal tract, and in the circulation it is 97% pro-tein-bound. A portion of it undergoes hepatic metabolism. The major portion is secreted via the proximal renal tubular organic-acid transport sites that can then be reabsorbed at more distal nephron sites via pH-dependent non-ionic diffusion (see Chapter 6).

**Torasemide** (Demadex), known as **torsemide** in the United States, is very well absorbed from the gastrointestinal tract and reaches peak plasma concentrations within 30 minutes. It is largely metabolized by the liver, only 20% being excreted unchanged in the urine, so it is less likely than the other drugs in this group to accumulate on repeated administration in patients with impaired renal function. It also has a longer half-life than the other agents of this class, so once-daily administration is sufficient.

**TABLE 37-2** Classification and Uses of Diuretic Agents

| Class | Relative Natriuretic Efficacy* | Chief Sites of Action | Major Indications | Major Complications |
|---|---|---|---|---|
| "Loop" diuretics | High (20–25%) | Thick ascending limb of loop of Henle | Pulmonary edema, resistant edema states | Vascular collapse, hypokalemia, metabolic alkalosis |
| Thiazide diuretics | Moderate (5–10%) | Distal convoluted tubule | Hypertension, edema | Hypokalemia, metabolic alkalosis, carbohydrate intolerance, hyponatremia |
| Carbonic anhydrase inhibitors | Low (1–3%) | Proximal tubule | Urinary alkalinization, glaucoma | Hypokalemia, metabolic acidosis |
| Potassium-sparing diuretics | Low (1–3%) | Cortical collecting duct | Potassium-sparing effects, ascites, congestive heart failure (spironolactone) | Hyperkalemia |
| Osmotic diuretics | Dose-dependent | Proximal tubule, loop of Henle | Cerebral edema | Acute volume overload |

*Maximum percent of filtered $Na^+$ load excreted (in parentheses).

The onset and duration of effect of these four drugs are summarized in Table 37-3.

## Pharmacological effects

Loop diuretics are highly potent natriuretic agents that have the capacity to inhibit the reabsorption of up to 20 to 30% of the filtered sodium load. This efficacy is related to the relatively large magnitude of sodium chloride transport occurring in this nephron segment and to the efficiency of the inhibition of the sodium transporter.

Loop diuretics increase potassium secretion through an increase in the delivery of sodium and water to the cortical collecting duct, where potassium is secreted, and through the stimulation of aldosterone secretion by release of renin from the kidney in response to increased sodium loss and reduction in ECF volume.

Since loop diuretics impair sodium chloride reabsorption in a water-impermeable segment of the nephron, they prevent the formation of medullary hypertonicity. Maximal urinary concentration is, therefore, impaired. Furthermore, in the presence of the diuretic, sodium chloride remains within the tubular lumen and "free water" cannot be formed. Thus, these agents also impair free water clearance (i.e., the renal capacity to form dilute urine).

The thick ascending limb is also an important site of calcium reabsorption. Inhibition of the sodium–potassium–2–chloride co-transporter indirectly inhibits calcium reabsorption and causes significant calciuresis. Thus, loop diuretics can be used in hypercalcemic states to increase urinary calcium excretion.

## Adverse effects and toxicity

The most commonly encountered adverse effects of loop diuretics are intravascular volume depletion (which can lower blood pressure excessively) and hypokalemia (which may be associated with cardiac arrhythmias and muscle weakness). Hypokalemia, in turn, can lead to metabolic alkalosis. When large doses of loop diuretics are used in patients with reduced glomerular filtration rates, the reduction in blood volume and blood pressure frequently reduces GFR further, seen clinically as an increase in serum creatinine.

Hyperuricemia is frequently observed and is primarily a consequence of enhanced proximal tubular reabsorption of solute (including uric acid) when intravascular volume contraction occurs. Loop and thiazide diuretics may thereby precipitate attacks of gout.

Carbohydrate intolerance is observed occasionally in patients with pre-diabetic states. Hyponatremia does not occur as commonly with loop diuretics as with thiazide diuretics because loop diuretics interfere with the renal concentrating mechanism (see "Thiazide Diuretics" below).

Acute administration of loop diuretics, usually when large doses are infused rapidly by the intravenous route, has produced deafness. The exact mechanism of this adverse effect is unknown, but there may be impairment of sodium extrusion from the endolymph to the perilymph in the inner ear. Although deafness is usually transient when caused by furosemide, there are reports of permanent hearing loss following ethacrynic acid administration. Allergic reactions to loop diuretics are uncommon, and these drugs are usually very well tolerated.

Of the drug interactions described with loop diuretics, the most common is the blunting of the natriuretic effect of the diuretics by most non-steroidal anti-inflammatory agents. Inhibition of intrarenal prostaglandin synthesis by the latter is thought to be the mechanism of this interaction.

FIGURE 37-3　Structural formulae of loop diuretics.

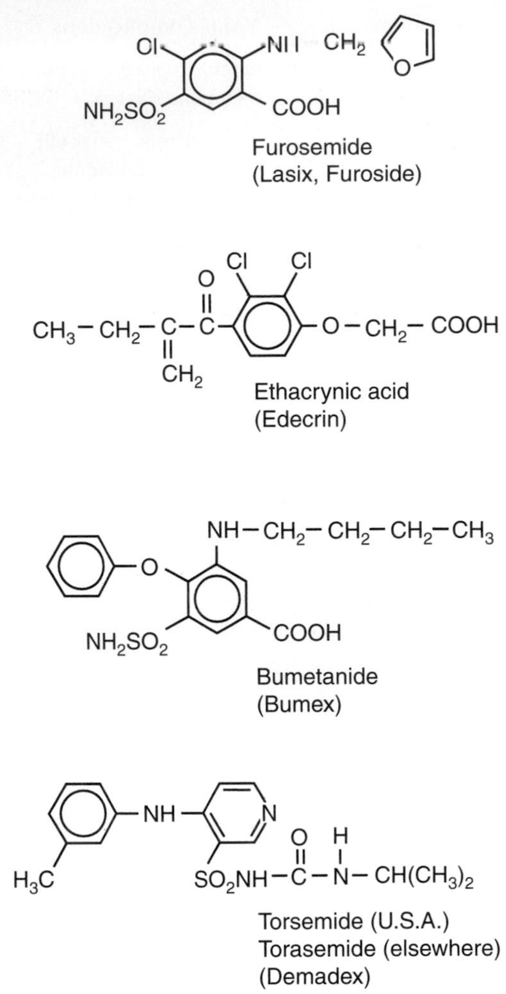

Furosemide
(Lasix, Furoside)

Ethacrynic acid
(Edecrin)

Bumetanide
(Bumex)

Torsemide (U.S.A.)
Torasemide (elsewhere)
(Demadex)

## Pharmacokinetics

Thiazide diuretics are rapidly absorbed from the gastrointestinal tract. The more substituted drugs (i.e., with hydrophobic side chain) are more highly bound to plasma proteins. As well, they are more lipid-soluble and have a greater apparent volume of distribution. Thiazides are weak acids and are secreted into the proximal renal tubular lumen by a transport system for organic acids. Protein binding decreases the rate of tubular secretion. Lipid solubility enhances reabsorption along the distal nephron. Most of these agents are excreted unchanged in the urine. The duration of action of the thiazide diuretics is noted in Table 37-4.

## Pharmacological effects

Thiazide diuretics are considered moderately efficacious natriuretic agents, capable of inhibiting reabsorption of about 5% of the total filtered sodium load. Thiazide diuretics, like loop diuretics, can cause hypokalemia by increasing sodium and water delivery to the cortical collecting duct and by indirectly stimulating the secretion of aldosterone, both of which enhance potassium secretion.

The distal convoluted tubule is relatively impermeable to water in the absence of antidiuretic hormone (ADH); inhibition of sodium chloride reabsorption by thiazide diuretics under conditions during which ADH is inhibited impairs urinary dilution and limits the amount of electrolyte-free water which can be excreted. Thus, thiazide diuretics impair urine dilution.

## Thiazide Diuretics

Currently available benzothiazide diuretics (Table 37-4; Fig. 37-4) were developed during attempts to synthesize more effective carbonic anhydrase inhibitors. The first member of this group to be studied extensively was **chlorothiazide** (Diuril); the basic pharmacological action of other analogues is similar to that of this agent. Somewhat different in structure, but with very similar pharmacological profiles, are agents such as **chlorthalidone** (Hygroton), **quinethazone** (Hydromox), and **metolazone** (Zaroxolyn).

## Mechanism and site of action

Thiazide diuretics inhibit reabsorption of sodium from the lumen of the distal convoluted tubule by blocking the neutral sodium–chloride co-transporter (sometimes called the thiazide-sensitive co-transporter).

| TABLE 37-3 | Loop Diuretics | | |
|---|---|---|---|
| **Drug and Route of Administration** | **Onset of Effect (minutes)** | **Peak Effect** | **Duration of Action (hours)** |
| Furosemide (Lasix, Furoside) | | | |
| PO | 15 | 1–2 hours | 4–6 |
| IV | 5 | 30 minutes | ~2 |
| Bumetanide (Bumex) | | | |
| PO | 30 | 1–2 hours | 2–6 |
| IV | 10 | 45 minutes | ~3 |
| Ethacrynic acid (Edecrin) | | | |
| PO | 20 | 2 hours | 6–8 |
| IV | 15 | 45 minutes | ~3 |
| Torasemide (torsemide; Demadex) | | | |
| PO | 10–15 | 1–2 hours | 12–16 |
| IV | 10–15 | 30 minutes | ~6 |
| IV = intravenously; PO = by mouth. | | | |

FIGURE 37-4    Structural formulae of thiazide diuretics and chlorthalidone.

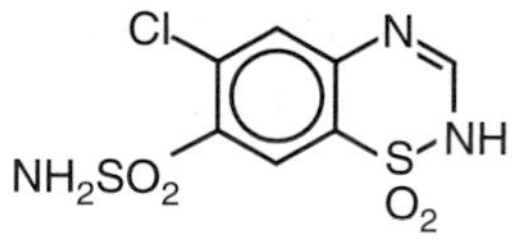

Chlorothiazide
(Diuril)

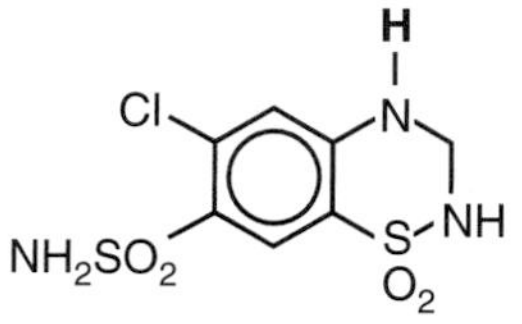

Hydrochlorothiazide
(HydroDiuril, Urozide
Esidrix, etc.)

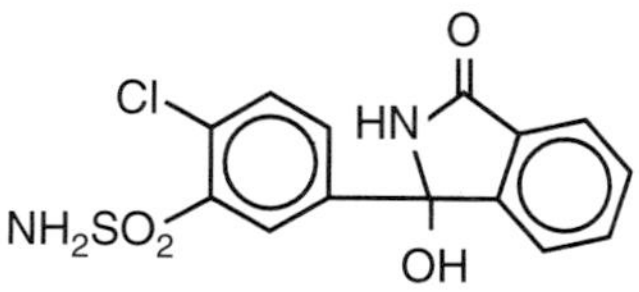

Chlorthalidone
(Hygroton, Uridon,
Novothalidone)

Thiazide diuretics decrease urine calcium excretion by two mechanisms: (1) they directly stimulate calcium reabsorption by the distal convoluted tubule, and (2) by reducing ECF volume, they stimulate passive calcium reabsorption along with sodium and water by the proximal tubule.

Therefore, thiazide diuretics are frequently used to treat hypercalciuria in patients with calcium-containing kidney stones.

## Adverse effects and toxicity

As with loop diuretics, thiazide diuretics frequently cause acute and chronic intravascular volume depletion and dose-related hypokalemia, metabolic alkalosis, and hyperuricemia.

Hyperglycemia and glucose intolerance have been observed with chronic use of thiazide diuretics. Controversy exists as to whether this occurs only in patients with pre-diabetic states. Recent studies suggest that this adverse effect may be common but that it is slowly reversible in up to 60% of patients once the diuretic is discontinued. When sustained fasting hyperglycemia occurs in patients receiving thiazide diuretics, the benefits of continued diuretic use must be carefully weighed against long-term risks of diabetes mellitus. Many factors are postulated to contribute to glucose intolerance, including direct or hypokalemia-related inhibition of insulin release, as well as inhibition of insulin release and enhancement of glycogenolysis due to reflex sympathetic activity caused by intravascular volume depletion.

Hyponatremia may arise as a complication of thiazide diuretic therapy, even when edema is still present. A combination of factors contributes to this untoward effect. In edema states with reduced effective circulating volume, intrarenal factors such as decreased GFR and increased proximal tubular sodium and fluid reabsorption diminish the delivery of tubular fluid to the diluting segments of the nephron. Inhibition of sodium chloride transport by the distal convoluted tubule, an important diluting segment, impairs its capacity to generate free water. Intravascular volume contraction increases ADH secretion, which increases water reabsorption by the collecting duct. Water

TABLE 37-4    Thiazide and Related Diuretics Available in North America

| Non-Proprietary Name | Trade Name | Approximate Relative Potency | Usual Oral Dose (mg/day) | Duration of Effect (hours) |
|---|---|---|---|---|
| Thiazides | | | | |
| Hydrochlorothiazide* | HydroDiuril, Esidrix, and others | 1 | 12.5–50 | 6–12 |
| Chlorothiazide | Diuril | 0.1 | 500–2000 | 6–12 |
| Bendroflumethiazide | Naturetin | 10 | 2.5–15 | 6–12 |
| Methyclothiazide | Duretic | 10 | 2.5–10 | 6–24 |
| Polythiazide | Renese | 10 | 2–15 | 24–48 |
| Sulfamoyl benzamides | | | | |
| Chlorthalidone* | Hygroton | 0.8 | 12.5–50 | 48 |
| Indapamide | Lozol, Lozide | 1 | 2.5 | 14–24 |
| Metolazone | Zaroxolyn | 10 | 2.5–10 | 12–24 |
| Quinethazone | Hydromox | 1 | 50–100 | 18–24 |

*Agents most frequently used, least expensive.

accumulates in both the intracellular and extracellular fluid compartments, and the sodium concentration decreases by dilution (hyponatremia).

In elderly patients receiving thiazide diuretics for non-edematous states such as essential hypertension, profound hyponatremia has been reported, with serum sodium values as low as 110 mmol/L. Patients with pre-existing mild renal failure seem to be at greater risk, possibly because they already have a significant impairment in diluting capacity.

Sustained hypercalcemia is very occasionally seen with thiazide diuretic use. This is partly due to the increased calcium reabsorption by the kidney. Its presence should alert the physician to pathological states that cause increased serum calcium (hyperparathyroidism, neoplastic disease; see also Chapter 65).

Thiazide diuretics occasionally produce gastrointestinal intolerance (nausea and vomiting), pancreatitis, and allergic manifestations (e.g., skin rashes). Thrombocytopenia and agranulocytosis are rare toxic phenomena. Thiazide diuretics are generally extremely well tolerated.

### Drug interactions

The major drug interaction currently recognized is the inhibition of the natriuretic and antihypertensive effects of the thiazide diuretics when non-steroidal anti-inflammatory agents are used concomitantly. Inhibition of intrarenal prostaglandin synthesis is felt to be part of the mechanism involved in this untoward effect.

## Carbonic Anhydrase Inhibitors: Acetazolamide

### Mechanism and site of action

A large fraction of proximal tubular sodium reabsorption occurs through the direct or indirect activity of the luminal sodium–hydrogen exchanger (Fig. 37-5). For this transporter to function normally, there must be an adequate supply of hydrogen ions within the cell and hydrogen ions secreted into the proximal tubular lumen must not accumulate there, or the adverse hydrogen ion gradient would inhibit the transporter. The enzyme carbonic anhydrase is located both in the cell cytoplasm and on the luminal brush border to facilitate the following reaction:

$$H^+ + HCO_3 \leftrightarrow H_2CO_3 \leftrightarrow CO_2 + H_2O$$

The enzyme is inhibited by drugs such as acetazolamide (Diamox, Acetazolam; Fig. 37-6). Carbonic anhydrase inhibition permits a buildup of hydrogen ions in the lumen of the proximal tubule and reduces bicarbonate reabsorption; the adverse hydrogen ion gradient across the cell membrane reduces the activity of the sodium–hydrogen exchanger, thus reducing sodium reabsorption as well. To the extent that carbonic anhydrase inhibitors enter the cell, they may also inhibit hydrogen ion generation within the cell, which may also limit the activity of the sodium–hydrogen exchanger. Carbonic anhydrase inhibitors tend to be weak diuretics, because the loop of

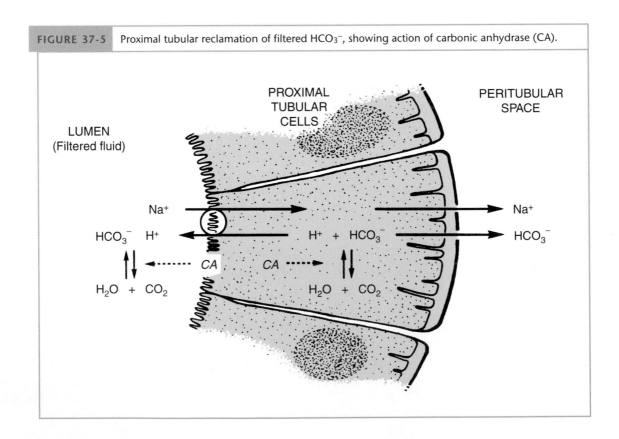

**FIGURE 37-5**     Proximal tubular reclamation of filtered $HCO_3^-$, showing action of carbonic anhydrase (CA).

FIGURE 37-6 | Structural formula of acetazolamide (Diamox, Acetazolam).

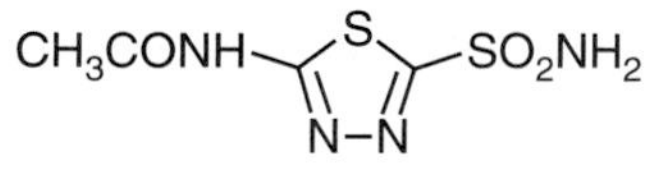

$$CH_3CONH - \underset{N-N}{\overset{S}{\diagup}} - SO_2NH_2$$

Henle has such a large capacity to reabsorb the additional sodium delivered to it from the proximal tubule.

## Pharmacokinetics

Carbonic anhydrase inhibitors, like thiazide diuretics, are well absorbed from the gastrointestinal tract and are excreted via proximal renal tubular secretion within 24 hours.

## Pharmacological effects

Acetazolamide is only a very mild natriuretic agent because of its proximal site of action, which does not alter sodium or water reabsorption in the more distal nephron.

Acutely, this drug increases urinary bicarbonate excretion. However, once sufficient bicarbonate losses accrue, a systemic metabolic acidosis occurs. Distal tubular secretion of $H^+$ is then sufficient to combine with the remaining luminal $HCO_3^-$ to ultimately form $H_2O$ and $CO_2$ and thus permit little $HCO_3^-$ to appear in the urine.

When carbonic anhydrase inhibitors acutely inhibit proximal sodium reabsorption, the sodium presented to distal sites (including the collecting duct) enhances kaliuresis and hypokalemia.

In the eye, carbonic anhydrase is responsible for the transport of sodium and bicarbonate ions, together with the osmotically equivalent amount of water, into the anterior chamber. Inhibition of carbonic anhydrase therefore decreases the formation of aqueous humor and can be used to treat some forms of glaucoma.

## Adverse effects

The most frequent adverse effects seen with carbonic anhydrase inhibitors are hypokalemia and metabolic acidosis.

Allergic and toxic effects are similar to those of thiazide diuretics. Acute renal failure caused by nephrolithiasis (acetazolamide may crystallize in acidic urine) has been described during chronic acetazolamide use in the treatment of glaucoma. A more recent congener, methazolamide (Neptazane), has not caused this side effect.

## Drug interactions

No recognizable adverse drug interactions have been described for these agents. When carbonic anhydrase inhibitors are combined with thiazide and loop diuretics, the natriuretic and kaliuretic effects of the drugs can be augmented.

## Potassium-Sparing Diuretics

### Aldosterone antagonists: spironolactone

*Mechanism and site of action.* Normally, aldosterone acts on the cortical collecting duct by increasing the number of open sodium channels (epithelial sodium channel). The movement of sodium through the channel from lumen to cell without an anion leaves the lumen negatively charged, which, in turn, can stimulate the secretion of potassium and, to a lesser extent, hydrogen ions by the cell. Spironolactone (Aldactone; Fig. 37-7) and its major metabolite, **canrenone**, inhibit the effect of aldosterone on the kidney. Both bind competitively to cytosolic receptor sites for aldosterone prior to translocation into the nucleus. By inhibiting aldosterone action on the cortical collecting duct cells, spironolactone reduces sodium entry into the cell from the lumen, reduces the lumen-negative potential difference, and thereby limits potassium secretion.

*Pharmacokinetics.* Spironolactone is well absorbed from the gastrointestinal tract and rapidly undergoes hepatic biotransformation to canrenone, the major metabolite. Canrenone is highly protein-bound and has an elimination half-life of approximately 18 hours, so it contributes to the total duration of action of spironolactone. Excretion occurs via the kidneys and the gastrointestinal tract.

*Pharmacological effects.* Aldosterone-stimulated sodium reabsorption in the cortical collecting duct accounts for only 1 to 3% of total sodium reabsorption. Spironolactone therefore causes only a mild natriuresis.

*Adverse effects.* The most potentially dangerous adverse effect of spironolactone is hyperkalemia. This occurs frequently when spironolactone is given to patients with impaired kidney function who may also be receiving other drugs that impair potassium excretion, such as ACE inhibitors, angiotensin receptor blockers, and nonsteroidal anti-inflammatory drugs. The current practice of using spironolactone together with an ACE inhibitor for treating congestive heart failure has led to a significant increase in hyperkalemic events in these patients.

Other frequent side effects of spironolactone include an unpleasant peppermint aftertaste and nausea/vomiting. Its steroid molecular structure has been implicated in painful gynecomastia, frequently noted in men. Other side effects related to the steroid structure include loss of libido, impotence, and menstrual irregularities.

### Other potassium-sparing diuretics: triamterene and amiloride

*Mechanism and site of action.* Triamterene (Dyrenium; Fig. 37-8) and amiloride (Midamor) inhibit sodium transport in the cortical collecting duct. They do not interact

FIGURE 37-7    Structural formulae of spironolactone (Aldactone) and its active metabolite, canrenone.

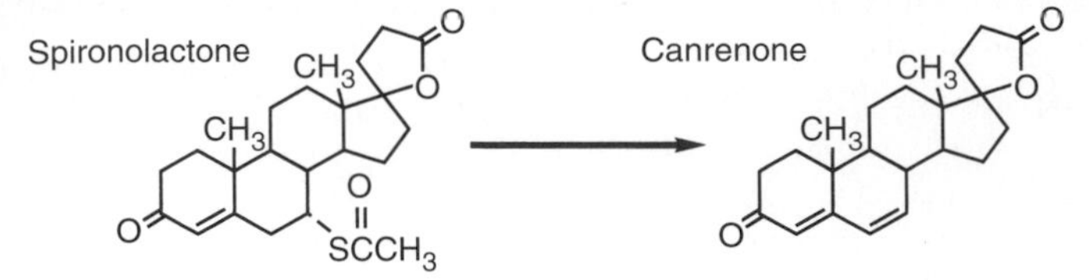

with aldosterone receptors. Both directly inhibit the epithelial sodium channel of the cortical collecting duct. Since sodium uptake enhances potassium secretion in the collecting duct, inhibition of sodium uptake reduces potassium loss.

*Pharmacokinetics.* Triamterene undergoes fast and essentially complete gastrointestinal absorption, whereas only 50% of amiloride is absorbed. Onset of diuretic effect is similar for the two drugs, occurring some 2 hours after ingestion. Duration of effect for triamterene is 7 to 9 hours and is up to 24 hours for amiloride.

*Pharmacological effects.* Since sodium uptake by the collecting tubules and ducts accounts for only 2 to 3% of total sodium reabsorption, only a mild natriuresis will occur with these potassium-sparing diuretics. The natriuresis is coupled with decreased potassium excretion.

*Adverse effects.* The major adverse effect is hyperkalemia, which frequently occurs because of inadvertent concurrent potassium supplementation, co-administration with ACE inhibitors or angiotensin receptor blockers, or because of moderate to severe renal insufficiency. Another frequent adverse effect is gastrointestinal intolerance.

*Drug interactions.* Although not extensively studied, nonsteroidal anti-inflammatory agents oppose the natriuretic effect of triamterene. Furthermore, use of indomethacin together with triamterene has been reported to cause reversible renal insufficiency.

## Osmotic Diuretics

**Mannitol** and **urea** have been utilized as osmotic diuretics. For this purpose, these agents are administered intravenously; they are rapidly and freely filtered by the glomerulus. The hyperosmolality caused by the high intratubular concentration of these solutes prevents sodium reabsorption by effectively diluting the intraluminal sodium concentration and by markedly increasing the tubular fluid flow rate. The overall effect is increased sodium and water excretion.

The adverse effects encountered with osmotic diuretics include hypokalemia and acute intravascular volume overload. The latter effect occurs because the osmotic agent increases the transfer of fluid to the intravascular compartment from interstitial sites. The principal indications for the use of mannitol are to reduce brain edema (e.g., after head trauma) and to acutely expand the intravascular volume (e.g., during cardiovascular surgery).

## THERAPEUTIC APPLICATIONS

## Hypertension

The most common indication for diuretics is essential hypertension, which affects up to 15% of the adult population. Thiazide diuretics have been used for the treatment of hypertension for decades. There was a period during the 1980s when diuretic use fell into relative disfavour for several reasons. First, doses of thiazide diuretics were too high, and the resultant potassium depletion was implicated in an increased risk of sudden death in patients with coronary artery disease. Second, newer classes of drugs were being developed, including ACE inhibitors and calcium-channel blockers, which were felt to be safer, better tolerated, and more effective. However, more recently, a large randomized controlled trial (The ALLHAT study) has shown that thiazide diuretics used in lower doses are as effective and safe as the newer agents and much less expensive. Currently, thiazide diuretics are indicated for first-line therapy of essential hypertension and are usually included in combination therapy with other drugs for

FIGURE 37-8    Structural formula of triamterene (Dyrenium).

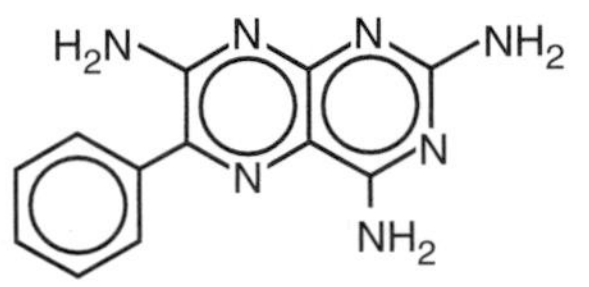

hypertension. Thiazide diuretics play such an important role in antihypertensive regimens that they are frequently marketed in combination with other agents as single formulations, primarily to improve compliance. For example, combinations of a thiazide with β blockers, ACE inhibitors, or angiotensin receptor blockers are available.

The mechanism of the antihypertensive effect of thiazide diuretics when used alone is not entirely clear. Initially, there is a small decrease in blood volume and cardiac output, but after days to weeks, blood volume and cardiac output return to normal, and arterial dilatation with reduced peripheral vascular resistance seems to be the mechanism for blood pressure lowering. Exactly how this occurs is not well understood. This antihypertensive effect requires low doses of thiazide, for example 12.5 to 25 mg daily of hydrochlorothiazide or chlorthalidone.

Many hypertensive patients require more than one agent to control blood pressure, and thiazides are almost always used in combinations. They are helpful in part because many other antihypertensives promote sodium retention, which is prevented by thiazide diuretics. Patients with significant renal failure will usually require a loop diuretic since thiazides are less effective in these patients.

The main complication of the use of thiazide diuretics for essential hypertension is potassium depletion and hypokalemia, which can trigger serious and even fatal arrhythmias in patients with coronary artery disease and myocardial ischemia. With the use of low-dose therapy, this risk is significantly reduced. Nevertheless, serum potassium must be monitored, and if hypokalemia develops, the addition of a potassium-sparing diuretic may be indicated. When thiazide diuretics are used in combination with either ACE inhibitors or angiotensin receptor blockers, hypokalemia is much less of a problem since both of these classes of drug inhibit aldosterone secretion by suppressing angiotensin II production or action.

## Edema States

Edema is a clinically detectable increase in the volume of the interstitial fluid. It is often very obvious but can be clearly demonstrated by the property of "pitting"; that is, when a finger is pressed and held for a few seconds in the area of swelling and then removed, the impression of the finger is left as a "pit." This is most commonly evident around the ankles or over the shins of an ambulatory patient, but in bedridden patients or when edema is very severe, it may be demonstrated in the thighs, trunk, or arms. Edema may also be associated with accumulation of ECF in other areas, such as the peritoneal cavity (ascites), pleural spaces (pleural effusions), or alveoli of the lungs (pulmonary edema). In all cases, edema represents an increase in the content of ECF sodium, with water retention being secondary. The causes of sodium retention will be discussed below. Other factors that contribute to edema include an increase in the hydrostatic pressure within capillaries, which forces more fluid across the capillaries into the interstitial space, and a low serum albumin concentration. Albumin provides an oncotic pressure, which serves to keep fluid within the vascular space; a reduction in serum albumin concentration reduces plasma oncotic pressure and favours a shift of salt and water into the interstitial space.

The general management of edema states includes treatment of the underlying cause, restriction of dietary sodium (which limits the amount of sodium which can be retained), and the use of diuretics. Generally, thiazides are used for mild edema when renal function is normal. For more severe and resistant edema, and particularly when renal function is impaired, loop diuretics such as furosemide are favoured.

### Congestive heart failure

Congestive heart failure (CHF) is a syndrome characterized by a decrease in cardiac output, which becomes inadequate to meet the body's needs. This reduction in "effective circulating volume" stimulates receptors in the carotid sinus and JGA to initiate a cascade of signals that ultimately results in sodium and water retention by the kidney. The "congestive" in the syndrome refers to accumulation of some of this retained sodium and water in the lungs, resulting in shortness of breath, orthopnea, or paroxysmal nocturnal dyspnea—all classic symptoms of CHF. Typically, patients with CHF have elevated circulating levels of angiotensin II, aldosterone, ADH, and catecholamines and have activation of the sympathetic nervous system. Over the past two decades, research has shown that the activation of these neurohormonal systems is a double-edged sword: although it raises blood pressure from low to normal values, it actually causes progression of the underlying heart dysfunction through increases in myocardial work and oxygen demand and increased myocardial fibrosis (scarring), which ultimately leads to death.

Modern treatment of CHF involves antagonism of the sympathetic nervous system and circulating catecholamines (β blockers) and of the renin–angiotensin system (ACE inhibitors and/or angiotensin receptor blockers). Diuretics have a major role to play in the therapy of CHF for the control of peripheral and pulmonary edema. Typically, thiazides would be used for patients with relatively mild edema and well-preserved renal function. For more severe heart failure, and particularly when heart failure leads to reduced renal blood flow and reduced GFR, a loop diuretic such as furosemide is preferred. For patients presenting with the dramatic and life-threatening syndrome of acute pulmonary edema, furosemide is given intravenously and may be life-saving. Given in high doses intravenously, furosemide not only causes a prompt and large diuresis, which helps eliminate the excess interstitial fluid, but acts as a venodilator, which reduces cardiac preload.

The major risk of diuretic therapy in patients with CHF is a reduction in GFR, manifested by an increase in serum creatinine concentration. This occurs if the diuretics reduce intravascular volume and cardiac preload to the point where blood pressure or cardiac output fall, and as a consequence, renal blood flow decreases. Faced with this complication, it may be a difficult decision whether to accept a modest decrease in renal function or reduce the diuretic dose and spare renal function but have significant edema.

Antagonism of aldosterone with spironolactone has recently been shown to improve survival in patients with advanced CHF. It is believed that aldosterone promotes myocardial fibrosis, which can impair cardiac function or precipitate arrhythmias. Spironolactone in a daily dose of 25 to 50 mg is now standard therapy for most patients with advanced CHF, along with an ACE inhibitor, a β blocker, and a diuretic. This combination of drugs can cause potentially life-threatening hyperkalemia in patients with underlying chronic renal disease and reduced GFR as both spironolactone and ACE inhibitors can suppress potassium secretion by the kidney.

## Cirrhosis with ascites

Hepatic cirrhosis frequently leads to accumulation of ECF in the abdominal cavity (ascites) and to peripheral edema. Cirrhosis causes profound changes in vascular tone in both the splanchnic and systemic circulations, typically resulting in reduced peripheral vascular resistance and increased cardiac output. However, the increase in cardiac output seems to be inadequate to meet the needs of the dilated arterial system so that the renin–angiotensin–aldosterone system, catecholamines, and ADH are all stimulated. Although the underlying cause of sodium retention is different, the effector mechanisms are much the same in cirrhosis as they are in CHF. The increased ECF tends to accumulate in the abdominal cavity as ascites because hepatic fibrosis (cirrhosis) obstructs the venous system in the liver, causing elevated pressure in the sinusoids of the liver and leading, in turn, to extravasation of plasma water and sodium into the peritoneal cavity.

The control of ascites by means of diuretics makes life more tolerable for patients. The diuretic of choice, in the absence of renal insufficiency, is spironolactone. Doses of 100 to 400 mg daily are recommended. Loop diuretics may be added if spironolactone is insufficient to control ascites.

Use of diuretics in people with cirrhosis can be associated with complications. Fluid shift from the peritoneal compartment into plasma is limited to about 700 to 900 mL/day. More rapid diuresis than that may lead to intravascular volume depletion and renal hypoperfusion. Occasionally patients with cirrhosis and ascites receiving high doses of diuretics develop irreversible acute renal failure, called hepatorenal syndrome, which is often ultimately fatal unless liver transplantation can be carried out.

## Renal diseases

Many types of kidney disease are associated with fluid retention, edema, and hypertension, so diuretic therapy is frequently required. There are two mechanisms for sodium retention in renal disease. The most common is called "primary" sodium retention, meaning that the kidney disease itself causes reduced sodium excretion, often by unknown mechanisms. Examples include acute glomerulonephritis (e.g., post-streptococcal glomerulonephritis), acute and chronic renal failure, and diabetic nephropathy.

The second mechanism for sodium retention in renal diseases is reduced effective circulating volume due to loss of albumin in the urine (nephrotic syndrome). This is a complex syndrome in which the primary abnormality is a change in the permeability of the glomerular capillary to protein, resulting in large losses of albumin in the urine. Serum albumin falls, and since plasma oncotic pressure also falls, fluid tends to shift from the plasma to the interstitial compartment. The reduction in plasma volume reduces effective circulating volume, and, through the effector mechanisms mentioned above, stimulates sodium and water retention, leading to edema. However, there appear to be a large number of patients with nephrotic syndrome whose sodium retention is primary (i.e., they do not have any indicators of reduced effective circulating volume). In these patients, it is speculated that proteinuria itself may promote increased sodium reabsorption by the tubules.

In patients with kidney disease, thiazide diuretics may be useful initially, but when GFR falls below about 40 to 50 mL/min, clinicians usually switch to loop diuretics. With advanced renal failure, doses of furosemide may have to be increased to as much as 250 mg/day.

## Diuretic resistance in edema states

In heart failure, nephrotic syndrome, and chronic renal disease, resistance to usual doses of loop diuretics is frequently seen. Renal failure itself reduces delivery of diuretics to the tubular site of action. Another mechanism of resistance to loop diuretics has been demonstrated in animal models. Chronic suppression of sodium reabsorption in the thick ascending limb of the loop of Henle by loop diuretics leads to profound functional and structural changes in the distal convoluted tubule and collecting ducts; these changes serve to dramatically increase the reabsorption of sodium and water in these segments. Since these segments are downstream from the loop, the natriuresis and diuresis anticipated with furosemide therapy may be blunted significantly. This basic science observation has helped explain and justify the combination of a loop diuretic and a thiazide-type diuretic, which is often remarkably effective in cases of resistant edema.

## Other Uses of Diuretics

### Calcium nephrolithiasis

In patients with idiopathic recurrent calcium nephrolithiasis, whether or not associated with abnormally elevated urine calcium (hypercalciuria), thiazide diuretics were demonstrated to be effective in preventing or significantly decreasing the frequency of stone formation. As reviewed earlier, this is due to both direct and reflex enhancement of urinary calcium reabsorption.

When thiazides are used for this purpose, moderate dietary sodium restriction is advised to maximize the hypocalciuric effect. States of hypercalcemia should be ruled out prior to the onset of therapy, and serum calcium should be monitored.

### Hypercalcemia

High serum calcium levels may be seen with hyperparathyroidism and malignancy, with or without bone metastases. If serum calcium rises above 3.0 mmol/L, profound neurological disturbances and dehydration supervene, requiring emergency therapy. Adequate intravenous fluid replacement is the mainstay of therapy, but loop diuretics may be added because of their calciuric effect. Great care must be taken to maintain electrolyte balance.

### Diabetes insipidus

Diabetes insipidus is a rare metabolic condition in which there is partial or complete lack of ADH secretion (see also Chapter 44). Nephrogenic diabetes insipidus (insensitivity of the renal collecting duct to ADH) is an equally rare condition. In both states, the kidneys are unable to reabsorb water from the collecting tubules and ducts. Consequently, large volumes (usually >10 L/day) of dilute urine are excreted, which requires replenishment through both oral and intravenous routes.

Thiazide diuretics have been used effectively to decrease urine volume in these conditions by causing natriuresis along with the water diuresis. Consequent intravascular volume contraction then enhances isotonic proximal and distal tubular sodium chloride reabsorption (i.e., accompanied by water). Less fluid reaches the collecting tubules and ducts, and urine volume decreases.

### Special uses of carbonic anhydrase inhibitors

Carbonic anhydrase inhibitors are rarely used as diuretic agents because of their low efficacy. They are used as urinary alkalinizing agents when it is desirable to maintain acidic substances in solution (e.g., uric acid, cysteine, hemoglobin, and myoglobin).

These diuretics have also been used to treat diuretic-induced metabolic alkalosis, to prevent acute mountain sickness, and to enhance urinary bicarbonate excretion in patients with chronic obstructive disease of the airways and $CO_2$ retention (chronic respiratory acidosis).

## SUGGESTED READINGS

Abdalla JG, Schrier RW, Edelstein C, et al. Loop diuretic infusion increases thiazide-sensitive Na/Cl cotransporter abundance: role of aldosterone. *J Am Soc Nephrol.* 2001;12:1335-1341.

ALLHAT Officers and Coordinators for the ALLHAT Collaborative Research Group. Major outcomes in high-risk hypertensive patients randomized to angiotensin-converting enzyme inhibitor or calcium channel blocker vs diuretic: The Antihypertensive and Lipid-Lowering Treatment to Prevent Heart Attack Trial (ALLHAT). *JAMA.* 2002;288:2981-2997.

Brater DC. Diuretic therapy. *N Engl J Med.* 1998;339:387-395.

De Bruyne LKM. Mechanisms and management of diuretic resistance in congestive heart failure. *Postgrad Med J.* 2003;79: 268-271.

Greger R. New insights into the molecular mechanisms of the action of diuretics. *Nephrol Dial Transplant.* 1999;14:536-540.

Jessup M. Aldosterone blockade and heart failure. *N Engl J Med.* 2003;348:14-16.

Moore KP, Wong F, Gines P, et al. The management of ascites in cirrhosis: report on the consensus conference of the international ascites club. *Hepatology.* 2003;38:258-266.

Murphy MB, Kohner E, Lewis PJ, et al. Glucose intolerance in hypertensive patients treated with diuretics: a fourteen-year follow-up. *Lancet.* 1982;2:1293-1295.

Okusa MD, Ellison DH. Physiology and pathophysiology of diuretic action. In: Seldin DW, Giebisch G, eds. *The Kidney: Physiology and Pathophysiology.* 3rd ed. Philadelphia, Pa: Lippincott Williams & Wilkins; 2000:2877-2922.

Shankar SS, Brater DC. Loop diuretics: from the Na-K-2Cl transporter to clinical use. *Am J Physiol Renal Physiol.* 2003;284: F11-F21.

Wilcox CS. New insights into diuretic use in patients with chronic renal disease. *J Am Soc Nephrol.* 2002;13:798-805.

# 38

# Drugs That Affect Hemostasis

## EL YEO

### Case 1

C.J.O'R., a 52-year-old Caucasian male, underwent bypass cardiac surgery for a prosthetic mitral valve replacement (MVR) because of rheumatic valve disease and developed persistent atrial fibrillation post-operatively. Both intra- and post-operatively, he was anticoagulated with unfractionated heparin. On post-operative day 7 he became acutely confused, and his platelet count, which had been in the 150 000 to 200 000/µL range, fell to 75 000/µL. There was no obvious cause for the thrombocytopenia and confusion state, and heparin-induced thrombocytopenia (HIT) was suspected. An urgent computed tomography (CT) scan of the head revealed no evidence of hemorrhagic or thrombotic stroke. A HIT ELISA assay was performed, the unfractionated heparin was stopped, and the direct anti-thrombin agent argatroban was started with a target value of 2.5 times control for the ecarin clotting time. Long-term coumadin, which had been started on day 4 for his prosthetic MVR and atrial fibrillation, was continued. The HIT ELISA test was positive. The confusional state cleared within 2 days of argatroban therapy. By day 10, the international normalized ratio (INR) had risen to 2.9, and on day 11, the argatroban was discontinued. The platelets gradually rose to normal over the next 10 days. He was discharged home on day 12 with a therapeutic INR between 2.5 and 3.5, a rising platelet count of 150 000/µL, and instructions never to be exposed to heparins in the future.

### Case 2

H.G., a 77-year-old man with chronic atrial fibrillation that has been treated with amiodarone, has been on long-term warfarin for stroke prophylaxis since the age of 65 years. His INR is checked monthly and is within the target range of 2 to 3 more than 90% of the time. His cardiologist has recently increased the amiodarone dose; 3 weeks later, his family physician noted that the patient's INR had risen to 5.5 and he was having significant bruising. At this time, the patient was given 1.0 mg of vitamin $K_1$ orally, the next day's dose of amiodarone was withheld, and the weekly dose was reduced by 25%. The next day, the INR was 3.2; a week later, it was 2.4 and the bruising had largely resolved. His discharge diagnosis was warfarin–amiodarone drug interaction resulting in decreased warfarin metabolism and increased INR.

## OVERVIEW OF HEMOSTASIS

### Stages of the Hemostatic Process

Hemostasis (the processes that collectively prevent or arrest the loss of blood from the vascular system) involves a tightly regulated interaction among cellular elements (platelets, endothelial cells) and hemostatic blood proteins. Under normal physiological conditions, these processes maintain a homeostatic balance between procoagulant (prothrombotic) and anticoagulant (anti-thrombotic) forces to prevent both excessive bleeding (hemorrhage) and intravascular clotting (thrombosis) at sites of vascular injury such as a cut or vessel trauma.

- When such injury occurs, the immediate reaction is vasoconstriction to diminish or shut off the blood flow to the injured site.
- Platelets are first recruited to form a *primary hemostatic plug.*

- Almost simultaneously, circulating procoagulant blood proteins are activated and complexed on local cell surfaces in a highly regulated sequence to form a protein mesh clot. Once the procoagulant activities are brought into play, anti-thrombotic proteins begin to down-modulate or inhibit the procoagulant enzymes. This procoagulant process with anticoagulant modulation is called *secondary hemostasis*.

- Any clot formed within a blood vessel must be removed through a process called *fibrinolysis*, in which the clot is digested and the vessel is remodelled to maintain patency and blood flow. This fibrinolytic activity is, in turn, down-regulated by anti-fibrinolytic proteins. There are drugs or agents that both promote (or emulate) and inhibit (or attenuate) each of the processes (primary hemostasis, secondary hemostasis, fibrinolysis) involved in hemostasis and clot formation.

When intimal injury and disruption of the endothelium occur, the platelets roll and adhere tightly to the exposed subendothelium (platelet adhesion) by direct binding of subendothelial adhesion molecules collagen, von Willebrand factor (vWF), and fibrinogen to their respective platelet receptors GP Ia/IIa, Ib/IX, and IIb/IIIa (Fig. 38-1) and primary hemostatis is initiated. Platelet adhesion triggers cell activation, leading to a series of cell surface and intracellular biochemical and physical alterations, including intracellular granule release, surface expression of activated ligand adhesion receptors, budding of the platelet membrane (microvesicle formation), and phospholipid membrane alterations that allow surface binding and formation of coagulation factor complexes, leading to thrombin generation. Thromboxane A2 is formed from arachidonic acid within the platelets (see Chapter 27), and adenosine diphosphate (ADP) and other substances including calcium, adrenaline, and serotonin are released from the intracellular platelet granules. These locally released platelet products directly activate and induce other locally recruited platelets to adhere and aggregate to the surface-attached platelets by cross-linkage of the bivalent molecule fibrinogen to the GP IIb/IIIa receptors of adjacent platelets, thus building up a platelet plug that blocks the disruption in the vessel wall (see Fig. 38-1, Fig. 38-2).

Almost simultaneously with primary hemostasis, secondary hemostasis is initiated. The protein tissue factor (TF) expressed in the exposed subendothelium initiates coagulation in the "extrinsic" pathway by binding factor VII to form the TF–FVIIa complex. This is followed by the interaction with a number of circulating, inactive, proenzymatic blood clotting molecules (zymogens) and their cofactors (factor V, VIII) to assemble them into active complexes localized at injury sites on cell surface phospholipid membranes. TF–FVIIa generates both tenase and prothrombinase complex formation, and through an orchestrated sequence of calcium-dependent enzymatic reactions, these protein–enzyme interactions

**FIGURE 38-1** Platelet adhesion, activation, and aggregation at sites of subendothelium exposed by a wound. The key platelet receptors engaged at each step in this process, and their respective protein ligands, are shown. This sequence of events ultimately leads to platelet clot formation and primary hemostasis. (Adapted from Clementson, 1999, with permission.)

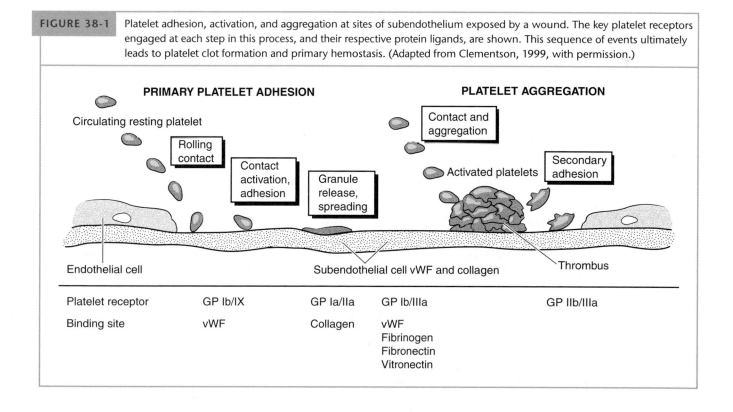

| Platelet receptor | GP Ib/IX | GP Ia/IIa | GP Ib/IIIa | GP IIb/IIIa |
|---|---|---|---|---|
| Binding site | vWF | Collagen | vWF<br>Fibrinogen<br>Fibronectin<br>Vitronectin | |

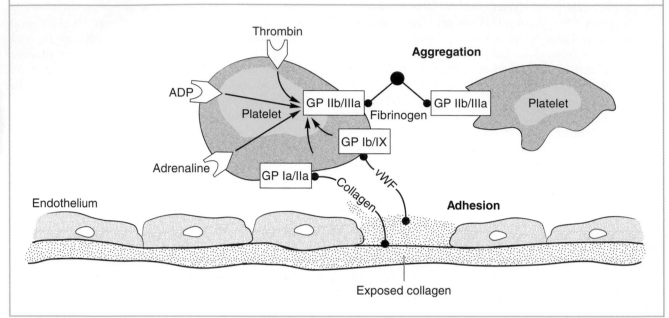

**FIGURE 38-2** Schematic representation of normal platelet responses, including receptor activation, at a site of exposed subendothelium. Platelet–agonist interaction (activation) and subendothelial and receptor–ligand binding (adhesion) are shown. Platelet–platelet interaction (aggregation) is brought about by a fibrinogen molecule linking to its receptors on two adjacent platelets, after these receptors have been activated by platelet agonists shown in the diagram. ADP = adenosine diphosphate.

lead to local thrombin generation. Thrombin then cleaves fibrinogen to form a fibrin mesh in and around the cellular hemostatic elements, forming a more stable clot with the action of factor XIII. Thrombin, once formed, also propagates its own generation by activating the "intrinsic" pathway directly at the levels of factors XI, VIII, and V. This sequence of steps is shown in greater detail in Figure 38-3.

The **anticoagulation proteins** regulate thrombin generation by inhibiting the active procoagulant enzyme complexes at critical steps in the coagulation process. The initiator of coagulation, TF–FVIIa, is inhibited by circulating tissue factor pathway inhibitor (TFPI). The serine protease factors XIa, IXa, and Xa and thrombin (IIa) are inhibited by antithrombin (AT). AT in the presence of endogenous heparins or heparinoids forms a 1:1 complex with the serine protease, thus inactivating it. Heparin is then released from this complex and the AT–serine protease complex is cleared. Finally, protein S, protein C, and thrombomodulin (TM) anticoagulant proteins play key roles in down-regulating activated factors V and VIII. At sites of vessel injury, tissue TM is expressed on cell surfaces and binds thrombin (IIa). This IIa–TM complex converts protein C from its inactive circulating form to activated protein C (APC). APC then complexes with its cofactor protein S, which is bound to cell surface phospholipid, and the protein S–APC complex then binds to and degrades factor VIIIa and factor Va, cofactors of the tenase

and prothrombinase complexes, respectively. These three major anticoagulant pathways play a key physiological role in anticoagulation, and deficiencies of antithrombin, protein C, or protein S lead to a hypercoagulable state and a significant increase in the risk of venous thrombosis. This sequence of steps is shown in Figure 38-4.

The **fibrinolytic process** of fibrin digestion and remodelling of the clot and injured vessel is triggered as soon as fibrin gets laid down at a site of vascular injury (Fig. 38-5). The fibrinolytic proenzyme plasminogen (PLA) binds selectively and with high affinity to fibrin at the site of clot formation and is converted to its active enzyme plasmin by fibrin-bound tissue-type plasminogen activator (t-PA) that has been released locally from the endothelium by thrombin stimulation. Plasmin has broad substrate specificity and digests not only fibrin but also fibrinogen, other plasma and clotting proteins, as well as cell membrane proteins within the clot. Both the plasminogen activators and plasmin are regulated by their respective rapidly inhibiting proteins, plasminogen activator inhibitors (PAI) and alpha-2-antiplasmin. Another important inhibitor of fibrinolysis is thrombin-activatable fibrinolysis inhibitor (TAFI). Upon activation by the thrombin–TM complex, TAFIa removes the PLA-binding lysine residues from fibrin, thus attenuating PLA incorporation within the clot and hence fibrinolysis.

Table 38-1 presents a list of agents that can be used to modify hemostasis.

FIGURE 38-3 Key procoagulant system and formation of a fibrin clot. Vascular injury initiates the coagulation process with exposure of tissue factor (TF). The TF pathway leads directly and indirectly to formation of the prothrombinase complex, resulting in thrombin generation. The dotted lines indicate the actions of thrombin in addition to clotting of fibrinogen. The intrinsic pathway extends from contact and factor XI activation through to factor Xa. The extrinsic pathway extends from TF through to factor Xa. The common pathway extends from the prothrombinase complex through to thrombin generation. PL = specific phospholipids; HMWK = high-molecular-weight kininogen; Pre-kal = prekallikrein.

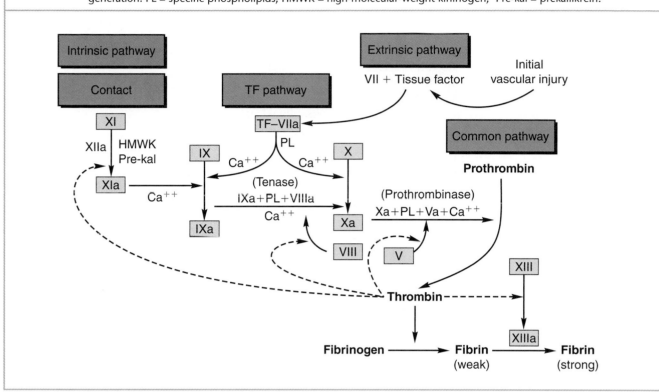

## Causes of Bleeding and Thrombosis

An increased risk of bleeding, and even frank hemorrhage, occur when there is a qualitative or quantitative defect in any of the procoagulant elements (cellular, protein) involved in hemostasis. Bleeding defects due to platelets, platelet adhesive proteins, and blood clotting factors may be hereditary, but they are more commonly acquired. Likewise, increased risk of thrombosis can be caused by qualitative and quantitative loss of function in the anticoagulant proteins or by increased function of key procoagulant proteins.

### Platelet defects

Platelets are synthesized in the bone marrow from progenitor cells called megakaryocytes. They are released into the vascular space in response to the megakaryocyte cytokine, thrombopoietin, and their numbers are physiologically maintained by thrombopoietin in five- to tenfold excess over the level necessary to maintain normal hemostasis. About 10% of the platelet mass is turned over daily. Platelet counts of less than 150 000/μL (i.e., thrombocytopenia) may be due to decreased production from megakaryocytes, as in chemotherapy-induced bone marrow suppression, or to excessive destruction of platelets within the vascular space, usually by immune, infective, or drug-related mechanisms. Common qualitative defects (thrombocytopathies) in which platelet function (but not number) is affected include the anti-platelet effect of non-steroidal anti-inflammatory drugs (NSAIDs), of which acetylsalicylic acid (ASA) is the prototypical example (see Chapter 28). Rare hereditary types of qualitative platelet defects are also recognized. Other common platelet abnormalities involve defects in key platelet adhesive proteins, including von Willebrand factor (vWF). Qualitative and quantitative defects in vWF protein are found in 1% of the population and are associated with a mild to severe bleeding disorder.

### Defects in blood clotting proteins

The blood clotting proteins (procoagulant, anticoagulant, and fibrinolytic) are synthesized in the liver, with the exception of factor VIII, plasminogen activators, and PAI. Qualitative or quantitative defects in the procoagulant proteins (coagulopathies) can be seen in a wide range of acquired, and more rarely hereditary, bleeding and

**FIGURE 38-4** The physiological blood coagulation regulatory system and sites of common anticoagulant drug action. Solid arrows indicate activation processes. Dashed arrows indicate inhibitory action at sites shown. Key regulatory systems include antithrombin, tissue factor pathway inhibitor (TFPI), and the thrombomodulin–protein S–protein C pathways: TF = tissue factor; TM = thrombomodulin; APC = activated protein C; PS = protein S. Small boxes with arrowheads show sites of action of the common anticoagulant drugs: UFH = unfractionated heparin; VKA = vitamin K antagonists; LMWH = low-molecular-weight heparin.

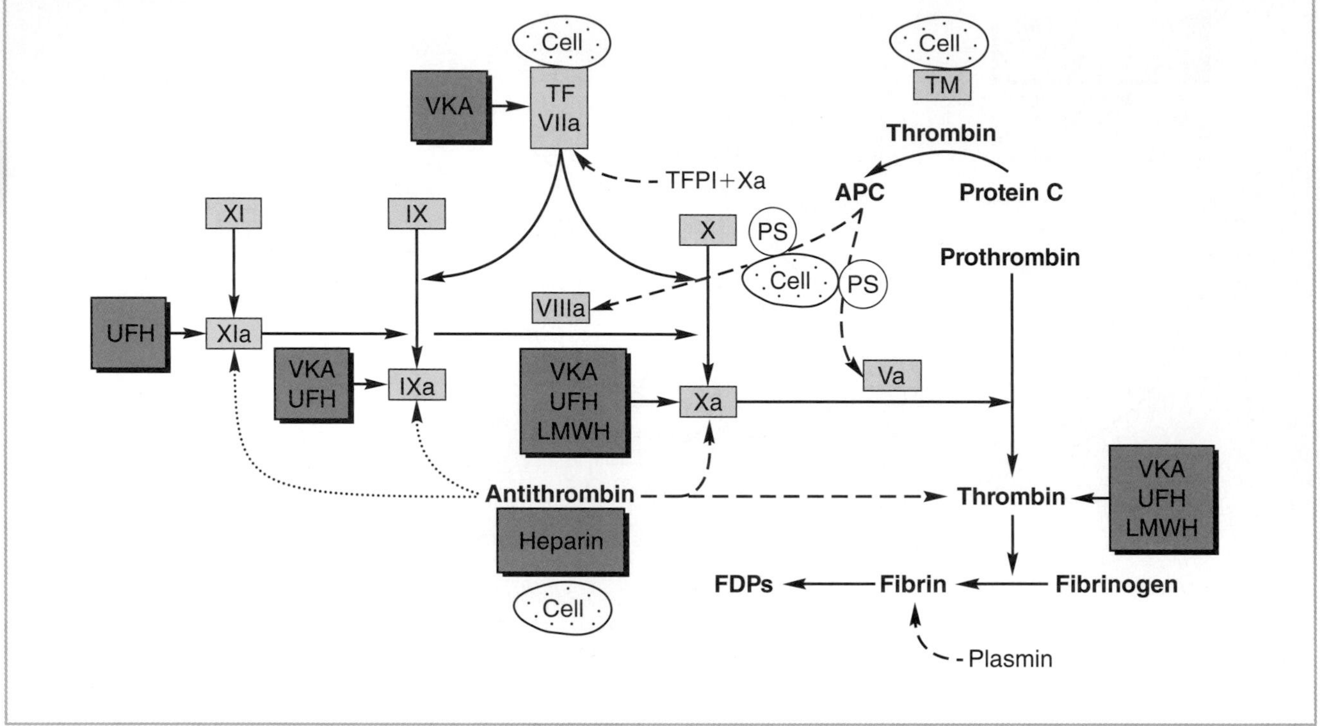

non-bleeding disorders. There are a number of common acquired coagulopathies, with or without bleeding, due to liver dysfunction, anticoagulant use, and disseminated intravascular coagulation (DIC). Anticoagulant drugs, acting on specific clotting proteins unique to each agent, are discussed later in this chapter. In DIC, unregulated activation of the clotting system triggered by pathological states such as sepsis, tissue damage, and inappropriate release of intracellular proteins and enzymes (e.g., by "ecstasy" [Chapter 26] or in malignant hyperthermia [Chapter 20]) results in consumption of platelets (thrombocytopenia), fibrinogen (hypofibrinogenemia), and clotting factors (coagulopathy).

Hereditary deficiencies of each of the blood clotting factors have been described and, depending upon the affected factor and level of the defect, can cause variable bleeding tendencies. Deficiencies in factors VIII, IX, and XI are most common. Bleeding is not seen with deficiencies of the contact factors (factor XII, high-molecular-weight kininogen, and prekallikrein).

While bleeding results from a loss of essential clotting factor activity, thrombosis results from either a loss of critical anticoagulant protein activity (protein S, protein C, AT) or a gain in procoagulant activity (factor V

and prothrombin gene defect, factor VIII). A biochemical hypercoagulable state can be found in 15 to 20% of the general population. Secondary causes of hypercoagulability, such as immobilization, pregnancy, estrogen use, surgery, cancer, trauma, anti-phospholipid antibodies, and hyperhomocysteinemia, are common and act by disruption of physiological anticoagulant pathways. Hereditary and acquired deficiencies in the anticoagulant proteins antithrombin, protein S, and protein C are well recognized. Other hereditary hypercoagulable states, characterized by increased procoagulant activity (factor V Leiden, prothrombin 20210, elevated factor VIII) lead to an increased thrombotic risk in 10% of the Caucasian population.

## Laboratory Assessment of Hemostasis

Laboratory tests to assess and monitor the ongoing integrity of the hemostatic system are essential in clinical medicine to ascertain bleeding risk, to diagnose causes of coagulopathies or clinical bleeding, and to direct therapies, including therapeutic use of hemostatic pharmacological agents. Laboratory hemostasis studies can be divided into screening and specific assays that character-

**FIGURE 38-5** The fibrinolytic system and molecular interactions determining fibrin specificity of thrombolytic agents. Solid arrows indicate activation; broken-line arrows indicate inhibition. Non-fibrin-specific agents (streptokinase, urokinase) activate plasminogen in the circulating blood as well as fibrin-bound plasminogen, whereas fibrin-specific agents (rt-PA, staphlokinase) preferentially activate fibrin-associated plasminogen. rt-PA = recombinant tissue-type plasminogen activator; FDPs = fibrin degradation products; PAI = plasminogen activator inhibitor; TAFI = thrombin-activatable fibrinolysis inhibitor.

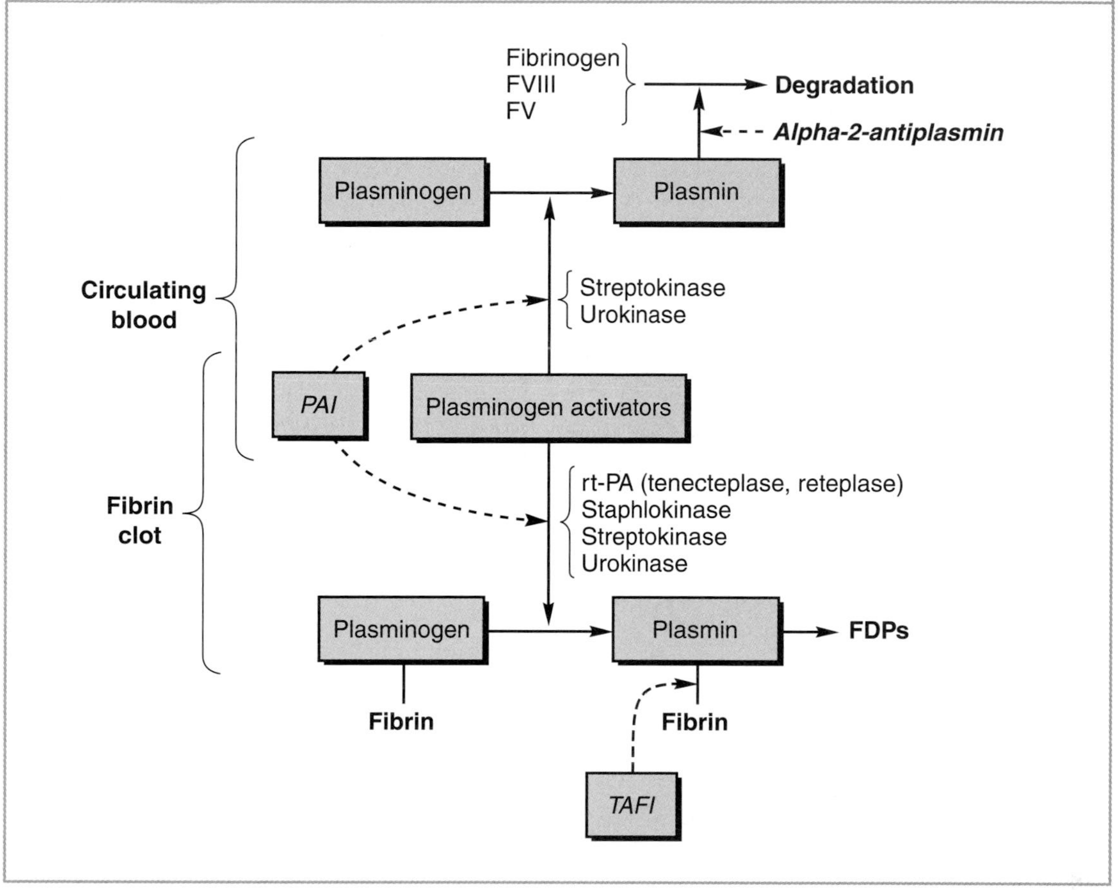


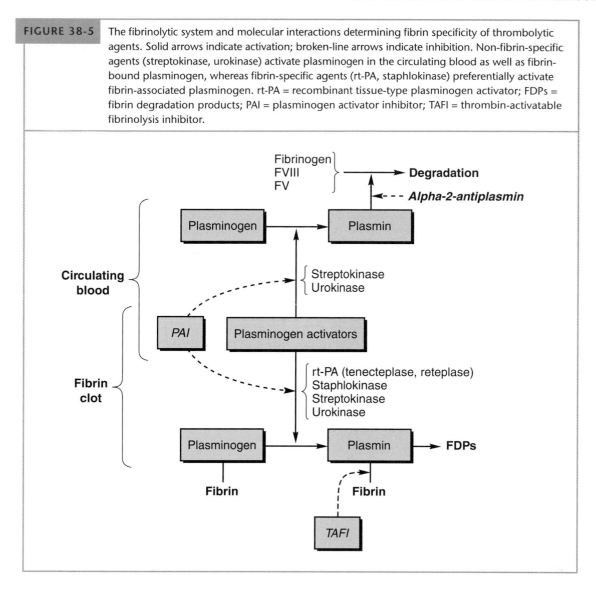

ize function of platelets, coagulation, and fibrinolytic and anticoagulant pathways.

### Laboratory testing of platelet function

The normal platelet count is 150 000 to 400 000/µL at all ages, and platelet count must be determined when hemostasis is being investigated. The platelet count is determined as part of the automated cellular blood count (CBC), together with the hemoglobin level and white blood cell count. If thrombocytopenia is noted, it must be confirmed by microscopic examination of a stained peripheral blood smear. Generally, the platelet count needs to fall below 50 000 to 80 000/µL before hemostasis is affected.

In addition to platelet number, tests of platelet function are also available, including bleeding time and platelet aggregation studies. However, in vivo bleeding time is a poor predictor of clinical bleeding risk and should not be used as a screening test for this purpose. More recently, several types of apparatus for measuring *ex vivo* platelet function have become commercially available. These instruments are both sensitive and specific for the identification of platelet function disorders, including moderate to severe von Willebrand's disease. A platelet aggregometer can be used to study the ability of platelets in platelet-rich plasma to aggregate in response to clinically relevant platelet agonists such as adrenaline, ADP, arachidonic acid, ristocetin, and collagen. The degree of platelet aggregation in response to the different agonists provides different patterns of aggregation that are associated with known platelet defects. Examples include ASA-like platelet storage defect in which aggregation response to all agonists is reduced, and the secondary but not the primary wave of aggregation by ADP is lost.

### Laboratory testing of coagulation pathways

Blood clotting factors in secondary hemostasis are assessed with two general types of assays: plasma-based

| TABLE 38-1 | Agents Modifying Hemostatic Mechanisms |
|---|---|

**Agents that prevent or treat thrombosis**
1. Anti-platelet drugs
   Acetylsalicylic acid (ASA)
   Clopidogrel (Plavix)
   Dipyridamole (Aggrenox)
   Abciximab (ReoPro)
   Eptifibatide (Integrilin)
   Tirofiban (Aggrastat)
2. Anticoagulant drugs
   Coumadin (e.g., Warfarin, Sintrom)
   Heparin
   Low-molecular-weight heparin (LMWH)
      (e.g., tinzaparin, dalteparin, enoxaparin)
   Danaparoid (Orgaron)
   Hirudin
   Lepirudin (Refludan)
   Argatroban
   Bivalrudin (Angiomax)
   Fondaparinux (Arixtra) and Idraparinux
   Ximelagatran (Exanta)

**Agents that prevent or treat bleeding**
1. Clotting factor concentrates
   Fibrinogen concentrate (Haemocomplettan)
   Prothrombin complex concentrate (e.g., FEIBA, Autoplex)
   FVII concentrate
   Factor VIIa (recombinant) concentrate (Novo-Seven, rFVIIA)
   Factor VIII concentrate (e.g., Alphante, Hemofil M,
      Humate-P, Koate-DVI, Monoclate-P)
   Factor VIII (recombinant Human) concentrate
      (e.g., Helixate, Kogenate, Recombinate)
   Factor VIII (Porcine) concentrate (Hyate-C)
   Factor IX concentrate (e.g., Mononine, Bebulin VH)
   Factor IX (recombinant) concentrate (e.g., BeneFix)
   Factor XI concentrate (e.g., Hemoeleven)
   Factor XIII concentrate (e.g., Fibrogammin)
2. Anti-fibrinolytic agents
   Aprotinin (Trasylol)
   Epsilon aminocaproic acid (EACA; Amicar)
   Tranexamic acid (Cyklokapron)
3. Desmopressin (DDAVP)
   Desmopressin acetate nasal spray (Stimate)

fering fibrinogen/fibrin degradation products; or, rarely, by specific antibody factor inhibitors and by deficiencies of factor XII.

The PT is measured in re-calcified citrated plasma in the presence of a preparation containing thromboplastin (TF). Prolongation of the PT indicates a deficiency of "extrinsic" pathway (see Fig. 38-3) proteins, including factors VII, X, V, prothrombin (at a level below 30 to 40% of normal), or fibrinogen (at a level less than 100 mg/dL). The PT result is usually converted to an **international normalized ratio (INR)**, which was developed specifically for the monitoring and dose adjustment of warfarin, because of the narrow therapeutic index of this drug. The **INR = [(patient PT)/control PT]$^{ISI}$**, that is, the ratio of the patient's PT to the laboratory's standard normal PT, raised to the power of an international sensitivity index (ISI) for the thromboplastin preparation that the laboratory uses. Human brain thromboplastins and recombinant thromboplastins have an ISI close to 1.0, whereas rabbit brain thromboplastins usually have an ISI of 1.5 to 2.0. Use of the INR greatly reduces the variability of PT results when a patient on warfarin therapy is tested in different laboratories.

The TT is measured by adding thrombin to re-calcified citrated plasma and measuring the time for thrombin to convert fibrinogen to fibrin. Prolonged TT is seen in patients with low levels of fibrinogen (<100 mg/dL) or prothrombin, dysfibrinogenemia, and interfering substances (including heparins, direct anti-thrombins, fibrin degradation products, and high levels of abnormal serum proteins, including the immunoglobulins).

More specialized clotting assays are used in coagulation laboratories to further clarify an abnormal screening test result or when there is strong clinical suspicion that a coagulation defect exists; these specialized tests include studies to differentiate a factor deficiency from inhibitory substances, and specific factor assays for each factor involved in hemostasis.

## Laboratory testing of fibrinolysis
The laboratory screening assay for the fibrinolytic system is the euglobulin clot lysis time (ELT). The ELT is a global assay for hyperfibrinolysis, and it is shortened with stress, desmopressin acetate (DDAVP) infusion, and hyperfibrinolytic states. Specific assays for all fibrinolytic proteins are also available.

## Laboratory testing of hypercoagulability
In thrombophilia, biochemical defects related to anticoagulant activity can frequently be found and identified by laboratory testing. Unlike coagulation assessment, there are no accepted screening tests for hypercoagulability, but assays for each of the specific genes and proteins involved are available. Molecular testing by polymerase chain reaction (PCR) for each of the common single gene defects

screening assays of clotting, and specific coagulation factor assays. The screening tests include the activated partial thromboplastin time (aPTT), prothrombin time (PT), thrombin time (TT), and fibrinogen activity level.

Prolongation of the aPTT indicates a deficiency or inhibition of one or more of the "intrinsic" clotting prekallikrein, high-molecular-weight kininogen, factor XI, IX, VIII, X, V, prothrombin, or fibrinogen (see Fig. 38-3). The aPTT is also prolonged by anticoagulant drugs such as unfractionated heparin, low-molecular-weight heparin, and direct thrombin inhibitors; by inhibitory immunoglobulins such as a lupus anticoagulant; by inter-involved in thrombophilia, factor V Leiden, and pro-thrombin 20210 disorders, is now widely available. Tests for levels of proteins S, protein C, AT, factor VIII, homo-cysteine, and anti-phospholipid antibodies are available through specialty laboratories.

## Hemostasis Drug Measurements

The blood levels of specific anticoagulant drugs and their effects on various aspects of hemostasis can be measured, both to determine the drug effect and to monitor ongoing drug utilization and dose adjustment. This monitoring is essential during treatment with unfractionated heparins, heparinoids, direct anti-thrombins, and warfarin. Labora-tory testing permits adjustment of drug dosage to main-tain the therapeutic index and to minimize the bleeding risk with all of these drugs. Other agents, such as low-molecular-weight heparins (LMWHs) and anti-platelet and pro- and anti-fibrinolytic agents, rarely require ongo-ing laboratory monitoring because they have predictable pharmacokinetics, lower bleeding risks, or a wide thera-peutic index that allows weight-based dosage. The specific laboratory tests used vary depending upon the specific drug and its mechanism of action. For some agents, unique assays have been created, such as anti–factor Xa assays for unfractionated heparin (UFH), heparinoids, and LMWH. For other drugs, widely available coagulation assays can be utilized for monitoring and dose adjust-ment, such as the aPTT for UFH and PT/INR for warfarin.

## ANTI-PLATELET AGENTS

Agents that interfere with the action of platelets play a key role in pharmacotherapy of coronary artery, cerebrovas-cular, and peripheral vascular diseases. There are four main classes of anti-platelet agents, according to their mechanisms of action:

1. ASA and related compounds (NSAIDs and sulfinpyra-zone) block cyclooxygenase (prostaglandin H/G syn-thase) and thus prevent biosynthesis of prostaglandins and thromboxane A2 (TXA2) from arachidonic acid.
2. Dipyridamole interferes with the breakdown of cyclic adenosine monophosphate (AMP) and prevents platelet activation by multiple mechanisms.
3. The thienopyridines (clopidogrel, ticlopidine) prevent platelet aggregation by blocking ADP binding to its specific platelet receptor, thus inhibiting activation of the platelet GP IIb/IIIa receptor for fibrinogen.
4. Platelet integrin GP IIb/IIIa antagonists and antibod-ies act by blocking the final common pathway of platelet aggregation. These GP IIb/IIIa agents inhibit the cross-bridging of platelets by fibrinogen binding and the initial adhesion to the injured vessel wall. Fig-

ure 38-6 shows the sites of action of anti-platelet drugs. All of these anti-platelet agents have bleeding as a common side effect, and all have efficacy in arterial but not venous thrombotic disease.

## ASA and Other NSAIDs

Acetylsalicylic acid (ASA; Aspirin) is a prototype of the family of NSAIDs. While it has analgesic, antipyretic, and anti-inflammatory properties (see Chapter 28), ASA is a major drug for the treatment and prevention of cardiovas-cular disease (CVD) because of its anti-platelet properties. CVD, including coronary artery disease and stroke, is the leading cause of death in North America. ASA has a major net benefit in decreasing the risk of CVD for a wide range of patients. Utilization of ASA for CVD indications in the elderly has risen from 60% in the 1990s to 75 to 85% in the last 5 years, but this still represents under-utilization.

### Mechanism of action

Small amounts of ASA (75 to 100 mg/day) irreversibly acetylate and inactivate cyclooxygenase (COX), thus blocking the first step in the conversion of arachidonic acid to TXA2 (see Chapter 28). ASA is a much more potent inhibitor of COX-1 than of COX-2. Platelets do not syn-thesize new COX enzyme, so the inhibition lasts for the life of the platelet or the bone marrow megakaryocyte. Through this action, ASA variably inhibits platelet aggre-gation. However, the degree of inhibition of aggregation does not correlate with the bleeding risk associated with ASA. After ASA therapy is discontinued, it takes approxi-mately 10 days for the effect of ASA to disappear as all cir-culating platelets are replaced.

### Pharmacokinetics

See Chapter 28 for a detailed account of the pharmacoki-netics of ASA.

### Adverse effects

The major side effect of ASA and other NSAIDs is hemor-rhage, and this bleeding risk is dose-dependent. Bleeding can occur at any site, although mucosal bleeding is most common. Bleeding risk is also dependent upon concur-rent use of other agents affecting hemostasis and on patient susceptibility factors, including age. Major bleed-ing is seen in 2 to 3% of patients, and transfusion is required in 1 to 2% at ASA doses up to 325 mg/day. Gen-erally, a lower dose is recommended (80 mg) for most anti-platelet indications, providing optimal efficacy while lim-iting toxicity.

Other adverse effects, including ASA sensitivity, gas-trointestinal (GI) damage, and metabolic and central nervous system (CNS) disturbances, are described in Chapter 28. Most patients who suffer GI side effects are able to tolerate a lower ASA dose, and ingesting the drug

**FIGURE 38-6** Schematic representation of the redundancy of normal platelet agonist responses and sites of anti-platelet drug interaction. Solid lines represent activation; dashed lines represent inhibition. ADP = adenosine diphosphate; ASA = acetylsalicylic acid; TXA2 = thromboxane A2.

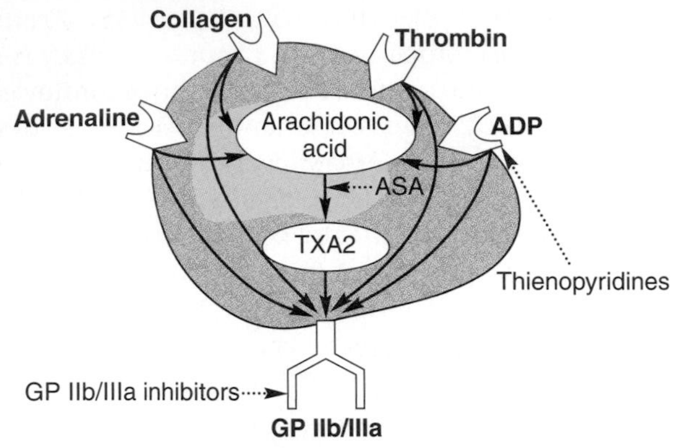

with food or a large volume of liquid may further ameliorate the gastric side effects. The use of enteric-coated ASA appears to cause less GI damage, although it does not protect against GI bleeding. Because of delayed absorption, enteric-coated ASA should be avoided in patients being treated for acute coronary syndromes, and the first dose should be crushed and chewed to ensure rapid absorption. ASA should be discontinued 7 to 10 days prior to any invasive procedure to reduce the risk of excessive bleeding.

### ASA resistance

The benefits of ASA in CVD are not observed in all patients, and biochemical ASA non-responders are well recognized. ASA resistance, or partial response, in which little or no ASA effect is seen on platelet aggregation, bleeding time, or TXA2 production, has been observed in a third to a half of treated individuals. In some, resistance seems to develop gradually over time and does not respond to increasing drug dose. While the clinical relevance of these observations is not clear, biochemical non-responders are at higher risk of poor vascular outcomes. Testing for ASA resistance is not currently indicated, nor is switching to alternative anti-platelet agents such as clopidogrel if ASA resistance is demonstrated.

### Other NSAIDs

NSAIDs are among the most commonly used drugs in the world. The reversible, non-selective cyclooxygenase (COX-1 and COX-2) inhibitor drugs, while exhibiting anti-platelet action, do not have a clinical role in the therapy of CVD. Indeed, there is evidence that when NSAIDs are co-administered with ASA they reduce the cardiovascular protective effect of ASA. The major indication for NSAIDs is for their anti-inflammatory, antipyretic, and analgesic properties (see Chapter 28).

### Mechanism of anti-platelet action

In general, when used in analgesic doses, NSAIDs other than ASA inhibit 70 to 90% of COX-1 activity. This level of COX inhibition may be insufficient to block platelet aggregation adequately in vivo because of the significant capacity of platelets to produce TXA2, which may explain the lack of therapeutic efficacy of these drugs in CVD. Ibuprofen is the only NSAID that has potent enough COX-1 inhibitory properties (>95%) to be comparable to ASA in standard doses and to be studied to any degree. None of the reversible COX inhibitors have been approved as anti-platelet drugs in North America, and there are no circumstances that warrant their use in place of ASA for this indication.

The *pharmacokinetics* and *adverse effects* of the NSAIDs are described in Chapter 28.

## Dipyridamole

Dipyridamole (Persantine), a pyrimidopyrimidine derivative, was originally used as a vasodilator but also has anti-platelet properties.

### Mechanism of action

Dipyridamole is a weak inhibitor of platelet function, by variably inhibiting ADP release from the platelets. Its precise mechanism of action is controversial. It inhibits cyclic nucleotide phosphodiesterase, resulting in accumulation of the platelet inhibitor cyclic AMP, and it also blocks adenosine uptake.

### Pharmacokinetics

Dipyridamole is absorbed quite variably by mouth, and its bioavailability is low with conventional preparations. An extended release (ER-DP) preparation has improved bioavailability. The peak concentration in serum is reached in 2 to 3 hours, and the serum half-life is 10 to 12 hours, so twice-a-day dosage is used. It is strongly protein-bound (90 to 99%). It is excreted primarily in the bile as a glucuronide conjugate and undergoes enterohepatic recirculation.

### Adverse effects

The major adverse effect is headache, seen in 20% of patients by 7 days of use. Bleeding with ER-DP was no greater than with low-dose ASA alone (2 to 4%). Other significant side effects include dyspepsia, abdominal pain, nausea, and diarrhea.

Because of its peripheral vasodilatory effect, dipyridamole should be used with caution in patients with stable angina because of the risk of myocardial ischemia during exercise.

# Thienopyridines

**Ticlopidine** (Ticlid) and **clopidogrel** bisulfate (Plavix) are structurally related thienopyridine derivatives with anti-platelet activity that have important therapeutic roles in secondary prevention of cardiovascular and cerebrovascular obstructive events. These drugs act by inhibiting ADP-induced platelet aggregation. Both drugs induce irreversible alterations in platelet receptor P2Y12, an ADP-binding receptor that activates platelet G proteins, thereby preventing activation of adenylyl cyclase and activation of the adhesion receptor complex GP IIb/IIIa and platelet aggregation. Ticlopidine and clopidogrel also inhibit platelet aggregation responses to collagen, thrombin, and arachidonic acid. Ticlopidine was the first oral anti-platelet agent shown to be as effective as ASA, and clopidogrel was the first one proven to be superior to ASA for the prevention of acute myocardial infarction and stroke in patients with known atherosclerotic disease. These drugs thus offered an alternative for patients with ASA resistance or failure.

## Ticlopidine

*Pharmacokinetics.* Ticlopidine is rapidly absorbed and 98% protein-bound, primarily to albumin. While a drug effect on platelet function can be seen within hours of an oral dose, the maximum inhibitory effect is not seen for up to 5 to 10 days. Thus, ticlopidine is not useful if a rapid anti-platelet effect is required. It is extensively metabolized and has an initial half-life of 24 to 36 hours, but after a week of drug administration, the apparent half-life is 96 hours.

*Adverse effects.* The major concern with ticlopidine is its toxicity, most of which is not seen with clopidogrel. GI side effects and mild elevations in transaminases are common (8%). Of major concern is the 2 to 3% incidence of neutropenia or agranulocytosis leading to a high risk of sepsis. Recovery of granulocytes upon discontinuation of the drug may take several weeks, but it is accelerated by the use of granulocyte colony-stimulating factor (G-CSF). This complication may appear anytime within the first 3 months of treatment. Ticlopidine has also been associated with thrombocytopenia, aplastic anemia, and thrombotic thrombocytopenic purpura (TTP). Although the risk of TTP is very low (<0.1%), it is 50 times greater in ticlopidine-treated patients than in the general population, and TTP carries a mortality of 20%. Because of these toxicities, patients on ticlopidine should be monitored with blood counts and liver function tests every 1 to 2 weeks for the first 3 months. These toxicities have led to general abandonment of ticlopidine in favour of ASA or clopidogrel.

Both ticlopidine and clopidogrel have a bleeding risk of approximately 2%. In the event of bleeding, the drug should be stopped, although the drug effect will not dissipate for several days. Desmopressin acetate and platelet transfusions may be required if the bleeding is unresponsive to local measures.

## Clopidogrel

*Pharmacokinetics.* The pharmacokinetics of clopidogrel differ from those of ticlopidine. Clopidogrel (75 mg/day) is rapidly absorbed, extensively metabolized by the liver, and transformed to a short-lived active metabolite with a half-life of 8 hours. The inhibition of ADP-induced platelet aggregation by clopidogrel is dose-dependent. Antiplatelet effect is seen in 2 hours and remains stable for 48 hours with larger loading doses (300 mg), but with standard dosage, the maximal inhibition is not seen for 3 to 7 days.

*Adverse effects.* Clopidogrel resistance, or non-response, as measured by ADP-induced platelet aggregation, is seen in 5 to 22% of individuals. Drug resistance may be a consequence of reduced activity of hepatic cytochrome P450 (which forms the active metabolite). There is some indication that this may be clinically relevant, as with ASA, since patients who were the poorest drug responders by platelet testing are at higher risk of recurrent cardiovascular events. These findings are too preliminary to warrant routine laboratory assessment for clopidogrel resistance.

Bleeding with clopidogrel is slightly less frequent than with ASA (2% versus 2.7%), although other side effects are more frequent. As with other anti-platelet agents, the drug should be used with caution in individuals at high risk of bleeding. The frequency of GI side effects is similar with clopidogrel and ticlopidine (10%), but cytopenias and TTP are not seen with clopidogrel. Dose adjustment may be necessary in patients with moderate to severe hepatic impairment. Clopidogrel should be stopped for at least 5 to 7 days before any procedure associated with an increased bleeding risk, to permit recovery of platelet function.

# GP IIb/IIIa Inhibitors

Given the redundancy of specific platelet pathways leading to platelet adhesion, activation, and aggregation (see Fig. 38-6), it is not surprising that ASA, ticlopidine, and clopidogrel have only partial clinical efficacy. These drugs do not interfere with the activity of thrombin, nor do they fully block the final step in platelet aggregation. The activated GP IIb/IIIa receptor on the surface of platelets is the final common pathway for platelet aggregation, regardless of the initiating stimulus, and is therefore a prime target for the development of anti-platelet agents.

GP IIb/IIIa inhibitors have had a major impact on the treatment and outcome of patients with acute CVD and those requiring coronary stents and angioplasties. While these drugs are quite different chemically, they share a common mechanism of action. They all bind to the activated platelet GP IIb/IIIa ligand receptor at the RGD (Arg-Gly-Asp) epitope and competitively inhibit the binding of the critical platelet adhesion proteins (fibrinogen, von Willebrand factor, and perhaps other ligands such as vitronectin and fibronectin) necessary for platelet aggregation. This group of inhibitors includes chimeric monoclonal antibodies, RGD-containing peptides, non-RGD peptidomimetics, and non-peptide RGD mimetics. These agents are all used intravenously and have very short half-lives in circulation, but their high affinity for the platelet receptor makes their effect essentially irreversible. Like other anti-platelet agents, the GP IIb/IIIa inhibitors act on both circulating platelets and bone marrow megakaryocytes, so any new platelets released from treated megakaryocytes have the same receptor blockade. Since 10% of the platelets are replaced daily, it takes up to 10 days to fully clear the effects of these drugs once they are discontinued.

## Abciximab

Abciximab (ReoPro) is an active fragment of a human–mouse chimeric monoclonal antibody originally raised against the GP IIb/IIIa receptor. After its intravenous injection, platelet function is immediately affected but recovers slowly over 48 hours. Inhibition of ADP-induced platelet aggregation is dose-dependent, and the bleeding time is prolonged. Abciximab also binds to the vitronectin receptor on platelets, endothelial cells, and smooth muscle cells and prevents platelet-mediated thrombin generation, clot retraction, and smooth muscle migration and proliferation. This effect on the vitronectin receptor may play an important role in abciximab actions, especially the decrease in the observed thrombin generation.

*Pharmacokinetics.* After intravenous bolus injection (0.25 mg/kg), abciximab has an initial half-life of 10 minutes, with a second-phase half-life of 30 minutes. At the highest doses, 80% of GP IIb/IIIa receptors are blocked by 2 hours. Blockade of more than 50% of GP IIb/IIIa is associated with significant inhibition of platelet aggregation. A more sustained GP IIb/IIIa inhibition is seen with prolonged infusions (10 µg/min) for 12 hours after bolus injection, and the effect can still be seen up to 10 days later. Within 24 hours of cessation of abciximab, platelet aggregation is back to 50% of normal. Within 12 hours, the bleeding time returns to less than 12 minutes.

*Adverse effects.* Complications include a significantly increased risk of bleeding, especially at the site of arterial puncture. Compared with standard therapy, abciximab carries a twofold increase in major bleeding and need for transfusion. Thrombocytopenia is seen in approximately 5.2% of patients, usually within 24 hours, and may be severe. It is critical to follow the platelet count at 2 and 4 hours after bolus injection and then daily thereafter. Treatment of thrombocytopenia involves discontinuing the drug and giving platelet infusions if clinical bleeding occurs or thrombocytopenia is severe (<10 000/µl.).

Pseudothrombocytopenia, an *apparent* reduction in platelet count due to platelet clumping in vitro, is seen in 2% of abciximab-treated cases. It is not associated with adverse outcomes or risk of bleeding. Abciximab carries a risk of stimulating formation of anti-abciximab chimeric antibodies that could theoretically result in allergic or anaphylactoid reactions upon drug re-exposure. Antibodies have been seen in up to 6% of exposed individuals. However, allergic reactions have not proved to be a clinical problem so far, and the incidence of thrombocytopenia (4.6%) was not any greater upon drug re-exposure.

## Tirofiban

Tirofiban HCl (Aggrastat) is a non-peptide derivative of tyrosine that selectively inhibits the GP IIb/IIIa complex and mimics the RGD sequence in geometry and stereotactic and charge characteristics. At standard doses, it inhibits ADP-induced aggregation by 90% by blocking fibrinogen binding to the active GP IIb/IIIa complex.

*Pharmacokinetics.* Tirofiban has a short half-life of 1.6 hours and is primarily cleared through the kidneys and biliary system. The standard infusion dosage is 0.4 µg/kg/min for 30 minutes and 0.1 µg/kg/min until chest pain subsides or for 12 to 24 hours post angiography. In the presence of renal insufficiency (renal clearance <30 mL/min), the dose should be reduced. After stopping tirofiban, the bleeding time returns to normal within 4 hours.

*Adverse effects.* Like other GPIIb/IIIa inhibitors, tirofiban results in a significant bleeding risk. Minor bleeding occurs in 10 to 20% of cases and major bleeding, in 1 to 2%. Thrombocytopenia occurs in 1.5% of tirofiban cases versus 0.6% and 5% with heparin and abciximab, respectively. Thrombocytopenia is due to the formation of antibodies against the conformational changes of GPIIb/IIIa induced by tirofiban binding. When bleeding occurs, stopping the drug usually proves effective, but if necessary, platelet transfusions and even hemodialysis to remove tirofiban are also effective.

## Eptifibatide

Eptifibatide (Integrelin) is a synthetic cyclic heptapeptide based on homology with the RGD sequence of the snake venom barbourin, isolated from the southeastern rattlesnake. It has high but not absolute specificity for GP IIb/IIIa and also inhibits the vitronectin receptor. It prolongs the bleeding time and inhibits platelet aggregation by all platelet agonists.

*Pharmacokinetics.* Eptifibatide has a rapid onset of action and is quickly reversible with a half-life of 10 to 15 minutes. It is predominantly cleared renally, and dosage must be adjusted in the face of renal insufficiency. The bleeding time returns close to normal within 1 hour of cessation of drug administration.

For acute coronary syndromes, a 180 µg/kg bolus is followed by continuous infusion of 2 µg/kg/min for up to 72 hours. For coronary angioplasty, a 135 µg/kg bolus is followed by continuous infusion of 0.5 µg/kg/min for up to 20 to 24 hours after the procedure.

*Adverse effects.* Eptifibatide had a bleeding risk of 5%, similar to that of placebo in the IMPACT-II trial. The majority of bleeding cases were at vascular puncture sites. The incidence of thrombocytopenia (2%) with eptifibatide is similar to tirofiban and less than with abciximab. Platelets should be monitored during eptifibatide treatment, just as for tirofiban and abciximab.

## Clinical Considerations in the Choice of Anti-platelet Agents

These agents are used to prevent thrombosis and vascular obstruction in a wide variety of vascular problems, including both primary and secondary prevention of coronary heart disease; acute myocardial infarction and acute coronary syndromes; various cardiovascular surgical interventions such as coronary artery bypass grafts, angioplasties, and stent placement; secondary prevention of transient ischemic attacks and strokes; peripheral vascular disease; and thromboembolic events due to atrial fibrillation. However, they are not all used equally for all these indications. ASA, clopidogrel, and dipyridamole all have a relatively slow onset of action and are therefore less suitable for treating acute emergencies such as acute myocardial infarction. On the other hand, their efficacy by oral administration and their long duration of action make them highly suitable for long-term use in prevention of heart attacks, strokes, and vascular re-occlusion after angioplasty or stent placement. ASA, when taken for such indications, produces a significant reduction in recurrent acute myocardial infarction and stroke, morbidity, and cardiovascular deaths.

The thienopyridines are also useful in the same situations as ASA, but because of its greater toxicity, ticlopidine has largely been replaced by clopidogrel. Clopidogrel has a modest advantage over ASA for the secondary prevention of stroke, acute myocardial infarction, and established arterial disease. The combination of ASA and clopidogrel has become standard therapy for 1 month after coronary stent placement. Clopidogrel is also indicated for primary treatment of acute coronary syndromes, secondary prevention of graft closure after coronary bypass surgery, and in cases of ASA intolerance.

In two major clinical trials, combination therapy with ASA and clopidogrel was not superior to clopidogrel alone and was associated with a significantly increased risk of bleeding. Thus, it did not offer any advantage over single-agent therapy for long-term secondary prevention in cardiovascular disease.

Dipyridamole is rarely used as a first-line anti-platelet agent today. Its current use is in a combined formulation of extended-release dipyridamole (ER-DP) and low-dose ASA (Aggrenox) for secondary stroke prevention in patients with a previous history of stroke or transient ischemic attacks. This combination was found to be superior to aspirin alone in only one study, and caution should be exercised in its use as a first-line agent for this indication. Dipyridamole is not currently being used in any other clinical situations.

In contrast to the foregoing agents, the new class of GP IIb/IIIa antagonists has almost immediate onset of action and rapid disappearance of effect after drug discontinuation. Therefore, they are especially suitable for use in emergencies such as acute myocardial infarction and during cardiovascular surgical procedures and the post-operative period. Abciximab, tirofiban, and eptifibatide, given by intravenous bolus injection followed by continued infusion, have all been found to reduce the incidence of death, post-operative vascular complications, and recurrent obstruction after angioplasty for up to 6 months after surgery. A small but significant mortality benefit was still seen at 3 years. When used as a single agent, tirofiban was similar to heparin (see below) in reducing adverse outcomes in acute coronary syndromes, but the combination of both agents resulted in a further 22% improvement of outcome at 1 and 3 months. The combination of tirofiban with heparin and ASA is commonly used in patients undergoing coronary angioplasty.

The requirement for intravenous administration of these agents is an obvious limiting factor in their longer-term use. However, their clinical success has led to the development of oral GP IIb/IIIa agents in hopes of improving the long-term benefits of anti-platelet agents. Unfortunately, all such oral agents (xemilofiban, orbofiban, sibrafiban, and lotrafiban) tested to date were no more effective than ASA and, in some cases, increased the mortality. None of these agents are available for current clinical use.

## ANTICOAGULANT AGENTS

Anticoagulants are used in the treatment and prevention of thromboembolic disease, both arterial (ATE) and venous (VTE). They interfere directly or indirectly with procoagulant proteins in the coagulation cascade, and, by doing so, they regulate thrombin generation. An ideal anticoagulant is one that has predictable pharmacokinetic properties, does not need ongoing laboratory monitoring, has no substantive side effects or toxicities, has a low risk of causing bleeding, is reversible in case bleeding does occur, and can be taken orally, subcutaneously, or intravenously depending on the need or circumstances. Many substances are capable of preventing blood clot formation but are unsuitable for clinical use because they lack too many of these qualities.

Anticoagulants can be classified according to the strategy by which they interfere with thrombin generation and resulting thrombus formation and include (1) direct anticoagulants that act directly on blood clotting proteins and interfere with their normal function (e.g., heparins, direct anti-thrombins, direct anti-Xa agents), and (2) indirect anticoagulants that interfere with the synthesis of specific clotting factors (e.g., vitamin K antagonists). Anticoagulants can also be grouped according to the steps where they act in the coagulation cascade: (1) initiation of coagulation (e.g., nematode anticoagulant protein c2), (2) propagation of coagulation (e.g., Factor Xa inhibitors), and (3) thrombin activity (i.e., direct anti-thrombins) (Fig. 38-7).

## Heparins

Heparin was discovered accidentally in the early twentieth century in acidic extracts of liver tissue (hence its name) and was found to have a dose-dependent in vitro anticoagulant effect. Unfractionated heparin (UFH) has been in wide use unchanged since the 1940s. **Heparans** are heavily sulfated mucopolysaccharides that line the inner surface of blood vessels. UFH is a heterogeneous group of heparan fragments obtained from porcine or bovine gut or lung. Low-molecular-weight heparins (LMWHs) were discovered in the 1980s and are made up of smaller fragments of heparin containing the anticoagulant activity. Two different structural features allow these fragments to bind to the naturally occurring anticoagulant protein, antithrombin (AT) and activate it.

1. The longer heparin fragments (>18 polysaccharide units) have a strong negative charge arising from their high density of sulfate and carboxylate groups that allows them to bind AT and thrombin and bring them into close apposition, preventing the thrombin from acting.
2. A unique pentasaccharide sequence is irregularly distributed in the smaller heparan chains, and is therefore found in only some of the heparin fragments. This sequence binds with very high affinity to AT and alters its conformation, markedly enhancing the ability of AT to bind covalently to the serine protease factors (serpins) IIa, IXa, Xa, and XIa, irreversibly inhibiting their procoagulant activity (see Fig. 38-4).

Thrombin and factor Xa are more sensitive to inhibition by heparin–AT than the other serine proteases are. Heparin inhibits thrombin (IIa) by both mechanisms

---

FIGURE 38-7    Steps in blood coagulation and sites of selective anticoagulant drug interaction. The coagulation pathway is broken into the following steps: (1) initiation, involving tissue factor and factor VIIa, (2) propagation of thrombin generation, involving factors IX/IXa and X/Xa and cofactors VIIIa and Va, and (3) thrombin activity. Drugs have been developed to target selective sites of interaction in each of these three compartments. Refer to the text for further details. TF = tissue factor; TFPI = tissue factor pathway inhibitors; NAPc2 = nematode anticoagulant protein c2; APC = activated protein C; sTM = soluble thrombomodulin.

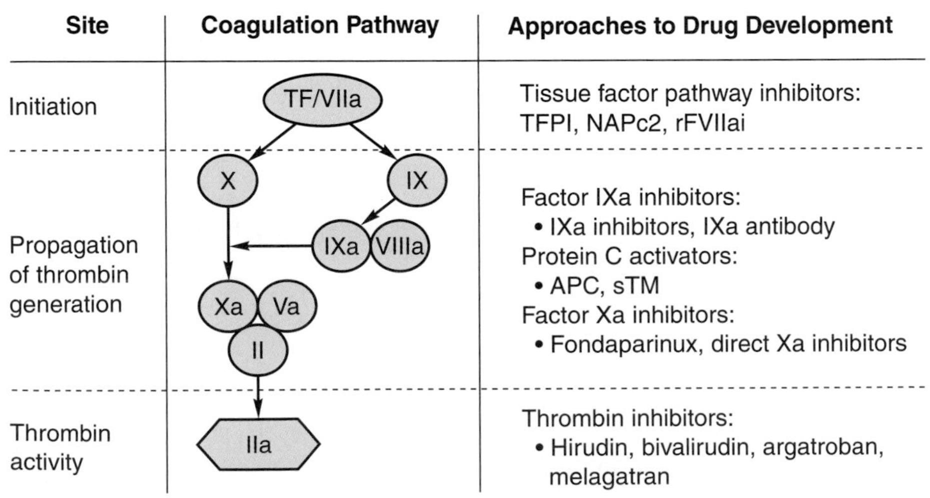

| Site | Coagulation Pathway | Approaches to Drug Development |
|---|---|---|
| Initiation | TF/VIIa | Tissue factor pathway inhibitors: TFPI, NAPc2, rFVIIai |
| Propagation of thrombin generation | X    IX    IXa  VIIIa    Xa  Va    II | Factor IXa inhibitors: • IXa inhibitors, IXa antibody  Protein C activators: • APC, sTM  Factor Xa inhibitors: • Fondaparinux, direct Xa inhibitors |
| Thrombin activity | IIa | Thrombin inhibitors: • Hirudin, bivalirudin, argatroban, melagatran |

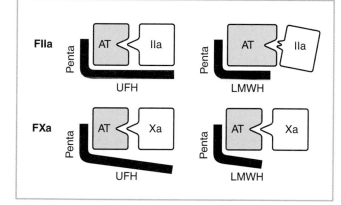

**FIGURE 38-8** Inactivation of clotting enzymes by unfractionated heparin (UFH) and low-molecular-weight heparin (LMWH). (Top) UFH inhibits thrombin (IIa) by binding to AT through the pentasaccharide group and to thrombin by a non-specific charge effect, thus allowing AT–IIa complex formation. LMWH lacks the longer fragments of UFH and fails to bring thrombin into the complex. (Bottom) In contrast, both UFH and LMWH are able to inhibit factor Xa because their binding to AT via the high-affinity pentasaccharide portion is sufficient to catalyze the binding of Xa to AT.

described above, while only the high-affinity pentasaccharide group in heparins inhibits factor Xa (Fig. 38-8).

## Unfractionated heparin (UFH)

*Mechanism of action.* UFH is heterogeneous with respect to size (5 000 to 30 000 Da), anticoagulant activity, and pharmacokinetics. Approximately one-third of the fragments are long enough to bind to AT by the first mechanism described above and are responsible for much of the anticoagulant activity of UFH (see Fig. 38-8). Heparin then dissociates from the AT–serpin complex and can be reutilized on another AT molecule, while the inactive AT–serpin complex is cleared from the circulation. By inactivating thrombin, UFH prevents not only fibrin formation but also further activation of platelets and activation of coagulation factors V, VIII, and XI. Clearance of UFH varies with chain length, with the higher molecular weight moieties being cleared more rapidly, so over time, there is accumulation of low-molecular-weight moieties with more anti-Xa activity. UFH inactivates free but not clot-bound factor IIa and Xa in a 1:1 ratio and inactivates the other serine proteases to a lesser extent.

*Pharmacokinetics.* UFH is administered either by continuous intravenous infusion or intermittent subcutaneous injection, but the latter is rarely used except for prophylaxis. The subcutaneous route requires a 10% larger dose than the intravenous route (35 000 units in divided doses) to compensate for the lower bioavailability. Once in the bloodstream, UFH binds to a number of endogenous heparin-binding proteins, such as vWF, fibronectin, and platelet factor (PF4), which reduces its anticoagulant activity since only free UFH is active. UFH is cleared rapidly from the plasma through a rapid saturation of vascular cells (endothelial cells, macrophages) followed by a slower non-saturable phase of clearance that is largely renal. Clearance is dose-dependent with an approximate half-life of 30 to 60 minutes.

*Indications.* Heparin is indicated for prophylaxis and treatment of VTE, ATE, and acute coronary syndromes and as adjuvant therapy in therapeutic fibrinolysis (see "Fibrinolytic Agents" below). The initial dose of UFH to treat VTE is an 80 U/kg bolus followed by an infusion of 18 U/kg/hr. Patients with acute coronary syndromes typically receive a 25% lower dose. Heparin is administered in a wide range of doses for other indications: 10 to 50 units for vascular catheter flushes, 5000 units subcutaneously twice daily for VTE prophylaxis, 20 000 to 50 000 U/day for the treatment of established ATE, VTE, and acute coronary syndromes, and even larger doses for cardiopulmonary bypass surgery.

*Bleeding risks.* The risk of bleeding increases with UFH dose and with any concomitant anti-platelet or thrombolytic agents. Because of the relationship between dose and bleeding risk, and because of variable levels of UFH binding proteins, close laboratory monitoring and UFH dose adjustment are necessary. While heparin will prolong the TT, PT, and aPTT, UFH has traditionally been monitored with the aPTT in the usual therapeutic dose range and with the activated clotting time (ACT) when higher UFH levels are required. For drug monitoring and adjustment of dose, the aPTT is kept at 1.5 to 2.5 times the aPTT control value. The aPTT is affected by a number of significant factors in the presence of UFH, including sensitivity of the aPTT laboratory reagent, levels of fibrinogen and factor VIII in the sample, levels of heparin-binding proteins, and the mechanical testing systems. These factors can make the aPTT unreliable in UFH monitoring and can lead to potential under-dosing or overdosing. The best current method of monitoring UFH is to measure free UFH plasma levels with an anti–factor Xa assay (therapeutic target 0.3 to 0.7 anti–factor Xa units/mL or 0.2 to 0.4 UFH units/mL). Despite the lack of reliability of the aPTT, it remains the most common method for monitoring UFH response because of its wide availability and long history of use. UFH should be measured (aPTT, UFH level) 4 to 6 hours after bolus injection and 4 to 6 hours after any adjustment of the rate of continuous infusion; the dose is then adjusted according to an institutional heparin dose adjustment nomogram. Heparin nomograms should be created individually for each institution on the basis of their laboratory aPTT control value and its relationship to UFH plasma levels as measured by anti–factor Xa assay.

*Heparin resistance* is recognized when an unusually high dose of UFH (>40 000 U/24 hr) is required to attain anticoagulation. Causes include AT deficiency, high levels of heparin-binding proteins, elevated levels of factor VIII or fibrinogen, and increased heparin clearance. When heparin resistance is suspected, heparin dosage should be based on an anti–factor Xa assay.

*Limitations of UFH* include the bleeding risk, pharmacokinetic and biophysical properties, risk of heparin-induced thrombocytopenia (HIT), and its long-term effect on bone metabolism. The bleeding risk with UFH depends upon the patient's age and UFH dose among other things, but it is generally around 2.5 to 3% for the uncomplicated treatment of venous thrombosis. In the hospitalized patient with medical and surgical problems, on multiple drugs and undergoing a variety of procedures, the risk is much higher. In these circumstances, fatal bleeding with UFH occurs at a rate of 0.5% per day, major bleeding at 0.8% per day, and all bleeding at 1.0 to 2.0% per day. Bleeding risk increases with age over 80 years; heart, liver, or renal disease; and aPTT of greater than 100 seconds.

Pharmacokinetic limitations are a result of the significant interaction of UFH with intravascular proteins released from platelets and endothelial cells and the requirement for available AT for full heparin function. AT plasma levels fall significantly during an acute thrombotic event, because AT is consumed in early clot formation and not enough is available for UFH binding. Heparin-binding proteins, such as the acute phase reactant vWF and PF4 released from activated platelets during clot formation, will rise during early UFH therapy, bind the drug, and reduce levels of free biologically active UFH. UFH has biophysical limitations because UFH–AT binds to free, but not to clot surface–bound, thrombin or factor Xa (within the prothrombinase complex), and thus UFH fails to inhibit procoagulant activity to its full theoretical extent.

HIT is an immunological disorder in which antibodies form against the heparin–PF4 complex bound to the platelet surface. These antibodies, in 1 to 3% of cases, upon binding to unique platelet Fc receptors and endothelial cells, are capable of activating these cells and causing thrombocytopenia and, paradoxically, given the degree of anticoagulation, arterial and venous thrombosis. HIT is associated with significant morbidity (stroke, coronary events, peripheral arterial occlusions) in 10 to 15% of cases. Therefore, any unexplained thrombocytopenia (fall in platelets of >50% from baseline or platelet count <100 000/μL) during UFH therapy requires investigation and elucidation of its etiology. If HIT is suspected, UFH must be stopped and replaced by an alternative anticoagulant not associated with HIT, such as hirudin, argatroban, or danaparoid, until the diagnosis is established.

All patients on UFH must be followed with platelet counts, and if HIT occurs, they should never be re-exposed to either UFH or LMWH.

***Protamine reversal of UFH effect.*** In the presence of bleeding associated with UFH, drug reversal may be necessary in addition to other supportive measures. The anticoagulant effects of UFH can be immediately antagonized with intravenous protamine. Protamine is a basic protein from fish sperm that forms an inactive salt complex upon binding to UFH. One milligram of protamine will neutralize 100 IU of UFH. Given the short half-life of UFH, only enough protamine is necessary to neutralize the heparin given in the last 2 to 3 hours. Protamine is associated with hypotension and bradycardia and should be infused slowly to minimize these side effects.

## Low-molecular-weight heparin (LMWH)

In the 1980s, it was discovered that heparin could be fractionated by a variety of physical or chemical methods to produce a much more homogeneous preparation of heparin fragments about one-third as long as those of native UFH that retained anticoagulant activity. LMWH has a molecular weight range of 3000 to 5000 Da. When compared with UFH, LMWH has a number of desirable pharmacological properties: (1) superior and predictable pharmacokinetic properties that allow once-daily subcutaneous dosing based on body weight and no laboratory monitoring, (2) more favourable benefit to risk ratio allowing home therapy, and (3) less anti-IIa and more anti-Xa activity.

Because of these properties, LMWH has replaced UFH for many clinical indications. It has allowed VTE therapy to be given in an outpatient setting, allowed outpatient bridging therapy for patients on warfarin, and has considerably simplified VTE therapy for inpatients. LMWH is indicated for the treatment and prophylaxis of VTE, including outpatient treatment of deep vein thrombosis and pulmonary embolism and treatment of acute coronary syndromes.

Like UFH, LMWH induces its major anticoagulant effect through AT binding and resulting AT conformational change that facilitates complex formation with factor Xa and, to a lesser extent, factor IIa (see Fig. 38-4). All of the LMWH fragments contain the high-affinity pentasaccharide necessary to bind AT and inactivate factor Xa, whereas only 25 to 50% of them have the appropriate chain length to form the tertiary complex with AT and factor IIa (see Fig. 38-8). This explains why the anti-IIa to anti-Xa ratio is 1:1 for UFH but is 1:2 to 1:5 for LMWH.

LMWH has a weak effect on the aPTT because the aPTT is much more sensitive to anti-IIa than to anti-Xa effects. A number of formulations are available in North America, including **nadroparin, enoxaparin, dalteparin,** and **tinzaparin.** They are prepared by different methods, resulting in slightly different pharmacokinetic and anticoagulant properties, but clinical efficacy is similar for all indications other than acute coronary sydromes. Bleeding risk is similar or slightly lower with LMWH than with UFH.

*Pharmacokinetics.* A major advantage of LMWH is that it exhibits very little binding to heparin-binding proteins or intravascular cells. This lack of protein binding results in more predictable pharmacokinetics and dose-response relationship, an increased plasma half-life, and a much lower incidence of HIT. The bioavailability of LMWH approaches 100%. Peak anticoagulant effect occurs at 4 to 6 hours after subcutaneous injection. Elimination half-life (3 to 5 hours) is longer than that of UFH and, unlike UFH, is not dose-dependent. Measurable anticoagulant effect of LMWH is largely gone by 24 hours. Depending on the formulations and supporting clinical evidence, LMWHs are administered either twice or once a day for specific indications. LMWHs are typically administered in a fixed dose for VTE prophylaxis but in weight-adjusted dosage for therapeutic indications. Unlike UFH, LMWHs are cleared renally and can accumulate in the presence of severe renal insufficiency. With renal failure, and in the presence of severe obesity, drug level monitoring with LMWH anti–factor Xa assay may be indicated to ensure adequate and not excessive LMWH activity.

Although anti-Xa levels above the therapeutic range are associated with an increased bleeding risk, there is not a close relationship between clinical outcomes (bleeding risk, re-thrombosis rates) and anti-Xa activity levels. Thus, routine monitoring of anti–factor Xa is not indicated other than in patients with renal failure or obesity.

*Adverse effects.* LMWH has far fewer adverse effects and lower overall mortality than UFH. The bleeding risk in the treatment of VTE (3%) is slightly less than with UFH. Unlike UFH, LMWH cannot be fully neutralized with protamine. Fortunately this is rarely necessary, but if bleeding is severe, 1 mg of protamine can be given for every 1 mg or 100 anti-Xa units of LMWH. HIT is much less common with LMWH than with UFH, although the precise incidence is not clear. Patients with known current or past HIT should not be exposed to either LMWH or UFH.

### Heparinoids

**Danaparoid** is a heparinoid rather than a heparin. It is a mixture of low-molecular-weight sulfated glucosamino-glucuronan fragments of heparan sulfate, dermatan sulfate, and chondroitin sulfate derived from porcine intestinal mucosa. It is devoid of heparin or heparin fragments. The major clinical indication for danaparoid is the treatment of HIT, although today the direct anti-thrombins argatroban and hirudin have largely supplanted it in this role other than in the outpatient setting.

Danaparoid has a much higher anti-Xa to anti-IIa ratio (approximately 28:1) than either UFH (1:1) or LMWH (3:1

to 5:1). As with UFH and LMWH, its anti-Xa activity is mediated by AT, and like LMWH, danaparoid activity is not neutralized by endogenous heparin-binding proteins. Danaparoid shows low, and generally weak, cross-reactivity with heparin-associated antibodies in the sera of patients with HIT, and it is unclear if this agent has caused any true cases of HIT.

*Pharmacokinetics.* The absolute bioavailability of danaparoid after subcutaneous administration approaches 100%. Onset of anticoagulation occurs immediately after an intravenous bolus dose, and peak plasma anti-Xa activity levels are reached in 4 to 5 hours. For patients with normal renal function, the half-lives of elimination of anti-Xa and thrombin generation–inhibiting activities are approximately 25 hours and 7 hours, respectively, after both subcutaneous and intravenous administration. Steady-state levels of plasma anti-Xa activity are usually reached within 4 to 5 days of danaparoid therapy (i.e., within 4 to 5 half-lives). Since danaparoid is mainly eliminated via the kidney, its half-life is significantly increased in patients with severely impaired renal function. Dosage reductions are recommended if creatinine clearance is less than 50 mL/min.

While danaparoid has predictable pharmacokinetics, measurement of drug activity levels is recommended on or after treatment day 3, especially in the presence of renal insufficiency. For therapeutic anticoagulation, the target anti-Xa level at 6 hours after subcutaneous administration of danaparoid should be in the range of 0.35 to 0.7 anti-Xa units/mL.

The major *adverse effect* of danaparoid is bleeding, which occurs with a frequency (3 to 5%) comparable to that seen with UFH. Other toxicities have included transient elevations of liver transaminases. There is no specific antidote for danaparoid, and protamine does not neutralize its anticoagulant activity.

### Direct Anti-thrombins

A number of drugs that act directly and selectively at the level of free and clot-bound thrombin are now available (see Fig. 38-7). The direct thrombin inhibitors (DTIs) **hirudin, argatroban,** and **bivalirudin** differ from the heparins and heparinoids in that they do not require AT as a cofactor. They selectively bind and neutralize all thrombin, both free and clot-bound. Further, they have the advantage that their activity is not interfered with by vascular drug binding proteins. Thus, their anticoagulant effect is much more predictable than that of UFH. DTIs also affect platelet adhesiveness and prolong the bleeding time slightly.

While the DTIs affect the ecarin clotting time (ECT), aPTT, PT, and thrombin time, they are monitored with the aPTT or ECT. Both of these coagulation tests show a good dose–response relationship in the target therapeutic drug range (1.5 to 2.5 times the aPTT or ECT control level). The aPTT should be kept below 100 seconds. The ECT is the more specific test since it is not affected by increased factor VIII or fibrinogen and the DTIs act directly upon the unique form of thrombin formed in this assay. While ECT is the preferred assay for DTIs, it is not widely available.

Hirudin and argatroban are approved for the treatment of HIT, and bivalirudin is approved as an alternative to UHF for coronary angioplasty. The disadvantages of all DTIs are high cost and lack of reversibility of anticoagulant effect.

## Hirudin

Hirudin is a 65-amino-acid polypeptide and naturally occurring anticoagulant isolated from the salivary gland of the leech (*Hirudo medicinalis*), but a recombinant form has been developed (lepirudin). Hirudin binds directly to the active enzymatic site of thrombin, forming an irreversible complex. The plasma half-life of hirudin is 60 to 90 minutes after intravenous infusion. Hirudin is largely cleared by the kidney; it should be used cautiously in patients with renal insufficiency, and frequent dose monitoring is recommended.

Hirudin (0.4 mg/kg bolus followed by intravenous infusion of 0.1 mg/kg/hr) is indicated for the acute treatment of HIT, including arterial and venous thrombotic complications, and as an alternative anticoagulant for patients intolerant of UFH. Hirudin is also as effective as UFH for adjuvant therapy after therapeutic fibrinolysis (see "Fibrinolytic Agents" below), and it may be superior to UFH for prevention of myocardial infarction and death in patients with acute coronary syndromes. Hirudin is also effective for prophylaxis of deep vein thrombosis after hip arthroplasty.

A major concern with hirudin is the formation of anti-hirudin antibodies in up to 40 to 60% of treated individuals. These antibodies have a major effect on the half-life of hirudin, increasing it from 1 hour to 24 hours by interfering with drug clearance. Thus, hirudin is frequently unsuitable for prolonged use, and when utilized, it requires close daily laboratory monitoring to avoid drug overdose.

The other major adverse effect of hirudin and its derivatives is bleeding, which occurs in about 3% of patients treated for VTE (the same as with UFH) and slightly more frequently than with UFH in patients treated for acute coronary syndromes. No instances of thrombocytopenia have been attributed to hirudin. The drug effect is irreversible and no direct antidote exists, so management of bleeding is a problem. If bleeding does occur, the drug must be stopped and supportive measures given. Given the short half-life, the antithrombin effect is quickly lost.

## Argatroban

Argatroban is a low-molecular-weight arginine derivative that is a competitive inhibitor of thrombin, with which it forms a reversible complex. Argatroban inhibits both free and clot-bound thrombin. It also decreases platelet adhesiveness, decreases smooth muscle proliferation, and blocks thrombin-induced platelet aggregation. It has a short plasma half-life of 35 to 55 minutes and reaches a steady state in 2 hours. Argatroban has predictable pharmacokinetics since it does not bind to vascular proteins such as acute phase reactants. It is metabolized in the liver and eliminated in the hepatobiliary system. Hepatic dysfunction has a significant effect on the normally short half-life; the dose should be reduced and the drug used with caution if liver dysfunction is present. Argatroban (2 μg/kg/min without bolus) is licensed for the treatment of HIT. For other indications, including acute coronary syndromes and coronary angioplasty, it has not been shown to be superior to UFH.

Bleeding with argatroban occurs with a frequency similar to that of UFH, at 2 to 3%. Rash is also seen in 2% of patients. If bleeding occurs, treatment with fresh frozen plasma may be useful, given the reversibility of argatroban inhibition.

## Bivalirudin

Bivalirudin is a 20-amino-acid synthetic polypeptide and analogue of hirudin that binds to thrombin and forms a 1:1 complex. However, unlike hirudin, thrombin activity can be recovered from this complex, which may explain the lower bleeding risk seen with this agent than with UFH. Bivalirudin has a half-life of 25 minutes; less than 20% is secreted renally and the rest is enzymatically metabolized. Like the other DTIs, it has a predictable anticoagulant response, and its short half-life makes it a useful agent. It is not approved for HIT but is used "off-label" for this indication (0.15 mg/kg/hr without bolus) because of its theoretical advantages over hirudin. In angioplasty treatment, bivalirudin is as effective as heparin but with a lower bleeding risk. As adjunct therapy to thrombolytics in acute myocardial infarction, bivalirudin was better than UFH in reducing the rate of re-infarction. Like the other anti-thrombins, bivalirudin requires monitoring with aPTT or ECT to maintain a target level of 1.5 to 2.5 times baseline control.

## Ximelagatran

Ximelagatran is an oral antithrombin that is the prodrug of the active site–directed thrombin inhibitor melagatran. This is the oral anticoagulant closest to clinical marketing, but it has not yet been released for uses other than prophylaxis in VTE. After absorption in the small intestine, ximelagatran undergoes rapid biotransformation to melagatran. It has a half-life of 3 to 4 hours and is orally administered twice daily. GI absorption does not appear to be affected by either food or other drugs. Ximelagatran has predictable pharmacokinetics and does not bind to intravascular proteins, so laboratory monitoring is not necessary. Clearance is through the kidney, and dose adjustments may be needed in renal insufficiency.

Ximelagatran is efficacious for prophylaxis of thrombosis in high-risk orthopaedic patients, for the treatment of VTE, for the prevention of cardioembolic events in atrial fibrillation, and for the prevention of recurrent ischemic events after myocardial infarction. In large trials, ximelagatran was shown to be as effective and safe as standard therapy with LMWH and warfarin for treatment of VTE and prevention of stroke in patients with atrial fibrillation. Patient acceptance of this oral anticoagulant was predictably very high.

However, ximelagatran elevated serum transaminases in 4 to 10% of patients on long-term therapy. This effect is usually asymptomatic and reversible on discontinuation of drug. For comparison, similar hepatic changes are seen in 4 to 8% of patients on UFH or LMWH and in 1% on warfarin. This drug has been approved only for prophylaxis of deep vein thrombosis because of concern about toxicity issues. Liver function will need to be monitored if this drug is released for therapeutic use.

Other oral anticoagulant agents targeting thrombin or factor Xa are undergoing early clinical trials and may be approved eventually for clinical use.

## Factor Xa Inhibitors

Another attractive target site for new anticoagulant agents is in the propagation of the clotting cascade, in which factor Xa and the prothrombinase complex play a key role (see Fig. 38-7). Various synthetic analogues of the heparin pentasaccharide chain form complexes with AT and selectively inhibit factor Xa without affecting any other serine proteases. Unlike the heparin–AT complex, these pentasaccharide factor Xa inhibitors inhibit both free and clot-bound factor Xa within the prothrombinase complex.

One such synthetic pentasaccharide, **fondiparinux**, has a half-life of 31 to 35 hours. The analogue **idraparinux** has a much longer half-life so that once-weekly subcutaneous injection is possible; it is now in clinical trials. These pentasaccharides are 100% bioavailable and immediately active upon administration. They are excreted renally without chemical change, and dose adjustments are recommended in the presence of renal insufficiency. The pentasaccharides are administered subcutaneously. They are indicated for prophylaxis and treatment of VTE. There is no evidence that they induce an HIT-like syndrome, and they are currently being used off-label in some countries for the treatment of HIT.

As with all anticoagulants, bleeding is the major adverse effect. Hemorrhage may occur at any site. Risk appears to be increased by a number of factors, including renal dysfunction, age (>75 years), and weight (<50 kg). Like most of the clinically available anticoagulants, they have a highly variable bleeding risk, but in the same range as UFH and LMWH. Other toxic effects have included fever and GI upset with nausea. Generally, laboratory monitoring of drug activity levels is not needed because of their predictable dosing and pharmacokinetics.

## New Emerging Anticoagulants

Discovery of new anticoagulants is accelerating, and an array of new drugs that target different specific steps in coagulation are in various stages of development and trial. Figure 38-7 outlines the sites of action and drugs involved. Agents targeting the initiation of the clotting pathway by the factor VIIa–TF complex that have reached clinical trials include recombinant tissue factor pathway inhibitor (TFPI), recombinant nematode anticoagulant peptide (NAPc2), and inactive factor VIIa (FVIIai), which blocks the action of factor VIIa. New agents that target propagation of the coagulation sequence, besides the pentasaccharides, include activated protein C (APC), which inactivates factors VIIIa and Va, and soluble thrombomodulin (sTM), which forms a complex with thrombin that catalyzes APC production.

Recombinant TFPI (Tifacogan) has been evaluated in a sepsis trial but was associated with a higher bleeding rate (6.5%) and showed no superiority over older drugs in reducing all-cause mortality. Further studies have been halted. NAPc2, an 85-amino-acid polypeptide originally isolated from a hookworm now available in a recombinant form, binds to factor X/Xa and the NAPc2–FXa complex, then inhibits the TF–FVIIa complex. NAP2c has a very long half-life of 50 hours after subcutaneous injection. Its bleeding risk and efficacy in prevention of VTE in orthopaedic thromboprophylaxis trials were similar to those of LMWH. Its utility in other cardiovascular indications is now under investigation. FVIIai binds to TF and interferes with initiation of coagulation by competitively blocking binding of FVII to TF. FVIIai has not been shown to be superior to UFH in clinical trials and is not under further current development.

APC already has a clinical role and has been licensed for the treatment of severe sepsis. A recombinant sTM analogue is being tested clinically for prophylaxis of VTE.

## Vitamin K Antagonists

Oral vitamin K antagonists remain the drugs of choice for long-term anticoagulation treatment for a wide range of indications because of their oral availability, clinically useful half-life, and reversibility of action. Dicumarol (bishydroxycoumarin) was first discovered in 1939 after cattle developed a bleeding disorder caused by eating sweet clover. In the 1940s, a dicumarol derivative, warfarin, was developed as an effective rodent poison that induced lethal bleeding. Since the 1950s, when reversal of the warfarin effect with oral or parenteral vitamin $K_1$ was first documented, warfarin has become the most widely used anticoagulant for short- and long-term anticoagulant therapy and prophylaxis.

## Warfarin

Warfarin induces a hypocoagulable state by interfering with the hepatic production of fully functional vitamin K–dependent blood clotting factors II, VII, IX, and X. Vitamin $K_1$ is an essential hepatic cofactor for the gamma carboxylation of glutamic acid residues in afunctional precursors of these clotting factors, converting them to their functional forms. Warfarin blocks the action of the essential vitamin $K_1$ by inhibiting vitamin K reductases (Fig. 38-9). This results in near-normal circulating levels of factors II, VII, IX, and X that have markedly reduced enzymatic potential. These vitamin K–dependent factors have quite variable half-lives (6 to 60 hours), and it is these half-lives that dictate the clinical efficacy and anticoagulant effect of warfarin. The anticoagulant efficacy of vitamin K antagonists most closely correlates with the functional level of prothrombin, which has the longest half-life (60 hours). Warfarin also affects two other vitamin K–dependent molecules, the anticoagulant proteins S and C. However, reduction of protein S and C function does not appear to be essential for the anticoagulant activity of warfarin.

*Pharmacokinetics.* Warfarin is rapidly absorbed from the gut. In the blood, 90% of the drug is bound to albumin, and only the free unbound warfarin is biologically active. The drug half-life is 36 to 48 hours. Hepatic metabolism by microsomal enzymes, including cytochrome P450 variants, partly explains the marked inter-individual variation in dosage required for adequate anticoagulant effect. Numerous factors affect the biologic activity of warfarin, including age, activity level, warfarin absorption, general state of health, and interfering drugs.

*Drug interactions.* Co-administration of other drugs, such as the anti-platelet agents, may alter the clinical effect and risks of warfarin by affecting hemostasis through different mechanisms. Other drugs may also induce or inhibit the action of hepatic cytochrome P450 enzymes, resulting in either potentiation or reduction of the active concentration of warfarin. Displacement of warfarin from albumin by competitive binding of other drugs can result in increased free biologically active warfarin. These two mechanisms are the most common causes of warfarin-drug interactions. The list of known interacting drugs that either potentiate or attenuate the anticoagulant effect is lengthy, and knowledge of their identity and expected interactions is important in view of the narrow margin of safety between overdose (bleeding risk) and under-dose (loss of efficacy).

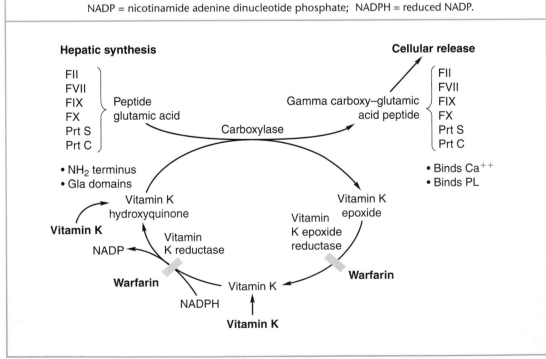

**FIGURE 38-9** The hepatic vitamin K cycle. Vitamin K is reduced to vitamin K hydroxyquinone by warfarin-sensitive K epoxide reductase and K reductase enzymes. The normal action of vitamin K hydroxyquinone is to gamma-carboxylate the amino-terminal glutamic acid domains of the afunctional vitamin K–dependent clotting proteins (II, VII, IX, X), making the proteins functional. Exogenous vitamin K can bypass the warfarin effect at the level of vitamin K hydroxyquinone. Prt S = protein S; Prt C = protein C; Gla = glutamic acid; PL = specific phospholipids; NADP = nicotinamide adenine dinucleotide phosphate; NADPH = reduced NADP.

*Diet* can also alter warfarin effect: ingestion of food-stuffs high in vitamin K can begin to counteract the effects of warfarin within 6 to 12 hours. Patients should be advised to be moderate and consistent in their diet with vitamin K food sources to minimize this effect on the INR.

*Management of therapy.* The optimal INR range for treatment and prophylaxis of most venous and arterial thromboembolic indications is 2 to 3. These indications include atrial fibrillation, cardiac tissue valve replacement, and VTE disease. For patients with mechanical heart valves, acute myocardial infarction, or high-risk venous thrombosis, the target INR range is 2.5 to 3.5 or higher. For any given indication, there is a trend to lower bleeding risk with no loss in clinical efficacy the lower the INR is within the therapeutic range. The aim should therefore be to keep the INR within the target range but towards the lower end of that range if feasible.

There is no reason to use a loading dose for the initiation of warfarin therapy. Given the long half-lives of both warfarin (36 hours) and factor II (60 hours), to attain the full anticoagulant effect of warfarin the INR must be within the therapeutic range for at least 4 to 6 days for all of the vitamin K–dependent proteins to decrease to 20 to 30% of normal (Fig. 38-10). The initial change in INR is most sensitive to the level of factor VII, which has the shortest half-life (4 to 6 hours). However, since the antithrombotic effect of warfarin is most closely dependent on the activity level of factor II and not factor VII, the initial drop in INR does not yet indicate the attainment of therapeutic anticoagulation. For this reason, when patients are being switched over from UFH or LMWH to warfarin, an overlap of treatments is required for a minimum of 2 to 3 days once the INR is in the target range, to ensure that prothrombin levels have been given enough time to fall and true anticoagulant effect is present. Similarly, any alteration in warfarin dose will not affect the INR for a number of days.

*Adverse effects.* Warfarin is generally well tolerated, with few side effects other than the bleeding risk. GI upset and hair thinning may be seen in 10 to 15% of cases. GI upset is seen more frequently in lactase-deficient individuals, and switching to preparations without lactose filler has proven useful. Other rare side effects include cholestatic jaundice and warfarin-induced skin necrosis. Warfarin-induced skin necrosis, a rare toxicity, is paradoxically due to microvascular thrombosis that occurs upon initiation of warfarin therapy and is felt to result from a transient hypercoagulable state induced by low levels of the vitamin K–dependent anticoagulant protein C, which has a very short half-life (<2 hours).

Warfarin is relatively contraindicated during pregnancy. Teratogenicity with midline birth defect is well described in 4 to 5% of pregnancies in which warfarin is used, but it is a risk only between the sixth and twelfth week of conception. A further bleeding risk to the fetus is caused by its immature liver, which results in supra-thera-

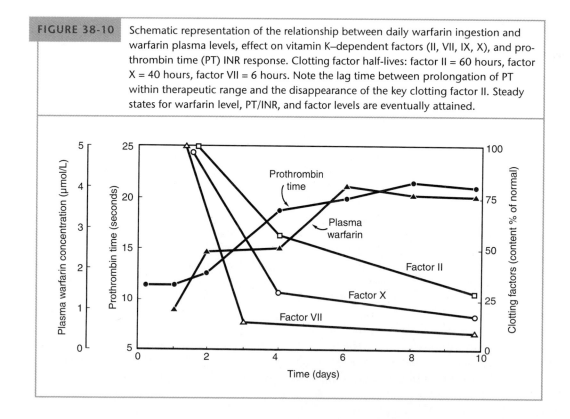

**FIGURE 38-10** Schematic representation of the relationship between daily warfarin ingestion and warfarin plasma levels, effect on vitamin K–dependent factors (II, VII, IX, X), and prothrombin time (PT) INR response. Clotting factor half-lives: factor II = 60 hours, factor X = 40 hours, factor VII = 6 hours. Note the lag time between prolongation of PT within therapeutic range and the disappearance of the key clotting factor II. Steady states for warfarin level, PT/INR, and factor levels are eventually attained.

peutic INRs in the fetus despite normal therapeutic maternal INRs. In North America, pregnant women requiring full anticoagulation are generally treated with LMWH or UFH throughout pregnancy.

As with other anticoagulants, the bleeding risk with warfarin varies greatly depending on associated risk factors, including age, nutritional status, concomitant medical conditions (e.g., tumour, mucosal injury), concurrent drugs, previous bleeding history, acquired or hereditary coagulopathies, and expertise of INR monitoring. Average annual frequencies of fatal, major, and minor bleeding are 0.6%, 3%, and 9.6% respectively. Patients with low, intermediate, and high risk for bleeding had a 3%, 12%, and 53% probability of bleeding, respectively. The bleeding risk is directly correlated with INR; it begins to rise quite markedly when the INR goes above 3.5, and an INR above 5 requires active intervention to lower the drug effect.

*Dosage.* The average dose of warfarin is 5 mg/day, and for patients over 70 it is 4 mg/day. There is great inter-individual variability in dosage, and 20% of individuals require a dose greater then 5 to 6 mg/day. As noted above, no loading dose is required. Initiation and maintenance warfarin dosing algorithms based on INR response should be utilized. During chronic treatment, the frequency of INR testing should be decreased to once every 4 to 6 weeks once a stable warfarin dose has been identified and as long as the INR remains stable.

Point of care testing of INR, analogous to glucose monitoring, has been developed for vitamin K antagonist therapy. A droplet of whole blood is placed on a test strip and inserted into a compact analyzer, and the time to clot is measured. A number of small hand-held home models are available, and results obtained with them correlate reasonably well with reference lab results in the INR range of 1.0 to 3.5. Above that range, correlation becomes less reliable.

Until recently, patients with conditions associated with high thrombotic risk (e.g., presence of a mechanical cardiac valve) for which they were receiving prophylactic long-term warfarin, and who then required invasive procedures associated with high bleeding risk, had to be hospitalized for up to 5 to 10 days to manage the transfer to and from the vitamin K antagonist and UHF. The advent of LMWH has made this problem much more manageable and cost-effective by eliminating hospital bed days. Many centres have adopted bridging therapy with LMWH as an outpatient procedure in high-risk thrombosis cases. For example, warfarin might be discontinued 5 days prior to scheduled biopsy, and subcutaneous LMWH is started on an outpatient basis 1 to 2 days later. The LMWH is last taken 24 hours prior to the procedure, making the patient hemostatically normal at the time of the procedure. On the day of the biopsy, warfarin is restarted at the previous dose. LMWH is restarted, as an outpatient, 24 to 48 hours after the procedure, depending upon the bleeding risk.

The LMWH is continued daily until the INR has returned to the target range for at least 48 hours. Outpatient INR testing is required to support this regimen. Patients have a very high acceptance and comfort level with this approach, and a specialized bridging program with over 2000 procedures in selected patients has had a bleeding risk of less than 1 to 2%.

*Reversal of anticoagulant effect.* If bleeding occurs during warfarin therapy, rapid therapeutic intervention to reverse this anticoagulant effect may be required. Depending on the clinical urgency, cessation of warfarin, oral or parenteral vitamin K therapy, fresh frozen plasma concentrate, and factor concentrates including recombinant VIIa may be used. Discontinuation of warfarin will not affect the INR for 1 to 3 days and is indicated for patients who are not bleeding but have an INR above the therapeutic range but less than 5. Vitamin K therapy, either oral, intravenous, or subcutaneous, is highly effective in reversing the warfarin effect in 6 to 12 hours. Caution is recommended in using large amounts of vitamin $K_1$ (5 to 10 mg) as this may render the patient warfarin-resistant for up to 2 weeks after administration. Generally, a low dose of vitamin $K_1$ (0.5 to 2 mg) is highly effective, especially for the patient who is not bleeding but has an INR greater than 5. Patients who are bleeding seriously, with or without a supra-therapeutic INR, require rapid reversal of the warfarin effect. This can be achieved only with rapid elevation of vitamin K–dependent proteins by intravenous administration of fresh frozen plasma (8 units will raise factor levels by 40 to 50%) or recombinant FVIIa (5 to 40 µg/kg).

# FIBRINOLYTIC AGENTS

Anticoagulant agents prevent new thrombus formation or extension of active thrombosis but do not remove already-formed clot. An integral physiological response to clot formation is the almost simultaneous initiation of the fibrinolytic process, with the release of endogenous tissue plasminogen activator (t-PA) and urokinase (UK) that lyse and remodel the active clot to reopen the vessel for blood flow. Agents that emulate this physiological fibrinolytic process, including recombinant tissue plasminogen activator (rt-PA), streptokinase (SK), and urokinase (UK), have had a major impact on the treatment of acute coronary artery thrombosis, VTE, ischemic stroke, and peripheral vascular thrombosis. However, thrombolytic therapy is associated with a very high risk of bleeding and re-thrombosis when blood flow through the vessel resumes. Adjunctive therapies such as UFH and antiplatelet agents are commonly used to minimize the risk of re-thrombosis after thrombolysis. New generations of thrombolytic agents are being developed with the goal of providing maximum clot lysis while lowering the bleeding and re-occlusion rates.

*Mechanism of action.* The fibrinolytic agents are specific plasminogen activator–like drugs that bind to plasminogen (PLA) and convert it to the enzyme plasmin that lyses fibrinogen and cleaves fibrin into soluble fibrin degradation products (FDPs), thus gradually digesting the clot (see Fig. 38-5). The available lytic agents vary in their mechanisms of action, fibrin (clot) specificity, pharmacokinetics, and therapeutic indications. However, all agents induce a systemic lytic state that results in marked impairment of hemostasis and a high bleeding risk.

The ideal fibrinolytic agent would be fibrin-specific and act only at the site of localized pathological occlusion of a vessel and not on any physiological hemostatic plugs. Such an agent does not exist, and different agents are either fibrin-specific or non-specific. SK is an example of a non-fibrin-specific drug that converts PLA to plasmin both in circulating blood and in the local clot, digesting both local fibrin and circulating fibrinogen. Agents such as t-PA are fibrin-specific, acting preferentially on clot-entrapped PLA, although some degree of systemic fibrinolysis occurs with their use (see Fig. 38-5).

Any circulating free plasmin, not neutralized by alpha-2 antiplasmin, destroys not only fibrinogen but also factors V and VIII, inducing a marked coagulopathy. The resulting FDPs are potent endogenous anticoagulants, able to interfere with new clot formation, resulting in an unstable clot. Platelet adhesion and aggregation are also compromised by fibrinolytics. Plasmin induces degradation of the platelet adhesion receptor GP Ib/IX and adhesion ligand vWF. FDPs also competitively interfere with the ability of fibrinogen to bind to GP IIb/IIIa and thus impair platelet aggregation. The lack of specific targeting of fibrinolytic agents to a pathological vessel occlusion results in lysis of not only the occlusive clot, but also of any normal physiological hemostatic plugs that may be present. This results in bleeding from vascular defects such as recent intravenous puncture sites or any sites of recent vascular injury or trauma. Thus, while these agents may result in life-saving re-opening of a critical occluded vessel, they can also lead to catastrophic bleeding from sites of physiological non-occlusive hemostasis.

*Clinical use.* Thrombolytics are for parenteral use only and are associated with a high bleeding risk. They can be administered systemically with large amounts of drug or by local catheter infusion of smaller doses directly into the clot bed to direct highest drug concentration to the site of occlusion and minimize systemic lysis and bleeding risk. Protocols vary and continue to evolve with experience, depending on the medical indication and the specific agent utilized. Both bolus and short-term infusions are given for acute coronary and cerebral artery occlusions and longer-term infusions, for venous thrombotic disease. Catheter-directed infusions are used in peripheral vascular disease and venous thrombosis.

Fibrinolytic agents are therapeutically effective only when used on an acute, fresh occlusion and not on a chronic or fully organized clot. Reperfusion rate varies greatly depending on the clinical indication and the time elapsed from occlusive event to drug delivery. Success of reperfusion correlates directly with time elapsed from onset of symptoms to drug delivery, regardless of which agent is used. Lytics must be delivered within 6 hours of acute coronary occlusion and 3 hours after cerebral occlusion for best clinical outcomes and maximal salvage of surrounding ischemic tissue. Failure to achieve vessel patency occurs in 15 to 20% of acute arterial occlusions. Lytic therapy can be successfully used up to 2 weeks after a venous or peripheral arterial thrombosis.

Thrombolytics have been in clinical use for at least 50 years. After their initial use, they fell rapidly out of favour because of unacceptable bleeding rates. Current uses for thrombolytics are well defined, as are the patient populations and vascular occlusion indications for which these agents are best suited and in which potential benefits outweigh bleeding risks. The major indications for thrombolytics are acute coronary, cerebrovascular, and peripheral vascular occlusions; acute, massive deep vein thrombosis with impending gangrene; and massive pulmonary embolism. When used according to the best current criteria, fibrinolytics can lower death rates by up to 50% in different indications. However, they also carry a 5 to 20% risk of major bleeding (this is three to five times greater than the risk for heparin) and can cause fatal intracranial hemorrhage in up to 1% of cases.

*Patient selection* is a critical issue in maximizing good outcomes while minimizing bleeding risk and morbidity and mortality. Inclusion and exclusion criteria for the use of thrombolytics must be followed closely.

*Adjuvant therapy.* Re-thrombosis, after the opening up and reperfusion of an occluded vessel, is a frequent complication of thrombolytics and is seen in 10 to 15% of successful thrombolytic studies in acute coronary occlusions. Re-occlusion occurs in spite of adjunctive anti-hemostatic therapies. While heparin and ASA are the mainstays of adjuvant therapy with fibrinolytics, other anticoagulants (DTIs, LMWH) and anti-platelet agents (clopidogrel, GP IIb/IIIa inhibitors) are sometimes given in combination. Newer agents and regimens that focus on reducing this significant re-occlusion rate are being tested. ASA or clopidogrel and a slightly lower dose of UFH or LMWH (see "Heparins" above) are given concomitantly with thrombolytics for indicated acute coronary events. GP IIb/IIIa agents are not recommended for use with thrombolytics, and DTIs should only be used in place of heparins if HIT is suspected. While concomitant therapy with anticoagulants or anti-platelet agents and thrombolytics improves patency rates, it comes with the increased risk of bleeding created by the combinations of these drugs. The benefits and risks must be weighed carefully in the use of these combinations.

*Treatment of bleeding* associated with thrombolytics requires the immediate cessation of the drug and use of local physical measures to control bleeding. If local measures fail or are not possible, administration of cryoprecipitate to raise the fibrinogen level above 100 mg/dL is indicated. Platelets and packed red cells are given as indicated by hemoglobin and platelet levels and by clinical condition. The use of anti-fibrinolytics should be reserved for uncontrolled life-threatening bleeding.

## Streptokinase

SK (Streptase) is a single-chain polypeptide derived from group C γ-hemolytic streptococci. It binds PLA directly, forming an active enzyme complex that cleaves a peptide bond in other PLA molecules to form plasmin. This agent and UK are not clot-specific. The onset of action of SK is immediate, the fibrinolytic effect lasts for several hours after cessation of drug administration, and the anticoagulant effect lasts for 12 to 24 hours. The half-life is relatively long (80 minutes). SK forms complexes with naturally acquired circulating antibodies, and these are cleared by the hepatic reticuloendothelial system. High doses of the drug may be required to overcome common anti-streptococcal antibodies formed as a consequence of streptococcal infections throughout life. SK is antigenic and results in both sensitization and allergic reactions, especially on repeat administration, and antibodies can remain for up to 7 years. The biological effects of SK are not reduced by allergic reactions. Anaphylaxis is uncommon, occurring in less than 0.5% of cases, but less severe symptoms including shivering, fever, and rash can be seen in up to 10% of individuals. Hypotension is also seen, especially if infusion rates are too rapid. Bleeding and stroke are common, with minor bleeding seen in 3 to 4% of cases, major bleeding in less than 1%, and stroke in less than 1% of all patients and 1.5 to 2% in those over 70 years of age.

## Tissue Plasminogen Activator

Recombinant t-PA (rt-PA; Activase, Alteplase) is a recombinant version of a naturally occurring serine protease produced by a number of cells including endothelial cells. Unlike SK, it binds specifically to fibrin, and once bound, it has increased affinity for PLA. Recombinant t-PA is a weak enzyme when not bound to fibrin. Thus, most of its effect is produced when it becomes entrapped in fresh clot along with PLA, resulting in lysis of the thrombus. The half-life of rt-PA is 3 to 4 minutes, much shorter than those of SK and UK. Its onset of action is immediate, and 80% is cleared within 8 minutes of termination of an infusion. Clearance is primarily hepatic. This agent is not associated with allergic reactions or hypotension and causes much less systemic fibrinogen depletion than SK. UFH is usually given as concomitant therapy to maintain vessel patency when rt-PA is used for coronary indications. Bleeding risk is similar to that of SK, while stroke risk is higher with rt-PA, particularly in patients aged over 70 years. However, death and morbidity related to stroke were lower with rt-PA than with SK. For acute coronary indications, accelerated administration of rt-PA has a 1% survival advantage over SK for all treated groups. rt-PA also produces more rapid, earlier, and sustained reperfusion than SK with lower re-occlusion rates.

## Urokinase

Urokinase (UK) is the second physiological plasminogen activator. It is present in high concentration in the urine since it is produced in the kidney. Many cell types secret UK in the form of prourokinase, also termed single-chain urokinase-type plasminogen activator (scu-PA). UK is cleared by the liver and has a half-life of 18 minutes. Like SK, UK is a non-fibrin-specific agent and directly binds to and activates all plasminogen, both free and fibrin-bound, converting it to plasmin. Bleeding risk with UK is the same as with other thrombolytics. UK is currently being used only in the management of pulmonary embolism.

## Newer Fibrinolytic Agents

Following the success of rt-PA, a number of mutant t-PA agents were developed. **Reteplase** (Retavase) is a mutated, non-glycosylated form of wild type t-PA with a half-life of 15 minutes and onset of action (as shown by a measurable fall in fibrinogen level) of 30 to 90 minutes. This is a longer half-life than that of rt-PA, and reteplase has less fibrin specificity. It has not been shown to be superior to rt-PA in cardiac indications. **Tenecteplase** (TNKase) is another mutated form of t-PA. It has an even longer half-life (90 to 130 minutes) and is metabolized primarily in the liver. Bolus injection of tenecteplase produces less major bleeding than alteplase but has similar clinical efficacy, and it is approved for the treatment of acute myocardial infarction in the United States. Staphylokinase, another new fibrinolytic, is no more effective than rt-PA and remains antigenic in spite of structural modifications. It has not been released in clinical practice.

## PROHEMOSTATIC AGENTS

Bleeding can be caused by single or, more commonly, combined hemostatic defects involving platelets, soluble clotting factors, and vessel wall and extra-vascular tissue defects and also by direct vascular injury (blunt or sharp trauma). Agents available for clinical use that have broad procoagulant activity and show good efficacy in achieving hemostasis in a wide number of clinical bleeding conditions include desmopressin (DDAVP), anti-fibrinolytics, conjugated estrogens, and recombinant factor VIIa. The etiology or mechanism of the hemostatic defect dictates the choice of agent(s) best suited for clinical use.

## Desmopressin (DDAVP)

Desmopressin (1-desamino-8-D-arginine vasopressin; DDAVP) is a synthetic analogue of the antidiuretic hormone L-arginine vasopressin (AVP). Unlike AVP, desmopressin acts largely on the $V_2$ receptor (antidiuretic and vascular cell stimulatory effect) and not the $V_1$ receptor (pressor and uterotonic effects). Its administration by nasal insufflation or subcutaneous or intravenous injection results in a series of prothrombotic events that generally enhance hemostasis and are seen within 5 to 30 minutes and last for 6 to 12 hours. Desmopressin primes and activates platelets either directly or indirectly, with the release of hemostatic platelet membrane microparticles. While not improving platelet aggregation, it does improve the bleeding time. Desmopressin causes endothelial cells to release large amounts of platelet adhesive protein vWF from storage granules, resulting in a three- to fivefold increase in vWF and factor VIII and a three- to fourfold increase in t-PA. The released vWF includes a preponderance of the high-molecular-weight forms that are highly prohemostatic.

Desmopressin is used for therapeutic and diagnostic indications. It is a major hemostatic therapy for mild hereditary and acquired hemophilia A and B and mild to moderate von Willebrand's disease. It is effective in hereditary and acquired thrombocytopathies including the ASA and NSAID defects, uremic platelets, and the exhausted platelets seen in bypass pump procedures. It enhances the activity of platelets and thus shortens bleeding times in thrombocytopenic and thrombocytopathic bleeding states and in unexplained prolongation of bleeding times. It is used diagnostically for the detection of hemophilia A carrier states and for acquired and hereditary defects in t-PA release. Controlled studies have demonstrated its efficacy in cardiovascular and orthopaedic surgery. It is frequently given as an empiric trial in post-operative bleeding if no surgical cause or coagulopathy is apparent to explain the bleeding. Desmopressin may be used in conjunction with anti-fibrinolytics if more significant bleeding is present. If desmopressin is being considered for future use for the common indications of mild hemophilia A and B and von Willebrand's disease, a desmopressin response trial is highly recommended. Appropriate baseline laboratory studies are done, the drug is given in controlled circumstances, and laboratory studies are repeated 60 minutes after infusion. This allows the confirmation of an appropriate hemostatic response and demonstrates that the drug will be clinically effective if used.

The effect of desmopressin is transient and gone in 12 hours. The dose can be repeated in 12 to 24 hours, but tachyphylaxis is not uncommon in von Willebrand's disease and hemophilia due to physiological exhaustion of protein stores in the endothelium. Repeated doses lead to an unpredictable response, especially beyond the second dose. When a predictable time response is required, as in preparation for surgery in patients with von Willebrand's disease, the dose should be administered 30 to 60 minutes before hemostatic challenge. The dose is 0.3 μg/kg (not to exceed 20 μg total) in 50 mL saline given over 20 to 30 minutes. Home therapy is available with insufflated desmopressin (Stimate) 150 μg per nostril (300 μg total) and is especially helpful for mild bleeding (e.g., in meningorrhagia) to avoid hospital visits for parenteral therapy. Drug monitoring includes following the factor VIII, IX, or vWF response as well as the bleeding time, as the indication dictates. For bleeding, the desmopressin is given empirically, and clinical response is assessed before further desmopressin intervention is considered.

Few significant adverse effects are seen with desmopressin; they include facial flushing, headaches, transient tachycardia, and minor alterations in blood pressure. Slowing the infusion rate or lowering the dose can modulate these side effects. Rare but serious hyponatremia can occur with repeated intravenous doses of desmopressin. No increased thrombotic episodes have been observed with this agent.

## Anti-fibrinolytics

Anti-fibrinolytics are used for two biological indications: blockade of systemic fibrinolysis and inhibition of local fibrinolysis at sites of local injury and clot formation. The three agents available are ε-aminocaproic acid (EACA), tranexamic acid (TA), and aprotinin.

The *clinical indications* for all three anti-fibrinolytics are the same and include the local and systemic treatment and prevention of fibrinolysis. Systemic fibrinolysis is seen in the rare hereditary defects of alpha-2 antiplasmin and plasminogen activator inhibitor (PAI) deficiency. After therapy with thrombolytic agents such as rt-PA, systemic fibrinolysis may persist, but anti-fibrinolytics are rarely needed because of the short half-life of thrombolytics. Systemic fibrinolysis can be seen as a complication of heat stroke, amniotic fluid embolism, and bleeding in some cancer patients. In acute promyelocytic leukemia, some patients have fibrinolysis with or without DIC due to the release of enzymatic products by cancer cells. In this circumstance, anti-fibrinolytics are contraindicated unless given together with heparin. One of the most common indications for these agents is cardiopulmonary bypass surgery. All three anti-fibrinolytics are effective in reducing both bleeding and transfusion requirements by 30 to 40% in cardiopulmonary bypass and are used widely.

At all sites of local bleeding and hemostatic plug formation, the normal physiological response involves local fibrinolysis. In the presence of a hemostatic defect, normal fibrinolysis accentuates bleeding or results in delayed bleeding. Local fibrinolysis can be blocked by either local application of anti-fibrinolytics (for example, oral mouth washes) or systemic administration. Oral anti-fibrinolytics are effective after dental procedures and other mucosal trauma in treated hemophiliacs, when given for 4 to 7 days.

Laboratory tests are not normally used to monitor the effectiveness of anti-fibrinolytics. The euglobulin lysis time, which is shortened by fibrinolysis, can be used, but this test is not widely available. Serial monitoring of fibrinogen levels and FDPs may be of some clinical benefit.

The major risk associated with anti-fibrinolytics is thrombosis, since these agents accelerate thrombus growth and allow a clot that is present to persist. Anti-fibrinolytics are contraindicated in DIC with bleeding because of the thrombotic pathophysiological process in this consumptive coagulopathy. The possibility of DIC, a common cause of bleeding in sick hospitalized patients, needs to be weighed each time use of an antifibrinolytic is considered. When an anti-fibrinolytic is used for surgical bleeding, thrombosis is not a significant complication.

### ε-Aminocaproic acid (EACA)

EACA (Amicar) is a lysine analogue that competitively inhibits the lysine-specific binding of plasminogen and t-PA to fibrin and fibrinogen. This inhibits the activation of plasminogen to plasmin and blocks fibrinolysis. EACA is a small molecule (131 Da) and reaches a peak concentration in 2 hours after oral ingestion. The onset of action is usually seen within 1 to 2 hours with appropriate dosing. EACA is rapidly cleared with a half-life of 2 hours and is excreted in the urine, where it reaches very high levels.

EACA is available in oral, topical, or intravenous preparations. EACA is much less frequently used today and has been largely replaced by tranexamic acid because of GI intolerance, dose size, and frequency of dosing. EACA is taken orally 50 to 60 mg/kg every 4 to 6 hours, or intravenously as a 100 to 150 mg/kg bolus followed by an infusion of 1 g/hr for 8 hours or until bleeding is controlled (maximum daily dose 30 g). Because it is cleared renally, EACA may accumulate in patients with decreased renal function. Rapid intravenous administration should be avoided since it may induce hypotension, bradycardia, or arrhythmia.

### Tranexamic acid

Tranexamic acid (TA; Cyclokapron) is a 157-Da lysine analogue that inhibits fibrinolysis with a mechanism of action identical to that of EACA. It reversibly binds to plasminogen and inhibits its binding to fibrin. TA is preferred to EACA as an anti-fibrinolytic and is much less expensive than aprotinin. TA has a longer half-life (2 to 10 hours) than EACA, but like EACA, it is excreted largely unchanged in the urine. TA dose is 10 mg/kg intravenously every 6 hours, starting immediately before surgery. The oral dose is 25 mg/kg three to four times a day for 2 to 8 days, even if

hemostasis appears to be attained. In the face of renal impairment, the dose should be reduced. GI side effects with TA are not uncommon (10%) but are less frequent than with EACA. The risk of both arterial and venous thrombosis needs to be considered when TA is used. Anti-fibrinolytics should be used with caution with infusions of activated factors such as FVIIa and activated prothrombin complex, and in individuals with a history of VTE, as TA may increase the risk of thrombosis.

### Aprotinin

Aprotinin (Trasylol) is a 6512-Da molecule extracted from bovine lungs that is a broad-spectrum inhibitor of several serine proteases, including kallikrein and plasmin. Its action does not affect platelet function. It also inhibits the contact phase activation of coagulation and preserves adhesive platelet glycoproteins, making them resistant to damage from increased circulating plasmin or mechanical injury occurring during bypass. Aprotinin is degraded to small polypeptides before excretion in the urine. It has a half-life of 2.5 hours and is available for topical and intravenous use. Hypersensitivity reactions are common (3%). A test dose is advised 10 minutes before loading dose, and re-exposure within 6 months should be avoided. Antibodies to this agent occur in about 50% of exposed individuals, but their significance is not known. Aprotinin is as efficacious as EACA, or slightly better, in reducing bleeding and transfusion requirements in major cardiac surgery. Cost is a major concern with aprotinin. Like other anti-fibrinolytics, aprotinin does not require laboratory monitoring during use. Aprotinin is unique in that it prolongs the aPTT and ACT. This latter effect can result in under-dosing of UFH when given concomitantly, as in bypass surgery.

## Conjugated Estrogens

Conjugated estrogens (CEs) have been used for many years as hemostatic agents in von Willebrand's disease and uremia. The exact mechanism of action of CEs is not clear, but they are known to increase levels of vWF and factor VIII, shorten bleeding times, and increase the reactivity of platelets. These effects are dose-dependent. Bleeding control can be achieved quickly with 0.6 mg/kg of CE intravenously, daily for five days, 2.5 to 25 mg of Premarin orally, or 50 to 100 µg of transdermal estradiol twice weekly. If an immediate effect is required, desmopressin is a superior agent. CE agents begin to act on the first day and reach peak effect in 5 to 7 days. This action persists for at least a week after cessation of therapy.

## Factor VIIa

Arguably, the single most significant advance in prohemostatic therapy in the last 5 to 10 years has been the development of a recombinant activated factor VII

**FIGURE 38-11** Recombinant factor VIIa mechanisms of action. Recombinant FVIIa acts through both tissue factor–dependent and tissue factor–independent pathways resulting in thrombin generation. Recombinant FVIIa binds to any available tissue factor (TF), at a wound site, initiating coagulation at the surface of TF-bearing cells and resulting in thrombin generation. Thrombin, among other things, activates platelets upon whose surface FVIIa can directly activate factor X, leading to TF-independent thrombin formation. (Adapted from Hoffman et al. Activated factor VIII activates factors IX and X on the surface of activated platelets: thoughts on the mechanism of action of high-dose factor VII. *Blood Coagul Fibrinolysis.* 1998;9(suppl 1): S61, with permission.)

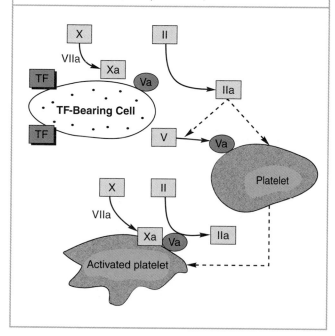

(rFVIIa) (Novo-Seven). Recombinant FVIIa, a vitamin K–dependent activated glycoprotein, was initially developed for bypassing acquired inhibitors to factors VIII and IX in patients with hemophilia A and B, respectively. Its intravenous administration results in a physiologically significant, dose-dependent burst of thrombin generation in both healthy volunteers and patients with bleeding syndromes. This thrombin burst can result in a dramatic cessation of clinical bleeding in a wide range of disorders involving both platelet defects and coagulopathies, even where traditional therapies have failed.

The mechanisms of action of rFVIIa are identical to those of natural FVIIa shown in Figure 38-11.

Clinical indications for the use of rFVIIa include the treatment of bleeding in patients with congenital or acquired deficiency of factor VII; all acquired factor inhibitors, especially those to factors VIII, IX, and vWF;

warfarin overdose associated with bleeding, when rapid reduction of anticoagulation is required; and the coagulopathy of severe liver dysfunction. Recombinant FVIIa is also effective in the treatment of bleeding in platelet disorders, including transfusion-refractory thrombocytopenia and thrombocytopathies, when platelet transfusions are either no longer feasible or need to be avoided. This agent has been shown to reduce perioperative blood loss in patients undergoing various types of surgery, including liver transplant and prostatectomy. The utility of rFVIIa for the treatment of uncontrolled hemorrhage in other situations including trauma, battlefield injury, and general surgery is less certain, but it has been successfully utilized in these situations when other measures have failed.

Recombinant FVIIa has a half-life of 2.3 hours (1 to 2 hours in children). Effective dosages have ranged from 35 to 120 µg/kg by intravenous bolus every 2 hours until hemostasis is achieved, or until the treatment is judged a failure. The dose and time interval may be adjusted, depending on the cause and severity of bleeding and the degree of hemostasis achieved. For major trauma, massive doses (200 to 400 µg/kg) have been successfully used. The optimum duration of therapy after attaining hemostasis is not well characterized, and one to two additional doses at 3- to 6-hour intervals may be appropriate. There are no laboratory measures for monitoring rFVIIa that correlate well with treatment efficacy, and the dosage remains empirical.

Because of its very high cost, FVIIa is reserved for use in clinical bleeding where other treatment modalities (surgical hemostasis, blood component therapy, anti-fibrinolytics) have failed and the bleeding is life-threatening. In this context, clinical concern about adverse drug reactions is tempered. In other circumstances, a major concern about this agent is its potential to induce an excessive prothrombotic response at non-bleeding sites, resulting in problems such as coronary thrombosis, stroke, and VTE. While these complications have been observed, they do not appear to be common.

## Other Prohemostatic Agents in Hemostasis

Other agents available to promote hemostasis are largely reserved for the replacement of specific deficiencies of various hemostatic factors. Fibrinogen is available in the blood product cryoprecipitate (250 mg fibrinogen/bag) and is indicated for use if fibrinogen levels are less than 60 to 100 mg/dL and active bleeding is present. Purified, sterilized human fibrinogen is used as a topical fibrin sealant at accessible sites in a two-vial process that combines soluble fibrinogen and human thrombin. This agent is best used for diffuse bleeding such as suture-related bleeding at anastomosis sites, open wounds, and general oozing in surgical vascular beds. Activated prothrombin complexes are available (Feiba, Autoplex) in which the purified vitamin K–dependent proteins (factors

II, VII, IX, and X) have been purposefully activated during isolation. These products are used in bleeding patients with acquired factor inhibitors and warfarin overdose. The well-described and significant risk of these agents is excessive clotting (VTE, DIC, myocardial infarction); moreover, they have been largely replaced by rFVIIa for the same indications. Purified prothrombin complex (factors II, VII, IX, and X) is also available for the treatment of FII and FX deficiency, coagulopathies of liver disease, and bleeding with warfarin overdose, and it has lower levels of activated clotting factors and lower thrombotic risk than activated prothrombin complex. Purified factor VIII, FIX, FXI, and vWF are available both as monoclonal purified plasma products and as recombinant proteins (except factor XI) for the treatment of their specific factor-deficient states. Prophylaxis and treatment regimens for individuals with deficiencies of these coagulation proteins depend on the specific defect, site and extent of bleeding, baseline factor levels, adjunctive prohemostatic therapies, and ongoing risk of re-bleeding.

These plasma products are not totally risk-free, but the risk of known viruses (HIV, hepatitis) is now negligible because of pre-collection screening and testing of plasma donors and the use of virus inactivation procedures in the preparation of the plasma products. Infections associated with recombinant protein concentrates have yet to be observed after many years of use, but it is possible that risks different from those of plasma products may eventually be recognized.

## SUGGESTED READINGS

Abshire T, Kenet G. Recombinant factor VIIa: review of efficacy, dosing regimes and safety in patients with congenital and acquired factor VIII and IX inhibitors. *J Thromb Haemost.* 2004;2:899-909.

Ansell J, Hirsh J, Poller L, et al. The pharmacology and management of the vitamin K antagonists: the Seventh ACCP Conference on Antithrombotic and Thrombolytic Therapy. *Chest.* 2004;126(3 suppl):204S-233S.

Antiplatelet Trialists' Collaboration. Collaborative overview of randomized trials of antiplatelet therapy—I, II, III. *BMJ.* 1994; 308:81-106, 159-168, 235-246.

Brown DL, Fann CS, Chang CJ. Meta-analysis of effectiveness and safety of abciximab versus eptifibatide or tirofiban in percutaneous coronary intervention. *Am J Cardiol.* 2001;87:537-541.

Choay J, Petitou M, Lormeau JC, et al. Structure-activity relationship in heparin: a synthetic pentasaccharide with high affinity for antithrombin III and eliciting high anti-factor Xa activity. *Biochem Biophys Res Commun.* 1983;116:492-499.

Clementson KJ. Primary hemostasis: sticky fingers cement the relationship. *Current Biol.* 1999;9:R110.

Collen D. The plasminogen (fibrinolytic) system. *Thromb Haemost.* 1999;82:259-270.

Dahlback B. Blood coagulation and its regulation by anticoagulant pathways: genetic pathogenesis of bleeding and thrombotic diseases. *J Intern Med.* 2005;257:209-223.

Fibrinolytic Therapy Trialists' (FTT) Collaborative Group. Indications for fibrinolytic therapy in suspected acute myocardial infarction: collaborative overview of early mortality and major morbidity results from all randomised trials of more than 1000 patients. *Lancet.* 1994;343:311-322.

Freedman MD. Oral anticoagulants: pharmacodynamics, clinical indications and adverse effects. *J Clin Pharmacol.* 1992;32: 196-209.

Hirsh J, Raschke R. Heparin and low-molecular-weight heparin: the Seventh ACCP Conference on Antithrombotic and Thrombolytic Therapy. *Chest.* 2004;126(3 suppl):188S-203S.

Kucher N, Connolly S, Beckman JA, et al. International normalized ratio increase before warfarin-associated hemorrhage: brief and subtle. *Arch Intern Med.* 2004;164:2176-2179.

Laupacis A, Fergusson D. Drugs to minimize perioperative blood loss in cardiac surgery: a meta-analysis using perioperative blood transfusion as the outcome: the International Study of Perioperative Transfusion (ISPOT) investigators. *Anesth Analg.* 1997;85:1258-1267.

Mahdy A, Webster NR. Perioperative systemic haemostatic agents. *Br J Anaesth.* 2004;93:842-858.

Sabatine MS, Jang IK. The use of glycoprotein IIb/IIIa inhibitors in patients with coronary artery disease. *Am J Med.* 2000;109: 224-237.

Schror K. Antiplatelet drugs. A comparative review. *Drugs.* 1995; 50:7-16.

Timmins GC, ed. *Thrombolytic Therapy.* Armonk, NY: Futura; 1999.

Turpie AG. Pharmacology of the low-molecular-weight heparins. *Am Heart J.* 1998;135(6 pt 3 suppl):S329-S335.

Weitz JI, Hirsh J, Samama MM. New anticoagulant drugs. *Chest.* 2004;126(3 suppl):265S-286S.

# 39

# Drugs (Agents) That Affect Erythropoiesis

EL YEO

## CASE HISTORIES

### Case 1

Mrs. M. is a 39-year-old Greek woman and mother of three who presented to her family physician complaining of symptoms of mild fatigue and lethargy. There is a family history of poorly defined anemia. She is on no medication other than the occasional multivitamin. On physical examination, there was little to note other than mild pallor. Her CBC revealed a hemoglobin of 99 g/dL, an MCV of 68 fL, and normal WBC and platelet counts. Review of the peripheral blood smear revealed hypochromic microcytosis with some target cells. Her ferritin level was 3 mg/L. There was no obvious source of iron loss other than that through menses. A diagnosis of iron deficiency was made, and she was given 6 months of oral ferrous gluconate, 300 mg orally three times a day. She felt much improved after treatment, and repeat blood work revealed that the hemoglobin had risen slightly to 102 g/dL and the MCV to 68 fL, but the peripheral blood smear was unchanged. The ferritin had risen to 55 mg/L. A diagnosis of resolved iron deficiency anemia superimposed on beta thalassemia minor was made.

### Case 2

Mr. A. is a 63-year-old man with progressive chronic renal failure due to diabetic nephropathy who has just begun hemodialysis three times a week. He has a normochromic, normocytic anemia with a hemoglobin of 82 g/dL, reticulocytopenia, and iron values consistent with anemia of chronic disease. His erythropoietin (EPO) level was 7 mU/mL, and he was started on recombinant EPO 100 µg/kg three times per week, folic acid 1 mg/day, and oral ferrous gluconate 300 mg/day. By the third week of therapy, his hemoglobin had risen to 11 g/dL, but he was markedly hypertensive, requiring therapeutic intervention. His EPO dosing regimen was decreased by 25%, the hypertension resolved, and his hemoglobin remained stable at 12.5 g/dL. A diagnosis of EPO-responsive anemia of chronic disease (chronic renal failure) complicated by hypertension was made.

## OVERVIEW OF ERYTHROPOIESIS AND HEMATOPOIESIS

Hematopoietic blood elements (erythrocytes, leukocytes, and platelets) are formed through the differentiation of precursor bone marrow cells. Under the influence of specific marrow-related cytokines, totipotent stem cells move through different stages of commitment and differentiation within the bone marrow and are ultimately released into the circulation as fully formed, functional, circulating blood elements (Fig. 39-1). Erythrocytes (red blood cells) develop, under erythroid non-specific and specific influences, through a multi-step process starting with commitment of the totipotent stem cells to primitive erythroid progenitors. Through differentiation, replication, and maturation, these progenitor cells in turn become morphologically identifiable erythroid precursors (proerythroblasts). During later stages of red blood cell (RBC) maturation, the nuclei and cytoplasmic organelles degenerate and disappear as increasing amounts of hemoglobin are synthesized and stored in the cytoplasm (see Fig. 39-1). The anucleated reticulocytes, both in the bone marrow and in circulation, then lose their RNA to become fully mature RBCs capable of transporting oxygen. The total mass of circulating RBCs and that part of the hematopoietic tissue from which they are derived are an inferred erythroid tissue concept called the *erythron*.

**FIGURE 39-1** Schematic representation of hematopoiesis. Totipotent primitive stem cells in the bone marrow, under the influence of cytokines called colony stimulating factors, undergo lineage commitment (erythroid, myeloid, megakaryocytic), differentiation, replication, and maturation. Under the lineage-specific cytokine erythropoietin (EPO), myeloid stem cells give rise to erythroid cells, which then undergo a series of maturation stages, losing their RNA and DNA while accumulating heme and globin and shrinking in size to ultimately emerge as mature red blood cells. Multi-CSF: multi-colony stimulating factor (CSF); GM-CSF: granulocyte–macrophage CSF; G-CSF: granulocyte CSF; M-CSF: macrophage CSF.

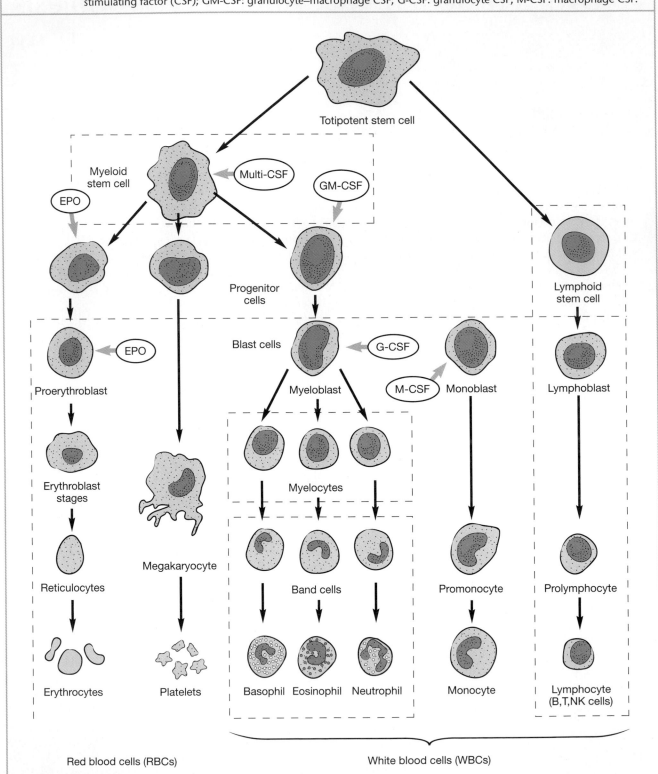

Each pronormoblast (earliest recognizable RBC precursor) can form 8 to 16 reticulocytes. The mean transit time from pronormoblast to circulating reticulocyte is approximately 5 days. Reticulocytes make up approximately 0.5 to 2% of RBCs, but this can be variably elevated or depressed depending upon stimulation or depression of the marrow portion of the erythron. RBCs have a 120-day life span in circulation. Decreased generation of adenosine triphosphate (ATP) initiates, through poorly understood mechanisms, the process by which these anuclear RBCs become senescent: membrane alterations occur, intracellular volume decreases, and all metabolic activity gradually shuts down. The senescent RBCs are then either primarily phagocytosed by the reticuloendothelial system (spleen) or undergo intravascular hemolysis.

## Hematopoietic Growth Factors

Erythropoiesis in the adult takes place within the bone marrow under the influence of the stromal bone marrow framework and a number of non-specific and specific cytokines, or hematopoietic growth factors (HGFs). The HGFs affecting the erythron include the erythroid non-specific cytokines granulocyte–macrophage colony stimulating factor (GM-CSF), thrombopoietin (TPO), interleukin-3 (IL-3), IL-9, and IL-11 and the erythroid specific growth factors erythropoietin (EPO), Steel factor (SF), and insulin-like growth factor 1 (IGF-1).

**EPO** is a critical erythron cytokine and plays a central role in erythropoiesis. It is a glycoprotein hormone produced by interstitial cells of the kidney and, to a lesser extent, of the liver. The production of EPO is induced by hypoxia (low tissue oxygenation) through mechanisms that involve activation of heme proteins that then stimulate EPO gene expression. EPO, by binding to its surface membrane receptors on erythroid progenitor cells, stimulates growth, proliferation, survival, and differentiation of the erythron, resulting in reticulocytosis. EPO production is a tightly regulated physiological process that maintains hemoglobin at levels adequate for tissue oxygenation. Deficiency of EPO (e.g., end-stage kidney disease) results in a hypoproliferative anemia. An excess of EPO, through either endogenous production (e.g., hypoxic states, EPO-producing tumours) or parenteral administration of recombinant EPO, results in erythrocytosis and increases of both circulating RBCs and red cell mass (RCM). Recombinant EPO-alpha, as a pharmacological agent, has revolutionized the clinical treatment of certain common forms of hypoproliferative anemia.

**SF** is another unique regulator of erythropoiesis. SF is constitutively expressed by endothelial cells, bone marrow stromal cells, and hepatocytes. By binding to its receptor c-kit, SF promotes the proliferation and differentiation of primitive erythroid precursors and acts synergistically with EPO. Deficiency of SF leads to anemia, underlining its important role in the erythron.

**IGF-1 (somatomedin C)** is a homologue of proinsulin that induces DNA synthesis in erythroid precursors and shares biological activities with EPO and SF.

## Red Cell Production (Essential Elements)

Critical nutritional elements are required for the development of a mature and fully functional RBC (Table 39-1). These include **vitamin B$_{12}$ (cobalamin)**, **folic acid**, and **iron** (see Chapter 63). Vitamin B$_{12}$ and folic acid are required for purine and pyrimidine synthesis, which, in turn, is necessary for DNA production as well as proper cell nuclear maturation and cell division. A deficiency in either of these vitamins will result in an anemia characterized by ineffective erythropoiesis, with faulty cell division and cell maturation defects. B$_{12}$ and folate deficiency lead to the appearance of megaloblasts (abnormally large RBC precursors with striking nuclear irregularities) in the bone marrow and of overly large (macrocytic) circulating RBCs. B$_{12}$ and folate have essential functions in other cells of the body, and their deficiency can lead to a spectrum of hematological and non-hematological findings.

Iron is critical in the normal production of hemoglobin, and iron deficiency anemia is the most common type of anemia. Iron regulation is a finely tuned and complex process directed at preserving this essential element needed by all cells for normal function while, at the same time, not allowing it to accumulate in toxic excess. Most functional iron in the body is in the form of hemoglobin and less, as myoglobin. Iron is essential both for the production of RBC hemoglobin and as the oxygen-carrying element within the RBC. Deficiency of iron leads to a slowing of erythropoiesis. The lack of iron results in increased mitotic division of erythroblasts, leading to smaller RBCs (microcytosis), a decrease in RBC hemoglobin (hypochromia), and a greatly reduced ability to carry oxygen (see below).

*Hemoglobin* is the main component of RBCs. It gives the RBC its red pigmentation and is the essential vehicle for transportation of oxygen and carbon dioxide to and from the tissues of the body. The hemoglobin molecule is a conjugated protein composed of four heme groups and a protein portion (two pairs of polypeptide chains) called globin. Each heme structure (protoporphyrin) carries an atom of ferrous iron (Fe$^{2+}$) that can reversibly combine with one molecule of oxygen or carbon dioxide. One molecule of hemoglobin, therefore, contains four atoms of iron and can carry four molecules of oxygen. When hemoglobin binds to oxygen, due in part to the structural alterations induced by 2,3-diphosphoglycerate, it is known as *oxyhemoglobin*. The amount of oxygen taken up by RBCs in the lungs, retained in circulation, and then released at the tissue level

| TABLE 39-1 | Nutritional Requirements for Effective Erythropoiesis | | | |
|---|---|---|---|---|
| | Daily Needs | Daily Loss | Special Needs (lactation, pregnancy) | Stores |
| $B_{12}$ (cobalamin)* | | | | |
| Men and post-menopausal women | 1–2 µg | 1.3 µg (0.1%) | | 2–5 mg |
| Women, pre-menopausal | 1–2 µg | 1.3 µg (0.1%) | 1.5–2.5 µg | 2–5 mg |
| Folic acid† | | | | |
| Men and post-menopausal women | 50 µg | | | 5 mg (0.5–10 mg) |
| Women, pre-menopausal | 50–100 µg | | 150–250 µg | 5 mg (0.5–10 mg) |
| Children | 25 | | | |
| Iron‡ | | | | |
| Men and post-menopausal women | 1 mg | 1 mg | | 1.5 g (2.5 g in circulating RBCs) |
| Women, pre-menopausal | 2 mg | 2 mg | 3–5 mg | 0.3 g (1.9 g in circulating RBCs) |

*Western diet $B_{12}$: 5–7 µg/day.

†Recommended daily intake of folic acid: 3 µg/kg/day.

‡Gut absorption of iron is 5–10% in normal circumstances; Western diet iron: 10 mg/day.

is dependent upon the partial pressure of oxygen present in immediate proximity to the RBC. Hereditary defects in globin result in anemias due to hemoglobinopathies such as sickle cell disease and thalassemia syndromes.

## Pathophysiology of Erythron States

Pathophysiological states involving the erythron tend to present as either anemia (loss of RCM) or erythrocytosis (excess of RCM). RCM can be truly measured only by isotope dilution studies, which are neither practical nor cost-effective for clinical use. Instead, circulating red cells are operationally screened and measured by an automated cell counter permitting evaluation of the red cell hemoglobin and/or hematocrit value. The hemoglobin value (Hb) is a measure of the concentration of the major oxygen-carrying pigment in whole blood and is expressed as grams of hemoglobin per 100 mL of whole blood (g/dL). The hematocrit value (Hct) is the percentage of a volume of whole blood that is occupied by intact red cells. The normal ranges (95% confidence limits) for Hb and Hct are 13.3 to 17.7 g/dL and 40 to 52%, respectively, in men and 11.7 to 15.7 g/dL and 35 to 47%, respectively, in women.

Other key automated measurements to assess the erythron include mean corpuscular volume (MCV) and mean corpuscular hemoglobin concentration (MCHC). The MCV (80 to 100 fL) is the average volume of the RBC measured in femtolitres (fL), while the MCHC (32 to 37 g/dL) is the average concentration of hemoglobin in RBCs. Reticulocyte percentage is a measure of bone marrow erythron activity. The circulating RBCs with remnant cytoplasmic RNA are identified by their staining characteristics, counted, and commonly reported as a percent of total RBC (normal value is 0.5 to 2%).

Microscopic morphological reviews of the RBCs in a stained peripheral blood smear and the erythroid precur-

sors in a bone marrow aspirate smear are also critical elements in the investigation of the erythron. Microscopic review of the peripheral blood smear is essential in any investigation of anemia, as there are characteristic morphological findings indicative of certain types of anemia.

## ERYTHRON ABNORMALITIES

A large number of drugs, through direct or indirect mechanisms, may affect the erythron at the level of the circulating RBCs and/or erythroid precursors. Many drugs directly exert known toxic effects on the RBC membrane, the hemoglobin, or the bone marrow. These are mentioned in the respective chapters in which these drugs are described. It must be understood that any drug with a known erythron effect (anemia or erythrocytosis) should not be administered without weighing the risks and benefits to the patient, and if it is administered, appropriate hematological surveillance must be put in place.

## Polycythemia (Erythrocytosis)

Erythropoietic erythrocytosis is the opposite of anemia. It is brought about by the overproduction of RBCs in the bone marrow and results in an increased RCM. The laboratory hallmark of erythrocytosis is an increased Hb (males: >18 g/dL; females >16 g/dL) or Hct (males: >52%; females >47%). Erythrocytosis may be a minor incidental finding or, at its extreme, may lead to hyperviscosity symptoms due to red cell sludging and tissue hypoxia. A finding of persistent erythrocytosis that is not due to contracted plasma volume (relative polycythemia) requires a detailed investigation and clear elucidation of cause in order to direct appropriate therapeutic interventions. Investigations include physical examination to look for cardiorespiratory disease and splenomegaly, laboratory studies of RCM, serum EPO level, and arterial $O_2$ saturation, and possibly a bone marrow aspiration and biopsy to direct further investigations. Table 39-2 outlines a pathophysiological approach to erythrocytosis.

The investigation of polycythemia has been greatly facilitated by the availability of a serum EPO assay. Whether the serum EPO is elevated, normal, or low, and whether this finding is deemed to be a clinically appropriate or inappropriate response, will help direct further investigations to fully characterize the underlying cause. Polycythemia may be a primary condition (e.g., polycythemia rubra vera) in which there is an acquired abnormality of the erythroid precursor leading to autologous overproduction of RBCs. The serum EPO level is low or normal for the degree of erythrocytosis in primary polycythemia. Treatment of primary erythrocytosis is directed at lowering RCM by regular phlebotomy or by erythroid suppression with agents such as **hydroxy urea** or **anagrelide**. Secondary polycythemia is due to high levels of plasma cytokines, usually EPO. The resulting erythrocytosis may be due to an appropriate EPO response stimulus (e.g., hypoxemia secondary to high altitude) or an inappropriate physiological response (e.g., tumour secretion of EPO).

## Anemia (Erythropenia)

Anemia is defined as a reduction, below the normal range, in the mass (number or content) of circulating RBCs. Anemia is indicated by an Hb or Hct value that is more than two standard deviations below the mean. Thus, an Hb <13.5 g/dL (men) or <12.0 g/dL (women), or an Hct <41.0% (men) or <36.0% (women) represent anemia. There are

many exceptions to these rules, including the following: a small percentage (2.5%) of the population will automatically be defined as anemic since the normal ranges for Hb and Hct are developed with only 95% confidence, and measurements of Hb and Hct depend not only on RBC mass but also on plasma volume. Thus, any condition that increases or decreases plasma volume can spuriously suggest or mask an anemia.

While there are many causes of anemia, the most common causes are iron deficiency, chronic disease, red cell destruction (hemolysis), or suppression of the bone marrow. The classification of anemias is approached both morphologically (average cell size) and pathologically (kinetically), depending on the clinical presentation. Table 39-3 provides a kinetic classification of anemias, including lack of RBC production, RBC destruction, and RBC loss. The multiplicity of different causes of anemia makes it evident that the first step in approaching this common clinical problem is to clearly define the underlying pathological process through clinical and laboratory investigations. This then naturally leads to a clear rationale for therapeutic intervention or specific therapy with the objective of fully correcting the anemia, if possible.

Table 39-4 is a commonly utilized morphological classification of anemia based on the red cell morphology (size) and the automated MCV measurement. This approach allows for the rapid identification of common subtypes of anemia that fall within the microcytic (low MCV) or macrocytic (high MCV) categories. This approach is especially useful clinically since the differential diagnostic alternatives within these two categories are limited and include the common forms of anemia. For example, a low MCV indicates iron deficiency anemia, thalassemia, anemia of chronic disease, or sideroblastic anemia.

### Iron deficiency anemia

Iron deficiency is the most common cause of anemia, affecting up to 30% of the population worldwide. A variable degree of iron deficiency is especially common in women of child-bearing age and in children. Even in North America, up to 25% of women have low or borderline low total body iron stores. Iron is an essential element for a number of cellular functions, of which the most important are the production and normal function of hemoglobin. Nutritional and physiological aspects of iron are discussed in Chapter 63.

Iron from dietary sources is absorbed in the small intestine. The amount of dietary iron absorbed depends on the amount of stored body iron, amount and type of iron in ingested food, status of the gastrointestinal mucosa, and pH of the gastric milieu. A healthy adult normally absorbs only 5 to 10% of ingested iron, while an iron-deficient individual absorbs 10 to 30% (see Table 39-1). If iron is not stored or utilized in the intestinal cell, it is transported across the basolateral membrane, oxidized back to $Fe^{3+}$ by ceruloplasmin (a copper-dependent enzyme), and bound

| TABLE 39-2 | Classification of Erythrocytosis (Polycythemia) |
|---|---|

**Relative** (isolated decrease in plasma volume) (e.g., dehydration)

**Absolute** (absolute increase in red cell mass)
  Primary
    Primary increase in erythropoiesis (appropriately low EPO levels)
      Clonal RBC or progenitor defect (e.g., polycythemia rubra vera)
  Secondary
    Primary increase in erythropoietin (inappropriately high EPO levels)
      EPO-producing neoplasms, renal lesions, exogenous EPO
    Secondary increase in erythropoietin (appropriately high EPO levels)
      Hypoxemia (e.g., high altitude, cardiorespiratory issue, RBC $O_2$ defect)
      Chronic carbon monoxide (CO) poisoning (e.g., smoking, work-related exposures)

| TABLE 39-3 | Etiological (Kinetic) Classification of Anemias |
|---|---|

**Decreased RBC production (hypoproliferative)**
- Disorders of bone marrow stem cell proliferation and differentiation (e.g., aplastic anemia, sideroblastic anemia, chemotherapy, irradiation therapy)
- Disorders of DNA synthesis (e.g., B12 deficiency, folic acid deficiency)
- Disorders of hemoglobin synthesis (e.g., iron deficiency, thalassemia)
- Disorders of erythron proliferation and differentiation (e.g., anemia of chronic disease, endocrine disorders, marrow infiltration, chemotherapy, irradiation therapy)

**Increased RBC destruction (hemolytic)**
- Intracorpuscular abnormalities
  Membrane defects (e.g., hereditary spherocytosis, paroxsysmal nocturnal hemoglobinuria)
  Enzyme defects (e.g., glucose-6-phosphate dehydrogenase [G-6-PD] deficiency, pyruvate kinase [PK] deficiency)
  Globin defects
  Hemoglobinopathies (e.g., sickle cell disease)
- Extracorpuscular abnormalities
  Mechanical (microangiopathic, or fragmentation, anemias)
  Infection (e.g., hemolytic anemia due to malaria, *Babesia* parasitic infection)
  Chemical or physical agent (e.g., drugs, toxins, burns, drowning)
  Antibody-mediated (acquired immune hemolytic anemia)

**Excessive RBC loss (bleeding)**
- Obvious or occult hemorrhagic anemia

Given the body's avidity for iron, most causes of iron deficiency are clinically apparent, including bleeding (occult or obvious), hemolysis followed by loss of free iron in the urine, and insufficient dietary intake to offset physiological loss. Clinical presentation is highly variable, from an asymptomatic laboratory finding to pallor, fatigue, lethargy, shortness of breath, headaches, cheilosis, and odd cravings resulting in the eating of ice, dirt, and clay (pica). Other symptoms include abnormalities in the oral and gastrointestinal mucosa, decreased resistance to infections, and difficulties of thermoregulation.

| TABLE 39-4 | Morphological Classification of Anemias* |
|---|---|

**Macrocytic (>100 fL)**
- Reticulocytosis (e.g., chronic hemolytic anemia, EPO therapy)
- Nucleic acid interaction (e.g., B12 deficiency, folic acid deficiency, antimetabolites such as hydroxyurea and cytosine arabinoside)
- Abnormal RBC maturation (clonal or chronic) (e.g., myelodysplastic syndromes, myeloproliferative disorder, acute leukemia)
- Other (e.g., alcohol abuse, chronic liver disease, hypothyroidism)

**Microcytic (<80 fL)**
- Reduced iron availability (e.g., iron deficiency, anemia of chronic disease)
- Reduced heme synthesis (e.g., lead poisoning, sideroblastic anemias)
- Reduced globin synthesis (e.g., thalassemia)

**Normocytic (80–100 fL)**
- Acute bleeding
- Splenomegaly
- Hemolytic anemias
  Intrinsic RBC defects
    Membrane (e.g., hereditary spherocytosis, elliptocytosis)
    Enzyme (e.g., G-6-PD deficiency, PK deficiency)
    Heme (e.g., porphyrias)
    Globin (e.g., sickle cell disease)
  Extrinsic causes
    Antibody-mediated
    Infective (e.g., malaria)
    Chemical or physical (e.g., drugs, toxins, burns)
    Mechanical (e.g., cardiac valves, thrombotic thrombocytopenic purpura, hemolytic uremic syndrome, disseminated intravascular coagulation)
- Bone marrow disease
  Acellular bone marrow (e.g., aplastic anemia)
  Hypercellular bone marrow (e.g., myeloma, myelofibrosis, primary refractory anemia)
  Normocellular bone marrow (e.g., marrow infiltration, uremia, anemia of chronic disease)

*The normal RBC has a mean corpuscular volume (MCV) of 80 to 96 fL ($1 \text{ fL} = 10^{-15}$ L) and a diameter of approximately 7 to 8 microns, equal to that of the nucleus of a small lymphocyte.

to its carrier protein, transferrin, a beta-globulin that transports it to the bone marrow. Most iron is stored in the liver, spleen, muscle, and bone marrow, predominantly as a ferritin complex but also as hemosiderin. Circulating serum ferritin is in equilibrium with stored tissue ferritin in normal physiological states; therefore, serum ferritin assays can be a useful measure of total body iron stores.

The transferrin surface receptor (Tfr) on red cell precursors facilitates the internalization of iron into erythroid cells for incorporation into hemoglobin. The level of serum transferrin receptor (sTfr), the soluble form of the membrane Tfr, reflects the total erythron activity. Therefore, the sTfR assay can be used as an indicator of erythron activity and iron stores. The production of these iron-regulating proteins is controlled by the tissue oxygen levels.

Iron is conserved tenaciously and is normally lost only through sweat, skin desquamation, and menstruation in females (see Table 39-1). It is because of this drive to conserve iron, without a mechanism for the body to rid itself of excess iron, that iron overload syndromes can occur (e.g., hemochromatosis, thalassemia). Since high levels of iron are toxic to cells, iron overload has serious clinical sequelae.

The modern laboratory offers several tests to assist in the assessment of iron stores. The gold standard is "stainable bone marrow iron" in a bone marrow aspirate, while the most sensitive and accessible laboratory assay is the serum ferritin. The serum ferritin directly reflects total body iron stores. However, ferritin is an acute-phase reactant protein that is elevated in inflammatory states. Thus, in inflammatory or chronic disease states with true iron deficiency, the serum ferritin result must be evaluated with care since it will be elevated, which leads to an incorrect indication of iron stores. Assays of iron stores that are not affected by inflammatory states, such as the sTfR, may be of value. Serum TfR is unaffected by inflammatory cytokines and directly reflects both erythroid activity and lack of iron stores. The ratio of sTfR to ferritin may be a more sensitive indicator of iron stores than sTfR alone in chronic inflammatory states and anemia of chronic disease.

Other traditional laboratory indicators of iron deficiency include low serum iron ($<50\,\mu g/dL$, compared with normal levels of 75 to 175 $\mu g/dL$ in males and 65 to 165 $\mu g/dL$ in females), increased total iron binding capacity (normal 230 to 430 $\mu g/dL$), and low percent transferrin saturation ($<5\%$, compared with normal 20 to 50%). In later stages of iron deficiency, when the hemoglobin is less than 100 $\mu g/dL$, the erythrocyte morphology becomes characteristically microcytic (low MCV) and then hypochromic with reticulocytopenia.

**Iron therapy** should never be administered to an individual without a clear evaluation of iron stores, given the toxicity of iron overload. Iron is available in a number of pharmacological preparations (oral, intramuscular, and intravenous). *Oral iron* provides a safe, cheap, and effective means of restoring iron balance in most clinical situations. Since iron is absorbed primarily in the proximal small bowel, the more expensive enteric-coated or sustained-release formulations that release iron further down the gastrointestinal (GI) tract are less efficacious. Acidification of the gastric milieu with 250 mg ascorbic acid at the time of oral iron intake is often recommended, since iron is best absorbed in the ferrous ($Fe^{2+}$) form, and this is facilitated by a mildly acidic medium. The cheapest iron preparation is ferrous sulfate, and a dose containing 300 mg of iron salts (60 mg elemental iron) should be taken three times daily between meals. A number of other ferrous iron preparations in common use are ferrous salts of organic acids such as fumarate, gluconate, and ascorbate.

A clinical reticulocytosis response to iron repletion is normally seen within 3 to 10 days and a rise in hemoglobin within 2 to 3 weeks. Failure to respond to iron therapy may be due to an incorrect diagnosis (e.g., thalassemia), presence of a coexisting disease interfering with response (e.g., anemia of chronic disease), failure of the patient to take the medication, or lack of absorption of the medication (e.g., enteric-coated tablets, concomitant use of antacids, malabsorption). Alternative parenteral routes for iron treatment are available but carry increased risks, including anaphylaxis. *Intramuscular or intravenous iron* (iron dextran, sodium ferric gluconate) is available for use in the rare patient who either cannot tolerate oral preparations or does not absorb iron (e.g., bowel resection, inflammatory bowel disease).

**Adverse effects** of oral iron are common ($>10\%$) and include GI irritation, epigastric pain, nausea, stomach cramping, and constipation. Almost all patients have dark or black stools due to oxidized iron. Other side effects include heartburn, diarrhea, and discoloration of urine. **Acute iron overdose** can lead to a constellation of symptoms, including acute GI irritation, erosion of GI mucosa, hematemesis, hepatic and renal impairment, acidosis, and coma. There are numerous reports of such toxicity in children who have ingested large amounts of iron or multi-mineral supplements. Severe toxicity (serum iron 300 $\mu g/mL$ or higher, or elemental iron 35 mg/kg or more) requires treatment with iron-chelating agents such as deferoxamine (see Chapter 72). **Chronic iron overload** leads to the condition of **hemochromatosis,** in which iron has saturated the normal storage sites and is then deposited in parenchymal tissues such as liver and heart. Iron is toxic to these cells and leads to tissue injury, inflammation, repair, and loss of organ function. The clinical manifestations of iron overload include liver disease, skin pigmentation, diabetes mellitus, arthropathy, impotence in males, and cardiac enlargement with or without heart failure or conduction defects.

A number of drugs may produce **drug interactions** that interfere with oral iron absorption, including antacids, $H_2$ blockers (cimetidine), levodopa, methyldopa, and penicillamine. Quinolones may decrease absorption by forming a non-absorbable, ferric ion–quinolone complex. The absorption of iron supplements is improved by ascorbic acid in orange juice, but it can be compromised if the supplements are taken together with beverages or foods containing polyphenols, phytate, oxalate, or calcium.

## Vitamin B₁₂ deficiency anemia

Vitamin $B_{12}$ (cobalamin) is an essential vitamin in animals, the lack of which leads to significant consequences, including neurological damage and anemia. Dietary sources of the cobalamins, and their absorption from the GI tract, are described in Chapter 63.

*Mechanism of action.* Cobalamin is a coenzyme for various cellular metabolic functions, including fat and carbohydrate metabolism and protein synthesis. It is critical for cell replication and hematopoiesis. Cobalamin is an essential coenzyme for two specific reactions in the body: the synthesis of methionine from homocysteine, and conversion of methyl malonyl coenzyme A (CoA) to succinyl CoA. A lack of adequate $B_{12}$ results in impaired DNA synthesis, since thymidylate synthesis is impaired and uridine triphosphate (UTP) accumulates, resulting in UTP misincorporation into DNA. Cobalamin deficiency is associated with increased serum levels of homocysteine, methyl malonyl CoA, and its metabolic product, methylmalonic acid (MMA). Homocysteine and MMA are both very useful adjunctive laboratory tests to assess true cobalamin deficiency.

*Deficiency syndrome.* An understanding of the multiple steps involved in $B_{12}$ intestinal transport, absorption, and delivery to tissues provides insight into the many potential causes that can lead to $B_{12}$ deficiency. Adequate $B_{12}$ uptake is dependent on (1) dietary intake, (2) acid–pepsin in the stomach to liberate $B_{12}$ from binding to proteins, (3) pancreatic proteases to free cobalamin from binding to R factors, (4) normal gastric parietal cell secretion of intrinsic factor (IF) to bind to cobalamin, and (5) an ileum with cobalamin–IF receptors. Causes of $B_{12}$ deficiency thus include gastric abnormalities (e.g., pernicious anemia due to antibodies to parietal cells and IF, gastrectomy, gastritis), small bowel disease (e.g., inflammatory bowel disease, malabsorption, ileal resection), pancreatitis, chronically inadequate diet, and agents that interfere with absorption (e.g., neomycin, biguanides, proton pump inhibitors). Body stores of cobalamin are substantial, amounting to 2 to 5 mg (see Table 39-1). The minimum daily requirement of $B_{12}$ is about 1 to 1.5 µg, while normal Western dietary intake is 5 to 20 µg/day. This means that dietary insufficiency is not likely to result in $B_{12}$ deficiency for years.

Mild or subclinical $B_{12}$ deficiency has been reported in 10 to 24% of the population, especially the elderly. The clinical hematological syndrome of $B_{12}$ deficiency ranges from asymptomatic to megaloblastic anemia with typical hypersegmented polymorphonuclear cells, mild neutropenia, and thrombocytopenia. Of particular concern is that cobalamin deficiency can lead to non-hematological syndromes, including neurological and/or neuropsychiatric manifestations. Neuropsychiatric problems may consist of paresthesias, numbness, weakness, loss of dexterity, impaired memory, and personality changes, especially in the elderly. Cobalamin deficiency can also lead to a unique pattern of irreversible demyelination termed subacute combined degeneration of the dorsal and lateral spinal columns. These non-hematological manifestations are particularly worrisome since they may occur prior to the development of an anemia. The neurological and neuropsychiatric manifestations of cobalamin deficiency are not seen in the other type of megaloblastic anemia, which is caused by folic acid deficiency.

*Laboratory diagnosis.* The normal range of serum $B_{12}$ concentration is 150 to 750 pg/mL, as commonly determined in a radioimmunoassay; the total amount in serum represents 0.1% of total body content. Levels below 150 pg/mL constitute a clear sign of deficiency. A significant problem is that clinically affected individuals with low-normal or even normal serum cobalamin values may be truly cobalamin deficient and respond to replacement therapy. The morbidity due to the non-hematological complications and the prevalence of $B_{12}$ deficiency have led authorities to recommend serum $B_{12}$ screening every 5 years starting at age 50, and yearly after age 65 years. False negative $B_{12}$ deficiency (i.e., elevated serum levels in the presence of deficiency) can occur in true deficiency, active liver disease, lymphoma, autoimmune disease, and myeloproliferative disorders. False positives (i.e., low levels in the absence of deficiency) can occur in folate deficiency, pregnancy, multiple myeloma, and excessive vitamin C intake.

The $B_{12}$ assays are quite specific for serum vitamin $B_{12}$ levels below 100 pg/mL, but they discriminate poorly when levels are between 100 and 300 pg/mL. In the latter case, other sensitive, albeit expensive, measures reflective of $B_{12}$ status, including serum homocysteine and serum MMA, should be used. MMA and homocysteine levels increase in vitamin $B_{12}$ deficiency. Homocysteine levels are also increased with age, folic acid and vitamin $B_6$ deficiency, renal failure, and hypothyroidism and in individuals with genetic defects involving the methionine pathways. MMA is elevated only in $B_{12}$ deficiency, renal failure, and hypovolemia. Other clinical laboratory findings in cobalamin deficiency include macrocytosis (elevated MCV >100 fL, although MCV >115 fL is more common; see Table 39-4) and peripheral blood morphology findings of oval macrocytes and hypersegmented neutrophils. The anemia seen in cobalamin deficiency is due to both ineffective erythropoiesis and intramedullary hemolysis or destruction (Table 39-3). Some physicians may proceed to a bone marrow aspiration, which will reveal characteristic changes of megaloblastosis. Anti-IF and anti-parietal cell antibodies may also be useful in clarifying the cause of the cobalamin deficiency. The classic Schilling test, involving administration of isotope-labelled $B_{12}$ with and without IF, helps determine whether there is a GI absorption problem and whether the deficiency is due to lack of IF.

*Treatment.* If cobalamin deficiency is confirmed, it must be treated because persistence of cobalamin deficiency for more than 3 months may result in neuropsychiatric problems or irreversible neurological damage. Treatment typically involves intramuscular $B_{12}$ injections since this route eliminates the need for IF. $B_{12}$ stores should be rapidly replaced, and then a maintenance schedule may be put in place. Treatment must be maintained for life unless the cause of $B_{12}$ deficiency is reversible and is corrected. The typical treatment regimen involves an initial dose of 1000 µg of $B_{12}$ given by intramuscular injection daily for 3 to 7 days, then weekly for 4 weeks, followed by a maintenance program of monthly injections of 100 to 1000 µg or quarterly injections of 1000 µg.

Oral $B_{12}$ should be given to patients with increased $B_{12}$ requirements due to pregnancy, thyrotoxicosis, hemorrhage, malignancy, or liver or kidney disease. Neomycin, colchicine, and anticonvulsants may decrease oral $B_{12}$ absorption. $B_{12}$ injections are generally well tolerated but can result in headache (2 to 10%), anxiety, dizziness, pain, nervousness, hypoesthesia, itching, and weakness (1 to 4%). Treatment of severe vitamin $B_{12}$ deficiency may result in hypokalemia as the anemia resolves because the rapid formation of new cells increases cellular potassium requirements. Oral potassium supplementation is recommended during the initial $B_{12}$ loading treatment.

## Folic acid deficiency anemia

Folic acid is essential for DNA synthesis and cell duplication. Normal daily requirements for adults are 200 to 400 µg/day, but recent research suggests that this is attainable only through the ingestion of supplemental folate. Since 1999, when all North American flour began to be supplemented with folic acid, the prevalence of folate deficiency has fallen markedly to well below 1% in the general population. Folate deficiency has become quite uncommon in North America, compared with $B_{12}$ deficiency (approximately 10 to 15% in those aged >65 years).

Dietary sources and absorption of folic acid are described in Chapter 63. Unlike $B_{12}$, folate stores (5 mg) are relatively small compared with the daily requirement, and stores will last only a few months with no dietary intake (see Table 39-1).

Folate exists in several forms in the body. Serum folate, at physiological levels, enters cells by binding to a folate receptor. Once inside the cell, folic acid is converted to the polyglutamate form, which is biologically active and cannot back-diffuse out of the cell into the plasma. Thus, RBC folate levels are a truer measure of long-term folate status and folate stores than are serum folate levels. Upon ingestion, dietary folate undergoes a series of chemical reactions, resulting in the formation of $N5$-methyl tetrahydrofolate (THF), which is then absorbed by the proximal small bowel (duodenum and jejunum). THF, attached to carrier proteins, is transported to the liver for storage. Distribution of folate from liver stores depends mostly upon enterohepatic recirculation, in which folate is reabsorbed from the bile into the serum.

THF is necessary for the formation of a number of coenzymes in many metabolic systems. THF is a critical coenzyme in the methylation of deoxyuridylate to thymidylate, which is an essential step in nucleoprotein synthesis and maintenance of erythropoiesis. Limitation of thymidylate synthesis impairs DNA synthesis, resulting in megaloblastic transformation. THF is also critical for the synthesis of methionine from homocysteine. Like $B_{12}$ deficiency, folate deficiency results in an increased serum homocysteine level, but unlike $B_{12}$, it does not affect MMA levels. Folate deficiencies are suspected with the clinical presentation of unexplained anemia or macrocytosis (MCV >100 fL). The hematological manifestations of folate deficiency are similar to those of cobalamin deficiency; however, neuropsychiatric and neurological manifestations are not found in folate deficiency as they are in $B_{12}$ deficiency, an important clinical distinction.

Folate deficiency may be due to inadequate dietary intake, malabsorption (small bowel disease or resection), drug interaction (methotrexate, trimethoprim, anticonvulsants, alcohol), or increased requirements (hemolysis, pregnancy, infancy). Laboratory diagnosis of folate deficiency hinges on the measurement of folic acid levels in serum, which reflect short-term dietary folate state, or in the red cells, long-term cellular stores. Macrocytosis occurs in folate deficiency before the hemoglobin decreases significantly. Peripheral blood and bone marrow red cell morphology in folate deficiency are similar to that seen in $B_{12}$ deficiency (see Table 39-4). Other common causes of macrocytosis include alcoholism, liver disease, and hemolytic anemias. As with $B_{12}$ deficiency, limitations in the specificity and sensitivity of the vitamin assay make other metabolic measurements helpful. In folate deficiency, the homocysteine level is elevated while the MMA is not. Elevated homocysteine needs to be interpreted carefully, and other causes for elevated homocysteine (including aging, renal disease, $B_{12}$ and $B_6$ deficiency, and hypothyroidism) should be ruled out. Before treatment with folic acid alone, $B_{12}$ deficiency must be unequivocally ruled out, given the morbidity associated with its potential neurological complications. Further, the treatment of a combined $B_{12}$ and folate deficiency or an isolated $B_{12}$ deficiency with folate alone can precipitate neurological damage.

**Treatment of folate deficiency** consists of either oral or parenteral administration of folic acid (1 to 5 mg/day) for 1 to 4 months, or until complete hematological recovery occurs. An oral dose of 1 mg/day is usually sufficient, even if malabsorption is present. Erythron response is seen within 3 to 7 days and a rise in hemoglobin, within 1 to 2 weeks.

There are a number of important **drug interactions** with folate. High-dose folic acid therapy (>15 mg/day) may increase phenytoin metabolism, while phenytoin, primidone, para-aminosalicylic acid, and sulfasalazine may decrease serum folate concentrations. Concurrent administration of chloramphenicol and folic acid may result in antagonism of the hematopoietic response to folic acid, and dihydrofolate reductase inhibitors (e.g., methotrexate, trimethoprim) interfere directly with folic acid utilization.

## Hemoglobinopathies

Hemoglobinopathies are inherited disorders in which a genetic mutation results in a qualitative (structural) or a quantitative abnormality of a particular globin chain. Commonly recognized hemoglobinopathies include the thalassemia syndromes and hemoglobin S (HbS). Sickle cell diseases (SSDs) are the most common hemoglobinopathies. Carrier status of HbS in Africa is between 20 to 40%, and the sickle cell trait is found in 8% of the American Black population. SSD is characterized by sickling (resulting from the development of hemoglobin liquid crystals due to polymerization of deoxy-HbS) and increased rigidity of the RBCs upon deoxygenation; these changes cause increased blood viscosity, sludging of blood in capillaries and arterioles, and infarction of surrounding tissues (vaso-occlusive events). Sickle cell crises include vaso-occlusion or infarction (painful crisis), aplastic crisis, sequestration crisis, and hemolytic crisis. The anemia of SSD is a chronic hemolytic anemia (see Table 39-3) that is normochromic, normocytic, and characterized morphologically by sickle cells in the peripheral blood smear. Diagnosis is confirmed by hemoglobin electrophoresis, in which the abnormal HbS is clearly differentiated from normal (Hb A, A2, F) and other forms of hemoglobin.

There is no specific treatment for SSD other than supportive measures, including hydration, folic acid, analgesia, oxygen treatment, and transfusion regimens. Transfusions are indicated in defined clinical circumstances, including crisis and pregnancy, and for long-term prevention of thrombotic complications such as stroke. Increased fetal hemoglobin (HbF) has a marked inhibitory effect on RBC sickling. *Newer drug treatment modalities* have been identified that reactivate the synthesis of HbF in the red cell. A number of drugs, including **hydroxyurea, 5-azacytidine,** and **butyric acid,** have been shown to reactivate HbF synthesis in SSD and result in increased concentrations of HbF in RBCs. Hydroxyurea is the only drug in common use in SSD and has been shown to improve the clinical course, outcome, and complications related to SSD. Treatment of sickle cell patients with hydroxyurea for at least 4 months results in a three- to fourfold increase in HbF (which can reach 15 to 20% of the total), a reduction in hemolysis, an increase in Hb concentration, and a significant decrease in crises and mortality.

Hydroxyurea is an anti-neoplastic and antimetabolite (see Chapter 57) that has a relatively non-toxic profile other than reversible myelosuppressive effects. Myelosuppression, primarily leukopenia, tends to recover within 7 days after the drug is stopped (but the platelet count may take 7 to 10 days to recover). Other hematological effects of hydroxyurea include megaloblastic erythropoiesis, macrocytosis, and decreased serum iron. Long-term tumourigenesis by hydroxyurea remains a concern with prolonged use of the drug, although all evidence to date indicates that this risk is very low.

### Hemolytic anemias

Anemias caused by the increased destruction of RBCs, both in circulation and within the bone marrow, are called hemolytic anemias (see Table 39-3). Drugs that induce hemolysis affect erythropoiesis indirectly by triggering an anemia that induces an appropriate increase in erythropoietin and a resulting physiological erythron response of reticulocytosis. The severity of anemia depends upon how adequately erythropoiesis (reticulocytosis) can compensate for the degree of hemolysis. Drugs and chemicals induce hemolytic anemias through immune and non-immune mechanisms.

*Non-immune hemolysis* by oxidizing agents occurs when the compound interacts directly with the hemoglobin molecule and either denatures the globin chains or oxidizes heme groups, causing methemoglobinemia and oxidative hemolysis. **Dapsone,** which is widely used in treating AIDS and leprosy, acts through this mechanism. Asymptomatic methemoglobinemia without anemia is more commonly found in subjects on dapsone. **Amyl nitrite** and butyl nitrite, used primarily via inhalation for relief of angina (or for arousal by some drug abusers) produce methemoglobinemia that may be so severe as to induce a coma. Resulting hemolysis with nitrites will be much more severe in individuals with inherited glucose-6-phosphate dehydrogenase (G-6-PD) deficiency (see Chapter 10). G-6-PD variants are X-linked hereditary enzymatic RBC disorders that affect 200 to 400 million people worldwide and 10 to 15% of people of African descent. **Lead intoxication** causes hemolysis by interfering with heme synthesis. Lead poisoning may be acute or result from a slow accumulation, and it is suggested by clinical history, clinical findings (gingival lead line), and characteristic RBC morphology (basophilic stippling). Treatment may require chelation therapy with ethylenediaminetetraacetic acid (EDTA; see Chapter 71). **Copper overload** also causes a potentially brisk hemolytic anemia, which is best illustrated by Wilson disease, a hereditary disease of cellular copper export, leading to inappropriate copper disposition in tissues with direct toxic cellular effects and high free serum copper (see Chapter 43). The mechanism of hemolysis is unclear but may be a direct oxidative injury to the RBC.

## ERYTHROPOIETIN

As described earlier in this chapter, erythropoietin (EPO, epoetin-alfa) is an essential hematopoietic growth factor and the primary cytokine stimulus for erythropoiesis. It promotes differentiation and proliferation of the erythron. The use of a **recombinant form (rHu-EPO)** of this glycoprotein has had a major impact on the management of a number of EPO-deficient and hypoproliferative anemias, including those associated with renal failure, chronic disease, bone marrow failure, myelodysplastic syndromes, cancer therapy, and AIDS. It is also used to mobilize RBCs for autologous red blood cell donations. In appropriate clinical circumstances, rHu-EPO has resulted in improved quality of life, decreased symptoms due to anemias, and decreased transfusion requirements.

rHu-EPO acts in a manner identical to that of the endogenous hormone. It induces erythropoiesis by stimulating the division and differentiation of committed erythroid progenitor cells and induces the early release of reticulocytes from the bone marrow into the bloodstream. There is a direct dose–response relationship between rHu-EPO and erythron up-regulation. Intravenous or subcutaneous administration of rHu-EPO results first in an increase in reticulocyte counts, followed by a rise in the hemoglobin level. Given the dose relationship between EPO and erythroid response, there is merit in measuring endogenous serum EPO levels to assist in determining the appropriateness of therapy with rHu-EPO. In individuals with normal hemoglobin, serum EPO ranges from 4.1 to 22.2 mU/mL. In anemia, endogenous EPO levels are typically inversely related to hemoglobin levels. The rHu-EPO hematological response (bone marrow erythroid hyperplasia and reticulocytosis) begins in several days, and the peak effect is seen in 2 to 3 weeks.

## Pharmacokinetics

After subcutaneous administration, bioavailability of rHU-EPO is about 21 to 31%. The drug is primarily excreted in the GI tract, with a half-life of 4 to 11 hours. EPO regimens vary depending upon the clinical indication and drug formulation. EPO is available in two human recombinant (rHu) forms: **epoetin-alpha** (EPO-alpha) or a much longer acting and newer form, **darbepoetin-alpha**. Darbepoetin has a threefold longer half-life and greater biological activity.

## Dosage

rHu-EPO should only be administered for those anemias that have been demonstrated to benefit from the drug. It should not be administered unless the Hb is less than 10 to 11 g/dL and no other coexisting causes of anemia, such as nutritional anemia, are present. For anemia in chronic renal failure, initial therapy with EPO-alpha is 50 to 120 µg/kg two to three times a week, and darbepoetin is 0.45 µg/kg once a week. Initial therapy may be given intravenously or subcutaneously, but the subcutaneous route is preferred since it requires a 30% lower drug dose. For maintenance therapy, the rHu-EPO dose is titrated to the hematological response to attain and maintain an Hb of 12 g/dL by 3 to 4 months. At 4 weeks of therapy, if the Hb has not risen by 1.2 to 2 g/dL, then the dose is increased by 25%. To attain this target hemoglobin level in chronic renal disease, the dosing range for EPO-alpha is 50 to 300 µg/kg. Targeting dosage adjustments to the hematocrit is not recommended since there is much greater inter-laboratory variability with hematocrit than with hemoglobin.

## Adverse Effects

The most common side effect of rHu-EPO is **hypertension**, usually diastolic, seen in 5 to 25% of individuals, especially if EPO is given intravenously. Other common side effects include headache (15%), fatigue (9 to 33%), dizziness (8 to 14%), edema (11 to 21%), arrhythmia (10%), fever (9 to 19%), diarrhea (16 to 22%), constipation (5 to 18%), vomiting (15%), nausea (14%), myalgia (21%), arthralgia (11 to 13%), and flu-like symptoms (5%). An excessive rate of rise in hemoglobin may be associated with an exacerbation of hypertension or seizures. Thus, blood pressure needs to be monitored closely in all individuals on rHu-EPO, and hypertension must be treated promptly. The rHu-EPO dose should be decreased if the Hb increase exceeds 1 g/dL in any 2-week period. rHu-EPO should be used with caution in patients at risk for thrombosis or with history of cardiovascular disease as increased thrombotic risk is a side effect of the drug. An uncommon but important complication of repeated or prolonged use of rHu-EPO is the development of pure red cell aplasia due to the production of anti-EPO antibodies. A complete failure to respond to rHu-EPO should result in a detailed investigation to rule out the cause, including other anemias and anti-EPO antibodies. Prior to and during rHu-EPO therapy, iron stores must be evaluated. Unless iron stores are in excess, oral iron supplementation is recommended during all forms of EPO therapy to provide for increased iron requirements during expansion of the RCM.

## Abuse in Sports

EPO has been used by athletes to improve athletic performance by increasing hemoglobin concentration and therefore the oxygen-carrying capacity of the blood. Both rHu-EPO administration and "blood doping" (RBC transfusions) are known to increase exercise performance. At the doses of rHu-EPO commonly used, no side effects have yet been reported. However, if the Hct is maintained above 50% with rHu-EPO and is further increased by dehydration during intense physical activity, thrombotic events might be expected with long-term use. Use of rHu-EPO by high-performance athletes should be suspected if the Hct is greater than 50% in males and 47% in females. rHu-EPO differs from endogenous EPO in its glycosylation patterns, and the recombinant form can be detected electrophoretically in serum. Surreptitious use of rHu-EPO is also suggested by elevation of the serum ratio of the soluble transferrin receptor to ferritin.

## ANDROGENS

Erythrocytosis is a common side effect of pharmacological doses of all androgens, probably due to direct androgenic stimulation of erythropoiesis. While testosterones are clinically indicated for hypogonadism, male impotency, breast cancer therapy, and replacement therapy in post-menopausal women, they are also frequently used as performance-enhancing agents by athletes and body builders. The pharmacology of androgens, including adverse effects and their misuse in competitive sports, is discussed in Chapter 46.

## SUGGESTED READINGS

Anthony AC. Megaloblastic anemias. In: Hoffman R, Benz E, Shattil S, et al, eds. *Hematology: Basic Principles and Practice.* 4th ed. New York, NY: Churchill Livingstone; 2005:519-556.

Brittenham GM. Disorders of iron metabolism: iron deficiency and overload. In: Hoffman R, Benz E, Shattil S, et al, eds. *Hematology: Basic Principles and Practice.* 4th ed. New York, NY: Churchill and Livingstone; 2005:481-498.

Carmel R, Green R, Rosenblatt DS, Watkins D. Update on cobalamin, folate, and homocysteine. *Hematology.* 2003;62-81.

Fisher JW. Erythropoietin: physiology and pharmacology update. *Exp Biol Med.* 2003;228:1-14.

Goodnough LT, Skikne B, Brugnara C. Erythropoietin, iron and erythropoiesis. *Blood.* 2000;96:823-833.

Meyron-Holtz EG, Ghosh MC, Rouault TA. Mammalian tissue oxygen levels modulate iron-regulatory protein activities in vivo. *Science.* 2004;306:2087-2090.

Wang WC. Sickle cell anemia and other sickling syndromes. In: Greer JP, Foerster J, Lukens JN, Rodgers GM, Paraskevas F, Glader B, eds. *Wintrobe's Clinical Hematology.* 11th ed. Philadelphia, Pa: Lippincott Williams & Wilkins; 2004:1272-1293.

# 40

# Immune System Organization, Modulation, and Pharmacology

## JW SEMPLE

A 26-year-old woman came to her physician with a 2-week history of easy bruising and a rash on her legs. She had also had several nosebleeds over the past week and had noticed gum bleeding when brushing her teeth. In addition, her last menstrual period 2 weeks ago had been heavier than usual. There was no hematuria, melena, or visible blood in the stools. She was otherwise in good health and was on no medications. She had not had a recent illness, and the past medical history and family history were unremarkable.

On examination, she appeared well, with no pallor or jaundice. Vital signs were normal. Conjunctivae and fundi were normal. There was slight oozing from her gums, and several petechial lesions were noted on her hard palate. There was no lymphadenopathy. Respiratory, cardiovascular, and abdominal examinations were normal; the liver and spleen were not enlarged. A number of ecchymoses were noted on her extremities, and numerous petechiae were present on both lower legs. The musculoskeletal and neurological examinations were normal.

A complete blood count (CBC) revealed RBC of $4.6 \times 10^{12}$/L (normal range 3.8 to $5.8 \times 10^{12}$/L), WBC of $5.4 \times 10^9$/L (normal range 4 to $11 \times 10^9$/L) with normal differential count, a hemoglobin of 125 g/L (normal range 115 to 163 g/L), and platelets of $8 \times 10^9$/L (normal range 150 to $400 \times 10^9$/L). The blood film confirmed the presence of marked thrombocytopenia with large platelets present. RBC and WBC morphology were normal. Prothrombin and partial thromboplastin times were normal. A bone marrow aspiration was normal with numerous megakaryocytes present.

A diagnosis of immune thrombocytopenic purpura was made. The patient was started on oral prednisone 80 mg daily and was advised to avoid products containing acetylsalicylic acid. After 5 days, the platelet count rose to $20 \times 10^9$/L, and no new bruising or bleeding was noted. The platelet count rose steadily thereafter and, 2 weeks later, was normal at $240 \times 10^9$/L. The prednisone was gradually tapered off over the following 6 weeks and then discontinued, with careful monitoring of the platelet count, which remained normal.

After treatment had been initiated, further investigations were performed to search for an etiology for the immune thrombocytopenia. Anti-nuclear antibody, rheumatoid factor, and HIV serology were negative. Abdominal ultrasound was normal, showing no lymphadenopathy and normal spleen size.

Six months after the cessation of prednisone, routine follow-up showed that the platelet count had dropped to $70 \times 10^9$/L. The patient was asymptomatic and had no evidence of bleeding by history or physical examination. No treatment was initiated. She was advised to have her blood counts monitored regularly, but she did not return for follow-up.

Three months later, the patient came to the emergency room with a 1-week history of bruising and petechiae. This time she had also had several episodes of melena over the previous 12 hours and was feeling increasingly weak. On examination, she appeared pale, blood pressure was 120/80 mmHg with a postural drop of 15 mmHg, and pulse was 110 beats/min. She again had extensive petechiae and ecchymoses on her skin. Stool was grossly black and was confirmed to be positive for blood.

Her CBC now revealed an RBC of $2.8 \times 10^{12}$/L, a WBC of $5.0 \times 10^9$/L, hemoglobin of 80 g/L, platelets of $3 \times 10^9$/L. The blood film again showed marked thrombocytopenia as well as red cell polychromasia.

The patient was admitted to hospital, cross-matched, and transfused with two units of packed red cells. She was also started on intravenous IgG 1 g/kg daily for 2 days. The morning after admission, her hemoglobin had increased to 100 g/L, and her vital signs had stabilized. Within 2 days, her platelet count had increased to $70 \times 10^9$/L and her melena had stopped. Her platelet count peaked at $250 \times 10^9$/L after 1 week and subsequently dropped to $50 \times 10^9$/L over the following 2 weeks. She was restarted on prednisone, vaccinated against pneumococcus, and referred for splenectomy, which was performed 10 days later. Following splenectomy, the platelet count increased to $300 \times 10^9$/L and has remained in the normal range on follow-up.

The body's **immune system** is generally divided into the innate system, which is the first line of defence against invading pathogens, and the adaptive system, which is composed of B and T cells and leads to long-term immunity against microbes. Many diseases and even their pharmacological treatments can lead to the disruption of the innate and adaptive immune systems. **Immunopharmacology** is a discipline that deals with the control (enhancement or suppression) of the immune response by chemical and/or biological mediators. The ultimate goal is to identify molecules that act on specific individual components of the immune system (preferably in an antigen-specific manner) to enhance or block the action of those particular components—the modern equivalent of Ehrlich's "magic bullet." **Immunosuppressant drugs** have been extensively studied and are effective in disorders in which the immune system is over-activated and is mediating pathology (e.g., autoimmune conditions or in transplantation settings). On the other hand, less is known about the nature of **immunostimulants**, although these types of drugs may be efficacious in treating immunosuppressive states such as primary immunodeficiencies, HIV/AIDS, or those associated with cancer.

## IMMUNE RESPONSE

The generation of an immune response by the adaptive immune system to a foreign antigen or antigens (e.g., a microorganism or heterologous transplanted organ) is a complex biological process involving the interaction of many cell types and their secreted products (Fig. 40-1). In general, initiation of the response occurs when the antigen (e.g., a bacterial protein) first interacts with an antigen-presenting cell (APC) of the innate immune system. An APC is a cell that is positive for major histocompatibility complex (MHC) class II; this can be a macrophage, dendritic cell, or B cell within a lymph node. The MHC is a series of genes located on chromosome 6 in humans that code for cell surface glycoproteins responsible for immune recognition. Class I MHC molecules are found on virtually all cell types (with the exception of red blood cells in humans). Class II molecules are more narrowly restricted in their expression on APCs. Once the APC interacts with an antigen and internalizes it, the cell can then "process" the antigen by proteolysis into smaller antigenic peptides and present them on its membrane, in association with class II molecules encoded by the MHC, to antigen-specific T-helper ($T_h$) cells of the adaptive immune system.

$T_h$ cells, in turn, become activated by signals passed via their T-cell receptor (TcR) complex, causing them to proliferate and secrete cytokines such as interleukin-2 (IL-2), IL-4, and interferon-$\gamma$ (IFN-$\gamma$). These events subsequently stimulate antigen-specific B cells to produce and secrete antibodies, which can ultimately either destroy the antigen or enhance its removal by the reticuloendothelial system.

$T_h$ cells are the critical cell type that will determine whether antibodies are produced against the foreign antigen. They exert fine control over the response by activating other regulatory cells (e.g., T-suppressor cells) or by secreting various regulatory agents (e.g., cytokines). Any defect in, or abnormal activation of, antigen-specific $T_h$ cells can thus alter the magnitude of the immune response. Furthermore, modulation of the components of T-cell recognition—the trimolecular complex of antigen, TcR, and MHC—is a potential avenue of immunotherapy.

Clusters of differentiation (CDs) are groupings of cell surface markers identified by specific groupings of antibodies, which serve to identify different types of lymphocytes and other leukocytes. Over 150 CDs have been identified, of which CD4 and CD8 are the most common in T-lymphocyte populations. During an immune response, CD4-positive $T_h$ cells can be subdivided into $T_h0$, $T_h1$, or $T_h2$ cells depending on the cytokines they secrete. In humans, $T_h0$ cells are thought to be less differentiated than $T_h1$ and $T_h2$ cells, since they can secrete most or all of the cytokines made by both the other cell types, particularly IL-2, IL-4, and IL-10. $T_h1$ activation usually results in the secretion of IL-2 and IFN-$\gamma$, whereas $T_h2$ cells secrete IL-4, IL-5, IL-6, IL-10, and IL-13 when activated. $T_h1$ and $T_h2$ cells respond differentially to different APCs; the site of exposure of the antigen and the physical nature of the antigen will influence which CD4-positive $T_h$ cell predominates in a given immune response. $T_h1$ responses generally mediate delayed-type hypersensitivity reactions and the development of complement-fixing immunoglobulin G (IgG) antibodies, whereas $T_h2$ responses generally mediate superior humoral immune responses, particularly IgE responses. It is becoming apparent that these $T_h$ responses critically influence immune reactivity, and modulation of these cell types through cytokine networks is a promising approach to immunopharmacology.

Immune system modulators are of two general types: (1) immunosuppressants, which usually suppress the immune response in a non-specific manner and are used to minimize the effects of autoimmune diseases or rejection of organ transplants; and (2) biological response modifiers or immunopotentiators, which can enhance the immune response and may be used in the treatment of conditions in which the immune response is depressed, such as cancer. Figure 40-2 is a simplified diagram showing components of the immune system and sites of action of some of the immune system modulators that are used as immunopharmacological agents.

## IMMUNOSUPPRESSANTS

Many immunosuppressive drugs in use today are also classed as anti-neoplastic agents, but the therapeutic plan differs for the two applications. For example, those cytotoxic agents that act primarily against proliferating cells

**FIGURE 40-1** The generation of a humoral immune response. (1) Antigen passes from the circulation into a regional lymph node. (2) B lymphocytes (with antigen-specific surface immunoglobulin) recognize the antigen and become "primed" for T-cell help (i.e., they increase the surface expression of IL-2 receptors). (3) Antigen is taken up (either by phagocytosis of a cell or by fluid-phase pinocytosis of a soluble protein) by an antigen-presenting cell (APC) and is processed by proteolysis within an endosomal compartment. (4) Antigenic peptides are re-expressed on the surface of the APC, within the antigen-binding groove of major histocompatibility complex (MHC) class II molecules. This complex can then be recognized by T-helper lymphocytes via their T-cell receptor (TcR); T-helper ($T_h$) cells become activated as a result. (5) $T_h$ cell activation causes secretion of cytokines (e.g., IL-2), which stimulate the antigen-primed B cells to differentiate into plasma cells and secrete antibodies.

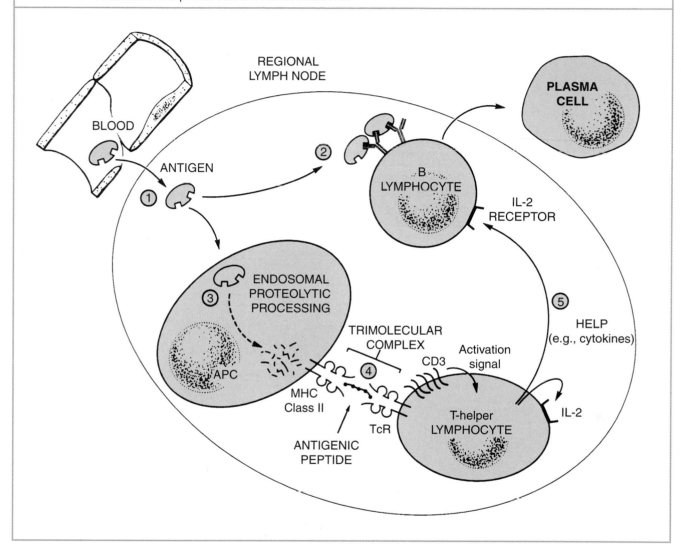

can act against both the proliferating cancer cells and normal immune cells. Cancer cell proliferation, however, is generally random, while immune cell proliferation is generally more "synchronized" in a burst of mitotic division after introduction of antigen. Therefore, when drugs are used at the time of a transplant or during treatment of an autoimmune disease, a large portion of the proliferating immune precursor cells can be destroyed by an initial high dose of immunosuppressant, and long-term immune suppression is maintained with a low-dose daily schedule thereafter. When the same drugs are used

against cancer (see Chapter 57), they are given in high-dose pulses every 3 to 6 weeks in order to allow immune rebound between treatments.

Immunosuppressant therapy from the 1960s to the present has consisted of combinations of various drugs such as corticosteroids and azathioprine to produce maximal immunosuppression while keeping adverse side effects to a minimum. Recently, a new wave of immunosuppressant therapy characterized by the selective regulation of defined subpopulations of lymphocytes has been used with such drugs as the cyclosporines and FK506. The future of immunosuppressant therapy will be the induction of antigen-specific depression of autoimmunity and allograft reactivity.

## Corticosteroids

The corticosteroids were the first group of agents recognized as having lympholytic properties. Corticosteroids inhibit the generation of arachidonic acid, thus preventing the production of various inflammatory mediators (e.g., prostaglandins) by the cyclooxygenase and lipoxygenase metabolic pathways (see Chapter 27). **Prednisone** is the most commonly used oral immunosuppressant, whereas **methylprednisolone** is used parenterally. Both preparations can reduce the size and lymphoid cell content of the lymph nodes and the spleen, although they

have no toxic effect on proliferating myeloid or erythroid stem cells in the bone marrow.

Prednisone suppresses the inflammatory response of cell-mediated immunity and may also directly suppress antibody synthesis. It is cytotoxic to certain subsets of T cells, and some of its diverse effects may be due to lysis of either suppressor or helper T cells. Continuous administration of prednisone increases the fractional catabolic rate of IgG, thus lowering the concentration of specific antibodies.

The corticosteroids also offset some effects of the immune response by reducing tissue injury from inflammation and edema. Prednisone is used in a wide variety of clinical conditions in which the immunosuppressant properties of the drug account for its beneficial effects. These include autoimmune disorders (e.g., autoimmune hemolytic anemia, autoimmune thrombocytopenic pur-

**FIGURE 40-2** Sites of action of some modulators that are used as immunopharmacological agents. Specific modulation: (1) Agents that can act on the trimolecular complex (e.g., anti-MHC or TcR antibodies, suppressive peptides). These agents are still used only experimentally. (2) Intravenous immunoglobulin (IVIg; anti-idiotypic antibodies). IVIg may be more appropriately classed as non-specific because it can affect all B cells; however, specific anti-idiotypes (for a B-cell clone) have been experimentally induced. Non-specific modulation: (3) Prednisone. (4) Azathioprine. (5) Cyclophosphamide. (6) Cyclosporine. (7) Anti-thymocyte globulin. (8) Cytokines. APC = antigen-presenting cell; CD = cluster determinant; CTL = cytotoxic T lymphocyte; IL-2 = interleukin-2; MHC = major histocompatibility complex. HELP (heavy arrows) can be in the form of cytokines, cell contact, etc. Light arrows represent differentiation pathways.

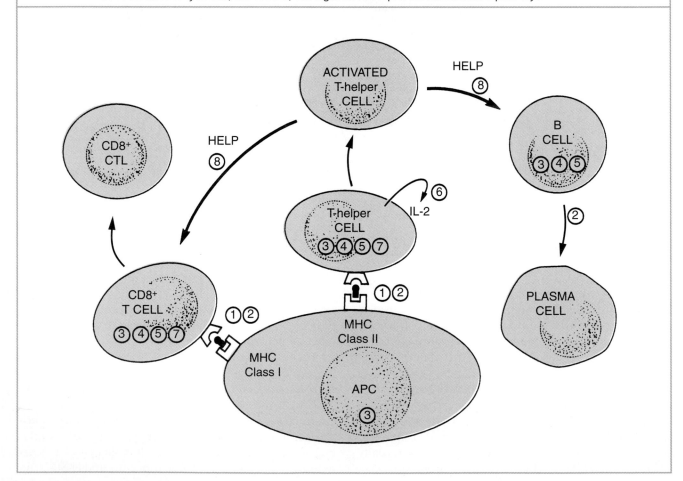

pura, systemic lupus erythematosus) and organ transplantation (e.g., kidney, bone marrow). Adverse side effects are usually attributed to the high doses used for immunosuppression and include hypertension, weight gain, hyperglycemia, euphoric personality changes, and cataracts (see Chapter 48).

## Anti-neoplastics

Until the development of cyclosporine A, **azathioprine** (Imuran) was the drug most often used for immunosuppression in relation to organ transplantation. It is now used as second-line immunosuppressant therapy in specific situations where corticosteroids have been found to have no beneficial effects (e.g., in one-third of patients with autoimmune thrombocytopenic purpura). Azathioprine is a precursor of mercaptopurine, which is the active molecule. Mercaptopurine, a structural analogue, or antimetabolite, of hypoxanthine, interferes with nucleic acid metabolism (purine synthesis) during the wave of lymphoid cell proliferation that follows antigen stimulation, and it is especially effective against T cells. Its toxic effects are primarily bone marrow depression and possible reactivation of viral hepatitis (see Chapter 57).

The alkylating agent **cyclophosphamide** is an antineoplastic drug that is also a potent immunosuppressant. It is used chiefly in patients who do not tolerate azathioprine. It is a modified nitrogen mustard that destroys proliferating lymphoid cells but also alkylates some resting cells, rupturing the DNA double helix and inducing lethal mutations. Cyclophosphamide (Cytoxan) was originally designed as an inactive nitrogen mustard precursor that would be converted to the active alkylating form at its site of action. Its adverse effects are those of the nitrogen mustards (see Chapter 57).

## Cyclosporine

This cyclic polypeptide is produced by the fungus *Tolypocladium inflatum* and has profound immunosuppressive effects on cell-mediated cytolysis in graft-versus-host reactions and on delayed-type hypersensitivity reactions. It has a remarkably specific affinity for T lymphocytes. Since its introduction in 1983, organ transplant survival rates have improved significantly. Although its therapeutic effects are palliative rather than curative, one of its great advantages is that the use of steroids can be greatly reduced or, in certain diseases, totally eliminated.

**Cyclosporine A** (Sandimmune) does not interfere with hematopoiesis, including the maturation of lymphoid stem cell precursors. Only when mature immunocompetent T cells have received an activation signal from antigen-presenting cells does cyclosporine block the ensuing cellular activation. The precise mechanism of action is still unclear. Cyclosporine blocks the activity of cyclophilin, a peptidyl-prolyl *cis-trans* isomerase that catalyzes protein unfolding. It has been postulated that through this mechanism, transcription of IL-2 and its receptor are blocked. Cyclosporine A can also suppress immune IFN-γ and other macrophage growth factors, resulting in a decrease of IL-1. Studies of the clinical pharmacology of the drug indicate a very large variation in bioavailability (ranging from 5 to 90%). Large amounts of the drug bind to erythrocytes and plasma proteins, and extensive biotransformation and elimination occur in the liver. Newer formulations of cyclosporin, such as microemulsions (e.g., Neoral), have improved oral absorption rates and increased half-lives.

The major adverse effects of cyclosporine are nephrotoxicity, hirsutism, and neurotoxicity, which can be potentiated when the drug is administered together with amphotericin B, aminoglycosides, and co-trimoxazole. Adverse drug interactions can occur because cyclosporine is able to inhibit the hepatic cytochrome P450 pathway. Other side effects such as elevated serum bilirubin, alkaline phosphatase, and transaminases and a risk of lymphomas have been reported.

## Macrolides

FK506 (**tacrolimus**) is a macrolide (similar in structure to that of erythromycin) derived from the fungus *Streptomyces tsukubaensis*. Its mechanism of action is similar to that of cyclosporine, except that it binds to a different protein that inhibits calcineurin (a phosphatase enzyme involved in gene transcription of IL-2, INF-γ, and other cytokines). In general, FK506 is more potent than cyclosporine in a number of experimental models of transplantation and autoimmunity. However, the two compounds have a similar spectrum of activity. **Sirolimus** (Rapamune) is a macrolide similar in structure to tacrolimus but exerts its activity at a different site of action than cyclosporine or tacrolimus; it binds to an immunophilin protein that binds to a key regulatory kinase required for T-cell activation. Adverse reactions include thrombocytopenia, hyperlipidemia, and rash, but, in contrast to cyclosporine, the molecule lacks direct end-organ toxicity.

## Mycophenolate Mofetil (CellCept)

CellCept is a derivative of mycophenolic acid that is known to inhibit inosine monophosphate dehydrogenase, an enzyme involved in *de novo* synthesis of purines within T and B cells. Thus, it inhibits the proliferative capabilities of these cells. It also stimulates phagocytosis by macrophages, which enhances their antigen-presenting capabilities. The molecule is absorbed orally and eliminated in the liver. Adverse side effects include diarrhea, leukopenia, cytomegalovirus infection, bacterial infections, and an increased incidence of lymphomas and other malignancies.

## Anti-thymocyte Globulin

The concentrated IgG fraction of plasma from hyperimmune rabbits immunized with human thymic lymphocytes (rabbit anti-thymocyte serum, or RATS) is primarily used today in patients undergoing kidney transplants. It reduces the number of T cells in the thymus-dependent areas of the spleen and lymph nodes and thus reduces the immune response. Since the human recipient can mount an immune response against the rabbit IgG, RATS is usually administered with other immunosuppressants such as azathioprine. Common adverse reactions include fever, chills, leukopenia, and skin reactions.

## Monoclonal Antibodies

An alternative to the use of polyclonal antibody preparations has been developed with the creation of monoclonal antibodies against individual leukocyte surface antigens, including CD3 (total T cells), CD4 (T-helper cells), and various T-cell activation markers (IL-2 receptor, CD25). In animal models, these agents have been shown to be effective in suppressing the immune response, probably via their ability to block the specific function of the cell surface molecules. For, example, the anti-CD3 drug **muromonab-CD3 (OKT3)**, given weekly by intravenous injection and in conjunction with cyclosporine, significantly inhibits the formation of cytotoxic T lymphocytes and effectively prevents acute rejection in renal transplant recipients.

Other monoclonal antibodies have recently been used successfully in the clinic. For example, **rituximab** recognizes the CD20 molecule on pre-B and mature B cells and is efficacious in treating non-Hodgkin's lymphoma and chemotherapy-resistant advanced follicular lymphoma. Infusion-related side effects (including cytokine release syndrome) are reported commonly with rituximab and occur predominantly during the first infusion; they include fever and chills, nausea and vomiting, allergic reactions (such as rash, pruritus, angioedema, bronchospasm, and dyspnoea), flushing, and tumour pain. Patients should be given an analgesic and an antihistamine before each dose of rituximab to reduce these effects. Premedication with a corticosteroid should also be considered.

**Abciximab** is specific for a cell surface receptor on activated platelets (see Chapter 38), and it is effective in preventing re-stenosis after coronary angioplasty. **Basiliximab (Simulect)** is a chimeric murine monoclonal antibody against the human IL-2 receptor alpha subunit of activated T cells that effectively blocks T-cell activation and inhibits clonal expansion of T cells. It is used to induce immunosuppression and, in combination with immunosuppressants, to prolong the life of transplanted organs. On the other hand, **daclizumab** (Zenapax) is a humanized immunoglobulin similar to basiliximab that blocks the IL-2 receptor, but it was formed by splicing complementary portions of light- and heavy-chain variable regions of a murine antibody into the human-derived Fab (antigen-binding fragment) framework and fusing the Fab to the Fc (crystallizable fragment) portion of human IgG. These latter chimeric and humanized antibodies have the advantage of being less immunogenic and allowing complement activation to occur, resulting in the activation of antibody-dependent cellular cytotoxicity and phagocytosis against the recipient's T cells. **Infliximab** (Remicade) is a chimeric human/murine anti-tumour necrosis factor (TNF) monoclonal antibody that effectively blocks TNF binding to its receptor and thus down-regulates the inflammatory properties of TNF. It has shown excellent results in patients suffering from rheumatoid arthritis and is also used in some cases of chronic inflammatory bowel disease (see Chapter 42). Newer monoclonal antibody preparations still in clinical trials include anti-CD40L, for a number of different autoimmune disorders.

## Intravenous γ-Globulin (IVIg)

Human immunoglobulin (Ig) preparations are of two types: normal immunoglobulins and specific immunoglobulins.

### Normal immunoglobulins

Normal intravenous immunoglobulin G (IVIg; Iveegam) is concentrated γ-globulin from the pooled plasma of thousands of blood donors that have been tested and found non-reactive for hepatitis B virus surface antigen and for antibodies against hepatitis C virus and human immunodeficiency virus (types 1 and 2). It thus represents a wide spectrum of naturally expressed and induced IgG antibodies with many different specificities, including autoantibodies. Figure 40-3 shows a schematic representation of a typical IgG protein molecule and its functional domains. These preparations have been used since the early 1950s as replacement therapy to treat primary and secondary immunodeficiency states. IVIg therapy has also been shown to be effective in treating bacterial and viral infections and in reducing lost plasma protein due to leakage in severely burned patients.

In 1981, IVIg was administered to a patient with Wiscott-Aldrich syndrome and concomitant immune thrombocytopenic purpura (ITP), and the child's platelet counts were found to be significantly raised the next day. Numerous subsequent clinical trials confirmed that IVIg therapy is an effective treatment for patients suffering from ITP. In adults, it is usually administered intravenously over several hours at a dose of 1 g/kg for 2 to 4 days; increases in platelet counts can be observed within 24 hours of the first dose. An IVIg dose of 400 mg/kg for 5 days is also effective in children with ITP. In the last 10 years, IVIg has also been used successfully to down-regulate the immune response in a number of other autoimmune diseases that are mediated primarily by auto-antibodies (e.g., myasthenia gravis, chronic inflammatory demyelinating polyneuropathy,

**FIGURE 40-3** Structure of an IgG molecule. The molecule consists of two light and two heavy chains. Each chain is made up of a series of highly conserved units of approximately 110 amino acids. The sites of proteolytic cleavage by papain and pepsin lie between conserved units. In the diagram, the conserved units are shown as outpouchings of the chain and are designated as C (constant) or V (variable). Membrane-bound forms possess a hydrophobic C-terminal extension for binding to the cell membrane but are otherwise identical in sequence to the secretory forms, which lack these extensions. Because of the inter-chain disulfide bridges located between their respective sites of cleavage, papain and pepsin yield quite different fragments. CHO = carbohydrate branched side chain; $C_H$, $C_L$ = constant units of heavy and light chains, respectively; $V_H$, $V_L$ = variable units of heavy and light chains, respectively; Fab = antigen-binding fragment; Fc = crystallizable fragment; FcR = crystallizable fragment receptor; SS = disulfide bridges, either within chains or between chains.

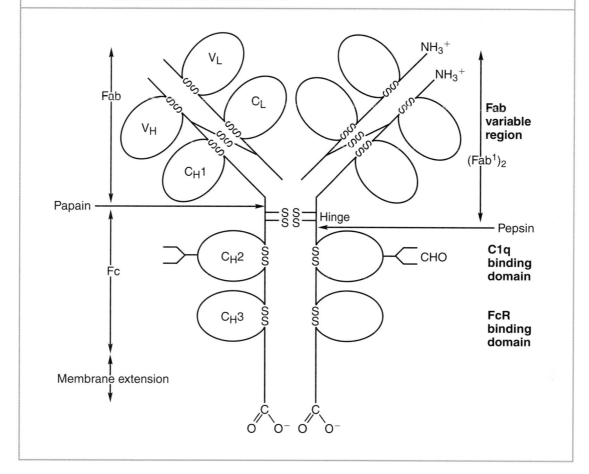

rheumatoid arthritis). This has resulted in significant off-label use of IVIg and has created occasional shortages of the product worldwide. Side effects of IVIg therapy may include chills, fever, and, rarely, anaphylactoid reactions.

While the mechanisms of the anti-inflammatory action of IVIg are complex and not fully elucidated, several theories that are probably not mutually exclusive have been proposed. In ITP, for example, there is experimental support for the theories that IVIg reduces platelet destruction by causing (1) reticuloendothelial Fc receptor–mediated blockade of the binding of opsonized platelets to macrophages, (2) Fc-mediated inhibition of opsonized platelet phagocytosis, or (3) Fc-mediated

cytokine alterations that affect reticuloendothelial system function and/or anti-idiotypic neutralization/regulation of anti-platelet auto-antibodies.

## Specific immunoglobulins

Specific immunoglobulins are prepared by pooling the plasma of selected donors with high levels of the specific antibody required. For example, specific hepatitis B immunoglobulin ("HBIG") is available for use in association with hepatitis B vaccine for the prevention of infection in laboratory and other personnel who have been accidentally inoculated with hepatitis B virus, and in infants born to mothers who have become infected with this virus in pregnancy or who are high-risk carriers. Other specific immunoglobulin preparations include anti-rabies, anti-tetanus, and anti-varicella zoster immunoglobulins.

## RhₒD Immune Globulin

**Anti-D** is classed as a specific or hyperimmune immunoglobulin preparation and is prepared from the pooled sera of RhₒD-negative male volunteers immunized with D+ erythrocytes. It is used to suppress the immune response in Rh– mothers after the delivery of an Rh+ baby. It is usually given to the mother within 72 hours after the birth of the baby to prevent hemolytic anemia of the newborn that may occur in subsequent pregnancies.

In 1984, it was demonstrated that anti-D administration can also raise the platelet counts of patients with ITP. Little is known about the mechanisms of action of anti-D, although the above theories for IVIg may apply. It has been suggested that anti-D opsonizes D+ red blood cells and blocks platelet destruction by adhering to the Fc receptors of leukocytes. Alternatively, it has been suggested that anti-D may cause immunosuppression by interacting with Fcγ receptor and stimulating the production of immunosuppressive cytokines. Anti-D is usually administered at a dose of 50 to 75 μg/kg for 2 to 4 days. This dosage significantly raises the platelet counts within 24 hours of the first administration. Side effects of anti-D therapy are similar to those of other antibody preparations and include chills, fever, and, rarely, anaphylactoid reactions.

## Cytokine Inhibitors

Cytokines are small, soluble protein molecules produced by a variety of cell types that are primarily concerned with cellular communication, particularly within the immune system. This communication is in the form of either activating events or suppressing events. Antagonists in the form of cytokine inhibitors have been cloned and are now being increasingly used to treat a variety of autoimmune disorders. For example, the tumour necrosis factor alpha (TNFα) inhibitor **etanercept** (Enbrel) is a recombinant form of the TNFα receptor that has shown some success in patients with rheumatoid arthritis. **Anakinra** (Kineret) is a human IL-1 receptor antagonist that is effective in treating rheumatoid arthritis and ITP.

## Future Considerations for Immunosuppressants

All the current immunosuppressant therapeutic strategies in autoimmune diseases and transplantation are aimed at inhibiting the emergence of pathological clones of lymphocytes. Unfortunately, they are generally non-specific in that the total immune response can be affected, and, therefore, the treatments eventually have to be discontin-

ued. Antigen-specific therapies that would inhibit only the clones responsible for the disease are still at an experimental stage. The majority of these therapies are aimed at the trimolecular complex: MHC, peptide, and T-cell receptor. Treatment with monoclonal antibodies specific for class II MHC molecules, blocking the function of the MHC with immunosuppressive competitor peptides, and idiotype-specific suppression are all examples of potential antigen-specific immunosuppression.

## IMMUNOPOTENTIATION

Immunopotentiation, or immunostimulation, can be defined as a process that directly or indirectly enhances immune functions. It can be classed as antigen-specific or non-specific, and each of these classes can be subdivided into active, passive, or adaptive events. Table 40-1 summarizes the classification scheme of immunopotentiation mechanisms.

## Vaccines

The most specific way to stimulate the immune system is to vaccinate (immunize) individuals to stimulate their immune system to produce long-lasting vaccine-specific immunity. Vaccines have probably increased world population survival rates more than any other drug. Vaccines can be administered as *live attenuated* forms of a virus (e.g., rubella or measles vaccine) or bacterium (e.g., BCG vaccine), as *inactivated* preparations of a virus (e.g., influenza vaccine), or as *extracts of exotoxins* or *detoxified exotoxins* produced by a microorganism (e.g., tetanus vaccine). They all stimulate production of antibodies and other components of the immune mechanism.

For live attenuated vaccines, immunization is generally achieved with a single dose (but three doses are required with oral poliomyelitis vaccine). Live attenuated

| TABLE 40-1 | Classification of Immunopotentiation Mechanisms |
|---|---|
| **Antigen-specific mechanisms** | |
| Active | Vaccination |
| Passive | Anti-tetanus or anti-rabies immunoglobulin |
| Adoptive | Tumour-infiltrating lymphocytes; sensitized lymphocytes |
| **Non-antigen-specific mechanisms** | |
| Active | Cytokines; synthetic chemicals |
| Passive | Intravenous γ-globulin (IVIg) therapy; plasmapheresis |
| Adoptive | Lymphokine-activated killer (LAK) cell therapy |

vaccines usually produce a durable immunity, but it is not always as long as that of the natural infection. When two live virus vaccines are required (and are not available as a combined preparation), they should be given either simultaneously at different sites or with an interval of at least 3 weeks. Inactivated vaccines may require a primary series of injections to produce adequate antibody response, and, in most cases, they also require booster (reinforcing) injections; the duration of immunity varies from months to many years. Exotoxin extracts and detoxified exotoxins are more immunogenic if adsorbed onto an adjuvant (such as aluminium hydroxide). They require a primary series of injections followed by booster doses.

## Levamisole

This drug is an anthelmintic agent that has been shown to potentiate immune responses in animals and humans. It is an imidazole derivative and is thought to act by inhibiting the production of an immunosuppressive substance by T-suppressor cells. A major side effect of this drug is arthralgia.

## Adjuvants, Cyclic Nucleotides, and Hormones

Adjuvants are molecules derived from bacterial cells, which have been known for many years to enhance immunity by attracting macrophages (APCs) and inducing inflammation at the site of injection. Most vaccine preparations have an adjuvant contained within them to enhance the immune response. **BCG** is derived from a viable strain of *Mycobacterium bovis* and significantly enhances macrophage activity. It has been routinely used in the treatment of bladder cancer and melanomas. Cyclic polynucleotides such as **Poly I:C** have also shown an immunostimulatory property, particularly enhancing natural killer (NK) cell activity. They have been used clinically to treat solid lymphomas. Thymic hormones have been used as purified proteins and recombinant products to improve primary immunodeficiency in children.

## Immunostimulatory Cytokines

The major cytokines associated with the immune system are the interferons and the interleukins. In addition, there are a number of specific factors which also play an important role in modulating the immune response (e.g., colony-stimulating factors, tumour necrosis factor, transforming growth factors).

### Interferons
**Interferons** (IFNs) are a group of glycoproteins first identified as compounds that inhibit intracellular viral replication (see Chapter 55). Currently, there are three major classes: α, β, and γ. IFNs are produced by stimulation of a variety of cell types, including lymphocytes, fibroblasts, and epithelial cells. As with many cytokines, they are now available through recombinant DNA technology. The IFNα and IFNγ are derived primarily from human lymphoblasts, and IFNβ from human fibroblasts. IFNγ is also referred to as immune interferon.

IFNα can modulate antibody responses by directly inhibiting B lymphocytes and enhancing NK cell activity. It has shown some anti-tumour effect in certain lymphomas and solid tumours, and it has given good results in the treatment of chronic hepatitis B and chronic hepatitis C. Currently, it is approved for use in hairy cell leukemia, malignant melanoma, and hepatitis C infection. It has been found in the serum of patients with a variety of autoimmune diseases and has been shown to be an effective treatment in certain autoimmune diseases and in Kaposi's sarcoma related to HIV infection.

Side effects are dose-related but commonly include anorexia, nausea, influenza-like symptoms, and lethargy. Ocular side effects and depression have also been reported. Myelosuppression may occur, particularly affecting granulocyte counts. Cardiovascular problems (hypotension, hypertension, and arrhythmias), nephrotoxicity. and hepatotoxicity have also been reported. Polyethylene glycol–conjugated ("pegylated") derivatives of IFNα (peginterferon alpha-2a and -2b) are available; pegylation increases the persistence of the interferon in the blood. They are licensed for use in the treatment of chronic hepatitis C, ideally in combination with ribavirin (see Chapter 55).

IFNβ causes a number of in vivo effects, including stimulation of expression of class I and class II human leukocyte antigen molecules and stimulation of NK cell activity. It has recently been approved for the treatment of relapsing forms of multiple sclerosis, although its mechanism of action in this illness is not yet known. Side effects reported most frequently include irritation at injection site (including inflammation, hypersensitivity, necrosis) and influenza-like symptoms (fever, chills, myalgia, or malaise), but these decrease over time; nausea and vomiting occur occasionally.

The biological activity of IFNγ is highly species-specific. It is a potent activator of NK cells and macrophage tumouricidal activity. Its interaction with other lymphokines can be either antagonistic (IL-4) or synergistic (IFNα and β). It may be effective in treating chronic granulomatous disease. Adverse effects have included fever, chills, hypotension, paresthesias, and altered mental state. Neutropenia and elevated serum transaminases are commonly observed.

### Interleukins
**Interleukins** (ILs) are small polypeptide hormones that are primarily associated with the immune system. They are produced by lymphocytes and have multiple effects on the

immune response. Their fine control is essential for adequate regulation of the immune response. In humans, probably the most important interleukin responsible for the stimulation of both humoral and cellular immunity is IL-2. Originally termed T-cell growth factor, it is produced primarily by T cells but acts on all lymphoid cells. Its major effects are the activation of T cells, B cells, and macrophages and the stimulation of secretion of other interleukins to further modulate the immune response. It has potent anti-tumour effects against metastatic melanoma and renal cell cancer. IL-2 has also been used as an *ex vivo* stimulus of lymphokine-activated killer (LAK) cells and tumour-infiltrating lymphocytes (TIL), which have been shown to be potentially therapeutic against certain tumours (e.g., lymphomas). **Aldesleukin** (recombinant IL-2) is licensed for treatment of metastatic renal cell carcinoma; it is usually given by subcutaneous injection. It is now rarely given by intravenous infusion because of its association with a capillary leak syndrome, which can cause pulmonary edema and hypotension. Aldesleukin produces tumour shrinkage in a small proportion of patients, but it has not been shown to increase survival. Bone marrow, hepatic, renal, thyroid, and central nervous system toxicity is common.

Various autoimmune diseases, including multiple sclerosis, rheumatoid arthritis, and systemic lupus erythematosus, have been found to be associated with increased serum levels of IL-2. Hypersecretion of endogenous IL-2 may lead to auto-aggression by a number of mechanisms, such as bypassing the need for T-cell co-stimulation, up-regulating co-stimulatory CD80 molecules on B cells, or inducing other cytokines such as IFNγ and IL-10. Thus, therapies that can regulate the production of IL-2 may have potential benefits in treating some autoimmune disorders.

## Hematopoietic Growth Factors

**Erythropoietin alpha** (epoetin-alpha; Procrit) is a growth factor cytokine critical for stimulation of the division and differentiation of erythroid progenitor cells (see Chapter 39). It is produced by recombinant DNA technology and is extensively used to treat the anemia associated with renal failure or cancer chemotherapy. Adverse effects include hypertension, headache, and, rarely, hypersensitivity reactions. The **colony stimulating factors** (CSFs) are cytokines derived from bone marrow and are involved in the stimulation of myeloid progenitor cells within the bone marrow. Granulocyte CSF (G-CSF, filgrastim; Neupogen) is currently used to treat neutropenia, and granulocyte–monocyte CSF (GM-CSF, sargramostim; Leukine) is used for myeloid recovery after bone marrow transplantation. Both have produced increased rates of immune recovery in bone marrow recipients.

## SUGGESTED READINGS

Klein M, Radhakrishnan J, Appel G. Cyclosporine treatment of glomerular diseases. *Annu Rev Med.* 1999;50:1-15.

Paul WE, ed. *Fundamental Immunology.* 5th ed. Philadelphia, Pa: Lippincott Williams & Wilkins; 2003.

Semple JW, Lazarus AH. Anti-inflammatory effects of intravenous immunoglobulin: FcγR inhibition/blockade and non-FcγR-mediated mechanisms. In: *Intravenous Immunoglobulins in the Third Millennium.* 5th International IVIG Symposium; Interlaken, Switzerland; September 25-27, 2003. Lancaster, United Kingdom: Parthenon Publishing; 2004:chap 30.

Sigal NH, Dumont F. Cyclosporine A, FK-506, and rapamycin: pharmacologic probes of lymphocyte signal transduction. *Annu Rev Immunol.* 1992;10:519-560.

von Mehren M, Adams GP, Weiner LM. Monoclonal antibody therapy for cancer. *Annu Rev Med.* 2003;54:343-369.

# Part VII

## Gastrointestinal System

# 41

# Pharmacotherapy of Acid–Peptic Disorders

## Y YUAN AND RH HUNT

### CASE HISTORY

A 38-year-old male office worker complained that he had been waking up in the middle of the night with abdominal pain for 3 weeks. The pain was located in the epigastrium and did not extend to his back, chest, or shoulders. It was not accompanied by other symptoms such as regurgitation, palpitation, sweating, or difficulty in breathing. This was occurring several nights a week, and he was also experiencing occasional discomfort in the middle of the afternoon. After taking a snack or eating food, he felt better. Symptoms were also initially relieved by liquid antacids, but these were not working anymore. Fatty foods did not precipitate the pain, but his appetite had suffered as a result of the pain and of the fear that eating might provoke the pain. Otherwise, he considered himself healthy. He smoked occasionally (<5 cigarettes per day) and did not drink more than once a week. He denied any history of hematemesis, melena, weight loss, or any other symptoms.

Physical examination showed a healthy, well-nourished male with stable vital signs. The abdomen was soft with only mild epigastric tenderness. Laboratory data showed a hemoglobin of 123 g/L (normal 130 to 180 g/L for males) and a normal platelet count. Endoscopy of the stomach and duodenum revealed a nodular gastritis and a 1.0-cm ulcer in the anterior wall of the duodenum. Biopsy from the site and the gastric antrum confirmed the presence of *Helicobacter pylori* infection.

The patient was prescribed triple therapy with the proton pump inhibitor omeprazole, 20 mg twice daily, and clarithromycin 500 mg and metronidazole 500 mg twice daily for 2 weeks. Within a few days, the patient's abdominal pain was relieved, but nausea with occasional vomiting occurred, especially soon after taking the medication. The metronidazole was replaced by amoxicillin 1000 mg twice daily, and his symptoms disappeared. He stopped the treatment after 14 days and felt well.

## DEVELOPMENT OF ACID–PEPTIC DISORDERS

Disorders of the gastrointestinal (GI) tract are numerous and diverse. The most common complaints of the upper GI tract are dyspepsia (including belching, nausea, early satiety, and abdominal bloating or distention), heartburn, and abdominal pain. At endoscopy, the most common organic diseases found are acid–peptic disorders, including peptic ulcer disease (PUD), gastroesophageal reflux disease (GERD), drug-induced mucosal injury, especially by non-steroidal anti-inflammatory drugs (NSAIDs), pathologic acid-hypersecretory conditions (e.g., Zollinger-Ellison syndrome), and acute stress ulcer. Peptic ulcer disease includes gastric ulcers (GUs), duodenal ulcers (DUs), and pyloric channel ulcers.

## Gastric Acid Secretion and Regulation

It has long been known that gastric acid plays a critical role in the development of these conditions. The human stomach has a capacity of about 1L, and the contents include hydrochloric acid, pepsinogens/pepsins, and mucus. The pH of the stomach in a normal healthy human fluctuates within the range of 1 to 3 for most of the time. High acidity hydrolyzes protein, destroys ingested bacteria (*H. pylori* survives by means of its urease survival mechanism), and activates pepsinogens to active pepsins, which initiate the digestion and breakdown of ingested proteins. The other major component of gastric juice is mucus, which protects the stomach lining from the acidic and proteolytic gastric contents.

Gastric acid is secreted by the parietal cells located in the fundus of the stomach. The parietal cell is regulated by paracrine, endocrine, and neural pathways. Five different types of cells are located in the gastric mucosa: (1) surface epithelial cells (secrete mucus), (2) mucous neck cells (secrete mucus and are the source of proliferating cells), (3) chief cells (secrete pepsinogens, which are converted to pepsin between pH 0.8 and 3.5), (4) G cells (gastrin-releasing cells in the antrum), and (5) parietal cells in the gastric fundus (secrete HCl and intrinsic factor). The physiological stimulus to acid secretion relies on three primary secretagogues—histamine, acetylcholine, and gastrin—acting via their receptors located on the basolateral membrane of the parietal cell (Fig. 41-1): (1) acetylcholine is released from cholinergic nerve fibres and binds to the muscarinic $M_3$ receptor on the cell surface, promoting release of $Ca^{2+}$ from intracellular stores; (2) gastrin binds to the cholecystokinin B (CCK-B) receptor on the cell membrane and releases intracellular $Ca^{2+}$; and (3) histamine is released from mast cells, binds to parietal cell sur-

**FIGURE 41-1** Schematic representation of the control of acid secretion by receptor-mediated pathways in the gastric parietal cell. Receptors for histamine, gastrin, acetylcholine (ACh), epidermal growth factor/transforming growth factor α (EGF/TGFα), prostaglandins (PGs), and somatostatin operate at the basolateral membrane through heterotrimeric G proteins, either stimulatory ($G_s$ or $G_q$) or inhibitory ($G_i$). The proton pump ($H^+/K^+$-ATPase) in the canalicular membrane of the parietal cell transports hydrochloric acid across the cell membrane to the lumen of the stomach by exchanging $H^+$ ions for $K^+$ ions, as the final step of acid production. $H^+/K^+\alpha\beta = H^+/K^+$-ATPase; ACase = adenylyl cyclase; EGF = epidermal growth factor; PKA = protein kinase A; PLC = phospholipase C; DG = diglyceride; PKC = protein kinase C; cAMP = cyclic adenosine monophosphate; CaM = calmodulin; CaMK = calmodulin-dependent kinases; MLCK = myosin light chain kinase; R = regulatory subunits; RII = type II regulatory subunits; SNARE = soluble N-ethylmaleimide-sensitive factor attachment protein receptor; Rab = the brain form of the oncogene *ras*; IP3 = inositol 1,4,5-trisphosphate. (From Urushidani T and Forte JG, 1997. Copyright © 1997 SpringerLink and Springer Verlag. Reprinted with permission.)

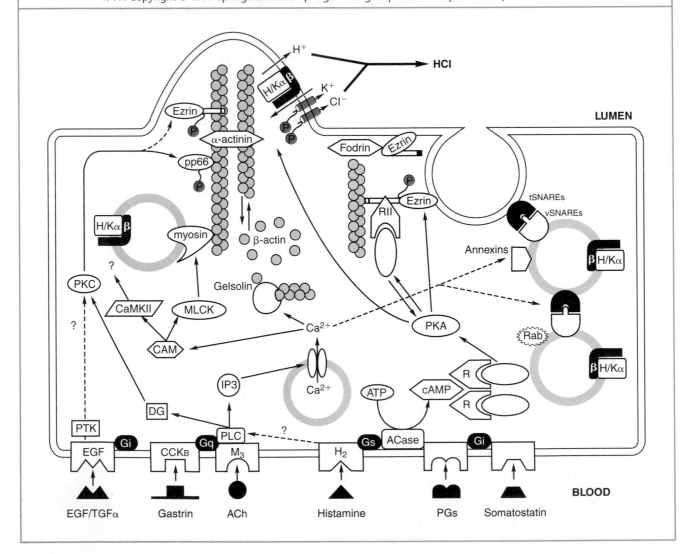

face $H_2$ receptors and activates adenylyl cyclase, increasing the intracellular production of cAMP, which is an important intracellular messenger (see Chapter 9). Histamine is stored in enterochromaffin-like (ECL) cells in the gastric mucosa, from which it is released upon stimulation and diffuses to the parietal cells.

Stimulation of gastric secretion occurs in three phases.

1. Cephalic phase: Taste, smell, and tactile sensations stimulate gastric acid secretion via the vagus nerve and cholinergic terminals, where acetylcholine is released and binds to the muscarinic $M_3$ receptors in the parietal cell membrane. Histamine and gastrin are also secreted during this stage.

2. Gastric phase: Distention of the stomach stimulates local reflexes and vagus nerve afferent signals to the medulla; gastrin is released from G cells, and this increases acid secretion. Gastrin acts as a local hormone that is carried in the blood to the gastrin receptors on the parietal cells.

3. Intestinal phase: The presence in the duodenum of chyme (the partly digested food passed from the stomach to the duodenum) with a pH >3.0 stimulates release of gastrin, which is carried in the blood to parietal cells. Also, some hormones act as secretogogue signals from the ileum. Stimulation of acid secretion typically involves an initial elevation of intracellular calcium and/or cAMP followed by activation of a cAMP-dependent protein kinase cascade that triggers the translocation and insertion of the proton pump, or $H^+/K^+$-ATPase, into the secretory canaliculus of the parietal cells (see Fig 41-1). Each secretagogue potentiates the effects of the others and contributes to more $H^+/K^+$-ATPase and more $Cl^-$ channels being inserted into the canalicular membrane, which is necessary for active acid secretion by the parietal cell (see Fig. 41-1).

There are also some inhibitory mechanisms controlling acid secretion. Acid at pH <2 directly inhibits acid secretion in the stomach, and acid in the duodenum leads to the release of secretin, which also inhibits gastric acid secretion. Fatty acids and peptides stimulate the release of gastric inhibitory polypeptide (GIP) and CCK. Somatostatin, prostaglandins of the $E_2$ class, and epidermal growth factor (EGF) are also inhibitors of HCl secretion by the parietal cell. They all act via the inhibitory $G_i$ protein to inhibit adenylyl cyclase and decrease cAMP levels in the cell (see Fig. 41-1).

The mucus bicarbonate barrier provides a mainly alkaline microenvironment over the surface of the gastric epithelium, which provides initial protection of the stomach against acid and peptic injury.

## Peptic Ulcer Disease

Peptic ulcer develops when there is an imbalance between the "aggressive" and "protective" factors at the luminal surface of epithelial cells. The aggressive factors include acid, pepsin, *H. pylori* infection and its consequences, and drugs such as NSAIDs. Peptic ulcers were formerly thought to be caused by an excess of gastric acid secretion as a consequence of greater parietal cell mass and a defect in the physiological inhibition of acid secretion in these patients. Therefore, anti-secretory medications and surgical operation were historically the most common therapeutic approaches to managing these patients.

Over the past 20 years, however, the roles of *H. pylori* infection and NSAIDs in acid–peptic disorders have raised great interest and promoted considerable basic research and clinical trials. It is now known that they each play an important role in the etiology of peptic ulcers and their complications. The treatment of patients with acid–peptic disorders has been revolutionized since that time. *H. pylori* infection is responsible for the majority of cases of duodenal and gastric ulcer that are not medication-related. *H. pylori* colonizes the mucus layer and secretes proteins that evoke both cellular and humoral immune responses, resulting in mucosal damage together with alteration of physiological regulatory mechanisms. Studies have shown that the abnormalities in acid secretion seen in patients with DU are primarily due to *H. pylori* infection. Therefore, *H. pylori* eradication therapy has largely superseded the suppression of acid as the backbone of ulcer treatment.

## Gastroesophageal Reflux Disease (GERD)

GERD comprises a group of conditions caused by the reflux of gastric contents from the stomach into the esophagus. Although acid is a primary factor in the cause of damage, it also involves other mechanisms, particularly the physiology of the lower esophageal sphincter (LES) and its incompetence. The drugs used for the treatment of GERD are essentially the same as for peptic ulcer, except that the promotility agents are also used for GERD, as described at the end of this chapter.

## DRUGS FOR ACID–PEPTIC DISORDERS

Over the past three decades, several classes of pharmacological agents have proved effective in the management of the acid–peptic disorders (Table 41-1). The main groups are (1) antacids that neutralize acid in the stomach, (2) acid-suppressing agents such as $H_2$ receptor antagonists ($H_2$-RAs) and proton pump inhibitors (PPIs), (3) agents that increase mucosal defence (e.g., sucralfate, prostaglandins), (4) antimicrobials that heal ulcers by the eradication of *H. pylori* infection (e.g., clarithromycin, amoxicillin, metronidazole, tetracycline, bismuth salt), and (5) prokinetic agents that promote motility of the esophagus (e.g., metoclopramide).

Antacids were the mainstay of ulcer treatment until the advent of the $H_2$-RAs in the 1970s. Since then, the suppression of gastric acid secretion with anti-secretory agents has been the primary medical treatment for patients with acid-related disorders. Although peptic ulcers are self-healing, suppression of gastric acid secretion can relieve the symptoms and also accelerate the healing rate. DU healing is significantly correlated with the degree and duration of acid suppression over 24 hours and with the duration of therapy. A sustained increase of gastric pH above 3 for 18 to 20 hours per day predicts a 100% ulcer healing rate at 4 weeks of therapy. Likewise, the percentage of time that intragastric pH is maintained above 4 over a 24-hour period is correlated with the healing rate of erosive esophagitis at 8 weeks. Other classes of agents also play a role in the therapy of acid–peptic disorders.

## Antacids

Antacids are readily available over the counter and are still used by primary care physicians as first-line therapy for controlling occasional mild to moderate heartburn or dyspepsia with "ulcer-like symptoms" as they are relatively safe and less costly than prescription medications. The commonly used antacids include salts of aluminum (aluminum hydroxide, dihydroxyaluminum aminoacetate), magnesium (carbonate, hydroxide, oxide, or magaldrate), calcium (carbonate), or sodium (bicarbonate) (Table 41-2). Sodium bicarbonate can cause belching, flatulence, and hypernatremia. Therefore, it is not useful for long-term treatment and is now rarely prescribed. Calcium carbonate is also used as a calcium supplement.

| TABLE 41-1 | Commonly Used Agents for the Treatment of Acid–Peptic Disorders |
|---|---|
| **Antacids** | |
| Calcium, magnesium, or aluminum-containing hydroxides or salts | |
| **Anti-secretory agents (acid-suppressing)** | |
| *Histamine H$_2$ receptor antagonists:* | |
| Cimetidine, ranitidine, famotidine, nizatidine | |
| *Proton pump inhibitors:* | |
| Omeprazole, lansoprazole, pantoprozole, rabeprazole, esomeprazole | |
| **Mucosal protective agents** | |
| Sucralfate | |
| *Prostaglandin E analogues:* Misoprostol | |
| Bismuth compounds | |
| **Antimicrobials** | |
| clarithromycin, metronidazole, amoxicillin, tetracycline | |
| **Promotility agents** | |
| metoclopramide, domperidone | |

### Efficacy

All antacids neutralize gastric acid and are appropriate for treating heartburn. In patients whose symptoms are relieved by antacids, relief typically occurs within 5 to 15 minutes after taking the drug. However, the relief may last for only 1 to 3 hours. The effect of antacids on acid–peptic disorders depends on the dose and dosing frequency. There are also major differences in how long the relief of symptoms will last after a maximum dose. The acid-neutralizing capacity (ANC) of antacids varies considerably depending on the amount of the active ingredients and the formulation. In vitro ANC studies show that calcium carbonate is very effective, but aluminum hydroxide is relatively ineffective. The effectiveness of magnesium-containing antacids varies with the preparation, depending on the particular combination and chemical formulation of the magnesium and other salts.

The effectiveness of an antacid in vivo is different from that in vitro, and the presence of food, other buffers in the stomach, and the rate of gastric emptying affect the in vivo neutralizing capacity. Generally, liquid antacids are more effective than tablets, but compliance may be less good. Some antacids contain simethicone to limit bloating and gas, or alginic acid or alginates to form a foam barrier to prevent refluxing from bringing acidic gastric contents into contact with the esophageal mucosa. More effective agents such as H$_2$-RAs and PPIs have replaced antacids for the treatment of peptic ulcer and GERD. Although their widespread use has declined, antacids are still commonly used for dyspepsia symptoms and minor episodes of heartburn.

### Adverse effects

The common unwanted effects of antacids differ from drug to drug, depending on their components. For example, aluminum can cause constipation and stomach cramps, render phosphate unabsorbable because of salt formation, and lead to osteomalacia. Magnesium salts can induce diarrhea, and they are sometimes used as a laxative. Calcium can give rise to constipation and hypercalcemia, which can cause renal failure. Antacids containing both magnesium and aluminum are often used to offset their individual effects on bowel function (e.g., combination products such as Mylanta and Maalox). Cation absorption is small, but aluminum or magnesium may accumulate to toxic levels in patients with renal problems. Patients with congestive heart failure, high blood pressure, or kidney disease, or who are on a sodium-restricted diet, should avoid sodium-containing antacids because of the risk of fluid retention.

All antacids are generally regarded as safe in pregnancy, although with respect to pregnancy risk, the U.S. Food and Drug Administration (FDA) categorizes them as class B (i.e., animal reproduction studies have not demonstrated a fetal risk, but there are no controlled studies in

| TABLE 41-2 | Some Commonly Used Antacids and Their Components in Canada | |
|---|---|---|
| **Brand Name** | **Formulation (Product Name)*** | **Principal Ingredients (mg per tablet, unless noted otherwise)†** |
| Amphojel | Tablets | Aluminum hydroxide (600 mg) |
| Brioschi | Powder, effervescent | Sodium bicarbonate (300 mg/g) |
| Diovol | Tablets (Plus Tablets) | Aluminum hydroxide-magnesium carbonate co-dried gel (300 mg), magnesium hydroxide (100 mg), simethicone (25 mg) |
| | Suspension (Ex Suspension) | Aluminum hydroxide (120 mg/mL), magnesium hydroxide (60 mg/mL) |
| Gaviscon | Tablets (Heartburn Relief Extra Strength Aluminum-Free) | Magnesium carbonate (63 mg), alginic acid (313 mg) |
| | Suspension | Aluminum hydroxide (20 mg/mL), sodium alginate (50 mg/mL) |
| Gelusil | Tablets (Extra Strength) | Aluminum hydroxide, magnesium hydroxide (400 mg each) |
| | Suspension | Aluminum hydroxide, magnesium hydroxide (40 mg/mL each) |
| Maalox | Tablets (Quick Dissolve tablets, chewable) | Calcium carbonate (600 mg) |
| | Tablets (TC tablets) | Aluminum hydroxide (600 mg), magnesium hydroxide (300 mg) |
| | Suspension (Quick Dissolve Extra Strength with AntiGas) | Magnesium hydroxide (40 mg/mL), aluminum hydroxide (45 mg/mL), simethicone (5 mg/mL) |
| Mylanta | Tablets (Double Strength) | Aluminum hydroxide (400 mg), magnesium hydroxide (400 mg), simethicone (30 mg) |
| Pepto-Bismol | Tablets, chewable | Bismuth subsalicylate (262 mg), calcium carbonate (350 mg) |
| Phillips Milk of Magnesia | Tablets | Magnesium hydroxide (311 mg) |
| | Suspension | Magnesium hydroxide (80 mg/mL) |
| Rolaids | Tablets (Extra Strength) | Calcium carbonate (750 mg), magnesium hydroxide (135 mg) |
| Tums | Tablets (Regular) | Calcium carbonate (500 mg) |

*There may be different preparations with different associated names under one brand name.
†Milligrams per dose may vary with different manufacturers or preparations.

women, or animal reproduction studies have shown an adverse effect that was not confirmed in controlled studies in women in the first trimester; e.g., aluminum hydroxide) or class C (i.e., studies in animals have revealed adverse effects on the fetus, but there are no controlled studies in women, or studies in women and animals are not available; e.g., calcium carbonate and simethicone). There are sporadic reports of fetal maldevelopment associated with prolonged use of high-dose aluminum-containing antacids. Some clinicians prefer the use of calcium-containing preparations in pregnant women.

## Interactions with other drugs

Antacids interact with a variety of prescription drugs when taken simultaneously. Antacids can affect absorption by reacting with the medication itself or by altering drug dissolution and absorption as a result of changes in gastric or intestinal pH. They can also alter drug elimination by changing urinary pH. An interaction is unlikely, however, if doses of the two drugs are taken at least 2 or 3 hours apart.

Important drugs with which antacids may interact and decrease drug levels or effect include the following:

angiotensin-converting enzyme (ACE) inhibitors, quinolone antibiotics (e.g., ciprofloxacin, ofloxacin), acetylsalicylic acid (aspirin; excretion increased in alkaline urine), chlordiazepoxide, digoxin, glyburide, isoniazid, levothyroxine, metronidazole, misoprostol, NSAIDs, penicillamine, phenytoin, sucralfate, and tetracyclines. In addition, magnesium trisilicate reduces the absorption of iron, nitrofurantoin, and proguanil; sodium bicarbonate interacts with lithium and reduces its plasma concentrations. In contrast, antacids may enhance the absorption of coumadin and L-dopa. Plasma quinidine concentrations are occasionally increased by alkalinization of the urine caused by antacids.

## Administration and dosage

It is best to take antacids 1 hour after meals, to take advantage of the natural buffering effect of food. Acidity is reduced for about 3 hours. Doses can be repeated if symptoms persist, typically up to four times a day, after meals and at bedtime. Maximum doses vary widely with different preparations (see Table 41-2), and maximum daily doses must not exceed those given in the mineral supplement labelling standard (e.g., for calcium, up to a maximum of 1500 mg/day). Antacids should not be taken continuously for more than 2 weeks. To help avoid or reduce drug interactions, other medications should not be taken within 1 to 2 hours of taking an antacid.

## H₂ Receptor Antagonists (H₂-RAs)

H₂-RAs were developed specifically to competitively and reversibly block the histamine H₂ receptor on the gastric parietal cell (see also Chapter 30). Cimetidine, the first H₂-RA developed for human use, was approved in 1977 and was more effective than placebo in inhibiting acid secretion and healing peptic ulcers. With the newer H₂-RAs, slightly better rates of symptom relief and ulcer healing have been achieved. High doses of H₂-RAs have also been used in pathological hypersecretory conditions such as Zollinger-Ellison syndrome. H₂-RAs are also prescribed to prevent gastrointestinal complications induced by long-term use of anti-inflammatory analgesic drugs (see Chapter 28). Four H₂-RAs are available in North America: cimetidine, ranitidine, famotidine, and nizatidine (Fig. 41-2, Table 41-3). Chemically, the H₂-RAs all resemble histamine but are slightly different from each other in structure, although there are many similarities in pharmacology among the four drugs.

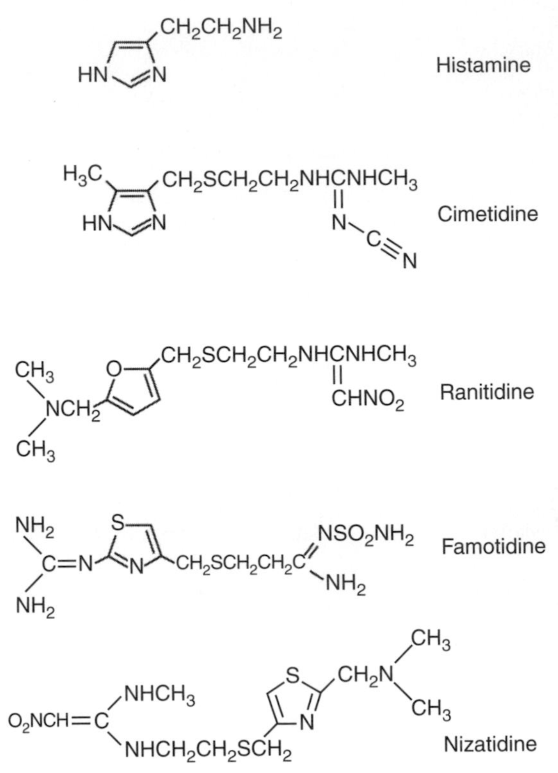

### Efficacy

The FDA has approved over-the-counter (OTC) sale for four H₂-RAs—cimetidine (Tagamet), ranitidine (Zantac), famotidine (Pepcid), and nizatidine (Axid)—for the relief and prevention of heartburn, acid indigestion, and sour stomach. With the exception of nizatidine, they are also available OTC in Canada. Under prescription use, they are also indicated for the treatment of active DU, GU, the maintenance treatment of healed DU, and treatment of GERD (see Table 41-3). Clinical trials have shown clear efficacy of H₂-RAs for peptic ulcer and GERD symptom relief and for DU healing. Because the longest period of basal acid secretion occurs at night, dosing with these agents after the evening meal or at bedtime is optimal for treatment of ulcer disease. However, they are relatively ineffective in increasing daytime intragastric pH sufficiently and cannot completely overcome food-stimulated acid secretion; that is why they have shown less benefit in GERD patients. Furthermore, many 24-hour pH-monitoring studies have shown that H₂-RAs are less effective in suppressing peptic activity.

**Cimetidine** (Tagamet) inhibits the acid secretion response to all known secretagogues and inhibits both daytime and nocturnal gastric acid secretion, although it is relatively less effective at suppressing daytime food-stimulated acid secretion. Cimetidine is best taken with or at the end of meals; it is rapidly absorbed after oral administration. Cimetidine is an inhibitor of cytochrome P450 (CYP). It inhibits enzymes in each of the CYP subfamilies,

**FIGURE 41-2** Structural formulae of histamine and H₂ receptor antagonists (H₂-RAs).

including CYP2C9, 2C19, 2D6, and 3A4, and this property underlies many of its drug interactions. Cimetidine may interact with warfarin and can increase blood levels of medications such as phenytoin, theophylline, lidocaine, diazepam, and metronidazole. Antacids may decrease the absorption of cimetidine. Long-term treatment with cimetidine can produce side effects, including elevated serum creatinine or aminotransferases. Reversible confusional states may occur, especially in elderly or severely ill patients. Impotence and gynecomastia have been rarely reported in some adult male patients receiving cimetidine because of its anti-androgen effect due to displacement of dihydrotestosterone from androgen binding sites. Information on the safety and effectiveness of cimetidine in children is limited, and it is not recommended for use in children under age 16, although gastroenterologists have used it in doses of 20 to 40 mg/kg/day for the management of GERD in children.

**Ranitidine** (Zantac) is a more potent blocker of H₂ receptors than cimetidine. The oral dosage forms include tablets, syrup, and effervescent formulations that must be dissolved in water before use (available in United States and Europe only); these are all considered bioequivalent. Ranitidine is 4 to 10 times as effective as cimetidine in suppressing gastric acid secretion in similar circumstances, while its duration of action is comparable. Ranitidine does not affect pepsin secretion and has little or no effect on fasting or postprandial serum gastrin levels. Propantheline slightly delays and increases peak blood levels of ranitidine, probably by delaying gastric emptying and prolonging drug transit time (see "Anticholinergics" below). Although ranitidine has been reported to bind weakly to cytochrome P450 in vitro, at the recommended doses

| TABLE 41-3 | Pharmacokinetic and Other Features of Major H₂-RAs Used in North America | | | |
|---|---|---|---|---|
| | **Cimetidine** | **Ranitidine** | **Famotidine** | **Nizatidine** |
| Ring | Imidazole | Furan | Guanidinothiazole | Thiazole |
| Preparation (may vary with manufacturer) | Tablets: 200, 300, 400, or 800 mg<br>Oral solution: 300 mg/5 mL<br>Intravenous injection: 300 mg/2 mL | Tablets: 75, 150, or 300 mg<br>Oral syrup: 15 mg/mL<br>Effervescent tablets: 25 or 150 mg<br>Intravenous injection: 25 mg/mL | Tablets/disintegrating tablets: 10, 20, or 40 mg<br>Oral suspension: 40 mg/5 mL<br>Intravenous injection: 10 mg/mL | Capsules: 150 or 300 mg<br>Tablets: 75 mg<br>Oral suspension: 15 mg/mL |
| Bioavailability (%)* | 60–70 | 50 | 40–45 | >70 |
| Time to peak plasma concentration (hours)* | 0.75–1.5 | 2–3 | 1–3 | 0.5–3 |
| Elimination half-life (hours)* | 2 | 2.5–3 | 2.5–3.5 | 1–2 |
| Duration of effect on gastric acid secretion after dose (hours)* | | | | |
|   Nocturnal | 8 | Up to 13 | Up to 10–12 | Up to 10 |
|   Meal | 3–4 | Up to 3 | Up to 3–5 | Up to 4 |
| Excretion of oral dose (%) | | | | |
|   Renal | >48 | >50 | 65–70 | >90 |
|   Hepatic | <52 | <50 | 30–35 | <6 |
| **FDA-approved label indications, dosage, and administration of oral preparations** | | | | |
| Active DU | 800 mg hs, or 400 mg bid, or 300 mg qid | 150 mg bid or 300 mg hs | 40 mg hs or 20 mg bid | 300 mg hs or 150 mg bid |
| Maintenance of healed DU | 400 mg hs | 150 mg hs | 20 mg hs | 150 mg hs |
| Active benign GU | 800 mg hs or 300 mg qid | 150 mg bid | 40 mg hs | 150 mg bid or 300 mg hs |
| Maintenance of healed GU | Not approved | 150 mg hs | Not approved | Not approved |
| GERD (relief of GERD symptoms and healing of EE) | 800 mg bid or 400 mg qid | 150 mg bid for symptoms; 150 mg qid for EE, 150 mg bid for maintenance of healed GERD | 20 mg bid for symptoms, 20 mg or 40 mg bid for EE | 150 mg |
| Pathological hypersecretory conditions (e.g., ZES)† | 300 mg qid, Max: <600 mg qid | 150 mg bid Max: 6g/day | 20 mg q6h Max: 160 mg q6h | Not approved |
| Probable side effects | Headache, diarrhea, dizziness, somnolence, reversible confusion status | Headache, constipation, diarrhea | Headache, dizziness, constipation, diarrhea | Headache, dizziness, diarrhea, urticaria |

*Average values after an oral dose.

†Dosage should be adjusted to individual patient needs.

DU = duodenal ulcer; GU = gastric ulcer; EE = erosive esophagitis; Max = maximum; ZES = Zollinger-Ellison syndrome; qid = four times daily; bid = twice daily; hs = at bedtime.

(Data summarized from FDA, from most recently approved individual product monograph/label. Available at: http:www.accessdata.fda.gov/scripts/cder/drugsatfda/. Accessed April 16, 2005.)

there is little interference with hepatic microsomal drug metabolism. At higher doses, however, it may interfere with the clearance and increase the effect of various drugs, including warfarin, triazolam, glyburide, and glipizide. The dose should be adjusted in patients with severely impaired renal function. Oral and intravenous ranitidine are approved for use in pediatric populations from 1 month to 16 years of age.

**Famotidine** (Pepcid) contains a guanidine-substituted thiazole ring, which gives it the greatest affinity for $H_2$ receptors. Its bioavailability is less than that of the other drugs in this group, and its plasma excretion half-life is longer. Bioavailability may be slightly increased by food or slightly decreased by antacids, but with no significant clinical consequence. Famotidine does not inhibit cytochrome P450 in the liver. Use of famotidine in pediatric patients is supported by well-controlled studies, but the dose must be adjusted on the basis of pediatric age (see Chapter 58) and indication.

**Nizatidine** (Axid) has the highest bioavailability of the $H_2$-RAs in adults (>70%), but antacids decrease its absorption by about 10%. The therapeutic response to nizatidine is not affected by age. However, this agent is largely excreted by the kidney (>90%), and the risk of toxic reactions to it may be greater in patients with impaired renal function, especially in the elderly. The dose and/or frequency of administration should be reduced in proportion to the severity of renal dysfunction. Nizatidine does not inhibit cytochrome P450; therefore, no drug interactions have been identified with warfarin or theophylline. Reported side effects include anemia and urticaria.

**Roxatidine** is administered as the prodrug roxatidine acetate, which has a high bioavailability. It has been evaluated at a dose of 75 mg in the evening or twice daily for treatment of DU, benign gastric ulcer, GERD, and the prevention of recurrent ulcers. It reduces total pepsin secretion in a dose-dependent manner and appears to have an independent mucosal protective effect. Roxatidine does not interact with hepatic cytochrome P450. Another new $H_2$-RA, **lafutidine**, which is reported to exhibit gastric mucosal protective action mediated by capsaicin-sensitive afferent neurons in addition to a potent anti-secretory effect, has been used in *H. pylori* eradication clinical trials. Neither roxatidine nor lafutidine has been approved in North America.

### Adverse effects and special therapeutic uses

Side effects of $H_2$-RAs are rare, usually of a minor nature, and generally rapidly reversible once the medication is stopped. The drug interactions between cimetidine and other drugs that are substrates for cytochrome P450 are of little clinical importance because of the wide therapeutic index of these drugs and the fact that their blood levels do not necessarily reflect the magnitude of their pharmacological effect. However, interactions may be significant with some medications that have a narrow therapeutic index, such as theophylline, phenytoin, and warfarin. In these cases, another $H_2$-RA can be substituted to avoid a possible drug interaction.

Urinary excretion is the principal route of elimination of $H_2$-RAs, and the dose should be modified in patients with renal impairment in whom the risk of toxicity may be increased. There are minor and clinically insignificant alterations in the half-life, distribution, clearance, and bioavailability of $H_2$-RAs in patients with hepatic dysfunction; however, the dosing schedule should be adjusted in patients with severely impaired hepatic function.

Tachyphylaxis may occur with chronic use of $H_2$RAs so that increasing the dose does not achieve the same anti-secretory effect as previously or keep patients in remission. Abrupt withdrawal of $H_2$-RAs may cause a temporary rebound increase in gastric acid secretion to above pre-treatment values, which may contribute to a rapid resurgence of symptoms and recurrence of ulcer or GERD. Such rebound is more marked in subjects treated with cimetidine, ranitidine, and nizatidine than with famotidine. The mechanism is unclear; a possible contribution may be the up-regulation of the parietal cell $H_2$ receptors. Rebound acid hypersecretion is a transient phenomenon, but it can be clinically important.

$H_2$-RAs should be used during pregnancy only if clearly indicated clinically. A small amount of the oral dose of $H_2$-RAs is secreted in human breast milk, and a decision should be made whether to discontinue nursing or discontinue the drug after taking into account the importance of the drug to the treatment of the mother.

The effectiveness of nizatidine in pediatric patients has not been established. Intravenous administration of $H_2$-RAs is indicated in some hospitalized patients with pathological hypersecretory conditions or intractable ulcers, or as an alternative for short-term treatment of patients who are unable to take oral medication. $H_2$-RAs are also widely used in the treatment of bleeding ulcer and in the intensive care unit to prevent stress ulcer.

## Proton Pump Inhibitors (PPIs)

Currently available PPIs are all substituted benzimidazoles (Fig. 41-3) and share the same mechanism of action. They bind to the gastric proton pump ($H^+/K^+$-ATPase) on the parietal cell membrane, inactivating the exchange of $H^+$ ions for $K^+$ ions. This prevents the transport of HCl across the cell membrane to the lumen of the stomach, thus blocking the final step of acid production. Both basal and stimulated acid secretion are inhibited regardless of the stimulus. The use of omeprazole was first approved in 1989, and there are now five PPIs approved for use (Table 41-4). They are omeprazole (Prilosec in the United States and Losec in Canada, Europe, and Asia), lansoprazole (Prevacid, Zoton), pantoprazole (Pantoloc, Protonix), esomeprazole (Nexium), and rabeprazole (Aci-

**FIGURE 41-3** Structural formulae of the protein pump inhibitors (PPIs).

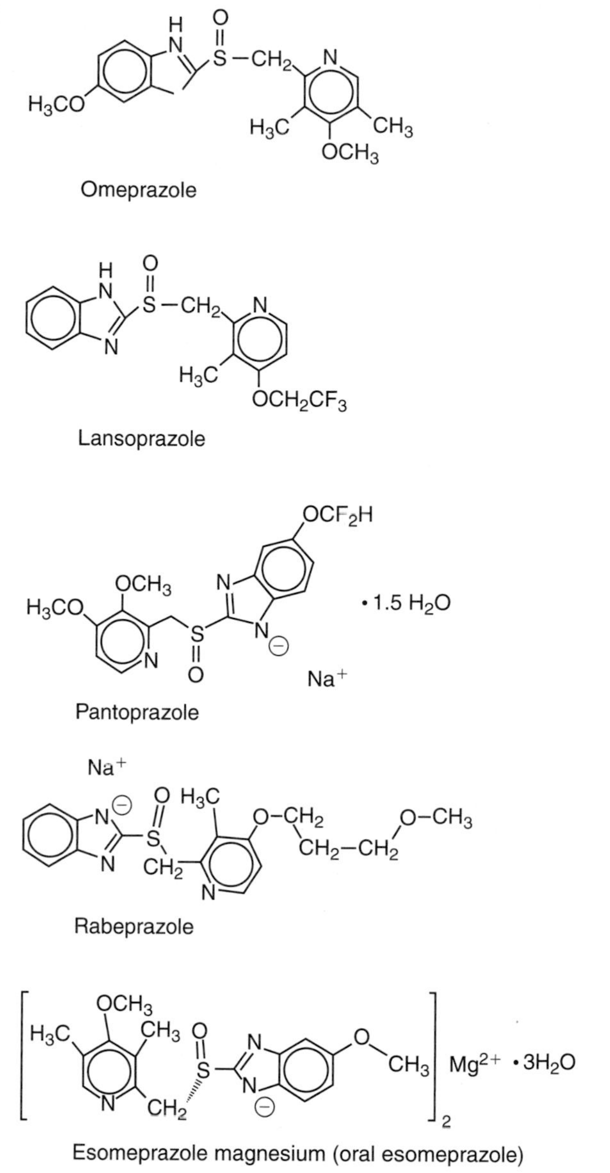

phex, not available in Canada). Esomeprazole is a second-generation PPI and is the *S*-isomer of omeprazole. It achieves a greater decrease in peak acid output than omeprazole when given at a similar dose.

## Efficacy

All PPIs show high efficacy in the treatment of symptoms and the healing of GERD and peptic ulcer disease, and they have been proven consistently to be more efficacious than the H2-RAs. For example, in severe reflux esophagitis, PPIs heal more than 80% of patients by 8 weeks, while H2-RAs heal approximately 60% over the same time. Indeed, PPIs heal a greater proportion of esophagitis patients by 2 weeks than H2-RAs do after 12 weeks. Therefore, the use of PPIs has dramatically altered the management of acid-secretory disorders. PPIs, except pantoprazole, are also approved for use in combination with one or more antibiotics in treatment regimens for the eradication of *H. pylori* infection. An eradication rate of ~90% is achieved with a PPI in combination with two antibiotics (triple therapy), or with two antibiotics plus bismuth (quadruple therapy), after 1 to 2 weeks of treatment.

Thus, PPIs are now the drugs of first choice for most gastric acid–related diseases. Although more expensive then H2-RAs, it is suggested that PPIs are most cost-effective in acid–peptic disorders. The indications approved by the FDA differ between PPIs, and at this time, lansoprazole has the largest number of approved indications.

However, there are some differences in pharmacokinetic and pharmacodynamic parameters for the PPIs. For example, lansoprazole 30 mg once daily achieves a maximal intragastric pH on day 1, and due to high oral bioavailability, it produces a faster onset and greater degree of acid inhibition than pantoprazole 40 mg or omeprazole 20 mg. The rapid onset explains the faster relief of acid-related symptoms, but the esophagitis or ulcer healing rates and recurrence rates are similar among all PPIs. Esomeprazole has higher bioavailability and is metabolized more slowly than omeprazole, and the area under the plasma concentration–time curve (AUC) for esomeprazole 20 mg is about 180% of that for omeprazole 20 mg. The plasma AUC is directly proportional to the amount of drug that has reached the systemic circulation and is available for binding to proton pumps in the parietal cell; thus, AUC is a direct indicator of the anti-secretory effect.

In studies, there was a statistically significantly higher healing rate of esophagitis in the esomeprazole groups (20 and 40 mg) than in the omeprazole group (20 mg) at 8 weeks. With esomeprazole 40 mg once daily, intragastric pH data show a further increase in control of gastric pH, with a lower rate of poor response for individual patients. It is still uncertain whether the statistically significant differences in GERD or ulcer healing rates seen in direct comparison trials of the PPIs are also clinically significant.

PPIs are rapidly absorbed once the drug enters the small intestine, and they undergo low rates of hepatic first-pass metabolism. The plasma elimination half-lives of PPIs are relatively short (<2 hours), but the drugs have a prolonged duration of acid suppression (>24 hours) because of covalent binding to the parietal cell H+/K+-ATPase. Thus, PPIs offer the convenience of once-daily dosing for most indications when given in the morning before breakfast. Once the PPI is bound to the acid pump, the binding usually lasts for the life of the parietal cell. PPIs only bind to the available pumps, and any newly synthesized proton pumps may secrete gastric acid after the PPI has left the circulation. The amount of unbound new pumps is small, but in a minority of patients they may

| TABLE 41-4 | Pharmacokinetic and Other Features of PPIs Used in North America | | | | |
|---|---|---|---|---|---|
| | **Omeprazole** | **Lansoprazole** | **Pantoprazole** | **Rabeprazole** | **Esomeprazole** |
| Preparation (may vary with manufacturer) | Delayed release capsules: 10, 20, or 40 mg Delayed release tablets: 20 mg | Delayed release capsules/disintegrating tablets: 15 or 30 mg Delayed release oral suspensions: 15 or 30 mg/packet Intravenous injection: 30 mg/vial | Delayed release tablets: 20 or 40 mg Intravenous injection: 40 mg/vial | Delayed release tablets: 20 mg | Delayed release capsules: 20 or 40 mg Intravenous injection: 20 or 40 mg/vial |
| Bioavailability (%)* | 30–40 | >80 | 77 | 52 | 64 Repeated once daily dose: 90 |
| Time to peak plasma concentration (hours)* | 0.5–3.5 | 1.7 | 2.5 | 2–5 | 1.5 |
| Elimination half-life in normal metabolizers (hours)* | 0.5–1 | 1.5 | 1 | 1–2 | 1–1.5 |
| Protein binding (%) | 95 | 97 | 98 | 96.3 | 97 |
| Route of elimination (%) Renal Biliary/feces | 77 23 | 33 66 | 71 18 | 90 10 | 80 20 |
| Metabolizing enzymes | CYP2C19 | CYP2C19, CYP3A4 | CYP2C19, CYP3A4 (minor: CYP2D6, 2C9) | CYP3A4, CYP2C19 | CYP2C19, CYP3A4 |
| **FDA-approved label indications, dosage, and administration of oral preparations** | | | | | |
| Active DU | 20 mg qd | 15 mg qd | Not approved | 20 mg qd | Not approved |
| Maintenance therapy of DU | Not approved | 15 mg qd | Not approved | Not approved | Not approved |
| Active benign GU | 40 mg qd | 30 mg qd | Not approved | Not approved | Not approved |
| For reduction of risk of GU associated with NSAIDs | Not approved | 15 mg qd for risk reduction, 30 mg qd for healing | Not approved | Not approved | 20 or 40 mg for up to 6 months |
| GERD (relief of GERD symptoms and healing of EE) | 20 mg qd | 15 mg qd for symptomatic GERD, 30 mg qd for EE | 40 mg qd | 20 mg qd | 20 mg qd for GERD, 20 or 40 mg qd for EE |
| Maintenance therapy of healing EE | 20 mg qd | 15 mg qd | 40 mg qd | 20 mg qd | 20 mg qd |
| Pathological hypersecretory conditions (e.g., ZES)[†] | 60 mg qd Max: 120 mg tid | 60 mg qd Max: 90 mg bid | 40 mg bid Max: 240 mg/day | 60 mg qd Max: 60 mg bid | Not approved |
| ***H. pylori* eradication for the reduction of DU recurrence** | | | | | |
| Triple therapy (with clarithromycin 500 mg bid and amoxicillin 1 g bid) | 20 mg bid × 10 days | 30 mg bid × 10–14 days | Not approved | 20 mg bid × 7 days | 40 mg qd × 10 days |
| Dual therapy | 40 mg qd × 14 days (with clarithromycin 500 mg tid) | 30 mg q8h × 14 days (with amoxicillin 1 g q8h) | Not approved | Not approved | Not approved |

*continued*

| TABLE 41-4 | continued | | | | |
|---|---|---|---|---|---|
| | Omeprazole | Lansoprazole | Pantoprazole | Rabeprazole | Esomeprazole |
| Drug interactions (excluding drugs affected by the change in gastric pH) | Diazepam, phenytoin, warfarin, clarithromycin, sucralfate | Theophylline, warfarin, sucralfate | None | Clarithromycin | Diazepam, clarithromycin |
| Pregnancy category | C | B | B | B | B |

*Average values after an oral dose.

†Dosage should be adjusted to individual patient needs.

DU = duodenal ulcer; GU = gastric ulcer; EE = erosive esophagitis; Max = maximum; ZES = Zollinger-Ellison syndrome; qd = once daily; bid = twice daily; tid = three times a day.

(Data summarized from FDA, from most recently approved individual product monograph/label. Available at: http:www.accessdata.fda.gov/scripts/cder/drugsatfda/. Accessed November 17, 2005.)

cause the persistence of acid secretion during PPI therapy at standard dose, underscoring the fact that there is substantial variation in the individual gastric anti-secretory response. Therefore, some patients may need to take their PPI twice daily to achieve optimal acid inhibition.

When the drug is discontinued, gastric secretory activity returns over 3 to 5 days and usually returns to pre-treatment levels within 2 weeks after withdrawal of omeprazole therapy. Some studies did not find acid rebound following discontinuation of omeprazole or other PPIs. Recent reports have suggested that H. pylori status can significantly affect the acid-inhibitory efficacy of PPI therapy. In one study, rebound acid hypersecretion occurred in H. pylori–negative patients after termination of an 8-week course of omeprazole 40 mg daily, and the degree of rebound increase in acid output was related to the degree of elevation of gastric pH during treatment. However, the clinical significance of any rebound hypersecretion following PPI therapy remains unclear. To reduce the risk of rebound hypersecretion, many physicians advise alternate-day therapy for a few days rather than an abrupt withdrawal of the PPI, although this approach is not based on evidence.

Prevacid NapraPAC is a combination package consisting of lansoprazole and naproxen, which is indicated for reduction in the risk of NSAID-associated GU in patients who require an NSAID.

All PPIs are acid-labile and thus rapidly degraded by gastric acid. Zegerid powder for oral suspension is an immediate-release formulation of omeprazole that is formulated with antacid (1680 mg sodium bicarbonate) to protect omeprazole from acid degradation. Zegerid is approved for treatment of DU, GERD, and maintenance of healing of EE. However, sodium bicarbonate is contraindicated in patients with metabolic alkalosis and hypocalcemia and should be used with caution in patients on sodium restriction.

OTC sale of omeprazole 20 mg has been approved for the treatment of frequent heartburn in patients older than 18 years. Treatment should be taken for a 2-week course. Intravenous lansoprazole, pantoprazole, and esomeprazole are available and approved for the treatment of erosive esophagitis in patients unable to take oral medications or with pathological acid hypersecretory states (pantoprazole only).

## Adverse effects and drug interactions

PPIs are generally well tolerated, and there are no significant differences among them with regard to adverse effects. The primary adverse effects are headache, nausea, abdominal pain, and diarrhea. PPIs are contraindicated in patients with known hypersensitivity to any product in the respective formulations. It is important to appreciate that symptomatic response to therapy with PPIs does not preclude the presence of a gastric malignancy, which may be masked by effective anti-secretory treatment. Atrophic gastritis has been noted occasionally in the gastric corpus biopsies from patients treated with long-term omeprazole, but it is now clear that this is related to underlying H. pylori infection. In rats, gastric ECL cell hyperplasia and carcinoid tumours have developed after high-dose PPI treatment for 24 months. Such results have not been seen in humans with any of the PPIs.

Reduced serum levels of vitamin $B_{12}$ have been found occasionally during long-term PPI therapy and are considered to be related to the presence of background atrophic gastritis rather than to be an effect of treatment. Most patients are unlikely to experience deficiency because of large body stores of vitamin $B_{12}$. However, vitamin $B_{12}$ level may be monitored in patients taking a PPI for longer than 3 years.

PPIs are mainly metabolized in the liver, and a dose reduction should be considered in patients with severe hepatic disease. Virtually no unchanged PPI is found in the urine, and PPI pharmacokinetics are not much affected by renal failure. No dose adjustment is necessary for patients with renal impairment or for the elderly. All of the PPIs are extensively metabolized to inactive metabolites by the hepatic cytochrome P450 isoenzymes and therefore can be expected to interact with other drugs that are substrates for that enzyme system.

Variation in the efficacy of PPIs occurs in different populations as a result of polymorphisms of the isoenzyme CYP2C19 (see Chapter 4). Slow metabolizers have a longer PPI plasma half-life. Poor metabolizers and heterozygous metabolizers exhibit greater acid inhibition and higher *H. pylori* eradication rates than homozygous rapid metabolizers of PPIs. In turn, genetic differences may cause difference in healing rates for GERD and PPI-based *H. pylori* eradication therapies, especially in Asian populations in whom there is a higher proportion of poor metabolizers. Rabeprazole and lansoprazole are reported to be less affected by CYP2C19 polymorphisms.

Clinically significant drug interactions are few for any of the PPIs in the general population. Omeprazole may inhibit the metabolism of diazepam, flurazepam, triazolam, phenytoin, and warfarin, so it is wise to monitor the clinical effect and dosing regimens of these drugs. Newer PPIs with different metabolic pathways may have fewer interactions than omeprazole. Co-administration of omeprazole, rabeprazole, or esomeprazole with clarithromycin has resulted in increased plasma levels of both the PPI and clarithromycin. The bioavailability of lansoprazole and omeprazole may be reduced when they are administered concomitantly with sucralfate, and the PPIs should be taken at least 30 minutes before the sucralfate. All the PPIs may interfere with the absorption of drugs requiring an acidic pH for optimal absorption, such as digoxin, ampicillin, ketoconazole, and iron salts. Concomitant administration of antacids does not affect the absorption of PPIs.

Because of the profound effect of PPIs on acid production, a marked rise in the serum gastrin levels occurs as an exaggerated pharmacological effect.

Omeprazole is listed as FDA pregnancy category C; lansoprazole, pantoprazole, rabeprazole, and esomeprazole are in pregnancy category B. It is not known whether omeprazole and lansoprazole are excreted in human breast milk, but they have been found in rat breast milk. PPIs should be used during pregnancy or in nursing mothers only if there is a clear clinical indication and the potential benefit exceeds the potential risk. The safety and effectiveness of omeprazole have not been established in patients less than 2 years old, or in patients under 1 year old for lansoprazole. Pantoprazole, rabeprazole, and esomeprazole have not been investigated in patients under 18 years of age.

## Mucosal Protective Agents

Mucosal protective medications protect the gastric and duodenal mucosa from damage by acid and pepsin.

Unlike H2-RAs and PPIs, gastric protective agents do not inhibit the secretion of acid.

### Sucralfate

**Sucralfate** (Carafate, Sulcrate) is a sulfated disaccharide complex of aluminum hydroxide that heals ulcers by mechanisms that are not fully understood. It is known to exert its effect through a local rather than a systemic action. It binds to tissue proteins and forms a protective barrier that may help maintain the integrity of the mucosa, thereby preventing access of bile salts and pepsin. It also enhances cell restitution and re-epithelization, allowing the ulcer to heal and preventing further damage by gastric acid. Sucralfate enhances epithelial proliferation by binding epidermal growth factor at the site of mucosal injury. It may also weakly inhibit *H. pylori* growth. Sucralfate is approved for short-term treatment (up to 8 weeks) and for maintenance treatment of DU at reduced dose. In some patients with ulcer, sucralfate is as effective as H2-RAs with respect to healing rates, but is less effective than PPIs.

Sucralfate is effective in various acid–peptic disorders and has few side effects. Sucralfate (tablets or suspension) is usually taken in a dose of 1 g four times a day, 1 hour before meals and at bedtime. Constipation and abdominal pain may occur. It blocks the absorption of some drugs, including digoxin, phenytoin, fluoroquinolone antibiotics, ranitidine, and PPIs, presumably as a result of sucralfate binding to the concomitant drug in the GI tract. Therefore, these drugs should not be taken at the same time as sucralfate. Sucralfate is in pregnancy category B, but it is considered relatively safe. It should not be used in pediatric patients.

### Prostaglandin E (PGE) analogues

Prostaglandin E (PGE) analogues (misoprostol, enprostil, arbaprostil, trimoprostil and rioprostil; see also Chapter 27) are synthetic prostaglandins similar to natural PGE produced by the body. These drugs protect the gastric mucosa by increasing mucus and bicarbonate secretion and by enhancing mucosal blood flow in the stomach; they also enhance epithelial regeneration. They bind to the PG receptors on the parietal cell and inhibit gastric acid secretion (see Fig. 41-1). PGE analogues are seldom used for the treatment of acute ulcer because of their poor symptom relief and modest healing effect, which is less than that of H2-RAs. They have a dose-dependent therapeutic effect on ulcer healing.

**Misoprostol** (Cytotec), a synthetic $PGE_1$ analogue, is the most common drug of this class; it is approved only for the prevention of NSAID-induced gastric ulcer in patients at high risk of complications from gastric ulcer. Its use is based on the fact that NSAIDs inhibit prostaglandin synthesis, thus contributing to mucosal damage. Misoprostol should be taken (200 µg four times daily) for the duration of NSAID therapy. It contains approximately equal amounts of the two diastereomers with their enantiomers (Fig. 41-4). It is rapidly absorbed after oral administration and has a half-life of 20 to 40 minutes. It undergoes some hepatic biotransformation but is mostly (80%) excreted via the kidney. The plasma concentration is reduced by use of concomitant antacids. Misoprostol does not affect the P450 enzyme system. The major side effects are diarrhea (13%) and abdominal pain (7%), which usually occur early in the course of therapy and are self-limiting, or which can be solved by slight dose reduction, but sometimes require discontinuation of misoprostol. Because of its abortifacient property, misoprostol is contraindicated in pregnant women or women with child-bearing potential (under pregnancy category X).

## Bismuth Compounds

Bismuth preparations have been used for the treatment of GI diseases for several centuries, but it is only recently that the mechanism of action of bismuth in accelerating the healing of peptic ulcer has become better understood. **Colloidal bismuth subcitrate** (CBS; De-Nol) and **bismuth subsalicylate** (Pepto-Bismol) have a mucosal protective effect and an antimicrobial effect against *H. pylori* infection. Bismuth subcitrate binds to proteins in the base of an ulcer and provides a protective coating that allows the ulcer to heal. It also inhibits peptic activity and stimulates local PG synthesis. CBS counteracts the adverse effects of *H. pylori* by inhibiting bacterial proteolytic enzyme activity. The healing rates of peptic ulcer in comparative trials were very similar between bismuth compounds and H2-RAs. CBS is more widely used than other bismuth compounds worldwide but is not available in North America. Bismuth subsalicylate is available OTC in North America for the treatment of traveller's diarrhea, indigestion, heartburn, nausea, and overindulgence. Bismuth subsalicylate is also prescribed for the eradication of *H. pylori* infection in patients with active DU or a history

of DU. It is used in combination with a gastric acid inhibitor (H2-RA or PPI) and two antibiotics (e.g., Helidac therapy includes bismuth subsalicylate 525 mg four times daily, metronidazole 250 mg four times daily, and tetracycline hydrochloride 500 mg four times daily for 14 days).

CBS remains largely in the intestinal tract; little of the bismuth in CBS is dissolved and absorbed. Any absorbed bismuth is excreted in the urine, and the bismuth in CBS is mainly excreted in feces. Pepto-Bismol reacts with hydrochloric acid in the stomach to form bismuth oxychloride and salicylic acid. Most of the salicylic acid, but very little bismuth, is absorbed. Possible side effects are harmless darkening of the tongue or stool (bismuth salts react with hydrogen sulfide to form bismuth sulfide, which turns the stool a black colour) and constipation. Serious adverse reactions are rare when bismuth is used at the recommended doses; however, an overdose can cause problems in some patients because of other GI disorders such as constipation. High-dose bismuth subsalicylate may cause salicylate accumulation. Like aspirin, bismuth subsalicylate may be associated with an increased risk of Reye syndrome, so it is contraindicated in children or teenagers who have, or are recovering from, influenza or chickenpox.

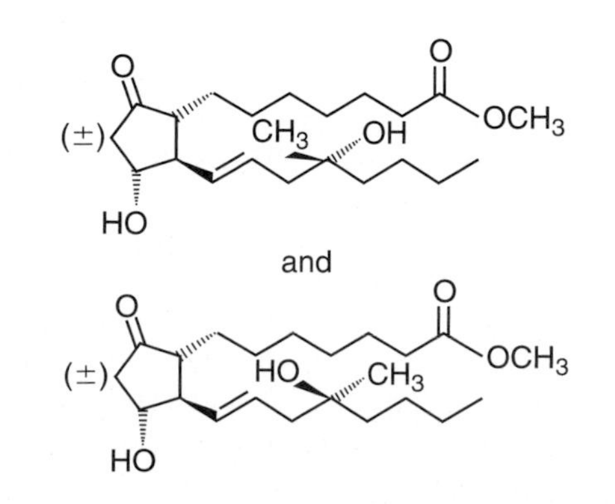

## Anticholinergics

Anticholinergics such as atropine and propantheline are anti-spasmodics but are not used for gastric acid suppression because of their adverse effects (see Chapter 12). **Pirenzepine** (Gastrozepin), a complex tricyclic compound, is a selective muscarinic M1 receptor antagonist and thus reduces both acid and pepsin secretion. It may also have mucosal protective properties. It is used for the prevention of stress ulcer in some European countries. Because of its low efficacy, use of pirenzepine for acid–peptic disorders was discontinued in Canada in 1996.

## Antimicrobials

The discovery of the link between peptic ulcer disease, particularly DU, and *H. pylori* infection has resulted in a dramatic change in treatment options. In addition to treatment aimed at decreasing the production of gastric acid, antibiotics are prescribed for patients with *H. pylori* infection. The most effective therapy is a 1- to 2-week triple drug treatment that eradicates the bacteria, heals the ulcer, and reduces the risk of ulcer recurrence in 90% of patients with DU. Patients with a gastric ulcer that is not associated with NSAIDs also benefit similarly from *H. pylori* eradication if, in fact, the infection is present.

Generally, two antibiotics (e.g., clarithromycin, amoxicillin, metronidazole) are used with a PPI, or tetracycline and metronidazole are used with bismuth subsalicylate (see Table 41-4). For example, a triple therapy includes a PPI (e.g., omeprazole 20 mg), plus amoxicillin 1000 mg and clarithromycin 500 mg (PPI+AC), or, less commonly,

| FIGURE 41-4 | Structural formula of misoprostol. |

plus clarithromycin 500 mg and metronidazole 250 mg (PPI+CM). An alternative triple therapy could be bismuth plus metronidazole 250 mg and tetracycline 500 mg (BMT); a quadruple therapy includes a PPI plus BMT. In cases where there is bacterial resistance to metronidazole, another antibiotic such as clarithromycin may be chosen. A PPI administered with clarithromycin and amoxicillin in triple therapy is active against most strains of *H. pylori* both in vitro and in the clinical setting. A combination (Prevpac) containing lansoprazole capsules (30 mg × 2), amoxicillin capsules (500 mg × 4) and clarithromycin tablets (500 mg × 2) together in a single daily administration pack provides for optimal patient adherence to *H. Pylori* eradication therapy.

*H. pylori* eradication regimens are complex and have several side effects and potential drug interactions with the antibiotics. For example, concomitant administration of clarithromycin with cisapride, pimozide, or terfenadine is contraindicated for there are reports of resulting cardiac arrhythmias with prolongation of the QT interval. Clarithromycin (pregnancy category C) is contraindicated in patients with a known hypersensitivity to macrolide antibiotics. Amoxicillin is contraindicated in patients with a history of an allergic reaction to any of the penicillins. Antibiotic resistance is another issue. For example, metronidazole resistance and clarithromycin resistance have been increasing in developed countries and occur in patients previously treated with the antimicrobials without successful eradication. Therefore, other antibiotics are being studied as alternative choices. Because of the measurable eradication failure rate, and the difficulty getting effective concentrations of antibiotics to the site of bacterial colonization, it is important to perform antibiotic susceptibility testing. Rescue regimens including antibiotics such as furazolidone, rifabutin, moxifloxacin, levofloxacin, doxycycline, and the quinolones are under investigation in clinical trials (for details of antibiotics see Chapters 50, 51, 52, 53).

## Promotility Agents

Promotility, or prokinetic, agents are designed to correct defects in gastrointestinal neuromuscular activity such as that occurring in pathological GERD and in patients with dyspepsia. Prokinetics may help to relieve reflux by accelerating gastric emptying and reducing the dwell time of acid in the distal esophagus. Prokinetics seldom work alone and are usually used in addition to antacid or antisecretory therapy in GERD. They can improve symptoms when used alone in mild GERD, but the effect on healing is modest, providing benefit only in mild erosive esophagitis. A more complete description of these drugs and their uses in lower gastrointestinal motility disorders is provided in Chapter 42.

**Cisapride** (Propulsid), though now withdrawn, was formerly the most commonly used drug in the prokinetic class. It acts as an agonist at muscarinic (M2) and some serotonergic (5-HT4) receptors, and as an antagonist at other serotonergic (5-HT3) receptors. It is a benzamide compound that increases LES pressure and promotes peristalsis, and it was used to treat nocturnal heartburn. However, it was withdrawn from the market in 2000 because of adverse cardiac effects, including prolongation of the QT interval leading to cardiac dysrhythmias. These effects appeared to be associated with concomitant use of drugs that affect the metabolism of cisapride by inhibition of hepatic cytochrome P450. Newer prokinetics in this class, such as the 5-HT4 receptor partial agonist tegaserod (Zelnorm), are being investigated in GERD patients and may have fewer adverse effects.

**Tegaserod** has both promotility and anti-nociceptive effects. In clinical trials, it improved esophageal acid exposure but has not been demonstrated to be an effective monotherapy in GERD. It is under investigation in combined therapy for a subset of GERD and functional dyspepsia patients.

**Metoclopramide** (Reglan, Maxeran) stimulates motility of the upper GI tract without stimulating gastric, biliary, or pancreatic secretion. It causes a dose-related increase in the LES resting tone and increases the amplitude of peristaltic contractions in the esophagus. It slightly increases their duration and speed of propagation, but it does not disturb synchrony of contractions. It does not interfere with LES relaxation in the course of swallowing. Its mode of action is unclear, but it seems to sensitize tissues to the action of acetylcholine. The principal beneficial effect is on symptoms of postprandial and daytime heartburn; there is less effect on nocturnal symptoms. Oral metoclopramide is approved only for short-term use (10 to 15 mg up to four times daily for 4 to 12 weeks) for adults with symptomatic proven GERD who fail to respond to conventional therapy.

Metoclopramide can pass the blood–brain barrier and has anti-dopaminergic side effects, including neurological and psychotropic reactions such as drowsiness, restlessness, or depression. Moreover, it has potentially severe adverse effects through extrapyramidal reactions, which may be irreversible (see Chapter 42). Thus, its side effects limit its use, and it is seldom used clinically these days.

**Bethanechol chloride** (Urecholine) is a cholinergic agonist, which is a synthetic ester structurally and pharmacologically related to acetylcholine. It acts principally by stimulation of the parasympathetic nervous system. It stimulates gastric motility, increases gastric tone, and may restore impaired peristalsis. Effects on the gastrointestinal and urinary tracts appear within 30 minutes after oral administration. It has been used as a prokinetic to treat GERD and gastroparesis in several studies. However, it is not approved for use in GERD, and it can cause abdominal cramping, blurred vision, shortness of breath, and other cholinergic symptoms.

**Domperidone** (Motilium) is primarily a peripheral dopaminergic antagonist acting on $D_2$ receptors in GI smooth muscle. It enhances gastric emptying, and this effect is more important than the effect on the LES. It helps to reduce reflux and the sensation of fullness. It has been used in GERD patients in clinical studies. It is used in Canada generally for nausea, vomiting, dyspepsia, and heartburn (10 mg three times a day), but it has not been approved by the FDA in the United States. It is excreted in breast milk, and its risk to an exposed breastfeeding infant is unknown.

Several drugs in this class are currently under development, especially those with a potential therapeutic role in altering fundic accommodation and enhancing antral emptying and antropyloroduodenal coordination. Particularly, the new 5-HT$_4$ agonists such as **mosapride**, GABA$_B$ agonists such as **baclofen**, and a dopamine $D_2$ antagonist, the benzamide derivative **itopride**, are under investigation and may be of value. For example, $\gamma$-aminobutyric acid (GABA) is a potent inhibitory transmitter in the central nervous system; it antagonizes the release of neurotransmitters from vagal nerve afferents through its action on the GABA$_B$ receptor. The GABA$_B$ agonist baclofen reduces the rate of transient LES relaxations and increases basal LES pressure; thus, it reduces symptoms and episodes of GERD and raises gastric pH. However, this agent has a relatively high rate of side effects, including seizures and drowsiness, and probably will not be routinely used in patients. Further research to find a baclofen-like agent with fewer and less troublesome side effects may yield a useful alternative treatment for GERD in the future.

## SUMMARY

Acid-related disorders include peptic ulcer disease and gastroesophageal reflux disease, and gastric acid plays a critical role in their development. *H. pylori* infection and NSAIDs play important etiological roles in peptic ulcers and ulcer complications. The suppression of gastric acid secretion with anti-secretory agents including H$_2$ receptor antagonists and proton pump inhibitors has been the mainstay of medical therapy of these disorders. With the widespread use of proton pump inhibitors, together with *H. pylori* eradication therapy or prokinetic agents, medical treatment is now successful in relieving symptoms, healing peptic ulcers and esophagitis, and preventing complications in most patients.

## SUGGESTED READINGS

Armstrong D, Marshall JK, Chiba N, et al. Canadian Consensus Conference on the management of gastroesophageal reflux disease in adults—update 2004. *Can J Gastroenterol.* 2005;19: 15-35.

Chong E, Ensom MH. Pharmacogenetics of the proton pump inhibitors: a systematic review. *Pharmacotherapy.* 2003;23: 460-471.

Ford AC, Delaney BC, Forman D, Moayyedi P. Eradication therapy in Helicobacter pylori positive peptic ulcer disease: systematic review and economic analysis. *Am J Gastroenterol.* 2004;99:1833-1855.

Hawkey CJ, Naesdal J, Wilson I, et al. Relative contribution of mucosal injury and Helicobacter pylori in the development of gastroduodenal lesions in patients taking non-steroidal anti-inflammatory drugs. *Gut.* 2002;51:336-343.

Howden C, Hunt RH. Guidelines for the management of Helicobacter pylori infection. *Am J Gastroenterol.* 1998;93: 2330-2338.

Huang JQ, Hunt RH. Pharmacological and pharmacodynamic essentials of H(2)-receptor antagonists and proton pump inhibitors for the practising physician. *Best Pract Res Clin Gastroenterol.* 2001;15:355-370.

Katz PO. Optimizing medical therapy for gastroesophageal reflux disease: state of the art. *Rev Gastroenterol Disord.* 2003;3:59-69.

Maton PN, Burton ME. Antacids revisited: a review of their clinical pharmacology and recommended therapeutic use. *Drugs.* 1999;57:855-870.

Qvigstad G, Waldum H. Rebound hypersecretion after inhibition of gastric acid secretion. *Basic Clin Pharmacol Toxicol.* 2004; 94:202-208.

Robinson M, Horn J. Clinical pharmacology of proton pump inhibitors, what the practising physician needs to know. *Drugs.* 2003;63:2739-2754.

Sachs G. Physiology of the parietal cell and therapeutic implications. *Pharmacotherapy.* 2003;23(10 pt 2):68S-73S.

Urushidani T, Forte JG. Signal transduction and activation of acid secretion in the parietal cell. *J Membr Biol.* 1997;159:99-111.

# 42

# Pharmacotherapy of Intestinal Motility Disorders and Inflammatory Bowel Disease

## SC GANGULI

### CASE HISTORY

A 30-year-old teacher developed a flu-like illness consisting of myalgias, fatigue, sore throat, and a low-grade fever, which lasted for 7 days. She seemed to recover completely, but about 10 days later, she noted the onset of progressive nausea. When seen 8 weeks later, she was experiencing nausea for 3 to 4 hours each day, was vomiting every 1 to 2 days, and had lost 10 kg (22 lbs), mainly due to decreased oral intake, especially of fatty foods. Except for mild epigastric tenderness and a succussion splash, physical examination (including neurological examination) was normal. Negative test results included those for CBC, electrolytes, thyroid studies, liver function tests, calcium, amylase, and glucose. Endoscopy and biopsies of the stomach and duodenum, as well as a small bowel follow-through, were also negative. A nuclear study of gastric emptying was carried out and showed significant delay. A diagnosis of postviral gastroparesis was made. Domperidone 20 mg orally four times a day (before meals and at bedtime) was started and resulted in marked improvement of her symptoms. She did well until a year later when she developed nipple tenderness and small amounts of milky discharge. Her prolactin level was checked and was found to be three times normal. Domperidone was stopped, and 2 weeks later, the prolactin level was within the normal range. Domperidone was then restarted at a lower dose, and it continued to control her symptoms.

## GASTROINTESTINAL MOTILITY

The physiology of gastrointestinal tract motility is currently an area of intensive research. The gastrointestinal tract has smooth muscle with intrinsic and variable contractions. There are sphincter-like structures at the gastroesophageal junction, the pylorus, and the ileocolonic junction. The various contractile functions should normally be smoothly coordinated throughout the gastrointestinal tract so that the contents are moved along as on a well-regulated conveyor belt. Muscular propulsive activity should also change with swallowing or with ingestion of food. Nervous system control of the enteric smooth muscle accounts for some of this adjustment. Hormonal factors also affect gastrointestinal tract motility. Motilin, a gastrointestinal hormone acting on specific motilin receptors in the enteric nerve plexuses, helps to initiate the "migrating myoelectric complexes" in the proximal bowel. Other external factors sometimes play a role (e.g., osmotic retention of excessive fluid in the lumen due to non-absorbable salts such as magnesium).

Several types of drugs are used to correct disturbances due to either decreased motility (e.g., gastroparesis, colonic inertia) or increased motility (diarrhea). These drugs include the so-called prokinetic agents, laxatives, and anti-diarrheals.

## PROKINETIC AGENTS

Metoclopramide, domperidone, and tegaserod (Table 42-1) are the major prokinetic agents that work by affecting neural control of enteric smooth muscle activity. A simplified version of this mechanism is shown in Figure 42-1. The final motor pathway of the enteric plexuses innervating smooth muscle is predominantly cholinergic. Thus, a prokinetic drug may work by enhancing the cholinergic effect directly (i.e., as a cholinergic agonist) or indirectly (either by enhancing acetylcholine release or by sensitizing the muscarinic receptors of the enteric smooth muscle so that the threshold for acetylcholine action is lower), or by interfering with the action of dopamine (i.e., as a dopamine antagonist). The overall outcome on smooth

| TABLE 42-1 | Prokinetic Agents | | |
|---|---|---|---|
| | Metoclopramide | Domperidone | Tegaserod |
| Structure | Benzamide class | Benzimidazole class | Aminoguanidine |
| Mechanism | Anti-dopaminergic (central and peripheral) Augments acetylcholine release | Anti-dopaminergic (peripheral) No cholinergic activity | 5-HT$_4$ partial agonist No cholinergic activity |
| Lower esophageal sphincter tone | Increase | Increase | No change |
| Gastric motility | Increase | Increase | Increase |
| Intestinal motility | ? Increase small bowel | No effect | Increase |
| Side effects | Many | Few | Few |

muscle activity varies from species to species and may vary somewhat from one part of the human gastrointestinal tract to another.

## Metoclopramide (Maxeran, Reglan)

This is a derivative of procainamide and is a central dopaminergic D$_2$ receptor antagonist and serotonergic (5-HT$_4$ receptor) agonist. At high doses, it is also a 5-HT$_3$ receptor antagonist. The structure of metoclopramide is shown in Chapter 12, Figure 12-6.

### Mechanism of action

Its mechanism of action is complicated. Its primary mechanism is to stimulate 5-HT$_4$ receptors and thereby enhance coordinated transmission in cholinergic nerve plexuses that finally release acetylcholine at muscarinic M$_2$ receptors on the muscle cells; its effect is abolished by atropine. Since it is a dopaminergic neuron antagonist in the central nervous system (CNS), it may possibly also have a direct influence on dopaminergic or other innervation of gastrointestinal smooth muscle.

In the upper gastrointestinal tract, metoclopramide raises the lower esophageal sphincter (LES) pressure (tone). It increases the amplitude of gastric (especially antral) contractions, relaxes the pyloric sphincter and the duodenal bulb, and increases peristalsis of the duodenum and jejunum, but does not influence gastric acid secretion. Metoclopramide increases the rate of gastric emptying in most people. It can be used for treatment of diabetic gastroparesis (10 mg four times a day for 2 to 8 weeks). Injectable metoclopramide can be used for the prevention of nausea and vomiting associated with cancer chemotherapy or occurring post-operatively. It has a good anti-emetic effect arising from its central D$_2$ and 5-HT$_3$ blocking actions.

### Pharmacokinetics

Metoclopramide is rapidly and well absorbed after oral administration and has an onset of action of 30 to 60 minutes. Peak plasma concentrations occur at about 1 to 2 hours after a single oral dose. Its excretion is predominantly renal, partly as the unchanged drug and partly as the sulfate or glucuronide. Approximately 85% of the oral dose is excreted in the urine within 72 hours. Its elimination half-life is 4 to 6 hours. It is not highly bound to plasma proteins, and it crosses the blood–brain barrier easily.

### Adverse effects

Metoclopramide has side effects (Table 42-2) such as fatigue, dizziness, faintness, and various extrapyramidal syndromes caused by its central anti-dopaminergic activity, including parkinsonism (reversible) and tardive dyskinesia, which may be irreversible. Increased irritability may be an important side effect in infants because the drug may aggravate gastroesophageal reflux in them. In children, the major extrapyramidal syndrome is an oculogyric crisis with torticollis and neck pain. Children who develop phenothiazine-induced oculogyric crisis may be more prone to this problem with metoclopramide. Phenothiazines, monoamine oxidase inhibitors, tricyclic antidepressants, and sympathomimetic drugs should not be given along with metoclopramide. With chronic use, metoclopramide may also cause increased serum prolactin levels in adults, which may result in gynecomastia and/or galactorrhea. Because it accelerates gastric emptying, it may increase the rate of absorption and the action of some other drugs.

## Domperidone (Motilium)

This benzimidazole derivative is a peripheral dopamine antagonist. It has no procholinergic effects. It is effective in reducing gastroesophageal reflux by increasing esophageal peristalsis and increasing lower esophageal sphincter pressure; it also increases gastric emptying rate in healthy indi-

**FIGURE 42-1** Mechanisms of action of prokinetic agents. Acetylcholine (ACh) from presynaptic neurons stimulates post-ganglionic primary motor neuron to release ACh, which acts on an ACh receptor on the smooth muscle cell. Atropine blocks the ACh receptor on a muscle cell. Dopamine stimulates $D_2$ receptors and inhibits release of ACh by the postsynaptic primary motor neuron. Tegaserod and metoclopramide stimulate serotonin receptors ($5-HT_4$), resulting in release of ACh by presynaptic neurons. Domperidone and metoclopramide antagonize the inhibitory effect of dopamine at $D_2$ receptors and augment postganglionic ACh release. NANC = non-adrenergic, non-cholinergic neuron. (Adapted from *Goodman and Gilman's The Pharmacological Basis of Therapeutics.* 10th ed. McGraw-Hill: New York; 2002:1024, with permission.)

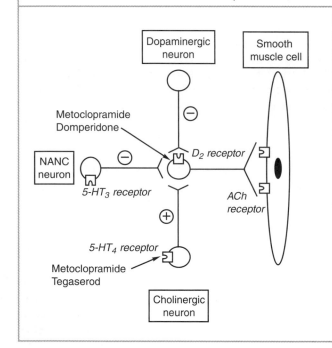

torrhea, menstrual irregularities, or impotence. Rare cases of prolongation of the QTc interval in the electrocardiograph (ECG) have been reported, and therefore this drug should be used with caution in patients on other QTc-prolonging drugs.

## Tegaserod (Zelnorm)

This aminoguanidine derivative of serotonin (Fig. 42-2) is a partial agonist at $5-HT_4$ receptors, including receptors located on modulatory cholinergic neurons along the gastrointestinal tract. It does not bind to human recombinant $5-HT_3$ or dopamine $D_2$ receptors. It is indicated in the short-term (up to 12 weeks) treatment of women with irritable bowel syndrome, in which constipation is the predominant symptom, or for chronic idiopathic constipation. In such cases, it has been shown to decrease global symptoms, abdominal discomfort, and bloating and increase stool frequency. Human studies have shown that in addition to accelerating colonic transit, tegaserod increases gastric emptying rate.

### Pharmacokinetics

Tegaserod is rapidly absorbed from the small intestine, having a $T_{max}$ of 0.8 to 1.3 hours and a bioavailability of $11 \pm 3\%$ if taken at least 30 minutes before meals. (If taken with meals, its bioavailability is decreased by 40 to 65%, and $C_{max}$ is reduced by 20 to 40%.) It is approximately 98% bound to plasma proteins and does not cross the blood–brain barrier in rats. Steady-state plasma levels are reached after 8 days. It is excreted primarily as inactive glucuronides. The elimination half-life is $8.6 \pm 5.4$ hours

viduals and in patients with gastroparesis. It relieves nausea by its effects on the chemoreceptor trigger zone. Absorption is prompt (time to peak serum concentration is 30 to 120 minutes). Domperidone is metabolized primarily by hepatic N-dealkylation. Plasma protein binding is high (93%), and the elimination half-life is 7 hours.

Unlike metoclopramide, domperidone has few side effects, though it can cause headache and abdominal cramps. It is thought to be well tolerated mainly because the quaternary nitrogen does not permit it to cross the blood–brain barrier as readily as metoclopramide does. Dystonic symptoms are rare; however, it may be associated with elevated serum prolactin in approximately 6% of patients, occasionally resulting in gynecomastia, galac-

| TABLE 42-2 | Estimated Frequency of Side Effects with Metoclopramide | |
|---|---|
| **Side Effects** | **Patients (%)** |
| Central nervous system | |
| Drowsiness, lethargy | 4–10 |
| Dizziness, faintness | 1–6 |
| Dystonic reactions | 1 |
| Increased prolactin secretion, galactorrhea | Occasional |
| Anxiety, agitation | Rare |
| Gastrointestinal | |
| Diarrhea, constipation, abdominal cramps | 1 |
| Other | |
| Rashes | <1 |
| Oropharyngeal edema | Rare |
| Hypertensive crisis with pheochromocytoma | 3 cases |
| Cardiac arrhythmia | Occasional |

for the recommended dose of 6 mg twice a day. The corresponding volume of distribution is 368 ± 223 L/70 kg, or approximately 5 L/kg, which implies a very high uptake into certain tissues where the drug accumulates. No adjustment in dose is needed for the elderly or for patients with mild to moderate renal or mild hepatic impairment.

### Adverse effects

Based on randomized clinical trials in over 11 000 patients and post-marketing surveillance for 3 years in 3 million patients, the main side effect was diarrhea (8.8% in patients vs. 3.8% for placebo), which was usually transient and led to discontinuation of the drug in only about 2% of patients in clinical trials. However, rare cases of severe diarrhea have been reported in 0.04% of patients and may result in dehydration or hospitalization. Approximately 20 cases of ischemic colitis have been reported in post-marketing surveillance, but since recent studies have shown that ischemic colitis is increased in patients with irritable bowel syndrome, it is unclear if these are really due to tegaserod. There is no evidence of rebound constipation upon termination of therapy, and careful analysis of over 11 000 ECGs has shown no changes in any electrocardiographic parameters.

Human studies have shown no clinically significant interactions with theophylline, dextromethorphan, warfarin, oral contraceptives, or digoxin. While tegaserod inhibits CYP1A2 and CYP2D6, this occurs at drug concentrations more than 100 times those seen with the 6 mg dose and is not clinically significant. The main metabolite does not inhibit cytochrome P450 enzymes. Tegaserod is contraindicated in cases of severe renal impairment and moderate to severe hepatic impairment and in patients with known or suspected bowel obstruction, symptomatic gallbladder disease, dysfunction of the sphincter of Oddi, or diarrhea.

## Macrolides

**Erythromycin,** a macrolide antibiotic (see Chapter 52), is representative of a new group of prokinetic agents that appear to work mainly through a unique mechanism. It increases gastrointestinal contractility mainly by acting as an agonist at the motilin receptor, for which it is a competitive ligand. It may also act at the neuromuscular junction. Current research is aimed at developing macrolides with predominant prokinetic activity and little antibiotic effect.

Erythromycin increases LES pressure and enhances esophageal contractility. It speeds gastric emptying and improves the coordination of antral and duodenal contractions. It appears to increase contractility of the gallbladder. In the colon, it induces migrating myoelectric complexes as motilin does. Its main clinical use (other than as an antibiotic) is in enhancing gastric emptying,

**FIGURE 42-2**  Structural formula of tegaserod.

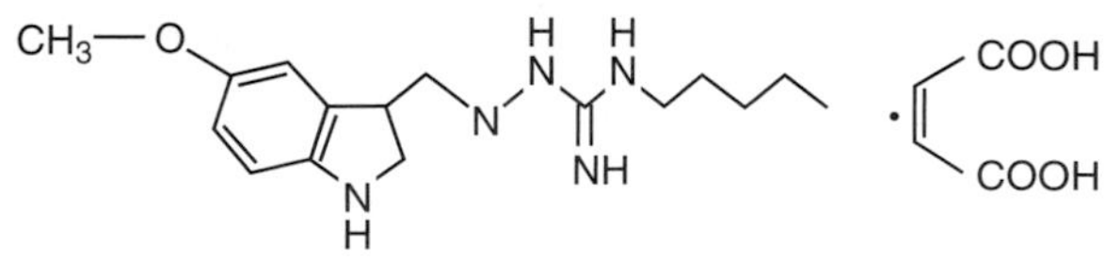

for which the liquid estolate form in doses of 1 to 3 mg/kg four times a day (before meals and at bedtime) appears to be most effective. It also can be used to treat constipation due to abnormal colonic motility, but it works best if there is some vestige of major migrating myoelectric complexes prior to treatment. It is clinically ineffective for treating disorders of esophageal motility.

Excretion is primarily hepatic; less than 5% is found in the urine. The half-life ranges from 60 to 150 minutes. Adverse reactions to erythromycin include rare but well-documented cases of hepatotoxicity as well as QT prolongation and torsades de pointes (see Chapter 33). In addition, dose-related symptoms of abdominal pain, cramps, nausea, vomiting, and diarrhea may occur. With prolonged use, there is, at least theoretically, a risk of selecting resistant bacterial strains. Tachyphylaxis develops for this and other prokinetic drugs. Since erythromycin is metabolized via CYP3A4, interactions with other drug substrates for CYP3A4 are possible.

## LAXATIVES

Laxatives can be considered prokinetic agents for the colon. Indeed, certain prokinetic agents enhance colonic motility. However, the mechanism of action of the laxative drugs is somewhat more complicated than simply affecting motility, because these drugs also lead to increased water content in the stool. Laxatives may promote colonic secretion of water by indirect or irritative effects or by modifying cellular processes for sodium and water secretion (Table 42-3). They may increase the excretion of water in the stool by either osmotic or bulk action. Certain laxatives retain water and block its colonic absorption. Colonic distension by hydrated luminal contents may then enhance colonic motility.

The average diet should contain sufficient nonabsorbable fibre to ensure regular bowel action. The average healthy person should not need or use chemical laxatives to obtain a daily bowel movement. Laxatives should not be given to anyone with abdominal pain because they may aggravate an undiagnosed bowel obstruction. Chronic routine use of chemical laxatives can lead to hypokalemia and to structural changes in the colon that

| TABLE 42-3 | Classification of Laxatives According to Effects on Intraluminal Fluid Accumulation |
| --- | --- |

| Laxative | Onset |
| --- | --- |
| Laxatives that increase secretion | |
| Anthraquinones | 6–8 hours |
| Castor oil (ricinoleic acid) | 2–6 hours |
| Diphenylmethane laxatives | 6–8 hours |
| Magnesium salts | 1–3 hours |
| Dioctyl sodium sulfosuccinate | 1–3 days |
| Plant resins | 1–3 days |
| Fibre | 1–3 days |
| Laxatives that decrease absorption | |
| Liquid petrolatum | 6–8 hours |
| Fibre | 1–3 days |
| Hydrophilic colloids | 1–3 days |
| Laxatives that work osmotically | |
| Magnesium salts | 1–3 hours |
| Polyethylene glycol electrolyte solution | 1–3 hours |
| Lactulose | 6–8 hours |
| Fibre | 1–3 days |

result in hypomotility. In contrast, patients with pseudo-obstruction syndromes may require multiple prokinetics to maximize colonic motility.

## Laxatives That Increase Secretion or Decrease Absorption

### Anthraquinones

Anthraquinones are found in the leaves, roots, or seed pods of various plants, such as aloe, cascara, and rhubarb, and they are present as glycosides as well as in the free forms. The glycoside conjugates are absorbed only after hydrolysis to the free anthraquinone and glucose. Hydrolysis occurs only in the large intestine by the action of the indigenous bacterial flora of the colon; this accounts, in part, for the delay in onset of action of these agents. The free anthraquinone is then reduced by the intestinal flora to the active anthral form. **Danthron** (1,8-dihydroxyanthraquinone) is a synthetic derivative that may be absorbed by the small intestine and may alter the function of this portion of the bowel. **Cascara sagrada**, in usual doses, is the mildest of the anthraquinone laxatives. It is effective in about 8 hours and seldom causes colic. **Senna** is more active, is effective in about 6 hours, and usually causes some colic. **Aloe** is the most irritating and can stimulate other visceral smooth muscles including the uterus. It acts in about 8 to 12 hours and usually causes considerable colic. **Rhubarb** is a relatively mild laxative that causes little discomfort.

These agents appear to work by inhibiting colonic mucosal $Na^+/K^+$-ATPase, leading to accumulation of salt and water in the lumen. At higher doses, they may stimulate colonic myenteric nerve fibres. Side effects include allergic reactions, fluid and electrolyte depletion, and melanosis coli.

### Castor oil (ricinoleic acid)

The active constituent of castor oil, extracted from the **castor bean** (*Ricinus communis*), is ricinoleic acid, an 18-carbon, aliphatic, monohydroxy fatty acid. It is present as a triglyceride that is hydrolyzed by pancreatic lipase to yield free ricinoleic acid. The laxative action takes place especially in the small bowel, the contents of which may be emptied into the colon within only 2 hours. A dose of castor oil is effective within 2 to 6 hours. Because the remaining unhydrolyzed oil is also eliminated, the effects tend to be self-limiting.

Ricinoleic acid acts rapidly on the small intestine and colon to increase the intraluminal fluid content. It inhibits mucosal $Na^+/K^+$-ATPase, thus decreasing the absorption of $Na^+$ and of the actively co-transported solutes (e.g., sugars, amino acids). It increases intracellular cyclic AMP in response to an increased synthesis of prostaglandin $E_2$ ($PGE_2$) that stimulates adenylyl cyclase activity, by a competitive inhibition of soluble cAMP-phosphodiesterase activity, or both. It damages enterocytes directly. On electron microscopy, disintegration of microvilli and damage to villus tips have been observed.

## Diphenylmethane Laxatives

### Phenolphthalein

This drug was widely used for many years in over-the-counter preparations but is no longer used because of concerns about carcinogenicity. Relevant points concerning its action are included in the following discussion of bisacodyl.

### Bisacodyl

This agent (Dulcolax) is chemically similar to phenolphthalein. It is an effective laxative, acting 6 to 8 hours after oral administration. It is active only after deacetylation, absorption from the small intestine, and excretion in the bile. When given in a rectal suppository, it is effective in 20 to 60 minutes. Like phenolphthalein, it is predominantly excreted in feces and has no laxative effect after bile duct ligation.

The mechanism of action of these drugs is essentially similar to that of ricinoleic acid. Both drugs inhibit $Na^+/K^+$-ATPase as well as increasing the synthesis and release of $PGE_2$, resulting in an indirect increase in cyclic AMP. The role of $PGE_2$ in the actions of phenolphthalein and bisacodyl explains the reduction of their laxative effect after pre-treatment with indomethacin. Bisacodyl may damage the intestinal mucosa, increasing its permeability, and it has been shown to cause a two- to threefold rise in $K^+$ efflux across the colonic mucosa. It has been proposed that this effect depends on raised levels of intracellular $Ca^{2+}$, and it probably reflects an increase in mucosal K+ permeability. There is evidence that both cyclic AMP and $Ca^{2+}$ may have a role in modulation of mucosal border K+ permeability.

## Dioctyl Sodium Sulfosuccinate (DSS)

This compound (Colace) was developed for use as a synthetic wetting agent. Its stool softening action is attributed to its ability to decrease surface tension and thus increase exposure of the stool surface to luminal water, resulting in fecal hydration. More recent studies have shown that DSS also acts through an increase in intraluminal water by mechanisms similar to those described for ricinoleic acid (inhibition of Na+/K+-ATPase, increase in cyclic AMP, and cellular damage).

## Liquid Petrolatum

Some oils literally "lubricate" the fecal mass, prevent excessive dehydration of the material, and may inhibit water reabsorption by coating the gut wall. The only oil preparation now in use is **liquid petrolatum (mineral oil)**, a mixture of liquid hydrocarbons. It is indigestible, but in some people, it is slightly absorbed. It interferes with the absorption of fat-soluble vitamins by retaining them in the intestinal lumen. It should always be taken at night on an empty stomach.

Mineral oil may leak past the anal sphincters. It has also been reported to interfere with healing of wounds in the anorectal area. It should not be used in very debilitated patients, the elderly, or patients with swallowing abnormalities because of the risk of aspiration and lipoid pneumonia.

## Hydrophilic Colloids, Bulk-Forming Laxatives

This group includes both natural and semi-synthetic polysaccharides and cellulose derivatives that dissolve or swell in water, forming a viscous solution or emollient gel. These gelatinous masses, of greatly increased bulk when moistened with water, exert a mildly laxative action. In addition, bulk-forming agents may actually promote colonic fluid accumulation by delivering bile acids and fatty acids to the colon, where they may interfere with water and electrolyte transport. Cases of esophageal obstruction, fecal impaction, and even intestinal perforation have occurred when these drugs are taken in the dry form. Fluids should always be administered concurrently. Somewhat paradoxically, these agents have also been used occasionally to provide relief in acute diarrhea, because they form an emollient intestinal mass and absorb water. **Agar, psyllium (*Plantago*), methylcellulose**, and **sodium carboxymethylcellulose** are examples of hydrophilic cellulose derivatives. Allergic reactions including asthma and anaphylaxis can occur in those who use or handle psyllium.

## Laxatives That Work Osmotically

### Magnesium salts

Laxatives such as **magnesium sulfate** (Epsom salts) and **magnesium hydroxide** (Milk of Magnesia) contain ions that are only slowly absorbed from the intestine, such as $Mg^{2+}$ and $SO_4^{2-}$. These ions retain fluid in the bowel lumen by virtue of their osmotic action and therefore increase the rate of transit in the small intestine and cause a larger volume of fluid to enter the colon. This distends the colon, thereby stimulating it so that catharsis occurs quickly. Magnesium laxatives may increase release of cholecystokinin (CCK), which in turn stimulates pancreatic and duodenal secretion and decreases water, sodium, and chloride reabsorption. CCK causes an increase in cyclic GMP without affecting cyclic AMP. As the kidneys normally handle whatever ions are absorbed, these laxatives can also act as diuretics. When absorbed in sufficient quantity, $Mg^{2+}$ can depress the CNS; however, this rarely happens unless there is impaired renal function or prolonged retention of the saline solution in the intestine.

### Lactulose (4-β-galactoside-(1,4)-D-fructose)

This disaccharide is resistant to hydrolysis by the small intestine disaccharidases. It has an osmotic effect in the small bowel, drawing water into the intestinal lumen. Thus, a large volume of fluid enters the colon. Once in the large intestine, lactulose is acted upon by the endogenous flora of the colon with the production of lactic acid and short-chain, volatile fatty acids. As these acids have low lipid solubility, their colonic absorption is very limited; therefore, they also have an osmotic effect. Like lactic acid, they increase colonic mucosal secretion. However, fermentation may produce bloating and excess flatus. Other non-digestible disaccharides and sorbitol work by a similar mechanism.

### Polyethylene glycol electrolyte solution

Polyethylene glycols are inert polymers of variable molecular weights, and those in the range of 3200 to 4000 Da are not absorbed (smaller molecules are absorbed and excreted unchanged in urine). They work by increasing the osmotic pressure of the intraluminal contents, thus retaining water and resulting in softer, more bulky stool; added electrolytes avoid the complications of electrolyte imbalance, water intoxication, or dehydration. In addition to being widely used as preparation for colonoscopy, in recent studies they have been shown to be efficacious for periods of up to 6 months in the treatment of fecal impaction and chronic constipation.

**Side effects** are rare and include abdominal cramps and fecal incontinence. In children, dehydration and hypokalemia have been reported. While no drug interactions have been noted, oral medications should not be administered within 1 hour of start of therapy because of possible decreased absorption.

## Side Effects of Laxatives

### Cathartic colon syndrome
Prolonged and excessive use of cathartics can cause diarrhea, abdominal pain, and cramps. In radiographs, the colon appears dilated, hypomotile, with few or absent haustral margins; sometimes, areas of pseudostricture are observed. Morphologically, there is mucosal inflammation, hypertrophy of the muscularis mucosae, thinning or atrophy of outer muscle layers, and damage to submucosal and myenteric plexuses. This entity is becoming rare and may have been due mainly to laxatives that are no longer in use.

### Laxative dependence
The desire to have a bowel movement every day may result in psychological dependence on laxatives, especially of the stimulant type. In addition, these laxatives, by emptying the distal colon prematurely, may lead the patient to misinterpret the absence of a daily bowel movement as constipation when in fact the rectum is merely empty. This results in the further use of stimulants, and a vicious cycle ensues.

### Hypokalemia
Excessive loss of Na$^+$ and water in stools results in a reduction of plasma volume, stimulation of the renin–angiotensin system, and increased serum levels of aldosterone. In the colon and kidney, aldosterone increases the reabsorption of Na$^+$ in exchange for K$^+$, which is then lost in stools and urine, respectively. Abnormal release of insulin and carbohydrate intolerance may occur as a consequence of hypokalemia.

### Malabsorption
Chronic and continuous use of laxatives can lead to malabsorption of xylose and other carbohydrates, fat, fat-soluble vitamins, and calcium and thus to the production of osteomalacia.

### Liver abnormalities
Chronic hepatitis has been reported after use of the combination of dioctyl calcium sulfosuccinate (Surfak) and the anthraquinone laxative danthron.

### Increased loss of proteins through the intestine
With the sole exception of fibre and lactulose, all laxatives have been reported to cause an excessive loss of proteins through the intestine.

## Indications for Laxatives

Most cases of constipation can be treated without the use of pharmacological agents simply by substituting whole wheat flour for white flour, by reducing the intake of food that contains no fibre, by eating plenty of fruits and vegetables, and by taking extra fibre in the form of unprocessed bran. In addition, an adequate daily intake of fluids, as well as regular physical activity or exercise, is necessary.

Laxatives should never be used on a regular basis simply to produce a daily bowel movement. Taking the above into consideration, the main indications for the use of these potentially risky pharmacological agents are to empty the bowel before elective colonic or rectal surgery or radiological or endoscopic examinations, to minimize straining at stool in patients with cardiovascular disease or with hernia, and to prevent hard abrasive bowel movements that elicit pain (the last of which may best be achieved with emollient laxatives). Other reasonable candidates for laxative use include patients taking drugs that inhibit bowel activity (e.g., narcotics) or those who are bedridden for an extended period. All laxatives should be avoided in persons with nausea, vomiting, cramps, colic, or other unexplained abdominal discomfort.

## Anti-diarrheals

Anti-diarrheals are a heterogeneous group of drugs used for the symptomatic relief of diarrhea. These agents have limited utility. The etiology of the diarrhea usually dictates specific, not symptomatic, treatment. In general, mild diarrhea due to enteric viral infections should be allowed to run its course. Bacterial enteric infections, if treated at all, should be treated etiologically. Cholestyramine, a resin which binds bile acids, has two uses: (1) the treatment of diarrhea due to the colonic spillage of bile acids, and (2) adjunctive therapy of diarrhea due to *Clostridium difficile* infection (cholestyramine binds the toxin produced by *C. difficile*). Giving opioids to a patient with diarrhea caused by ulcerative colitis may precipitate toxic megacolon. In general, anti-diarrheals are reserved for patients who cannot cope anatomically with their colonic contents because of a short gut, altered rectal or anal tone, or other problems, as in Crohn's disease.

## Opioid Analogues

Diphenoxylate (Lomotil) and loperamide (Imodium) are the opioid analogues used most specifically as anti-diarrheals (Fig. 42-3). Both are synthetic opioids of the piperidine group, which act on peripheral μ-opioid receptors, and diphenoxylate is closely related to meperidine (see Chapter 19).

These drugs resemble morphine in their effect on the small intestine and colon. They are thought to decrease fluid secretion by the small intestine and decrease intestinal motor activity in general.

### Diphenoxylate
Diphenoxylate acts as an agonist at μ-opioid receptors at two locations in the gastrointestinal tract. Receptors on

**FIGURE 42-3** Structural formulae of diphenoxylate, difenoxin, and loperamide. (Common elements are emphasized in bold.)

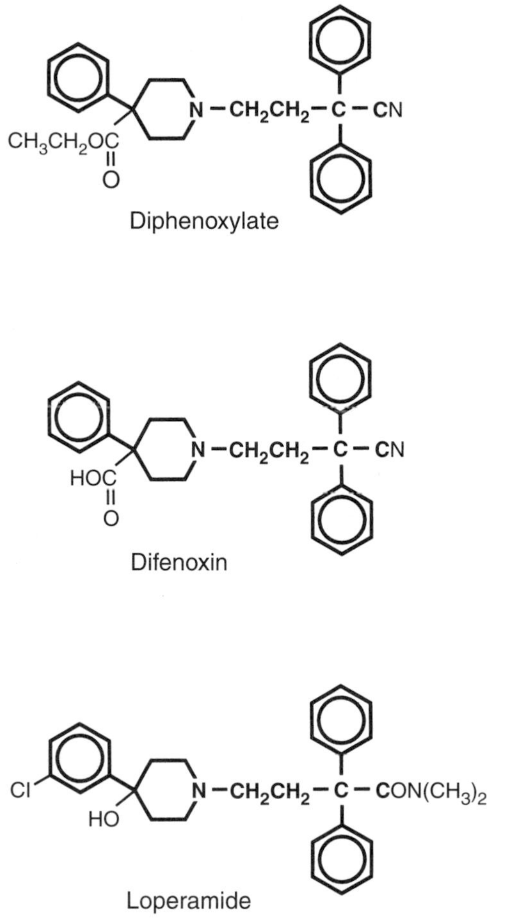

The elimination half-life of diphenoxylate is about 12 hours, but the drug is biotransformed in the liver to the active metabolite **difenoxin,** which is more potent than diphenoxylate (see Fig. 42-3). Therefore, overdose effects can occur after many hours have passed and the concentration of difenoxin has risen.

### Loperamide

Loperamide has largely replaced diphenoxylate as the drug of choice. It is effective, non-habituating, and safe. It is chemically similar to both diphenoxylate and haloperidol. Loperamide has high affinity for both peripheral and central opioid receptors but enters the brain even less readily than diphenoxylate. It acts in the intestinal tract, principally in the jejunum, via opioid μ receptors, and its effects can be blocked by naloxone. In addition, it increases anal sphincter tone, which is beneficial in patients with fecal incontinence. It is demethylated in the intestinal wall, and little is absorbed systemically. It is highly protein-bound. Its elimination half-life is about 10 to 15 hours. About 7% of the drug is excreted in the urine; significant hepatic biotransformation and biliary excretion occur, and substantial amounts of the unchanged drug and metabolites are found in the feces.

Loperamide is two to three times more potent than diphenoxylate, and its action is more rapid in onset and more prolonged. It has no analgesic effects. It has not been reported to have CNS or cardiovascular effects. Side effects are uncommon but include dizziness, dry mouth, and fatigue.

## INFLAMMATORY BOWEL DISEASE

Crohn's disease is an idiopathic disorder characterized by inflammation that extends across the bowel wall. Classically it involves the terminal ileum and colon, but in a minority of cases it may extend to the proximal gastrointestinal tract. Ulcerative colitis is a related disease with more superficial mucosal involvement that is limited to the colon. The predominant symptom of ulcerative colitis is diarrhea that is often bloody, whereas Crohn's disease may also cause significant pain and be complicated by fistulas or abscesses. While some patients respond satisfactorily to 5-aminosalicylates (see below), others require immunosuppression with corticosteroids or more potent immunomodulators.

## SALICYLATES

### Sulfasalazine (Salazopyrin)

Sulfasalazine (Fig. 42-4, Table 42-2) is the name commonly used for salicylazosulfapyridine (i.e., salicylate linked to a sulfonamide via an azo linkage). The salicylate

cholinergic terminals inhibit the release of acetylcholine and thus decrease propulsive contractions of the longitudinal muscle. Those on presynaptic terminals of inhibitory neurons inhibit the release of vasoactive intestinal peptide, thus *disinhibiting* the sphincter-like segmental contractions of circular muscle. Both effects contribute to decreased propulsive motility of the gastrointestinal tract.

Diphenoxylate is well absorbed after oral administration but does not cross the blood–brain barrier as easily as most opioids do and therefore is relatively selective for peripheral opioid receptors. However, at high doses or when used for more than a few days, it can produce drowsiness, depression, and potentiation of the effects of ethanol, barbiturates, benzodiazepines, and other CNS depressants. Overdose can cause respiratory depression that is reversible by naloxone. It can also produce an opioid-like euphoria, and a small amount of atropine is therefore added to the diphenoxylate preparation (Lomotil) to prevent abuse by causing disagreeable symptoms if too much is taken.

FIGURE 42-4 Structural formula of sulfasalazine. The azo bond between 5-ASA and sulfapyridine is split by intestinal bacterial action, liberating the active anti-inflammatory component, 5-ASA.

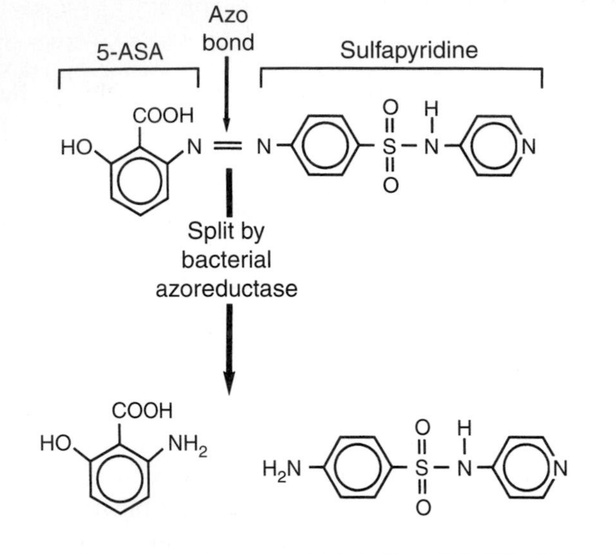

is 5-aminosalicylic acid (5-ASA), an anti-inflammatory agent that was invented in the 1940s as a possible treatment for rheumatoid arthritis, for which it proved to have rather limited utility. It is valuable in the chronic treatment of ulcerative colitis and for initial treatment of Crohn's disease with a prominent colonic involvement.

Sulfasalazine is a good example of a **prodrug**. The 5-ASA, which is in fact the active ingredient, is linked to the sulfonamide so that it can be delivered to the colon. Sulfasalazine is not absorbed in the stomach; what is absorbed in the small intestine is subject to enterohepatic circulation and ends up in the colon eventually. In the colon, the bacteria cleave the azo bond and thus separate the 5-ASA from the sulfapyridine. The sulfapyridine is absorbed, biotransformed in the liver, and excreted. The 5-ASA is mostly retained locally in the colon, where it exerts its anti-inflammatory effect.

The mechanism of this anti-inflammatory effect has been the subject of much research. The inflammatory response in ulcerative colitis and Crohn's disease includes such diverse features as cellular infiltration, increased vascular permeability, and variable local tissue damage. Increased concentrations of soluble mediators of inflammation can be detected. Principal among these are the products of arachidonic acid metabolism: prostaglandins, thromboxanes (via the cyclooxygenase pathway), and leukotrienes (via the 5-lipoxygenase pathway) (see Chapter 27). Prostaglandins have numerous effects: They are vasodilators and enhance the effects of other inflammatory mediators, such as histamine, but they also decrease phagocyte activa-

tion and cytokine production. Thromboxane $A_2$ is a vascular constrictor. Leukotriene $B_4$ has potent chemotactic effects, and other leukotrienes increase smooth muscle contraction and vascular permeability. With respect to these agents, the main action of 5-ASA is inhibition of leukotriene (e.g., LTB4) and prostaglandin production, as well as scavenging free radicals and decreasing production of cytokines such as interleukin-1 (see Chapter 40). 5-ASA also appears to neutralize activated oxygen species produced in the inflammatory response. It may also inhibit leukocyte adhesion to endothelial cells. 5-ASA blocks the pro-inflammatory transcription factor NF-κB and the synthesis of lymphocyte DNA, and thus stops the proliferation of potentially harmful B-cell and T-cell populations. Which of these actions is most important for its intestinal anti-inflammatory effect remains to be established.

The problem with sulfasalazine is that the sulfapyridine component causes significant toxicity; as a result, sulfasalazine may be poorly tolerated in up to 30% of patients. Nausea and dyspepsia affect about 1 in 6 patients and can be avoided by using enteric-coated formulations, while diarrhea occurs in another 7% of patients. Rare side effects include hemolytic and other anemias, rashes, Stevens-Johnson syndrome, pancreatitis, fibrosing pulmonary disease, hepatitis, and even acute liver failure. These tend to be worse in slow acetylators (see Chapter 10). Sulfasalazine has been shown to impair male fertility; fortunately, sperm morphology and motility revert to normal when the drug is stopped. Known hypersensitivity to sulfonamides or the presence of glucose-6-phosphate dehydrogenase deficiency precludes the use of sulfasalazine.

## 5-Aminosalicylic Acid (5-ASA)

Since 5-ASA (or a metabolite) is the active component, and the sulfonamide portion of sulfasalazine causes most of the side effects, it seemed reasonable to link two molecules of 5-ASA together via an azo bond and exclude sulfapyridine altogether. The resulting drug is called **olsalazine** (Dipentum; see Table 42-4). Olsalazine and sulfasalazine both have some predictable problems because they are dependent on bacterial degradation. Whenever intestinal transit is too fast, there is less bacterial degradation. If a patient is treated with broad-spectrum antibiotics that reduce the bacterial flora, olsalazine and sulfasalazine are ineffective.

A second strategy to avoid the need for sulfapyridine is to develop special formulations of 5-ASA to favour delivery to the distal ileum or colon. These are collectively called **mesalazine** in Canada and **mesalamine** in the United States. These drugs are unusual in that the pharmaceutical preparation itself is important in determining the pharmacological characteristics, and thus it is often necessary to refer to these drugs by trade name, rather than by the official or non-proprietary name. Likewise, each required separate clinical testing. These drugs are effective at inducing and maintaining remission in ulcerative colitis and Crohn's disease, and they have greater efficacy at doses of 3 g/day or more. Side effects in randomized controlled trials are comparable to those of placebo. When compared with sulfasalazine in clinical trials, 5-ASA has similar response rates, but the overall adverse event rate for mesalamine is significantly lower (12% vs. 28%), as is the rate of drug discontinuation (5% vs. 14%).

Current formulations of mesalamine are detailed in Table 42-4. Some preparations consist of 5-ASA coated with an acrylic resin that disintegrates at a fixed pH. When the acrylic coating is Eudragit S (Asacol), the resin breaks down at pH >7, releasing 5-ASA in the distal ileum or right colon. When the acrylic coating Eudragit L is used (Salofalk), the resin breaks down at pH >6, and the 5-ASA is released in the proximal ileum and onward. When 5-ASA is packaged in microgranules coated with an ethylcellulose membrane (Pentasa), it acts as a timed-release preparation and is gradually released throughout the entire small intestine and colon. Theoretically, these drugs have the same efficacy as salazopyrine but none of the toxicity associated with sulfapyridine.

Pure 5-ASA preparations are not, however, entirely free of adverse side effects, although the incidence is much lower than with salazopyrine. Watery diarrhea is an adverse effect of olsalazine; it occurs at higher doses and with severe or more extensive disease, in approximately 10% of subjects. This problem occurs at a lower rate with other forms of 5-ASA. The probable mechanism is promotion of ileal fluid secretion, which is not reabsorbed by the inflamed right colon. 5-ASA may also cause nephrotoxicity in about 1 in 4000 patients per year. The most common form of such toxicity is chronic interstitial nephritis. This is generally reversible, especially if the patients have been treated for less than 12 months. For this reason, renal function should be regularly monitored (by measurement of serum creatinine) in these patients, especially during the first year of treatment.

Less common side effects of 5-ASA include myocarditis, blood dyscrasias, pericarditis, pneumonitis, and pancreatitis. Occasionally, patients have identical adverse reactions to sulfasalazine and 5-ASA; therefore, 5-ASA should be used cautiously in patients who do not tolerate sulfasalazine, although the general experience is that approximately 80% will tolerate 5-ASA.

Pure 5-ASA is also formulated as suppositories and enemas. These are effective treatment for ulcerative proctitis and distal ulcerative colitis. In distal colitis, 5-ASA enemas are superior to steroid enemas.

# IMMUNE SYSTEM AGENTS

## Infliximab

This drug was developed after both animal and human studies suggested an independent role for tumour necrosis factor alpha (TNFα) in Crohn's disease. It is currently indicated for the induction and maintenance of remission of active and fistulizing Crohn's disease refractory to conventional medical therapies, or in steroid-dependent Crohn's disease. Structurally, it is a chimeric IgG$_1$ monoclonal antibody consisting of a mouse-derived antigenic portion (25%), while the rest of the molecule is of human origin (75%). Its presumed mechanism of action is neutralization of membrane-bound and soluble TNFα, although induction of T-cell apoptosis, complement activation, and antibody-mediated cytotoxicity may be additional mechanisms.

| TABLE 42-4 | Preparations of 5-Aminosalicylate Used in the Treatment of Inflammatory Bowel Disease | | | | |
|---|---|---|---|---|---|
| Non-Proprietary Name | Trade Name | Formulation | Release Mechanism | Site of Release | Systemic Absorption |
| Sulfasalazine | Salazopyrin | Sulfapyridine + 5-ASA | Bacterial action on azo bond | Colon | 20–30% of 5-ASA |
| Olsalazine | Dipentum | Two 5-ASA moieties joined via azo bond | Bacterial action on azo bond | Colon | 20–40% |
| Mesalamine (United States) | Asacol | Acrylic resin coating (Eudragit S) | pH-dependent from resin | pH >7, distal ileum onward | 34–44% |
| Mesalazine (Canada) | Salofalk, Claversal | Acrylic coating (Eudragit L) | pH-dependent from resin | pH >6, proximal ileum onward | 44% |
| | Pentasa | Microgranules with ethylcellulose membrane | Timed-release | Entire small intestine, colon | 60% |

Administration is by intravenous infusion and requires observation of the patients for 4 hours. Serum levels correlate with the duration of clinical response, are undetectable in 50% of patients 14 weeks after infusion, and are lower in patients who develop antibodies to the drug or have an infusion reaction.

Infusion of a dose of 5 mg/kg is associated with an initial remission rate of 31 to 80% and response rate of 65 to 90% in luminal disease compared with 24 to 55% and 66 to 78%, respectively, in fistulizing disease; the duration of response ranges from 8 to 12 weeks. Current dosing regimens consist of induction doses at 0, 2, and 6 weeks and maintenance therapy every 8 weeks, and they result in remission rates of 39% at 1 year in subjects with luminal disease who have responded to an initial dose. The overall response rate is approximately 25% but is likely higher in subjects on concomitant treatment with azathioprine or other immunosuppressants.

Common adverse events include headaches, abdominal pain, and respiratory tract infections. Infusion reactions occur in 5 to 23% of patients and are usually mild (e.g., urticaria, sweating, skin erythema) but may also be serious (bronchospasm, stridor) in 0.5% of cases. Infusion reactions usually respond to slowing of the infusion rate and administration of antihistamines, but it may be necessary to stop therapy and give intravenous hydrocortisone or adrenaline. Myalgia, rashes, and arthralgia are examples of delayed hypersensitivity-like reactions and seem to be less common in patients treated regularly with infliximab (i.e., every 8 weeks) than in those who are re-treated after a drug-free period of many months.

Human anti-chimeric antibodies develop in 27% of patients treated with infliximab and are associated with a decreased duration of response to the drug and an increased incidence of infusion reactions. These antibodies seem to be less common in patients on concomitant immunosuppressive therapy and may be prevented by pre-medication with intravenous hydrocortisone. Antinuclear antibodies develop in 9 to 44% of subjects, new antibodies against double-stranded DNA develop in 22%, and a lupus-like syndrome develops in 0.4 to 3.0%. While infections are common and occur in approximately one-third of patients on infliximab, serious infection occurs in only 4%. Tuberculosis reactivation has been reported in 101 patients treated with infliximab; before treatment, latent infection must be excluded by PPD (purified protein derivative) skin tests (which are unreliable, as Crohn's patients often have cutaneous anergy) or chest X-ray. Infliximab should not be given to patients with a known or suspected active infection. In a recent retrospective case series of 500 patients treated with infliximab at the Mayo Clinic, 5 deaths (mortality rate of 1%) were felt to be possibly related to infliximab. While concern has been raised that infliximab treatment may predispose patients to develop malignancy, no increase in incidence has been noted in clinical trials. Since infliximab is partly derived from mice, known hypersensitivity to any murine proteins is a contraindication to its use.

## Other Immunosuppressive Medications

Azathioprine and its metabolite 6-mercaptopurine are antimetabolites with potent immunosuppressive actions (see Chapter 40). They are given orally in doses of up to 2.5 mg/kg and 1.5 mg/kg, respectively, and are effective at inducing remission in about 1 in 5 patients with severe Crohn's disease. They may also be used as steroid-sparing agents, to treat fistulizing disease, and to maintain remission in chronic Crohn's disease. They are also effective in ulcerative colitis.

Methotrexate, a folate anti-metabolite (see Chapter 57), has been shown in a single large randomized trial to be effective at inducing remission in some patients with chronic, steroid-dependent Crohn's disease when given intramuscularly at a dose of 25 mg/week.

## SUGGESTED READINGS

Alfadhli AAF, McDonald JWD, Feagan BG. Methotrexate for induction of remission in refractory Crohn's disease. *Cochrane Database Syst Rev.* 2004;(4):CD003459.

Arnott IDR, Watts D, Satsangi J. Azathioprine and anti-TNF therapies in Crohn's disease: a review of pharmacology, clinical efficacy, and safety. *Pharmacol Res.* 2003;47:1-10.

Baert F, Noman M, Vermeire S, et al. Influence of immunogenicity on the long-term efficacy of infliximab in Crohn's disease. *N Engl J Med.* 2003;348:601-608.

Colombel JF, Loftus EV Jr, Tremaine WJ, et al. The safety profile of infliximab in patients with Crohn's disease: the Mayo Clinic experience in 500 patients. *Gastroenterology.* 2004;126:19-31.

Greiff JM, Rowbotham D. Pharmacokinetic drug interactions with gastrointestinal motility modifying agents. *Clin Pharmacokinet.* 1994;27:447-461.

Hasler WL, Schoenfeld P. Safety profile of tegaserod, a 5-HT$_4$ receptor agonist, for the treatment of irritable bowel syndrome. *Drug Saf.* 2004;27:619-631.

Marshall JK, Irvine EJ. Rectal corticosteroids versus alternative treatments in ulcerative colitis: a meta-analysis. *Gut.* 1997;40:775-781.

Muller AF, Stevens PE, McIntyre AS, et al. Experience of 5-aminosalicylate nephrotoxicity in the United Kingdom. *Aliment Pharmacol Ther.* 2005;21:1217-1224.

Nielsen OH. Sulfasalazine intolerance. *Scand J Gastroenterol.* 2003;17:389-393.

Pearson DC, May GR, Fick G, Sutherland LR. Azathioprine for maintenance of remission in Crohn's disease. *Cochrane Database Syst Rev.* 1998;(4):CD000067.

Sandborn WJ, Hanauer SB. Infliximab in the treatment of

Crohn's disease: a user's guide for clinicians. *Am J Gastroenterol.* 2002;97:2962-2972.

Sandborn WJ, Sutherland L, Pearson D, et al. Azathioprine or 6-mercaptopurine for induction of remission in Crohn's disease. *Cochrane Database Syst Rev.* 1998;(3):CD000545.

Schiller LR. Review article: the therapy of constipation. *Aliment Pharmacol Ther.* 2001;15:749-763.

Smith DS, Ferris CD. Current concepts in diabetic gastroparesis. *Drugs.* 2003;63:1339-1358.

Stein RB, Hanauer SB. Medical therapy for inflammatory bowel disease. *Gastroenterol Clin North Am.* 1999;28(2):297-322.

Sutherland L, MacDonald JK. Oral 5-aminosalicylic acid for induction of remission in ulcerative colitis. *Cochrane Database Syst Rev.* 2003;(3):CD000543.

Sutherland L, Roth D, Beck P, et al. Oral 5-aminosalicylic acid for maintenance of remission in ulcerative colitis. *Cochrane Database Syst Rev.* 2002;(4):CD000544.

Wingate D, Phillips SF, Lewis SJ, et al. Guidelines for adults on self-medication for the treatment of acute diarrhea. *Aliment Pharmacol Ther.* 2001;15:773-782.

Xing JH, Soffer EE. Adverse effects of laxatives. *Dis Colon Rectum.* 2001;44:1201-1209.

# 43

# Drugs, Alcohol, and the Liver

## H KALANT AND EA ROBERTS

### CASE HISTORY

During routine examination, a 14-year-old girl was found to have a moderately enlarged liver and a palpable spleen. She was well and had never been jaundiced. She denied fatigue, pruritus, or easy bruisability. Slit-lamp examination of the eyes revealed definite Kayser-Fleischer rings. Neurological examination was normal.

The hemoglobin was 110 g/L (slightly low), with a mildly elevated reticulocyte count. The direct Coombs' test was negative; serum haptoglobin was low at 0.22 g/L. Abnormal liver function tests included elevated AST (92 U/L) and ALT (56 U/L), low albumin (29 g/L), and prothrombin time prolonged to 5 seconds beyond normal control. Serum copper was 8.2 μmol/L, and ceruloplasmin was 68 mg/L (both subnormal). Basal 24-hour urinary copper excretion was greatly elevated at 8.4 μmol/day. Serological tests for viruses commonly causing hepatitis were negative. The patient was diagnosed as having Wilson's disease, and treatment was begun with penicillamine 500 mg twice daily. To minimize side effects, the drug was started gradually, and the full dose was reached within 10 days. The patient's only complaint was that some foods now tasted peculiar.

The complete blood count showed no abnormalities over the first several weeks of treatment. However, after approximately 2 months, the child developed a vasculitic rash on her arms. White blood cell and platelet counts were normal, but urinalysis revealed proteinuria. Quantified 24-hour urine collection showed the urine protein to be twice normal for her age. There was no urinary tract infection. Serum creatinine was normal. The most likely explanation, therefore, was penicillamine nephrotoxicity.

The occurrence of vasculitis and nephrotoxicity made it necessary to stop the penicillamine. However, continuous treatment with a chelating agent is mandatory in Wilson's disease. Therefore, the patient was treated with trientine, which she tolerated well. The rash disappeared spontaneously, and the proteinuria resolved over the next few weeks.

Interactions between drugs and the liver are of pharmacological interest in relation to three questions: (1) How do variations in liver function affect the fate of drugs? (2) How do drugs (including ethanol) affect liver function? and (3) How are drugs used in the treatment of liver disease? The first question is dealt with in several other chapters of this book and will therefore be mentioned only briefly in the present context. The second question will be covered in greater detail, in particular as it relates to drug-induced liver disease. The third question is partly covered in several other chapters, and only certain drugs that are used specifically in some types of liver disease are dealt with here.

## EFFECTS OF LIVER FUNCTION ON PHARMACOKINETICS

### Basic Liver Functions Relevant to Drug Metabolism

#### Circulation

In keeping with its major metabolic role, the human liver normally receives a large blood supply, amounting to about 25 to 30% of the cardiac output. However, this comes from two different sources: the portal vein supplies about 70 to 75% of the liver blood flow, and the hepatic artery about 25 to 30%. Since the portal venous blood has already passed through the intestinal circulation, it is a low-pressure flow with a Po2 of about 55 mmHg, compared with 95 mmHg in the hepatic arterial blood.

In the normal liver architecture seen in a two-dimensional microscopic section, illustrated schematically in Fig. 43-1, terminal branches of the hepatic artery and portal vein merge to form the sinusoids, which, at their distal ends, flow into the terminal hepatic venules. The sinusoids are surrounded by cell cords made up of hepatocytes and reticuloendothelial cells. Two alternative three-dimensional interpretations of this architecture are based on the concepts of the *liver lobule* and the *liver acinus.* The lobule is pictured as having a terminal hepatic venule at its centre, into which flow sinusoids from all the surrounding liver tissue; the portal venules and terminal hepatic arterioles are pictured as feeding into the lobule from the periphery. In contrast, the acinus is pictured as being centred on the incoming portal venule and hepatic

arteriole, which merge to form sinusoids radiating out in all directions and terminating in hepatic venules on the periphery of the acinus. The embryological development of the liver as an outcropping of the intestine, accompanied by the hepatic artery and portal vein, which all divide and subdivide into smaller and smaller branches, lends some support to the acinar concept.

The normal oxygen tension at the confluence of the hepatic arterial and portal venous flows at the proximal end of the sinusoid (zone I of the liver acinus) is therefore about 65 to 70 mmHg. As the blood moves along the sinusoid and oxygen is removed by the surrounding liver cells, the Po2 falls steadily to about 30 to 35 mmHg at the venous end (zone III of the liver acinus). This is still high enough to meet the basic needs of the last liver cells along the sinusoid. However, zone III is normally in a state of relative hypoxia. If the arterial Po2 falls because of conditions such as anemia, congestive heart failure, or anaesthesia, or if the oxygen requirement of the liver is

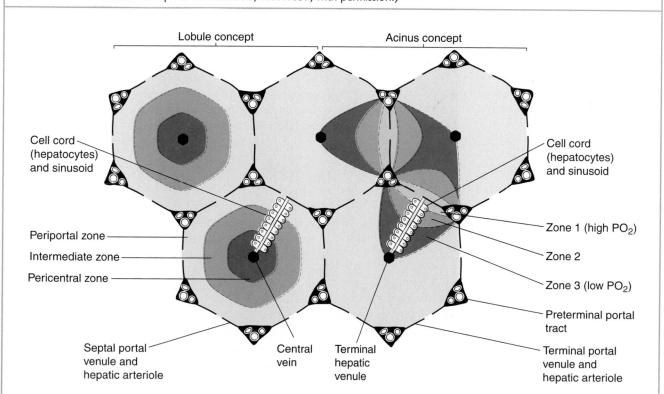

**FIGURE 43-1** Simplified schematic representation of hepatic vascular architecture according to the concepts of liver lobule and liver acinus. Left: hypothetical lobule with terminal hepatic venule at its centre; Right: hypothetical acinus with portal triad of hepatic arteriole, portal venule, and bile canaliculus at its centre; I, II, and III indicate periportal zone, midzone, and perivenular zone, respectively, of liver cell cords. (Adapted from Wanless IR. Anatomy and developmental anomalies of the liver. In Feldman M, Scharschmidt BF, Sleisenger MH, eds. *Sleisenger and Fordtran's Gastrointestinal and Liver Disease.* 6th ed. Philadelphia: WB Saunders; 1997:1059, with permission.)

increased by conditions such as fever or hyperthyroidism, there may be insufficient oxygen left at the venous end. Unless the increased oxygen demand is met by a corresponding increase in oxygen delivery, the further reduced $P_{O_2}$ in zone III could result in **focal damage or necrosis** of liver cells.

The liver also has low-resistance shunts that connect the junction of the portal venous and hepatic arterial flows directly to the terminal hepatic venule (central vein), bypassing the sinusoid. These shunts probably serve to permit portal venous blood to reach the systemic circulation when the perfusion pressure is too low to ensure flow through the sinusoids. The cost of this safeguard is that blood passing through the shunts is not exposed to the hepatocytes. Variations in blood flow and in intrahepatic shunting, therefore, markedly affect the delivery of drug to the liver. The importance of this factor in drug clearance is explained in Chapter 6.

### Cellular uptake mechanisms

Free drug can enter the hepatocyte by passive diffusion or active transport; protein-bound drug can be taken up by pinocytosis. More than one mechanism may be involved in the uptake of the same drug. For example, free *d*-tubocurarine, which is actively transported across the cell membrane into the cytoplasm, is secreted into the bile, but protein-bound tubocurarine, which is taken up by pinocytosis, finds its way into lysosomes, where it is stored and from which it can be displaced by quinacrine and other competing drugs. Mathematical analysis of hepatic uptake of drugs is considered in Chapter 6.

### Storage

Storage can occur in lysosomes, as mentioned above, or by binding to intracellular proteins, as in the case of the antimalarial drugs. It seems likely that highly lipid-soluble drugs can also be stored within intracellular fat droplets.

### Biotransformation

This is dealt with in detail in Chapter 4. As noted there, biotransformation can inactivate many drugs, but it can activate others and convert them into toxic compounds. The latter process will be of special interest later in this chapter.

### Biliary secretion

Bile secretion is driven mainly (about 75%) by the uptake of bile salts from the blood into the hepatocytes and their secretion into the bile canaliculi; the remaining 25% is driven by secretion of $HCO_3^-$ and reduced glutathione. Uptake of bile salts into the hepatocyte is carried out by two types of transport protein in the basolateral (sinusoidal) membrane: NTCP ($Na^+$-dependent taurocholate co-transporting polypeptide) and the OATPs (a family of $Na^+$-independent organic anion transport proteins). $Na^+/K^+$-ATPase maintains the transmembrane sodium ion gradient required for the functioning of the NTCP. At the canalicular surface of the hepatocyte, two other types of ATP-dependent transport protein actively secrete the bile salts into the biliary canaliculus: the MDR (multidrug resistance) P-glycoprotein and the BSEP (bile salt export pump). This active secretion is the rate-limiting step in bile formation.

Once the bile reaches the biliary ductules, movement of electrolytes and water across the bile duct epithelium, under endocrine control, regulates the concentration and volume of the bile and therefore its rate of flow down the duct system.

Biliary secretion may be an important factor in the fate of some drugs and of negligible significance to others.

## Effects of Disturbed Liver Function on Pharmacokinetics

### Circulation

Shock causes a fall in visceral blood flow and portal pressure, and within the liver, the blood is diverted from the sinusoids to the low-pressure shunts. This reduces the delivery of drug to the liver cells and also decreases the supply of oxygen needed for most drug biotransformations. Both effects tend to prolong the half-life of the drug in the body. The same results can be produced by an extrahepatic portacaval shunt or by intrahepatic obstruction of blood flow due to swelling of the liver cells (e.g., inflammation, fat accumulation, hypertrophy of endoplasmic reticulum, osmotic swelling) or fibrosis (e.g., portal cirrhosis). Similar effects can be produced temporarily by vasoconstrictor drugs such as catecholamines and vasopressin, which can therefore alter the hepatic uptake of other drugs. In congestive heart failure, similar functional alterations are produced by increased venous pressure in the inferior vena cava and hepatic vein, which is transmitted backwards through the sinusoids to the terminal branches of the hepatic artery and portal vein, reducing blood flow to the liver.

While the major effect of such circulatory disturbances is to reduce the rate of drug delivery to the liver, they can also decrease the rate of absorption of drug from the intestinal lumen. Increased intrahepatic pressure, with corresponding decrease in hepatic blood flow, also results in back pressure in the splanchnic vasculature, which decreases the rate of flow through submucosal capillaries in the gastrointestinal tract and thus decreases the concentration gradient that maintains diffusion of drug from the lumen to the blood. For example, in one study of patients with portal hypertension, the time to reach peak plasma concentration after an oral dose of the anti-inflammatory agent sulindac (see Chapter 28) was increased to 2.5 hours from a normal time of 1.2 hours.

The effect of such changes in drug delivery depends on the relative importance of hepatic biotransformation versus other routes of elimination for the individual drug in question. For example, the fate of digoxin will be unchanged because it is eliminated by renal excretion, while the half-life of digitoxin will be prolonged because it depends primarily on hepatic biotransformation. Similarly, the fate of ether will not be affected appreciably because it is primarily cleared by the lung, whereas halothane and methoxyflurane will have a longer sojourn in the body because they undergo a substantial degree of biotransformation in the liver. For most drugs, the effect of decreased hepatic circulation will be a decreased rate of elimination from the body and, therefore, an increased risk of toxicity. However, this same effect can be protective in the case of a drug that is transformed into a toxic agent in the liver.

### Hepatocellular uptake

A reduction in functional liver cell mass can have two competing effects on the hepatic uptake of drugs:

1. Decreased plasma protein concentration, which often results from liver disease, can cause a significant increase in the free fraction of a drug that is normally extensively protein-bound, and this, in turn, can result in increased hepatic uptake. Many different types of drugs are affected in this way. Some well-studied examples are amobarbital, cefoperazone, diazepam, morphine, phenytoin, propranolol, tolbutamide, and various non-steroidal anti-inflammatory drugs. The increase in hepatic uptake of the drug is sometimes greater than the reduction in plasma albumin concentration; this suggests that a qualitative change in the albumin may result in lower drug-binding affinity.

2. The decreased liver cell mass can mean a decreased uptake capacity. The actual result in any given case depends on the balance between the effects of reduced liver cell mass and decreased plasma protein binding. Usually, in severe liver disease, the effect of reduced cell mass predominates, and drug uptake is diminished. Several studies of patients with severe liver disease have shown a significant decrease in the clearance of antipyrine that is closely correlated with the decreased clearance of indocyanine green (a marker of liver cell function) and with decreased liver size as estimated by ultrasonic scan. Severe cirrhosis also greatly prolongs the serum half-life for phenobarbital, amobarbital, and hexobarbital.

Severe liver disease may also be accompanied by an increase in the apparent volume of distribution (see Chapter 3) for some drugs. This can be due to reduced plasma protein binding or to the accumulation of ascitic fluid, into which the drug can equilibrate.

### Biotransformation

The effect of liver disease on the biotransformation of drugs after their uptake depends on the stage and severity of the disease. In mild disease, during the stage of recovery, there may be proliferation of liver cells to replace those previously damaged. In this regeneration phase, all constituents of the cytochrome P450 pathway (see Chapter 4) may be increased, and the rate of biotransformation of barbiturates and many other drugs may actually be greater than normal.

However, in severe liver disease, punch biopsies have shown a 40 to 50% reduction in the cytochrome P450 content and in the activities of $N$- and $O$-demethylases, pseudocholinesterase, and glucose-6-phosphate dehydrogenase (G-6-PD). Such changes are found in alcoholic hepatitis and active cirrhosis, but not in uncomplicated fatty liver or mild viral hepatitis. These factors may require a decrease in dosage for some drugs. For example, patients with active liver disease may require a 15 to 65% reduction in the dosage of various opioid analgesics, non-steroidal anti-inflammatory agents, long-acting benzodiazepines, digitoxin, β blockers, and verapamil.

Similar decreases in drug biotransformation by the liver may result from endocrine or other factors affecting the liver secondarily. For example, progesterone and synthetic progestogens used in oral contraceptive pills prolong the sleeping time after a test dose of hexobarbital in the rat. Experimental kidney disease, in the stage of uremia, causes a fall in the hepatic content of cytochrome P450 and a decrease in drug-metabolizing activity. The mechanism of this effect is not clear; it may be due to endocrine disturbances or possibly result from the accumulation of some hepatotoxic material that is normally excreted in the urine.

### Bile flow

The importance of a reduction in the rate of bile flow varies greatly from drug to drug. Some drugs (e.g., $d$-tubocurarine) or drug metabolites, (e.g., hydroxybarbiturates) are secreted in high concentration in the bile and are significantly affected by changes in bile flow rate. For example, in one study an infusion of saline or sodium taurocholate, which increased the canalicular bile formation, resulted in a 40% increase in biliary excretion of pentobarbital and its metabolites. Since the ratio of pentobarbital to pentobarbital metabolites was not altered, the effect must have been exclusively on the flushing out of the biliary tree rather than on the biotransformation reactions in the liver cell. Ligation of the bile duct caused the opposite change: the duration of action of thiopental, hexobarbital, and zoxazolamine was doubled 24 hours after bile duct obstruction. In contrast, other drugs (e.g., digitoxin) are biotransformed in the liver, but the metabolites are passed back into the circulation and excreted by the kidney. Neither biliary obstruction nor bile flow stimulation affects their duration of action.

Very closely related drugs may differ markedly with respect to their biliary excretion pattern. For example, after a test dose of the anti-cancer drug doxorubicin (see Chapter 57), only 20% of the drug appeared in the bile in 24 hours, mainly as unaltered drug; with the analogue trifluoroacetyldoxorubicin, over 80% appeared in the bile, mainly as metabolites.

A general problem in such studies is that biliary excretion of a drug is normally investigated in animals or surgical patients with bile duct drainage via a catheter to the exterior. Therefore, the results do not indicate what would happen in the normal subject when the bile reaches the intestine. If there is a significant degree of enterohepatic recirculation (see Chapter 1), the half-life for whole-body clearance might not be appreciably altered by a change in biliary secretion rate.

## MECHANISMS OF DRUG-INDUCED LIVER DISEASE

Drugs can cause pathological changes in liver histology and liver function by at least three different mechanisms. The type of damage, the speed of onset, and the dose–effect relations all differ according to the mechanism involved.

### Indirect Extrahepatic Mechanisms

Drugs that produce major effects on circulation or respiration can cause liver damage by sharply decreasing the blood or oxygen supply to the liver, even temporarily. For example, a massive release of noradrenaline or adrenaline causes a temporary **constriction of the splanchnic arterial bed,** including the hepatic artery. Production of shock by an overdose of drugs that **impair myocardial contractility** (e.g., quinidine) can produce an equivalent effect by decreasing the perfusion pressure. **Respiratory depression,** by large doses of barbiturates or other hypnosedative drugs, causes poor oxygenation of the blood, so oxygen supply to the liver is decreased even if the blood flow is not markedly affected.

All of these disturbances can lead to hypoxia of the liver. If severe enough, this may result in degenerative changes or necrosis of liver cells. Because of the special features of hepatic circulation described above, the damage tends to be mainly in zone III (i.e., in the region of the terminal hepatic venule).

Drugs can also reduce hepatic blood flow by producing lesions of the intrahepatic blood vessels themselves. Oral contraceptives (see Chapter 46) and various anti-cancer chemotherapeutic agents (see Chapter 57) have been incriminated in **thrombosis** of the large hepatic veins (Budd-Chiari syndrome) and in **veno-occlusive disease** of the small intrahepatic veins. The latter is a gradual constriction of the small veins by deposition of connective tissue around them. The same drugs, as well as a number of metallic poisons and vinyl chloride, have also been linked to perisinusoidal fibrosis and to gradual fibrous occlusion of the branches of the portal vein (hepatoportal sclerosis). Intravenous use of methamphetamine has been reported to cause necrotizing angiitis, a condition characterized by the formation of inflammatory nodules and micro-aneurysms in the walls of arterioles in the liver, brain, kidney, and other organs. These drug-induced vascular lesions are relatively rare but can be fatal when they do occur.

### Indirect Intrahepatic Mechanisms

Many drugs can cause liver injury by **interfering with an important metabolic pathway** and depriving the liver cell of an essential product. For example, tetracyclines and chloramphenicol (see Chapter 52) are antibiotics that can interfere with the synthesis of cell proteins, including the very-low-density lipoproteins that normally transport triglycerides out of the hepatocyte. Anti-cancer drugs (e.g., methotrexate, urethane, 6-mercaptopurine) can inhibit the synthesis of nucleic acids in normal cells as well as in malignant ones.

These metabolic disturbances typically lead to the production of fatty liver and other degenerative changes, and only occasionally (in severe cases) to liver cell necrosis. The effects are generally dose-dependent but exhibit a high degree of variability that possibly reflects differences in the degree of metabolic activity in the liver at the time the drug was given. The latency between the administration of the drug and the appearance of the damage ranges from several hours to several days. The percentage of exposed individuals who actually suffer liver damage is relatively low.

Indirect cell damage can also be caused by **cholestasis** (obstruction of bile flow by precipitation of bile within the bile canaliculi). Several steroids that are alkylated at C-17, such as the anabolic steroids and the synthetic estrogens and progestins used in oral contraceptives (Fig. 43-2), can inhibit the uptake of bilirubin from the plasma into the liver cell and its secretion into the bile. In addition, these steroids inhibit the $Na^+/K^+$-ATPase of the liver cell membrane and thus decrease active secretion of $Na^+$ into the bile. They also increase the permeability of the canalicular membrane to back-diffusion of water and some solutes from the bile canaliculi into the liver cell. Other compounds, such as halogenated hydrocarbons and chlorpromazine and a number of its derivatives, increase the permeability of the ductal epithelium, thus reducing the volume and the rate of bile flow along the canaliculi, permitting the conjugated bile components to precipitate and form solid plugs. These plugs block the canaliculi and lead to obstructive jaundice and mild degenerative changes in the liver cells. These effects are reversible when the drug is stopped. Other drugs, such as the insulin sensitizer troglitazone (see Chapter 47) and the endothelin receptor antagonist bosentan (see Chapter 31), can produce cholestatic liver disease by inhibiting the function of the bile salt export pump, thus causing accumulation of cytotoxic bile salts within the hepatocyte.

Jaundice can also be caused by drugs that **interfere with the uptake of unconjugated bilirubin** from the cir-

**FIGURE 43-2** Examples of C-17 alkylated steroids capable of causing cholestatic jaundice.

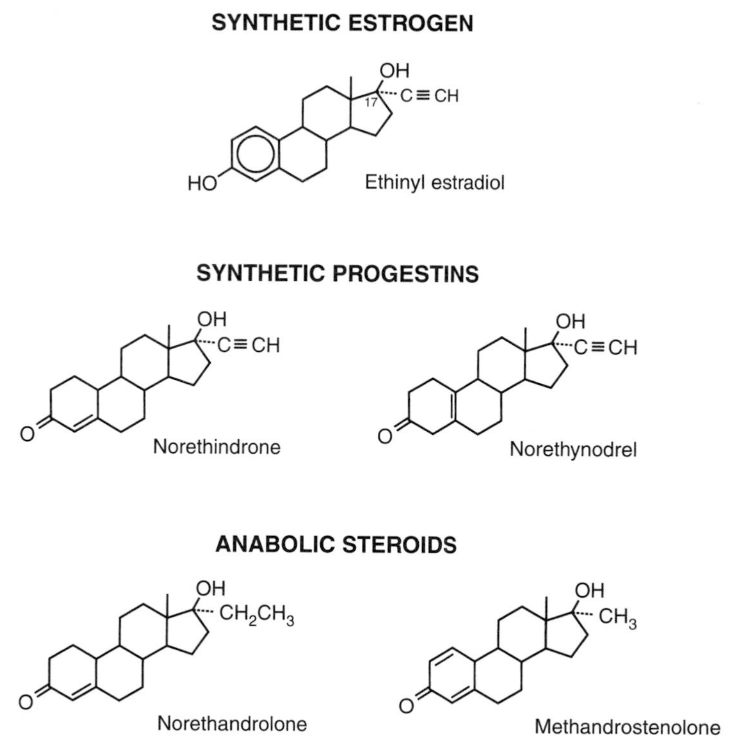

SYNTHETIC ESTROGEN

Ethinyl estradiol

SYNTHETIC PROGESTINS

Norethindrone

Norethynodrel

ANABOLIC STEROIDS

Norethandrolone

Methandrostenolone

culating blood into the hepatic parenchymal cells. Examples include the antibiotics novobiocin and rifampin and various radiopaque dyes used for X-ray visualization of the gallbladder. Since the bilirubin is prevented from being taken up into the liver and conjugated, they remain poorly water-soluble, are not readily excreted by the kidney, and remain largely bound to serum proteins, where they can compete against the binding of other drugs.

## Direct Hepatic Toxicity

A number of agents, including chloroform, carbon tetrachloride, furosemide, phenacetin, and acetaminophen, are directly toxic to the liver cell. Unlike the indirect hepatotoxins, these direct-acting compounds show **strict dose dependence** with very **high reproducibility** experimentally and with a very **high incidence of damage** in exposed individuals. There is a **very short latency** between drug administration and onset of damage, on the order of a few hours.

Some drugs appear to cause direct damage to the cell membrane and mitochondrial membranes. For example, the anti-seizure drug valproate causes mitochondrial membrane damage, with leakage of mitochondrial enzymes, consequent failure of β-oxidation of fatty acids, and microvesicular fat accumulation in the cytoplasm. Acetaminophen-induced hepatotoxicity in the rat was reported to cause a selective 52% drop in hepatocyte membrane $Na^+/K^+$-ATPase 3 hours after drug administration, whereas leakage of alanine aminotransferase and microscopic signs of necrosis were not found until 24 hours later. However, the typical lesion associated with direct hepatotoxicity is **necrosis** (rather than fatty change, as caused by the indirect mechanisms). It tends to be widespread throughout the liver and indiscriminately located, although with a few of these drugs it may be zonal (periportal with some drugs, and surrounding the terminal hepatic venule with others).

For a number of the direct hepatotoxins, there is a **threshold dose** necessary to cause damage. For example, acetaminophen does not cause liver cell necrosis until the dose exceeds 300 mg/kg; beyond that, the damage is proportional to the dose. The reason for this appears to be that the damage is caused by a minor but highly reactive oxidized metabolite (Fig. 43-3) that is produced by cytochromes P450 and that can be inactivated by glutathione conjugation (see Chapter 4) to yield a mercapturic acid derivative that is excreted harmlessly in the urine. No damage occurs until the available glutathione is insufficient, at which time the toxic material is then free to react with a variety of essential constituents of the cell, including microsomal glutamine synthetase, cytosolic glutamate dehydrogenase, mitochondrial carbamyl phosphate synthetase, aldehyde and glutamate dehydrogenase, and nuclear lamin A. The inactivation of these cellular constituents impairs oxidative phosphorylation, the trapping of ammonia and its conversion to urea, and transcription of various genes. In addition, the cytochrome P450 activity generates superoxide radicals that react with nitric oxide to form peroxynitrite, which is also highly reactive with macromolecules. The damage is increased by metabolic factors that reduce the cellular content of reduced glutathione and thus prolong the half-life of the toxic metabolite. Damage is also increased by drugs that induce CYP1A2, 2E1, and 3A and thus increase production of the toxic metabolite of acetaminophen.

Numerous other drugs can produce direct hepatocellular damage by mechanisms involving the production of reactive intermediates by cytochrome P450 reactions. For example, α-**methyldopa** is converted to an epoxide intermediary metabolite, which acts as an arylating agent. **Halothane** is generally a safe anaesthetic, but a certain number of patients, especially those who undergo repeated exposure to it, develop fever, muscle and joint pains, nausea, anorexia, abdominal discomfort, and jaundice, which progresses to a zone III hepatocellular necrosis. The explanation again appears to be the formation of a reactive metabolite. Under normoxic conditions, the cytochrome P450 system oxidizes the halothane to trifluoroacetate, but under hypoxic conditions, it acts as a reducing system (see Chapter 4) and produces a toxic free radical (Fig. 43-4).

The mechanism of damage in all these cases appears to involve covalent bonding of the toxic metabolite to a vital cell constituent, possibly a membrane protein or a nucleic acid. Extent and severity of damage are proportional to the amount of covalent binding, which can be shown to occur about 1 to 2 hours before the appearance of cytological damage. Glutathione can protect against such damage in at least three different ways: (1) detoxification of $H_2O_2$ and organoperoxides by a glutathione peroxidase reaction, (2) non-catalyzed nucleophilic reaction of glutathione and drug to form stable adducts, and (3) the glutathione transferase reaction (see Chapter 4). Cell destruction can be prevented if reducing substances, such as cysteine or dimercaprol, are given early enough after the hepatotoxic drug. These substances can react with the toxic metabolite and prevent it from bonding to the target constituents in the cell. In the case of CCl₄ poisoning, the toxic metabolite is the free radical, CCl₃·, which can be "mopped up" by N-acetyl-cysteine or cysteamine given up to 12 hours after the CCl₄. In contrast, drugs such as pyrazole or aminotriazole, which prevent the free radical formation, are protective only if given before or together with the CCl₄, but they can do nothing against the CCl₃· if given after it has formed.

After covalent binding has occurred, two different mechanisms may be responsible for immediate versus delayed cell damage. **Immediate damage,** as in the case of halothane, appears to be due to altered ion permeability. Covalent binding of reactive intermediates to membrane proteins renders the membrane permeable to $Ca^{2+}$, which floods in along a concentration gradient and is the agent that finally kills the cell. In tissue culture, cell death can be

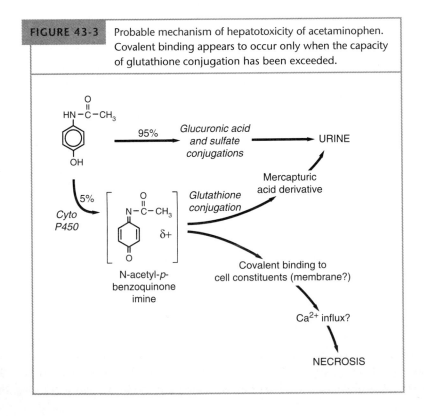

FIGURE 43-3   Probable mechanism of hepatotoxicity of acetaminophen. Covalent binding appears to occur only when the capacity of glutathione conjugation has been exceeded.

**FIGURE 43-4** Postulated mechanism of hepatotoxicity by halothane. Pathway 1 would be the mechanism of necrosis produced by a single exposure to halothane; pathway 2 is the suggested explanation of the increased risk upon subsequent exposures. Both occur only under conditions of hypoxia in the liver, when the cytochrome P450 functions as a reductase.

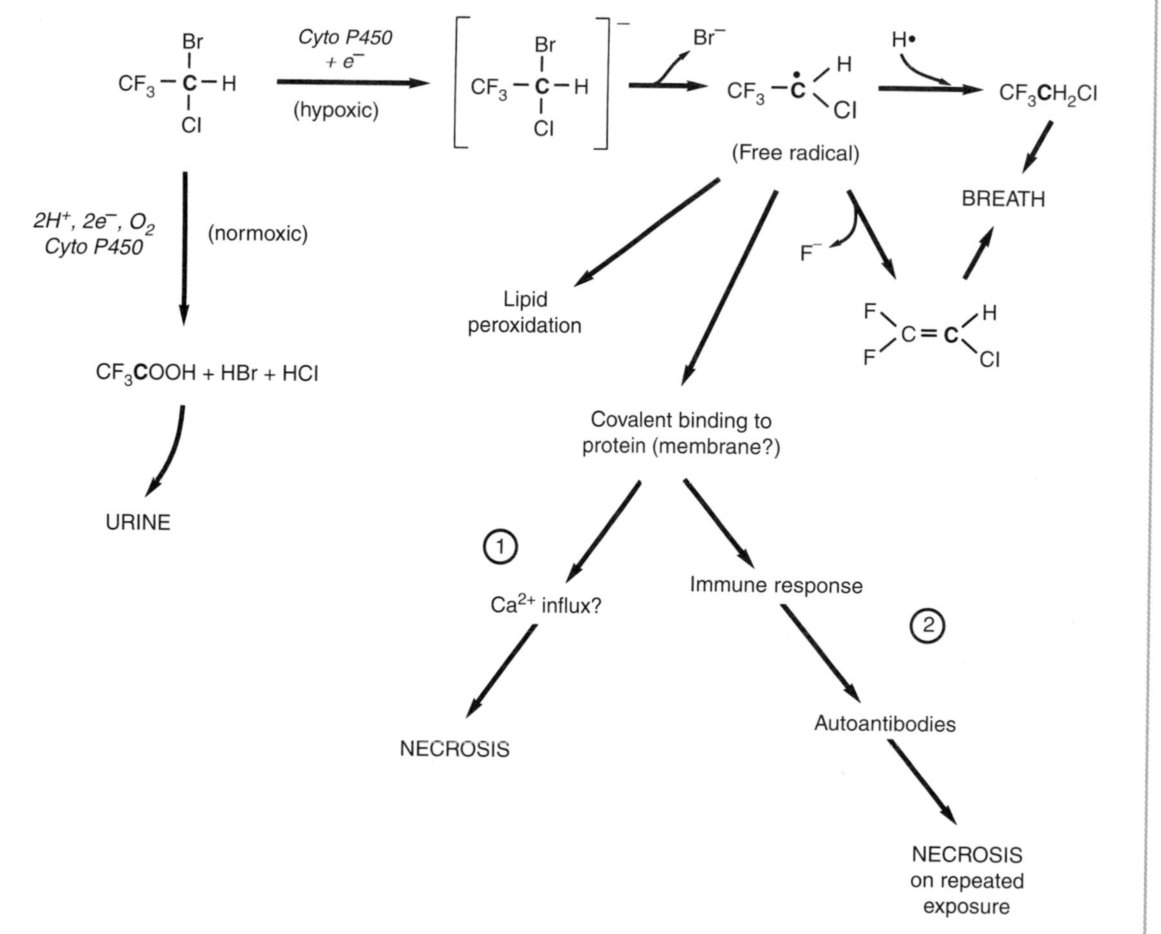

prevented (even after covalent binding has occurred) by using a very-low-calcium medium. Chlorpromazine, which hinders $Ca^{2+}$ entry into the cell, also has a protective effect, but it is not used clinically for this purpose.

**Delayed cell death,** however, appears to be the result of an autoimmune reaction. The proteins that have been altered by covalent binding of the reactive drug metabolites can serve as antigens, giving rise to antibodies that may be able to attack the native proteins in previously undamaged cells. There is evidence that this may explain the increased risk of hepatotoxicity with repeated exposure to halothane, as well as the relatively long latent period. Similarly, tienilic acid (ticrynafen, a diuretic and uricosuric agent now removed from the market because of hepatotoxicity) gives rise to a reactive intermediate that can alkylate a specific cytochrome P450 enzyme, converting it into an antigen. This gives rise to an antibody that reacts specifically with that cytochrome P450 and decreases its ability to carry out hydroxylation of tienilic acid and of various other drugs. This antibody was found in the plasma of patients with ticrynafen hepatitis but not in the plasma of patients who also received the drug but did not develop hepatitis. It is believed that the hepatitis was caused by the antibody attacking the native cytochrome P450 in previously undamaged cells.

Since the damage in these cases is done by a **reactive metabolite** of the original drug, it can be prevented by inhibitors of the cytochrome P450 system or be increased by inducers of this system. **Zonal distribution** of damage is seen with those drugs for which the biotransformation is localized to a specific zone (Fig. 43-5). The damage tends to occur at the point where the toxic metabolite is produced. For example, allyl alcohol is converted to acrolein in the periportal zone (zone I) and produces necrosis there. In contrast, with acetaminophen, the biotransformation and damage are essentially in zone III. **Genetic variations** in drug biotransformation may also affect susceptibility to liver damage by the metabolites.

## Drug Hypersensitivity Hepatitis

Other drugs can cause jaundice as a result of a hypersensitivity reaction, with accompanying signs such as rash, eosinophilia, and severe hepatitis with cholestasis. The reaction can sometimes be severe enough to cause death. The drugs that can give rise to it are quite diverse, chemically and pharmacodynamically (e.g., the antiviral agent nevirapine and the $H_2$ receptor blocker ranitidine). This type of jaundice is fortunately relatively rare and is considered to be dose-independent.

# MECHANISMS OF ETHANOL-INDUCED LIVER PATHOLOGY

Alcoholic liver disease (ALD) is a major cause of liver-related death in the Western world. In 1999, for example, more than two million adults in the United States were estimated to have ALD. Mortality estimates for the United States range from 12 000 to 40 000 deaths a year. In 1999, in the United Kingdom, 19 200 hospital admissions were attributed to ALD. Worldwide, the death rate due to this disease correlates quite well with the mean per capita alcohol consumption in a population (see Chapter 70).

Traditionally, ALD has been classified into three categories according to morphological criteria: (1) fatty liver, (2) alcoholic hepatitis (liver cell necrosis and inflammation), and (3) cirrhosis, in which the normal lobular architecture of the liver is replaced by irregular nodules surrounded by thick, fibrous septa. In the context of this chapter, ALD serves to illustrate how all three mechanisms of drug-induced liver damage described above can be activated by the same drug.

## Fatty Liver

This abnormality results mainly from the change of NAD (nicotinamide adenine dinucleotide) to NADH (the reduced form of NAD) during the metabolism of ethanol

---

**FIGURE 43-5**   Zonal distribution of necrosis in the liver acinus, produced by various hepatotoxic agents.

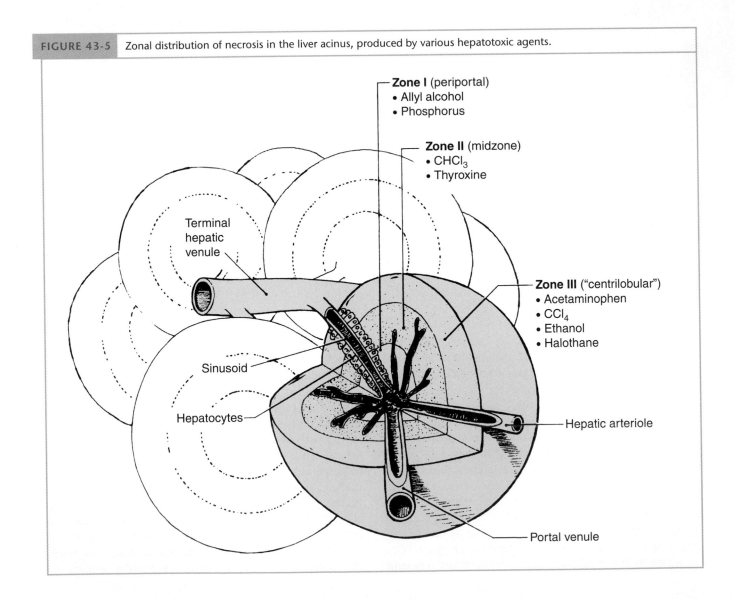

and acetaldehyde (see Chapter 22). The increase in hepatic NADH inhibits the oxidation of both glycerophosphate and free fatty acids, raising their levels in the cytoplasm and stimulating formation and accumulation of neutral triglycerides in the liver. The process can be accentuated by a high dietary intake of lipids, especially polyunsaturated fatty acids, and by obesity. This is an *indirect intrahepatic* mechanism of liver damage. For other examples of ethanol-induced disturbances of intermediary metabolism in the liver, see Chapter 22. Fatty liver, itself, probably does not lead directly to cell death, hepatic fibrosis, or cirrhosis, because if the intake of ethanol is stopped, the fat accumulation in the hepatocytes is fully reversible. However, if ethanol intake is continued, the accompanying metabolic disturbances in the liver give rise to oxidative stress and cytokine activation, which contribute directly to cell damage and fibrosis, as described in greater detail below.

## Alcoholic Hepatitis

Alcoholic hepatitis is characterized by clusters or foci of necrotic liver cells, surrounded or infiltrated by inflammatory cells. Enzymes and other molecules that are normally confined within the liver cells are released into the circulation as the damaged cells break down, and they serve as diagnostic markers of the disease process. Several different effects of ethanol or its metabolism have been implicated in the production of necrosis and inflammation.

### Hypoxia

As described above, the special features of hepatic blood flow make the liver very susceptible to hypoxic damage in zone III of the acinus. Both acute and chronic ingestion of ethanol lead to increased oxidative activity of the liver mitochondria and thus increase the hepatic oxygen consumption. This does not usually result in liver cell damage because of a compensatory increase in portal blood flow induced by ethanol. However, if this increase is prevented by other factors, the degree of hypoxia in zone III can become sufficient to cause cell death. Among such factors encountered in chronic heavy drinkers are anemia, pulmonary insufficiency, and reduced oxygen-carrying capacity of hemoglobin due to heavy smoking (carbon monoxide).

In addition, hepatomegaly is a nearly constant finding in the early stages of ALD in humans, and it is due to an increase in hepatocyte size rather than in the number of hepatocytes. The cell swelling is largely due to an increase in intracellular water caused by the osmotic effect of raised levels of intracellular $K^+$ and protein, secondary to disturbances of transport functions. The enlarged hepatocytes compress the sinusoids, resulting in increased resistance to blood flow and, after a threshold cell size is exceeded, in increased intrahepatic and portal venous pressure. In humans with ALD, biopsies also reveal a marked reduction in the calibre of the sinusoids and in total sinusoidal cross-sectional area. The compression of the sinusoids decreases blood flow through them and reduces delivery of oxygen to the hepatocytes.

The increase in oxygen consumption induced by both acute and chronic administration of ethanol requires thyroid hormone function as a permissive factor. Both thyroidectomy and the administration of the anti-thyroid drug propylthiouracil (PTU; see Chapter 45) markedly suppress or abolish the hypermetabolic state induced by alcohol. PTU administration markedly protected rats against liver necrosis induced by ethanol in the presence of low atmospheric oxygen tensions. Prolonged administration of PTU to patients with ALD resulted in an important decrease in mortality during a 2-year period of observation. However, PTU has not found general acceptance as a treatment for ALD in humans.

### Acetaldehyde

Acetaldehyde, the initial product of alcohol oxidation, is a highly reactive metabolite that can bind to a number of molecules of biological importance, including proteins (such as hemoglobin, tubulin, and albumin), DNA, phospholipids, and serotonin. Also, it can interact with dopamine and noradrenaline, yielding pharmacologically active and potentially cytotoxic compounds.

Acetaldehyde per se can become a hapten when bound covalently to amino acid residues in macromolecules. The antibodies generated are directed against acetaldehyde-modified proteins, independently of the nature of the carrier protein. Increased antibody titres against acetaldehyde-containing epitopes have been found predominantly in those alcoholics with alcoholic hepatitis characterized by cell necrosis and polymorphonuclear infiltration. Acetaldehyde might also contribute to the predominantly zone III localization of cell necrosis since it is formed in the metabolism of ethanol along the sinusoid and is present in higher concentration in blood leaving zone III than in zone I.

### Oxidative stress

As described in Chapter 22, ethanol is oxidized not only by alcohol dehydrogenase but also by CYP2E1, especially at high alcohol concentrations and in regular heavy drinkers. This pathway generates a variety of highly reactive oxidizing species, including superoxide free radicals, hydroxyl radical, and $H_2O_2$. In addition, the increase in the ratios of NADPH (reduced nicotinamide adenine dinucleotide phosphate) to NADP and NADH to NAD mobilizes free $Fe^{3+}$, which acts as a catalyst for the peroxidation of lipids. Normally, these oxidizing factors are scavenged by glutathione and other intracellular reducing agents, but ethanol tends to decrease the protection afforded by these agents. Acutely, ethanol decreases the synthesis of glutathione and increases its efflux from liver cells. Chronically, it decreases the mitochondrial content of both vitamin E and glutathione, thus decreasing the protection against superoxide radicals formed during the electron transport process.

The consequence of this loss of protection is referred to as *oxidative stress,* which includes increased risk of cell membrane lysis by lipoperoxides formed by the peroxidation of fatty acids. Mitochondrial membranes are also damaged by the reactive oxygen species, becoming abnormally permeable and allowing leakage of cytochrome c and other mitochondrial macromolecules into the cytoplasm, where they initiate changes leading to apoptosis. Among these changes is the formation of Mallory bodies, which are intracytoplasmic clumps of collapsed organelles and filaments of cytokeratin protein. The Mallory bodies and lipoperoxides, as well as interleukin-8 (see below), act as chemotactic factors for polymorphonuclear leukocytes, thus accounting for the leukocytic infiltration that is seen in alcoholic hepatitis.

### Cytokines and ALD

In the intestine, alcohol increases the permeability of the mucosa to bacterial lipopolysaccharides (LPS), which can thus enter the portal venous circulation and be carried to the liver, where they act on the nuclear factor NF-κB in Kupffer cells and circulating monocytes to cause excessive release of a variety of cytokines and other pro-inflammatory molecules, including tumour necrosis factor alpha (TNFα), interleukins (IL-1, -6, and -8), and eicosanoids (see Chapters 27 and 40). The oxidative stress resulting from CYP2E1 oxidation of ethanol (primarily in zone III) also stimulates excessive release of these inflammatory factors. Ordinarily, glutathione and other antioxidants protect against the excessive production of these cytokines, but, as noted earlier, alcohol reduces the glutathione levels in the hepatocytes, rendering them more susceptible to TNFα. In addition, ethanol inhibits production of RNA and proteins in the hepatocyte, and this inhibition also increases the susceptibility of the hepatocyte to TNFα. At low concentrations, TNFα stimulates hepatocyte growth and proliferation, but this effect is prevented by the ethanol inhibition of protein synthesis. At higher concentrations, TNFα favours apoptosis, and at still higher levels it causes necrosis of the hepatocytes. Increased iron content in the hepatocytes, which is favoured by alcohol, also sensitizes the hepatocyte to the action of TNFα. This sequence of events is summarized in Figure 43-6.

### Cirrhosis

This is the end stage of alcoholic liver disease and develops in about 10% of persons taking alcoholic beverages in excess. The condition is characterized by a loss of the normal architecture of the liver, formation of fibrous septa bridging the portal veins, and formation of regenerative nodules. As a consequence of these abnormalities, hepatic vasculature is grossly distorted: sinusoids are transformed into capillary-like structures, and blood is shunted from the portal venules to the hepatic vein. Much of the portal blood therefore bypasses the hepatic parenchymal cells, and there is a progressive loss of the liver's important role as a filter for substances entering the circulation from the gastrointestinal tract.

The mechanism by which prolonged heavy intake of alcohol leads to cirrhosis probably includes all of the processes described above, in addition to others that may be described as self-aggravating "vicious cycles." For example, constriction of the sinusoids and swelling of the hepatocytes cause increased portal venous pressure, which, in turn, results in upper gastrointestinal bleeding, increase in collateral circulation bypassing the liver, increased collagen deposition in the space of Disse, reduced functional blood perfusion of the liver, hypersplenism, and secondary anemia. All of these reduce oxygen availability to the liver, and therefore, in the presence of continued alcohol intake, they increase the risk of further hypoxic necrosis of the liver. The immediate stimulus to collagen formation again appears to involve hypoxia (via production of lactic acid), oxidative stress, cytokines, and possibly acetaldehyde adducts with cell surface proteins. Ethanol stimulates the excessive release not only of TNFα, as noted above, but also of a transforming growth factor, TGFα. All of these factors activate the Ito (stellate) cells, a type of fibroblast, causing them to lay down collagen in the space between the sinusoidal endothelium and the hepatocytes (space of Disse). As hepatocyte death and collagen deposition become more marked, the collagen that originally formed fine deposits around the sinusoids becomes converted into coarse bands of fibrous tissue that totally distort the liver architecture and compress the hepatic blood vessels, causing ascites, edema, and other characteristic clinical signs of cirrhosis.

The risk of development of cirrhosis is related to the degree and duration of excessive alcohol use. Most people with cirrhosis have consumed more than 250 mL of distilled spirits (equivalent to more than 80 g of absolute ethanol) daily for more than 10 years. Absolute alcohol intake seems to be the important factor, regardless of the type of beverage consumed: beer, wine, and distilled spirits are all capable of causing ALD and cirrhosis if enough is drunk.

## LIVER DISEASES AND THEIR DRUG TREATMENTS

In recent years, the drug treatment of hepatic disease has expanded extensively. Antiviral agents such as interferon-α and lamivudine, corticosteroids, and immunosuppressive drugs figure prominently in the treatment of various hepatic diseases (discussed elsewhere in this textbook). Specific treatments for Wilson's disease and cholestasis

FIGURE 43-6 Schematic summary of the mechanisms involved in the production of alcoholic hepatitis and cirrhosis. EtOH = ethanol; Fe = iron; GSH = reduced glutathione; LPS = bacterial lipopolysaccharides; NF-κB = nuclear factor κB; ROS = reactive oxygen species; TGFβ = transforming growth factor beta; TNFα = tumour necrosis factor alpha; IL-1, IL-8 = interleukin-1 and -8; ↑ = increased; ↓ = decreased. (Adapted from Figs. 8.3 and 8.4 by Laso, Madruga, and Orfao. In: Sherman, Preddy, and Watson, eds. *Ethanol and the Liver: Mechanisms and Management.* London: Taylor & Francis; 2002:212-213, with permission.)

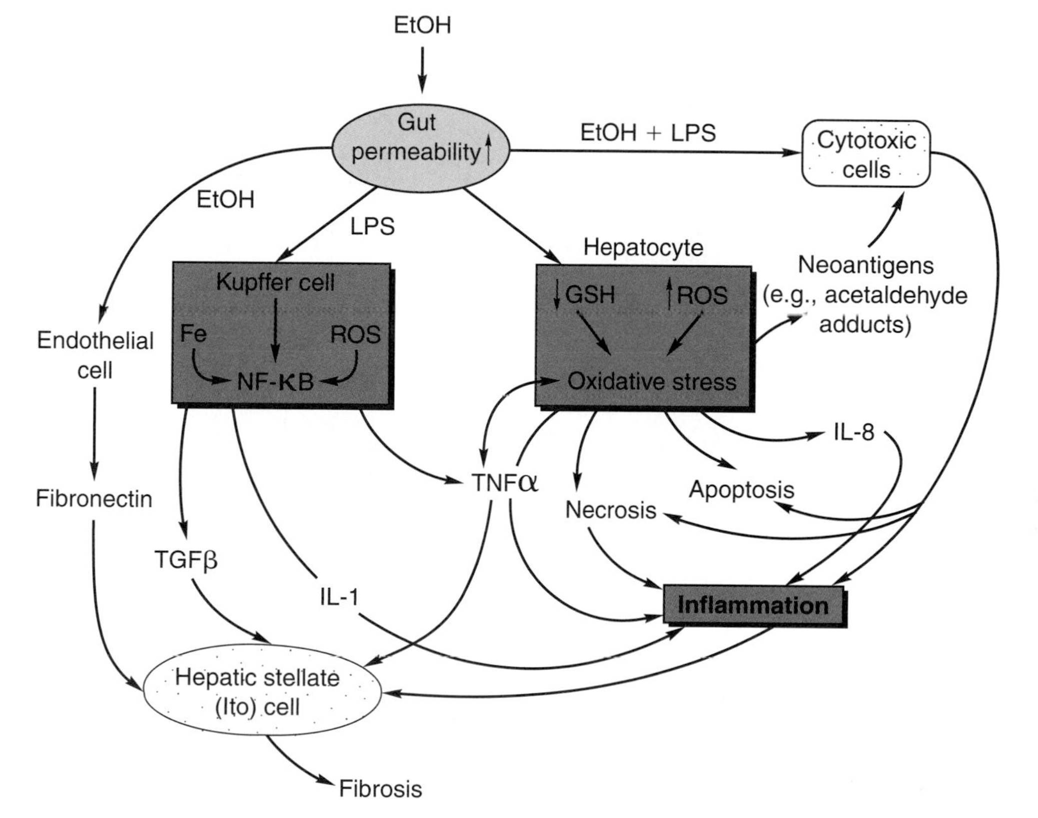

## Wilson's Disease

Wilson's disease is an autosomal recessive inherited disorder of hepatic copper metabolism. In this disease, hepatic incorporation of copper into the ferroxidase ceruloplasmin and excretion of copper into bile are abnormal. The gene that is abnormal in Wilson's disease, identified in 1993, encodes an intracellular metal-transporting P-type ATPase. Nevertheless, the biochemical mechanisms defective in Wilson's disease remain poorly understood. Patients with this disorder accumulate copper in the liver; this leads to liver damage and later to systemic, principally central nervous system (CNS), damage when the copper begins to spill out of the liver and accumulate in

are important. The former include penicillamine, trientine, and zinc; the bile acid ursodeoxycholic acid is used for cholestasis.

other organs such as the brain and eyes (Kayser-Fleischer rings). Wilson's disease is treatable with chelating agents. If it is diagnosed before there is major organ damage, the patient may remain asymptomatic indefinitely after treatment is begun. Untreated Wilson's disease is fatal, with progressive hepatic and/or neurological damage.

### Penicillamine

This drug chelates copper and can be taken orally. It is a sulfur-containing amino acid in which the thiol group and the amino group play similar roles to those of the two thiol groups in the classic chelator dimercaprol (Fig. 43-7). Penicillamine is quite toxic. However, the D-isomer is less toxic than the L-isomer, and D-penicillamine is the routine treatment modality. Penicillamine can bind lead, mercury, iron, arsenic, and copper. It can bind cystine and is used to treat cystinuria. Because it inhibits collagen cross-linking and exerts an anti-inflammatory effect, it has been used for

FIGURE 43-7 Structural formulae of dimercaprol (BAL), D-penicillamine, and triethylene tetramine (trientine), and the formation of metal chelates.

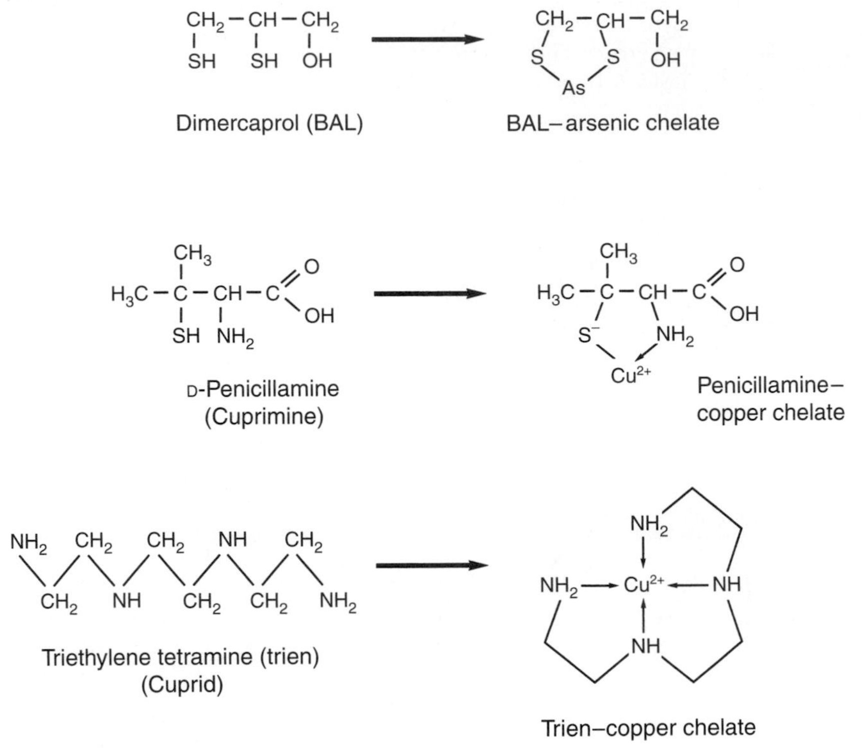

Dimercaprol (BAL) → BAL–arsenic chelate

D-Penicillamine (Cuprimine) → Penicillamine–copper chelate

Triethylene tetramine (trien) (Cuprid) → Trien–copper chelate

the treatment of rheumatoid arthritis. It is an anti-vitamin for pyridoxine, lowering its plasma and tissue levels; therefore, this vitamin is given along with penicillamine.

Penicillamine is fairly rapidly absorbed from the gastrointestinal tract. Approximately 50% of the oral dose is absorbed, and a peak blood concentration is reached in 2 hours. The mechanism of absorption is unusual: penicillamine binds to the enterocyte membrane and then is absorbed through the enterocyte, perhaps by pinocytosis. The overall bioavailability is 40 to 70%. A meal taken with penicillamine decreases absorption of the drug by approximately one-half. Once absorbed, 80% circulates bound to plasma proteins; of the 20% unbound, 6% is free penicillamine, and the rest consists of inactive disulfides. Excretion of penicillamine is largely renal; fecal excretion accounts for approximately 16%. S-methylation of penicillamine occurs in the liver, but this metabolite (S-methyl-D-penicillamine) is more common in patients with rheumatoid arthritis than in those with Wilson's disease. The elimination half-life of penicillamine varies widely between 1.7 and 7 hours. Some metabolites of penicillamine remain detectable in the urine months after the drug is stopped.

Adverse side effects of penicillamine are said to be more common in patients without Wilson's disease, but the incidence in Wilson's disease is as high as 30%. Severe degenerative skin changes may develop over time due to changes in collagen formation. Adverse cutaneous reactions include various rashes, pemphigus, and elastosis perforans serpiginosa. The sense of taste may change (dysgeusia). Adverse hematological reactions (leukopenia or thrombocytopenia) are common but are usually reversible if identified early. Rarely, severe global bone marrow failure (aplastic anemia) develops, which may not be reversible. Perhaps the worst problems are autoimmune-like syndromes: nephrotic syndrome, systemic vasculitis resembling lupus erythematosus, Goodpasture's syndrome affecting the lungs, or a myasthenia gravis–like syndrome. Severe hematological or systemic side effects always require cessation of treatment. If penicillamine treatment in Wilson's disease is stopped because of adverse side effects, a different chelator must be substituted.

Some patients develop an early hypersensitivity reaction to penicillamine in the first 7 to 10 days of taking it. They develop rash, fever, anorexia, lymphadenopathy, leukopenia, and thrombocytopenia. Proteinuria may also occur. In general, another chelator (trientine) is then substituted. Alternatively, the penicillamine is stopped and then reintroduced gradually, and these patients may develop tolerance for the drug. Occasionally, steroids must be given briefly.

## Trientine

The usual alternative treatment for patients with Wilson's disease who develop severe toxicity from penicillamine is triethylene tetramine dihydrochloride (2,2,2-tetramine), known as trientine, or by its official short name trien (see Fig. 43-7). Trientine does not contain sulfhydryl groups. It chelates copper by forming a stable complex with its four constituent nitrogens in a planar ring. Trientine increases urinary copper excretion and may interfere with its intestinal absorption.

Little is known about the pharmacokinetics of trientine. It is poorly absorbed from the gastrointestinal tract; what is absorbed is biotransformed and inactivated. Chronic treatment may lead to iron deficiency. Trientine may rarely cause severe gastritis, dysgeusia, and rashes. However, adverse effects due to penicillamine resolve and do not recur during treatment with trientine. Although it may be intrinsically a somewhat weaker chelator than penicillamine, the dose can be increased as necessary for clinical effectiveness.

## Zinc

Although zinc was used to treat Wilson's disease in the early 1960s, it has only recently received wider attention as an alternative treatment modality for this disease. Some treatment regimens are unwieldy. For adults, the most practical and effective regimen is 50 mg elemental zinc orally at least 30 minutes from meals, three times daily. Half of this dose is used for smaller children. The dosage regimen must be individualized by titrating against its effect on non-ceruloplasmin-bound serum copper.

This drug therapy is important because the mechanism of action of zinc in Wilson's disease is entirely different from that of chelators. Zinc treatment interferes with the uptake of copper from the gastrointestinal tract. It is postulated that excess zinc induces the formation of metallothionein in enterocytes; however, this metallothionein has greater affinity for copper than for zinc, and it preferentially binds copper present in the gastrointestinal tract. Once bound, the copper is not absorbed but instead is lost into the fecal contents as enterocytes are shed in the course of normal cellular turnover. Since copper enters the gastrointestinal tract from saliva and gastric secretions, zinc treatment can remove stored copper. An unresolved problem with respect to long-term safety of zinc therapy is the effect on hepatic copper. Patients treated chronically with zinc have been found to have higher concentrations of hepatic copper late in the treatment, despite being clinically well. Possibly, this copper is complexed to hepatic metallothionein and is thus detoxified.

The major adverse effect of zinc treatment has been epigastric pain, probably due to gastritis. Acetate or gluconate salts of zinc may be less irritating than the sulfate. The effectiveness of zinc is the same irrespective of which salt is used. Abdominal pain is probably less likely to occur if zinc is taken with food, but food interferes greatly with zinc absorption. Other long-term effects in humans remain unknown. Studies in laboratory animals suggest that high doses of zinc may be immunosuppressive. Patients regularly develop elevated serum zinc levels, and the long-term effects on body tissues, notably the kidney, are uncertain.

## Cholestasis and Cholelithiasis: Ursodeoxycholic Acid

Ursodeoxycholic acid (UDCA; ursodiol) is a hydrophilic epimer of one of the primary bile acids, chenodeoxycholic acid (CDCA). As shown in Figure 43-8, the difference is in the position of one hydroxyl group. In pharmacological doses, UDCA displaces more toxic bile acids from the bile acid pool, partly by decreasing intestinal absorption of the primary bile acids CDCA and cholic acid. UDCA appears to have three main pharmacological effects: (1) increasing cholesterol saturation in bile, (2) causing increased bile secretion (choleresis), and (3) providing hepatic cytoprotection. The choleresis appears to be due to increased biliary bicarbonate secretion and increased contractility of the smallest bile duct radicles. UDCA was originally used for the treatment of cholesterol gallstone disease, but more recently, it has been used for other types of chronic liver disease involving damage to any bile ducts.

UDCA, administered orally as unconjugated bile acid, is rapidly absorbed from the small intestine. It is conjugated with glycine or taurine in the liver and enters the enterohepatic circulation. With repeated dosing, UDCA becomes a major constituent of the bile acid pool. Excretion is ultimately via the feces. The elimination half-life for exogenously administered UDCA is estimated to be 3 to 6 days.

UDCA is well tolerated when taken orally. It may cause transient itching. Unlike CDCA, it does not cause diarrhea to any great extent because it does not stimulate colonic water secretion. It is not hepatotoxic; however, it should not be given to patients with complete blockage of bile drainage because in this situation liver damage may ensue.

With respect to gallstone dissolution, its original use, UDCA is effective in dissolving pure cholesterol gallstones that are not calcified. It is more likely to work when the stone is small (<1 cm diameter) and floating on the gallbladder contents. It is not effective if the gallbladder is so diseased that it does not concentrate the bile or if the cystic duct is blocked. The mechanism of dissolution is that UDCA increases the effectiveness of micelle formation, supports cholesterol liquid crystal formation within these micelles, and increases the amount of cholesterol that can be solubilized.

As a therapy, gallstone dissolution by UDCA will not replace cholecystectomy, especially laparoscopic cholecystectomy, but it may have a role in patients who cannot undergo surgery, in hepatolithiasis, or as an adjunct to

**FIGURE 43-8** Structural formulae of ursodeoxycholic acid (UDCA) and chenodeoxycholic acid (CDCA).

Ursodeoxycholic acid (UDCA)
3α, 7β-dihydroxy-5β-cholanic acid

Chenodeoxycholic acid (CDCA)
3α, 7α-dihydroxy-5β-cholanic acid

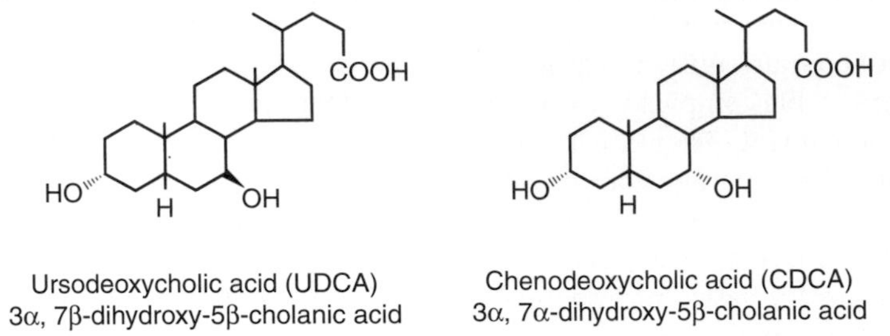

lithotripsy. Chronic administration of UDCA can dissolve cholesterol gallstones without producing the diarrhea or hepatotoxicity that are major side effects of CDCA, which has also been used for gallstone dissolution. Compared with CDCA, UDCA is safer and more effective, but surface calcification of the gallstone is more likely to develop. UDCA enhances micelle formation in the bile to a greater extent than CDCA, thus increasing the cholesterol-carrying capacity, but it does not suppress hepatic bile acid synthesis as much as CDCA does.

In the course of studying the use of UDCA for gallstone dissolution, its beneficial effects in chronic cholestasis were discovered. Treating cholestatic liver disease has become the main indication for UDCA treatment. UDCA has been tried in nearly every chronic cholestatic disease and may be beneficial in some of them. In primary biliary cirrhosis, biochemical abnormalities improve with UDCA treatment, and the overall outcome is improved. UDCA appears to improve liver function in children with liver disease associated with cystic fibrosis, and it decreases cholestasis in children with Alagille's syndrome, improving pruritus and lowering serum cholesterol levels. UDCA improves liver function in babies with certain rare inborn errors of bile acid metabolism.

Several mechanisms of action have been proposed to explain the beneficial effect of UDCA in chronic cholestatic disease. Its action as a choleretic may be important. Also, it prevents damage to hepatocyte and bile duct epithelial cell membranes by more hydrophobic bile acids. This cytoprotective effect has been demonstrated in vitro. UDCA also inhibits apoptosis. It affects some immune functions, including decreased expression of class I human leukocyte antigens (HLAs) on hepatocytes. It has been shown to inhibit proliferation of peripheral blood mononuclear cells in vitro.

## Viral Hepatitis

Viral hepatitis exists in three forms, designated hepatitis A, B, and C. Hepatitis A, the most common form, is also usually the most benign, and it typically resolves spontaneously without the need for antiviral chemotherapy. In contrast, hepatitis B and C are more severe and tend to become chronic and potentially fatal. Antiviral chemotherapy has therefore become a central part of their treatment. The drugs used for this purpose include **lamivudine, interferon-α**, and **pegylated interferon-α**. Please see Chapter 55 for detailed descriptions of the pharmacology of these drugs.

## SUGGESTED READINGS

Arias IM, Jakoby WB, Popper H, Schachter D, Shafritz DA, eds. *The Liver: Biology and Pathobiology.* New York, NY: Raven Press; 1988.

Cameron RG, Feuer G, de la Iglesia FA, eds. *Drug-Induced Hepatotoxicity.* Berlin, Germany: Springer-Verlag; 1996.

Cohen SD, Pumford NR, Khairallah EA, et al. Selective covalent protein binding and target organ toxicity. *Toxicol Appl Pharmacol.* 1997;143:1-12.

Farrell GC. *Drug-Induced Liver Disease.* Edinburgh, United Kingdom: Churchill Livingstone; 1994.

Fattinger K, Funk C, Pantze M, et al. The endothelin antagonist bosentan inhibits the canalicular bile salt export pump: a potential mechanism for hepatic adverse reactions. *Clin Pharmacol Ther.* 2001;69:223-231.

Israel Y, Kalant H, Orrego H, et al. Experimental alcohol-induced hepatic necrosis: suppression by propylthiouracil. *Proc Natl Acad Sci USA.* 1975;72:1137-1141.

Israel Y, Orrego H. Hypermetabolic state, hepatocyte expansion and liver blood flow: an interaction triad in alcoholic liver injury. *Ann NY Acad Sci.* 1987;492:303-323.

Jaeschke H, Knight TR, Bajt ML. The role of oxidant stress and reactive nitrogen species in acetaminophen hepatotoxicity. *Toxicol Lett.* 2003;144:279-288.

Jerrells TR, ed. Symposium on role of fatty liver, dietary fatty acid supplements, and obesity in the progression of alcoholic liver disease [special issue]. *Alcohol.* 2004;34:1-87.

Kelly DA. *Diseases of the Liver and Biliary System in Children.* 2nd ed. Oxford, United Kingdom: Blackwell Science; 2004.

Meeting Report. Current progress in studies on alcohol-induced organ injury. *Alcohol.* 1993;10:437-484.

Mitchell JB, Russo A. The role of glutathione in radiation and drug induced cytotoxicity. *Br J Cancer Suppl.* 1987;8:96-104.

Poupon RE, Lindor KD, Cauch-Dudek K, Dickson ER, Poupon R, Heathcote EJ. Combined analysis of randomized controlled trials of ursodeoxycholic acid in primary biliary cirrhosis. *Gastroenterology.* 1997;113:884-890.

Schilsky ML. Wilson disease: genetic basis of copper toxicity and natural history. *Semin Liver Dis.* 1996;16:83-95.

Sherlock S, Dooley JS. *Diseases of the Liver and Biliary System.* 11th ed. Oxford, United Kingdom: Blackwell Science; 2002.

Sherman DIN, Preedy VR, Watson RR, eds. *Ethanol and the Liver: Mechanisms and Management.* London, United Kingdom: Taylor & Francis; 2002.

Spahr L, Negro F, Rubbia-Brandt L, et al. Acute valproate-associated microvesicular steatosis: could the $[^{13}C]$-methionine breath test be useful to assess liver mitochondrial function? *Dig Dis Sci.* 2001;46:2758-2761.

Trauner M, Boyer JL. Bile salt transporters: molecular characterization, function, and regulation. *Physiol Rev.* 2003;83:633-671.

Trauner M, Graziadei IW. Mechanisms of action and therapeutic applications of ursodeoxycholic acid in chronic liver diseases. *Aliment Pharmacol Ther.* 1999;13:979-996.

Tsukamoto H, Takei Y, McClain CJ, et al. How is the liver primed or sensitized for alcoholic liver disease? *Alcohol Clin Exp Res.* 2001;25(5 suppl):171S-181S.

Zafrani ES, Pinaudeau Y, Dhumeaux D. Drug-induced vascular lesions of the liver. *Arch Intern Med.* 1983;143:495-502.

Zimmerman HJ, Maddrey WC. Toxic and drug-induced hepatitis. In: Schiff L, Schiff ER, eds. *Disease of the Liver.* 5th ed. Philadelphia, Pa: JB Lippincott; 1987:591-667.

# Part VIII

## Endocrine Systems

# 44

# Vasopressin, Oxytocin, and Uterotonic Drugs

## SR GEORGE AND BP SCHIMMER

### CASE HISTORY

A 32-year-old male race car driver crashed during a race and sustained a skull fracture with severe contusions of the head and loss of consciousness. In hospital, his urinary output was noted to be excessive, at a rate of 500 mL/hr. The urine was pale and dilute with a specific gravity of 1.005. The serum sodium was elevated, with a value of 149 mmol/L (normal range 132 to 145 mmol/L), and there was serum hyperosmolality. A diagnosis of diabetes insipidus secondary to trauma was made. He was given desmopressin 1 μg subcutaneously, and the signs of diabetes insipidus diminished within a few hours. The treatment was repeated every 12 hours. After 3 days, his general condition, including consciousness, reflexes, and movement, improved markedly, and he was switched from parenteral desmopressin to the nasal spray, 10 μg twice daily.

After 5 weeks on this treatment, during which time his injuries continued to steadily improve, he began to complain of headache and some flushing of the face. Two days later, he became rather confused and suffered a generalized tonic–clonic seizure. His plasma sodium was found to be 115 mmol/L. The desmopressin was stopped and fluid intake was restricted. Over the next 3 days, he recovered fully and was able to maintain normal water and electrolyte balance without reinstatement of desmopressin therapy.

Vasopressin and oxytocin are related nonapeptides that differ by only two amino acids. Both hormones may have evolved from a single ancestral peptide, vasotocin, through molecular processes involving mutation and gene duplication. Vasotocin is the form found in primitive species such as elasmobranchs and bony fishes, and it has biological activities intermediate between those of vasopressin and oxytocin when tested in mammalian systems. Du Vigneaud is credited with determining the structure of these peptide hormones and with synthesizing them. He was awarded the Nobel Prize in 1955.

Because of their structural similarities, the two peptides have similar pharmacological activities, but these are expressed to different degrees. For example, vasopressin has greater antidiuretic and pressor activities and less uterotonic and milk-ejecting activities than oxytocin.

Following the pioneering work of du Vigneaud, a large number of synthetic hormone analogues have been prepared and tested for separation of various pharmacological activities. Some of the analogues have markedly selective actions and have become clinically important drugs.

## BIOSYNTHETIC AND ANATOMICAL RELATIONSHIPS

The hypothalamus and the posterior lobe of the pituitary gland function together as a neurosecretory unit. The anatomical relationships of this unit are shown in Figure 44-1.

### Site of Synthesis

Vasopressin and oxytocin are synthesized in the cell bodies of specialized neurons of the hypothalamus and are transported to the nerve terminals in the posterior lobe (pars nervosa) of the pituitary gland by axonal transport. **Vasopressin** is synthesized in neural cell bodies that are localized predominantly in the **supraoptic nucleus**, while **oxytocin** is synthesized in neural cell bodies that are predominantly in the **paraventricular nucleus**.

### Synthesis and Processing

Both peptides have molecular weights of approximately 1100 Da but are synthesized as larger precursor proteins

**FIGURE 44-1** Anatomical structure and relationships of the hypothalamus and pituitary gland.

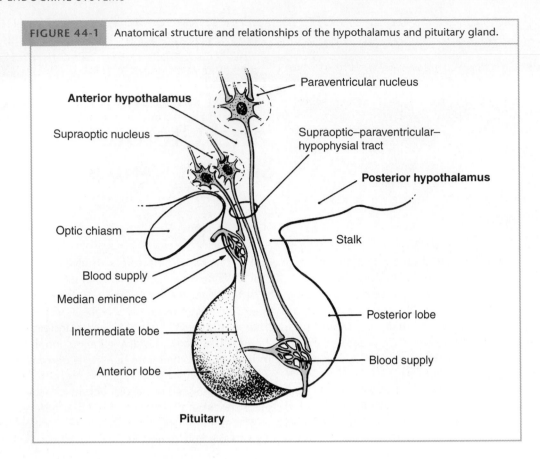

(prohormones). The prohormones also give rise to two distinct neurophysins (approximately 10 000 Da), which serve as carriers for vasopressin and oxytocin. The prohormones are synthesized on membrane-bound ribosomes, packaged into secretory granules, and then enzymatically cleaved so that the hormones remain associated with the neurophysins through electrostatic forces. The hormone-containing granules are transported to nerve terminals via unmyelinated axons. Most axons pass through the pituitary stalk and end in the posterior pituitary. Some axons only extend to the median eminence.

## Secretion

Inputs from peripheral signals and from the central nervous system (CNS) converge on the hypothalamic nuclei. These signals trigger electrical impulses that travel down the axons of the neurosecretory fibres to the nerve terminals and stimulate hormone secretion. The secretory response is thought to involve (1) influx of calcium to the cytosol, (2) fusion of secretory granules with the membranes of the nerve terminals, (3) emptying of the granule contents into surrounding capillaries, and (4) recapture of empty granules (as small vesicles) from the cell surface. Although vaso-

pressin and oxytocin are synthesized in separate neurons, most stimuli for secretion may cause the release of both peptides. The type of stimulus, however, does determine the relative proportions of the secreted mixture. For example, thirst or hemorrhage causes preferential release of vasopressin; suckling stimulates the preferential release of oxytocin.

## Role of the Posterior Pituitary Gland

The posterior pituitary serves as a storage site for vasopressin and oxytocin. It is a physical, as well as functional, extension of the nervous system, organized into a specialized secretory apparatus. The posterior pituitary is composed of swollen, granule-filled nerve terminals in juxtaposition to blood capillaries (see Fig. 44-1) and supported by pituicytes (glial cells). Lesions in the hypothalamic nuclei or in the hypothalamic–neurohypophysial tract destroy the capacity for vasopressin and oxytocin synthesis. Removal of the posterior pituitary or transection of the pituitary stalk, however, generally causes only a transient deficiency because the nerve fibres terminating in the median eminence remain functional and release amounts of these hormones sufficient for normal physiological requirements.

# CHEMICAL STRUCTURE

The structures of vasopressin and oxytocin are shown in Figure 44-2. In both hormones, six of the amino acids form ring structures by closure of the S–S bond between cysteines at positions 1 and 6; attached to the ring of each peptide is a tail of three amino acids with an amide at the carboxyl terminus. Opening the S–S bond results in a linear nonapeptide that is devoid of hormonal activity. For vasopressin activity, the tail must contain a basic amino acid (arginine in most mammals, lysine in the pig) at position 8 (see Fig. 44-2).

# VASOPRESSIN (ADH)

## Physiology and Pharmacology

### Receptors

Vasopressin acts through different types of G protein–coupled receptors, designated $V_1$, $V_2$, and $V_3$ (an isoform of $V_1$, also called $V_{1b}$). The $V_1$ and $V_3$ receptor acts through $G_{q/11}$ to increase the inositol trisphosphate cycle and results in a large increase in intracellular $Ca^{2+}$ (see Chapter 9). The $V_2$ receptor, acting through the stimulatory

FIGURE 44-2 Amino acid sequences for vasopressin and oxytocin. The hormones differ in sequence at positions 3 and 8.

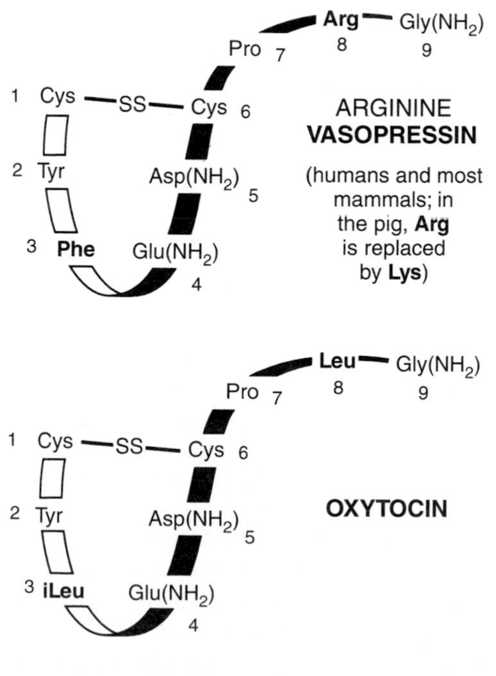

guanine nucleotide–binding protein ($G_s$), activates adenylyl cyclase and increased cAMP-dependent signalling. $V_1$ is found predominantly in vascular tissue, $V_2$ is in the kidneys, and $V_3$ is primarily in the pituitary. Synthetic peptides have been produced that act as specific agonists or specific antagonists for each receptor so as to permit a more selective activation or blockade of the different physiological effects of vasopressin.

## Antidiuretic action

In humans, the major physiological action of vasopressin is stimulation of the reabsorption of water by the collecting ducts of the kidney. Therefore, vasopressin is also known as antidiuretic hormone (ADH). ADH increases the permeability of the tubular epithelium to the passage of water. Water, together with sodium and urea, moves from the tubular lumen into the interstitial fluid in response to an osmotic gradient, leaving solutes behind in more concentrated urine. The antidiuretic effect is extremely potent. Less than 0.1 µg/hr, administered by slow intravenous infusion, suppresses human urine flow completely.

The mechanism of action of ADH on the collecting duct is shown in Figure 44-3. ADH, in sequential fashion, (1) interacts with a $V_2$ receptor ($V_2$R), (2) activates $G_s$, (3) activates adenylyl cyclase and causes cyclic adenosine monophosphate (cAMP) to accumulate, and (4) activates cAMP-dependent protein kinase, increasing the phosphorylation of specific proteins. There is some evidence that one of the consequences of ADH-stimulated protein phosphorylation is the appearance of cell-surface water channels (aquaporins), thus increasing the permeability of the luminal membrane to water. Since this process is sensitive to microtubule poisons (colchicine, vinca alkaloids), microtubules are probably involved. As part of its action, ADH also stimulates the synthesis of prostaglandin $E_1$ ($PGE_1$), which serves to locally inhibit ADH action in a negative feedback loop. The adenylyl cyclase system appears to be the target of the inhibitory influence of $PGE_1$. Atrial natriuretic peptide antagonizes the ADH effect on water permeability in the collecting ducts and promotes diuresis through a cyclic guanosine monophosphate (GMP) mechanism (see Chapter 37).

Secretion of ADH can be stimulated or inhibited by osmotic, volemic, or neural stimuli reaching cells in the supraoptic nucleus (Fig. 44-4).

**ADH secretion is stimulated by the following:**

- Hyperosmolality of plasma: Secretion is responsive to as little as 1 to 2% change in osmolality. This action is exerted through **osmoreceptors** located in the hypothalamus and other brain regions.
- Volume depletion: This may include hemorrhage or pooling of blood in the extremities while standing. As little as 6 to 10% change in blood volume affects

**FIGURE 44-3** Mechanism of action of ADH on water reabsorption (see text for abbreviations).

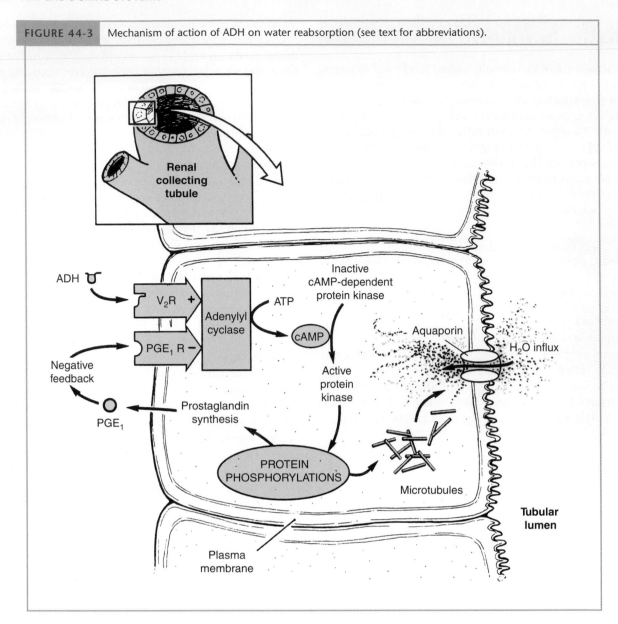

ADH release by an action mediated through stretch receptors and baroreceptors in the left atrium, carotid bodies, aorta, and pulmonary vessels.

- Drugs: These include cholinergic agonists (e.g., nicotine), clofibrate, tricyclic antidepressants, and cyclophosphamide.
- Noxious stimuli: These include pain and nausea.

**ADH secretion is inhibited by the following:**

- Hemodilution: Hypo-osmolality and increased blood volume are the operative factors.
- Nervous stimuli: These include cold exposure and emotional stress.
- Drugs: These include alcohol, some antipsychotics such as haloperidol, and glucocorticoids.

In addition to stimulating and inhibiting ADH secretion, drugs can affect the antidiuretic action of ADH in a variety of ways, as shown in Table 44-1.

### Smooth muscle contraction

At high dose, vasopressin causes the contraction of smooth muscle fibres in a number of tissues through an action on vasopressin $V_1$ receptors located on vascular and other smooth muscle cells:

- It causes pronounced vasoconstriction; the effect is general and includes coronary blood vessels.
- The motility of intestinal smooth muscle, especially in the lower bowel, is increased.
- It stimulates uterine and cervical contractions, particularly in circular smooth muscle. It causes short,

frequent contractions without distinction between pregnant and non-pregnant uterus.

## Blood coagulation

Vasopressin increases the levels of clotting factor VIII and von Willebrand factor. These effects may have implications in the management of some blood clotting diseases and in prophylactic control of bleeding during surgery in patients with factor VIII deficiency.

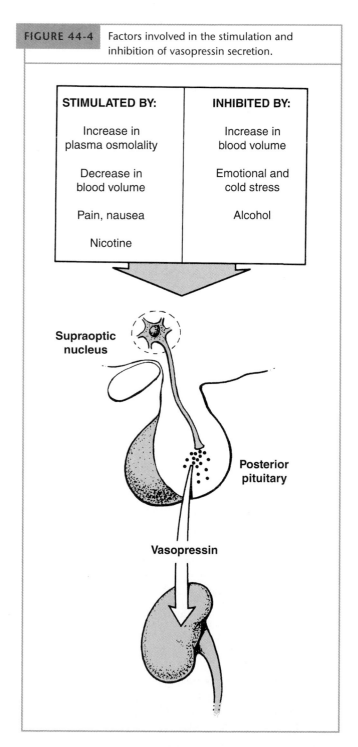

**FIGURE 44-4** Factors involved in the stimulation and inhibition of vasopressin secretion.

| STIMULATED BY: | INHIBITED BY: |
|---|---|
| Increase in plasma osmolality | Increase in blood volume |
| Decrease in blood volume | Emotional and cold stress |
| Pain, nausea | Alcohol |
| Nicotine | |

**Supraoptic nucleus**

**Posterior pituitary**

**Vasopressin**

## ACTH secretion

Vasopressin stimulates adrenocorticotropic hormone (ACTH) release from the anterior pituitary through the $V_3$ receptors present on corticotrophs. This effect is synergistic with corticotropin-releasing hormone (CRH), which is the principal releasing factor for ACTH.

## CNS function

Vasopressin is found in other parts of the brain in association with both $V_1$ and $V_2$ receptors; this fact suggests that vasopressin has neurotransmitter or neuromodulator activity and may play various physiological roles in the CNS (see Chapter 16). When administered through normal routes, vasopressin improves the ability to learn new information and enhances long-term memory. These effects are being explored in the treatment of amnesia and in the improvement of attention and memory in the elderly. Vasopressin also has effects on autonomic function mediated via the CNS, including actions that decrease body temperature, slow the heart rate, and increase the respiratory rate.

## Synthetic Analogues

Both vasopressin and oxytocin have short half-lives in the circulation (approximately 10 minutes), principally due to proteolytic degradation. An important site in both hormones for proteolytic inactivation is between the first two amino acids (Cys–Tyr). Cleavage of peptide bonds in the tail also contributes to loss of activity. The rapid turnover of these peptides limits their duration of action. Hence, synthetic analogues of vasopressin with increased duration of action have been developed and are more important clinically.

Another important rationale for the development of synthetic analogues is to achieve greater separation of the antidiuretic and pressor actions of vasopressin. As shown in Table 44-2, four modifications are important for enhanced antidiuretic activity. Combinations of these four modifications produce synergistic results. For example, 1-desamino-8-D-arginine vasopressin (DDAVP, desmopressin) has an antidiuretic activity that is 2000 times greater than its pressor effect. The analogue 1-desamino-4-valine-8-D-arginine vasopressin (DVDAVP) is even more selectively potent but has been used only experimentally so far. Deamination at position 1 also renders the peptide more resistant to proteolysis, as does the substitution of D-arginine at position 8.

Other modifications can selectively increase the pressor effect of vasopressin, yielding derivatives with clinical potential as local hemostatic agents during surgery. One such analogue is 2-phenylalanine-3-isoleucine-8-ornithine vasopressin. It has a pressor to ADH ratio of 255:1; it is used for experimental purposes only.

| TABLE 44-1 | Drugs Affecting Antidiuretic Action of ADH |
|---|---|
| **Drug** | **Mechanism of Action** |
| Potentiators of ADH action<br>  Acetylsalicylic acid (aspirin)<br>  Chlorpropamide<br>  Indomethacin | Inhibit renal prostaglandin synthesis; chlorpropamide also stimulates ADH secretion |
| Inhibitors of ADH action<br>  Lithium carbonate $\big\}$<br>  Prostaglandin $E_1$ | Inhibit adenylyl cyclase |
|   Colchicine $\big\}$<br>  Vinca alkaloids | Microtubular poisons |
| Demeclocycline | Inhibits ADH action on the collecting ducts: used to treat SIADH |
| Diuretics<br>Thiazides<br>(e.g., hydrochlorthiazide) | Unknown and paradoxical; effects may result from systemic depletion of electrolytes, which in turn causes enhanced resorption of salt and water from the proximal tubule (see also Chapter 37); useful in treatment of nephrogenic or partial hypothalamic diabetes insipidus |

SIADH = Syndrome of inappropriate antidiuretic hormone secretion.

## Preparations

**Desmopressin** (DDAVP), the 1-desamino-8-D-arginine synthetic analogue, has a longer half-life than vasopressin. Since it is selective for $V_2$ vasopressin receptors, it has greater ADH potency and less pressor activity than vasopressin. It has to be administered in high doses when given by mouth because it is broken down by intestinal peptidases. Preparations are supplied in isotonic saline as the acetate salt (0.1 mg/mL) and are administered intranasally. DDAVP for injection (4 µg/mL) also is available. Its duration of action is 8 to 12 hours. An oral formulation is also available.

**Arginine vasopressin** (Pressyn) is an aqueous solution for intravenous or intramuscular injection; the standard dosage formulation provides a 10 IU/0.5-mL ampoule. (The international unit of vasopressin is defined by the pressor activity, in rats, of 0.5 mg of a USP standard posterior pituitary powder. One unit of activity corresponds to approximately 3 µg of purified arginine vasopressin.) The active agent may be purified from animal posterior pituitary (in which case it may have some contaminating oxytocic activity); more often, it is chemically synthesized. It acts for 3 to 4 hours.

## Therapeutic Uses

### Diabetes insipidus

This disease, caused by insufficient endogenous ADH, is characterized by excretion of large volumes of dilute urine (specific gravity about 1.002), serum hyperosmolality, extreme thirst, and copious intake of water. Diabetes insipidus can be congenital or can result from *lesions*—caused by, for example, tumours, surgery, or head trauma—affecting the hypothalamus, posterior pituitary, or pitu-

itary stalk. The treatment of choice is desmopressin (DDAVP) administered intranasally, orally, or by injection. The dose depends on the severity of the symptoms and ranges from 2.5 to 20 µg intranasally two or three times a day, 0.1 to 0.2 mg orally twice a day, or 1 to 2 µg twice a day by subcutaneous, intramuscular, or intravenous injection. The main adverse effect of nasal administration is local irritation (rhinitis).

The existence of polyuria and polydipsia is not a priori due to diabetes insipidus of hypothalamic origin. For example, similar symptoms are seen in diabetes insipidus of nephrogenic origin (i.e., failure of the kidney to respond to ADH). Small doses of desmopressin are very effective in decreasing polyuria, polydipsia, and restoring serum osmolality in hypothalamic diabetes insipidus; desmopressin is ineffective in nephrogenic diabetes insipidus.

| TABLE 44-2 | Modifications Affecting the Ratio of Antidiuretic to Pressor Activity of Vasopressin | |
|---|---|---|
| **Modification** | | **ADH/Pressor Ratio*** |
| Deamination at position 1 | | 4 |
| Substitution of Phe for Tyr | | 3 |
| Substitution of Val or Thr for Glu ($NH_2$) | | 23 |
| Substitution of D-Arg for L-Arg | | 28 |
| 1-Desamino plus 8-D-Arg | | 2000 |
| 1-Desamino-8-D-Arg plus 4-Val | | >150 000 |

*Results are compared with arginine vasopressin, which is assigned a normalized value of 1.0.

### Enuresis (bedwetting)

Desmopressin has also been used to treat children with primary enuresis by administering a single bedtime dose to increase nocturnal renal concentrating ability. However, the high probability of spontaneous disappearance of the problem, and the possibility of side effects of the treatment, limit the value of this therapy.

### Local hemostasis

Arginine vasopressin is used for hemostasis in the treatment of bleeding esophageal varices and in the control of active gastrointestinal bleeding. It is administered by local arterial infusion to cause splanchnic vasoconstriction.

### Coagulation disorders

Desmopressin is used to treat von Willebrand's disease and hemophilia associated with factor VIII deficiency, particularly before elective surgery.

### Ventricular fibrillation

Arginine vasopressin has been added to the advanced cardiac life support protocol for the resuscitation of patients with ventricular fibrillation or pulseless ventricular tachycardia. In this setting, the vasoconstrictor effects are used to treat underlying systemic vasodilation and an accompanying decrease in circulating endogenous hormone. Arginine vasopressin has been shown to be as effective as adrenaline, but its effect on long-term outcomes has yet to be established.

## Toxicity

Symptoms of toxicity (which may occur from overdose) result from a mixture of effects at vasopressin $V_1$ and $V_2$ receptors and include hypertension, headache, cerebral or coronary arterial spasm, water intoxication, hyponatremia, pallor, nausea, abdominal cramps from increased intestinal activity, uterine cramps, and peripheral arterial vasospasm that may result in gangrene.

## Other Conditions Involving ADH

### Syndrome of Inappropriate Antidiuretic Hormone Secretion (SIADH)

SIADH results from the pathological overproduction of ADH as a result of CNS disorders or ectopic production by tumours. This condition is treated by demeclocycline (a tetracycline), which inhibits ADH action in the collecting ducts of the kidney.

### Treatment of chronic heart failure

Data from small clinical studies suggest that ADH antagonists may reduce water retention and improve hemodynamics in patients with chronic heart failure. Two small-molecule antagonists, called vaptans, are currently under evaluation: the $V_2$ receptor-selective antagonist **tolvaptan** and the $V_1/V_2$ antagonist **colvaptan**.

## OXYTOCIN

## Physiology and Pharmacology

### Milk ejection

Milk ejection appears to be the major physiological function of oxytocin. Oxytocin stimulates the contraction of myoepithelial cells of the breast during the postpartum period. These cells surround the channels of the glandular system and serve to squeeze milk out of the alveoli and ducts into larger sinuses. This is called "milk letdown" and is different from milk secretion. Suckling at the nipple of the breast is an important stimulus for the release of oxytocin.

### Uterine contraction

Sensitivity of the uterus to oxytocin increases rapidly during the last trimester of pregnancy because of a dramatic increase in uterine oxytocin receptors. Thus, when labour is imminent, sensitivity to oxytocin is much greater than to vasopressin. Oxytocin stimulates slow, long-lasting peristaltic contractions of the upper uterine segment and relaxes the cervix. This is a useful type of contraction for the expulsion of uterine contents. Estrogen increases the sensitivity of the uterus to oxytocin; progesterone renders uterine tissue more resistant but this effect of progesterone wanes in late pregnancy. The effect of oxytocin on the non-pregnant uterus is slight.

The physiological importance of oxytocin in the initiation of labour or in delivery is debatable. Arguments against the involvement of oxytocin include the observations that blood levels of oxytocin do not increase until labour is well advanced and that parturition still proceeds in the absence of oxytocin (although prolonged labour has been reported).

### Effects on the corpus luteum

Oxytocin may also regulate the lifespan of the corpus luteum and thus may play a role in the regulation of fertility. Evidence for this includes the observations that oxytocin administered to experimental animals shortens the lifespan of the corpus luteum and hastens the onset of estrus, while active immunization of animals against oxytocin has the opposite effect.

### Vascular effects

Oxytocin tends to relax circular fibres of smooth muscle and, in large doses, will lower blood pressure. Deep anaesthesia or concurrent use of ganglionic-blocking drugs increases the likelihood of this potentially dangerous effect.

## Mechanism of action

The hormone exerts its action through specific G protein–coupled receptors at the cell surface. Activation of the receptor is associated with increased phospholipase C activity and consequent mobilization of intracellular calcium. Activation of voltage-sensitive calcium channels has also been demonstrated.

## Preparations

**Oxytocin injection** (Pitocin, Syntocinon) contains synthetic, pure oxytocin and is provided as an aqueous solution for intramuscular or intravenous injection, containing 10 IU/mL. (One unit is equivalent to about 2 μg of pure oxytocin. Oxytocic activity is bioassayed by measuring the drop in blood pressure in chickens; uterotonic activity parallels the decrease in blood pressure.) **Oxytocin nasal solution** is a nasal spray containing 40 IU/mL of synthetic oxytocin.

## Therapeutic Uses

### Stimulation of labour at term

Oxytocin is used primarily to induce labour. The aim is to determine the dose that just initiates labour without producing overly strong contractions, thereby avoiding damage to the fetus or uterus in the early stages. Preferably, oxytocin is administered by slow intravenous infusion. Initial doses are small (2 mU/min) and are gradually increased to a maximum of 20 mU/min if necessary. Throughout this treatment, the resting uterine tone; the force, duration, and frequency of uterine contractions; and the fetal heart rate should be carefully monitored. The short half-life (minutes) of oxytocin permits effective control through changes of the infusion rate. Oxytocin may be used in select cases to resume labour if the uterus shows inertia during the first stage.

Contraindications for the use of oxytocin include a predisposition to uterine rupture, signs of fetal distress, or situations that preclude normal vaginal delivery.

### Control of postpartum bleeding

Bleeding may occur if the uterus relaxes too much during the interval of placental expulsion. Administration of oxytocin (approximately 5 IU) after the head is delivered will prevent excessive relaxation of the uterus during this stage. If oxytocin is administered again *after* the placenta is expelled, it will cause strong tetanic contraction of the uterus and prevent postpartum bleeding.

### Stimulation of milk ejection

Oxytocin is sometimes useful in relieving breast engorgement or in facilitating breastfeeding when milk letdown is a problem. For these purposes, oxytocin is administered as a nasal spray a few minutes before feeding. Oxytocin is of no value if there is inadequate milk production.

## Adverse Effects

The toxicity of oxytocin is an extension of its physiological effects and may include tetanic uterine contractions, which may result in fetal hypoxia. β2-Adrenergic agonists may be used to reverse the sustained (tetanic) uterine contractions. Hypotension occurs as a result of relaxation of vascular smooth muscle. Symptoms of water intoxication may be elicited because of the structural similarity between oxytocin and vasopressin.

# ERGOT ALKALOIDS AND OTHER OXYTOCIC DRUGS

A number of other agents, though chemically unrelated to oxytocin, are used clinically because of their ability to stimulate contraction of uterine muscle. Some of these agents are described briefly in this section.

## Ergot Alkaloids

These compounds are derived from a fungus commonly known as ergot that grows on grain. For centuries, crude extracts of ergot were used by midwives as an obstetrical aid to hasten the onset and progress of labour. Their effects on uterine contraction, however, were vigorous and sustained. As a consequence, fetal anoxia and uterine rupture occurred with unacceptable frequency. In high concentrations, the extracts caused ergot poisoning, characterized by marked vasoconstriction and burning sensations in the extremities ("St. Anthony's Fire") and sometimes by gangrene and CNS irritation (leading to convulsions).

With the isolation and purification of the various alkaloids of ergot, **ergonovine** and **methylergonovine** were identified and found to have a highly selective action on the uterus while causing minimal vasoconstriction. Structurally, they are simple amide derivatives of lysergic acid (Fig. 44-5).

The ergot alkaloids are never used in the early stages of labour; however, because they are so effective in "clamping down" the uterus, they are used to control postpartum hemorrhage. The actions of the two ergot alkaloids are rapid and are exerted directly on the uterus. Effects are observed 8 to 10 minutes after an oral dose and almost immediately after intravenous or intramuscular injection. In very high doses, the toxic symptoms of ergot poisoning become evident.

Ergonovine differs from both vasopressin and oxytocin in its effects on the uterus (Table 44-3). In the nonpregnant uterus, it stimulates short, rapid contractions of the body of the uterus and contraction of the cervix. It has a preferential action on the pregnant uterus, stimulating sustained contractions, and has a longer duration of action than oxytocin.

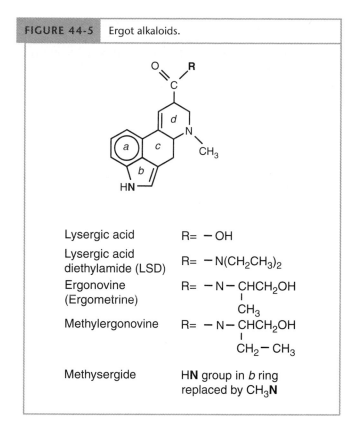

| | |
|---|---|
| Lysergic acid | R= −OH |
| Lysergic acid diethylamide (LSD) | R= −N(CH₂CH₃)₂ |
| Ergonovine (Ergometrine) | R= −N−CHCH₂OH \| CH₃ |
| Methylergonovine | R= −N−CHCH₂OH \| CH₂−CH₃ |
| Methysergide | HN group in *b* ring replaced by CH₃N |

**Ergonovine maleate** ("ergometrine maleate"; Ergometrine, Ergonovine, Ergonovine Maleate Injection USP) and methylergonovine maleate (Methergine, not available in Canada) are strong uterotonic agents used to control excessive uterine bleeding. They are available as injectables and as tablets.

**Ergotamine tartrate** is an amino acid–substituted alkaloid with prominent vasoconstrictor activity. It is a partial agonist at α-adrenergic and 5-HT receptors and is used to relieve migraine headaches, which have a vascular component. The drug is used in combination with caffeine (Cafergot; ergotamine tartrate 1 mg and caffeine 100 mg), in combination with caffeine and diphenhydramine (Ergodryl; ergotamine tartrate 1mg, caffeine 100 mg, and diphenhydramine HCl 25 mg), or in combination with belladonna alkaloids and pentobarbital (Bellergal Spacetabs; ergotamine tartrate 0.6 mg, belladonna alkaloids 0.2 mg, and phenobarbital 40 mg). The addition of caffeine facilitates the absorption of the alkaloid from the gastrointestinal tract, while the additions of diphenhydramine, belladonna alkaloids, and phenobarbital help relieve nausea and promote relaxation. It is used only in the early-onset phase of the migraine, not for routine maintenance therapy. The most serious adverse effects are due to systemic vasoconstriction and may include angina and stroke. **Methysergide maleate** (Sansert) is an ergot alkaloid used in the prophylactic treatment of severe, recurring migraine at doses ranging from 2 to 6 mg per day. It possesses the same serious vascular side effects as the other ergot alkaloids and, in addition, can lead to retroperitoneal fibrosis. See Chapter 29 for other drugs used in the treatment of migraine headaches.

**Bromocriptine mesylate** (Parlodel) is a semisynthetic ergot alkaloid that functions as a specific dopamine D₂–like receptor agonist. It suppresses the production of prolactin and reverses effects of hyperprolactinemia, including amenorrhea, galactorrhea, and infertility in women as well as impotence and infertility in men. In patients with prolactin-secreting pituitary tumours, bromocriptine can cause tumour regression. Usual therapeutic doses range from 2.5 to 7.5 mg. It is available as 2.5-mg tablets and 5-mg capsules.

Bromocriptine is also used in the treatment of acromegaly, suppressing growth hormone production in

**TABLE 44-3** Comparison of the Effects of Oxytocic Agents

| Agent | ADH Activity | Smooth Muscle Blood Vessels | Gut | Non-pregnant Uterus | Pregnant Uterus | Onset | Duration |
|---|---|---|---|---|---|---|---|
| Oxytocin (injection) | + | − | 0 | ± (cervix −) | +++ | Quick | Short |
| Ergonovine (injection, oral) | 0 | + | 0 | ++ | +++ | Quick | Long |
| Ergotamine (for migraine) | 0 | ++ | 0 | + | ++ | Quick | Variable |
| Prostaglandin E₂, F₂α (injection) (local) | 0 0 | ++ 0 | ++ 0 | ++ ++ (cervix −) | +++ +++ | Slow | Medium |
| Vasopressin (injection) | ++++ | ++ | ++ | ++ | ++ | Quick | Short |

Effects: + = positive; − = negative; 0 = none.

doses ranging from 7.5 to 40 mg/day. It is also employed as an adjunct in the treatment of Parkinson's disease in doses that may range up to 100 mg/day (see Chapter 17).

The use of bromocriptine is associated with a high incidence (68%) of mild side effects, including nausea, headache, postural hypotension, nasal stuffiness, and dizziness. At the higher doses cited above for acromegaly and Parkinson's, additional side effects are seen, including abnormal involuntary movements, hallucinations, and mental confusion.

**Pergolide mesylate** (Permax) is another semi-synthetic ergot alkaloid that is a dopamine receptor agonist. It is primarily used in the treatment of Parkinson's disease. It is supplied as tablets of 0.05, 0.25, and 1 mg. The adverse effects of pergolide are similar to those of bromocriptine but also include instances of sinus tachycardia and sudden onset of sleep.

**Cabergoline** (Dostinex) is a dopamine $D_2$ receptor agonist used in the treatment of hyperprolactinemia. In patients with prolactin-secreting pituitary tumours, cabergoline can cause tumour regression. Because it has a four-fold higher potency and a longer half-life (63 to 69 hours) than bromocriptine, it is effective in a dose range of 0.25 to 0.5 mg administered once or twice per week. Doses can be increased to 1.5 to 2.0 mg twice weekly if serum prolactin levels remain elevated. Cabergoline has a lower tendency to cause nausea than bromocriptine and is better tolerated; however, it can still cause headache and dizziness.

## Prostaglandin $E_2$

**Dinoprostone** (Prostin $E_2$) is used as an alternative to oxytocin, to induce labour when vaginal delivery is intended or to induce abortion. It is available as tablets of 0.5 mg, vaginal suppositories of 20 mg, or a gel of 1 to 2 mg. The objective is to aim for the minimum effective concentration of prostaglandin by gradual administration of drug. Prostaglandin $E_2$ is equally effective on the pregnant and non-pregnant uterus; it generally has a slow onset of action and a short half-life once absorbed. Other actions include stimulation of gastrointestinal smooth muscle, leading to nausea, vomiting, and diarrhea (see Table 44-3). See Chapter 27 for more information on prostaglandin $E_2$.

## SUGGESTED READINGS

Brindley BA, Sokol RJ. Induction and augmentation of labour: basis and methods for current practice. *Obstet Gynecol Surv.* 1988;43:730-743.

Chen P. Vasopressin: new uses in critical care. *Am J Med Sci.* 2002; 324:146-154.

Howl J, Wheatley M. Molecular pharmacology of $V_{1a}$ vasopressin receptors. *Gen Pharmacol.* 1995;26:1142-1153.

Manning M, Bankowski K, Sawyer WH. Selective agonists and antagonists of vasopressin. In: Gash DM, Boer GJ, eds. *Vasopressin: Principles and Properties.* New York, NY: Plenum Press; 1987;335-368.

Margolis B, Angel J, Kremer S, Skorecki K. Vasopressin action in the kidney—overview and glomerular actions. In: Cowley AW, Liard JF, Ausiello DA, eds. *Vasopressin: Cellular and Integrative Functions.* New York, NY: Raven Press; 1988:97-106.

Mitchell BF, Schmid B. Oxytocin and its receptor in the process of parturition. *J Soc Gynecol Investig.* 2001;122-133.

North WG. Biosynthesis of vasopressin and neurophysins. In: Gash DM, Boer GJ, eds. *Vasopressin: Principles and Properties.* New York, NY: Plenum Press; 1987:175-209.

Russell SD, DeWald T. Vasopressin receptor antagonists: therapeutic potential in the management of chronic heart failure. *Am J Cardiovasc Drugs.* 2003;3:13-20.

# 45

# Thyroid Hormones and Antihyperthyroid Drugs

## BP SCHIMMER AND SR GEORGE

### CASE HISTORY

A 47-year-old woman consulted her physician because of heart palpitations, tremulousness, weight loss of 3.18 kg (7 lb.), and heat intolerance, all of which had started 6 weeks previously. Physical examination revealed a resting heart rate of 110 bpm, BP of 150/70 mmHg, and a diffusely enlarged thyroid gland. She had a fine tremor of her outstretched hands, a wide-eyed stare, and "lid lag." She was started on treatment with propranolol, 20 mg three times daily, and was sent for laboratory tests. The results showed a free thyroxine (T4) level of 40 pmol/L and a free triiodothyronine (T3) level of 10.6 pmol/L. Thyroid-stimulating hormone (TSH) was undetectable, but thyroid-stimulating globulins were markedly elevated, confirming the diagnosis of Graves' disease.

The patient was started on propylthiouracil, 200 mg twice daily, and the propranolol was continued. She became euthyroid in 6 weeks, and the propranolol dose was gradually reduced and finally discontinued. She continued receiving a maintenance dose of propylthiouracil (50 mg twice daily) for 1 year, after which the drug was discontinued. She remained well for 3 years, but the symptoms of hyperthyroidism then recurred. Treatment with propranolol and propylthiouracil was reinitiated in the same dosages as before to normalize the thyroid hormone levels and provide symptomatic relief. However, after 7 weeks she developed an itchy, red, maculopapular rash over her whole body. The propylthiouracil and propranolol were therefore discontinued, and she was given Na$^{131}$I by mouth in a dose of 370 mBq (10 mCi) for definitive control of her hyperthyroidism.

Three months later, the patient returned, complaining of lethargy, tiredness, a feeling of coldness at normal room temperature, puffiness around the eyes, and constipation. Laboratory tests showed a free T4 level of 8 pmol/L, free T3 level of 3.0 pmol/L, and a TSH level of 25 mU/mL, confirming a diagnosis of hypothyroidism. She was started on levothyroxine, 0.1 mg daily. Six weeks later, a blood test showed a TSH level of 3.2 mU/mL, and the patient's complaints had disappeared. She has remained well on this therapy for the past 2 years.

The thyroid gland synthesizes and secretes thyroid hormones, which are required for the integration of normal body function. Abnormalities of thyroid hormones can lead to impairment of growth, development, metabolic regulation, central nervous system (CNS) function, and adaptive responses, including acclimatization to heat and cold. This chapter deals with drugs used in the management of thyroid hormone deficiency and thyroid hormone excess.

## SYNTHESIS AND METABOLISM OF THYROID HORMONES

Figure 45-1 shows the principal features of the biosynthesis and metabolism of thyroid hormones, which are discussed in detail below.

## Hypothalamic–Pituitary–Thyroid Unit

Thyrotropin-releasing hormone (TRH) is a hypothalamic peptide that functions via a specific G protein–coupled receptor, the TRH receptor, to stimulate the release of thyrotropin (thyroid-stimulating hormone, TSH) from the anterior pituitary (see Fig. 45-1). TRH is a tripeptide with the structure L-pyroglutamyl-L-histidyl-L-prolinamide (Fig. 45-2).

TRH also stimulates the release of prolactin and growth hormone; its effect on prolactin secretion provides the basis for diagnostic testing of lactotroph function in hyperprolactinemic patients. TRH has other effects within the CNS itself; for example, it increases the sense of well-being and motivation and has been postulated to have a role in depression and other psychiatric disorders. Factors that increase TRH levels include circadian rhythms

**FIGURE 45-1** Principal features of the biosynthesis and metabolism of thyroid hormones (see text for abbreviations).

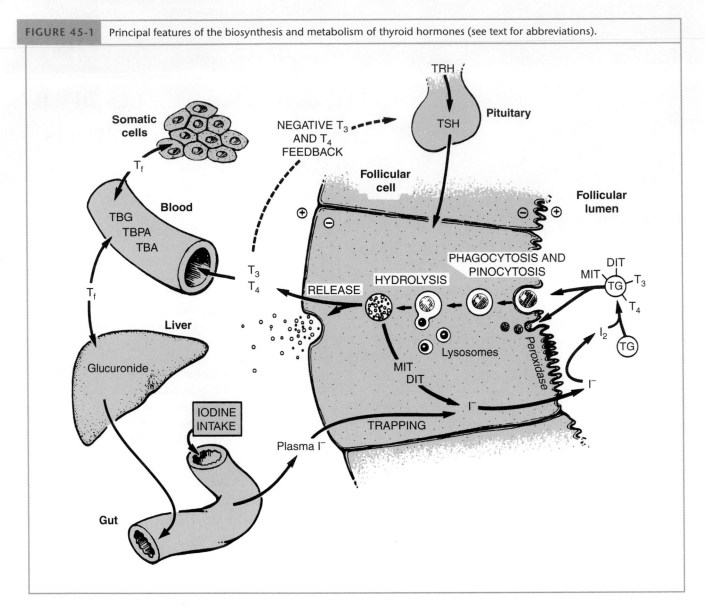

(highest during sleep), low ambient temperature, and noradrenaline. Non-specific stress (e.g., trauma, anaesthesia) reduces the level of TRH.

TSH is a pituitary glycoprotein (molecular weight about 28 000 Da) made up of two chains designated α and β. The α chain is identical to the α chains of FSH and LH (see Chapter 46). TSH stimulates the production of thyroid hormones through interactions with a specific G protein–coupled TSH receptor at the thyroid cell surface that activates adenylyl cyclase and phospholipase C. Cyclic AMP, $Ca^{2+}$, and diacylglycerol serve as the intracellular second messengers for the hormone. TSH stimulates the synthesis and secretion of thyroid hormones through actions on virtually every step of the pathway (see Fig. 45-1). TSH also stimulates the growth of thyroid cells (excess TSH causes thyroid enlargement, i.e., goiter) and maintains cellular structure. Circulating thyroid hor-

mones exert a negative-feedback inhibition of TSH production by inhibiting transcription of the TSH β gene. Thyroid hormones also decrease the level of TRH receptors in the pituitary and decrease TRH secretion from the hypothalamus (see Fig. 45-1).

Recombinant TSH (thyrotropin alfa, Thyrogen) stimulates thyroglobulin secretion and iodine uptake and is used diagnostically for the early detection of well-differentiated thyroid cancer recurrence.

## Structure of Thyroid Hormones

The two active hormones produced by the thyroid gland are **thyroxine** (tetraiodothyronine, $T_4$) and **triiodothyronine** ($T_3$). Their structures are shown in Figure 45-3.

The triiodinated hormone $T_3$ has 4 to 10 times the activity of the tetraiodinated compound $T_4$. The basic

FIGURE 45-2 Thyrotropin-releasing hormone (TRH; L-pyroglutamyl-L-histidyl-L-prolinamide).

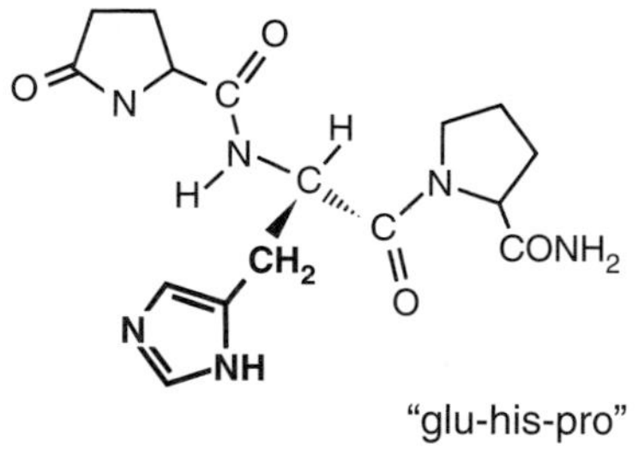

"glu-his-pro"

structural requirements for thyroid hormone activity include two aromatic rings with an aliphatic side chain (an alanine side chain gives optimum activity). The iodine atoms and the oxygen bridge maintain the two aromatic rings in the proper spatial alignment necessary for optimal interaction with the thyroid hormone receptor. A similar spatial alignment with resultant hormonal activity can be achieved by using other bulky groups (e.g., methyl, isopropyl) in place of iodine. For example, dimethyl-isopropyl-thyronine (DIMIT; see Fig. 45-3) has about 20% of the activity of $T_4$.

## Biosynthesis of Thyroid Hormones

The points to be noted regarding the biosynthesis of thyroid hormones are illustrated in Figure 45-1:

1. Iodine (150 µg/day) is ingested in food and water and is absorbed into the blood as iodide ($I^-$).
2. Iodide is "trapped" in the thyroid gland by an active transport process leading to concentrations within the gland that are 20 to several hundred times higher than in plasma. Iodide not taken up by the thyroid is readily excreted by the kidneys.
3. In the follicular lumen near the apical cell membrane, iodide is oxidized to a more reactive hypoiodate form by thyroid peroxidase.
4. In successive stages, the reactive iodine combines with tyrosine residues in the glycoprotein thyroglobulin (TG) to form monoiodinated and diiodinated tyrosine residues. In a subsequent oxidation reaction involving the same peroxidase, the iodotyrosine residues are condensed to form the iodothyronine precursors for $T_3$ and $T_4$.
5. The iodinated thyroglobulin is stored in the acini of the gland.
6. The release of thyroid hormones from the gland is initiated by endocytosis of thyroglobulin from the lumen into the cells of the follicle. Within the cells,

thyroglobulin is hydrolyzed to amino acids by lysosomal enzymes; $T_4$ and some $T_3$ are released into the circulation. The iodine associated with monoiodotyrosine (MIT) and diiodotyrosine (DIT) is reutilized. With a normal dietary intake of iodine, $T_4$ is the major hormone produced. When the dietary intake is low, the proportion of $T_3$ is increased.

## Transport and Metabolism

1. Most of the thyroid hormone in the circulation (about 90%) is in the form of $T_4$; 5% circulates as $T_3$. Both hormones are tightly bound to certain plasma proteins, with only a small fraction circulating as "free" hormone. The free hormone is considered to represent the physiologically active fraction. Unbound, or free, thyroxine ($T_f$) accounts for approximately 0.05% of the total $T_4$. $T_3$ is bound more loosely than $T_4$ (0.5% is free). Since the free hormone is metabolized more rapidly than the bound, it follows that the half-life of $T_3$ in the circulation (about 2 days) is shorter than that of $T_4$ (about 7 days).
2. Thyroxine-binding globulin (TBG) acts as a carrier for approximately 75% of the thyroid hormone. The remainder is bound to thyroxine-binding prealbumin (TBPA, or transthyretin) and to albumin.
3. Measurements of free thyroid hormones and TSH levels are used as indicators of thyroid function. Normal

FIGURE 45-3 Agents with thyroid hormonal activity.

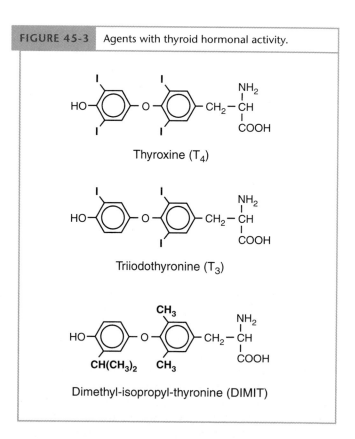

Thyroxine ($T_4$)

Triiodothyronine ($T_3$)

Dimethyl-isopropyl-thyronine (DIMIT)

values are as follows: free $T_4$, 11 to 24 pmol/L; free $T_3$, 3.3 to 6.5 pmol/L; TSH, 0.5 to 5.0 mU/mL.

4. Thyroid hormones circulate to all tissues and are taken up in varying amounts. Thyroxine is metabolized by deiodination, about 35% to the more potent $T_3$ and about 45% to "reverse" $T_3$ ($rT_3$; monodeiodinated at the inner α-benzene ring rather than the outer ring; metabolically inactive). Further metabolism results in acetic and propionic acid derivatives of $T_3$ (metabolically active), various deiodinated derivatives, and iodotyrosines. The second major pathway for disposal of thyroid hormones is via glucuronic acid conjugation in the liver and excretion in the feces (20 to 40% of the total amount).

5. Although the thyroid gland secretes some $T_3$, most of the active hormone (at least 70%) arises from deiodination of $T_4$ in peripheral tissues by the selenoprotein enzyme iodothyronine 5-deiodinase, for which three isoforms (types 1, 2, and 3) exist. The type 1 enzyme is found in the thyroid gland, liver, and kidney, exhibits both 5- and 5′-deiodinase activity, and is responsible for the formation of most of the circulating $T_3$ and reverse $T_3$. The type 2 and type 3 enzymes have only 5-deiodinase activity and are responsible for the formation of $T_3$ at specific sites, such as brain, muscle, pituitary gland, certain reproductive tissues, and other endocrine sites. Since $T_3$ is considerably more potent than $T_4$, it has been suggested that $T_4$ functions as a circulating "prohormone" for $T_3$.

## ACTIONS

Thyroid hormones are essential for normal function of all body tissues. They have profound influences on integrated processes such as differentiation and development, growth, and adaptation to environmental stress. The importance of these actions is apparent from the signs and symptoms of hyper- and hypothyroidism.

With thyroid hormone deficiency (**hypothyroidism**), there is impairment of the following:

- Growth of skeletal tissues
- Growth, development, and function of the central nervous system
- Protein synthesis
- Carbohydrate absorption
- Lipid metabolism
- Adrenocortical and gonadal functions
- Cardiac and renal functions
- Overall tissue metabolism

With excessive function (**hyperthyroidism**; thyrotoxicosis), the principal effect is an increase in metabolism of most (if not all) tissues, causing an increased basal consumption of oxygen (BMR) and an increase in the amount of energy expended as heat. Other manifestations of hyperthyroidism include increased appetite, weight loss, rapid pulse, high systolic blood pressure, increased water turnover by sweating, dyspnea, and fine tremor of skeletal muscles. Many of these changes resemble those of excessive activity of the sympathetic nervous system.

The diverse actions of thyroid hormones result from the actions of $T_3$ binding to specific receptors in the cell nuclei of many tissues. Thyroid hormone receptors are members of the superfamily of nuclear hormone receptor transcription factors and are encoded by two genes that give rise to multiple alternately spliced variants. The thyroid hormone receptors function as dimers or as heterodimers with retinoid X receptors. These complexes recognize DNA sequences (thyroid hormone response elements, TREs) in the promoter regions of specific genes to alter transcription either positively or negatively. This results in altered synthesis (increased or decreased) of several important proteins. Among these are nerve growth factors (CNS development) and β-adrenergic receptors (potentiation of cardiovascular and metabolic effects of catecholamines). In addition to these nuclear receptor-mediated actions, thyroid hormones also may have non-genomic actions.

## Autoimmunity and Thyroid Function

**Graves' disease** (Basedow's disease; diffuse toxic goiter; exophthalmic goiter) is the major cause of thyroid hyperactivity (hyperthyroidism) in humans; the incidence of Graves' disease is at least three times greater in women than in men. In Graves' disease, the circulating $T_4$ is high and TSH is suppressed. Autoimmune disease is the underlying cause of this disorder, in which circulating antibodies to the TSH receptor (thyroid-stimulating immunoglobulins, TSIs) are present. These antibodies bind to and activate the TSH receptor, resulting in thyroid enlargement and hormone overproduction. As might be expected, the elevated thyroid hormones do not suppress the action of TSIs. Circulating antibodies to thyroglobulin and to microsomal antigens are also increased in this disease. A significant number of cases of Graves' disease undergo spontaneous remission but often relapse.

A distinctive disorder often associated with Graves' disease is exophthalmos (Graves' ophthalmopathy), a protrusion of the eyeballs and widening of the palpebral fissures. It is produced by an enlargement of external ocular muscles and associated connective tissue; however, there is no agreement as to its cause. Exophthalmos cannot be produced experimentally by administering thyroid hormone, nor does it occur in all hyperthyroid patients. Immune mechanisms, both cell-mediated and humoral, are currently regarded as likely pathogenic factors.

**Hashimoto's disease** (chronic thyroiditis) belongs to the spectrum of autoimmune thyroid disorders and is usually characterized by hypothyroidism due to autoimmune destruction of the thyroid gland.

## Thyroid Hormones in Pregnancy

Pregnancy or estrogen treatment increases the concentration of thyroxine-binding globulin, resulting in increased amounts of thyroid hormones in the bound form. Feedback regulatory mechanisms compensate, however, and thyroid hormone synthesis increases enough to maintain a normal level of free hormone.

$T_4$ and $T_3$ are rapidly degraded by a highly active deiodinase (type 3) in the placenta, so only small amounts of maternal thyroid hormones reach the fetus. The amount of thyroid hormone necessary for normal development of the fetus is open to debate. Body growth is not affected in the athyreotic fetus, but proper brain development is at risk. There is agreement that after birth, prompt and vigorous replacement treatment is essential in the management of **neonatal hypothyroidism.** Failure to treat this condition will result in severe mental retardation, growth retardation, and other manifestations of cretinism. Even prompt treatment after birth may not reverse all the effects of hypothyroidism on brain development. **Hyperthyroidism** also is of concern in pregnancy. While the placenta represents an enzymatic barrier that restricts the transfer of thyroid hormone to the fetus, the maternal thyroid hormone that does cross the placenta is critical for fetal neural development. Therefore, it is essential to maintain maternal thyroid hormones in the normal range throughout pregnancy. In maternal hyperthyroidism due to Graves' disease, thyroid-stimulating immunoglobulins will traverse the placenta and stimulate the fetal thyroid gland. In addition, labour and delivery may precipitate "thyroid storm" in the mother, an extreme and life-threatening state of hyperthyroidism. Treatment is designed to maintain the euthyroid status of the mother.

## CLINICAL USE OF THYROID HORMONES

The administration of thyroid hormones is indicated as replacement therapy for treatment of hypothyroidism. The goal is to achieve a euthyroid state as established by laboratory tests of TSH and thyroid hormones (i.e., free $T_3$ and free $T_4$). Thyroid hormone deficiency may present with symptoms ranging from severe hypothyroidism (e.g., cretinism, myxedema), to mild hypothyroidism in which only one, or at most a few, symptoms are present. Thyroid hormones, specifically L-triiodothyronine, is sometimes used as adjunctive therapy with antidepressants in the treatment of refractory depression. Though the underlying mechanism is not well understood, it may

involve the desensitization of $5\text{-HT}_{1A}$ receptors with a resultant increase in serotonin release.

## Preparations

### Levothyroxine sodium (sodium L-thyroxine, USP, BP; Eltroxin, Levothroid, Levoxine, Synthroid)

This is a synthetic crystalline compound prepared in oral tablets in strengths ranging from 0.025 to 0.3 mg; it is also available in sterile lyophilized form for injection after reconstitution. Because of its chemical purity and uniform bioavailability, levothyroxine has replaced thyroid powders and extract (e.g., desiccated thyroid).

Levothyroxine is well absorbed by mouth but is influenced by intestinal contents; bioavailability ranges from 40 to 75%. In the plasma, more than 99% is protein-bound. The normal half-life is 6 to 7 days, but it is increased in myxedema and pregnancy and during treatment with estrogens (that increase the level of thyroid-binding globulin). Conversely, the half-life is shortened if protein binding is decreased by disease (e.g., hepatic cirrhosis, nephrotic syndrome) or by drugs (e.g., salicylate, dicumarol, phenytoin, carbamazepine).

### Liothyronine sodium (L-triiodothyronine; Cytomel, Triostat)

This is a synthetic crystalline compound available in oral tablets of 5 and 25 µg or in an injectable form. A dose of 25 µg is equivalent to 0.1 mg of levothyroxine.

### Liotrix (Thyrolar, Euthyroid)

This is a combination of synthetic $T_4$ and $T_3$ in a ratio of 4:1; this ratio is thought to closely resemble the physiological secretion ratio. The value of this combination is not clear since $T_3$ is readily derived from circulating $T_4$. The mixture is supplied as tablets in several strengths. It is available in the United States but is not currently available in Canada.

## Therapy of Hypothyroidism

The drug of choice in the treatment of hypothyroidism is levothyroxine, and the goal is to achieve a euthyroid state as determined by laboratory tests of TSH and free thyroid hormone levels. If the patient is otherwise healthy, it is usual to begin with a dose (e.g., 0.075 to 0.1 mg daily) that is sufficient to render the patient euthyroid. The full effect takes several weeks to develop; therefore, because of the long half-life of levothyroxine, the dose should not be adjusted upward for 4 to 6 weeks. In the elderly or in the presence of cardiac disease, the initial dose and subsequent increments should be low and the intervals between them extended. By successive increments (0.025 to 0.05 mg L-thyroxine), the dose is eventually brought up to a maintenance level based on normalization of the TSH level. If there is concomitant adrenal steroid deficiency, glucocorticoid replacement therapy should be started before thyroid hormone replacement.

In infants and children, the dosage is related to age and body weight and is adjusted to normalize TSH. Adequate dosage is extremely important for normal growth and mental development.

Triiodothyronine is much more rapid in action and more potent than L-thyroxine. Effects start to occur in 4 to 8 hours, reach a maximum in 24 to 48 hours, and wear off in a few days if medication is stopped. In contrast, thyroxine has a prolonged action that takes up to 3 months to wear off completely. Therefore, the "evenness" of effect of triiodothyronine depends more closely on regularity of dosage, which makes it a difficult agent for routine use. It is also more expensive than thyroxine. The value of triiodothyronine lies in its relatively short duration of action; in certain cases, repeated thyroid function tests may be desirable, and these can be done a few weeks after stopping triiodothyronine medication.

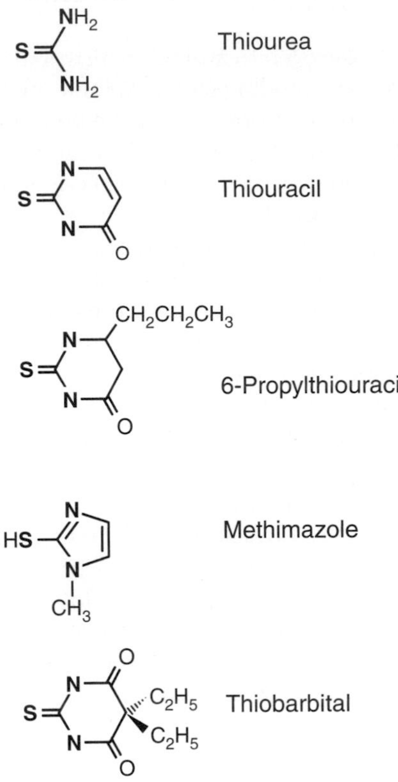

## THERAPY OF HYPERTHYROIDISM

When the thyroid gland is overactive, secreting excessive (thyrotoxic) amounts of thyroid hormones, the therapeutic objective is to interrupt synthesis and/or release. Several methods are available.

## Inhibition of Thyroid Hormone Synthesis by Thionamides

The thionamides are ringed structures derived from thiourea (Fig. 45-4). They inhibit thyroid peroxidase and in this way block the iodination of tyrosyl groups and the coupling of iodotyrosines in thyroglobulin. The resultant effect is to block thyroid hormone synthesis.

They do not interfere with the processing of stored iodinated thyroglobulin or the release of thyroid hormones; therefore, the onset of clinical effect is slow and depends on depletion of the stored hormone precursor. Several weeks are usually required to produce a maximal effect. These drugs may also have immunosuppressive effects in patients with autoimmune thyroid disease. Propylthiouracil, but not methimazole or carbimazole, inhibits the type 1 iodothyronine deiodinase and hence the conversion of $T_4$ to $T_3$ in tissues. Some clinicians feel this is an added benefit; however, it also inhibits the deiodination (inactivation) of $T_3$.

### Propylthiouracil (PTU; Propyl-Thyracil)

Propylthiouracil (PTU) is well absorbed orally (bioavailability 60 to 90%), reaches peak plasma concentration within 1 hour, and is rapidly distributed. It is partly biotransformed and inactivated in the liver, and both the

**FIGURE 45-4**  Thiourea and derivatives.

original drug and the metabolites are excreted by the kidneys. The normal half-life is approximately 1 to 1.5 hours. The initial dosage usually is 200 to 600 mg/day in divided doses; maintenance doses range from 50 to 200 mg/day. It is provided as 50- and 100-mg tablets.

### Methimazole (thiamazole; Tapazole)

Methimazole has a plasma half-life of approximately 6 hours, which is longer than the half-life of PTU and is approximately 10 times as potent. It is well absorbed orally and excreted by the kidneys. Initial dosage is 15 to 60 mg/day depending on severity; maintenance doses are 5 to 15 mg/day. It is provided as 5-mg tablets.

## Toxic Effects of Thionamides

All drugs of this group are capable of causing toxic effects (in about 3% of patients taking propylthiouracil and 7% taking methimazole). These effects include the following:

- Agranulocytosis (most serious, reported in 0.5% of cases)

- Drug rash, arthralgia, edema (in over 2% of cases), drug fever (very rare), alopecia, hair depigmentation
- Rare cases of hepatitis, lymph node swelling, loss of taste

Physiologically, the level of free thyroid hormone determines the secretion of TSH by feedback regulatory mechanisms. With thionamides, inhibition of thyroid hormone synthesis may cause a gradual increase in the output of TSH, making the gland larger.

Thionamides cross the placenta (<1% of the dose) and are also secreted in breast milk in small amounts. Therefore, in the treatment of maternal hyperthyroidism, and during the perinatal period, one uses the lowest possible dose so as to avoid symptoms of hypothyroidism in the neonate. Propylthiouracil is the preferred drug of choice in nursing mothers since the small amount of anti-thyroid drug that appears in breast milk does not affect thyroid function of the infant.

## Inhibition of Thyroxine Release

**Iodide** is thought to inhibit the lysosomal protease that releases thyroid hormones from thyroglobulin; treatment with iodide therefore causes large amounts of colloid to accumulate in the gland. It also inhibits other steps in the regulation of thyroid hormone synthesis, including iodide transport and iodination of thyroglobulin (Wolff–Chaikoff effect). Symptoms of hyperthyroidism are relieved rapidly, making iodide useful in the treatment of thyroid storm.

Iodide is not suitable for long-term therapy because the gland escapes the inhibitory effect of $I^-$, and the release of thyroid hormones is resumed. Therefore, it is used only for a few weeks. The available form is **potassium iodide** (Lugol's solution; saturated KI solution). Enough is used to provide 60 mg of $I^-$ per day.

**Lithium carbonate** is also effective in preventing release of thyroid hormones from the thyroid gland. It most likely acts by inhibiting the thyroid adenylyl cyclase. It is used as an adjunct in the treatment of the severe hyperthyroidism in thyroid storm.

## Radioactive Iodine

Radioactive iodine is used to diagnose the etiology of hyperthyroidism and to achieve non-surgical ablation of thyroid tissue in hyperthyroidism or in thyroid cancer. $Na^{131}I$ is taken up and concentrated by the gland in the same way as ordinary $I^-$. For diagnostic purposes, a tracer dose of $^{131}I$ is used—less than 25% of an administered dose is taken up by a normal gland, whereas the hyperactive one may take up 80% or more. Higher doses are used therapeutically (e.g., 6 to 15 mCi for Graves' disease, 75 to 200 mCi for thyroid cancer). The accumulation of $^{131}I$ within the thyroid causes intense local β-irradiation that destroys glandular epithelium; apart from the salivary glands, which may become transiently inflamed, other tissues are not damaged. The most common side effect is hypothyroidism. The effectiveness of $^{131}I$ in the treatment of thyroid carcinoma, including metastases, depends upon the integrity of the $I^-$ trapping mechanism (i.e., the degree of differentiation of the carcinoma).

If the thyroid gland has a large store of colloid, surgical manipulation or destruction of thyroid tissue by $^{131}I$ may release a flood of thyroid hormones into the circulation and cause thyroid storm. Therefore, one usually tries to block hormone synthesis first with a thionamide, allowing the gland to become depleted; the thionamide is withdrawn for a period of 10 to 14 days before using radioablation. $^{131}I$ is not used in pregnant women because it crosses the placenta and can have potentially harmful effects on fetal tissues, especially thyroid. It also is not generally used in children.

## Symptomatic Relief

β-Adrenergic receptor blockers such as propranolol (see Chapter 13) can be administered to block the sympathetic effects of excess thyroid hormone, such as tachycardia, tremor, and systolic hypertension. Propranolol acts quickly and is well tolerated. The usual contraindications for use of propranolol should be kept in mind (e.g., bronchial asthma, chronic obstructive lung disease, congestive heart failure).

Calcium channel blockers also may be used to control tachycardia and reduce arrhythmias.

Glucocorticoids may be used for the rapid treatment of severe hyperthyroidism or thyroid storm; they inhibit the conversion of $T_4$ to $T_3$ in peripheral tissues.

## SUGGESTED READINGS

Cooper DS. Hyperthyroidism. *Lancet.* 2003;362:459-468.

Harvey CB, Williams GR. Mechanism of thyroid hormone action. *Thyroid.* 2002;12:441-446.

Hernandez D, St. Germain D. Thyroid hormone deiodinases: physiology and clinical disorders. *Curr Opin Pediatr.* 2003;15: 416-420.

Pearce EN, Farwell AP, Braverman LE. Thyroiditis. *N Engl J Med.* 2003;348:2646-2655.

Shi YB, Ritchie JW, Taylor PM. Complex regulation of thyroid hormone action: multiple opportunities for pharmacological intervention. *Pharmacol Ther.* 2002;94:235-251.

Streetman DD, Khanderia U. Diagnosis and treatment of Graves disease. *Ann Pharmacother.* 2003;37:1100-1109.

# 46

# Gonadotropic and Gonadal Hormones

## SR GEORGE AND BP SCHIMMER

### CASE HISTORY

A 55-year-old woman who had been experiencing gradual lengthening of her menstrual cycles consulted her physician after 4 months of amenorrhea. She complained of severe and debilitating hot flashes, sleep disturbance, and vaginal dryness. She was given a prescription for conjugated estrogen 0.3 mg daily, plus medroxyprogesterone 2.5 mg daily. This treatment resolved her symptoms. Initially she felt slightly nauseated and gained 1.4 kg (3 lb.) in weight, but the discomfort disappeared after three cycles of treatment.

Four years later, the patient noticed a small mass, 1 cm in diameter, in her left breast. Radiological investigation and a needle aspiration biopsy revealed carcinoma of the breast. The estrogen and progestin were discontinued, and the patient underwent a lumpectomy and received a course of post-operative radiation treatments. The carcinoma proved to be strongly positive for estrogen receptors, and she was therefore started on tamoxifen 40 mg daily. She remained well on this treatment and showed no signs of recurrence or metastasis during the next 5 years. The tamoxifen was then replaced with letrozole 2.5 mg daily; she has continued to feel well.

Gonadal hormones are important for conception, embryonic development, development at puberty (primary and secondary sex characteristics), and for the desire and ability to procreate. While not essential for life, they are essential for an individual's well-being. Their use in fertility control has had significant impact both socially and economically.

The production and release of the gonadal steroid hormones (estradiol, progesterone, testosterone) are controlled by the gonadotropins (luteinizing hormone, LH; follicle-stimulating hormone, FSH) of the anterior pituitary, and these are, in turn, under the influence of gonadotropin-releasing hormone (GnRH) from the hypothalamus.

The principal features of these relationships are shown in Figures 46-1 and 46-2.

## GONADOTROPIN-RELEASING HORMONE

Gonadotropin-releasing hormone (GnRH) is a decapeptide with the following structure:

PyroGlu-His-Trp-Ser-Tyr-Gly-Leu-Arg-Pro-GlyNH$_2$

In the human, this peptide acts through a specific G protein–coupled receptor linked to G$_{q/11}$ to stimulate phospholipase C and increase intracellular calcium. These effects result in the release of both LH and FSH from the gonadotrophs in the anterior pituitary. The quantal release of FSH is less than that of LH. This quantitative discrepancy is related to differential responses of gonadotrophs to stimulation by GnRH and to feedback modulation by gonadal steroids, and by two types of polypeptide hormones (activin and inhibin) produced in the gonad.

There is evidence that endogenous opioids exert a central inhibitory regulation of GnRH secretion that may be relieved by adrenergic influences. Higher dopaminergic pathways may also be involved, but their role is less well defined.

The secretion of GnRH is pulsatile, the frequency and amplitude of the pulse being of major importance in the effects it produces on secretion of LH and FSH during the menstrual cycle (see Fig. 46-2). Single bolus injections of synthetic GnRH (**gonadorelin hydrochloride**, Factrel) are used diagnostically for testing the responsiveness and function of pituitary gonadotrophs. Pulsatile administration of gonadorelin maintains receptor sensitivity, and gonadorelin acetate (Lutrepulse) has been used successfully in this manner to increase fertility in males and females. Factrel is no longer available in Canada, and Lutrapulse has been discontinued in the United States. Continuous administration of GnRH or its agonist analogues initially stimulates release of LH and FSH, but then inhibits it due to desensitization of the GnRH receptors on the gonadotrophs.

**FIGURE 46-1** Physiological relationships of gonadotropins and gonadal hormones and their influences on the ovary, uterus, and breast. PRL = prolactin.

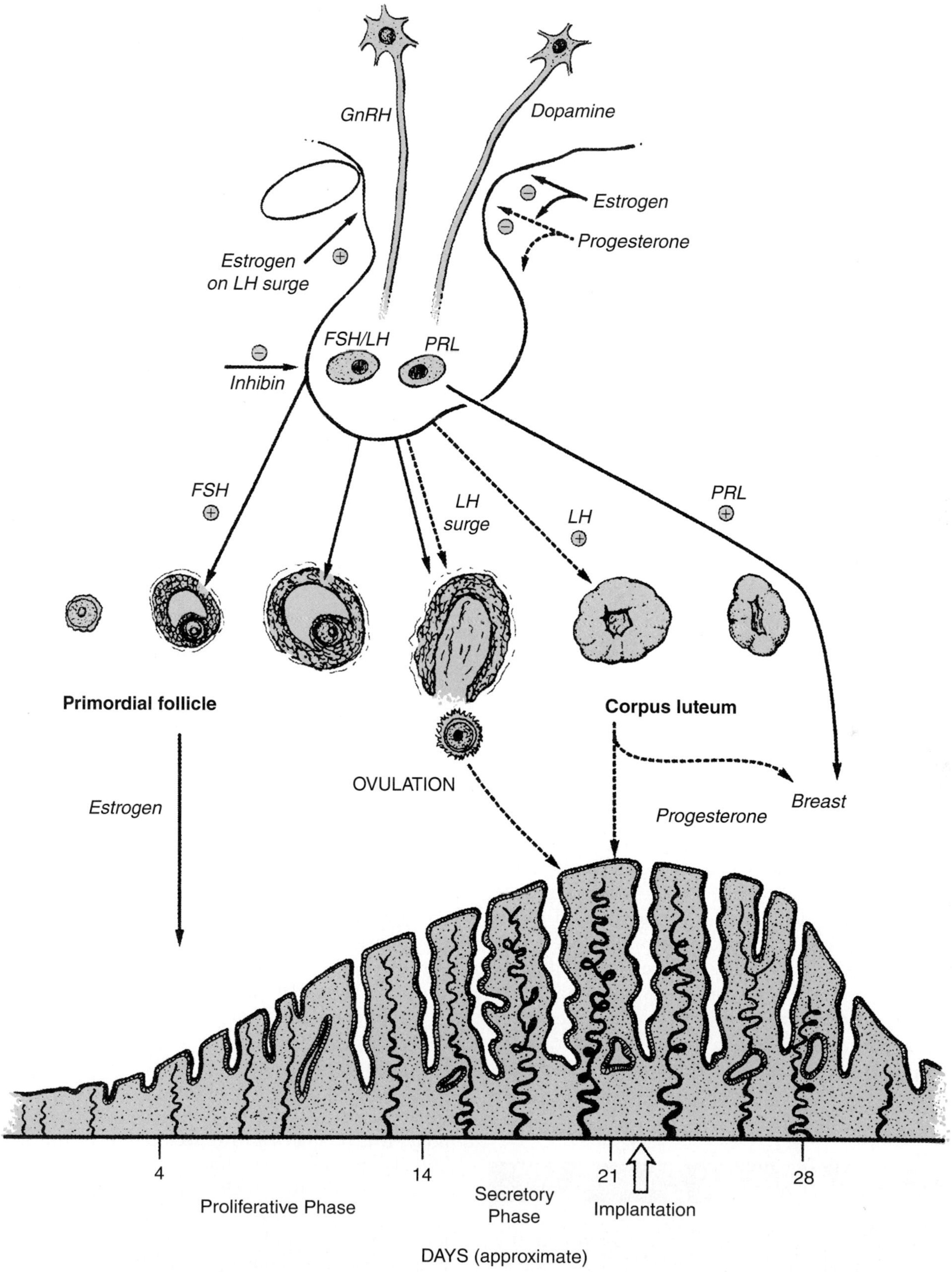

**FIGURE 46-2** Pulsatile release of GnRH and approximate plasma concentrations of ovarian hormones and gonadotropins during a normal menstrual cycle. The change in body temperature throughout the cycle is also shown.

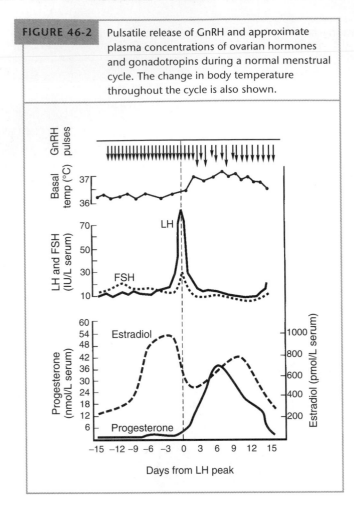

distinct β subunits (LH-β, FSH-β) that confer specificity. The hormones are synthesized within the same cells, the gonadotrophs of the anterior pituitary, although there is heterogeneity in the relative amounts of LH and FSH produced in each gonadotroph. FSH induces development of ovarian follicles in the female and initiates and maintains spermatogenesis in the male. LH induces estrogen and progesterone synthesis and continued follicular development, followed by ovulation and corpus luteum formation. In the male, LH stimulates androgen formation by the Leydig cells of the gonad. Each of these hormones interacts with specific G protein–coupled receptors to generate cyclic adenosine monophosphate (cAMP) and other second messengers.

An LH-like gonadotropin (human chorionic gonadotropin, or hCG) is found in the chorion of the placenta. It is detectable in plasma as early as 7 days after conception and forms the basis for the test to confirm pregnancy.

## Preparations

- **Human chorionic gonadotropin** (hCG; Profasi HP, Pregnyl) has predominantly LH activity and is derived from the urine of pregnant women. It can be used in infertile women to promote ovulation by duplicating the LH "surge," in infertile men to promote spermatogenesis, in male children to stimulate Leydig cells in the treatment of undescended testicles, and as an adjunct in in vitro fertilization treatment programs. A recombinant form of hCG (Ovidrel) also is available.
- **Menotropin** (hMG; Pergonal, Humegon, Repronex) is a combination of LH and FSH purified from the urine of post-menopausal women. It is used to mimic the LH surge and produce ovulation.
- **Urofollitropin** (FSH; Fertinorm, Fertinex, Metrodin) is FSH immunopurified from the urine of post-menopausal women. It is used to stimulate ovulation, particularly in women with relatively low FSH levels (e.g., in polycystic ovarian disease).
- **Follitropin** (recombinant FSH; Follistim, Gonal-F, Puregon) is used to stimulate ovulation. It comes in two forms, alpha and beta, that are differentiated by their glycosylation patterns but that are functionally equivalent.

Whereas the biological half-life of GnRH is short, the GnRH agonist analogues are more metabolically stable and function as inhibitors via desensitization. These long-acting GnRH agonists (Fig. 46-3) have proven useful as GnRH inhibitors in the treatment of hormone-dependent tumours (prostate, breast, uterine fibroids) and other conditions such as precocious puberty and endometriosis. They are available as subcutaneous injectable, nasal spray, and intramuscular depot forms. Antagonists of GnRH (**ganirelix**, Orgalutran, Antagon; **cetrorelix**, Cetrotide; **abarelix**, Plenaxis) also have been developed. Unlike the long-acting agonists, the antagonists do not cause an initial stimulation of gonadotropin production; they are used to prevent a premature LH surge in women undergoing fertility treatment. Abarelix is used for the palliative treatment of prostate cancer and is not indicated for use in women because it can cause birth defects.

## GONADOTROPINS

In the human, there are two pituitary gonadotropins that act on the ovary and testis. Chemically, they are complex glycoprotein hormones that consist of a common α and

## Related Hormones

**Prolactin** is chemically closely related to growth hormone. It is produced in the lactotrophs of the anterior pituitary. Its release is under inhibitory dopaminergic control from the hypothalamus. Overproduction of prolactin can occur from pituitary adenomas, loss of dopaminergic control (e.g., pituitary stalk section), or drugs with anti-dopaminergic activity, such as morphine, metoclopramide, haloperidol, and estrogen.

| FIGURE 46-3 | Gonadotropin-releasing hormone (GnRH) analogues. Names in parentheses are trade names for these preparations. |

**AGONISTS**             **STRUCTURE**

Gonadorelin
(acetate – Lutrepulse)
(hydrochloride – Factrel)

PyroGlu – His – Trp – Ser – Tyr – Gly – Leu – Arg – Pro – GlyNH$_2$

Goserelin acetate
(Zoladex)

PyroGlu – His – Trp – Ser – Tyr – **D-Ser** – Leu – Arg – Pro – **azaGlyNH$_2$**
                                          |
                                  **(O-terbutyl)**

Buserelin acetate
(Suprefact)

PyroGlu – His – Trp – Ser – Tyr – **D-Ser** – Leu – Arg – Pro – **ethylNH$_2$**
                                  |
                                  **(O-terbutyl)**

Leuprolide acetate
(Lupron, Eligard, Viadur)

PyroGlu – His – Trp – Ser – Tyr – **D-Leu** – Leu – Arg – Pro – **ethylNH$_2$**

Nafarelin acetate
(Synarel)

PyroGlu – His – Trp – Ser – Tyr – **D-Ala** – Leu – Arg – Pro – GlyNH$_2$
                                  |
                               **[3-(2-naphthyl)]**

**ANTAGONISTS**

Ganirelix acetate (Orgalutran, Antagon)

Acetyl-D-Ala —— D-Ala —— D-Ala —— Ser —— Tyr —— N,N-diethyl-D —— Leu —— N,N-diethyl-D —— Pro —— D-AlaNH$_2$
        |             |          |                       |                          |
[3-(2-napthyl)]   pCl-phenyl   3-pyridy1                      homoArg                     homoArg

Cetrorelix acetate (Cetrotide)

Acetyl-D-Ala —— D-Ala —— D-Ala —— Ser —— Tyr —— D-Cit —— Leu —— Arg —— Pro —— D-AlaNH$_2$
        |             |          |
[3-(2-napthyl)]   pCl-phenyl   3-pyridy1

Prolactin, along with other hormones (e.g., ovarian and adrenal steroids, placental lactogen, thyroid hormones), plays a major part in the growth and development of the breasts during pregnancy and lactation. Prolactin also inhibits the secretion of GnRH, and this action contributes to the infertility seen with hyperprolactinemia. Drugs used to treat hyperprolactinemia are agonists of dopamine receptors and are discussed in detail in Chapter 44.

# ESTROGENS

## Metabolism and Pharmacokinetics

The principal naturally occurring estrogen is 17-β-estradiol. It is formed from androstenedione or testosterone and is produced predominantly in the ovaries and placenta, but small amounts may be secreted from testes, adrenals, and adipose tissue. Estradiol circulates in the plasma strongly bound to an $\alpha_2$ globulin called sex hormone–binding globulin (SHBG) and less avidly bound to albumin. The free estradiol (unbound hormone) is the fraction available for hormone action in target cells. The levels of urinary estrogen metabolites may be used as an index of endogenous estrogen production.

Estrogens are readily absorbed from the skin, mucous membranes, and gastrointestinal tract. After oral administration, a high proportion is biotransformed and partly inactivated during passage through the liver (first-pass metabolism). Estradiol exists in equilibrium with its oxidation product, estrone. Estradiol and estrone are irreversibly hydroxylated by a hepatic microsomal 16-α-hydroxylase, leading to the formation of estriol (Fig. 46-4). Estrone and estriol retain some estrogenic activity but are much less potent than estradiol. A fraction of the estriol is conjugated with sulfuric and glucuronic acids. Estriol and its metabolites are excreted by the kidney. The conjugated

FIGURE 46-4    Natural estrogens and their metabolic interconversions.

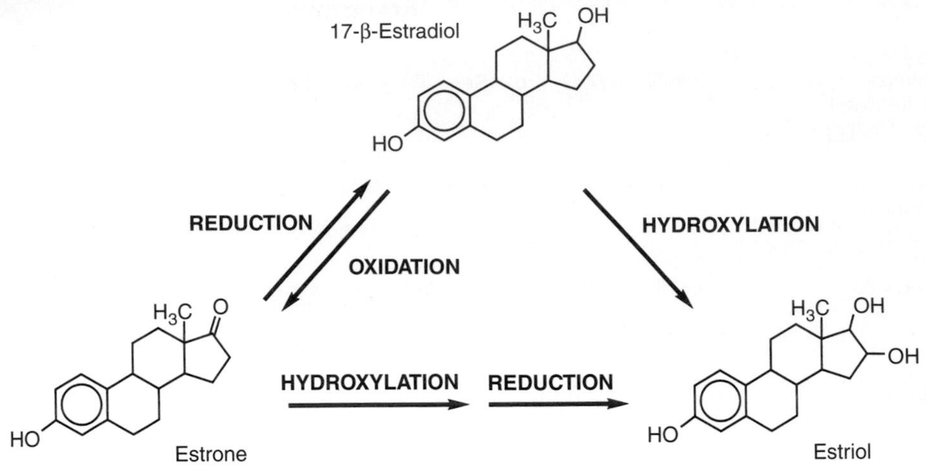

estrogens are also excreted into the bile and may be recycled by bacterial hydrolysis and reabsorption from the gut (enterohepatic recirculation).

Estradiol is only very slightly soluble in water and is therefore formulated as transdermal, oral, and injectable preparations to maximize its bioavailability. Estradiol has enough polarity to be quickly absorbed from the site of delivery. Esters of estradiol (e.g., valerate, cypionate) become less polar as the size of the ester substituent is increased, and the rate of absorption from oily solutions is decreased accordingly, leading to a less intense but longer-lasting action.

The synthetic analogues 17-α-ethinyl estradiol and mestranol (Fig. 46-5) are well absorbed after oral administration, but unlike estradiol they are inactivated very slowly in the liver and peripheral tissues. This slow inactivation is responsible for their high potency and prolonged action.

## Non-Steroidal Estrogens

Certain non-steroidal substances are highly estrogenic. These compounds sufficiently resemble natural estrogens in structure or spatial arrangement to stimulate estrogen receptors in target tissues. The first example was the stilbene derivative **diethylstilbestrol** (DES; Honvol; Fig. 46-6). Once a widely used estrogen substitute, DES is currently limited to palliative treatment of inoperable prostatic carcinoma.

## Actions

Estradiol binds to specific estrogen receptors, ERα and ERβ, that have distinct patterns of anatomic distribution. These receptors reside in the nuclei of cells of estrogen-sensitive target tissues (e.g., brain, pituitary, breast, uterus,

and bone), where they act as nuclear transcription factors either by binding directly to estrogen response elements (EREs) or to other transcription factors. In these tissues, the specific estrogen receptor binds the steroid hormone and undergoes an activation process that permits interaction with specific estrogen-responsive DNA elements and with co-activators of transcription in order to alter the transcription of certain genes. As a consequence, the expression of messenger RNA is either stimulated or inhibited, leading to changes in the production of various proteins. Estrogen also has non-nuclear actions mediated by specific G protein–coupled receptors.

FIGURE 46-5    Structural formulae of ethinyl estradiol and mestranol, the C-3 methoxy derivative of ethinyl estradiol.

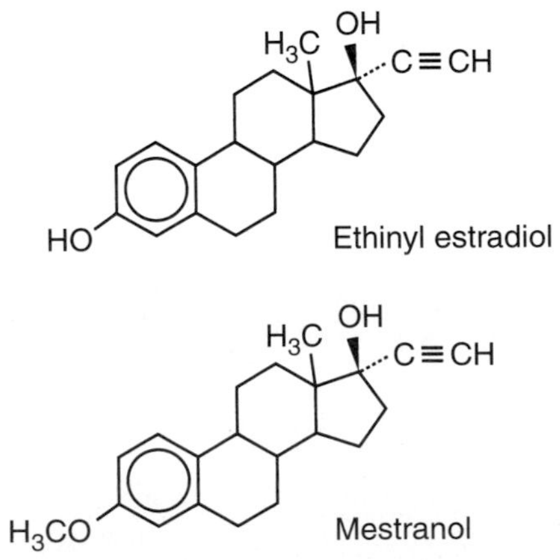

**FIGURE 46-6** Formulae of diethylstilbestrol: (upper) structural formula; (lower) theoretical spatial arrangement (steroid-like form).

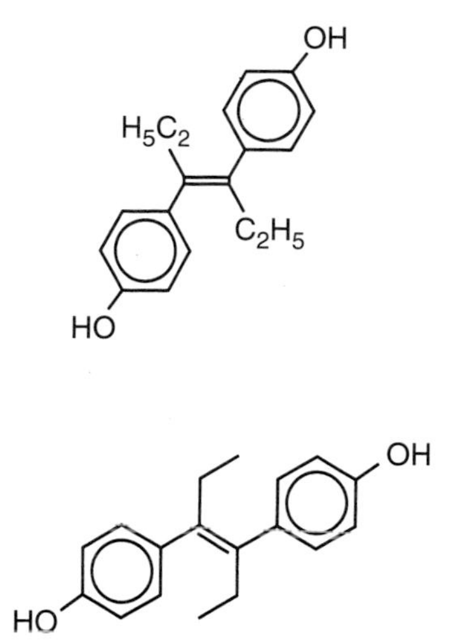

The **physiological functions** of estrogens may be summarized as follows:

- Growth and development of reproductive organs in females
- Development of female secondary sex characteristics
- Linear bone growth, prevention of bone resorption, and hastening of epiphyseal closure
- Behaviour (sexual, maternal)
- Sensitization of tissues to progesterone by induction of progesterone receptors
- Feedback regulation of gonadotrophs, including stimulation of the pre-ovulatory LH surge
- Other metabolic effects include increases in high-density lipoprotein (HDL) levels, synthesis of hepatic proteins, and secretion of corticosteroid-binding globulin (CBG), thyroid-binding globulin (TBG), SHBG, renin substrate, and clotting factors.

## Preparations

- **17-β-Estradiol** is available as dermal patches for absorption through the intact skin (Estraderm) or as micronized tablets (Estrace) and vaginal creams.
- **Conjugated estrogens** are extracted from pregnant mare's urine (Premarin, CES). This preparation contains estrogen conjugates, principally sodium estrone sulfate (60%) and sodium equilin sulfate (30%). They are effective orally or by injection.
- **Estropipate** (piperazine estrone sulfate; Ogen) is an orally active, water-soluble preparation of estrone sulfate, stabilized with piperazine.

- **Esters of 17-β-estradiol** (estradiol valerate; Delestrogen) are given by intramuscular injection for slow absorption from the site, resulting in prolonged action.
- **Ethinyl estradiol** is a synthetic estrogen with an ethynyl group at C-17 that makes this compound orally active. It is the estrogen most commonly used in oral contraceptive preparations.
- **Mestranol** (17-α-ethynyl estradiol 3-methyl ether) is inactive until it is converted to ethinyl estradiol in the liver.

Equivalent replacement doses for selected estrogens are as follows: 17-β-estradiol transdermal 25 to 50 μg; 17-β-estradiol oral micronized 0.5 to 2 mg; conjugated estrogens 0.3 to 1.25 mg; and ethinyl estradiol 5 to 20 μg.

## Clinical Uses

### Hypogonadism
An estrogen is used in replacement therapy for estrogen-deficient patients. Cyclical administration, in combination with a progestin, is recommended if the uterus is intact in order to prevent endometrial carcinomas (see below).

### Menopause
Following natural menopause or surgical castration, many patients show varying degrees of vasomotor instability, headache, emotional lability, sleep disturbances, and atrophy of estrogen-dependent tissues. Estrogens are effective in alleviating these symptoms. A recent large-scale multicentre clinical trial (Women's Health Initiative) showed that the long-term use of estrogen in post-menopausal women was associated with increased risk of coronary heart disease, breast cancer, and thromboembolic events. This has radically changed the approach to long-term estrogen replacement therapy. When symptoms of vasomotor instability are particularly severe, estrogens may be used for a brief period to provide relief; however, the doses should be low. Estrogens may still be used for a few years in severe osteoporosis in young post-menopausal women, in conjunction with calcium, vitamin D, bisphosphonates, and, rarely, with androgens (see Chapter 65).

### Senile atrophic vaginitis
Local therapy, in the form of vaginal creams, may be used to avoid systemic effects.

### Dysmenorrhea
In severe cases, a combination of an estrogen and a progestin is used cyclically to control endometrial proliferation and shedding. Withdrawal of these drugs is followed by painless menstruation.

### Carcinoma of the prostate
Estrogens (e.g., DES) have been used, either alone or in combination with surgical castration, for metastatic carci-

noma of the prostate. In prostatic cancer, estrogen decreases androgen synthesis by shutting off the release of LH. The use of estrogen in this condition has largely been replaced by GnRH analogues and anti-androgens, which have fewer side effects.

### Contraception

Estrogens, given together with a progestin, inhibit the production of gonadotropins and GnRH and thus prevent ovulation (see "Fertility Control").

### "Morning after" contraceptive pill

For this use, ethinyl estradiol is given within 72 hours, in two doses (100 µg each), 12 hours apart, usually in an oral contraceptive formulation. Postulated actions include acceleration of passage of the fertilized ovum along the fallopian tube as well as induction of withdrawal bleeding.

### Hirsutism

Hirsutism resulting from excess androgens of ovarian origin may respond to estrogen therapy, which inhibits the hypothalamic–pituitary–ovarian axis. The estrogen-induced increase in SHBG also serves to effectively decrease circulating concentrations of free androgens (i.e., the fraction that is not protein-bound).

## Adverse and Toxic Effects

- **Gastrointestinal upset** (nausea and vomiting) is the most common disturbance.
- **Breast engorgement, endometrial hyperplasia**, and **vaginal bleeding** may occur. The risk of endometrial carcinoma consequent to endometrial hyperplasia is increased if the estrogen is not combined with progestin.
- **Retention of Na$^+$ and water** and an increase in plasma renin substrate also occur. Hypertension, weight gain, edema, or heart failure may occur. Caution is advisable in older patients.
- The use of estrogen predisposes, in a dose-related fashion, to **thromboembolic events** such as thrombophlebitis, pulmonary embolism, myocardial infarction, stroke, and mesenteric and retinal thromboses. The risk is increased in smokers, those over age 35, and the obese.
- DES has been implicated as the likely cause of the rare clear cell **vaginal or cervical adenocarcinoma** and of the more frequent benign abnormalities of the genital tract that have been reported in a number of young women whose mothers received DES during early pregnancy. In the male offspring, an increased incidence of genital abnormalities has been reported. The use of any exogenous estrogen in pregnancy is not recommended.
- **Cholestatic jaundice** and an increased incidence of gallstones (**cholelithiasis**) have been reported in patients taking estrogens (see Chapter 43). The formation of hepatic adenomas in long-term users is recognized.
- **Carbohydrate tolerance** may be impaired during estrogen therapy. Diabetics or patients with positive family histories of diabetes should be followed closely.
- Onset of **migraine headaches** or exacerbation of migraine is experienced by some patients. Other non-specific headaches may also occur.
- **Hyperprolactinemia** results from estrogen interference with the tonic dopaminergic inhibition of prolactin secretion. In some women, this may result in galactorrhea.
- Many other **secondary effects** have been documented, including appetite stimulation, depression, chloasma or hyperpigmentation, loss of scalp hair, rashes, pancreatitis, vaginal candidiasis, and post-pill amenorrhea.

## Anti-estrogens

The term anti-estrogen refers to estrogen-receptor antagonists, such as clomiphene and tamoxifen (Fig. 46-7). These compounds have weak estrogenic activity and inhibit the action of potent estrogens by competing for access to receptor sites.

**Clomiphene** citrate (Clomid, Serophene) interferes with the "negative feedback" of estrogens on the hypothalamus and pituitary, resulting in an increase in the secretion of GnRH and gonadotropins. A short course of administration stimulates ovarian function and leads to maturation of multiple follicles, ovulation, and luteinization. It has been used successfully to treat infertility, often in conjunction with a gonadotropin (hCG or menotropin) to induce ovulation. There have been reports, considered controversial, suggesting that the use of this drug may be associated with an increased risk of ovarian cancer. In addition, the possibility of multiple births or ovarian hyperstimulation must be kept in mind when clomiphene is employed.

**Tamoxifen** citrate (Nolvadex, Tamofen) has a greater blocking effect on peripheral target tissues than does clomiphene. For this reason, it is used in the adjunctive treatment of carcinoma of the breast provided that estrogen receptors are present in the tumour tissue. Clinical trials indicate that the maximum benefit of tamoxifen is obtained in the first 5 years, after which the prognosis worsens with continued use. Trials to evaluate the use of tamoxifen in the prophylaxis of breast cancer were discontinued because of an associated increase in the incidence of endometrial carcinoma, probably due to its weak estrogenic activity.

**Raloxifene** (Evista) is a selective estrogen receptor modulator (SERM) that has estrogen-like activity on bone

Clomiphene

Tamoxifen

Raloxifene

which are used in the treatment of estrogen-dependent breast cancer either instead of, or after treatment with, tamoxifen. They are used in post-menopausal women to prevent the formation of estrogens (from androgen precursors) at peripheral sites such as muscle and fat tissue.

# PROGESTINS

The chemical structure of **progesterone**, the natural hormone of the corpus luteum, is shown in Figure 46-9. It is also produced by the placenta, testis, and adrenal cortex.

For therapeutic use, progesterone is available as a micronized oral form (Prometrium) or as an injectable in an oil-based solution. Synthetic progesterone esters (e.g., medroxyprogesterone acetate; Provera) and 19-nor derivatives of testosterone (Fig. 46-10) also are available for use as progestational agents. The latter compounds are the progestational component of combination oral contraceptive pills. These 19-nor derivatives have undergone three phases of development. Norethisterone and norethyn-

and is used in the treatment of osteoporosis. Like other estrogens, it poses a risk for thromboembolic disease, but it is devoid of estrogenic activity on the breast and endometrium and acts as an antagonist at these sites. The selective activity of raloxifene, like that of other SERMs, results from many factors, including its partial agonist activity at ERA, antagonist activity at ERB, tissue-specific distribution of the ER subtypes, and differential recruitment of co-regulators of transcription by the SERM-occupied receptor.

# AROMATASE INHIBITORS

Aromatase is the enzyme in the estrogen biosynthetic pathway that converts androgen precursors to estradiol. Aromatase inhibitors (Fig. 46-8) include **anastrozole** (Arimidex), **letrozole** (Femara), and **exemestane** (Aromasin),

FIGURE 46-8 | Structural formulae of aromatase inhibitors.

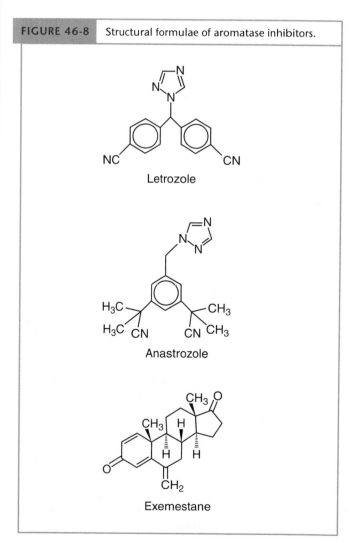

Letrozole

Anastrozole

Exemestane

**FIGURE 46-9** Structural formula of progesterone.

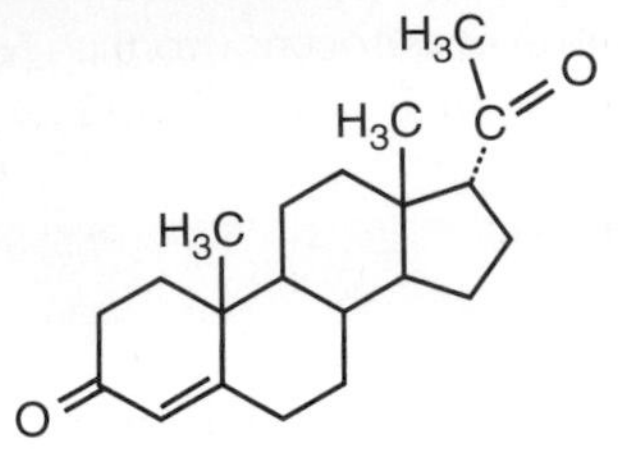

Progesterone, with estrogen, prolactin, and other hormones, is important in breast development and lactation. It is also responsible for the rise in body temperature that occurs close to the midpoint of the menstrual cycle, corresponding with the time of ovulation.

odrel were among the first derivatives generated, followed by norgestrel, levonorgestrel, and norgestrienone. Third-generation compounds include desogestrel and gestodene. These latter compounds have been associated with a somewhat greater risk of venous thromboembolic events than second-generation compounds.

Newer compounds (e.g., drospirenone) have pure progestational activity compared with the 19-nortestosterone derivatives and, therefore, do not have androgenic (acne, hirsutism) and mineralocorticoid-like (edema, weight gain) side effects. They are used as the progestational agent in a newer oral contraceptive formulation (Yasmin).

## Metabolism and Excretion

Progesterone in the circulation is bound to albumin and CBG and is almost entirely metabolized in its first passage through the liver. Progesterone is biotransformed to pregnanolone and pregnanediol. The latter is conjugated with glucuronic acid in the liver and excreted via the kidney. The 19-nor compounds (ethinyl-substituted) are more stable.

## Actions and Uses

Progesterone interacts with a specific nuclear steroid hormone receptor to influence gene transcription and protein synthesis.

In the uterus, progesterone converts the proliferative endometrium (estrogen effect) to a secretory state in preparation for implantation of a fertilized ovum. In the hypothalamus and pituitary, progesterone suppresses the production of gonadotropins and thus prevents further ovulation and follicular maturation. The abrupt fall in progesterone levels (associated with the end of the menstrual cycle or cessation of administration of exogenous progestin) produces vascular changes in the endometrium that result in shedding, resulting in menstrual flow. If a fertilized ovum is implanted before this series of events takes place, hCG from the placenta supports the corpus luteum of pregnancy. The secretion of progesterone thus continues, and the uterine endometrium is maintained, permitting the pregnancy to continue.

**FIGURE 46-10** Synthetic progestins used in oral contraceptive preparations.

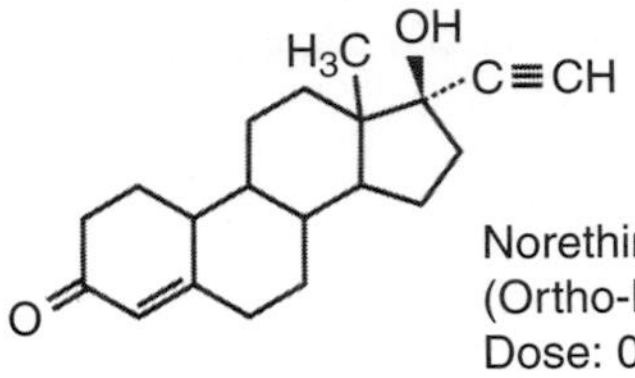

Norethindrone
(Ortho-Novum)
Dose: 0.5–10mg

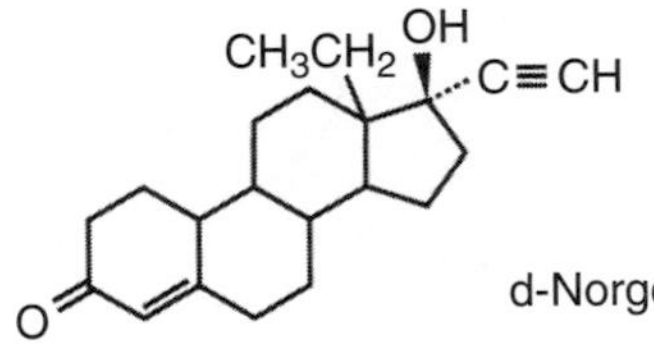

d-Norgestrel
(30–100 times the progestational activity of norethindrone)

Usual dose: *dl*-form 0.3mg; *d*-form 0.15mg

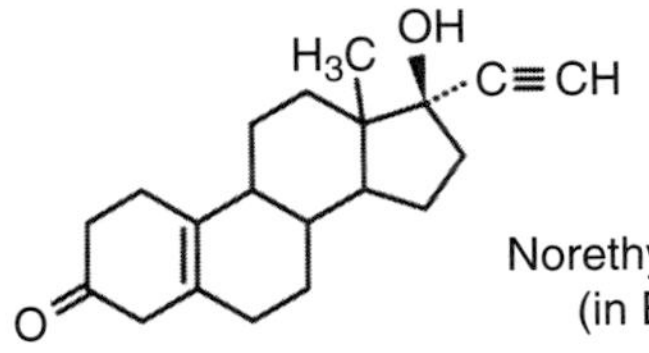

Norethynodrel
(in Enovid)

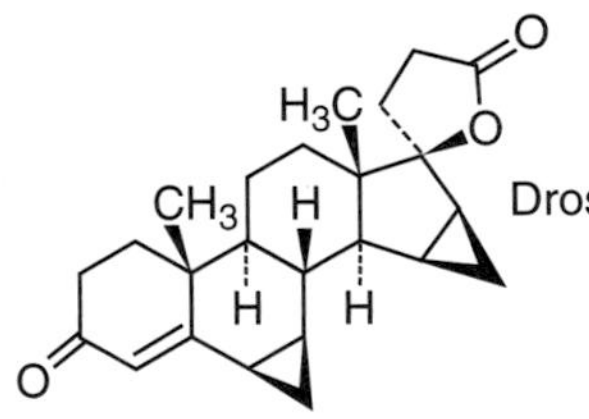

Drospirenone

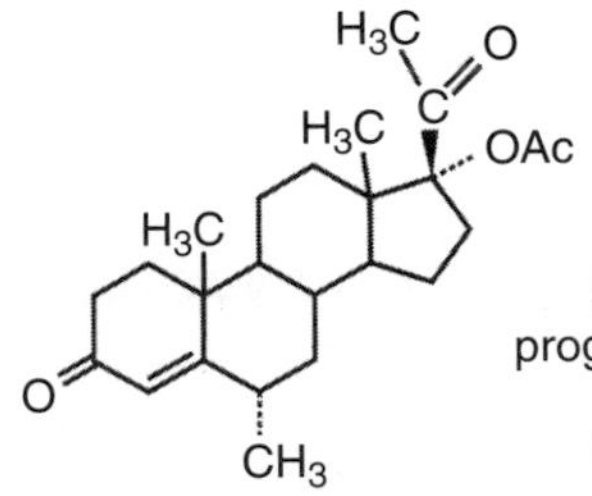

Medroxy-progesterone acetate
(Provera)

By far the greatest clinical use of progestins is as a component of **oral contraceptive pills** in combination with estrogen (discussed below in connection with "Fertility Control"). The availability of inexpensive oral progestins has also greatly extended the range of therapeutic uses, some of which are listed below:

*Dysfunctional uterine bleeding.* A short period of daily administration of a progestin, followed by sudden withdrawal, causes rapid shedding of the endometrium and helps to control anovulatory bleeding.

*Endometriosis.* When progestins are given for prolonged periods, the ectopic endometrial tissue undergoes some involution and develops areas of necrosis, thus presenting a decidua-like reaction.

*Metastatic cancers.* Progestins are used as adjunctive or palliative treatment of certain metastatic cancers originating from endometrial, breast, renal, and other primary cancers.

*Amenorrhea.* Progesterone can be used diagnostically to test for endogenous estrogen production and endometrial proliferation. If sufficient estrogen has been produced to cause endometrial proliferation, a short period of daily administration of progesterone followed by sudden withdrawal causes menstrual flow.

*Emergency contraception.* Progestins (levonorgestrel; Plan B) prevent ovulation, fertilization, and implantation of the fertilized ovum and are 99% effective if used within 72 hours of intercourse. Plan B is available without a prescription (over the counter) in Canada. They are only for emergency use because they are a less effective substitute for routine contraception than the combination oral contraceptive formulations.

## Adverse Effects

- Atherogenic effects may occur. Progestins reduce HDL and elevate low-density lipoprotein (LDL). Thromboembolic events have been reported as noted above.
- Edema and weight gain may result from fluid retention.
- Miscellaneous effects, such as break-through bleeding, skin rashes, breast tenderness, and headache, have been associated with progestins.

## ANTI-PROGESTINS

**Mifepristone** (RU-486; Mifeprex) is a 19-nortestosterone derivative that functions as a progesterone antagonist, although it has weak partial agonist activity. Administra-

tion of this agent prevents ovulation by a central action that suppresses the pre-ovulatory LH surge, and it can terminate early pregnancy by causing endometrial shedding. RU-486 also binds to glucocorticoid receptors to block cortisol action, but it does not bind to estrogen or mineralocorticoid receptors.

RU-486 is approved as an abortifacient in some countries, including the United States, but it is not yet approved for use in Canada. It is effective in disrupting pregnancy if given within the first 49 days of gestation and is administered together with a prostacyclin to stimulate uterotonic activity.

## FERTILITY CONTROL

A decrease in fertility can be achieved in many ways:

- Interfering with fertilization by non-pharmacological means (e.g., behavioural control, mechanical barriers, tubal ligation, vasectomy)
- Interfering with maturation of gametes (e.g., by gossypol, a phenolic compound from cottonseed, which has been used in China as a male fertility inhibitor)
- Impairing gametogenesis (e.g., by mitotic damage caused by alkylating agents, radiation, chemotherapy, or elevation of testicular temperature)
- Preventing ovulation (suppression of gonadotropins by the use of 19-norprogestins, alone or in combination with estrogens; prevention of follicular maturation by continuous dosage of long-acting analogues of GnRH)
- Interfering, before or at implantation, by mechanical means (e.g., intrauterine device) or alteration of the endometrium by hormones (e.g., very low dosage of a progestin)
- Interfering with gestation (abortion)

All these methods have been examined, but at present, preventing ovulation is the most widely used.

## Preparations

The available commercial oral preparations (commonly known collectively as "the pill") include a synthetic estrogen (ethinyl estradiol or mestranol) together with a progestin. They are administered for the first 21 days of each 28-day cycle.

Currently used oral contraceptive preparations (Table 46-1) consist of a combination of estrogen and progestin in a fixed daily dose or in a phasic formulation. In the fixed-dose preparation, the estrogen dose is usually 20 to 50 μg, and the progestational agent varies depending on its potency. In the phasic preparation, the concentration of the estrogen and/or progestin is varied through phases in the cycle to maintain optimal gonadotropin suppression and prevent break-through bleeding. When the oral contraceptive is discontinued, the endometrium sheds, and menstrual flow usually results.

Combinations containing lower doses of estrogen are preferable as they offer a low but effective dose with a usually acceptable level of side effects. With low-dose estrogen, break-through bleeding may occur due to incomplete suppression of gonadotropins or suboptimal maintenance of the endometrium; other possible explanations of bleeding in patients using the pill are worth considering. For instance, the concurrent administration of substances such as tetracycline, rifampin, and ampicillin may induce hepatic cytochrome P450 and related enzymes and so accelerate the biotransformation of estrogens, thus reducing their effectiveness.

The effectiveness of the combination oral contraceptives is due to suppression of ovulation (primary action), creation of an endometrium that is unfavourable for implantation of the ovum, and a thickening of cervical mucus that impairs sperm penetration. This technique is almost 100% effective. Generally, the incidence of side effects is low, and their nature depends to a large extent on the quantities and composition of the two components in the combination pill together with patient factors such as age, obesity, and whether the person smokes.

Other combination estrogen–progestin contraceptives include a transdermal formulation of ethinyl estradiol, 750 µg, and norelgestromin, 6 mg (Evra). The formulation

| TABLE 46-1 | Representative Oral Contraceptive Preparations | |
|---|---|---|
| **Estrogen** | **Progestin** | **Product** |
| Monophasic | | |
| Ethinyl estradiol | Norethindrone | |
| 20 µg | 1 mg | Minestrin 1/20, Loestrin 1/20 |
| 30 µg | 1.5 mg | Loestrin 1.5/30 |
| 35 µg | 0.5 mg | Brevicon 0.5/35, Ortho 0.5/35, ModiCon |
| 35 µg | 1.0 mg | Ortho 1/35, Brevicon 1/35, Select 1/35 |
| 50 µg | 1 mg, 2.5 mg | Norlestrin 1/50, 2.5/50 |
| Ethinyl estradiol | Norgestrel | |
| 20 µg | 0.1 mg (levo-isomer) | Alesse |
| 30 µg | 0.15 mg (levo-isomer) | Minovral |
| 50 µg | 0.5 mg (racemate) | Ovral |
| Ethinyl estradiol | Norgestimate | |
| 35 µg | 0.25 mg | Cyclen |
| Ethinyl estradiol | Ethynodiol | |
| 30 µg | 2 mg | Demulen 30 |
| 35 µg | 1 mg | Demulen 1/35 |
| 50 µg | 1 mg | Demulen 1/50 |
| Ethinyl estradiol | Desogestrel | |
| 30 µg | 0.15 mg | Marvelon, Ortho-Cept |
| Ethinyl estradiol | Drospirenone | |
| 30 µg | 3.0 mg | Yasmin |
| Mestranol | Norethindrone | |
| 50 µg | 1 mg | Ortho-Novum 1/50 |
| Triphasic | | |
| Ethinyl estradiol | Norethindrone | |
| 35 µg | 0.5 mg, then 0.75 mg, then 1.0 mg | Ortho 7/7/7 |
| 35 µg | 0.5 mg, then 1 mg, then 0.5 mg | Synphasic |
| Ethinyl estradiol | Norgestrel | |
| 30 µg, then 40 µg, then 30 µg | 0.05 mg, then 0.075 mg, then 0.125 mg | Triphasil, Triquilar |
| Ethinyl estradiol | Norgestimate | |
| 35 µg | 0.18 mg, then 0.215 mg, then 0.25 mg | Tri-Cyclen, Ortho Tri-Cyclen |
| Progestins | | |
| None | Norethindrone | |
| – | 0.35 mg | Micronor |

is applied as a patch weekly for the first 3 weeks (21 days) of each 28-day cycle. Seasonale (30 µg ethinyl estradiol, 0.15 mg levonorgestrel) is an extended-cycle oral contraceptive that is taken for 84 consecutive days over a cycle of 91 days. While this regimen reduces the number of menstrual cycles to four per year, users experience a relatively high incidence of break-through bleeding. The "minipill" (Micronor), consisting of norethindrone 0.35 mg, is taken continuously but does not appear to be as effective as the combination.

Implants of a progestin (medroxyprogesterone; Depo-Provera) are effective for 3 months or more.

## Side Effects and Contraindications

The estrogens and progestins in these preparations contribute to the production of side effects. The most serious of the common side effects is an increase in the incidence of **thromboembolic disease** (thrombophlebitis, pulmonary emboli, cerebrovascular disease). Common but less severe side effects include weight gain, mild edema, nausea, fullness of the breasts, headache, dizziness, and depressed mood.

Among young women, these hazards and the mortality associated with them are much lower than the risks associated with pregnancy or abortion. These risks, however, increase with age and with smoking tobacco. An upper limit of 35 years is recommended for use of these drugs in women who smoke.

Thromboembolic side effects may be related to the increases in clotting factors, decrease in antithrombin III, and acceleration of platelet aggregation, and they are largely estrogen dose–dependent. Other factors, such as the progestational agent and genetic factors (e.g., blood groups A, B, and AB), may play a role.

Other side effects include changes in carbohydrate metabolism, with a decrease in glucose tolerance; adverse changes in the lipid profile; occasional alteration in liver function tests; increased incidence of gallbladder disease and hepatic adenoma; and acceleration of closure of epiphyses in the adolescent.

Several studies have suggested a link between estrogen use and an increased risk of breast carcinoma. While these reports remain controversial, they suggest that the risk is small among current and recent users and eventually disappears after oral contraceptives have been discontinued.

The side effects of oral contraceptives are offset by some desirable features, including lack of fear of pregnancy and reduced frequency of ovarian cysts, benign breast lesions, heavy and irregular periods, anemia, and dysmenorrhea. A decreased incidence of ovarian and endometrial carcinoma has been reported in users and previous users of the pill who are over the age of 40 years.

In terms of effectiveness and aesthetic acceptance, no method of contraception compares with the use of the combination pill. It seems clear that its benefits must be balanced against the costs involved. The costs are likely to be too high in the presence of the following conditions, which are considered to be **absolute contraindications:**

- Thromboembolic disease
- Cerebrovascular or oculovascular disease
- Myocardial infarction or coronary arterial disease
- Deep vein thrombosis
- Impaired liver function or liver disease
- Carcinoma of the breast or other estrogen-dependent neoplasia
- Undiagnosed vaginal bleeding
- Pregnancy or suspected pregnancy
- Classical migraine

Other conditions such as uncontrolled hypertension, cardiovascular disease, diabetes mellitus with vascular complications, a history of gestational diabetes, or prospects of major surgery are indications for caution in the use of these agents.

# ANDROGENS

## Physiology

Testosterone (Fig. 46-11) is the principal natural androgen produced in the Leydig cells of the testis. Androstenedione and dehydroepiandrosterone are weaker androgens that serve as precursors for testosterone. In some tissues, testosterone acts directly, while in others it is first converted to the more potent derivative dihydrotestosterone (DHT). As discussed above, testosterone may also be converted to 17-β-estradiol. After binding to the specific androgen receptor, testosterone and dihydrotestosterone localize in the nuclei of target tissues (a similar mechanism to that of estrogens) to alter gene transcription. Testosterone plays an essential role in spermatogenesis (initiated by FSH) and has a variety of other physiological effects on male genital development (prostate, external genitalia), secondary sex characteristics (hair distribution,

**FIGURE 46-11**  Structural formula of testosterone.

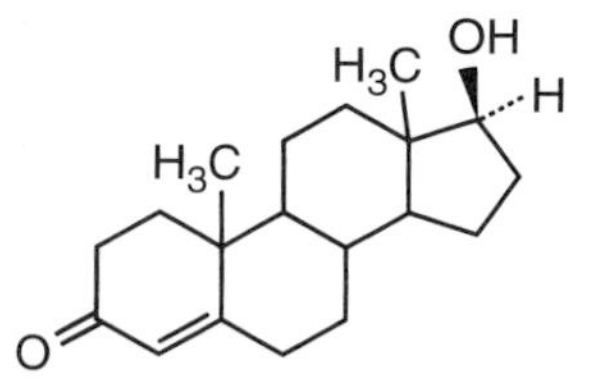

voice), and somatic development in general (skeletal muscle, organic matrix of bone).

Most modifications of the testosterone molecule affect all these activities in equal proportions; for example, stanolone (androstane-17-ol-3-one), which resembles testosterone except that the 4,5 double bond is saturated, is a much weaker androgen and also a weaker anabolic hormone. All the modifications have a $CH_3$ group at C-19 and are often referred to as C-19 steroids.

Like estrogens, testosterone in blood is largely bound to the carrier protein SHBG. Examples of the actions of testosterone and its metabolites on various tissues are shown in Table 46-2.

## Metabolism

In various tissues, but chiefly in the liver, testosterone is biotransformed to the compounds shown in Figure 46-12. The most important metabolic changes are the following:

1. Oxidation of the 17-OH group to a keto group
2. Reduction of the 3-keto group to OH
3. Saturation of the 4,5 double bond to yield 5α and 5β stereoisomers

These metabolites are much less potent androgens than testosterone. They are the main urinary excretion products of testicular origin; however, they represent only about 30% of total urinary androgen metabolites (17-ketosteroids). In the normal male, 70% of the urinary ketosteroids are derived from the adrenal cortex, the most important being dehydroepiandrosterone. In the female, almost all (98%) are from the adrenal cortex.

## Modified Testosterones

Testosterone is readily absorbed from the gastrointestinal tract but is inactivated by first-pass metabolism in the liver. Since these natural modifications all result in loss of activity, synthetic changes for pharmacological purposes are of two different types: those that modify solubility and susceptibility to enzymatic breakdown and, hence, affect route and duration of action; and those intended to give some separation of androgenic and anabolic effects. The half-life of testosterone is generally 10 to 20 minutes. In order to delay absorption and prolong its duration of action, testosterone has been converted to esters that are much less polar. Esterification with propionic acid (Testex) at the 17-OH position yields a product that has a steady effect when injected at 2- to 3-day intervals. The cyclopentylpropionate (Depo-Testosterone C) and enanthate (Delatestryl) esters are effective for periods of up to 3 weeks. The undecanoate (Andriol) is an orally active testosterone ester that bypasses the liver via absorption through the lymphatic system. A transdermal patch (Androderm) and a topical gel (AndroGel) are formulations of unmodified testosterone that are administered once daily.

## Uses

### Androgen replacement therapy
In cases of testicular hypofunction, whether primary or secondary to pituitary failure, androgens maintain the secondary sexual characteristics and muscular development and prevent the development of anemia. In older patients, it is used to treat symptoms of "andropause," including loss of libido and loss of muscle and bone mass.

### Anabolic effects
Androgens produce an increase in the mass of skeletal muscle, an increase in the organic matrix of bone, and retention of nitrogen. These anabolic actions may be useful as adjunctive therapy to promote bone matrix formation and calcification in senile osteoporosis; to reverse acutely catabolic conditions, such as burns and chronic debilitating diseases; and to counter the catabolic effects of adrenal cortical hormones. They are also used by athletes to increase muscle mass; however, only long-term use of anabolic steroids can be expected to improve competitive athletic performance, and there are significant risks of side effects attendant on such use. National and international athletic federations strongly disapprove of the use of anabolic steroids. For all of these purposes, androgenic effects are undesirable but unavoidable side effects. A selective anabolic activity is claimed for synthetic testosterone analogues, such as **nandrolone** (19-nortestosterone decanoate; Deca-Durabolin), but significant androgenic effects persist.

### Carcinoma of the breast
Androgens are sometimes used in pre-menopausal women to suppress the growth of carcinoma of the breast. Most often, these are cases with extensive metastases, especially to the skeleton.

| TABLE 46-2 | Examples of the Actions of Testosterone and Its Derivatives |
|---|---|
| Intracellular Product | Examples of Actions |
| Testosterone | Development of structures derived from Wolffian duct; erythropoietin synthesis; pectoral muscle development; kidney hypertrophy |
| 5-α-DHT | Growth of genital tubercle, hair |
| Estradiol | Behavioural effects; gonadotropin secretion; anabolic effects on some muscle types |
| 5-β-DHT | Red blood cell production in bone marrow |

FIGURE 46-12 | Metabolic products of testosterone.

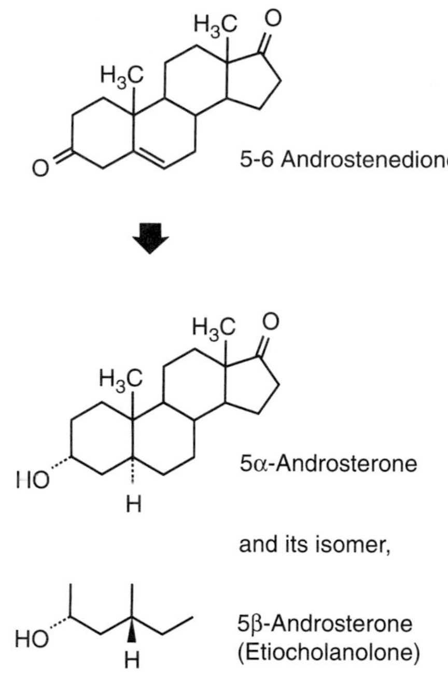

## Treatment of anemias

The mild anemia associated with hypogonadism is corrected by administration of androgens. Large doses have been observed to cause polycythemia. Androgens are used in the treatment of aplastic anemia and sometimes for other anemias refractory to other treatments. Androgens stimulate erythropoietin production from the kidney and have stimulatory effects on other cells of the bone marrow.

## Side Effects

Virilization is the most common side effect. All androgens can cause salt and water retention due to mineralocorticoid-like activity and should be used cautiously if heart failure is a threat. Androgens adversely alter the lipid profile by raising LDL cholesterol and lowering HDL cholesterol (see Chapter 35). Gynecomastia may occur, secondary to the aromatization of testosterone to estrogen in peripheral tissues.

Androgens with a methyl or ethyl group on C-17 cause hepatic dysfunction and cholestatic jaundice. This appears to be a direct effect on the liver, related to dose, and not a sensitivity reaction (see Chapter 43). A high dose or prolonged use may cause dilatation of biliary ducts, cholestasis, obstructive jaundice, and hepatic adenoma. Anabolic androgenic steroids also reduce output of testosterone and gonadotropins, thus causing a reduction in spermatogenesis.

## ANTI-ANDROGENS

Potential anti-androgens are compounds that block the synthesis or action of androgens. Continuous administration (see "Gonadotropin-Releasing Hormone" above) of GnRH or its analogues effectively inhibits the whole axis and shuts off testicular production of androgens.

**Cyproterone acetate** (Androcur) is a progestin that antagonizes androgen action by competitive inhibition of the binding of androgen to its receptor. It is used as a palliative treatment for advanced prostate cancer and for androgen-dependent disorders in women such as hirsutism and acne. Cyproterone acetate also is formulated together with ethinyl estradiol (Diane-35) for use in women. **Flutamide** (Euflex), **bicalutamide** (Casodex), and **nilutamide** (Anandron, Nilandron) are nonsteroidal anti-androgens that prevent androgen uptake and inhibit the binding of androgen to its receptor. However, by blocking the feedback of testosterone on LH secretion, these drugs markedly elevate LH and testosterone levels. Thus, to be effective, they have to be co-administered with a GnRH analogue to completely block androgen action.

These classes of compounds that function as anti-androgens have clinical utility in the treatment of carcinoma of the prostate (see Chapter 57). In addition, some of these drugs have potential value for the treatment of prostatic hypertrophy, male pattern baldness, acne, hirsutism, male precocious puberty, and for reduction of libido in male sex offenders.

**Finasteride** (Proscar) and **dutasteride** (Avodart) are type II 5-$\alpha$-reductase inhibitors that block the conversion of testosterone to dihydrotestosterone and are used in the treatment of benign prostatic hypertrophy. In a lower dose finasteride (Propecia) is used to treat mild to moderate hair loss in male pattern baldness.

## SUGGESTED READINGS

Anderson GL, Limacher M, Assaf AR, et al, for the Women's Health Initiative Steering Committee. Effects of conjugated equine estrogen in postmenopausal women with hysterectomy: the Women's Health Initiative randomized controlled trial. *JAMA.* 2004;291:1701-1712.

Bagatell CJ, Bremmer WJ. Androgen and progestagen effects on plasma lipids. *Prog Cardiovasc Dis.* 1995;38:255-271.

Byrne M, Nieschlag E. Testosterone replacement therapy in male hypogonadism. *J Endocrinol Invest.* 2003;26:481-489.

Chlebowski RT, Hendrix SL, Langer RD, et al, for the WHI Investigators. Influence of estrogen plus progestin on breast cancer and mammography in healthy postmenopausal women: the Women's Health Initiative Randomized Trial. *JAMA.* 2003; 289:3243-3253.

Evans RM. The steroid and thyroid hormone receptor superfamily. *Science*. 1988;240:889-895.

Gustafsson JA. What pharmacologists can learn from recent advances in estrogen signaling. *Trends Pharmacol Sci*. 2003; 24:479-485.

Hanstein B, Djahansouzi S, Dall P, et al. Insights into the molecular biology of the estrogen receptor define novel therapeutic targets for breast cancer. *Eur J Endocrinol*. 2004;150:243-255.

Hasbi A, O'Dowd BF, George SR. A G protein–coupled receptor for estrogen: the end of the search? *Mol Interv*. 2005;5:158-161.

Hillier SG. Gonadotropic control of ovarian follicular growth and development. *Mol Cell Endocrinol*. 2001;179:39-46.

Ingle JN. Endocrine therapy trials of aromatase inhibitors for breast cancer in the adjuvant and prevention settings. *Clin Cancer Res*. 2005;11:900s-905s.

Johnston SR, Dowsett M. Aromatase inhibitors for breast cancer: lessons from the laboratory. *Nat Rev Cancer*. 2003;3:821-831.

Jordan VC. Antiestrogens and selective estrogen receptor modulators as multifunctional medicines. 2. Clinical considerations and new agents. *J Med Chem*. 2003;46:1081-1111.

Katzenellenbogen BS, Frasor J. Therapeutic targeting in the estrogen receptor hormonal pathway. *Semin Oncol*. 2004;31:28-38.

Kiesel LA, Rody A, Greb RR, et al. Clinical use of GnRH analogues. *Clin Endocrinol (Oxf)*. 2002;56:677-687.

Larsen PR, Kronenberg HM, Melmed S, Polonsky KS, eds. *Williams Textbook of Endocrinology*. 10th ed. Philadelphia, Pa: WB Saunders; 2002.

Martinelli I, Battaglioli T, Mannucci PM. Pharmacogenetic aspects of the use of oral contraceptives and the risk of thrombosis. *Pharmacogenetics*. 2003:13:589-594.

McConnell JD, Roehrborn CG, Bautista OM, et al. The long-term effect of doxazosin, finasteride, and combination therapy on the clinical progression of benign prostatic hyperplasia. *N Engl J Med*. 2003;349:2387-2398.

McDonnell DP. Mining the complexities of the estrogen signaling pathways for novel therapeutics. *Endocrinology*. 2003;144: 4237-4240.

Molitch ME. Medical management of prolactin-secreting pituitary adenomas. *Pituitary*. 2002;5:55-65.

Morley JE, Perry HM III. Androgen treatment of male hypogonadism in older males. *J Steroid Biochem Mol Biol*. 2003;85: 367-373.

Nelson HD, Humphrey LL, Nygren P, Teutsch SM, Allan JD. Postmenopausal hormone replacement therapy: scientific review. *JAMA*. 2002;288:872-881.

Rossouw JE, Anderson GL, Prentice RL, et al, for the Writing Group for the Women's Health Initiative Investigators. Risks and benefits of estrogen plus progestin in healthy postmenopausal women: principal results from the Women's Health Initiative randomized controlled trial. *JAMA*. 2002;288:321-333.

Schneider HP. Androgens and antiandrogens. *Ann N Y Acad Sci*. 2003;997:292-306.

Shlipak MG, Chaput LA, Vittinghoff E, et al, for the Heart and Estrogen/progestin Replacement Study Investigators. Lipid changes on hormone therapy and coronary heart disease events in the Heart and Estrogen/progestin Replacement Study (HERS). *Am Heart J*. 2003;146:870-875.

Warren MP. A comparative review of the risks and benefits of hormone replacement therapy regimens. *Am J Obstet Gynecol*. 2004;190:1141-1167.

Wassertheil-Smoller S, Hendrix SL, Limacher M, et al, for the WHI Investigators. Effect of estrogen plus progestin on stroke in postmenopausal women: the Women's Health Initiative: a randomized trial. *JAMA*. 2003;289:2673-2684.

# 47

# Insulin and Other Anti-diabetic Drugs

## BP SCHIMMER AND SR GEORGE

### CASE HISTORY

A 45-year-old man first consulted his physician because of nocturia, mild thirst, and some fatigue. At the time, he was somewhat overweight and sedentary in his habits. Laboratory tests showed an elevated fasting blood glucose level of 15 mmol/L (normal 4 to 6.5 mmol/L), glucose but no ketones in the urine, normal plasma electrolytes, and normal anion gap. Type 2 diabetes mellitus was diagnosed, and he was placed on a diabetic diet low in free sugar and fat and on a program of regular exercise. He also was referred to a diabetes education program. After 2 months on this diet, he had a fasting blood glucose level of 9.5 mmol/L, a 2-hour, post-lunch glucose value of 12.8 mmol/L (normal <8.5 mmol/L), and a glycosylated hemoglobin (HbA1C) level of 10.5% (normal <6%). He was therefore started on glyburide (5 mg) and metformin (500 mg) before breakfast and dinner, and this achieved a good result.

After 3 years on this regimen, he developed unstable angina pectoris, and the blood glucose and HbA1C levels were again found to be elevated. He showed glycosuria, and urinary microalbumin excretion exceeded normal levels. His weight had fallen to a level that yielded a normal body mass index, and his blood pressure was normal. His physician therefore decided to transfer him to insulin therapy and added an angiotensin-converting enzyme (ACE) inhibitor, ramipril 5 mg, to his drug regimen.

The patient was extremely reluctant to start insulin but was convinced to take Humulin insulin 70/30 premix, 22 units every morning before breakfast. His 8:00 A.M. blood glucose was found to be 10 mmol/L, and there was continued glycosuria. In an attempt to normalize blood sugar levels, the dose of insulin was raised gradually to 35 units. As a result, his 4:00 P.M. blood glucose level fell to 3 mmol/L, rising to 13 mmol/L by the next morning at 8:00 A.M., before breakfast. A second dose of Humulin 70/30 was added at suppertime, and glycemic control improved significantly. The patient's blood sugar levels ranged from 4.5 to 8 mmol/L before breakfast and before dinner, and from 6.5 to 13 mmol/L 2 hours after meals. During the next year, he had three mild hypoglycemic reactions. He was found to have stable background retinopathy, mild diabetic nephropathy, and mild numbness and tingling in both feet, but blood pressure remained normal.

In the following year, during three routine visits to his family physician, his blood pressure readings were 140/90, 145/95, and 150/100 mmHg. His physician added propranolol to his antihypertensive medication and increased the dose of ramipril. Three weeks later, the patient was found at home in a semiconscious state resulting from severe hypoglycemia, having taken an unusually long walk earlier in the day. After being revived, he denied feeling any of his usual symptoms of hypoglycemia.

Diabetes mellitus has been recognized for centuries as a debilitating and life-threatening disease. It is a metabolic disturbance that is characterized by hyperglycemia, resulting in the excretion of large volumes of urine (containing sugar) and in excessive thirst. Other features include altered metabolism of lipids and carbohydrates and wasting of tissue (loss of nitrogen). In severe insulin deficiency as seen in type 1 diabetes mellitus, ketoacidosis develops, leading to coma and, if uncorrected, death. Type 2 diabetes is characterized by insulin resist- ance with eventual insulin hyposecretion. The long-term complications include vascular disease, retinopathy and other microvascular disease, atherosclerosis, nephropathy, dermopathy, and neuropathy.

An extract of pancreas prepared by F.G. Banting and C.H. Best at the University of Toronto in 1921 contained an active principle (insulin) capable of controlling the hyperglycemia of diabetes. The very first diabetic patient treated with Banting and Best's pancreatic extract was a 14-year-old boy named Leonard Thompson at the Toronto General

Hospital. Thompson continued the use of insulin until he died of bronchopneumonia at age 27. This discovery dramatically improved the lifespan of diabetic patients. However, the long-term complications secondary to diabetes continue to cause significant morbidity. In North America, diabetes mellitus is prevalent in 6% of the population and has a hereditary component. The high prevalence of obesity in today's population is also a major risk factor.

The disease is categorized into two major classes: type 1, insulin-dependent diabetes mellitus, and type 2, non-insulin-dependent diabetes mellitus. Type 1 diabetes mellitus often occurs in juveniles and is characterized by destruction of β cells of the pancreas, possibly triggered by viral and autoimmune mechanisms. This results in severe insulin deficiency leading to ketoacidosis. Type 2 diabetes mellitus typically exhibits a slow onset and occurs predominantly in older age groups. The hyperglycemia is thought to result from resistance of target tissues to insulin, which is caused by defects at different points in the signal transduction pathway that mediates insulin action and by a failure of pancreatic β cells to produce sufficient insulin in response to glucose. Insulin resistance also is correlated with visceral obesity. In obese patients, increased levels of free fatty acids and changes in levels of tumour necrosis factor alpha (TNFα), resistin, and adiponectin reduce sensitivity to insulin. Therefore, type 2 diabetes represents a heterogeneous group of genetic disorders with similar clinical manifestations.

The objective of treatment is the same for both type 1 and type 2 diabetes—to maintain blood glucose within normal limits so as to prevent the development of complications associated with this disease.

## INSULIN

Insulin is a protein with a molecular mass of about 6000 Da, and it is made up of two polypeptide chains (an A-chain consisting of 21 amino acids and a B-chain of 30 amino acids) linked by two disulfide bonds (Fig. 47-1). It is produced in the β cells of the islets of Langerhans, initially as a single precursor molecule, proinsulin (formed from a larger precursor, pre-proinsulin), that is cleaved by proteolytic enzymes to form insulin. Porcine insulin differs from human insulin by only one amino acid, whereas bovine insulin differs from human insulin by three amino acids.

Most of the insulin in the β cells of the human pancreas (approximately 200 units) is contained in secretory granules. Under appropriate stimulation, the contents of the granules are secreted by exocytosis. Connecting peptide (C-peptide) and some proinsulin are released into the circulation along with insulin, but they do not contribute significantly to hormone activity.

The molecule contains a high proportion of dicarboxylic acids, which enables it to combine readily with basic proteins without affecting its fundamental structure. This property is utilized in the preparation of long-acting insulin for clinical use. In an acidic medium, it tends to polymerize into insoluble fibrils.

## Physiology

Glucose produces a rapid release of insulin, as well as a secondary slower release that raises blood levels of insulin for about 1 hour. The rapidly released insulin is from the pool stored in the secretory granules present in the β cells; the slow release is attributed to release of newly synthesized insulin. Glucose taken orally has a greater effect on insulin secretion than glucose by injection, the explanation being that glucose taken orally concurrently stimulates the secretion of ileum-derived glucagon-like peptide 1 and gastric inhibitory polypeptide (GIP). These, in turn, additively stimulate the release of insulin from the islet cells. Other factors that may enhance the release of insulin include some amino acids (arginine, leucine) and free fatty acids (FFA), secretin, pancreozymin, gastrin, and glucagon.

Autonomic mediators also influence insulin secretion. Adrenaline and noradrenaline (acting through α2-adrenergic receptors) inhibit the secretion of insulin induced by a rise in blood glucose. Cholinergic drugs enhance the release of insulin. Growth hormone stimulates the synthesis of insulin but probably does not have a direct effect on its release. Drugs of the sulfonylurea group (e.g., glyburide, gliclazide, glipizide) and the glitinides (e.g., repaglinide, nateglinide) also stimulate release of insulin (Fig. 47-2).

Somatostatin, produced by the δ cells of the pancreatic islet, inhibits the secretion of both insulin and glucagon by direct actions on islet β and α cells. The physiological importance of this action is not clear. Somatostatin is also produced in the gastrointestinal (GI) tract, where it inhibits the secretion of gastrin, secretin, cholecystokinin, pepsin, and HCl, and in the hypothalamus, where it regulates growth hormone secretion. Therefore, its physiological role in glucose homeostasis may be very complex.

## Mechanism of Insulin Action

Insulin exerts its actions by binding to specific receptors on the surface of target cells. The insulin receptor is made up of α and β subunits and exists as an α2–β2 dimer. The α subunits have extracellular domains that provide the binding site for insulin. The β subunits are transmembrane proteins that anchor the α subunits and have intracellular tyrosine kinase activity. The binding of insulin to the α-chains leads to activation of the β subunit tyrosine kinase and consequent intracellular phosphorylation of other substrate proteins. These events initiate a complex cascade of enzymatic reactions and changes in gene expression that impact glucose homeostasis, the utilization and storage of nutrients, and cell proliferation (Fig. 47-3).

**FIGURE 47-1** Structure of human insulin (A-chain = 21 amino acids, B-chain = 30 amino acids). The two chains are connected by two of three disulfide bridges, at positions A7–B7 and A20–B19). The proinsulin molecule contains a "C-peptide" of 31 amino acids, which is removed by proteolysis to form insulin.

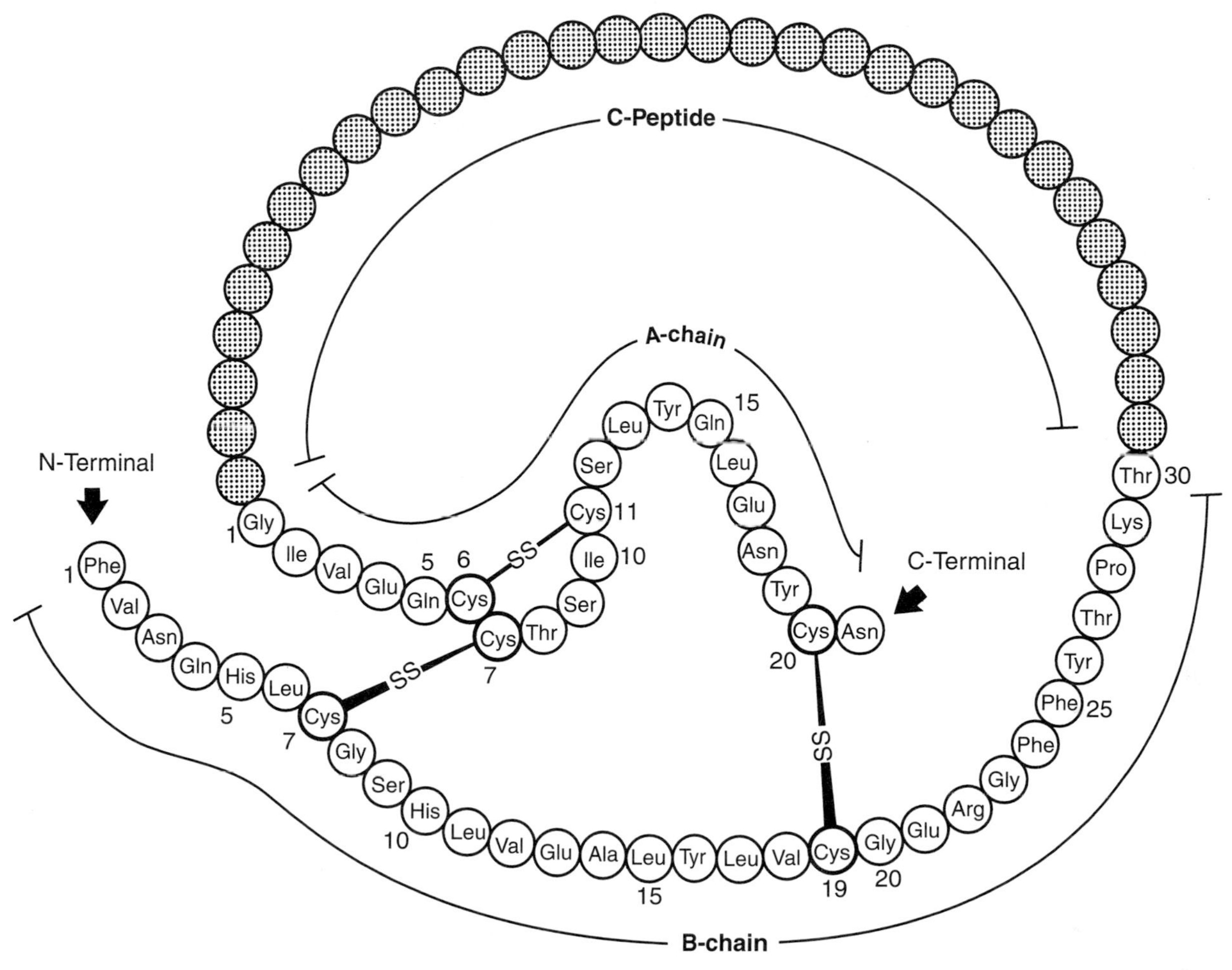

Insulin receptor activation results in the mobilization of the type 4 glucose transporter (GLUT-4) in muscle and adipose tissue, which promotes the uptake of glucose. Glucose uptake in certain tissues (neuron, erythrocyte, intestinal mucosa, kidney) is mediated by different glucose transporters that are not dependent on insulin. In liver and muscle, insulin stimulates glycogen synthase activity and inhibits glycogen phosphorylase activity, leading to increased deposition of glycogen. In liver tissue, insulin also inhibits the synthesis of glucose (gluconeogenesis) and increases glucose uptake, in part by stimulating glucokinase activity. In muscle, insulin promotes protein synthesis by facilitating amino acid uptake. In adipose tissue, insulin promotes triglyceride synthesis and inhibits lipolysis. Therefore, insulin is an anabolic and anti-catabolic hormone.

Insulin increases glucose uptake and oxidative metabolism by muscle and other tissues. This prevents breakdown of tissue protein and conversion of residual amino acids into glucose by the liver. Insulin thus prevents gluconeogenesis and glycogenolysis and consequently reduces glucose release from the liver. It also prevents mobilization of fatty acids from fat depots and the consequent breakdown of these fatty acids by the liver; therefore, insulin prevents the formation of ketone bodies. Indeed, fat synthesis from glucose is promoted by insulin. In the diabetic subject, these actions result in a lowering of blood sugar, disappearance of glycosuria and polyuria, and disappearance of ketone bodies from the blood and urine.

## Preparations and Properties

For many decades following the discovery of insulin, the world's supply for therapeutic use was derived from extracts of bovine and porcine pancreases. Human insulin has since become available and is used more widely, while the use of bovine insulin has waned, in part because of concerns over bovine spongiform encephalopathy (BSE, mad cow disease). Human insulin is produced by means of recombinant DNA (rDNA) technology in which human proinsulin is expressed in bacteria or yeast and then hydrolyzed to yield insulin (Table 47-1 and see Fig. 47-1). Human insulin is more polar than insulin from animal sources and is therefore absorbed more quickly from its site of injection. Recombinant insulin has provided an assured supply of hormone in the face of a worldwide increase in the incidence of diabetes.

A large variety of formulations have been developed that affect the onset time, the time to maximal activity (peak time), and the duration of action of insulin. These are summarized below and in Table 47-2.

### Crystalline zinc insulin (regular insulin)

Pure insulin is crystallized as a zinc salt and then re-dissolved to give a clear solution (1 mg of crystalline human insulin equals 27.5 units). It is usually given subcutaneously, but the intravenous route is used in emergencies and other circumstances such as during surgery. When administered subcutaneously, it lowers plasma glucose within minutes, and its effects last for 8 to 12 hours; however, the exact duration and magnitude of effect depend on the dose and the individual patient. The plasma half-life of intravenous insulin is only a few minutes. Regular insulin is prepared from recombinant human insulin or from pork insulin, which is purified from porcine pancreas.

### NPH insulin (neutral protamine; Hagedorn)

NPH insulin is formed by treating regular insulin (human or pork) with protamine and zinc at neutral pH (7.2), causing a fine precipitate of protamine zinc insulin. This fine suspension can only be given subcutaneously and is absorbed slowly and evenly. Its onset of action is 1 to 2 hours, its peak action occurs at 6 to 12 hours, and the effect wears off 18 to 24 hours after administration.

### Insulin mixtures

These are premixed formulations containing crystalline zinc insulin and NPH insulin in different ratios (e.g., 30% regular: 70% NPH). These mixtures combine the benefits of rapid onset and prolonged duration of action.

**FIGURE 47-2** Factors involved in the stimulation (+) and inhibition (−) of insulin production and release.

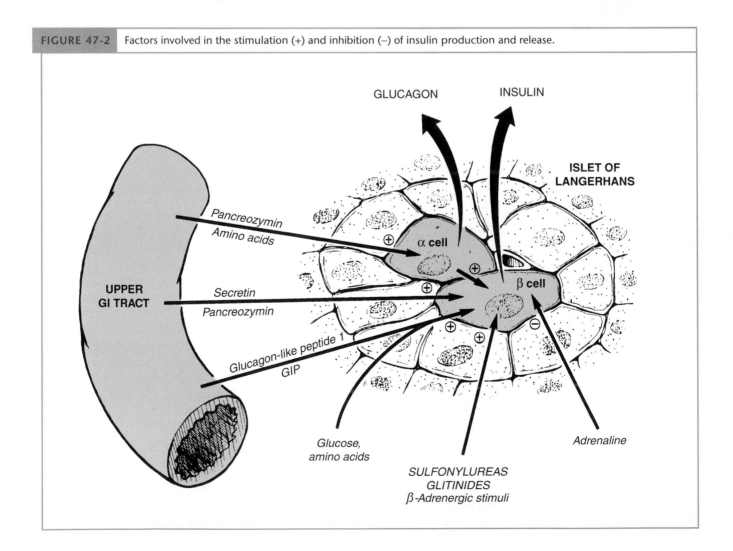

**FIGURE 47-3** Mediators of insulin action. Akt = thymoma viral oncogene homologue (also known as protein kinase B); αPKC = protein kinase C– alpha; Cb1 = Cas-Br-M (murine) ecotropic retroviral transforming sequence; CAP = cadherin-associated protein; Grb2 = growth factor receptor-bound protein 2; GSK3 = glycogen synthase kinase 3; G-6-P = glucose 6-phosphate; IRS = insulin receptor substrate; MAP kinase = mitogen-activated protein kinase; MEK = mitogen-activated protein kinase kinase; PDK = pyruvate dehydrogenase kinase; PI-3 K = phosphatidylinositol 3 kinase; PTP 1B = protein tyrosine phosphatase type 1B; PP1 = pyrophosphate phosphatase 1; p70S6k = ribosomal protein S6 kinase, 70kDa; Ras = murine sarcoma virus oncogene product; SOS = son of sevenless; SHC = Src homology 2 domain containing protein. (Adapted from Zhang B. Insulin signaling and action: glucose, lipids, protein. In: Goldfine ID, Rushakoff RJ, eds. *Diabetes and Carbohydrate Metabolism*. Available at: http://www.endotext.org/diabetes/diabetes4/diabetesframe4.htm. Accessed November 20, 2005. Adapted with permission.)

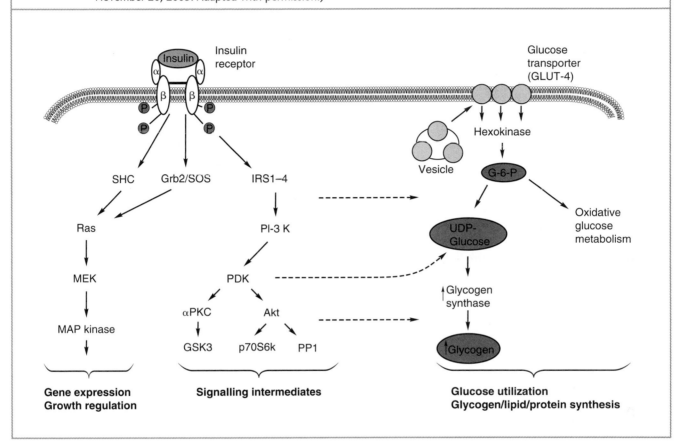

## Lente insulins

These are suspensions of insulin in acetate buffer at neutral pH. The physical state and crystal size influence the rate of absorption from the site of injection. Lente insulins are provided as intermediate-acting (lente) or long-acting (ultralente) formulations made from recombinant human insulin or pork insulin. Lente insulin (insulin zinc suspension USP) has an onset of action of 2.5 hours, reaches a peak of activity in 7 to 15 hours, and lasts for ~22 hours. Ultralente insulin (insulin zinc suspension extended USP) has an onset of action of 4 hours, peak activity from 8 to 24 hours, and duration of action of 28 hours.

## Insulin Pharmacokinetics

Insulin, like many proteins, can be hydrolyzed and inactivated in the gastrointestinal tract. Therefore, insulin is administered by injection, most commonly by the subcutaneous route. When regular insulin is injected subcutaneously, it is absorbed and distributed rapidly, and within minutes, it can be detected in the cells of liver, kidney, and muscle. These tissues (particularly liver and kidney) contain an enzyme, insulinase, which is of primary importance in degrading the hormone. After intravenous injection, the plasma half-life of insulin is less than 9 minutes. Its volume of distribution approximates that of extracellular fluid. Attempts to modify the time of onset and duration of action of injected insulin are all based on influencing the rate at which it reaches the bloodstream from the site of injection.

The fate of injected insulin is different from that of secreted insulin. About 50% of insulin secreted into the portal vein is destroyed in the liver and never reaches the general circulation. This creates a marked differential concentration gradient between the liver and the periphery,

| TABLE 47-1 | Structural Differences among Insulins from Different Species and Recombinant Analogues* | | | | | | | |
|---|---|---|---|---|---|---|---|---|
| | Amino Acid Differences at the Indicated Positions on the A- and B-Chains | | | | | | | |
| Type of Insulin | A8 | A10 | A21 | B28 | B29 | B30 | B31 | B32 |
| Human | Thr | Ile | Asn | Pro | Lys | Thr | | |
| Pig | Thr | Ile | Asn | Pro | Lys | Ala | | |
| Ox | Ala | Val | Asn | Pro | Lys | Ala | | |
| Insulin lispro | Thr | Ile | Asn | Lys | Pro | Thr | | |
| Insulin aspart | Thr | Ile | Asn | Asp | Lys | Thr | | |
| Insulin glargine | Thr | Ile | Gly | Pro | Lys | Thr | Arg | Arg |

* See also Figure 47-1.

resulting in a greater effect of secreted insulin on hepatic function. Attempts to control hepatic gluconeogenesis with injected insulin therefore do not mimic the effects of secreted insulin because there is no concentration gradient. Adequate levels of insulin for hepatic effect may result in peripheral hyperinsulinemia.

The different time relations of various insulin preparations are idealized in Figure 47-4. These profiles assume a constant level of glycemia. In normal subjects, a regular eating pattern consists of taking three or four meals about 4 to 5 hours apart, followed by a long overnight period with little or no food intake. Therefore, there usually are three main peaks of hyperglycemia: in mid-morning, mid-afternoon, and early evening. These increases in plasma glucose stimulate peaks of insulin secretion. Plasma glucose is lower overnight and lowest in the early morning. During the overnight (fasting) period, insulin secretion is at a low basal level.

In insulin-dependent diabetic patients, combinations of regular insulin together with an intermediate or long-acting form can be administered in various proportions to approximate the normal endogenous patterns of insulin secretion. The regular insulin provides rapid, short-term effect; the longer-acting preparations provide sustained effects with peak action at later times.

All preparations in North America are standardized at 100 U/mL. The standard mode of insulin administration is via a needle and calibrated 1-mL syringe. For convenience, portable injector pens with a retractable needle are available that contain cartridges of insulin sufficient for multiple injections.

## Insulin Analogues

Recombinant DNA technology has facilitated the development of insulin analogues with different profiles of action. **Insulin lispro** (Humalog, Novalog; an analogue with $Pro^{28}$ and $Lys^{29}$ in reverse order on the B-chain) and **insulin aspart** (NovoRapid; an analogue in which Asp replaces

$Pro^{28}$) have less tendency to form aggregates in solution and thus have faster times of onset (30 to 45 minutes), sooner peak action (0.75 to 2.5 hours), and shorter durations of action (3 to 5 hours). Because of their improved kinetic profiles, these insulin analogues can be administered to diabetics just before meals and pose less risk of hypoglycemia. Insulin lispro is also available in combination with protamine (Humalog Mix25; a mixture of 25% Insulin lispro/75% protamine suspension) to extend its duration of action.

**Insulin glargine** (Lantus; an analogue with Gly replacing $Asn^{21}$ in the A-chain and two additional Arg residues added to the end of the B-chain) has a higher isoelectric point than human insulin. This results in a preparation that is soluble when dispensed in an acidic solution and that precipitates at the higher pH found at the injection site. The microprecipitate dissolves slowly from the site of injection, providing a continuous basal supply of insulin (over approximately 24 hours after a 70-minute delay) without a peak effect.

## Clinical Uses

### Diabetes mellitus

The principal use of insulin is for replacement therapy in insulin-dependent diabetes mellitus, in which the patient's own insulin supply is deficient. The therapeutic objective is to maintain plasma glucose concentrations in the normal range. This involves administering sufficient insulin to control the hyperglycemia associated with food intake as well as maintaining a basal level of insulin to prevent excessive mobilization of fuels between meals.

Several different insulin treatment regimens are used to achieve these objectives, usually by means of a combination of intermediate or long-acting insulin with a rapidly acting insulin such as regular insulin, insulin lispro, or insulin aspart. In a typical regimen of insulin administration, an intermediate-acting insulin (lente or NPH) in combination with regular insulin is given twice daily, usu-

| TABLE 47-2 | Summary of Available Insulin Preparations | | | | |
|---|---|---|---|---|---|
| Insulin Preparation | USP Official Name | Common Synonyms and Proprietary Names | Action (hours) | | |
| | | | Onset | Peak | Duration |
| **Rapid action** | | | | | |
| Insulin lispro (biosynthetic analogue) | | Humalog | 0.5–0.75 | 0.75–2.5 | 3–5 |
| Insulin aspart (biosynthetic analogue) | | NovoRapid | 0.5–0.75 | 0.75–2.5 | 3–5 |
| **Short action** | | | | | |
| Insulin regular* (human biosynthetic) | | Humulin-R Novolinge Toronto Insulin regular | 0.5 | 3–5 | 6–8 |
| Insulin regular (pork) | | Iletin II Pork Regular | 0.5 | 3–5 | 6–8 |
| **Intermediate action** | | | | | |
| Insulin NPH (pork) | Isophane insulin suspension USP | Iletin II Pork NPH | 2.5 | 4–12 | 12–24 |
| Insulin NPH (human biosynthetic) | | Humulin-N Novalinge NPH (these insulin NPH preparations are also provided premixed with insulin regular in various combinations) | 1.5 | 4–12 | 12–24 |
| Insulin lispro protamine suspension 75% / insulin lispro 25% (biosynthetic) | | Humalog Mix25 | 0.25–0.5 | 0.5–1.5 | 8–12 |
| Insulin lente (pork) | Insulin zinc suspension USP | Iletin II Pork Lente | 2.5 | 7–15 | 12–24 |
| Insulin lente (human biosynthetic) | | Humulin-L | 1–3 | 7–15 | 18–24 |
| **Prolonged action** | | | | | |
| Insulin ultralente (human biosynthetic) | | Humulin-U | 4 | 8–24 | 28 |
| Insulin glargine (biosynthetic) | Insulin glargine USP | Lantus | 4 | none | 24 |

*For intravenous use, regular insulin is the preferred preparation; insulin lispro may also be used. All other formulations are unsuitable.

ally before breakfast and before the evening meal. Additional fine adjustments to glucose homeostasis can be achieved by altering meal times to correspond better with peak insulin concentrations or by delaying the evening injection of intermediate-acting insulin until bedtime. For more precise regulation of blood sugar, intensive regimens of insulin can be used (e.g., intermediate-acting insulin at bedtime and doses of short-acting insulin—regular insulin or insulin analogue—before each meal; or continuous delivery of a rapid-acting insulin with pulses at mealtime via a pump).

In type 2 diabetes, dietary control and weight reduction, where necessary, together with regular exercise are often sufficient. Insulin may be used in these patients if they remain hyperglycemic in spite of diet and exercise.

Infections, uremia, surgical trauma, other serious illnesses, and even anxiety tend to increase insulin require-ments because of increased secretion of counter-regulatory hormones (hormones that oppose the action of insulin), such as cortisol, adrenaline, glucagon, and growth hormone. With appropriate treatment of the underlying condition, the insulin requirements decrease.

As indicated earlier, insulin has dramatically increased the life expectancy of diabetics, but the complications of diabetes mellitus—cardiovascular, renal, neural, and ocular—remain major contributors to morbidity and accelerated mortality. Large clinical trials in North America and the United Kingdom have shown that good control of blood sugar prevents such complications or slows their progression in both type 1 and type 2 diabetics. Achieving rigid control of blood sugar, however, is not without attendant difficulties, including poor patient compliance, cost, and increased frequency of hypoglycemic reactions from intensive therapy.

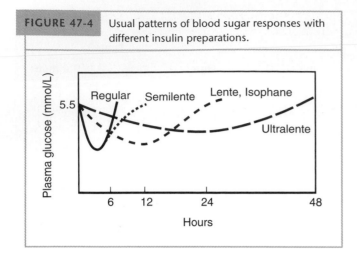

**FIGURE 47-4** Usual patterns of blood sugar responses with different insulin preparations.

## Diabetic coma

This is an emergency situation associated with severe dehydration and acidosis, which may be fatal. Intravenous fluid and regular insulin are the mainstays of treatment. The soluble short-acting type of insulin is needed to achieve rapid and flexible therapy, since the condition of the patient can change rapidly with massive administration of intravenous fluid and electrolytes. The usual recommended dose of insulin in this case is 0.1 U/kg/hr by infusion, preceded by an initial bolus that is equivalent to the dose in the first hour. This dosage approximates the normal rate of endogenous insulin delivery to the periphery and produces a level of venous plasma insulin (about 100 μU/mL) close to that seen after a carbohydrate meal. However, the dosage has to be titrated to individual patient requirements. As blood glucose levels fall toward normal, the rate of insulin infusion can be slowed, and intravenous glucose can be started to prevent insulin-induced hypoglycemia.

## Diagnostic test

Insulin-induced hypoglycemia stimulates the output of releasing factors from the hypothalamus that, in turn, release growth hormone and adrenocorticotropic hormone (ACTH) from the anterior pituitary. Injection of insulin is therefore used as a diagnostic test of the integrity of these hypothalamic and pituitary responses.

## Undesired Side Effects

### Hypoglycemic reactions

Mild hypoglycemic reactions are common and are seen when a meal is missed, when an overdose of insulin has been taken, or when strenuous muscular work has been done. The typical symptoms include sweating, tachycardia, tremor, weakness, hunger, "being ill at ease" (adrenergic symptoms resulting from a compensatory increase in the secretion of adrenaline), blurred vision, and mental confusion; severe cases may develop into convulsions or coma. If the latter occurs, it is important to differentiate it from diabetic coma.

Laboratory tests or capillary glucose monitoring provide conclusive differentiation. If these are not available and diagnosis is uncertain, intravenous glucose will cure hypoglycemic coma in minutes and will not do much harm to diabetic coma. On the other hand, insulin administration in hypoglycemic coma may kill the patient. When intravenous glucose is unavailable, glucagon injection (purified glucagons from bovine/porcine pancreas; Glucagon Emergency Kit or recombinant glucagon; GlucaGen) is used for the immediate treatment of severe hypoglycemia. Glucagon acts through its specific G protein-coupled receptor to stimulate adenylyl cyclase activity, increase cyclic adenosine monophosphate (cAMP), and thereby increase blood glucose via hepatic glycogenolysis. The glucagon is administered by injection (1 mg intravenously, intramuscularly, or subcutaneously); the route of administration affects time of onset and duration of action. Glucagon will not be very effective in patients with chronic hypoglycemia or other conditions that result in inadequate glycogen stores. Treatment with glucagon should be followed by intravenous glucose and the ingestion of complex carbohydrates to maintain blood sugar levels and replete liver glycogen.

### Local lipodystrophy

Irregular atrophy and lumpiness of subcutaneous fat may occur if insulin injections are given repeatedly in the same place. To prevent this occurrence, the sites of injection should be varied.

### Insulin presbyopia

This visual disturbance is due to osmotic changes in ocular fluids; it occurs early in therapy but is usually transient.

### Edema

Edema lasting for a few weeks may occur on initiation of insulin therapy. This effect results in part from insulin-dependent sodium retention by the kidney.

### Insulin allergy

The most common manifestation of insulin allergy is a cutaneous reaction at the site of injection (e.g., rash or hives due to IgE-mediated histamine release from mast cells). Severe allergy, with urticaria, angioneurotic edema, and anaphylaxis, occurs in only a small percentage of patients. The allergic reaction is often due to traces of other proteins present, but it may also result from reactions to denatured or aggregated insulin. In cases of allergy to human insulin, pure pork insulin may be used. Treatment of insulin allergy may also require the use of antihistamines and glucocorticoids and a desensitization regimen.

### Insulin resistance

A totally insulin-deficient diabetic usually requires from 30 to 50 units of insulin per day for control. A requirement of 200 units or more per day indicates that the patient is "resistant" to insulin. Occasionally, 1000 or more units fails to control hyperglycemia and the frequent attendant ketoacidosis. Several factors may cause insulin resistance.

Genetic mutations in components of the insulin-signalling pathway, such as insulin receptor, insulin receptor substrate 1 (IRS-1), glucokinase, GLUT-4, and so forth, occur rarely but have been implicated as a cause of variability in response to insulin, including insulin resistance.

Fewer insulin receptors are present in the cells of obese type 2 diabetics, and adipocyte products such as free fatty acids, cytokines, and adipokines are produced that reduce sensitivity to insulin and interfere with insulin action. As a consequence, these individuals have relatively high blood insulin levels accompanying their hyperglycemia. This resistance is often reversible through weight loss and exercise.

## Problems and Prospects

It is very important that insulin-dependent diabetics monitor plasma glucose so that periods of hyperglycemia and hypoglycemia do not go undetected. Since reliable methods are now available for monitoring blood glucose at home, using a drop of capillary blood, such monitoring has vastly improved diabetic control.

Measurements of glycosylated hemoglobin (HbA$_{1C}$) provide another index of glycemic control. Fractions of hemoglobin are slowly and irreversibly glycosylated in erythrocytes by a non-enzymatic glycation reaction. Therefore, the levels of glycosylated hemoglobin reflect the glucose concentrations encountered over the lifespan of the erythrocyte (about 120 days) and provide a time-averaged measurement of plasma glucose levels. The normal HbA$_{1C}$ level is less than 6% of total hemoglobin. In poorly controlled diabetics, values may range upwards from 15%.

Along with these means of assessing the degree of control, attempts have been made to develop systems for the continuous delivery of insulin from portable or implanted pumps in amounts determined by metabolic need. Two principal methods have been explored: the "closed loop," in which delivery is controlled by frequent automated measurements of blood glucose, and the "open loop" used in ambulatory patients, in which delivery is controlled by a pre-set schedule based on times of food intake and physical activity.

Efforts also have been made to find more acceptable routes of insulin administration and achieve more physiological profiles of blood glucose. The nasal route of administration may offer an alternative to the parenteral route, but further work is required to identify agents that will safely increase the bioavailability of insulin from the nasal passages.

Finally, some success has been achieved with islet cell transplants from human donors.

## ORAL ANTI-DIABETIC DRUGS

## Sulfonylureas

Soon after the discovery of insulin, the search began for anti-diabetic drugs that could be taken by mouth. In 1942, French workers Janbon, Loubatières, and colleagues found that some antibacterial sulfonamides lowered blood sugar. This discovery led to subsequent modifications of the sulfonamide molecule that enhanced hypoglycemic activity and removed the antibacterial effect (Fig. 47-5).

These modified drugs, termed sulfonylureas, appear to act by binding to adenosine triphosphate (ATP)–dependent potassium channels in pancreatic β cells, thereby inhibiting potassium efflux. This action leads to the intracellular accumulation of positive charges and consequent cellular depolarization, calcium influx, and

**FIGURE 47-5** Sulfanilamide and selected sulfonylureas.

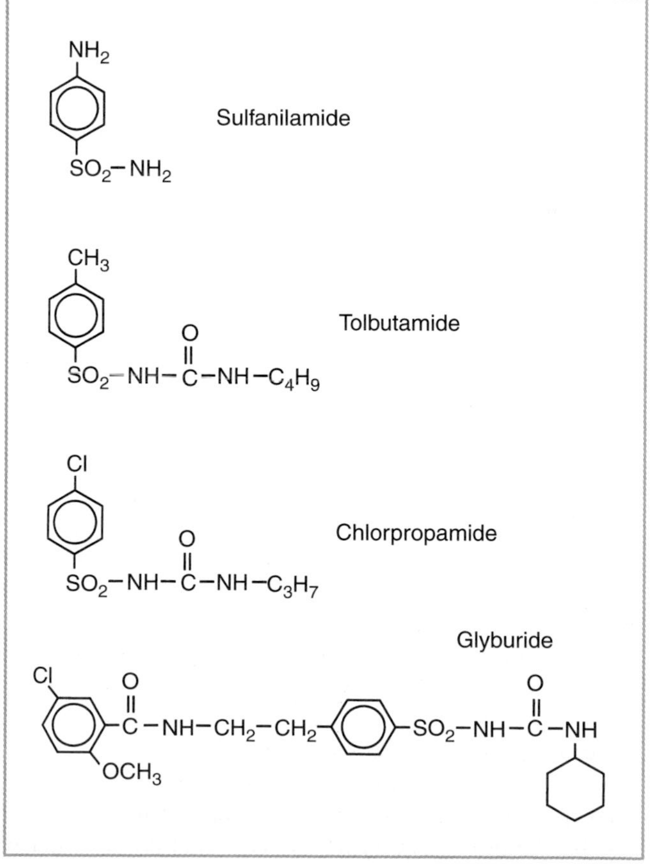

calcium-stimulated release of insulin from the pancreas. Second-generation derivatives (e.g., glyburide) also seem to potentiate the peripheral and hepatic actions of insulin and are now preferred over the first-generation drugs (e.g., tolbutamide, chlorpropamide). Because these drugs act as hypoglycemic agents only in patients whose pancreases can produce insulin, they cannot be used as insulin substitutes in patients with type 1 diabetes. The main use of the oral hypoglycemic drugs is in moderately severe cases of type 2 diabetes that do not respond adequately to a regimen of diet and exercise.

### Preparations of first-generation drugs

**Tolbutamide** (Orinase, Mobenol) is available in 0.5- and 1.0-g tablets. The dose is 1 to 6 tablets daily.

**Chlorpropamide** (Diabinese) is available in 0.1- and 0.25-g tablets. The usual dose is 1 to 2 tablets daily.

**Acetohexamide** (Dimelor) is available in 0.5-g tablets. The dose is 1 to 3 tablets daily.

### Preparations of second-generation drugs

**Glyburide** (glibenclamide; Diaβeta, Euglucon, Micronase) is available in 2.5- and 5.0-mg tablets. The usual dose is 5 to 10 mg daily.

**Gliclazide** (Diamicron) is available in 80-mg tablets. The usual dose is 40 to 320 mg daily.

**Glimepiride** (Amaryl) is available in 1-, 2-, and 4-mg tablets. The usual maintenance dose is 1 to 4 mg daily.

**Glipizide** (Glucotrol) is available in 5-mg tablets. The usual dose is 5 to 40 mg daily; however, it is not available in Canada.

### Pharmacokinetics

All of the sulfonylureas are well absorbed from the small intestine, but rates of absorption vary. Glyburide is the most slowly absorbed and therefore is prepared as a micronized powder to reduce particle size and facilitate uptake. These agents are mainly converted to hydroxylated derivatives and are excreted; in contrast, 5% of glipizide is excreted unchanged. For the most part, the sulfonylurea metabolites have no activity; one of the metabolites of glimepiride is an exception since it retains one-third of the activity of the parent compound. Some of the major pharmacokinetic data are shown in Table 47-3.

There are few significant drug interactions involving these agents. Barbiturates and rifampin have been reported to decrease the effect of some sulfonylureas by inducing their biotransformation in the liver. β-Adrenergic receptor blockers may increase the risk of hypoglycemia by preventing the adrenergic response to a fall in blood sugar.

### Untoward effects and toxicity

Since these drugs cause release of endogenous insulin, they can cause **hypoglycemic reactions**; these reactions may be insidious in onset and therefore hard to recognize.

**Adverse reactions** most commonly encountered are nausea and vomiting, which may be severe enough to prevent use; occasional hematological and dermatological effects have been reported. Intolerance to alcohol (disulfiram-like), a common occurrence with chlorpropamide, is much less likely to occur with the newer-generation sulfonylureas.

Patients receiving chlorpropamide may occasionally develop hyponatremia and water retention, resembling the syndrome of inappropriate antidiuretic hormone (ADH) secretion (SIADH). This is probably due to an effect on renal tubular cells, increasing their sensitivity to endogenous ADH. An increased formation and release of ADH has also been reported.

About 75% of cases show good initial response to these drugs, but about 5 to 10% later stop benefiting from them. Some will show a response if switched to another drug, but most do not, indicating a loss of insulin reserves. Therefore, if secondary failure occurs, the patient should be switched to insulin therapy.

## Glitinides

**Repaglinide** (GlucoNorm, Prandin; Fig. 47-6) and **nateglinide** (Starlix) are amino acid derivatives with essentially the same mechanism of action as the sulfonylureas. They bind to and inhibit ATP-dependent potassium channels on pancreatic β cells, promoting membrane depolarization, $Ca^{2+}$ entry, and stimulation of insulin release. Compared with the sulfonylureas, the glitinides have much faster onsets and shorter durations of action and are usually taken within 15 minutes of a meal. This allows for a prompt action with reduced risk of hypoglycemia. They are used either as monotherapy or in combination with other anti-diabetic agents. Repaglinide is contraindicated for use in combination with the lipid-lowering drug gemfibrozil because, in this combination, the hypoglycemic effects of repaglinide are enhanced and prolonged. Repaglinide is supplied as 0.5-mg, 1-mg, or 2-mg tablets; nateglinide is supplied as 60-mg, 120-mg, or 180-mg tablets.

## Biguanides

Biguanides act directly on muscle to increase glucose uptake and utilization. They also reduce hepatic glucose production and divert intestinal glucose into lactic acid production. Since these effects require the presence of insulin, biguanides are effective only in non-insulin-dependent diabetics. Biguanides do not cause hypoglycemia, and they tend to lower the levels of plasma lipids, especially very-low-density lipoproteins.

**Metformin** (Glucophage; see Fig. 47-6) is a biguanide closely related to phenformin. Phenformin was taken off the market in 1978 because it caused serious lactic acidosis

| TABLE 47-3 | Some Pharmacokinetic Features of Sulfonylureas and Metformin | | | |
|---|---|---|---|---|
| Agent | Oral Bioavailability (%) | $T_{max}$ (hours) | Half-Life (hours) | Excretion in Urine* |
| **Sulfonylureas** | | | | |
| Glyburide | 60–100 | 2–3 | 6–10 (terminal half-life 15–20) | Negligible |
| Gliclazide | 100 | 4–8 | 10 | Negligible |
| Glipizide | 95 | 1–2 | 4–7 | <5% |
| Glimepiride | 100 | 2–3 | 1–2 | Negligible |
| **Glitinides** | | | | |
| Repaglinide | 100 | 1 | 1–1.4 | Negligible |
| Nateglinide | 73 | 1 | 1.5 | <16% |
| **Biguanide** | | | | |
| Metformin | 50–60 | 2 | 1.5–4 | 100% |

*Percentage excreted unmetabolized.

in some patients. Metformin is still in use and has a much lower incidence of lactic acidosis. However, the risk of lactic acidosis is increased when renal or hepatic disease coexists.

The mechanism of action of metformin has recently been clarified. In the liver an enzyme called LKB1 phosphorylates and activates an AMP-activated protein kinase (AMPK), which in turn phosphorylates a cytoplasmic protein named TORC2. In the unphosphorylated state, TORC2 can enter the nucleus and stimulate genes that lead to increased production of glucose. When phosphorylated, however, TORC2 cannot enter the nucleus. Metformin has been shown to increase the action of LKB1 on the AMPK and thus prevent the increased output of glucose by the liver, as well as increase glucose uptake by muscle.

Metformin accumulates in the gastrointestinal tract and salivary glands, and its most common side effects are nausea, vomiting, epigastric distress, and diarrhea. It is reported to decrease the risk of vascular complications of diabetes by reducing platelet aggregation and increasing fibrinolytic activity. The usual dose is 1 to 2 g/day. Metformin may be especially useful as a first-choice treatment if insulin resistance is a marked feature of the clinical presentation. It is also used to promote ovulation and regular menstrual cycles in select patients with polycystic ovarian syndrome accompanied by insulin resistance.

## Thiazolidinediones

The **thiazolidinediones** rosiglitazone (Avandia) and pioglitazone (Actos; see Fig. 47-6) act as insulin sensitizers. They bind to and activate the transcription factor peroxisome proliferator–activated receptor γ (PPARγ) to promote adipocyte differentiation, to regulate the expression of specific genes in adipocytes that mediate insulin resistance, and to improve insulin sensitivity of muscle and liver. The effects in adipocytes decrease the release of TNFα, leptin, and resistin, and increase adiponectin secre-

tion. Hepatic glucose production is reduced as a result. These drugs are used in the treatment of diabetes mellitus as monotherapy or in combination with other agents. The usual dose of rosiglitazone is 4 to 8 mg/day and pioglitazone is 15 to 45 mg/day. These drugs have also been shown to have a role in the prevention of type 2 diabetes mellitus, the treatment of insulin resistance (associated with obesity or polycystic ovarian syndrome), and the mobilization of fat from visceral sites. Side effects may include weight gain, fluid retention, and hepatotoxicity.

## Glucosidase Inhibitor

**Acarbose** (Precose) is an oligosaccharide that competitively inhibits the activity of intestinal α-glucosidases, such as α-glucoamylase, maltase, and sucrase. This action results in inhibition of carbohydrate digestion and delay of glucose uptake. By slowing the formation and absorption of glucose following a meal, acarbose reduces the peaks of hyperglycemia following food intake.

The major side effects are gastrointestinal since the drug is not systemically absorbed. Dose is 150 to 300 mg/day.

## Lipase Inhibitor

**Orlistat** (Xenical) is used to reduce caloric intake from fats, thereby assisting in weight control in patients at risk for type 2 diabetes and other weight-related co-morbidities. Orlistat is a lipophilic beta-lactone, which acts by covalently binding to residues within the active sites of gastric and pancreatic lipases, thereby inhibiting their activities and preventing the hydrolysis of dietary fat in the stomach and small intestine. As undigested fats are not absorbed, caloric intake is reduced. The recommended dose of 120 mg three times a day inhibits dietary fat absorption by 30%. The most common side effects are gastrointestinal, with fatty stools, oily spotting, and

**FIGURE 47-6** Structural formulae of a glitinide, a biguanide, and two thiazolidinediones.

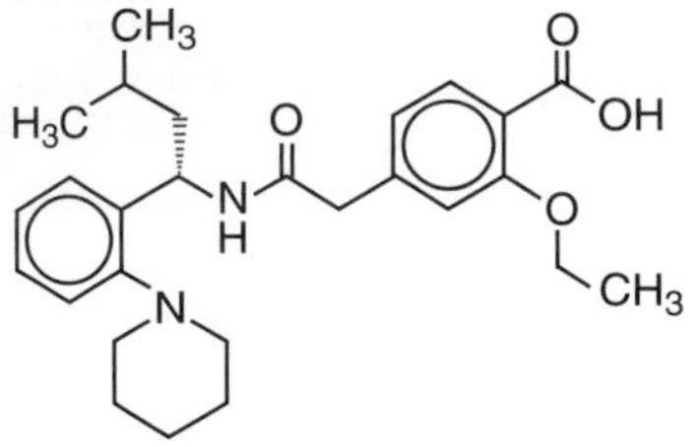

abdominal discomfort. The drug may also reduce absorption of some fat-soluble vitamins.

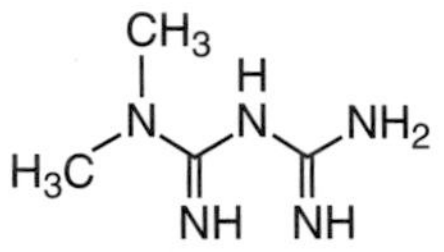

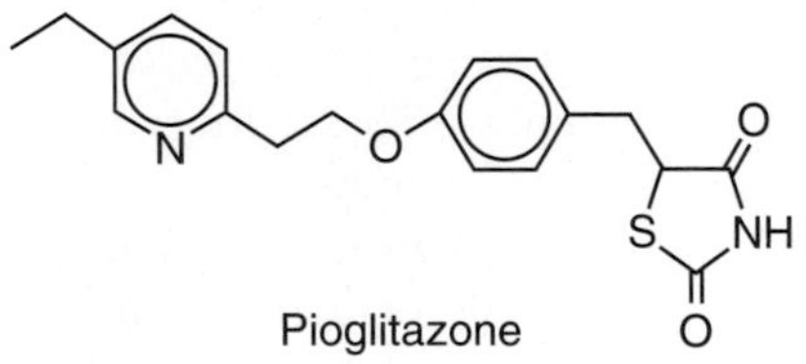

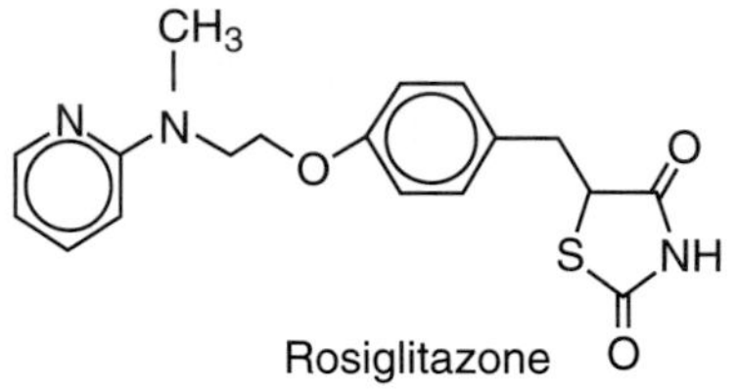

## Diabetic Peripheral Neuropathic (DPN) Pain Medication

**Duloxetin.HCI** (Cymbalta) is a selective serotonin and noradrenaline reuptake inhibitor approved for use in patients with DPN pain. The drug is provided as enteric-coated, delayed-release capsules of 20 mg, 30 mg, or 60 mg. The usual total dose is 60 mg per day, though a lower dose could be considered. This drug is not recommended for patients with renal or hepatic impairment and should be used with caution in elderly patients and in pregnant women during the third trimester.

**Pregabalin** (Lyrica) is an analogue of gamma aminobutyric acid (GABA), but its mechanism of action as a DPN pain medication is unknown. It is supplied as capsules of various doses from 25 mg to 300 mg. The usual total dose is 150 mg to 300 mg. Lower doses are recommended in patients with reduced renal function. Side effects include dizziness, drowsiness, peripheral edema, and weight gain.

## COMBINED THERAPY

The combinations of two or more drugs with different mechanisms of action often have greater efficacy in type 2 diabetics than drugs used as monotherapy. Examples include a sulfonylurea or a glitinide in combination with a biguanide and/or a thiazolidinedione. A glucosidase inhibitor may also be added to this regimen. Insulin is sometimes used at bedtime to augment the effect of some of the oral anti-diabetic agents when maximal doses of the latter are inadequate to control hyperglycemia.

## SUGGESTED READINGS

Bailey CJ, Turner RC. Metformin. *N Engl J Med*. 1996;334:574-579.

Baker DE, Campbell RK. The second generation sulfonylureas: glipizide and glyburide. *Diabetes Educ*. 1985;11:29-36.

Bergman RN, Steil GM, Bradley DC, Watanabe RM. Modeling of insulin action in vivo. *Annu Rev Physiol*. 1992;54:861-883.

Bunn HF, Gabbay KH, Gallop PM. The glycosylation of hemoglobin: relevance to diabetes mellitus. *Science*. 1978;200:21-27.

Goldstein BJ. Insulin resistance as the core defect in type 2 diabetes mellitus. *Am J Cardiol*. 2002;90(suppl):3G-10G.

Muller-Wieland D, Streicher R, Siemeister G, Krone W. Molecular biology of insulin resistance. *Exp Clin Endocrinol*. 1993;101: 17-29.

Nathan DM. Initial management of glycemia in type 2 diabetes mellitus. *N Engl J Med*. 2002;347:1342-1349.

Proks P, Reimann F, Green N, Gribble F, Ashcroft F. Sulfonylurea stimulation of insulin secretion. *Diabetes*. 2002;51(suppl 3): S368-S376.

Saltiel AR. Putting the brakes on insulin signaling. *N Engl J Med*. 2003;349:2560-2562.

Setter SM, Iltz JL, Thams J, Campbell RK. Metformin hydrochloride in the treatment of type 2 diabetes mellitus: a clinical review with a focus on dual therapy. *Clin Ther*. 2003;25:2991-3026.

Stumvoll M, Haring HU. Glitazones: clinical effects and molecular mechanisms. *Ann Med*. 2002;34:217-224.

The Diabetes Control and Complications Trial Research Group. The effect of intensive treatment of diabetes on the development and progression of long-term complications in insulin-dependent diabetes mellitus. *N Engl J Med*. 1993;329:977-986.

UK Prospective Diabetes Study Group. Tight blood pressure control and risk of macrovascular and microvascular complications in type 2 diabetes: UKPDS 38. *BMJ*. 1998;317:703-713.

# 48

# Adrenocortical Steroid Hormones

## BP SCHIMMER AND SR GEORGE

### CASE HISTORY

A 35-year-old woman with a 6-year history of Hashimoto's thyroiditis (autoimmune thyroiditis) with hypothyroidism, who had been well and stable on treatment with levothyroxine 0.125 mg daily, came to see her physician with complaints of fatigue, lethargy, and loss of appetite over the preceding 3 to 4 months. She had lost 6.8 kg (15 lb.) in that time. She also complained of intermittent nausea and dizziness upon standing up from a recumbent position. Physical examination revealed a lean person with a BP of 115/70 mmHg in the supine position and 90/60 mmHg when standing. She said that she had not been in the sun for at least a year, yet her skin was tanned and there was increased pigmentation in the creases of her palms and on the gum margins. The thyroid gland was at the upper range of normal size, and she was clinically euthyroid on her usual dose of levothyroxine. She had developed areas of hypopigmentation over her hands compatible with vitiligo.

Laboratory investigations revealed a mild normochromic normocytic anemia, normal $T_4$ and $T_3$ levels, but elevated serum $K^+$. A random plasma sample showed a cortisol level of 100 nmol/L (normal range 170 to 660 nmol/L) and an adrenocorticotropic hormone (ACTH) level of 330 pmol/L (normal <22 pmol/L). A presumptive diagnosis of Addison's disease was made. The patient was quickly stabilized with intravenous hydrocortisone hemisuccinate and was rehydrated with intravenous saline. Subsequently, a 3-day infusion of ACTH was given to test adrenal cortical function, but no adrenal response to ACTH was found.

She was therefore started on long-term replacement therapy with prednisone 5 mg each morning and 2.5 mg each evening, together with fludrocortisone acetate 0.1 mg twice daily. She has felt well and completely symptom-free on this therapy.

## THE HYPOTHALAMIC–PITUITARY–ADRENAL AXIS

Certain neurons in the hypothalamus produce corticotropin-releasing hormone (CRH). These CRH-producing neurons of the hypothalamus, the corticotropin-producing cells of the anterior lobe of the pituitary gland, and the adrenal cortex constitute a closely integrated functional system that is often referred to as the hypothalamic–pituitary–adrenal (HPA) axis. This axis acts as a regulatory mechanism for maintaining normal levels of adrenal cortical hormone activity, but it also permits sudden increases in the output of these hormones in response to stressors of various types, including inputs from the immune system. The normal physiological relationships of the hypothalamic–pituitary–adrenal axis and the immune system are summarized in Figure 48-1.

The adrenal cortex is divided into histologically and functionally distinct zones. The outermost zone, the zona glomerulosa, is the site of mineralocorticoid (aldosterone) synthesis. The inner zones, the zonae fasciculata and reticularis, produce glucocorticoids (cortisol) and weak androgens (dehydroepiandrosterone).

*Glucocorticoid* production is stimulated by adrenocorticotropic hormone (ACTH) secreted from the anterior pituitary gland. Secretion of ACTH is stimulated by the hypothalamic peptide CRH acting via type 1 receptors located on the pituitary corticotrophs and is inhibited by feedback effects of the glucocorticoids, which act at the level of the hippocampus, hypothalamus, and pituitary. The immune system also plays important roles in the positive and negative regulation of glucocorticoid production.

*Mineralocorticoid* secretion is governed primarily by the renin–angiotensin system and circulating potassium concentrations. ACTH has only a minor role.

FIGURE 48-1 Functional relationships in the hypothalamic–pituitary–adrenal axis. (+) indicates stimulation of release; (−) indicates inhibition.

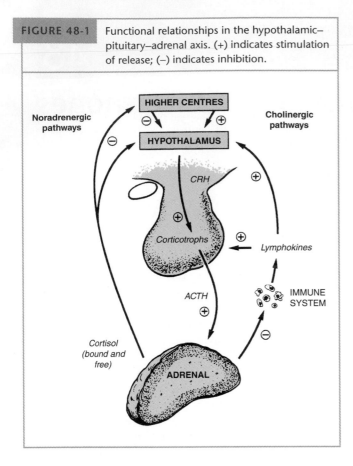

The functional differences of the adrenocortical zones can be related to different patterns of gene expression. For example, the zona glomerulosa expresses angiotensin II receptors at high levels, whereas the inner zones express angiotensin II receptors only at low levels. Additionally, the zona glomerulosa expresses aldosterone synthase (P450aldo), the P450 enzyme uniquely responsible for aldosterone synthesis, whereas the inner zones do not express aldosterone synthase but do express enzymes required for glucocorticoid synthesis, that is, 17-α-hydroxylase (P450c17) and 11-β-hydroxylase (P450c11β).

# CORTICOTROPIN-RELEASING HORMONE

CRH is a 41 amino acid peptide present in high concentrations in neurosecretory cells in the paraventricular and periventricular nuclei of the hypothalamus. Cholinergic and serotonergic pathways stimulate CRH release, whereas specific noradrenergic pathways are inhibitory. The release of CRH varies in a circadian pattern under basal conditions, resulting in the occurrence of diurnal rhythms of ACTH and cortisol levels in the blood (high in the morning, low in the evening). Neural stimuli brought about by stress, trauma, infection, hypoglycemia, and anxiety override the basal controls and increase the release of CRH.

Vasopressin also stimulates ACTH release from pituitary corticotrophs and potentiates the action of CRH on ACTH release. In contrast to CRH, vasopressin appears not to stimulate ACTH synthesis.

# ADRENOCORTICOTROPIC HORMONE

ACTH is a protein composed of 39 amino acids that is synthesized in the corticotrophs of the anterior pituitary. The first 24 amino acids of ACTH are responsible for the hormonal activity of the peptide. The basic amino acids at positions 15 to 18 provide a high-affinity recognition site for the ACTH receptor, and amino acids 6 to 10 participate in receptor activation. Species variation occurs in the region from the 25th to the 33rd residue.

ACTH is derived from a larger precursor protein, proopiomelanocortin (POMC), by the proteolytic activity of prohormone convertase 1. Cleavage of POMC also liberates other important regulatory peptides, as shown in Figure 48-2. These include α-, β-, and γ-MSH (melanocyte-stimulating hormones), a lipid-mobilizing factor (β-lipotropin), and the opioid peptide β-endorphin (see Chapter 19).

Neural control of ACTH is demonstrated by the wide variety of stimuli that increase ACTH secretion and therefore plasma cortisol levels. Those factors that regulate the secretion of ACTH similarly regulate the production of the other peptides associated with POMC. These stimuli include both physical and psychological stresses, which can override the usual feedback control. Interleukins produced by macrophages, monocytes, and lymphocytes also stimulate ACTH secretion as part of the immune system's contribution to the stress response; cortisol suppresses lymphokine production (see Fig. 48-1).

The most important physiological effect of ACTH is to stimulate the biosynthesis and output of adrenal steroid hormones. Its basic action is to stimulate the first step in the adrenal steroid hormone biosynthetic pathway, that is, the oxidative cleavage of cholesterol to pregnenolone in adrenal mitochondria. The further metabolism of pregnenolone and the secretion of steroid products occur rapidly and are not under acute hormonal influence. The translocation of cholesterol from the cytoplasm to the inner mitochondrial membrane (where the oxidative cleavage occurs) is rate-limiting for steroidogenesis. ACTH exerts its effects through the ACTH receptor, which activates adenylyl cyclase, thereby increasing cyclic adenosine monophosphate (cAMP) formation and stimulating cAMP-dependent protein kinases. The subsequent intervening steps between the cAMP-dependent protein kinase and cholesterol metabolism are not fully elucidated but include the involvement of a protein known as StAR (steroid acute regulator) that binds to and participates in the delivery of cholesterol to the inner mitochondrial membrane.

ACTH also maintains the structural integrity of the zonae fasciculata and reticularis of the adrenal cortex and

> **FIGURE 48-2** Biologically important peptides derived from proopiomelanocortin. The first 24 amino acids of ACTH are shown. This sequence is invariant among species and is responsible for the biological activity of the hormone. MSH = melanocyte-stimulating hormone; CLIP = corticotropin-like intermediate lobe peptide.

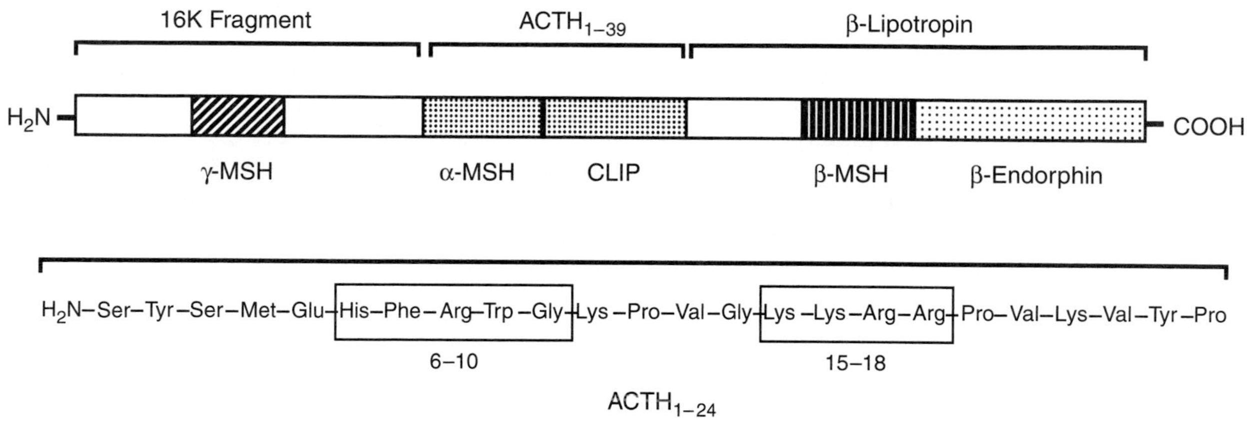

the levels of the adrenal steroidogenic enzymes through actions on gene expression. When ACTH levels are suppressed for prolonged periods (e.g., following hypophysectomy or feedback inhibition by exogenous glucocorticoids), the inner zones of the cortex lose their steroidogenic machinery, atrophy, and secrete less steroid.

Regulation of aldosterone production involves a different mechanism. Angiotensin II and potassium are the major regulators of aldosterone production by the zona glomerulosa. Aldosterone secretion from the glomerulosa is stimulated by high levels of ACTH (equivalent to the levels encountered in response to stress), but secretion is not maintained.

## MINERALOCORTICOID ACTIONS

Mineralocorticoids are corticosteroids with greater action on water and electrolyte ("minerals") metabolism than on carbohydrate and protein metabolism. They cause the renal tubule to retain $Na^+$, $HCO_3^-$, and water and to excrete more $K^+$; these actions ordinarily help to maintain normal concentrations of plasma $Na^+$ and $K^+$. Mineralocorticoid deficiency results in the loss of $Na^+$ and water by the kidney, leading to dehydration and vascular collapse. Mineralocorticoid excess results in elevated plasma $Na^+$, decreased plasma $K^+$, and retention of water, leading to elevated blood volume and blood pressure.

## GLUCOCORTICOID ACTIONS

Glucocorticoids are corticosteroids with greater effect on carbohydrate metabolism than on water and electrolyte metabolism. Glucocorticoid receptors are found in virtually every cell in the body. As a consequence, glucocorticoids exert a wide range of physiological actions affecting every organ system. Glucocorticoids are so named because of their actions on intermediary metabolism of glucose; however, they affect many other metabolic activities as well.

### Metabolic Effects

Many of the physiological effects of the adrenal steroid hormones have been known for years; classically, they were deduced from the pathological states of adrenal insufficiency associated with Addison's disease and their reversal by steroid hormone replacement therapy, and from the symptoms of adrenocortical excess associated with Cushing's syndrome.

Under the influence of glucocorticoids, proteins in muscle, bone, and other tissues are broken down to amino acids (catabolic actions). The amino acids are carried to the liver, deaminated, and converted to glucose (gluconeogenesis). The net effect is to *increase* liver glycogen concentration, fasting blood sugar levels, and urinary nitrogen output. The proportions of carbohydrate and fat utilized by muscle are altered (increased mobilization and oxidation of depot fat; decreased utilization of glucose).

### Effects on Blood and Lymphoid Systems

Erythrocyte and hemoglobin levels are increased in response to glucocorticoids. Circulating lymphocytes and eosinophils are decreased, mainly due to redistribution of these elements away from blood into other body compartments such as bone marrow, spleen, and lymph nodes and, to a lesser extent, due to lymphocytolysis. The intensity of inflammatory responses is dampened by multiple actions. These include decreased production of vasoactive substances (e.g., prostaglandins and leukotrienes) and chemoattractants (e.g., cytokines), decreased secretion of lipolytic and proteolytic enzymes (e.g., phospholipases, collagenase, elastase), and inhibition of fibroblast growth.

## Renal and Cardiovascular Effects

The ability of the kidney to excrete water is maintained by permissive effects of glucocorticoids on renal tubular free water clearance and maintenance of the glomerular filtration rate. Generally, a shift of water into cells is prevented, and extracellular volume is maintained. Cardiac contractility and vascular tone are enhanced in response to glucocorticoids, in part as a result of increasing sensitivity to vasoactive substances such as catecholamines and angiotensin II.

## Other Physiological Effects

Central nervous system (CNS) effects of glucocorticoids include regulation of mood and an increased sense of well-being as a result of direct actions in the brain and via supportive metabolic effects.

The ability of muscles to do prolonged work is maintained and includes effects on the circulatory system (independent of effects on carbohydrate and fat metabolism).

The production of gastric acid is increased.

Glucocorticoids decrease total body calcium by inhibiting uptake from the intestine (competitive inhibition of the action of vitamin D3) and stimulating renal calcium excretion.

## MECHANISM OF ACTION

Most if not all of the effects of the adrenal steroid hormones are produced by the activation of intracellular mineralocorticoid and glucocorticoid receptors. In the absence of corticosteroids, the receptors are complexed with other regulatory proteins (e.g., heat-shock proteins and immunophilin) that restrict the receptors to the cytoplasm in an inactive state. In the presence of corticosteroids, the receptors dissociate from the inhibitory proteins, migrate to the nucleus, and act as transcription factors for specific genes to either stimulate or inhibit their expression (see Chapter 9). These actions on gene expression account for the pharmacological effects of the corticosteroids.

Glucocorticoid and mineralocorticoid receptors are structurally related and have extensive similarities in amino acid composition. Whereas the glucocorticoid receptor is highly selective for glucocorticoids, the mineralocorticoid receptor interacts equally well with both glucocorticoids and mineralocorticoids. Since the circulating levels of glucocorticoids are much higher than the circulating levels of mineralocorticoids, mineralocorticoid-responsive tissues must contain additional mechanisms that provide for the specific effects of the mineralocorticoid hormones. One such mechanism seems to be the formation of an enzymatic barrier that selectively inactivates glucocorticoids before they reach the mineralocorticoid receptor. A key enzyme forming this barrier is the type 2 11-β-hydroxysteroid dehydrogenase (11-β-HSD2). This enzyme inactivates cortisol by oxidizing the 11-β-hydroxyl group (Fig. 48-3) to an 11-keto group. The 11-β-hydroxyl group on the mineralocorticoid may be protected from oxidation through the formation of a cyclic hemiacetal structure (see Fig. 48-6). Individuals with an inherited deficiency of 11-β-HSD2 exhibit symptoms of apparent mineralocorticoid excess due to the glucocorticoids acting inappropriately to activate the mineralocorticoid receptor. Interestingly, glycyrrhetinic acid, the active pharmacological ingredient of licorice, which inhibits the activity of the 11-β-HSD2, also produces similar symptoms.

## CHEMISTRY, KINETICS, AND SYNTHETIC ANALOGUES

### Structural Requirements

The structure of cortisol is shown in Fig. 48-3. Important features that determine glucocorticoid activity are the keto group at C-3, the double bond between C-4 and C-5, and the three hydroxyl group substitutions at C-21, C-17α, and C-11β. The 11-β-OH is essential for glucocorticoid activity. In its absence, the adrenal corticoids exhibit only mineralocorticoid activity (e.g., 11-deoxycorticosterone; Fig. 48-4). A keto group at C-11 (e.g., cortisone or prednisone) also supports glucocorticoid activity but only when it is metabolized to an 11-β-OH by the type 1 isoform of 11-β-HSD (11-βHSD1; see Fig. 48-3). The 17-α-OH is not as critical, although it does have a quantitative influence; in its absence, corticosteroids exhibit weaker glucocorticoid activity (e.g., corticosterone; Fig. 48-5). The 21-OH is required for both glucocorticoid and mineralocorticoid activity. However, in some synthetic glucocorticoids, other functional groups such as Cl may be substituted for OH at C-21.

Aldosterone also has an OH at C-11 but has negligible glucocorticoid activity because of its relatively lower affinity for the glucocorticoid receptor and its very low levels in the circulation (100 to 1000 times lower than cortisol).

### Transport and Metabolism

The daily rates of secretion of adrenal steroids and their normal levels in plasma are given in Tables 48-1 and 48-2. The cortisol secretion rate is about 10 mg/day, and cortisol concentrations in plasma are in the range of 10 µg/100 mL (280 nmol/L); 90 to 95% is bound to proteins. Most is bound with high affinity to a specific globulin called cortisol-binding globulin (CBG); the remainder is bound

Structural formulae of cortisol and cortisone. The four rings that constitute the steroid nucleus are virtually coplanar. Chemical substitutions to the steroid molecule that reside above the plane of the rings are designated β and are conventionally represented by solid lines; substitutions made below the plane of rings are designated α and are conventionally represented by broken lines, as shown here and in subsequent figures. Features that are important for glucocorticoid activity are shown in bold. The interconversion of cortisol to cortisone is catalyzed by the type 1 and type 2 isoforms of 11-β-hydroxysteroid dehydrogenase (11-β-HSD) as indicated.

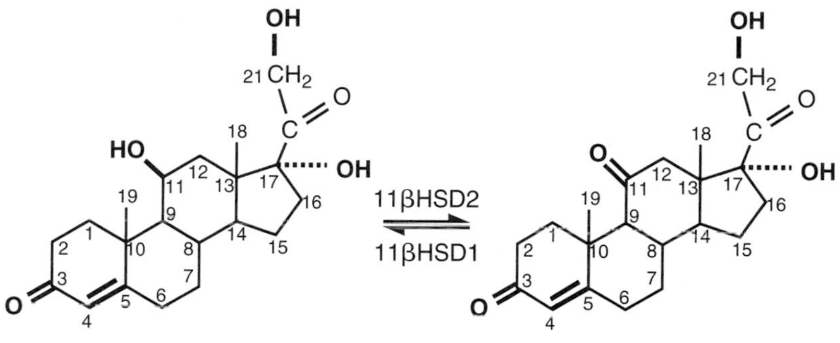

Cortisol          11βHSD2 / 11βHSD1          Cortisone

non-specifically, and with low affinity, to albumin. Free cortisol, the active fraction, is in equilibrium with the bound forms. Aldosterone is present in plasma at much lower levels (see Table 48-2) and circulates primarily in the free form, not bound to plasma proteins.

Cortisol has a plasma half-life of about 90 minutes, and to a large extent it is inactivated in the liver by reduction of the 3-keto, 4,5-double bond and subsequent conjugation with sulfate or glucuronate. Aldosterone is metabolized somewhat more rapidly, chiefly to glucuronides.

## Synthetic Analogues

Selective modifications of the corticosteroid structure decrease the rate of metabolic inactivation of corticos-

teroids in the body. Analogues with a double bond between C-1 and C-2 or with a fluorine atom introduced into the molecule are biotransformed much more slowly, and the half-life is correspondingly increased. More importantly, these modifications enhance affinity for the glucocorticoid receptor, increase selective action as glucocorticoids, and reduce mineralocorticoid activity. The relative effectiveness of several synthetic analogues is given in Table 48-3, and their structures are shown in Figure 48-7. Specific modifications include the following:

1. Insertion of a double bond between C-1 and C-2: This changes cortisol (hydrocortisone) to prednisolone, and cortisone to prednisone; the resulting molecules are four times more potent than their respective pre-

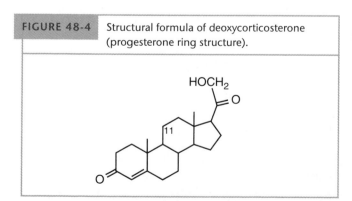

Structural formula of deoxycorticosterone (progesterone ring structure).

Structural formula of corticosterone.

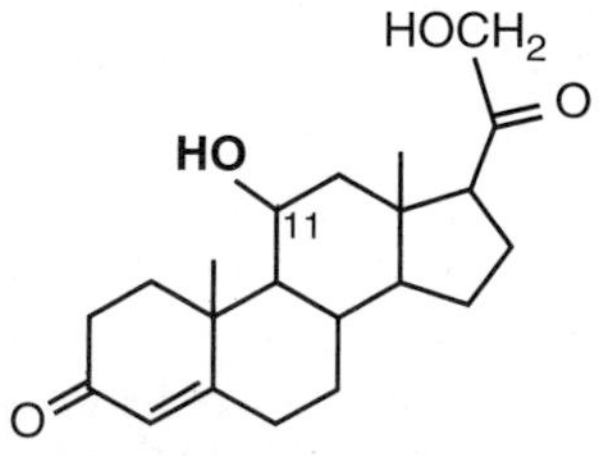

FIGURE 48-6    Aldehyde (left) and hemiacetal (right) forms of aldosterone.

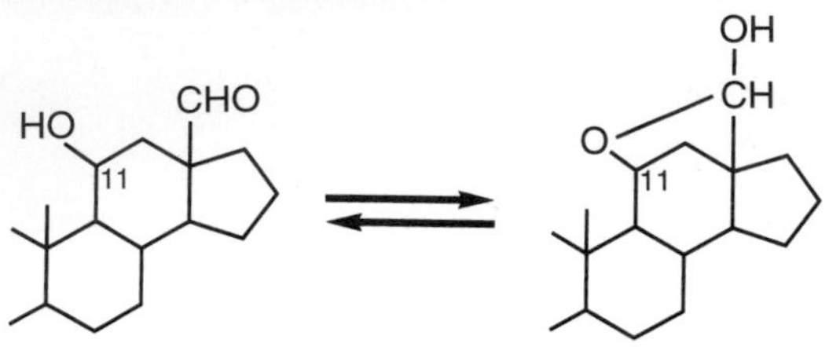

cursors. Neither has appreciable mineralocorticoid activity. Prednisone has a half-life of 3 to 4 hours, is converted to prednisolone in the liver, and is ultimately degraded via the same pathways as cortisol.

2. Addition of a methyl group to C-6 of prednisolone: This gives methylprednisolone, which has slightly greater glucocorticoid potency than prednisolone.

3. Addition of fluorine to C-9 of cortisol: This gives fludrocortisone. This addition markedly increases both glucocorticoid and mineralocorticoid potencies, but the increase in mineralocorticoid activity is far greater, so fludrocortisone is used therapeutically as a mineralocorticoid. Fludrocortisone is 70 to 80% bound to proteins in the plasma and has a half-life of 6 to 8 hours, although its biological effects are longer lasting. It is biotransformed by reactions similar to those of other corticosteroids.

4. Combining the 9α-fluoro substitution, the C-1, C-2 double bond insertion, and additions at C-16: This yields very potent glucocorticoids with minimal mineralocorticoid activity. Included in this group of C-16 modified derivatives are triamcinolone (OH), dexamethasone (α-CH3), and betamethasone (β-CH3).

5. Addition of fluorine at C-6 of triamcinolone: This yields fluocinolone and increases glucocorticoid activity still further. Fluocinolone is used topically.

6. Formation of the 9α-chloro analogue of betamethasone: This yields beclomethasone, which is used topically and as an aerosol for the treatment of asthma. Its effectiveness by the latter route makes it possible to reduce (or even eliminate) systemic therapy in severe chronic asthma.

7. Formation of a prednisolone derivative with butyraldehyde in a C-16, C-17 cyclic acetal linkage: This yields budesonide, which is used orally or rectally in the treatment of inflammatory bowel disease (e.g., Crohn's disease). Its poor absorption from the gastrointestinal (GI) tract preserves local actions while reducing suppression of the HPA axis and other systemic effects. It is also used in inhalers for allergic rhinitis and asthma.

## CLINICAL USES

### Replacement and Substitution Therapy

Primary or secondary adrenocortical insufficiency as well as congenital adrenal hyperplasia (CAH) are effectively treated with substitution of adrenocorticosteroids. Although secondary adrenal insufficiency due to pituitary or hypothalamic defects could be treated with ACTH, responses are not always predictable and are difficult to titrate. Therefore, ACTH is not used, and the treatment of choice is the administration of adrenal steroids.

CAH is caused in 95% of cases by 21-hydroxylase insufficiency. As a consequence of this defect, cortisol synthesis (and sometimes aldosterone synthesis) is impaired, and precursor steroids, including the adrenal androgens, rise. Depending on the nature and severity of the enzyme defect, the clinical manifestations will vary and may include virilization and salt wasting. The second most common cause of CAH is 11-β-hydroxylase deficiency, which results in impairment of cortisol synthesis, with accumulation of androgens and steroids with mineralocorticoid activity. Treatment with synthetic glucocorti-

TABLE 48-1    Steroid Secretion by the Human Adrenal Gland

| Steroid | Daily Secretion Rate* |
|---|---|
| Cortisol (hydrocortisone) | 10–20 mg |
| Corticosterone | 2–4 mg |
| Aldosterone | 50–200 μg (100 μg) |
| Dehydroepiandrosterone | 15–30 mg (20 mg) |
| Progesterone | 0.4–0.8 mg |
| Androstenedione | 1–10 mg |
| Testosterone | Trace |
| Estradiol | Trace |

*Average values for the most significant steroids are given in parentheses. Values selected are approximate and vary in different reports.

TABLE 48-2    Normal Steroid Plasma Levels

| Steroid | Plasma Level (per 100 mL) | |
|---|---|---|
| | Total | Free |
| Cortisol (hydrocortisone) | 5–20 μg | 1000 ng |
| Corticosterone | 1 μg | 100 ng |
| Aldosterone | 3–15 ng | 3 ng |
| Dehydroepiandrosterone | 65 μg | 65 μg |

coids suppresses ACTH production by feedback regulation of the pituitary, shutting off abnormal steroid production and substituting a normal level of glucocorticoids.

Mineralocorticoid deficiency is the more acute threat to life because of salt wasting, hypotension, and vascular collapse. Therefore, replacement therapy with adrenal steroid hormones must take into account both glucocorticoid and mineralocorticoid status. These must be treated separately since no single corticosteroid analogue provides sufficient activity for both.

FIGURE 48-7 Structural formulae of synthetic corticoid analogues. Features shown in boldface indicate important differences from hydrocortisone.

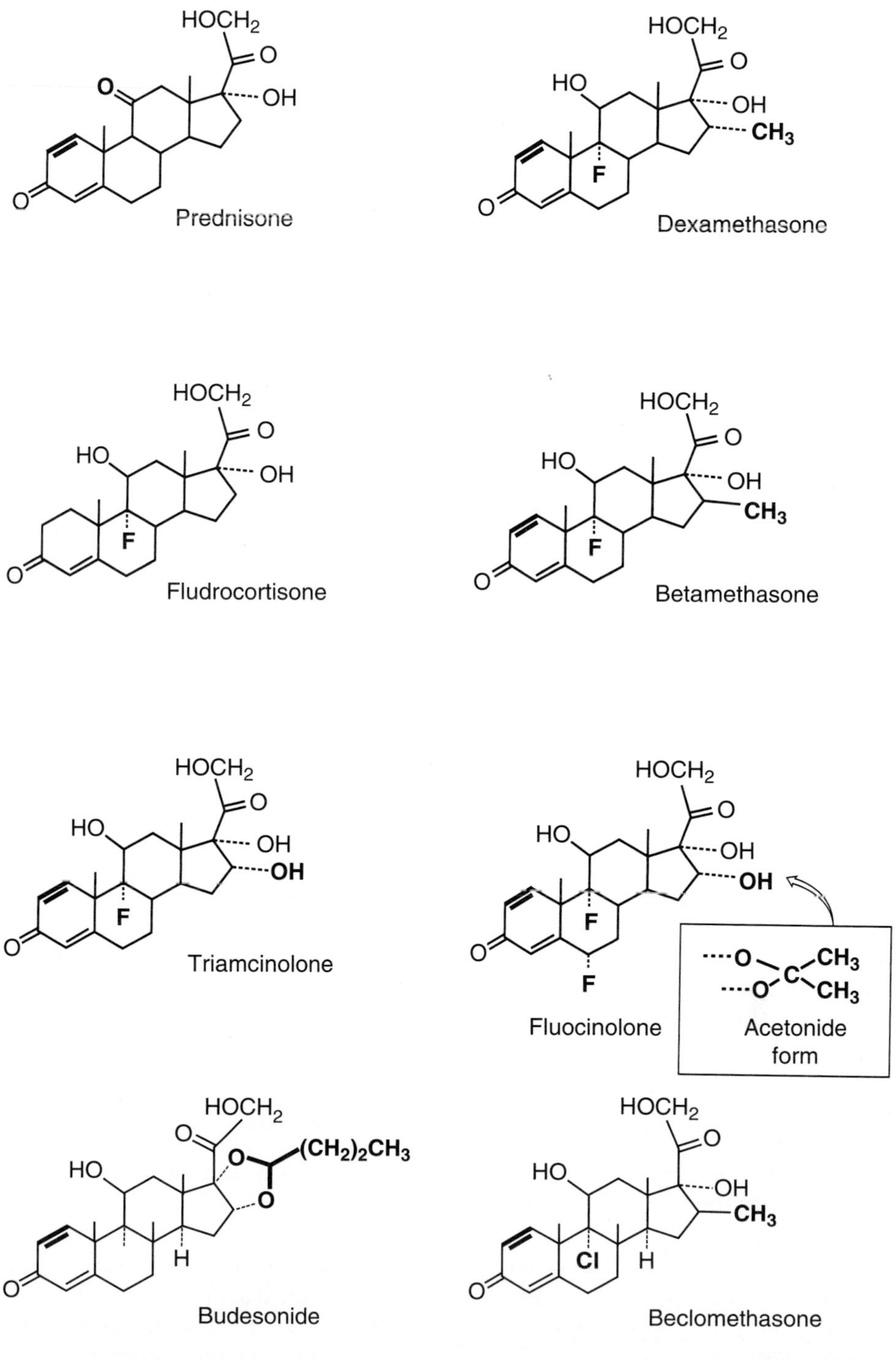
HOCH2
O
OH
Prednisone
HO
CH3
F
Dexamethasone
Fludrocortisone
Betamethasone
Triamcinolone
Fluocinolone
Acetonide form
(CH2)2CH3
H
Budesonide
Cl
Beclomethasone

| TABLE 48-3 | Relative Potencies of Various Synthetic Analogues as Glucocorticoids (GC) and Mineralocorticoids (MC) | | | |
|---|---|---|---|---|
| | | Equivalent Dose | Relative GC Activity | Relative MC Activity |
| Cortisol (hydrocortisone) (Cortate, Cortef, others) | | 20 mg | 1 | 1 |
| Cortisone (Cortone) | | 25 mg | 0.8 | 0.8 |
| Prednisone (Deltasone, Winpred) | | 5 mg | 4 | 0.3 |
| Prednisolone (Delta-Cortef, others) | | 5 mg | 4 | 0.8 |
| Methylprednisolone (Medrol) | | 4 mg | 5 | 0.5 |
| Triamcinolone (Aristocort) | | 4 mg | 5 | 0 |
| Dexamethasone (Decadron, Dexasone) | | 0.75 mg | 25 | 0 |
| Betamethasone (Beben, Betnovate, Celestone, Diprosone, others) | | 0.5 mg | 40 | 0 |
| Fludrocortisone (Florinef) | | Not applicable | 10 | 250 |

# Anti-allergic and Anti-inflammatory Therapy

The anti-allergic and anti-inflammatory effects were discovered when Hench and Kendall reported, in 1949, that one of the adrenal steroids, now known as cortisone (compound "E"), relieved pain, inflammation, and disability in rheumatoid arthritis. This finding led to one of the most important clinical uses of the glucocorticoids, that is, as anti-inflammatory, anti-allergic, and immunosuppressive agents.

By far the most frequent use of corticosteroids today is in the treatment of inflammatory and allergic conditions in doses that range from the physiological to the pharmacological. Antibody titres seem not to be affected; instead, suppression of each stage of the inflammatory response seems to underlie both the anti-inflammatory and anti-allergic actions of the glucocorticoids. Among the known components of the anti-inflammatory and anti-allergic actions are decreases in capillary and leukocytic responses to local injury, inhibition of secretion of proteolytic and lipolytic enzymes, stabilization of lysosomes, inhibition of fibroblast growth, and inhibition of scar formation. For these reasons, corticosteroids are used in the treatment of many conditions, including the following:

- Allergic conditions such as serum sickness, urticaria, bee stings, and drug reactions
- Rheumatic diseases such as rheumatoid arthritis, rheumatic fever, and the collagen-vascular disorders (e.g., systemic lupus erythematosus, polyarteritis nodosa, and giant cell arteritis)
- Respiratory diseases such as asthma and infant respiratory distress syndrome
- Dermatological disorders such as contact dermatitis, pemphigus, psoriasis, and eczema
- Ophthalmological diseases such as allergic conjunctivitis and acute uveitis
- Conditions as varied as nephrotic syndrome secondary to minimal change glomerulonephritis, inflammatory bowel disease, cerebral edema, and organ transplantation

# Malignancies

**Lymphosarcoma, lymphatic leukemia, multiple myeloma,** and **Hodgkin's disease** may respond to corticosteroid therapy, with remissions lasting from weeks to many months. These effects are in part due to lytic actions of pharmacological doses of glucocorticoids on lymphatic and related tissues.

Glucocorticoids also have been used to treat hypercalcemia associated with tumour **metastases to bone**, though bisphosphonates are currently preferred. These metastases put out a parathyroid hormone–like substance that stimulates osteoclastic resorption of bone and releases calcium into the blood. Glucocorticoids lower blood calcium by decreasing calcium uptake from the intestine (anti–vitamin D$_3$ effect). Glucocorticoids are also used to reduce cerebral edema swelling due to metastases, surgery, or radiation to the brain.

# General Considerations for Therapeutic Uses

It must be stressed that the actions of corticosteroids against allergic and inflammatory disorders are not curative but merely palliative and aimed at relieving symptoms. Because these steroids act largely at the level of transcription, most actions are not immediate.

In the case of an acute allergic or inflammatory reaction, initial therapy may require administration of glucocorticoids at high doses (5 to 10 times the replacement dose). If therapy is stopped abruptly, the disease may recur in full force; hence, the glucocorticoid dose is tapered gradually. In the case of diseases requiring chronic glucocorticoid therapy, the objective is to provide the lowest dose of glucocorticoid necessary to keep the symptoms under control. Prolonged use of glucocorticoids (longer than a few weeks) can suppress ACTH production. Therefore, withdrawal of exogenous glucocorticoid must be gradual to avoid precipitation of adrenal insufficiency. (Complete withdrawal may require 1 year or longer.)

Extreme caution must be exercised in the use of glucocorticoids because latent infections may be reactivated (see later section on "Toxic Effects"). Systemic glucocorticoids should not be used for minor conditions, but may be used for (1) relief of acute allergic reactions, (2) relief of severe or potentially fatal symptoms, and (3) prevention of tissue and organ damage.

In patients with adrenal insufficiency or glucocorticoid-induced ACTH suppression, stressful conditions such as trauma, surgery, or infections necessitate an increase in the glucocorticoid dosage to approximate the increased glucocorticoid output of the normal stressed adrenal.

## Diagnostic Uses

CRH is used diagnostically to release ACTH and thereby test the adequacy of pituitary corticotroph function. Insulin hypoglycemia is a stimulus for endogenous CRH release and thus is used as a test for the integrity of the entire HPA axis.

ACTH is used diagnostically to assess the integrity of the HPA axis for the purpose of identifying those patients needing supplemental glucocorticoid in stressful situations. ACTH stimulation also is used diagnostically to distinguish primary from secondary adrenal insufficiency. ACTH is not the preferred treatment for adrenal hormone replacement because of difficulty with dose titration, inconvenience of administration, and stimulation not only of glucocorticoid but also of mineralocorticoid and adrenal androgen secretion.

Dexamethasone is used to test the suppressibility of the HPA axis in patients with elevated levels of cortisol. Because dexamethasone is a potent glucocorticoid, low doses (1 mg) will inhibit the release of ACTH from the anterior pituitary in normal individuals. In some depressed or psychotic patients, ACTH and cortisol production is not suppressed on the 1-mg dexamethasone dose, and a higher dose may be required. In patients with elevated cortisol due to Cushing's syndrome, low doses of dexamethasone (0.5 mg every 6 hours for 48 hours) do not suppress ACTH or cortisol levels effectively. Higher doses of dexamethasone (2 mg every 6 hours for 48 hours) are used to distinguish pituitary-dependent Cushing's disease

(suppressible) from adrenal tumours and ectopic ACTH-producing tumours (not suppressible).

## PREPARATIONS

Synthetic ACTH (cosyntropin; Cortrosyn, Synacthen) is a peptide containing the first 24 amino acids of the natural hormone and is available as a purified powder to be reconstituted for intramuscular or intravenous injection.

All glucocorticoids named in Table 48-3 are in clinical use. They are available in many forms, including oral tablets, ointments, lotions, ophthalmic drops, aqueous suspensions for intramuscular use, and solutions for intravenous and inhalational administration. The choice of one glucocorticoid over another is not clear-cut. Perhaps the most important consideration is the degree of separation of desired glucocorticoid effects from undesired mineralocorticoid effects.

In replacement therapy, the morning dose is generally twice as large as the evening dose in order to mimic the normal diurnal rhythm of cortisol secretion. The usual daily replacement doses have been 30 mg hydrocortisone or 7.5 mg prednisone or 37.5 mg cortisone acetate. The recognition that patients on these "standard" doses may exhibit signs of mild glucocorticoid excess has resulted in consideration of lower daily replacement doses—20 mg hydrocortisone or 5 mg prednisone or 25 mg cortisone acetate. Fludrocortisone (Florinef) is a potent, orally active mineralocorticoid. The daily replacement doses are in the range of 0.05 to 0.2 mg.

## TOXIC EFFECTS

The adrenal cortical steroids show toxic effects that are exaggerations of their physiological actions and relate to the potency, dose, and duration of treatment. Side effects may include the following:

- Salt and water retention can lead to edema, hypertension, and congestive heart failure. Excessive $K^+$ loss in urine at the same time may cause hypokalemia, resulting in muscular weakness and cardiac arrhythmias. Excessive $HCO_3^-$ retention may cause hypochloremic alkalosis. This is most likely to occur with mineralocorticoids, cortisone, or hydrocortisone (cortisol).
- Metabolic effects, including negative nitrogen balance and impaired glucose utilization, may cause myopathy and induce a diabetic state in predisposed subjects. Redistribution of fat from the periphery to central locations results in truncal obesity, moon facies, buffalo hump, and supraclavicular fat pad enlargement.

- Osteoporosis and impaired wound healing, including impaired synthesis of collagen, result from a catabolic effect on protein metabolism. The inhibition of growth in children receiving corticosteroids over long periods probably falls into this same category.

These first three groups of toxic effects make up most of the clinical picture of "iatrogenic Cushing's syndrome" caused by exogenous adrenal steroids. The following are also important adverse effects:

- Masking of infections may result from inhibition of inflammatory and immune responses. Susceptibility to infection may be increased. In the presence of infection, the use of glucocorticoids may precipitate a fulminating course. Latent infections may become activated (e.g., tuberculosis). In herpetic keratitis, for instance, glucocorticoids may allow the infection to spread and cause blindness unless effective antiviral chemotherapy is used concurrently (see Chapter 55). Therefore, in the presence of infection, glucocorticoids should be used together with appropriate and effective antibiotic/antiviral therapy.
- Peptic ulceration, GI bleeding, and perforation may occur. The association of glucocorticoids with these effects is debatable, but increased secretion of HCl and pepsin by the stomach, together with impaired healing, may contribute.
- Precipitation of mood disorders, ranging from euphoria to depression, and psychoses in certain individuals have been reported.
- Adrenal insufficiency may result from inhibition of ACTH secretion. As a consequence, the adrenal cortex loses steroidogenic capacity and undergoes atrophy. Therefore, therapy cannot be stopped abruptly, and dosage should be reduced gradually. There is some evidence that administration of glucocorticoids on alternate days in the treatment of chronic diseases may result in less suppression by negative feedback.
- Avascular necrosis of bone (also referred to as osteonecrosis), most notably of the femoral head, has been reported. This is more likely to occur with long-term use or higher doses of glucocorticoids.
- Posterior subcapsular cataracts and increased intraocular pressure may occur.

# INHIBITORS OF ADRENOCORTICOSTEROID BIOSYNTHESIS

This group of drugs is used clinically in the treatment of glucocorticoid overproduction caused by diseases such as Cushing's disease, ectopic ACTH production, and adrenal carcinoma. These agents interfere with the cytochrome P450 hydroxylases required for steroid hormone biosynthesis. They not only affect adrenal steroid hormone production but also may inhibit the biosynthesis of gonadal steroid hormones.

## Aminoglutethimide

Aminoglutethimide (Cytadren) is a reversible inhibitor of P450scc, which catalyzes the oxidative cleavage of cholesterol to pregnenolone, the first step in the biosynthesis of glucocorticoids, mineralocorticoids, and gonadal steroids. In addition, aminoglutethimide inhibits the adrenal 11-β-hydroxylase as well as the aromatase that converts androgens to estrogens. Aminoglutethimide has been used to reduce glucocorticoid overproduction and also to reduce estrogen production (e.g., in the treatment of breast carcinoma).

## Ketoconazole

The principal use of ketoconazole (Nizoral) is as an antifungal agent that inhibits the synthesis of sterols required for fungal cell membrane integrity (see Chapter 51). At higher doses, ketoconazole inhibits P450c17 and P450scc, enzymes required for the synthesis of both the adrenal and gonadal hormones.

## Metyrapone

Metyrapone (Metopirone) inhibits 11-β-hydroxylase, the enzyme responsible for the final step in the synthesis of cortisol. Consequently, the precursor of this hormone (11-deoxycortisol, compound S), which is biologically inactive as a glucocorticoid and does not inhibit ACTH secretion, is excreted in the urine. Because *less* cortisol is formed, the blood level falls, and in the normal person, this causes an increased release of ACTH. The increased levels of ACTH stimulate further steroid synthesis so that an increased amount of 11-deoxycortisol is synthesized (and excreted). Although metyrapone also inhibits aldosterone synthase, one of the enzymes required for aldosterone synthesis, the mineralocorticoid-dependent activities are maintained by the elevated levels of 11-deoxycortisol.

Metyrapone has been used as a test of pituitary function, since a fall in the blood level of cortisol is expected to induce ACTH secretion. This drug is currently available both in Canada and the United States for therapeutic use only on a compassionate basis.

## Mitotane

Mitotane (o,p'-DDD; Lysodren) is an organic insecticide derivative that is cytotoxic to the adrenal cortex. It is used for the treatment of inoperable metastatic adrenocortical carcinoma.

# SUGGESTED READINGS

Chrousos GP. The hypothalamic-pituitary-adrenal axis and immune-mediated inflammation. *N Engl J Med.* 1995;332: 1351-1362.

Cronstein BN, Weissman G. Targets for anti-inflammatory drugs. *Annu Rev Pharmacol Toxicol.* 1995;35:449-462.

Dooms-Goossens A. Sensitisation to corticosteroids. Consequences for anti-inflammatory therapy. *Drug Saf.* 1995;13:123-129.

Eastell R. Management of corticosteroid-induced osteoporosis. UK Consensus Group meeting. *J Intern Med.* 1995;237:439-447.

Ellershaw JE, Kelly MJ. Corticosteroids and peptic ulceration. *Palliat Med.* 1994;8:313-319.

Funder JW, Krozowski Z, Myles K, et al. Mineralocorticoid receptors, salt and hypertension. *Recent Prog Horm Res.* 1997;52: 247-260.

Funder JW, Pearce PT, Smith R, et al. Mineralocorticoid action: target tissue specificity is enzyme, not receptor, mediated. *Science.* 1988;242:583-585.

Hanania NA, Chapman KR, Kesten S. Adverse effects of inhaled corticosteroids. *Am J Med.* 1995;98:196-208.

Imura H. Control of biosynthesis and secretion of ACTH: a review. *Horm Metab Res Suppl.* 1987;16:1-6.

Jusko WJ. Receptor-mediated pharmacodynamics of corticosteroids. *Prog Clin Biol Res.* 1994;387:261-270.

Larsen RP, Kronenberg HM, Medmed S, Polonsky KS, eds. *Williams Textbook of Endocrinology.* 10th ed. Philadelphia, Pa: WB Saunders; 2003.

Taylor AL, Fishman LM. Medical progress: corticotropin-releasing hormone. *N Engl J Med.* 1988;319:213-222.

Weisman MH, Wenblatt ME, Louie JS. *Treatment of the Rheumatic Diseases: A Companion to Kelley's Textbook of Rheumatology.* Philadelphia, Pa: WB Saunders; 2001.

# Part IX

## Anti-infective and Anti-neoplastic Chemotherapy

# 49

# Principles of Antimicrobial Therapy

## J UETRECHT, EJ PHILLIPS, AND SL WALMSLEY

One of the greatest achievements of medical science has been the control and management of infectious diseases. The role of microbes in causing severe infections was not appreciated until Louis Pasteur (1822–95) formulated the germ theory in the years 1853 to 1867. Between 1880 and 1910, dozens of pathogenic bacteria were discovered. It was, however, not until the twentieth century that therapy directed specifically against these microbes was developed.

## THE ERA OF PRE-ANTIBIOTIC SYNTHETIC COMPOUNDS

Paul Ehrlich (1854–1915) was responsible for establishing a basic principle of chemotherapy. The importance of drug distribution as a determinant of drug action had been realized in the latter part of the nineteenth century. Struck by the observation that certain chemicals show a remarkable affinity for various materials (e.g., the affinity of dyes for the proteins of wool), Ehrlich reasoned that if chemicals with antimicrobial activity could be targeted to be taken up in certain human tissues, they would exert a chemical action there against infecting microbes. Unfortunately, Ehrlich's search for such "magic bullets" was initially rather non-specific. He utilized chemicals that fix to specific biological macromolecules; therefore, these chemicals interfered not only with the infecting microbes, but also with host tissues. Ehrlich realized that a useful antimicrobial drug would have to be selectively toxic to the microbes, and he therefore began to investigate chemical modifications that would cause the toxic materials to be selectively taken up by the pathogens. This led to the introduction in 1909 of an arsenic derivative, **arsphenamine (Salvarsan)**, for the treatment of syphilis. Although this drug had considerable toxicity, it and its successor **Neosalvarsan** were the standard treatments for the disease throughout the world for over 40 years, until superseded by penicillin. Ehrlich not only developed an important chemotherapeutic agent, but he also began the systematic exploration of the molecular basis of antibacterial chemotherapy.

Within about three decades of Ehrlich's original work, Domagk and others found that a red tissue dye had antibacterial action. This substance, **Prontosil**, was the forerunner of the sulfonamides, which are still among the most important of the synthetic antibacterial compounds.

## THE ERA OF ANTIBIOTICS

The term antibiosis was coined in 1889 by Vuillemin and originally meant the antagonism between living creatures. This terminology was refined by Waksman, who, in 1942, defined antibiotics as substances produced by microorganisms that are, even in high dilution, antagonistic to the growth or life of other microorganisms. The first clinically useful antibiotic was **penicillin**, a product of a *Penicillium* mould. It was discovered by Fleming in 1928, and it initiated the antibiotic era, which extends to the present. Innumerable microbial products have been investigated since the discovery of penicillin, and a great variety of them have proven to be useful antibiotic substances. Pharmaceutical companies have been extremely active in the search for these products and have made fundamental contributions to the development of antibiotic drugs.

Much work has been done in modifying the natural products (by removing some chemical groups and adding others) in attempts to enhance the beneficial effects while minimizing the toxic effects. The resultant modified end product is termed a semi-synthetic antibiotic. Most antibiotics currently used in clinical practice are semi-synthetic. Some of the desirable pharmacological characteristics cultivated in these semi-synthetic agents are stability, solubility, diffusibility, activity in the complex environment of the body, and slow excretion. In addition, these agents are designed to possess as large a therapeutic index as possible (i.e., the amount of drug causing toxicity exceeds by as much as possible the amount of drug necessary for a therapeutic response).

The relationships among patient, infecting pathogen, and antimicrobial agent are illustrated in Figure 49-1. The therapeutic usefulness of a given chemotherapeutic agent is usually determined by its selective toxicity to the pathogen.

## MECHANISMS OF ACTION

The mechanisms of action of antimicrobial agents are based upon an attack on targets present in bacteria and other organisms but either absent or less vulnerable in human cells (i.e., **selective toxicity**, a term formally introduced by Adrien Albert in 1951). These microbial targets include the cell wall, the cytoplasmic membrane, cellular proteins, cellular nucleic acids, and intermediary metabolism. It is traditional to classify antimicrobial agents by their mechanism of action, a system that is used throughout this section on anti-infective chemotherapy. In the following chapters, the drugs will be described in relation to their sites of action, including the following:

- Cell wall: penicillins, cephalosporins, carbapenems, monobactams, vancomycin, bacitracin, cycloserine, isoniazid, ethambutol, echinocandins
- Cell membrane: polymyxins, nystatin, amphotericin B, imidazoles, triazoles, allylamines
- Cellular proteins: aminoglycosides, spectinomycin, tetracyclines, chloramphenicol, clindamycin, macrolides, streptogramins, oxazolidinones

- Cellular nucleic acids: griseofulvin, 5-fluorocytosine, rifampin, pyrazinamide, para-aminosalicylic acid, quinolones, sulfonamides, trimethoprim, pyrimethamine, sulfones

The individual mechanisms of action are described in detail in the respective chapters.

## BACTERIOSTATIC VERSUS BACTERICIDAL ANTIMICROBIALS

Bacteriostatic antimicrobial agents such as chloramphenicol, the tetracyclines, and erythromycin inhibit bacterial cell replication but do not kill the organisms; that is, they stop bacterial growth and allow the host's immune system to ultimately clear the infection. Therefore, if host immunity is suppressed, or if the infection is in an area of poor immunological surveillance (e.g., cerebrospinal fluid or vegetations of subacute bacterial endocarditis), bacteriostatic drugs may not suffice as the sole therapeutic agent.

Bactericidal antimicrobial agents such as the penicillins and cephalosporins cause microbial death by lysis. They therefore rely less on host immunity for clearing bacterial infections.

Some antimicrobial agents, such as the sulfonamides and tetracyclines, are indeterminate in the extent of their action. They are bacteriostatic or bactericidal depending on the concentration of drug, the nature of the environ-

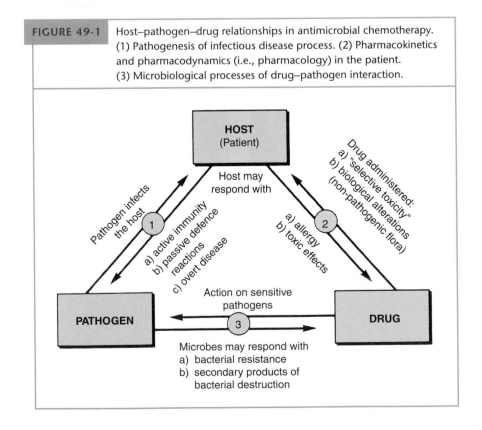

**FIGURE 49-1**   Host–pathogen–drug relationships in antimicrobial chemotherapy. (1) Pathogenesis of infectious disease process. (2) Pharmacokinetics and pharmacodynamics (i.e., pharmacology) in the patient. (3) Microbiological processes of drug–pathogen interaction.

ment, and the specific microorganisms against which they are employed.

## ANTIBIOTIC RESISTANCE

Most, if not all, microorganisms are capable of developing resistance to the action of antimicrobial agents. For example, when penicillin was first introduced, almost all *Staphylococcus aureus* organisms were sensitive; however, resistant strains that produce penicillinase (an enzyme that inactivates penicillin) have increased over time to the point that *S. aureus* is now generally resistant to penicillin. Newer penicillins were synthesized that are resistant to penicillinase; however, some strains of *S. aureus* have developed resistance to these newer agents through a different mechanism. Some strains of *Neisseria gonorrhoeae* and *Streptococcus pneumoniae,* which were previously very sensitive to penicillin, have also developed resistance. Thus, there is a constant evolution of bacteria with changing patterns of antibacterial sensitivity. The parallel development of new antibiotics requires constant re-evaluation to determine the optimal drug for the treatment of a given bacterial infection.

Despite the recognition that bacteria can develop resistance, the steady stream of new antibiotics made it appear as if we were gaining the upper hand against bacterial infections, and work on the development of new antibiotics almost came to a stop. But the ability of bacteria to develop resistance was underestimated, and we have actually lost ground over the last decade. Among contemporary pathogens, especially those that are hospital-acquired (nosocomial), resistance to a specific drug is often part of a larger package of resistance factors located on bacterial plasmids or transposons. This can result in simultaneous resistance to more than one antibiotic. Also, the use of a certain antibiotic may select for the emergence of bacterial strains that are resistant to another antibiotic. Changing the pattern of antibiotic use would not end the selective pressure unless all relevant drugs were withdrawn.

There are now several bacteria, such as vancomycin-resistant enterococci, methicillin-resistant *S. aureus* (MRSA), and multidrug-resistant mycobacteria, that are more difficult to treat. The additional antibiotic pressures created by these multi-resistant bacteria (e.g., MRSA) have in turn led to new problems of resistance, such as the emergence of vancomycin-intermediate *S. aureus* (VISA) and, more recently, vancomycin-resistant *S. aureus*. This has renewed efforts by pharmaceutical companies to develop new agents. Among the promising ones that have become available are oxazolidinones (linezolid), which inhibit protein synthesis, and more recently, the lipopeptides (daptomycin), which aid in the treatment of multi-resistant, Gram-positive infections. However, resistance to even these newer agents has now been described and presumably will strengthen with the increasing use of these drugs.

## Mutation

A mutation is a rare, spontaneous, "normal" event that is not usually induced (although it may be selected for) by antimicrobials. However, the actions of antimicrobials may be affected by a variety of mutations, including the following:

- Alterations of cell walls or cell membrane components that prevent the entry of drugs into the cell or actively exclude them
- Alteration of the target or binding site for an antimicrobial agent inside the cell
- Other indirect mechanisms (such as chromosomal mutations affecting the regulation of antibiotic resistance genes, including those encoding for β-lactamase) by which previously susceptible cells may become non-responsive to the action of drugs

Mutationally altered cells are often metabolically inferior to wild-type cells; they tend to be suppressed and diluted out in competitive growth of a bacterial population. Thus, they rarely give rise to a resistant strain. However, mutants may become a threat when selective antibiotic pressure on the wild-type organisms is maintained by suboptimal antibiotic exposure, extensive topical use of the drug, or other factors that allow resistant mutants to gain the competitive advantage.

## Inheritance

Inheritance is the most common way for microbes to acquire resistance to antimicrobials. It is selected for by exposure to antimicrobial agents, and it is transferable within a microbial population.

The genetic agents that confer antimicrobial resistance are the resistance plasmids (**R plasmids**), which may encode for resistance to as many as six or seven antimicrobial agents. Plasmids are extra-chromosomal genetic elements in bacteria, ranging in size from a few daltons to more than a million daltons. Their main role is to allow bacterial evolution under greatly varying environmental conditions. They code for genetic properties that confer selective advantages for bacterial survival under particular conditions, such as the presence of antibiotics. Thus, plasmid-determined functions include bacterial replication, fertility, metabolism, virulence, and resistance to toxic metals, in addition to resistance to antimicrobials.

Resistance plasmids are believed to arise from collections of foreign genes that are not normally part of a bacterium's chromosomes. These genes may have come from a variety of unrelated microorganisms (such as antibiotic-producing bacteria or fungi ). The fact that they have been assembled into resistance plasmids that have propagated implies that the genes must have experienced strong selective pressure (such as that which may have been created by exposure to metals, halogens, and similar antibacterial agents of the pre-antibiotic era). Since the description of R plasmids by Watanabe in 1963, R-plasmid activity and dissemination have been recognized as the major threat to continued antibiotic effectiveness.

Examples of the products of R plasmid–coded factors include the following:

- Products produced in cell walls or cell membranes that interfere with transport systems or block pores so that antibiotics cannot enter the cell
- Enzymes produced by microbes that modify the site of drug action in such a way that even though the antibiotic enters the cell, the drug-binding site is lacking
- Enzymes produced by microbes that destroy the antibiotic (i.e., no active antibiotic remains)
- Substitute enzymes produced by microbes that are resistant to antibiotic action and replace antibiotic-sensitive essential enzymes, permitting cell growth in the presence of the antibiotic
- Active transport systems that remove the antibiotic from the bacterial cell

## Dissemination of Resistance

Most R plasmids are transferable and conjugative; that is, they possess the sex-factor activity necessary to initiate conjugation between resistance-positive (R+) and resistance-negative (R−) bacteria. This conjugation leads to a direct transfer of complete R plasmids from one bacterial cell to another.

R plasmids can also spread among microorganisms via a bacteriophage vector. This process, called **transduction**, is limited to R plasmids that can be accommodated in a bacteriophage chromosome (i.e., plasmids of smaller size).

R plasmids may be carried between microorganisms by direct DNA transfer, a process called **transformation**. This is the basis of recombinant DNA technology and "genetic engineering" with *Escherichia coli*. Although unproven in nature, it conceivably occurs through the contact of plasmid DNA from lysed bacteria with recipient cells.

Resistance determinants can be transferred independently of R plasmids by a process called **transposition** (i.e., hopping from one plasmid to another, or to a chromosome, or to a bacteriophage). This is thought to be the "natural" means of construction of R plasmids from various genetic sources; the new resistance is then permanently transferred with its new vector. This process allows previously non-transferable factors to be joined to transferable R plasmids, which may be the most common basis of resistance in hospital environments.

Some known mechanisms of antibiotic resistance, relative to the mode of action of the respective drugs, are shown in Table 49-1.

## LABORATORY MONITORING

As a general rule, it is best to use a single agent that is specific for the organism involved, rather than "shotgun" therapy with a combination of agents, or a specific agent with a very broad spectrum of activity. Specific therapy usually decreases toxicity and reduces the emergence of resistant strains of bacteria. Nevertheless, there are exceptions to this rule. Although the use of multiple antibiotics leads to the overall risk that bacteria will develop resistance in the treatment of a specific infection, it may decrease the probability that some of the organisms in that infection will be resistant to the multiple antibiotics. This can be an important concept in the treatment of serious infections in which there is a high incidence of resistant organisms, such as tuberculosis. The tubercle bacillus is very polymorphic, and there is a high probability that a given infection will contain organisms that are resistant to any one anti-tubercular drug. These resistant organisms can proliferate and become the dominant organism of infection. The use of two or more anti-tubercular drugs decreases the risk of such an occurrence.

Another exception is the use of synergistic combinations such as penicillin and an aminoglycoside in the treatment of enterococcal endocarditis, which is a life-threatening infection that is difficult to treat with a single agent. The combination of sulfamethoxazole and trimethoprim is also said to be synergistic, but the evidence is not compelling, and since sulfamethoxazole is associated with a relatively high incidence of serious adverse reactions, the routine use of this combination is now being questioned. A final example is an infection in an immunosuppressed patient, in which it is often difficult to culture the responsible organism; therefore, one is forced to employ broad-spectrum therapy.

The rational use of antimicrobial agents requires careful laboratory monitoring. One important aspect of this monitoring is determination of the degree of activity of the selected antimicrobial agent against the infecting bacterial strain. This is termed sensitivity testing. Though most bacteria have a predictable sensitivity pattern (to be discussed in subsequent chapters for specific antimicrobial agents), there is sufficient variation that the degree of activity of a specific antibiotic against an organism causing a serious infection should always be assessed. Knowledge of local patterns of resistance is very important because patterns can vary considerably between geographical regions and from one hospital to another.

The principle at work in sensitivity testing is that the activity of the antibiotic against one or several specific

| TABLE 49-1 | Known Mechanisms of Antibiotic Resistance | |
|---|---|---|
| Agent | Mode of Antibacterial Action | Microbial Resistance Mechanism |
| Sulfonamides | Block synthesis of tetrahydrofolic acid and cell-linked metabolic pathways | R plasmid–coded, sulfonamide-resistant dihydrofolic acid synthetase |
| Trimethoprim | Competitive inhibition of dihydrofolic acid reductase; blocks synthesis of tetrahydrofolic acid | R plasmid–coded, trimethoprim-resistant dihydrofolic acid reductase |
| Penicillins and cephalosporins | Interfere with cell wall biosynthesis by interacting with penicillin-binding proteins | Hydrolysis of the antibiotic's β-lactam ring by β-lactamase enzyme |
| Tetracyclines | Inhibit protein synthesis by interaction with 30S and 50S ribosomal subunits | Interference with transport of drug into cell; cell unable to maintain drug |
| Aminoglycosides | Bind to 30S (and 50S) ribosomal subunit, cause translational misreading, inhibit peptide elongation | Enzymatic modification of drug by R plasmid–coded enzyme; drug has reduced affinity for ribosome; reduced drug transport into cell |
| Erythromycin and lincomycin | Bind to 50S ribosomal subunit; inhibit protein synthesis at chain elongation step | Enzymatic modification of ribosomal DNA of sensitive cells renders ribosome drug-resistant |
| Chloramphenicol | Inhibits protein synthesis by interacting with 50S ribosomal subunit | Drug inactivated by acetylation of –OH groups by chloramphenicol transacetylase; interference with drug transport into cell |
| Rifampin | Binds to bacterial RNA polymerase and blocks RNA synthesis (transcription) | Resistance arises by spontaneous mutation (no plasmid-coded mechanism known) |

bacteria can be determined in vitro under conditions that simulate the environment of the bacteria in the host. The two methods of performing sensitivity testing are the disk-diffusion method and the dilution method.

## Disk-Diffusion Method

This was the earliest available method and is currently the most extensively used worldwide. Commercially available paper disks impregnated with specific amounts of antimicrobial agents are placed onto agar plates containing a standardized number (inoculum) of the bacteria to be tested. The antibiotic diffuses out of the disk into the agar, establishing a linear concentration gradient from the centre of the disk to some peripheral point in the agar. Bacteria growing on the agar are therefore presented with a continuous concentration gradient of antibiotic that inhibits or kills them for a variable distance around the disk. This resulting zone of antibacterial effect, the diameter of which is determined after an overnight incubation, is called the zone of inhibition.

The exact size of the zone (expressed in millimetres) reflects the degree of susceptibility or resistance, but the interpretation of the results is based upon prior studies using dilution tests (see below), which have correlated zone sizes with the minimum amount of antibiotic required to inhibit the growth of the bacterium. Results are expressed in only three susceptibility categories: sensitive, intermediate, and resistant. These categories are based upon observations

of clinical outcomes in a large number of cases in which (1) the infection being treated was in the bloodstream or in tissues having approximately the same antibiotic concentrations as those in the bloodstream, (2) the patient was receiving a "standard dose" of the antibiotic in question, and (3) the dosage produced the usual concentration of the antibiotic in the bloodstream. Therefore, the categories are meaningful only in cases in which the same criteria apply. If the infection is in the urinary tract, for example, it is necessary to use a different set of disks that release different concentrations of antibiotic that reflect those found in the urine in order to generate corresponding sensitivity categories.

Although it is recognized that the disk-diffusion method of sensitivity testing is rather imprecise, in general it provides sufficient information to permit choice of the appropriate antibiotic.

## Dilution Method

This method of sensitivity testing can be carried out in agar or broth. A standardized inoculum of bacteria is exposed to varying concentrations (usually successive twofold dilutions) of an antimicrobial agent. The minimum concentration of antibiotic required to inhibit the growth of the bacteria can then be determined. This **minimum inhibitory concentration (MIC)** can then be compared with the measured or predicted concentration of antibiotic at the site of infection, be that blood, urine, cerebrospinal fluid, or other site.

In addition to the MIC, the **minimum bactericidal concentration (MBC)** can also be determined, especially if the original dilutions were done in broth. To measure the MBC, aliquots of broth from tubes showing no visible growth after overnight incubation are subcultured onto antibiotic-free agar. The MBC is represented by the lowest concentration of antibiotic that completely prevents the growth of bacteria in the subculture. In general, the MIC and MBC of a bactericidal agent will be equal, whereas a bacteriostatic drug will have a large difference between the MIC and MBC. The clinical significance of the difference between MIC and MBC is unclear, and most reporting is in terms of the MIC. (MBCs are performed in hospital laboratories only under special circumstances.)

Many laboratory variables may affect the results of a sensitivity test, such as size of the inoculum, the temperature of incubation, and the pH and cation content of the culture medium. These and other important variables are usually controlled in a consistent fashion by the laboratory providing this critically important information to clinicians; but clinicians must realize that, as with any test, extraneous factors (such as the immune status of the host, site of infection, extent of plasma protein binding, etc.) may influence the observed results. Newer methods have been developed in hospital microbiology laboratories for the automation and semi-automation of antibiotic sensitivity testing. In some cases, the results are expressed as sensitive or resistant, while in other circumstances, actual MIC values are reported. These automated methods may decrease the time required for the performance of sensitivity testing and allow for large numbers of organisms to be tested.

Another important aspect of sensitivity testing relates to assessing the in vitro **interactions of a combination of antibiotics.** Two antimicrobial drugs acting together in vitro may be indifferent, antagonistic, additive, or synergistic. When their combined action is no greater than that of the more active drug alone, they are said to be **indifferent.** When the activity of one is reduced by the presence of the other, they are said to be **antagonistic.** When their combined effect is equal to the sum of their individual effects, they are said to be **additive.** When their combined effect is significantly greater than that of either drug individually or the sum of their individual effects, they are said to be **synergistic.** Description of the precise mathematical definitions of these combined actions and of the methodologies available to test for these effects is beyond the scope of this chapter.

As early as 1952, it was suggested that the type of interaction of two drugs could be predicted on the basis of whether the component drugs were bactericidal or bacteriostatic. Two bacteriostatic drugs together would be additive, two bactericidal drugs together would be synergistic, and the combination of one of each type would be antagonistic. It has become clear, however, that those general-izations do not apply to all combinations of antimicrobial agents. When a clinician deals with serious infections, especially those caused by relatively resistant microbes, the type of interaction can only be ascertained by direct synergy testing.

## Determinations of Antimicrobial Concentrations

Another aspect of laboratory monitoring in the rational use of antimicrobial agents involves the determination of the concentrations of these agents. Although the approximate concentrations that will be attained in various body sites after standard therapeutic doses can be predicted from the literature, there is considerable inter-patient variability. The only way of knowing what concentrations are attained after a given dose is to measure the plasma or serum levels. This is not so important for relatively non-toxic agents, which, at usual doses, generally attain concentrations several hundred times greater than the MIC of the bacteria being treated (e.g., penicillin in *S. pneumoniae* bacteremia). Here the permissible margin for error is wide; however, for other agents that may attain concentrations only three to four times higher than the MIC of the bacteria being treated (e.g., aminoglycosides in enteric aerobic infections), determining the attained concentrations is more important. In addition, the aminoglycosides have a low therapeutic index (i.e., narrow margin of safety), so the determination of concentrations is also important for limiting concentration-related toxic reactions.

## Serum Bactericidal Titres

The ultimate control of infection not only depends on the action of the antimicrobial agents but also reflects the resultant effect of many host factors, primarily immunological. Therefore, a meaningful test of therapeutic activity should take all of these factors into account. Such a test is the measurement of serum bactericidal titre (SBT). Serum samples are obtained to coincide with anticipated maximum (peak) and minimum (trough) antimicrobial drug levels. The test is performed by adding a known inoculum of the bacterium isolated from the patient to serial twofold dilutions of the serum. The minimum concentration (highest dilution) of the serum capable of inhibiting and ultimately killing the inoculated bacteria is determined. This test, which has been most widely used for the determination of therapeutic effectiveness in bacterial endocarditis and other serious infections, permits monitoring of therapeutic response and allows modification of the choice and dosage of various antimicrobial agents. Although there is controversy about this point, for the highest probability of clinical improvement, the peak SBT should represent a dilution of at least 1:8. Trough SBTs and other tests, such as the area under the concentration–time curve above the MIC, are being evaluated as methods of predicting clinical outcome.

## DETERMINANTS OF RESPONSE TO ANTIMICROBIAL THERAPY

Several factors must be considered when an antimicrobial agent is prescribed if therapy is to be successful. Antimicrobial agents are of no value in treating viral infections or in treating non-infectious ailments. Presuming that an established bacterial infection is being treated, the antibiotic must be active against the infecting bacteria. This implies knowledge of the most likely pathogens causing a specific disease or syndrome and knowledge of the spectrum of activity of the selected antimicrobial agent. If a bacterium has actually been isolated, then in vitro sensitivity testing is appropriate. The appropriate dose, route of administration, and duration of therapy must be selected for the specific patient, keeping in mind the specific site of infection. This is intended to maximize the chance of attaining adequate concentrations of the antimicrobial agent at the site of infection. For certain antibiotics, especially those with a low therapeutic index, the actual drug concentrations attained should be measured. Finally, successful therapy requires an assurance of compliance with the prescribed agents and dosage regimens, a factor that must be remembered in outpatient therapeutics.

Successful outcome may also require the employment of ancillary modes of therapy to assist antibiotic action. This might include surgical drainage of abscesses, removal of obstructions to urinary flow, or removal of foreign bodies such as intravascular catheters.

## PHARMACOKINETIC FACTORS ESSENTIAL FOR OPTIMAL ANTIMICROBIAL THERAPY

The rational use of antibiotics requires some knowledge of their pharmacokinetics. Although it may not be necessary to know all kinetic details for each agent, the following are essential:

1. The *anticipated concentration of the antibiotic that the selected dose will yield at the site of infection.* This implies knowledge of the serum concentration attained and the diffusion characteristics (distribution) of the antibiotic into the infected tissue. The anticipated concentration can then be related to the sensitivity of the infecting bacterium. It is generally desirable to attain antibiotic concentrations at the site of infection at least two to four times in excess of the MIC for the infecting organism.

2. The *elimination half-life of the antibiotic.* This allows an approximation of the dosing interval that will result in maintenance of the desired concentration range.

3. The *sources of pharmacokinetic variation.* This implies some knowledge of biotransformation and elimination. If an agent is excreted primarily by the kidneys and the patient is in renal failure, it is necessary to recognize the need for dose adjustment. Similarly, if the agent is biotransformed in the liver and the patient is in hepatic failure, or if, on the contrary, the biotransforming enzymes have undergone induction by another agent, the dose may have to be adjusted.

Some of the host variables influencing the kinetics of antibiotics, with examples from clinical practice, are outlined in Table 49-2. In the chapters that follow, these variables will not be specifically considered for each antibiotic; rather, the discussion will refer to normal adult patients. It is important, however, to always consider sources of pharmacokinetic variation, for no patient will behave precisely in textbook fashion.

## NEW ANTIMICROBIALS IN DEVELOPMENT

The rapid emergence of drug resistance, particularly in Gram-positive cocci such as methicillin-resistant *S. aureus* (MRSA) and vancomycin-resistant *Enterococcus* (VRE), as well as the threat of vancomycin-resistant *S. aureus* (VRSA), has become a crisis in North American hospitals. It has spurred the development of a number of new drugs and drug classes with activity against multi-resistant, Gram-positive cocci (Table 49-3). These drugs act by various mechanisms:

- Elaboration of a novel penicillin-binding protein 2a renders MRSA resistant to *all* β-lactams currently on the market (see Chapter 50) since these agents have no affinity for the altered protein and hence cannot inhibit bacterial cell wall synthesis. However, **ceftobiprole** is a novel, broad-spectrum cephalosporin currently in development that is able to bind with high affinity to penicillin-binding protein 2a and hence has activity against MRSA.
- The **glycylcyclines** are newer derivatives of tetracyclines that share a common ribosomal binding site with the tetracyclines and work similarly by inhibiting protein synthesis (see Chapter 52). However, the glycylcyclines have a fivefold greater ribosomal binding affinity, which may be responsible for their increased activity against tetracycline-resistant organisms.
- Although drugs in the **lipoglycopeptide** class inhibit cell wall synthesis by the same basic mechanism of

| TABLE 49-2 | Some Variables Influencing the Kinetics of Antimicrobial Agents | |
|---|---|---|
| **Variable** | **Mechanism of Effect** | **Example** |
| Age | Decreased renal function early in life and late in life | Need to decrease dose of aminoglycosides in neonates and elderly |
| Renal function | Important for drugs dependent on renal excretion | Need to decrease dose of aminoglycosides in patients with compromised renal function |
| Liver function | Important for drugs biotransformed in the liver | Need to decrease dose of chloramphenicol in patients with compromised liver function (e.g., premature newborns) |
| Fever/burns | Increased excretion or increased $V_D$ of some drugs | Need to increase dose of aminoglycosides |
| Acetylation status | Important for drugs being acetylated | Need to increase dose of isoniazid in rapid acetylators on regimen of once- or twice-weekly dosage |
| Diabetes mellitus | Reduced absorption of certain drugs after intramuscular dosing | Need to increase dose of intramuscular penicillins in diabetics |
| Cystic fibrosis | Increased clearance and $V_D$ of some drugs Altered absorption of some drugs | Need to increase dose of aminoglycosides in these patients Chloramphenicol palmitate malabsorbed because of lipase deficiency |
| GI surgery | Altered absorption of drugs in patients with short bowel (e.g., ileal bypass) | Ampicillin bioavailability is 15% of normal after small bowel bypass |

$V_D$ = volume of distribution.

action as glycopeptides such as vancomycin (see Chapter 50), they have better activity against *S. aureus*. The hydrophobic substituents of these lipoglycopeptides may be responsible for their increased binding affinity for bacterial cell walls. In addition, more recent evidence suggests that some of these drugs (e.g., **televancin**) may act via a second mechanism by interacting with, and increasing the permeability of, the bacterial cell membrane (see Chapter 51).

• In addition to drugs, **S. aureus vaccines** have been developed and, in phase II/III studies, have shown promise in preventing or reducing the incidence of *S. aureus* infections. This is a potential new weapon in the fight to clear MRSA from hospital wards.

| TABLE 49-3 | New Antimicrobials in Clinical Development | | | | |
|---|---|---|---|---|---|
| **Drug Class** | **Drug** | **Target** | **Stage of Development** | **Company** | **Spectra of Activity** |
| Cephalosporin | Ceftobiprole | Cell wall | Phase II | Basilea | Active against many multi-resistant, Gram-positive organisms (MRSA, VRSA, PRSP) |
| Glycylcycline | Tigecycline | Protein synthesis | Phase III | Wyeth | Multi-resistant, Gram-positive organisms (MRSA, PRSP, VRE); enteric and nosocomial Gram-negative organisms |
| Lipoglycopeptides | Dalvavancin Oritavancin Telavancin | Cell wall Cell wall | Phase III Phase III Phase III | Vicuron InterMune Thervance | VRSA, not Van A VRE VRSA/VRE VRSA/VRE |
| Quinolone and non-quinolone topoisomerase inhibitors | Garenafloxacin | Topoisomerase | Phase III | Toyama/ Schering-Plough | Improved Gram-positive activity (*S. pneumoniae*) |

VRSA = vancomycin-resistant *Staphylococcus aureus*; VRE = vancomycin-resistant *Enterococcus*; Van A VRE = *Enterococcus* resistant to vancomycin because of the Van A phenotype; MRSA = methicillin-resistant *Staphylococcus aureus*; PRSP = penicillin-resistant *Streptococcus pneumoniae*.

## SUGGESTED READINGS

Albert A. *Selective Toxicity: The Physicochemical Basis of Therapy.* 7th ed. London, United Kingdom: Chapman & Hall; 1985.

Burns JL. Mechanisms of bacterial resistance. *Pediatr Clin North Am.* 1995;42:497-508.

Cockerill FR III. Conventional and genetic laboratory tests used to guide antimicrobial therapy. *Mayo Clin Proc.* 1998;73: 1007-1021.

Cossart P, Sansonetti PJ. Bacterial invasion: the paradigms of enteroinvasive pathogens. *Science.* 2004;304:242-248.

Dalhoff A, Schmitz F. In vitro antibacterial activity and pharmacodynamics of new quinolones. *Eur J Clin Microbiol Infect Dis.* 2003;22:203-221.

Estes L. Review of pharmacokinetics and pharmacodynamics of antimicrobial agents. *Mayo Clin Proc.* 1998;73:1114-1122.

Fattom AI, Horwith G, Fuller S, et al. Development of StaphVAX, a polysaccharide conjugate vaccine against S. aureus infection: from the lab bench to phase III clinical trials. *Vaccine.* 2004;17:880-887.

Goldfarb J. New antimicrobial agents. *Pediatr Clin North Am.* 1995;42:717-733.

Jacoby GA, Archer GL. New mechanisms of bacterial resistance to antimicrobial agents. *N Engl J Med.* 1991;324:601-612.

Koren G, Prober CG, Gold R, eds. *Antimicrobial Therapy in Infants and Children.* New York, NY: Marcel Dekker; 1988.

Page MG. Cephalosporins in clinical development. *Expert Opin Investig Drugs.* 2004;13:973-985.

Rosenblatt JE. Laboratory tests used to guide antimicrobial therapy. *Mayo Clin Proc.* 1991;66:942-948.

Samaha-Kfoury JN, Araj GF. Recent developments in β-lactamases and extended spectrum β-lactamases. *BMJ.* 2003;327:1209-1213.

Sanders CC. Beta-lactamases of Gram-negative bacteria: new challenges for new drugs. *Clin Infect Dis.* 1992;14:1089-1099.

Service RF. Antibiotics that resist resistance. *Science.* 1995;270: 724-727.

Stager CE, Davis JR. Automated systems for identification of microorganisms. *Clin Microbiol Rev.* 1992;5:302-327.

Timmis KN, Gonzales-Carrero MI, Sekizaki T, Rojo F. Biological activities specified by antibiotic resistance plasmids. *J Antimicrob Chemother.* 1986;18(suppl C):1-12.

Thompson RL, Wright AJ. General principles of antimicrobial therapy. *Mayo Clinic Proc.* 1993;73:995-1006.

Van Bambeke F. Glycopeptides in clinical development: pharmacological profiles and clinical perspectives. *Curr Opin Pharmacol.* 2004;4:471-478.

Virk A, Steckelberg JM. Clinical aspects of antimicrobial resistance. *Mayo Clinic Proc.* 2000;75:200-214.

Zhanel GG, Homenuik K, Nichol K, et al. The glycylcyclines: a comparative review with the tetracyclines. *Drugs.* 2004;64: 63-88.

# 50

# Antimicrobial Agents That Act on Microbial Cell Wall Formation

## EJ PHILLIPS, J UETRECHT, AND SL WALMSLEY

### CASE HISTORY

A 65-year-old man with a history of chronic obstructive lung disease and non-insulin-dependent diabetes mellitus saw his physician for complaints of increasingly hesitant urination, nocturia, and post-void dribbling. On physical examination, his prostate gland was palpably enlarged. He was referred to a urologist and was booked for an elective transurethral prostatectomy.

Three weeks before the date of surgery, he developed dysuria and hematuria. A urine culture confirmed *Escherichia coli* cystitis, sensitive to ampicillin and the quinolones and resistant to trimethoprim–sulfamethoxazole. This infection was treated with oral ampicillin, 250 mg four times daily for 7 days, and full recovery occurred. Three weeks later, the patient was admitted for prostatectomy, which was performed under intravenous perioperative antibiotic prophylaxis with 1 g ampicillin and 80 mg gentamicin given once before and again 6 hours after surgery. He recovered well from this procedure.

One week after discharge, he was seen by his urologist in follow-up. A VDRL (Venereal Diseases Research Laboratory) test and confirmatory test, which had been performed as part of a routine hospital admission screen, had been reported positive. The patient could not recall a history of syphilis, but he had had intercourse with prostitutes as a young soldier in World War II. There was no clinical evidence of tertiary cardiovascular or central nervous system (CNS) syphilis. Although a false-positive VDRL test could not be ruled out, he was treated with benzathine penicillin G, 2.4 million units weekly for 3 weeks, because of the possibility of untreated late latent syphilis.

Three years later, he came to the local emergency room with a 3-hour history of crushing retrosternal chest pain. A diagnosis of unstable angina pectoris was made. Following an urgent coronary catheterization that confirmed triple-vessel disease, a coronary artery bypass procedure was performed, during which he received intravenous antibiotic prophylaxis with cefazolin, 1 g before and 1 g every 6 hours after surgery for 48 hours. Surgery was uneventful, but 48 hours later he developed fever and elevation of his white blood cell count as well as infiltration on his chest X-ray. A diagnosis of nosocomial pneumonia was made, and he was treated with intravenous cefotaxime, 1 g every 8 hours. This decision was based on the assumption that Gram-negative organisms are the usual pathogens in nosocomial pneumonia. A third-generation cephalosporin was chosen in this case because the patient had experienced an elevation of serum creatinine to 300 µmol/L post-operatively and his physician wished to avoid the nephrotoxicity of the aminoglycosides. Forty-eight hours later, sputum cultures were reported positive for *Klebsiella pneumoniae* resistant to ampicillin and sensitive to cefotaxime, and a strain of *Pseudomonas aeruginosa* sensitive to tobramycin and imipenem and resistant to cefotaxime and ceftazidime. Cefotaxime was therefore changed to imipenem, 500 mg every 6 hours for 48 hours.

Despite continued antibacterial treatment, the incision at the site of the vein removal became red and warm. A swab was taken from the purulent exudate and methicillin-resistant *Staphylococcus aureus* was cultured. Intravenous vancomycin, 1 g every 12 hours, was added to the antibiotic regimen and the patient was placed in contact isolation. The wound healed, the pneumonia resolved, and the patient was discharged from hospital after 2 more weeks of therapy.

A ll living cells, including bacteria as well as mammalian cells, have *cell membranes* (plasma membranes) that are necessary for the functional integrity of the cells. These membranes have complex lipid structures that can be disrupted by surfactants (detergents). Surfactants can therefore have antibacterial action, but they will also damage mammalian cells.

However, bacteria have much higher internal osmotic pressure than mammalian cells, and they require a *rigid outer cell wall*, external to the cell membrane, to prevent osmotic rupture in the isotonic medium of mammalian blood and tissues. These cell walls also maintain the shape of the bacteria. Mammalian cells do not have such cell walls.

During bacterial cell growth and division, the original cell wall must enlarge and form a new septum (cross wall) between the two daughter cells so that, when they separate, each has a complete outer wall. This requires the synthesis of new wall material. Inhibitors of bacterial cell wall biosynthesis will therefore render growing bacteria vulnerable to osmotic rupture, without affecting mammalian cells (Fig. 50-1). Since cell wall biosynthesis is complex, inhibitors can act at different points in the sequence.

## MECHANISMS OF ACTION

The process of cell wall formation begins in the bacterial cytoplasm with conversion of L-alanine into D-alanine. Two D-alanine molecules are then linked together. **Cycloserine** competitively inhibits the conversion of L-alanine into its D-form and the linking of the two D-molecules. Since the D-ala–D-ala unit is needed for the synthesis of all bacterial cell walls, cycloserine is effective against Gram-positive and Gram-negative bacteria alike, as well as against the tubercle bacillus. However, other antibiotics are superior in treating infections caused by most organisms; the use of cycloserine is limited to the treatment of infections caused by the tubercle bacillus resistant to first-line agents, and even that use is uncommon.

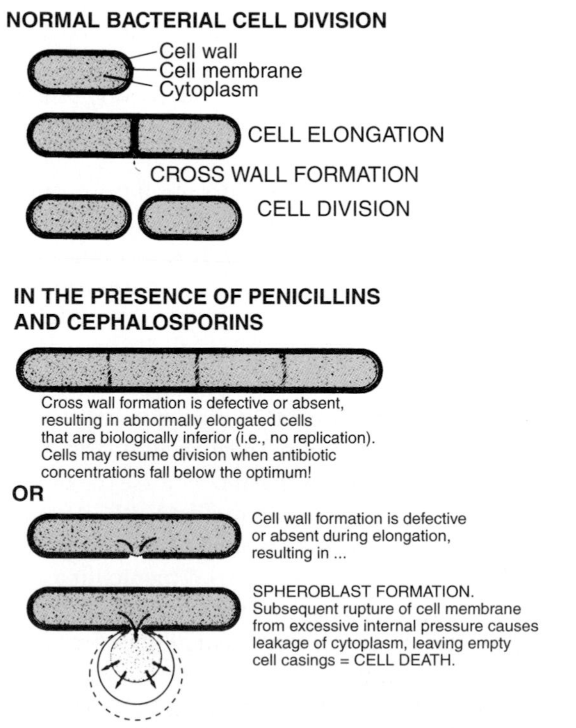

The next step in cell wall synthesis is the linkage of the D-ala dipeptide to three other amino acids and an amino sugar, *N*-acetylmuramic acid, to form a sugar–pentapeptide. This, in turn, is coupled to a molecule of another amino sugar, *N*-acetylglucosamine (Fig. 50-2). The whole sugar–peptide structure, linked to a lipid carrier molecule, isoprenyl phosphate, is then transported from the cytoplasm to the exterior of the cell membrane, where the sugar–peptide unit is added on to the lengthening polymer chains (peptidoglycan strands) from which the new cell wall is being built. **Bacitracin** interferes with this process by binding to the isoprenyl phosphate to form an unusable complex inside the bacterial cell. **Vancomycin** prevents the transfer of the sugar–pentapeptide from the carrier molecule to the growing polymer chain on the outside of the cell membrane.

The terminal event in cell wall synthesis is a cross-linking of the peptidoglycan strands by connecting a D-ala of a sugar–peptide in one strand to a diaminopimelic acid unit in a sugar–peptide of an adjacent strand (Fig. 50-3). This is a transpeptidation reaction, which is catalyzed by various enzymes that differ in different bacterial species. **Penicillins** and **cephalosporins** bind to the active site of the enzyme (in susceptible species) and prevent the formation of the cross-links.

The specificity of penicillins and cephalosporins for the transpeptidase involved in cell wall synthesis is due to the similarity of the antibiotic's three-dimensional structure to that of D-alanyl-D-alanine, which is the site on the peptidoglycan strand to which these enzymes bind. These transpeptidases are actually part of a group of proteins in bacterial cell walls called **penicillin-binding proteins (PBPs)**, which have a high affinity for penicillins and cephalosporins. The degree to which the binding of β-lactams to other penicillin-binding proteins contributes to their antibacterial activity is unknown but is probably very important for the action against Gram-negative organisms. One such penicillin-binding protein cross-links lipoprotein to peptidoglycan in the wall of Gram-negative bacilli. In addition, penicillins and cephalosporins have been reported to activate an endogenous autolytic system in some bacteria, which initiates cell lysis and death.

## PENICILLINS

The penicillins are the most diverse and probably the most important group of antibiotics used for the treatment of infection. In 1928, Alexander Fleming fortuitously isolated penicillin from a sample of the mould *Penicillium notatum* that was growing in his laboratory. However, it was not introduced into clinical medicine

---

**FIGURE 50-1** | Principal structural effects of penicillins and cephalosporins on bacterial (*E. coli*) replication.

**NORMAL BACTERIAL CELL DIVISION**

- Cell wall
- Cell membrane
- Cytoplasm

CELL ELONGATION

CROSS WALL FORMATION

CELL DIVISION

**IN THE PRESENCE OF PENICILLINS AND CEPHALOSPORINS**

Cross wall formation is defective or absent, resulting in abnormally elongated cells that are biologically inferior (i.e., no replication). Cells may resume division when antibiotic concentrations fall below the optimum!

**OR**

Cell wall formation is defective or absent during elongation, resulting in ...

SPHEROBLAST FORMATION. Subsequent rupture of cell membrane from excessive internal pressure causes leakage of cytoplasm, leaving empty cell casings = CELL DEATH.

| FIGURE 50-2 | Sites of action of bacitracin and vancomycin as inhibitors of cell wall synthesis. UDP = uridine diphosphate; UMP = uridine monophosphate; MurNAc = N-acetylmuramic acid; GluNAc = N-acetylglucosamine. |
| --- | --- |

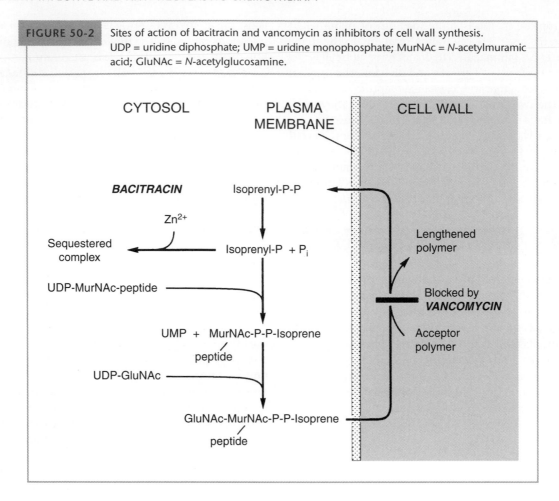

until 1941, when Florey, Chain, and associates devised suitable methods for large-scale culture of the mould and extraction of the penicillin. Since its original production, extensive chemical manipulation of the natural product has been carried out, resulting in a large number of natural and semi-synthetic congeners with diverse pharmacokinetic characteristics and altered spectra of activity.

## Chemistry

The basic structure of penicillin consists of a nucleus (6-aminopenicillanic acid, 6-APA) and side chains (acyl groups in amide linkage with 6-APA). The 6-APA nucleus has a thiazolidine ring connected to a β-lactam ring (Fig. 50-4). In the natural penicillin, penicillin G, the R group is benzyl; in the semi-synthetic penicillins, other R groups are substituted for the benzyl group (Fig. 50-5).

These agents contain a β-**lactam ring** that is chemically unstable (and therefore reactive) because of ring strain (i.e., the normal bond angle for carbon atoms is 109 to 120° but is forced by the ring to be 90°). The chemical reactivity of the β-lactam ring, which confers antibacterial activity by ring opening and covalent bonding to the target enzyme, is also responsible for the pencillins' *instability in an acid medium* (Fig. 50-6). The R group has a major

effect on acid stability; an electron-withdrawing atom close to the β-lactam, such as the oxygen in penicillin V or the nitrogen in ampicillin, confers relative acid stability. Cloxacillin and dicloxacillin are also relatively resistant to acid hydrolysis because of the electron-withdrawing effect of the heterocyclic ring.

The R group also controls susceptibility of the molecule to the **penicillinases**, produced by most *S. aureus* and some other bacteria, which hydrolyze the β-lactam ring and inactivate penicillins, causing the microorganisms to be resistant to the action of these antibiotics. Large, bulky groups, such as those found in methicillin, prevent binding of penicillinases and, therefore, inactivation by these enzymes. Other penicillins that are resistant to penicillinase are oxacillin, cloxacillin, dicloxacillin, and nafcillin. Unfortunately, these bulky groups decrease the binding of penicillins to the transpeptidases and other penicillin-binding proteins, which is responsible for the antibacterial activity of penicillins. In general, penicillinase-resistant penicillins are less active than penicillin G against organisms that do not produce penicillinase (see Fig. 50-5 and Table 50-1).

While most of the clinically significant microbial resistance to β-lactam antibiotics is due to bacterial β-lactamase activity, a new type of non-enzymatic penicillin resistance

**FIGURE 50-3** Sites of action of cross-linking and unlinking enzymes in *E. coli* cell wall synthesis. (1) Transpeptidase cleaves terminal D-ala and connects remaining D-ala to *m*-dap in peptide side chain on adjacent peptidoglycan strand. (2) Carboxypeptidase cleaves terminal D-ala from side chain of second strand, preventing further cross-linkage at that site. (3) Endopeptidase splits cross-link, providing site for transverse wall formation before the dividing bacteria separate. Penicillins and cephalosporins prevent transpeptidation (see text). D-ala = D-alanine; L-ala = L-alanine; D-glut = D-glutamate; *m*-dap = *m*-diaminopimelate; GluNAc = *N*-acetylglucosamine; MurNAc = *N*-acetylmuramic acid.

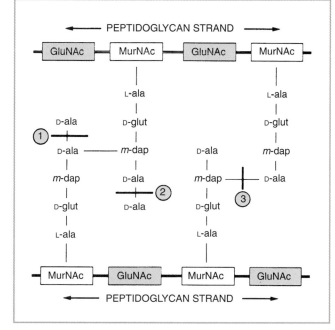

## Bacterial Susceptibility

The penicillins can be divided into three groups on the basis of their antibacterial spectra. These groups are narrow spectrum, β-lactamase sensitive; broad spectrum, β-lactamase sensitive; and β-lactamase resistant.

The antibacterial activity of penicillins representative of each of these groups is outlined in Table 50-1. The attainable serum concentrations of these antibiotics that can be related to the MICs are discussed below.

**Narrow-spectrum, β-lactamase-sensitive penicillins**
**Penicillin G** is the prototype of this group. The oral formulation representing this group is phenoxymethyl penicillin (**penicillin V**). As outlined in Table 50-1, penicillin G is very active against many Gram-positive bacteria, both aerobes and anaerobes, with the exception of penicillinase-producing *S. aureus*. Unfortunately, the majority of *S. aureus* strains encountered in clinical practice are now penicillinase producers. Penicillin G is also very active against the Gram-negative anaerobes, with the exception of β-lactamase-producing strains of *Bacteroides fragilis*. However, this antibiotic is not active against enteric Gram-negative organisms such as *E. coli*, hence the designation of narrow spectrum. Although penicillin is very active against *Neisseria* species, many strains of *N. gonorrhoeae* are now resistant, and this drug is no longer considered the drug of choice for gonorrhea in some metropolitan areas.

The basis for the lack of activity of penicillin G against Gram-negative enteric organisms lies in the nature of the cell wall. Although Gram-negative organisms also have a cell wall composed of peptidoglycan and its synthetic enzymes, these organisms are surrounded by an additional membrane of lipopolysaccharide and a capsule, which are relatively impermeable to penicillin. Furthermore, Gram-negative organisms have β-lactamases in the periplasmic space that contribute to the failure of penicillin to reach its site of action.

has been described in which one or more of the penicillin-binding proteins in the bacterial cell membrane are changed by mutation, rendering them less sensitive targets for penicillins. For example, some strains of staphylococci (called methicillin-resistant) possess an altered penicillin-binding protein. This protein has decreased affinity for methicillin and confers resistance to that antibiotic. These resistant bacteria require several-thousandfold increases in minimal inhibitory concentration (MIC) values for the β-lactam antibiotics, and the newly resistant bacteria emerge as a significant fraction of the respective pathogenic flora.

Penicillin can also be reacted, via its free carboxyl group, with amines such as **procaine** and **benzathine** to form salts that have a low solubility. These salts are given by intramuscular injection and slowly release penicillin to provide a sustained level of antibiotic. A single injection of benzathine penicillin provides therapeutic levels for almost 1 month and measurable levels for about 3 months.

**FIGURE 50-4** Structure of penicillin nucleus: A = thiazolidine ring; B = β-lactam ring. Sites of penicillinase action: (1) = amidase; (2) = β-lactamase.

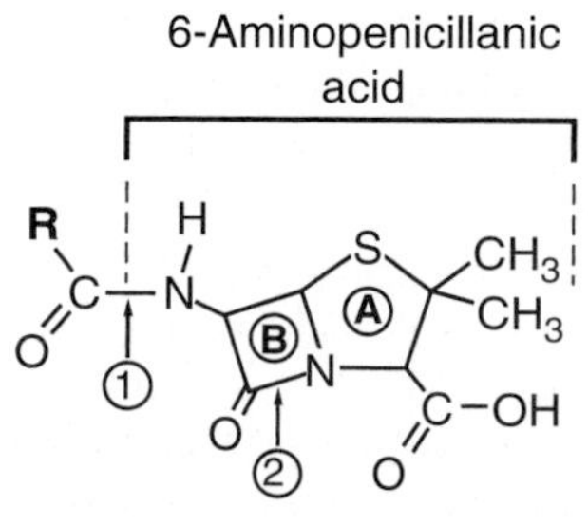

6-Aminopenicillanic acid

**FIGURE 50-5**  Chemical structures of R side chains and names of various penicillins.

| R SIDE CHAIN | CHEMICAL NAME | NON-PROPRIETARY NAME | PROPRIETARY NAMES |
|---|---|---|---|
| 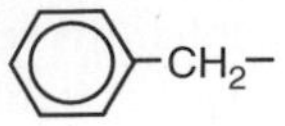 $CH_2-$ (benzyl) | Benzyl penicillin | Penicillin G | Megacillin, others |
| 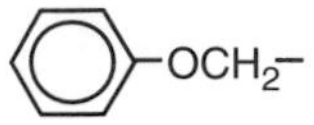 $OCH_2-$ (phenoxymethyl) | Phenoxymethyl penicillin | Penicillin V | Pen-Vee, others |
| 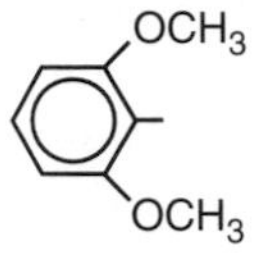 dimethoxyphenyl ($OCH_3$, $OCH_3$) | Dimethoxyphenyl penicillin | Methicillin | Staphcillin |
| 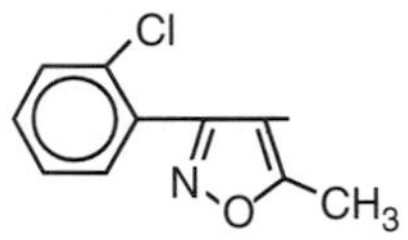 5-methyl-3-o-chlorophenyl-4-isoxazolyl ($Cl$, $CH_3$) | 5-Methyl-3-o-chloro-phenyl-4-isoxazolyl penicillin | Cloxacillin | Orbenin |
| 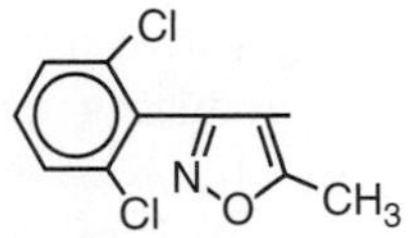 5-methyl-3-(2,6-dichlorophenyl)-4-isoxazolyl ($Cl$, $Cl$, $CH_3$) | 5-Methyl-3-(2,6-dichloro-phenyl)-4-isoxazolyl penicillin | Dicloxacillin | Dynapen |
| 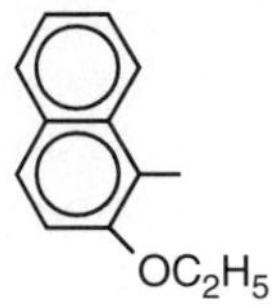 2-ethoxy-1-naphthyl ($OC_2H_5$) | 2-Ethoxy-1-naphthyl penicillin | Nafcillin | Unipen |
| 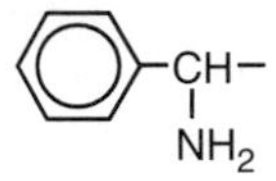 $CH-$, $NH_2$ (α-aminobenzyl) | α-Aminobenzyl penicillin | Ampicillin | Ampicin, Penbritin, others |
| 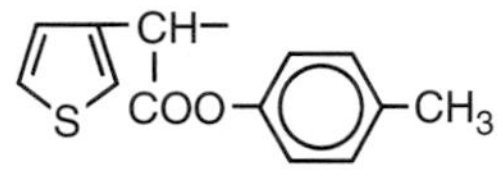 $CH-$, $COO-$...$CH_3$ (thienyl, cresylcarbonyl) | α-p-Cresylcarbonyl-3-thienylmethyl penicillin | Ticarcillin | Ticar |
| 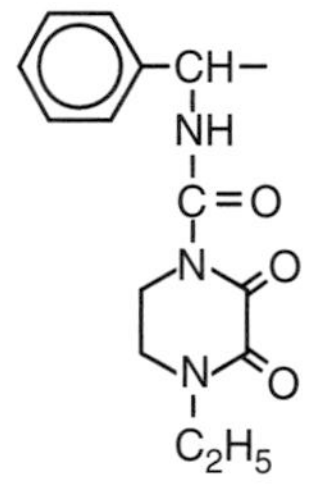 $CH-$, $NH$, $C=O$, piperazinedione, $C_2H_5$ | α-[(4-Ethyl-2,3-dioxo-1-piperazinyl)-carbonyl-amino] benzyl penicillin | Piperacillin | Pipracil |

## Broad-spectrum, β-lactamase-sensitive penicillins

Modification of the R group (e.g., adding an amino group to make **ampicillin** and **amoxicillin**) leads to activity against some enteric Gram-negative organisms. As described earlier, this also increases stability in acid, does not significantly decrease activity against Gram-positive organisms, and does not prevent hydrolysis by penicillinases. These agents also have increased activity against *Enterococcus* species and *Haemophilus* species, although the emergence of penicillinase-producing *Haemophilus* species has made these agents inappropriate as the sole therapy for severe infections due to *Haemophilus*.

Adding a carboxyl group (i.e., to form **carbenicillin** and **ticarcillin**) markedly increases activity against *Pseudomonas* but decreases activity against Gram-positive organisms. The newer ureidopenicillins (**azlocillin**,

**FIGURE 50-6** Inactivation of penicillin by β-lactamase, acid, and reaction with protein to form the major determinant causing penicillin hypersensitivity reactions.

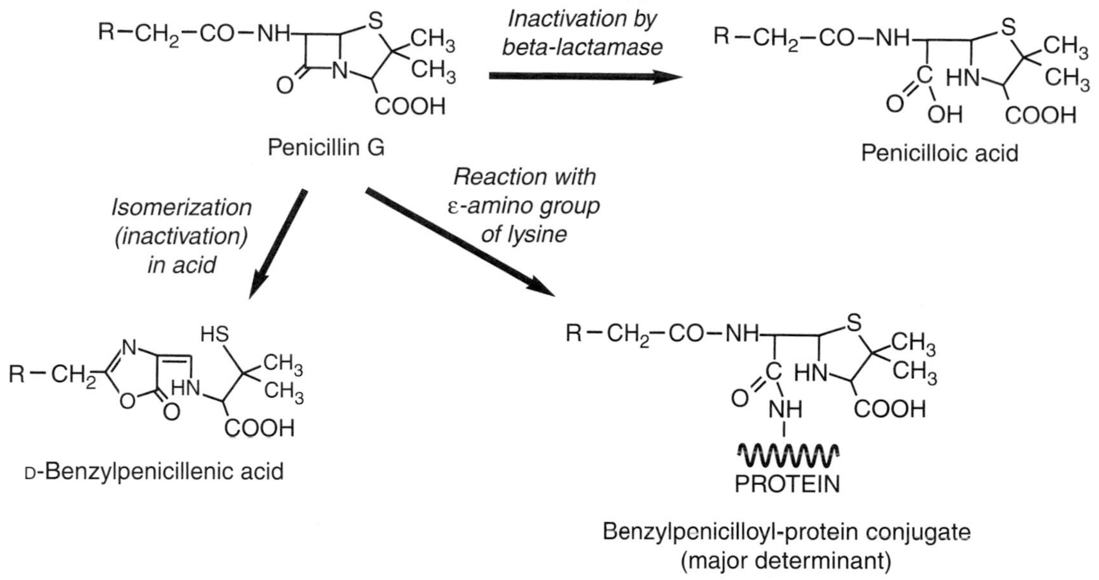

mezlocillin, and piperacillin) have even greater activity against *Pseudomonas* and other Gram-negative organisms and also have significant activity against *Klebsiella.*

These β-lactamase-sensitive antibiotics can be made resistant to β-lactamase by combination with β-lactamase inhibitors such as clavulanic acid, as discussed later.

### β-Lactamase-resistant penicillins

**Cloxacillin** is the representative of this group (see Table 50-1). Other members include **methicillin, oxacillin, nafcillin,** and **dicloxacillin.** The principal bacteriological advantage of this group of antibiotics is their high degree of activity against the penicillinase-producing staphylococci. They are, however, much less active than penicillin G against the other Gram-positive bacteria and are totally inactive against Gram-negative enteric organisms. Some strains of *S. aureus* have developed resistance to these agents through a different mechanism. As mentioned previously, these bacteria have penicillin-binding proteins that have a much lower affinity for penicillins.

## Pharmacokinetics

The degree of absorption of the various penicillin preparations from the gastrointestinal (GI) tract is variable and most dependent upon their relative susceptibility to acid hydrolysis in the stomach (see Fig. 50-6). Penicillin V, ampicillin, cloxacillin, dicloxacillin, and oxacillin, are quite acid-stable, and therefore a large fraction of an oral dose of any of these is absorbed from the GI tract. Peni-cillin G, methicillin, nafcillin, carbenicillin, ticarcillin, and piperacillin are more acid-labile, and hence only a small fraction of an oral dose is absorbed. These latter penicillins are, therefore, preferably administered parenterally. Of this group, only penicillin G is available in an oral formulation. Serum concentrations of the penicillins after representative doses are outlined in Table 50-2.

The volumes of distribution for the penicillins range from 0.1 to 0.3 L/kg (or 7 to 21 L/70 kg). Their degree of protein binding is quite variable, as noted in Table 50-2. The penicillins spread widely throughout the body and enter all body fluids. Concentrations in brain and cerebrospinal fluid (CSF), however, vary depending upon the specific penicillin and the degree of meningeal inflammation present at time of dosing, which increases permeability of the blood–brain barrier. The approximate concentrations attained in the CSF during treatment for meningitis are 25 to 30% of serum concentrations with penicillin G, ampicillin, carbenicillin, and ticarcillin. Methicillin, oxacillin, cloxacillin, and nafcillin, however, penetrate the CSF poorly.

The penicillins are not significantly biotransformed but are administered, distributed, and excreted in a biologically active form. Free penicillins are rapidly eliminated in the urine, with serum half-lives of less than 1 hour. They are mainly excreted by glomerular filtration and renal tubular secretion. In addition, there is significant excretion of nafcillin, oxacillin, and the ureidopenicillins in the bile. Renal tubular secretion takes place through the organic anion transport system and can be blocked, and

| TABLE 50-1 | Median MICs (in µg/mL) of Some Penicillins | | | | |
|---|---|---|---|---|---|
| Bacterium | Penicillin G | Cloxacillin | Ampicillin | Ticarcillin | Piperacillin |
| **Gram-positive** | | | | | |
| *Staphylococcus aureus*, penicillinase (–) | 0.03 | 0.25 | 0.05 | 1.25 | 0.8 |
| *Staphylococcus aureus*, penicillinase (+) | 25 to >800 | 0.5 | 125.0 | 25.0 | 25.0 |
| *Streptococcus* group A | 0.007 | 0.1 | 0.05 | 0.5 | 0.05 |
| *Streptococcus viridans* | 0.01 | — | 0.012 | 0.2 | 1.2 |
| *Enterococcus faecalis* | 2.0 | 25.0 | 0.38 | 34.0 | 4.0 |
| *Streptococcus pneumoniae* | 0.015 | 0.5 | 0.05 | 0.25 | 0.05 |
| *Listeria* | 0.1 | — | 0.1 | 2.5 | 1.25 |
| *Clostridium* | 0.06 | — | 0.05 | 0.5 | — |
| **Gram-negative** | | | | | |
| *Neisseria meningitidis* | 0.05 | 0.5 | 0.02 | 0.1 | 0.05 |
| *Neisseria gonorrhoeae* | 0.06 | 1.0 | 0.125 | 0.1 | 0.05 |
| *Haemophilus influenzae* | 0.16 | — | 0.05 | 0.5 | 0.25 |
| *Salmonella* | 5.0 | >250 | 2.0 | 4.0 | 4.0 |
| *Shigella* | 16.0 | >250 | 6.0 | — | — |
| *Klebsiella* | 50.0 | >250 | 50.0 | 50.0 | 4.0 |
| *Escherichia coli* | 64.0 | >250 | 5.0 | 5.0 | 2.0 |
| *Pseudomonas aeruginosa* | >400 | >250 | >400 | 25.0 | 10.0 |
| *Proteus mirabilis* | 32.0 | >250 | 1.25 | 1.25 | 1.25 |
| *Bacteroides fragilis* | 32.0 | — | 25.0 | 37.5 | — |
| Other *Bacteroides* | 0.12 | — | 6.2 | 2.0 | — |

the action of the penicillins prolonged, by probenecid. Probenecid may also increase serum concentrations by blocking distribution into tissues. In theory at least, therapeutic efficacy might be compromised by this action.

## Adverse Reactions

Penicillins are of very low toxicity. Their specificity of action as antibiotics is such that they have little effect on mammalian cells. However, all penicillins have the potential to cause hypersensitivity reactions, neurotoxicity, nephrotoxicity, and hematological toxicity.

**Hypersensitivity reactions** are the major type of toxicity seen with penicillin, and they occur in about 5% of patients. The most serious of these occur immediately after exposure (in less than 30 minutes) and are mediated by IgE (anaphylaxis). The incidence of anaphylaxis is about 0.01% of treatment courses. The mechanism of the immediate reactions is thought to involve the chemical reactivity of the β-lactam ring. Penicillins are a classic example of haptens (i.e., small molecules that are not immunogenic but bind to larger molecules, making them immunogenic) and react with the γ-amino group of lysine in proteins to make them immunogenic (see Fig. 50-6). This is the so-called major determinant because it is the major reaction leading to protein conjugates that can lead to a hypersensitivity reaction. There are also minor determinants composed mainly of penicilloic and penilloic acids. Although these determinants are quantitatively minor and are less commonly responsible for hypersensi-

tivity reactions, a high percentage of the life-threatening, immediate, hypersensitivity reactions (i.e., anaphylaxis) are due to the minor determinants.

Accelerated reactions (occurring within 1 to 48 hours) are usually manifested by rash and sometimes by fever. Delayed reactions (beginning more than 48 hours after exposure) can consist of skin reactions or other systemic reactions such as nephritis or serum sickness. In addition to these reactions, ampicillin and amoxicillin are commonly associated with a characteristic non-urticarial, maculopapular rash. The mechanism of this rash is not understood, but it is not an "allergic reaction." It usually starts 3 to 4 days after the onset of therapy. For reasons not understood, this reaction is much more frequent in patients with viral infections, especially mononucleosis, or when penicillin is taken together with allopurinol.

In deciding on therapy for a patient with a history of **penicillin allergy,** several facts should be kept in mind. The vast majority of patients who have been labelled as having a penicillin allergy will not have a reaction if given penicillin. This can be because the patient really was never allergic to penicillin and the adverse event was due to some other factor or a combination of factors. Examples of such factors include a viral infection causing a rash, for which antibiotic was inappropriately prescribed; some other drug or allergen to which the patient was exposed at the same time; or, in cases that occurred many years before, impurities in earlier preparations of penicillin. Other patients incorrectly refer to other types of adverse reactions, such as nausea, vomiting, or diarrhea, as an allergy. The other pos-

| TABLE 50-2 | Serum Concentrations and Protein Binding of Different Penicillins | | | |
| --- | --- | --- | --- | --- |
| | Dosage | | Serum Concentration | Protein Bound |
| Agent | (mg) | Route | (μg/mL) | (% at therapeutic concentrations) |
| Ampicillin | 1000 | IV | 40 | 20 |
| | 500 | PO | 4–6 | – |
| Cloxacillin | 500 | PO | 8 | 95 |
| Dicloxacillin | 250 | PO | 8 | 95 |
| Methicillin | 1000 | IV | 20–40 | 35–40 |
| Nafcillin | 15/kg | IV | 20–40 | 90–95 |
| Oxacillin | 1000 | IV | 40 | 90 |
| | 500 | PO | 4 | – |
| Penicillin G | ~670 | IV | 10 | 65 |
| | 500 | PO | 2 | – |
| Penicillin G procaine | 800 | IM | 3 | – |
| Penicillin G benzathine | 800 | IM | 0.1 | – |
| Penicillin V | 250 | PO | 2–3 | 80 |
| Carbenicillin | 5000 | IV | 200–300 | 50 |
| Ticarcillin | 3000 | IV | 150–200 | 50 |
| IV = intravenously; PO = by mouth. | | | | |

sibility is that the patient did have an allergic reaction to penicillin but has since lost the sensitivity to penicillin. About 10% of patients per year who have been previously positive on penicillin skin testing will lose their reactivity. Despite this fact, *the possible consequences make a past history of a severe reaction to penicillin a contraindication to its use unless skin testing (which includes the minor determinant) indicates that the patient is no longer allergic to penicillin.*

Alternatively, if the infection is life-threatening and can be adequately treated only with a penicillin (e.g., bacterial endocarditis), a program of **desensitization** is indicated. Unfortunately, there is not a good correlation between the nature of the penicillin reaction history and the probability of a severe adverse reaction on re-exposure; therefore, most physicians would *elect to use an alternative antibiotic* irrespective of the nature of the past history of penicillin allergy. Although adequate skin testing would solve most of these problems, the minor determinant is unstable and is not commercially available; therefore, penicillin skin testing that includes the minor determinants is, at present, available in only a few centres.

Convulsions and other forms of **encephalopathy** may occur with extremely high doses of penicillin. These reactions are more likely to occur in patients with renal insufficiency, a condition that predisposes to high serum concentrations of the penicillin. In addition, renal failure can lead to the accumulation of organic anions, which, like probenecid, inhibit the active anion transport system that pumps penicillin out of the CSF. These reactions are most closely related to the concentration of the penicillin in the CSF and have occurred more frequently in patients with meningeal inflammation.

**Interstitial nephritis** can occur during the course of therapy with any penicillin, although it is most frequently associated with the administration of methicillin. Hypokalemia may be a side effect of high-dose parenteral penicillin therapy because the penicillins act as non-reabsorbable anions.

Coombs' test–positive **hemolytic anemia** may occur with excessive doses, or on an allergic basis, with any of the penicillins. **Neutropenia**, which is reversible upon discontinuation of the drug, is also seen in some patients, especially those receiving methicillin, nafcillin, or cloxacillin. **Decreased platelet aggregation** has been noted at high concentrations of most penicillins but has been most marked with carbenicillin and ticarcillin. This may predispose to a bleeding diathesis.

## Drug Interactions

Penicillins in high concentrations bind to and inactivate aminoglycoside antibiotics (see Chapter 52) in vitro and in vivo. Therefore, penicillins and aminoglycosides should not be mixed in intravenous infusions, and when administered to the same patient, their infusions should be separated in time.

Penicillins and bacteriostatic drugs are often antagonistic in vitro, especially if the bacteria are exposed to the bacteriostatic agents first. The only in vivo example of this antagonism is the poorer outcome of *Streptococcus pneumoniae* meningitis treated with both penicillin and tetracycline than treated with penicillin alone.

Probenecid, indomethacin, sulfinpyrazone, and high-dose acetylsalicylic acid (>3 g/day) can block the tubular secretion of penicillins and may lead to prolonged high serum levels. Probenecid may also block the active transport of penicillin out of the CSF and thereby potentially lead to neurotoxicity, as described above.

## Dosage Regimens and Routes of Administration

Penicillins may be administered by the oral, intramuscular, or intravenous route. The choice of dosage, route, and regimen is dependent upon the specific agent, the infecting pathogen, and the seriousness and site of infection. The approximate daily dose of the penicillins that can be administered orally (penicillin V, ampicillin, cloxacillin, and oxacillin) ranges from 20 to 30 mg/kg. This amount is usually divided into four equal doses. The approximate daily dose of the penicillins that can be administered intravenously or intramuscularly (as in the treatment of serious infections requiring high blood levels of the antibiotic) is between 50 and 200 mg/kg for ampicillin, cloxacillin, methicillin, nafcillin, and oxacillin; 300 mg/kg for ticarcillin; 400 to 500 mg/kg for carbenicillin; and 100 000 to 200 000 IU/kg for aqueous benzyl penicillin G. (Penicillin G is prescribed in international units, 1 unit being equivalent to 0.6 µg.) The parenteral penicillins are usually administered in four to six equal doses per day. The longer-acting penicillin G preparations (procaine and benzathine) are administered as a single daily dose or as a single weekly to monthly dose, respectively. The approximate unit dose for these penicillins is 1.2 million units.

It must be emphasized that these are only broad guidelines. Considerable variation is observed among clinicians and institutions, even for similar indications.

## Therapeutic Applications

The penicillins belong to perhaps the most frequently prescribed class of antimicrobial agents.

Penicillins G and V are used for a variety of mild-to-severe infections proved or presumed to be caused by sensitive organisms. Examples of mild infections for which oral penicillin V would be indicated include pharyngitis and skin and soft tissue infections caused by group A *Streptococcus*. Moderate-to-severe infections treated with parenteral penicillin G include streptococcal pneumonia, meningitis caused by *S. pneumoniae* and *Neisseria meningi-*

*tidis,* gonorrhea, and syphilis, to name a few. However, the increasing incidence of penicillinase-producing *N. gonorrhoeae* has resulted in the replacement of penicillin by ceftriaxone for empirical (i.e., in the absence of bacterial diagnosis or sensitivity testing) treatment of gonorrhea. There are increasing reports from many parts of the world of strains of *S. pneumoniae* that have developed resistance to penicillin. In these areas, vancomycin or a third-generation cephalosporin is used to treat infections caused by these organisms.

Ampicillin has been used to treat mild-to-severe, Gram-negative, urinary tract infections, but the development of significant antibiotic resistance (25 to 30%) in common organisms such as *E. coli* has limited its widespread use of late.

Carbenicillin, ticarcillin, and piperacillin are used almost exclusively for *Pseudomonas* infections of the urinary tract, lung, and blood. These drugs should not be used in monotherapy because of the rapid development of resistance and are typically administered together with an aminoglycoside.

Cloxacillin, oxacillin, nafcillin, and methicillin are used almost exclusively for infections caused by staphylococci, including skin and soft tissue infections, pneumonia, osteomyelitis, endocarditis, and septicemia.

# CEPHALOSPORINS

*Cephalosporium acremonium,* the first source of the cephalosporins, was isolated from the sea near a sewer outlet off the Sardinian coast. Crude filtrates from cultures of this fungus inhibited the growth of *S. aureus* in vitro and cured staphylococcal infections in humans.

Since the original isolation of *C. acremonium* and the identification of its active product, cephalosporin C, many semi-synthetic derivatives and structurally related analogues have been developed. The newer derivatives possess an increasing spectrum of activity and diverse pharmacokinetic characteristics.

## Chemistry

The nucleus of cephalosporin C (7-aminocephalosporanic acid; Fig. 50-7), which formed the basis for all early cephalosporins, is closely related but not identical to the penicillin nucleus, 6-aminopenicillanic acid. It also contains a β-lactam ring, the chemical reactivity of which is responsible for the antibacterial activity, acid instability, susceptibility to β-lactamase hydrolysis, and hypersensitivity reactions to the cephalosporins. The diversity of the cephalosporins is based on the $R_1$ and $R_2$ substituents placed on the parent structure (see Fig. 50-7). As with penicillin, the presence of electron-withdrawing substituents on $R_1$ near the ring increases the stability in acid.

| FIGURE 50-7 | Structure of 7-aminocephalosporanic acid, the parent structure of cephalosporins, which are differentiated by substitutions at R₁ and R₂. A = dihydrothiazide ring; B = β-lactam ring. |
|---|---|

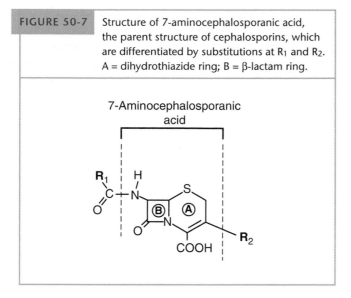

two representative agents from each generation are discussed, unless important differences exist for other members. The antibacterial activity of cephalosporins representative of each of the three generations is outlined in Table 50-4. The attainable serum concentrations of these antibiotics that can be related to the MICs are discussed below.

Resistance to the first-generation cephalosporins can be mediated by plasmid-encoded β-lactamase enzymes. These are typically found in certain strains of the Enterobacteriaceae, including *E. coli* and *Klebsiella*, and resistance is mediated by an enzyme called TEM. Resistance to third-generation cephalosporins may be due to either plasmid- or chromosome-mediated β-lactamase enzymes. Plasmid-mediated resistance is very uncommon, but it has been described in strains of *E. coli* and *Klebsiella* in which mutations have occurred in the amino acid structure of the TEM β-lactamase enzyme. Resistance is more commonly seen in certain strains of *Pseudomonas*, *Serratia*, and *Enterobacter*, in which high levels of chromosome-mediated β-lactamase activity are expressed.

## Bacterial Susceptibility

The evolution of cephalosporins and diversity of their properties have led to their division into three "generations." The original agents are referred to as first-generation cephalosporins, and the most recently introduced are referred to as third-generation cephalosporins. (Fourth-generation cephalosporins are currently being studied.) In general, with each new generation, the activity against Gram-negative organisms increases while that against Gram-positive organisms decreases. A list of representative cephalosporins from each generation is provided in Table 50-3. In the following account, the details of only one or

### First-generation cephalosporins

The prototype of this group of cephalosporins is **cephalothin,** which has a low oral bioavailability because of instability in acid. The acid-stable orally administered representative of this group is **cephalexin.** As outlined in Table 50-4, this antibiotic is very active against staphylococci, pneumococci, and streptococci except enterococci. Activity against aerobic and anaerobic Gram-negative organisms is limited, whereas there is good activity against *Clostridia* species and many of the other Gram-positive anaerobes. **Cefazolin,** another member of this generation,

| TABLE 50-3 | Generations of Cephalosporins | | |
|---|---|---|---|
| | First | Second | Third |
| Compounds for parenteral use | Cephalothin (Keflin) Cefazolin (Ancef, Kefzol) Cephaloridine (Ceflorin) | Cefamandole (Mandol) Cefoxitin (Mefoxin) Cefuroxime (Ceftin) Cefotetan (Cefotan) | Cefotaxime (Claforan) Cefoperazone (Cefobid) Ceftazidime (Captaz, Tazidime) Ceftizoxime (Cefizox) Ceftriaxone (Rocephin) |
| Compounds for oral use | Cephalexin (Keflex) Cephaloglycin (Kefglycin) Cephradine (Cefradex) Cefadroxil (Duricef) | Cefaclor (Ceclor) Cefuroxime axetil (Ceftin) | Cefixime (Suprax) |

| TABLE 50-4 | Median MICs (in µg/mL) of Some Cephalosporins | | | |
|---|---|---|---|---|
| Bacterium | Cephalothin | Cefamandole | Cefoxitin | Cefotaxime |
| Gram-positive | | | | |
| Staphylococcus aureus, penicillinase (–) | 0.2 | 0.25 | 3.1 | 2.0 |
| Staphylococcus aureus, penicillinase (+) | 0.4 | 0.5 | 3.1 | 2.0 |
| Streptococcus group A | 0.1 | 0.06 | 0.4 | 0.01 |
| Streptococcus viridans | — | 0.5 | 1.6 | 0.125 |
| Enterococcus faecalis | 50.0 | 32.0 | 100.0 | >128 |
| Streptococcus pneumoniae | 0.1 | 0.25 | 3.12 | 0.03 |
| Listeria | 4.0 | 6.0 | 25.0 | 25.0 |
| Clostridium | 0.4 | 0.12 | 1.0 | 0.25 |
| Gram-negative | | | | |
| Neisseria meningitidis | 0.5 | <0.125 | 0.12 | 0.004 |
| Neisseria gonorrhoeae | 3.1 | <0.125 | 0.12 | 0.015 |
| Haemophilus influenzae | 6.3 | 0.5 | 8.0 | 0.03 |
| Salmonella | 2.0 | 1.0 | 2.0 | 0.25 |
| Shigella | 125.0 | 2.0 | 25.0 | 0.25 |
| Klebsiella | 10.0 | 1.0 | 12.5 | 0.25 |
| Escherichia coli | 20.0 | 0.5 | 8.0 | 0.25 |
| Pseudomonas aeruginosa | >200 | >125 | >400 | 16.0 |
| Proteus mirabilis | 10.0 | 1.0 | 6.3 | 0.1 |
| Bacteroides fragilis | <25 | 64.0 | 16.0 | 8.0 |
| Other Bacteroides | 12.5 | 1.0 | 1.0 | — |

has somewhat more activity against aerobic Gram-negatives, especially against *E. coli* and *Klebsiella* species.

## Second-generation cephalosporins

**Cefuroxime, cefoxitin,** and **cefotetan** are three representative members of this group. Their Gram-positive spectrum is similar to that of the first-generation cephalosporins, but they possess increased activity against Gram-negative organisms. They are, however, inactive against *Pseudomonas* species. The principal advantage of cefuroxime is its activity against *H. influenzae* and its ability to penetrate the CNS, whereas that of cefoxitin and cefotetan is their broadened activity against anaerobic organisms. Strictly speaking, cefoxitin is not a cephalosporin derivative but rather a cephamycin, a fermentation product of *Streptomyces*. **Cefaclor** and **cefuroxime axetil** are the prototypical oral preparations of this group, with similar activity.

## Third-generation cephalosporins

**Cefotaxime, ceftriaxone,** and **ceftazidime** represent this rapidly increasing group of antibiotics. This generation retains most of the activity of the first two generations against Gram-positive bacteria but also possesses a remarkable amount of activity against Gram-negative organisms. Ceftazidime also has activity against many isolates of *Pseudomonas*. **Cefixime** is an oral agent belonging to this group. Although it has activity against the Enterobacteriaceae, the antibacterial activity is inferior to that of the intravenous members of this group.

## Pharmacokinetics

Cephalosporins designated for parenteral administration must be given by that route because they are poorly absorbed from the gastrointestinal tract. Cephalosporins designated for oral use, however, are almost completely absorbed, and serum concentrations are similar to those obtained after equivalent doses of the parenteral preparations. Serum concentrations of some of the cephalosporins after representative doses are outlined in Table 50-5.

The apparent volumes of distribution for the cephalosporins range from 0.1 to 0.4 L/kg, and their degree of plasma-protein binding at therapeutic concentrations ranges from 17 to 90% (see Table 50-5). The cephalosporins distribute widely throughout the body. The first- and second-generation derivatives (except cefuroxime), however, do not penetrate well into the CSF even in the presence of meningitis and, hence, must never be used to treat CNS infections. At least three of the third-generation cephalosporins (cefotaxime, ceftazidime, and ceftriaxone) do penetrate into the CSF to a sufficient degree (10 to 30%) to be the drugs of choice in the treatment of Gram-negative meningitis.

In general, the cephalosporins are not extensively biotransformed but are distributed and excreted principally in a biologically active form. The primary route of excretion for most of the cephalosporins is renal (60 to 100%), although there are exceptions. Ceftriaxone is excreted through both the biliary and urinary tracts.

Both glomerular filtration and tubular secretion are involved in the excretion of cephalosporins, although with some (e.g., cephaloridine, ceftriaxone, and ceftazidime), the amount of drug undergoing tubular secretion is negligible.

The elimination half-lives of the cephalosporins range from 0.5 to 8 hours depending on the specific agent, as noted in Table 50-5.

## Adverse Reactions

As with most antibiotics, the full spectrum of **hypersensitivity reactions**, including rash, hives, fever, eosinophilia, serum sickness, and anaphylaxis, may occur. It is estimated that primary allergic reactions to the cephalosporins are seen in approximately 5% of cases. Reversible neutropenia and thrombocytopenia, both of which may have an allergic basis, have been observed occasionally.

The incidence of allergic reactions to the cephalosporins is increased in patients known to be allergic to penicillins. The precise frequency of such cross-reactions is, however, unclear. Although traditional estimates have varied from 5 to 16% based on non-consecutive case reports and early formulations of cephalosporins, more recent estimates have been closer to 2% or lower. Whether or not these reactions are due to cross-sensitivity is unknown because the sensitivity to penicillin was not confirmed by skin testing, and, in addition, it may be that patients with a sensitivity to penicillin have a higher incidence of reactivity to immunologically unrelated drugs. It is generally held, however, that *all cephalosporins probably should be avoided in patients with a clear past history of anaphylaxis or immediate-type hypersensitivity to any of the penicillins.* It is reasonable, however, to consider their use in patients with a less severe type of reaction to the penicillins, such as a delayed skin rash, if they are otherwise the agents of choice against a particular infection.

Adverse reactions related to the route of administration are also common with the cephalosporins. These reactions include pain after intramuscular injection, phlebitis with intravenous administration, and minor gastrointestinal complaints with oral preparations.

Therapy with the cephalosporins may lead to the development of a positive direct Coombs' reaction, although it is not commonly associated with hemolytic anemia. The incidence of positive Coombs' test is approximately 3%.

Some of the cephalosporins (e.g., cephaloridine) have been withdrawn from use because of **dose-related nephrotoxicity**, probably resulting from proximal tubular damage. Interstitial nephritis has been described with some of the other cephalosporins (e.g., cephalothin); however, the risk of nephrotoxicity with currently available cephalosporins is very low.

The third-generation cephalosporins have also been associated with transient elevations of aspartate aminotransferase and alanine aminotransferase levels, reversible elevation of the blood urea nitrogen, and disturbances of vitamin K–dependent clotting function. This latter reaction is seen with cefamandole, cefotetan, and cefoperazone, which contain a methylthiotetrazole (MTT) ring. The MTT group competitively inhibits vitamin K–dependent carboxylase that is responsible for converting clotting factors II, VII, IX, and X to their active forms (see Chapter 38). The MTT group may also inhibit vitamin K–2,3-epoxide

| TABLE 50-5 | Serum Concentrations, Half-Lives, and Protein Binding of Different Cephalosporins | | | | |
|---|---|---|---|---|---|
| | Dosage | | Serum Concentration | Protein Bound (% at therapeutic | Half-Life |
| Drug | (mg) | Route | (µg/mL) | concentrations) | (hours) |
| Cephalothin | 1000 | IV | 40–60 | 60–70 | 0.5 |
| Cefazolin | 1000 | IV | 90–120 | 85 | 1.5 |
| Cephalexin | 500 | PO | 15–20 | low | 0.5–1.0 |
| Cefoxitin | 1000 | IV | 60–80 | 70 | 1.0 |
| Cefamandole | 1000 | IV | 60–80 | 70 | 1.0 |
| Cefaclor | 200 | PO | 6 | — | 0.5 |
| Cefotaxime | 1000 | IV | 41 | 40 | 1.1 |
| Ceftriaxone | 1000 | IV | 145 | 90 | 8.0 |
| Cefoperazone | 1000 | IV | 125 | 90 | 2.0 |
| Ceftazidime | 1000 | IV | 83 | 17 | 1.8 |

IV = intravenously; PO = by mouth

reductase that converts inactive vitamin K to its active form. This same structure also inhibits aldehyde dehydrogenase and can lead to a disulfiram-like reaction when the patient drinks alcohol (see Chapter 22).

## Drug Interactions

Although it was once believed that cephalosporins enhanced the nephrotoxicity of aminoglycosides, more recent studies have found no evidence for such an interaction.

Cephalosporins may produce a "false-positive" glycosuric reaction with Clinitest.

Uricosuric agents such as probenecid may decrease the clearance of some cephalosporins by blocking renal tubular secretion.

## Dosage Regimens and Routes of Administration

Cephalosporins may be administered by the oral, intramuscular, or intravenous route, depending on the specific agent and the therapeutic indications (see Table 50-3). In general, however, the intramuscular agents are avoided as they tend to cause pain upon injection. The approximate daily dose of the cephalosporins that can be administered orally ranges from 25 to 50 mg/kg. This amount is usually divided into two to four equal doses. The approximate daily dose of the cephalosporins that are administered intravenously is 50 to 200 mg/kg. This amount is usually divided into two to six equal doses depending on the half-life of the individual agents (see Table 50-5). Agents with the longest half-lives (e.g., ceftriaxone) may be administered every 24 hours, whereas those with short half-lives (e.g., cephalothin) must usually be administered every 4 to 6 hours.

As emphasized with the penicillins, these are only broad dosing guidelines, and considerable variation is common in clinical practice.

## Therapeutic Applications

The therapeutic applications of the cephalosporins are different for each of the three generations, and, therefore, each will be considered separately.

**First-generation cephalosporins** are rarely the antibiotics of first choice; however, they are useful for infections caused by penicillin-resistant staphylococci, *Klebsiella* species, and urinary tract infections resistant to penicillins and sulfonamides. This group of antibiotics, particularly cefazolin, is also useful for short-term perioperative prophylaxis for certain operations carrying a high risk of infections caused by Gram-positive organisms but in which Gram-negative organisms cannot be ruled out. They may also be useful in patients with a history of minor penicillin allergy but should not be administered to patients who have had immediate or accelerated penicillin reactions.

The broadened spectrum of activity of **second-generation cephalosporins** increases their range of potential therapeutic applications, although they also are rarely the antibiotic of first choice. The activity of cefuroxime against Gram-positive cocci as well as against β-lactamase-producing *H. influenzae* makes it a theoretically attractive agent for infections that might be caused by one or more of these organisms. It is particularly useful in pediatric infections, including otitis media and pneumonia.

Cefoxitin and cefotetan, with their effectiveness against anaerobic and Gram-negative organisms, are potentially useful single agents for short-term perioperative prophylaxis for pelvic or abdominal operations. Increasing resistance of *Bacteroides fragilis* to the cefamycins has been worrisome, and they should not be relied upon as the sole treatment for these infections.

The most important indication for the **third-generation cephalosporins** is the treatment of meningitis caused by Gram-negative aerobes. Although they have not replaced aminoglycosides, the third-generation cephalosporins can sometimes be used instead of the more toxic combination of a penicillin and an aminoglycoside. Their indications also include the treatment of hospital-acquired, Gram-negative aerobic infections or those otherwise rendered resistant to multiple antibiotics, empirical treatment in neutropenic patients, and some intra-abdominal infections. Single-dose ceftriaxone is effective for the treatment of gonorrhea, even when the organism is resistant to penicillin.

## β-LACTAMASE INHIBITORS

The resistance of many bacteria to penicillins is due to their production of β-lactamase; therefore, the co-administration of an agent that inhibits β-lactamase would extend the antibacterial spectrum of the penicillins. Examples of such agents are **clavulanic acid, sulbactam,** and **tazobactam.** These compounds act as "suicide" inhibitors by irreversibly binding to the bacterial β-lactamases that would otherwise inactivate the penicillins.

Clavulanic acid (Fig. 50-8) is a naturally occurring β-lactam isolated from *Streptomyces clavuligerus*. Sulbactam and tazobactam are semi-synthetic penicillanic acid sulfones. None of these agents has significant antibacterial activity when used alone; they are used solely to extend the activity of penicillins or cephalosporins. Current examples of such combinations are amoxicillin–clavulanic acid, ticarcillin–clavulanic acid, ampicillin–sulbactam, piperacillin–clavulanic acid, and piperacillin–tazobactam. The β-lactamase inhibitors have pharmacokinetic parameters similar to those of penicillin; their major route of elimination is renal. Their half-lives are about 1 hour but are increased in neonates and the elderly. Unlike the penicillins, however, their half-lives are not increased by probenecid.

The combination of amoxicillin–clavulanic acid is useful for the oral treatment of otitis media, sinusitis, and infections of the lower respiratory tract caused by β-lactamase-producing strains of pathogens. The combination of ticarcillin–clavulanic acid increases the activity of ticarcillin against β-lactamase-producing strains of *S. aureus, H. influenzae, N. gonorrhoeae, E. coli, Klebsiella,* and *B. fragilis.* The combination of ampicillin–sulbactam has broad-spectrum activity in the treatment of infections caused by β-lactamase-producing strains of *H. influenzae, Branhamella catarrhalis, Neisseria,* many anaerobes, *E. coli, Proteus, Klebsiella, S. aureus,* and *S. epidermidis.* The combination of piperacillin–tazobactam increases the activity of piperacillin against β-lactamase-producing strains of *E. coli, Klebsiella, Bacteroides,* and *Haemophilus.*

## CARBAPENEMS

**Imipenem** is the first of a new class of β-lactam antibiotics, the carbapenems (see Fig. 50-8). It is a more stable derivative of the natural product, thienamycin. Imipenem is inactivated by a dehydropeptidase in the brush border of the kidney, and therefore it is given in combination with an inhibitor of this enzyme, **cilastatin,** which increases tissue and urinary levels of active drug. **Meropenem** is a newer carbapenem with a similar spectrum of activity to imipenem, but it does not have to be administered with

cilastatin. It is also easier to administer in patients with abnormal renal function. All carbapenems currently available have poor oral bioavailability and are only used intravenously. A newer carbapenem called **ertapenem** is also available for intravenous use but lacks activity against *P. aeruginosa.* There are newer carbapenems in development that will be formulated for oral administration.

## Bacterial Susceptibility

Imipenem has the broadest spectrum of all antibacterial agents that are presently available for clinical use. It is active against most Gram-positive and Gram-negative bacteria, including anaerobes; however, methicillin-resistant staphylococci are usually resistant to imipenem, and it is not active against *Chlamydia* and *Mycoplasma.* Although it is active against *Legionella* in vitro, it may not be useful clinically because *Legionella* are intracellular organisms. It is active against most anaerobes, including *B. fragilis,* but has low activity against *Clostridium difficile.* Imipenem is active against *P. aeruginosa,* but resistant strains have already emerged. When resistance appears, it is usually due to a modification of the cell wall that prevents penetration of the drug. Less commonly, resistance results from modification of penicillin-binding proteins or from the induction of β-lactamases that are capable of inactivating the β-lactam ring of imipenem. Imipenem is a potent inducer of cephalosporinases, which do not hydrolyze imipenem itself, but do hydrolyze a broad range of other β-lactam antibiotics; therefore, it is irrational to combine imipenem with other β-lactam antibiotics.

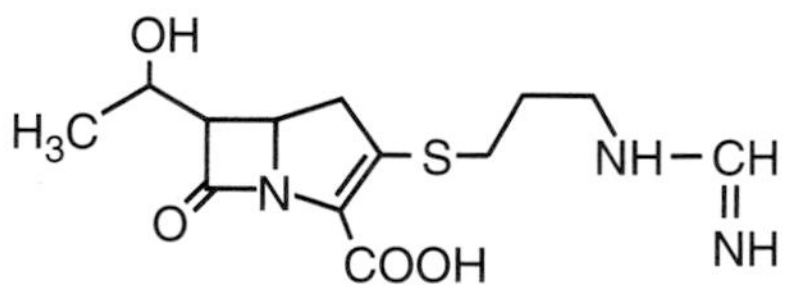

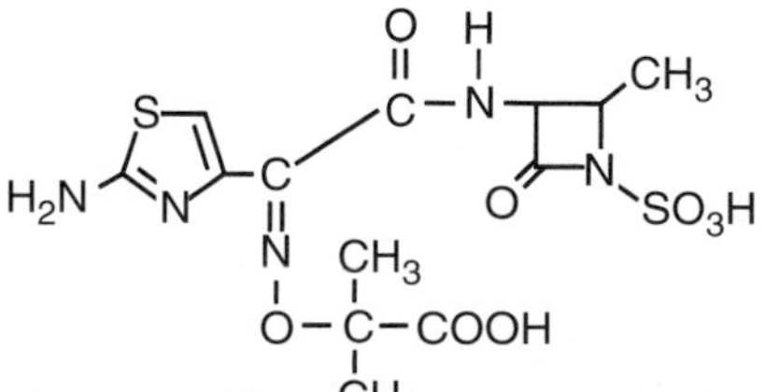

## Pharmacokinetics

Imipenem is administered intravenously. Its clearance is renal, and cilastatin increases the proportion of the intact drug that is cleared from 20 to 70%. The average half-life is 1 hour. Penetration of the CNS is variable, but because imipenem can cause seizures, it is not usually used for the treatment of meningitis. Meropenem has less of a propensity to cause seizures, particularly in patients with abnormal renal function.

## Adverse Reactions

The most common adverse reactions are pain at the site of infusion, nausea and vomiting, and diarrhea. In one study, a rash or drug fever occurred in 2.7% of patients, and seizures in 1.5%. When seizures occur, they are usually associated with use of imipenem in patients with CNS abnormalities or renal failure. The degree of cross-reactivity between carbapenems and penicillins has not been accurately determined, but it appears to be even higher than that between penicillins and cephalosporins, so carbapenems should not be used in patients with a clear history of an anaphylactic reaction to penicillin.

**FIGURE 50-8** Structures of other β-lactams.

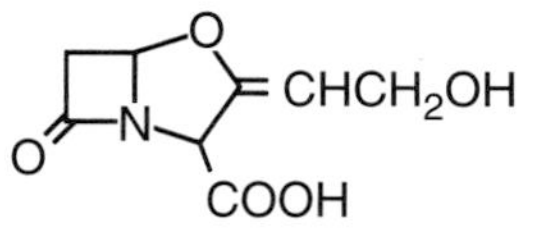

## Therapeutic Applications

Its broad spectrum of activity makes imipenem most useful for severe infections with mixed bacterial flora. The number of well-controlled studies comparing it with other therapy is limited, and for many indications, such as intra-abdominal infections, pneumonia, and empirical therapy of febrile patients with cancer and neutropenia, imipenem is probably not significantly better than conventional therapy, although it may have fewer side effects. In order to slow the emergence of resistant bacteria, its use should be limited to those infections for which less broad-spectrum (and less costly) agents cannot be used.

## Dosage and Routes of Administration

Imipenem is available only for intravenous administration in combination with cilastatin (Primaxin). The dose depends on the susceptibility of the organism and the type of infection being treated; however, the usual daily dose for patients with normal renal function is 2 g divided into four doses. For patients with glomerular filtration rates less than 30 mL/min, the dose should be decreased by 50%.

## MONOBACTAMS

As the name suggests, the monobactams have a β-lactam ring, which, unlike that of penicillins and cephalosporins, is not fused to a second ring. The first of the monobactams to be marketed, **aztreonam** (Azactam; see Fig. 50-8), contains a sulfonic acid group attached to the N of the β-lactam ring, which activates the β-lactam ring but also limits oral absorption. Aztreonam is therefore used only parenterally, usually by intramuscular injection. This agent is not universally available.

## Bacterial Susceptibility

Although the mechanism of action of the monobactams is similar to that of other β-lactams, aztreonam does not bind to the penicillin-binding proteins of Gram-positive bacteria or anaerobic organisms; therefore, activity is limited to aerobic Gram-negative organisms. Aztreonam is not hydrolyzed by most β-lactamases, but it is destroyed by those that hydrolyze cefotaxime or ceftazidime. It is active against most Enterobacteriaceae and all isolates of *N. gonorrhoeae, N. meningitidis,* and *H. influenzae.* Although it has activity against *P. aeruginosa* and *Enterobacter* species, some strains may be resistant.

## Therapeutic Applications

Except for its lack of activity against Gram-positive organisms, aztreonam has a spectrum of activity similar to that of the aminoglycosides. It has been demonstrated to be effective in the treatment of urinary tract infections due to Enterobacteriaceae, *P. aeruginosa,* and *Providencia,* some of which were resistant to penicillins, first- and second-generation cephalosporins, and aminoglycosides. It has also been used to treat urinary tract, pelvic, and peritoneal infections; pneumonia; and osteomyelitis, either as a single agent or in combination with other drugs. Dosage can range from 0.5 to 1.0 g every 8 to 12 hours to as much as 2 g every 6 to 8 hours in life-threatening infections.

## Pharmacokinetics

Aztreonam is almost completely absorbed from injection sites and distributes into virtually all body fluids. After an intravenous dose of 2 g, aztreonam reaches CSF concentrations of 2 µg/mL at 1 hour and 3.2 µg/mL at 4 hours. Its plasma half-life is 1.5 to 2 hours, and elimination is mainly by excretion in the urine by both glomerular filtration and tubular secretion. Dosage may therefore have to be reduced if renal function is impaired.

## Adverse Reactions

Aztreonam is usually well tolerated, and the pattern of adverse effects is similar to that of other β-lactam antibiotics. Despite having a β-lactam ring, aztreonam shows little cross-reactivity to antibodies against penicillins and cephalosporins, and it has been used safely in some patients with positive skin test reactions against penicillin.

## VANCOMYCIN

Vancomycin (Vancocin) was isolated from *Streptomyces orientalis,* an actinomycete found in soil samples from Indonesia and India. It was purified and characterized in 1956. The agent is not chemically related to any of the other antimicrobial agents in present use. It is an unusual glycopeptide containing a chlorinated polyphenyl ether and has a molecular mass of about 1500 Da.

## Bacterial Susceptibility

The primary activity of vancomycin is against Gram-positive bacteria. The importance of this agent has increased with the emergence of organisms resistant to the anti-staphylococcal penicillins and with better purification techniques that have reduced its toxicity. The vast majority of staphylococcal species, including penicillinase-negative and -positive strains, and streptococcal species, including enterococci, are killed by less than 1.6 µg/mL of this antibiotic. Gram-positive bacilli, including *Clostridium* species, are also very sensitive to vancomycin. Gram-negative bacteria are invariably resistant. Recently, strains of enterococci resistant to this agent have been reported. This is of great concern, as there are now no effective antibiotics available to treat these strains.

## Pharmacokinetics

Vancomycin is not absorbed from the gastrointestinal tract. A single intravenous dose of 10 mg/kg in adults produces serum concentrations of 20 to 30 µg/mL at 1 to 2 hours after the infusion.

The volume of distribution of vancomycin is 0.5 to 0.9 L/kg. The drug is less than 10% protein-bound. It appears in various body fluids, and 20 to 30% is detectable in the CSF when the meninges are inflamed.

Vancomycin is normally not biotransformed in the body. It is excreted by the kidneys, and about 80 to 90% of a dose can be recovered from the urine during the first 24 hours. Its serum half-life is 6 to 9 hours.

## Adverse Reactions

Sustained high serum concentrations of vancomycin, in excess of 60 to 80 µg/mL, have been associated with hearing loss. Nephrotoxicity is rare at recommended doses and when vancomycin is used without other nephrotoxins. The early reports of this complication may have been due to an impurity in the formulation. Both ototoxicity and nephrotoxicity are more common when the drug is used together with an aminoglycoside. A "red man" syndrome consisting of flushing and a maculopapular rash on face, neck, trunk, and extremities may occur during, or shortly after, intravenous administration. It is believed to be caused by histamine release, and although not an allergic reaction, it may lead to hypotension, tachycardia, shock, and, rarely, cardiac arrest. This syndrome is most likely to occur if vancomycin is administered rapidly as an intravenous bolus; therefore, the dose should be infused over a period of 45 to 60 minutes.

## Drug Interactions

Cholestyramine can bind vancomycin *if the two drugs are administered together orally.* Heparin also binds to vancomycin and inactivates it if the two are mixed in the same intravenous line. The ototoxicity and nephrotoxicity of vancomycin may be increased by co-administration with aminoglycosides and other drugs associated with these toxicities.

## Dosage and Routes of Administration

Because vancomycin is not absorbed from the gastrointestinal tract, it should be administered orally only if high concentrations in the intestinal lumen are desired (see below). The recommended daily intravenous dose is 20 to 30 mg/kg divided into two or three doses.

## Therapeutic Applications

The primary clinical use of vancomycin is the treatment of severe staphylococcal and streptococcal (including enterococcal) infections in patients who are allergic to penicillin. In addition, some recently isolated staphylococci and *S. pneumoniae* with multiple resistance to other antibiotics are sensitive only to this antibiotic.

Vancomycin is administered orally in the treatment of antibiotic-associated pseudomembranous colitis but is used only as a third-line drug for this purpose. This illness is caused by the toxin produced by *C. difficile.*

## BACITRACIN

In contrast to the penicillins and cephalosporins, which act on the *outside* of microbial cells, inhibit transpeptidation and cross-linking of peptidoglycan strands, and thus interfere with bacterial cell wall synthesis in susceptible microorganisms, bacitracin acts *intracellularly* by binding to, and rendering unusable, the isoprenyl phosphate lipid carrier responsible for transport of cell wall precursors from the bacterial cytoplasm to the exterior of the cell membrane (see Fig. 50-2). Bacitracin therefore lacks the high degree of selective antibacterial toxicity of the majority of antibiotics classified as cell wall inhibitors, and it is capable of also causing damage to susceptible mammalian cells.

Because of an unacceptably high degree of nephrotoxicity when administered systemically, the use of bacitracin in anti-infective therapy is confined to topical administration in the form of ophthalmic and skin ointments and as a powder for specialized topical applications, from which it cannot be absorbed.

Bacitracin inhibits a variety of Gram-positive cocci and bacilli and some *Neisseria* and *Haemophilus* species. Because of its limitations in treating superficial skin infections when used alone, it is available for topical use in mixtures with neomycin and/or polymyxin. Its other main clinical use is in the eradication of nasal carriage of *S. aureus.*

Hypersensitivity reactions to bacitracin are very rare.

## CYCLOSERINE

Cycloserine (Seromycin), an antibiotic isolated from *Streptomyces orchidaceus,* interferes with the *intracellular* synthesis of glycopeptides that are required, after transfer to the outside, for the construction of bacterial cell walls. As noted at the beginning of this chapter, cycloserine inhibits the conversion of L-alanine to D-alanine and the linking of two D-molecules (see Fig. 50-3).

The antibiotic has marked in vitro inhibitory activity against *Mycobacterium tuberculosis,* without cross-resistance between cycloserine and other anti-tubercular agents. Resistance develops, however, because of bacterial enzyme adaptation and altered pathways in cell wall synthesis.

Cycloserine is well absorbed after oral administration, is well tolerated by the GI tract, and is distributed widely in tissues, body fluids, and the CSF. About two-thirds of a dose is excreted unchanged in the urine, and the remainder is biotransformed to unknown metabolites. Peak plasma concentrations of the drug are reached in about 3 to 4 hours, with a plasma half-life of about 10 hours. The usual adult dose of cycloserine is 250 mg twice a day, which is associated with a negligible risk of toxicity.

The most common adverse reactions, such as excitement, aggression, confusion, depression, hyperreflexia, and focal or tonic–clonic seizures, result from the drug's considerable CNS toxicity. This CNS toxicity can be minimized by limiting peak plasma concentrations to less than 30 μg/mL. A history of epilepsy, severe depression, or severe anxiety are contraindications to the use of cycloserine.

Cycloserine is considered a second-line, anti-tubercular drug, useful for re-treatment or in the presence of microbial resistance to other drugs, and it must always be given in combination with other effective drugs, as outlined in Chapter 53. Although its use had decreased, it is increasing again for the management of infections caused by multidrug-resistant strains of *M. tuberculosis* (MDRTb) encountered in prisons, hospitals, and shelters in various parts of the world.

# ISONIAZID (INH)

Isoniazid (INH; Fig. 50-9) was discovered in 1952. It is the hydrazide of isonicotinic acid and has proved to be the most useful antimicrobial agent for the treatment and prophylaxis of tuberculosis.

INH is bactericidal against actively replicating *M. tuberculosis* and bacteriostatic against non-replicating organisms. Resting organisms resume multiplication when drug contact is ended. The minimal tuberculostatic concentration is 0.025 to 0.05 μg/mL.

Among the variety of proposed mechanisms of action, there is strong evidence that the primary action of INH is inhibition of oxygen-dependent synthetic pathways of mycolic acid, an important and unique constituent of mycobacterial cell walls. The inhibition of mycolic acid synthesis by INH produces very rapid effects on mycobacteria (in 60 to 90 minutes), whereas the inhibition of DNA synthesis is slow (10 to 12 hours). The effects on mycolic acid synthesis are obtained with the lowest effective con-

centration of isoniazid, and they are seen in INH-sensitive mycobacteria, but not in INH-resistant strains.

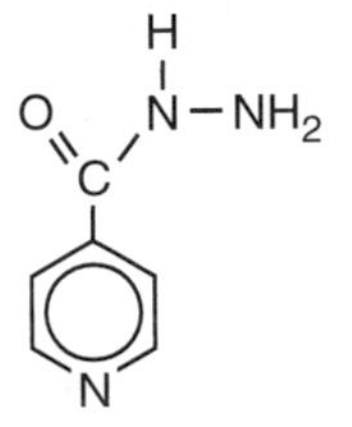

## Pharmacokinetics

Isoniazid is readily absorbed after oral administration. Peak plasma levels of 1 to 5 μg/mL are attained 1 to 2 hours after an oral dose of 5 mg/kg.

The volume of distribution of INH is approximately 0.6 L/kg. It is poorly protein-bound, diffuses readily into all body fluids and cells, and is present, in varying concentrations, in all body organs. Cerebrospinal fluid penetration is variable, but CSF concentrations may be nearly equal to those in serum. Isoniazid penetrates well into the caseous material in the central parts of the tubercles from which the disease gets its name. Infected tissues retain the drug for long periods of time in quantities well above those required for tuberculostasis.

The main method of inactivation of the drug is acetylation in the liver by the enzyme *N*-acetyltransferase, which converts INH to acetylisoniazid. This, in turn, is partly hydrolyzed to isonicotinic acid and acetylhydrazine. Non-acetylated INH is excreted in the urine in its unchanged form or as its hydrazone conjugates. The rate of INH acetylation is genetically controlled. The amount of INH acetylation metabolites in the urine reflects the acetylator status of the patient. About 90% of Asians are rapid acetylators, compared with about 45% of Caucasians and Blacks (see Chapter 10).

Approximately 70% of administered INH is excreted via the kidneys, but most of this is in an inactive form. Slow acetylators excrete about 10 times more active INH in the urine than do rapid acetylators. The half-life of INH is 0.5 to 1.5 hours in rapid acetylators, compared with 2 to 3 hours in slow acetylators.

## Adverse Reactions

Neurotoxicity and hepatotoxicity are the two most important side effects of INH. The incidence of neurotoxicity is higher in slow acetylators, but acetylator phenotype probably has no bearing on the incidence of hepatotoxicity. It was once thought that patients with the rapid acetylator phenotype had the highest risk of hepatotoxicity because the mechanism appears to involve an acetylhydrazine intermediate; however, although acetylhydrazine is formed more rapidly in rapid acetylators, it is also converted rapidly to non-toxic diacetylhydrazine.

**Neurotoxic manifestations,** including psychosis, confusion, convulsions, and coma, may occur with overdosage. Peripheral neuropathy may occur at therapeutic doses, but it is more common with larger doses than smaller ones and in older or malnourished patients with pyridoxine deficiency. The administration of pyridoxine prevents this toxicity.

| FIGURE 50-9 | Structural formula of isoniazid. |

**Hepatotoxicity** is an age-related occurrence more prevalent in patients over 35 years old. Hepatitis may progress to hepatocellular necrosis with jaundice if the drug is not discontinued. Alcoholics are more prone to this liver injury. An early asymptomatic transient rise in serum transaminases is noted in about 20% of INH recipients, but this does not, in itself, necessitate discontinuance of INH.

A significant number of INH recipients develop antinuclear antibodies, and some develop a lupus-like syndrome. This is reversible with discontinuation of the drug. The incidence of this adverse reaction is probably higher in slow acetylators.

## Drug Interactions

Aluminum hydroxide or other antacids may interfere with the absorption of INH. Also, isoniazid may inhibit the cytochrome P450–mediated metabolism of phenytoin or anticoagulants, thereby causing excessively high serum concentrations and related toxicity of these drugs.

## Dosage Regimen, Route of Administration, and Therapeutic Applications

Isoniazid is usually administered orally as a single daily dose of 5 to 10 mg/kg. If pyridoxine is given concomitantly, its dose is 10 mg for every 100 mg of INH.

Isoniazid is a first-line tuberculocidal drug. It is used in combination with various other anti-tubercular drugs for the treatment of all types of tuberculosis (TB). Isoniazid is also used as a prophylactic agent in persons infected with *M. tuberculosis* but who do not have active disease. Isoniazid prophylaxis (300 mg/day for 6 to 12 months) is recommended for persons with a positive tuberculin skin test, without evidence of active disease, who (1) are under 35 years of age; (2) have demonstrated TB skin test conversion; (3) have household contacts of active cases of pulmonary TB; (4) are over 35 years of age with an increased risk of reactivation, especially those with silicosis, immunosuppression, dialysis, or gastrectomy; (5) are co-infected with HIV; or (6) have old fibrotic scars on chest X-ray. If the person is thought to be infected with an INH-resistant strain, either INH plus rifampin or rifampin alone (see Chapter 53) can be considered.

It is important to remember that approximately one in $10^6$ tubercle bacilli is resistant to isoniazid and one cavitary lesion usually contains $10^7$ to $10^9$ bacilli; therefore, combination therapy (e.g., isoniazid and rifampin) must be used to treat active disease to prevent the emergence of a resistant infection. This is in contrast to prophylactic therapy in patients with a positive TB skin test, where there are only a few dormant tubercle bacilli present, and treatment with isoniazid as a single agent is appropriate.

## ETHAMBUTOL

Ethambutol (Myambutol) was discovered in 1961 when randomly selected compounds were being tested for anti-tubercular activity. It is a relatively simple molecule, consisting of two residues of aminobutanol connected by an ethylene bridge. Ethambutol is bacteriostatic against *M. tuberculosis,* with in vitro activity against about 75% of strains at a concentration of 1 μg/mL.

Ethambutol does inhibit RNA synthesis, but it simultaneously inhibits the transfer of mycolic acid into the cell walls of mycobacteria. Ethambutol was also shown to break the "exclusion barrier" in cell walls, thus enabling other drugs to penetrate into cells.

## Pharmacokinetics

Ethambutol is well absorbed after oral administration. Peak serum concentrations of approximately 5 μg/mL are attained about 4 hours after a 15 mg/kg dose.

The apparent volume of distribution of ethambutol approximates 1.5 L/kg. It is 20 to 30% protein-bound in plasma. There are no data available on its distribution to various body tissues. However, it is known that levels equal to 25 to 50% of the serum concentration are attained in the CSF when the meninges are inflamed.

Between 8 and 15% of absorbed ethambutol is converted to various inactive metabolites, which are excreted in the urine together with approximately 80% of absorbed drug in its active unchanged form. About 20% of an oral dose is unabsorbed and excreted unchanged in the feces.

## Adverse Reactions

The most important adverse reaction to ethambutol is a **reversible retrobulbar neuropathy,** which results in defective red–green vision and eventual field constriction or blindness. The incidence of this reaction increases with increasing doses, reaching approximately 5% of patients at 25 to 50 mg/kg/day. Patients should have baseline visual acuity tests and then be monitored regularly every 4 to 6 weeks. They should be instructed to promptly report optic symptoms.

## Dosage Regimen, Route of Administration, and Therapeutic Applications

Ethambutol is administered orally as a single daily dose of 15 to 25 mg/kg. Its main use is in combination with other antimicrobial agents to treat infections caused by *M. tuberculosis.* It is also increasingly used in combination with other agents to treat *Mycobacterium avium* and *Mycobacterium intracellulare* infections in patients with AIDS.

FIGURE 50-10 | Structural formula of caspofungin.

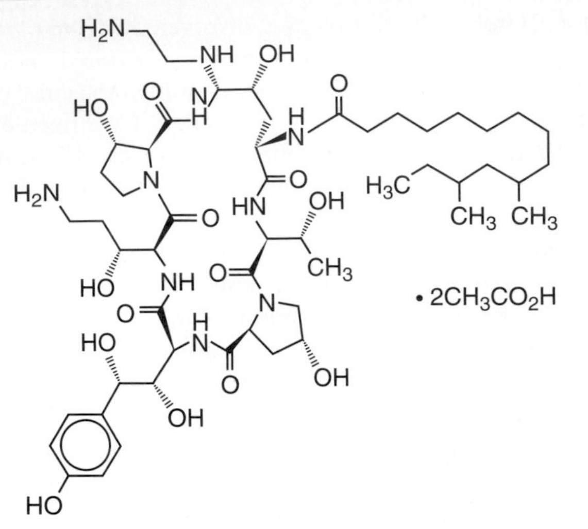

and mild adverse events at usual human doses, and they do not interact with cytochrome P450, so they have only a minimal tendency for interactions with other drugs.

## SUGGESTED READINGS

Boucher HW, Groll AH, Chiou CC, Walsh TJ. Newer systemic antifungal agents: pharmacokinetics, safety and efficacy. *Drugs.* 2004;64:1997-2020.

Cunha BA. Vancomycin. *Med Clin North Am.* 1995;79:817-832.

Denning DW. Echinocandin antifungal drugs. *Lancet.* 2003;362: 142-151.

Drobniewski F, Balabanova Y, Coker R. Clinical features, diagnosis, and management of multiple drug-resistant tuberculosis since 2002. *Curr Opin Pulm Med.* 2004;10:211-217.

Hellinger WC, Brewer NS. Carbapenems and monobactams: imipenem, meropenem and azteronam. *Mayo Clin Proc.* 1999; 74:420-434.

Joumana N, Araj GF. Recent developments in β lactamases and extended spectrum β lactamases. *BMJ.* 2003;327:1209-1213.

Klein NC, Cunha BA. Third-generation cephalosporins. *Med Clin North Am.* 1995;79:705-720.

Marshall WF, Blair JE. The cephalosporins. *Mayo Clin Proc.* 1999; 74:187-195.

Nagarajan R. Antibacterial activities and modes of action of vancomycin and related glycopeptides. *Antimicrob Agents Chemother.* 1991;35:605-609.

Neu HC. Beta-lactam antibiotics: structural relationships affecting in vitro activity and pharmacologic properties. *Rev Infect Dis.* 1986;8(suppl 3):S237-S259.

Neu HC. The crisis in antibiotic resistance. *Science.* 1992;257: 1064-1072.

Norrby SR. Carbapenems. *Med Clin North Am.* 1995;79:745-760.

Rastogi N, David HL. Mode of action of antituberculous drugs and mechanisms of drug resistance in *Mycobacterium tuberculosis. Res Microbiol.* 1993;144:133-143.

Sahm DF, Kissinger J, Gilmore US, et al. In vitro susceptibility studies of vancomycin-resistant *Enterococcus faecalis. Antimicrob Agents Chemother.* 1989;33:1588-1591.

Sensacovic JW, Smith LG. Beta-lactamase inhibitor combinations. *Med Clin North Am.* 1995;79:695-704.

Swanson DS, Starke JR. Drug-resistant tuberculosis in pediatrics. *Pediatr Clin North Am.* 1995;42:553-582.

Tan JS, File TM. Antipseudomonal penicillins. *Med Clin North Am.* 1995;79:679-694.

Tomasz A. Penicillin-binding proteins and the antibacterial effectiveness of beta-lactam antibiotics. *Rev Infect Dis.* 1986; 8(suppl 3):S260-S278.

Zhang Y. The magic bullets and tuberculosis drug targets. *Annu Rev Pharmacol Toxicol.* 2005;45:529-564.

## A NEW CLASS OF ANTIFUNGALS: ECHINOCANDINS

The targets of most antifungal drugs are either the fungal *cell membrane* or the synthesis of fungal *nucleic acids*; those drugs are described in detail in Chapters 51 and 53, respectively. However, a new class of antifungal drugs, known as the echinocandins, targets the fungal *cell wall* and therefore belongs appropriately in this chapter. The echinocandins are large, cyclic, hexapeptide molecules with lipophilic side chains that inhibit 1,3-β-D-glucan synthase, an enzyme that catalyzes a key step in fungal cell wall synthesis. Currently, three echinocandin drugs exist: **caspofungin, anidulafungin,** and **micafungin.** Caspofungin (Fig. 50-10) was the first one in clinical use. All echinocandins currently available have poor oral bioavailability and are for intravenous use only.

The echinocandins have a narrower spectrum of antifungal activity than amphotericin B; they are active mainly against *Aspergillus* and *Candida* species. In particular, the activity of caspofungin is fungicidal against *Candida.* and clinical evidence suggests that it is equivalent to amphotericin B in the treatment of invasive candidal infections. Combination therapy with caspofungin and voriconazole appears to be particularly effective against invasive *Aspergillus* and *Candida* infections in patients with compromised immune systems. One advantage of the echinocandins is that they cause only uncommon

# 51

# Antimicrobial and Antifungal Agents That Act on Cell Membranes

## J UETRECHT, EJ PHILLIPS, AND SL WALMSLEY

## CASE HISTORY

A 35-year-old gay man who was HIV-positive and had a CD4 count of $150 \times 106/L$ saw his physician because of complaints of dry mouth and sore throat. Clinical examination showed that he had developed oral thrush (candidiasis), which was successfully treated with "swish and swallow" nystatin, 500 000 IU three times daily for 7 days. Six months later, he had a recurrent episode of thrush, which responded to similar treatment.

Three months later, the patient saw his physician with a complaint of retrosternal discomfort on swallowing. Endoscopy confirmed the diagnosis of esophageal candidiasis. The patient was therefore treated with oral ketoconazole, 200 mg/day for a period of 2 weeks, and showed improvement. Because the patient tolerated the drug well, it was decided to continue oral ketoconazole, 200 mg/day, as secondary prophylaxis.

One year later, the patient came to the emergency room with a 5-day history of bifrontal headache, fever, and chills. The headache increased when he bent over or coughed, and he had vomited on four occasions. On physical examination he looked unwell and had a temperature of 39°C. There were no focal neurological deficits and there was no neck stiffness. A lumbar puncture was performed, and India ink examination of the cerebrospinal fluid (CSF) showed budding yeast cells that were confirmed on culture as *Cryptococcus neoformans*. A cryptococcal antigen test of the CSF was reported positive with a titre of 1:5096. The patient was admitted and was treated with intravenous amphotericin B at a dose of 1 mg/kg/day. After 2 weeks, he had improved significantly and treatment was changed to oral fluconazole at a dose of 400 mg/day. After a total of 6 weeks of treatment, the lumbar puncture was repeated, and the CSF cultures for cryptococci were reported negative. Therefore, the dose of fluconazole was decreased to 200 mg/day, which was continued indefinitely as secondary prophylaxis against cryptococci.

## MECHANISMS OF ACTION

Cytoplasmic membranes maintain the intracellular contents, both by controlling passive diffusion and by providing the mechanisms of active transport. Human and microbial cell membranes are similar in that they both possess lipid and protein structural elements. However, bacterial lipids are primarily phospholipids, and fungi contain sterols. These differences in lipid composition give rise to differences in the sensitivity of human, bacterial, and fungal cell membranes to the actions of relatively selective detergent compounds.

**Polymyxins** and **colistin** are large cyclic polypeptides with amino and carboxyl groups providing a polar face and hydrocarbon chains providing a non-polar face. Thus, they act as cationic detergents, reacting with the phosphate groups of cell envelope phospholipids. Disorganization of the cytoplasmic membrane follows, with leakage of the intracellular contents and cell death. Unfortunately, these agents can affect mammalian cell membranes in the same way, especially in the renal tubule, where they are concentrated after excretion; therefore, they are used mainly as topical agents for superficial infections. Less commonly, they have been used in the face of multi-resistant, Gram-negative infections such as those due to *Pseudomonas aeruginosa*, which are resistant to less toxic antibiotics.

Common antifungals in use today have the fungal cell membrane as their target site of action. Unlike human cell membranes, which have cholesterol as their main sterol, fungal cell membranes have ergosterol as the primary sterol. This difference, in part, allows for the selective toxicity of antifungal drugs against the fungal versus human cell membrane. **Amphotericin B** (Fig. 51-1) and **nystatin** have an analogous action on fungal cell membranes. Both of these antifungal agents have multiple conjugated double bonds (i.e., they are "polyenes;" see Fig. 51-1), which

| FIGURE 51-1 | Structural formula of amphotericin B. |

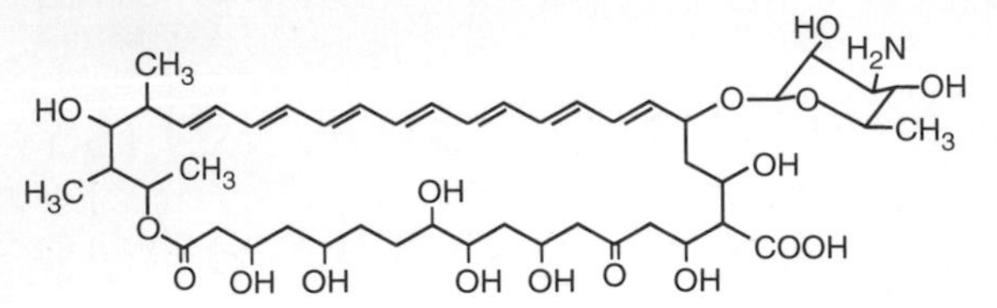

cause them to interact preferentially with ergosterol. They produce hydrophilic channels through the fungal membrane, permitting leakage of essential cell contents, including potassium.

The azole antifungals also exploit the requirement for ergosterol in the fungal cell membrane, but do so by inhibiting a specific cytochrome P450 enzyme that demethylates lanosterol, which is the precursor of ergosterol. This leads to an accumulation of 14-α-methylsterols and reduced concentrations of ergosterol, a sterol necessary for a normal fungal cell membrane. The **imidazoles,** such as **miconazole** and **clotrimazole,** were among the earliest drugs developed in the azole class. Newer azoles, which have a triazole ring instead of an imidazole ring (and are therefore called **triazoles**), have an antifungal spectrum and mechanism of action similar to those of the imidazoles, but they have less effect on human steroid metabolism and therefore fewer adverse effects. Examples of this class are **fluconazole** and **itraconazole.** More recently, so-called second-generation triazoles have been developed, of which **voriconazole, posaconazole,** and **ravuconazole** are the available examples.

The **allylamines,** a new class of synthetic antifungal drugs, also inhibit the synthesis of ergosterol; in this case, the target enzyme is squalene epoxidase. This inhibition not only leads to a decrease in ergosterol, but also to a buildup of squalene, which is toxic to the fungal cell. The major drug in this class at the present time is **terbinafine,** which has a minimum inhibitory concentration (MIC) of 0.001 to 0.01 µg/mL for *Trichophyton rubrum,* a common fungal pathogen in skin, hair, and nails. The squalene pathway is also involved in the synthesis of cholesterol in mammalian cells, but the basis for the selective toxicity to fungi is that terbinafine is 10 000 times more active against the fungal enzyme than against the mammalian enzyme.

## POLYMYXINS AND COLISTIN

The polymyxins were discovered as antimicrobial agents in 1947. Polymyxin is a generic term for a group of closely related antibiotic substances (polymyxins A, B, C, D, and E) that are relatively simple basic polypeptides with molecular masses of about 1000 Da. They were elaborated by various strains of an aerobic spore-forming rod, *Bacillus polymyxa,* which is found in soil. Polymyxin B (Polysporin), in the form of its sulfate, is the least toxic to humans. Colistin (Methacolymycin) is identical to polymyxin E but is supplied as the sulfomethyl derivative (methane sulfonate).

## Bacterial Susceptibility

The activity of the polymyxins is related to a detergent action on the bacterial cell membrane, resulting in lysis of the organisms even in hypertonic media. This action is restricted to Gram-negative bacteria. *Enterobacter, Escherichia, Haemophilus, Klebsiella, Pasteurella, Salmonella, Shigella,* and *Vibrio* are sensitive to concentrations of 0.02 to 2 µg/mL. Most strains of *P. aeruginosa* are inhibited by less than 4 µg/mL. Most strains of *Proteus* and some *Neisseria* are resistant to the drug. In general, the antibacterial activity of colistin is inferior to that of the methane sulfonate derivatives.

## Adverse Reactions

The same detergent action that is responsible for the bactericidal effect can also be exerted on mammalian cell membranes, especially in the renal tubule, where the drug is concentrated during excretion. Neurotoxicity and nephrotoxicity are the major severe adverse effects of these antimicrobials.

## Drug Interactions

Neuromuscular blockade from muscle relaxants or general anaesthetics may be potentiated by the neurotoxic effects of these drugs.

## Dosages and Routes of Administration

Polymyxin B is administered intramuscularly at a dose of 25 000 to 40 000 units/kg/day, divided into two or three doses (10 000 units = 1 mg).

Colistin is administered intramuscularly or intravenously at a dose of 3 to 5 mg/kg/day, divided into two or three doses.

The polymyxins are also available in numerous topical preparations such as creams, ointments, solutions, sprays, and eye drops. They are usually combined in these preparations with other antibiotics such as neomycin and bacitracin (see Chapters 50 and 52).

## Therapeutic Applications

At present, the parenteral preparations of these agents have largely fallen into clinical disuse because of the availability of more efficacious, less toxic substances. Occasionally, however, they are still used in the treatment of infections caused by organisms that are resistant to all other available antibiotics (e.g., *P. aeruginosa*). The topical preparations of polymyxin B are widely used because of its excellent activity against Gram-negative organisms, its lack of absorption, and, hence, its lack of toxicity when applied superficially. Oral colistin has been used successfully as part of an oral decontamination regimen to prevent systemic infections in patients with acute leukemia and chemotherapy-induced neutropenia.

# NYSTATIN

Nystatin (Mycostatin, Nilstat) is an antifungal antibiotic that was isolated from *Streptomyces noursei* in 1950. It belongs to the group of polyene antibiotics. Its large, conjugated, double-bond ring system is linked to an amino sugar, mycosamine.

## Fungal Susceptibility

Nystatin is fungicidal against *Candida, Cryptococcus, Histoplasma, Blastomyces, Trichophyton, Epidermophyton,* and *Microsporum audouinii* in vitro at concentrations ranging from 1.5 to 6.5 µg/mL.

## Pharmacokinetics

In its current form, nystatin is too toxic for parenteral administration; it is therefore used only for the treatment of superficial mycotic infections. For this reason, the pharmacokinetics and toxic effects of parenteral nystatin need not be described. Very little, if any, nystatin is absorbed after topical or oral administration of pharmacological doses.

## Adverse Reactions

There are virtually no side effects related to the topical use of nystatin. The drug may cause irritation or allergic reactions when applied to skin or mucous membranes. Nausea and diarrhea may occur following the administration of large oral doses.

## Dosage Regimens and Routes of Administration

Many preparations of this drug (1 mg = 3500 units) are available, including oral tablets (500 000 units), oral suspension (100 000 units/mL), and vaginal tablets (100 000 units). Vaginal and skin creams are also available containing nystatin either alone or in combination with other antimicrobials (e.g., bacitracin, neomycin, polymyxin B) or anti-inflammatory agents (principally steroids). Usually, one tablet (orally or vaginally) or 5 mL of the suspension

(swished in the mouth and swallowed) is administered two to four times a day. Topical application is usually made two or three times a day.

## Therapeutic Applications

Nystatin is used almost exclusively for the treatment of mucosal or cutaneous candidal infections, including oral and vaginal candidiasis. However, some cases of oral candidiasis, especially those appearing as superinfections during the use of an antimicrobial agent, or in patients with advanced HIV infection, may fail to respond.

# AMPHOTERICIN B

Amphotericin is an antifungal compound that was isolated from *Streptomyces nodosus* in 1956. It exists in two forms, A and B: the latter, being more active, is used clinically. Amphotericin B (Fungizone) is another polyene antibiotic; the basic moiety is aminodesoxyhexose, an aminomethyl pentose. It is closely related chemically to nystatin.

## Fungal Susceptibility

*Candida* species, *Histoplasma capsulatum, Cryptococcus neoformans, Coccidioides immitis, Rhodotorula, Blastomyces dermatitidis, Paracoccidioides brasiliensis, Sporotrichum schenckii, Aspergillus, Cladosporium* species, *Phialophora* species, *Mucor,* and *Rhizopus* are usually killed by less than 1.0 µg/mL of amphotericin B. The drug acts by binding to ergosterol in the fungal cell membrane, leading to formation of channels through which potassium, other ions, and essential metabolites are lost, a mechanism of action that is identical to that postulated for nystatin.

## Pharmacokinetics

As would be expected from its structure (it is a large hydrophobic molecule; see Fig. 51-1), amphotericin B is poorly absorbed from the gastrointestinal tract. The intravenous injection of 0.5 to 1 mg/kg yields peak plasma concentrations of 1.5 to 2 µg/mL.

Data on the distribution of amphotericin B in both humans and animals are very limited. It is very lipophilic and apparently distributes to cholesterol-containing membranes. This gives it a large volume of distribution of approximately 4 L/kg. For intravenous injection, amphotericin B is made more water soluble by addition of sodium deoxycholate. In serum, the deoxycholate separates from amphotericin B, and more than 95% of the latter binds to plasma proteins, primarily β-lipoprotein, presumably on cholesterol moieties. The drug leaves the circulation promptly. Amphotericin B is stored in the liver and other organs, and it re-enters the circulation slowly. Only small quantities enter the CSF.

The primary route of elimination of amphotericin B is unclear. Most of the drug is degraded, and only a small amount is excreted in urine and bile. Only 2 to 5% of a given dose is excreted in biologically active form in the urine. Blood levels are not influenced by renal or hepatic function or by hemodialysis.

The elimination of this agent is biphasic with an initial half-life of 24 hours, followed by a terminal half-life of 15 days, reflecting slow release from the large peripheral compartment.

## Adverse Reactions

The main adverse reactions to amphotericin B are those that occur in the short term during intravenous infusion or later as renal and hematological toxicity.

Infusion reactions include fever, chills, headache, anorexia, nausea, vomiting, and thrombophlebitis. These reactions may be due to deoxycholate used to form a colloidal solution of the drug, or to the colloidal solution itself. They may be ameliorated by analgesics, antiemetics, antipyretics, heparin (to prevent thrombophlebitis), or hydrocortisone.

Nephrotoxicity is a common and most important side effect of amphotericin B. Impairment of renal function and nephrotoxic reactions often limit the total amount of drug that can be administered. Early manifestations caused by the disruption of renal tubular cell membranes include hypokalemia, hypomagnesemia, and renal tubular acidosis. The degree of hypokalemia is often great enough to require potassium replacement. This drug also causes progressive impairment of renal function that is probably mediated by ischemia induced by renal artery spasm. This is manifested by rises in blood urea and serum creatinine, a decrease in creatinine clearance, and the appearance of red and white blood cells, albumin, and casts in the urine. Such renal damage is usually reversible; however, permanent impairment and irreversible renal failure can occur and appear to be related to the total dose of drug used. Some degree of renal impairment has been demonstrated in 40% of adults who have received more than 4 g of amphotericin B. Recent evidence suggests that progression of amphotericin-induced nephrotoxicity may be limited by sodium loading to prevent proximal tubular uptake of the drug.

Hematological toxicity includes a normochromic, normocytic anemia that may be associated with amphotericin B therapy. This is usually reversible and may be related to suppression of erythropoietin. Thrombocytopenia has also been noted occasionally.

## Drug Interactions

Caution must be taken to monitor for hypokalemia in patients receiving digitalis preparations. Any drug that is renally excreted may accumulate as a consequence of the renal damage seen in most patients receiving amphotericin B. For example, the toxicity of 5-fluorocytosine (see Chapter 53), which is commonly administered with amphotericin B, may be augmented.

## Dosage Regimens and Routes of Administration

Amphotericin B is administered intravenously, although it is occasionally used topically, intraperitoneally, intrathecally, or by direct instillation into the bladder. There is no universal agreement on the method of intravenous administration. It is, however, common practice to treat fungal infections on the basis of a total dose of amphotericin B. That is, anywhere between 200 mg and 3 to 4 g of amphotericin B will be administered to treat a specific infection. The total dose will depend upon the specific infecting organism, the host, the site of infection, and the anticipated and observed responses to treatment. In general, a daily dose of 0.5 to 1 mg/kg will be administered for as many days as it takes to attain the desired total dose. Some prefer to give this on alternate days, using a similar unit dose. Amphotericin B is the only anti-infective agent that is administered on the basis of a total cumulative dose rather than on the basis of a daily dose administered for a specified period of time. The rationale for this method of administration is not entirely clear.

## Therapeutic Applications

Parenteral amphotericin B is used for proven or highly suspected systemic fungal infections caused by susceptible organisms. The major infections treated with this drug in North America are disseminated candidiasis, aspergillosis, coccidioidomycosis, histoplasmosis, mucormycosis, blastomycosis, and cryptococcosis. The topical formulations of amphotericin B are useful for the treatment of cutaneous or mucosal candidiasis. Intraperitoneal amphotericin B has been used successfully for the treatment of fungal peritonitis. Because of poor distribution to the CSF, it is frequently combined with 5-fluorocytosine to treat fungal infections of the central nervous system (e.g., cryptococcal meningitis). Bladder instillation has been used to treat lower urinary tract infections (cystitis) caused by *Candida*.

Other formulations of amphotericin include a complex of the drug with a lipid carrier. The rationale for this preparation is that the drug will concentrate in cells of the reticuloendothelial system and avoid the cells where end organ toxicity can occur (e.g., kidney). Existing formulations include amphotericin B colloidal dispersion (ABCD), amphotericin B lipid complex (ABLC), and liposomal amphotericin B. These three formulations are less nephrotoxic than amphotericin B itself, and higher daily doses can be administered. Clinical efficacy superior to that of amphotericin B has not been consistently demonstrated.

## TOPICAL IMIDAZOLE ANTIFUNGAL AGENTS

The topical imidazole antifungal agents are synthetic compounds that bind to the heme of the fungal cytochrome P450 and inhibit ergosterol synthesis. Two major drugs in this class are **miconazole** (Micatin, Monistat) and **clotrimazole** (Canesten, Myclo), but there are a number of others with similar properties, such as **oxiconazole** (Oxistat), **econazole** (Ecostatin), and **bifonazole** (Mycospor). They are lipophilic compounds with low water solubility at neutral pH, but the imidazole ring is ionized under acidic conditions, and this greatly increases water solubility.

### Fungal Susceptibility

These agents have a broad spectrum of activity including *Epidermophyton, Microsporum, Trichophyton, Pityrosporon orbiculare,* and *Candida albicans.* They can be either fungistatic or fungicidal, depending on the concentration.

### Adverse Reactions

Topical imidazoles seldom lead to adverse reactions although they can cause erythema, stinging, blistering, pruritus, and even urticaria at the site of application.

### Therapeutic Applications

The topical imidazoles are used to treat superficial fungal infections of the feet, nails, perineum, vagina, and mouth. In general, they are very effective and represent the treatment of choice for such infections. One limitation in the treatment of fungal infections of the nails is that penetration of topical agents into the nails is poor, because of the very tight cross-linkage between keratin strands.

## SYSTEMIC IMIDAZOLE ANTIFUNGAL AGENTS

**Ketoconazole** (Nizoral; Fig. 51-2) is an imidazole used for systemic antifungal therapy.

### Fungal Susceptibility

Ketoconazole is usually active against *C. immitis, C. neoformans,* and *H. capsulatum* at levels less than 0.5 μg/mL. Activity against *Candida, Aspergillus,* and *Sporothrix* usually requires levels from 6 μg/mL to more than 100 μg/mL.

### Pharmacokinetics

Absorption of ketoconazole after oral administration is good; however, an acidic environment is necessary for dis-

**FIGURE 51-2** Structural formula of ketoconazole.

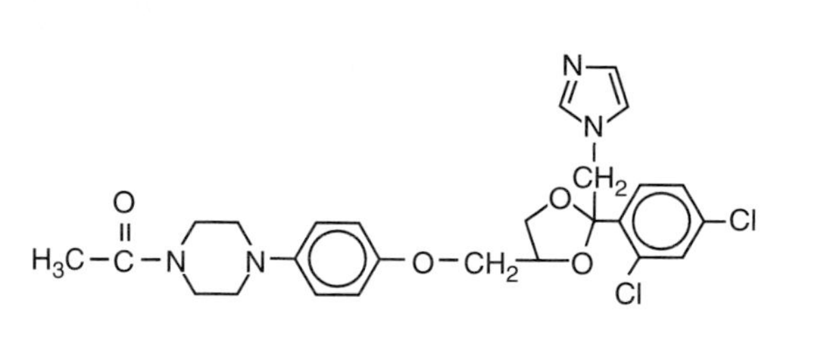

solution of the drug, and absorption is markedly decreased by antacids and histamine $H_2$ receptor blockers, or in patients with achlorhydria. Rifampin causes a substantial lowering of ketoconazole blood levels, probably by accelerating its biotransformation. The drug is highly protein-bound (90%). Distribution is limited, and the level reached in the CNS is very low.

Elimination of ketoconazole is primarily by hepatic biotransformation. The kinetics of ketoconazole appear to be dose-dependent; the half-life increases from 90 minutes after a 200-mg dose to almost 4 hours after an 800-mg dose. This implies the participation of more than one enzymatic pathway, with different kinetic parameters (see Chapter 28, on acetylsalicylic acid).

### Adverse Reactions

The most common side effects of ketoconazole are nausea and vomiting. Mild, asymptomatic elevation of transaminases is observed in 5 to 10% of patients, and serious **hepatotoxicity** occurs with an incidence of approximately one in 15 000.

Although ketoconazole has some selectivity for the cytochrome P450 that is involved in the synthesis of ergosterol, it also inhibits the metabolism of several other drugs by hepatic cytochrome P450 in a manner similar to that of cimetidine (also an imidazole). It also inhibits the testicular synthesis of androgens; this is the probable mechanism for the observed association of ketoconazole with gynecomastia in some patients. Cyclosporine drug levels should be monitored during combined therapy with ketoconazole because these levels usually increase, causing nephrotoxicity.

### Dosage and Route of Administration

Ketoconazole is available in 200-mg tablets for oral administration. The usual dose is 200 to 400 mg/day. In cases of achlorhydria, the drug may be dissolved in dilute hydrochloric acid and sipped through a straw to avoid contact with the teeth. Alternatively, patients are advised to take the drug with a cola drink or orange juice.

## Therapeutic Applications

Ketoconazole is used most commonly to treat oral or esophageal candidiasis that is resistant to nystatin. It is also used in the treatment and prophylaxis of vaginal candidiasis. Clinically resistant strains of *Candida* have been noted in patients with HIV. The drug is effective in the treatment of non-meningeal histoplasmosis involving the lungs, bones, skin, or soft tissue, and in disseminated disease, but it is less effective than itraconazole (see below). It is effective in non-meningeal cryptococcal disease, but penetration of the CNS is not sufficient for the treatment of cryptococcal meningitis. It is also useful in the treatment of paracoccidioidomycosis, blastomycosis, and certain dermatomycoses. Its major limitation is its slow onset of action; therefore, amphotericin B is usually the drug of choice in severe acute fungal infections, especially in immunocompromised hosts.

# TRIAZOLE ANTIFUNGAL AGENTS

## Pharmacokinetics

Absorption of **fluconazole** (Diflucan; Fig. 51-3) is very good; oral bioavailability is greater than 90%. Oral absorption is not decreased in patients taking histamine $H_2$–blocking agents. The average half-life is 30 hours. Distribution is to total body water, and the major route of elimination is renal, with about 80% of the administered dose appearing in the urine as unchanged drug. Only 11% of serum fluconazole is protein-bound. Concentrations in the CSF are approximately 70% of simultaneous blood levels, whether or not the meninges are inflamed. Rifampin lowers fluconazole blood levels by about 25%.

**Itraconazole** (Sporanox) is an analogue of ketoconazole, and its oral absorption is also increased by gastric acidity. The peak blood levels are lower than those of ketoconazole, but tissue levels are higher. The major route of elimination is hepatic biotransformation, and the drug is highly protein-bound (99%).

**Voriconazole** and **ravuconazole** are closely related to fluconazole, and **posaconazole** is a close structural relative of itraconazole.

## Adverse Reactions

The two most common adverse effects associated with fluconazole appear to be an increase in serum transaminase levels, and skin rashes. Nausea, vomiting, abdominal pain, and diarrhea occur in less than 2% of patients. Hepatic necrosis has been observed but appears to be uncommon. Dose-related nausea and vomiting can complicate itraconazole use. Unlike ketoconazole, itraconazole does not suppress adrenal or testicular function.

| FIGURE 51-3 | Structural formula of fluconazole. |

Voriconazole has a number of potentially serious adverse effects, including elevation of serum levels of hepatic enzymes, skin reactions, visual effects, and drug interactions.

## Therapeutic Applications

**Fluconazole** is currently available in 50-, 100-, and 150-mg tablets and as an intravenous formulation. The drug is used in the management of oral and esophageal candidiasis in patients who are unresponsive to nystatin or ketoconazole or in patients who do not have the gastric acidity required for absorption of ketoconazole. A single dose of 150 mg is as effective as topical therapy of vulvovaginal candidiasis. Because of enhanced CNS penetration, fluconazole is also used in the treatment of cryptococcal meningitis. In general, treatment is initiated with amphotericin B but may be completed with fluconazole. It is very useful for the long-term maintenance therapy of cryptococcal meningitis in patients with AIDS. There are increasing reports in the literature of cases of oral thrush clinically resistant to fluconazole. These are described almost exclusively in patients with advanced HIV infection on long-term use of the drug.

Fluconazole has recently been demonstrated to be equivalent to amphotericin B in the management of systemic candidiasis in non-neutropenic hosts. It has also been shown to be effective in the treatment of *Candida* endophthalmitis.

Fluconazole as prophylactic therapy has been shown to lower the incidence of superficial, deep, and systemic fungal infections (primarily candidiasis) in recipients of bone marrow transplants. An effect on survival has not been demonstrated. Although used prophylactically in febrile neutropenic patients, it has been shown only to decrease the incidence of superficial candidal infections (not invasive fungal infections) in this patient population.

Fluconazole has emerged as the drug of choice in coccidioidal meningitis.

**Itraconazole** has recently been released for clinical use. It is marketed as a 100-mg capsule. An oral suspension in cyclodextrin is under clinical trial. This may have the advantage of increased local effect. An intravenous formulation is under development.

Itraconazole is useful for the treatment of candidiasis. It has excellent activity against histoplasmosis, sporotrichosis, and blastomycosis, for which it has become the drug of choice. There are increasing reports that it is active in invasive *Aspergillus* infections, but its activity in relation to amphotericin B remains uncertain. It appears to be very useful as long-term maintenance therapy against histoplasmosis in AIDS.

The advantages of **voriconazole** are its good activity against *Aspergillus* spp. (unlike fluconazole) and its good penetration of the CNS, so it is becoming standard therapy for invasive aspergillosis.

## Drug Interactions

Simultaneous ingestion with antacids and buffered didanosine (ddI; see Chapter 55) decreases absorption of both itraconazole and ketoconazole. Rifampin, phenytoin, and carbamazepine decrease itraconazole and ketoconazole levels. Like ketoconazole, itraconazole is a potent inhibitor of cytochrome P450 3A4 and increases blood levels of cyclosporine, digoxin, terfenadine, astemizole, and loratidine. The last three can lead to torsades de pointes (see Chapter 33). Fluconazole, when given in doses of 200 mg/day or more, is an inhibitor of the cytochrome P450 2C9 isoform; hence, caution must be used when co-administering it with CYP2C9 substrates such as warfarin and phenytoin. Terbinafine is an inhibitor of CYP2D6 and should be administered with caution in patients taking drugs that are substrates for that isoform (e.g., some psychotropic drugs, β blockers).

## Dosage and Route of Administration

Fluconazole is available for both intravenous and oral administration, and the dosage is the same for both routes. For oral candidiasis, the usual dose is 100 mg/day, but for more serious infections, the usual dose is 200 to 400 mg/day as a single dose. For serious infections, a loading dose of double the normal daily dose is recommended. In patients with impaired renal function, the daily dose should be decreased. Resistant isolates are increasingly recognized, especially in HIV patients on long-term therapy.

Itraconazole is available for oral administration. The usual dose is 200 mg/day for oral and esophageal candidiasis. For more serious infections, a dose of 400 mg/day is used.

Voriconazole, the first available second-generation triazole, can be administered either by mouth or intravenously, as can the newer agent ravuconazole. Posaconazole is available only for oral use, and it must be administered four times daily.

---

**FIGURE 51-4**  Structural formula of terbinafine.

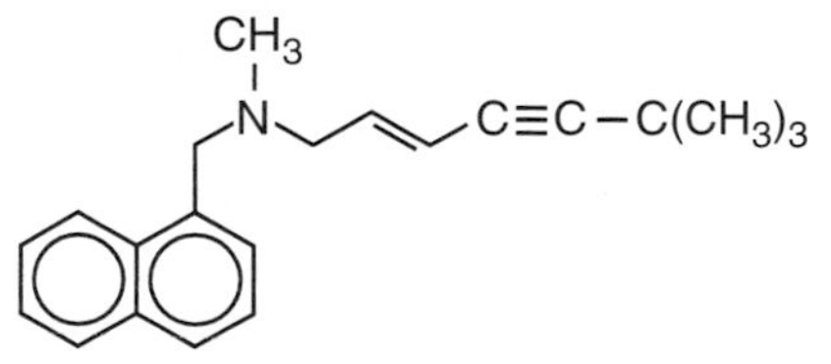

## ALLYLAMINE ANTIFUNGAL AGENTS

### Fungal Susceptibility

Although the present allylamines have some activity against yeasts, they are fungistatic and require doses that are a hundred times higher than those required for activity against dermatophytes; therefore, at present, their use is limited to the treatment of dermatophyte infections.

### Pharmacokinetics

The first antifungal allylamine to be developed was **naftifine** (Naftin). It is available as a topical cream. **Terbinafine** (Lamisil; Fig. 51-4) is available in topical and oral forms. Its bioavailability after oral administration is approximately 70%. It is found in the stratum corneum as early as 24 hours after administration but requires from 3 to 18 weeks to reach therapeutic levels in the nails. After steady state has been achieved, therapeutic levels of terbinafine remain in the skin for 2 to 3 weeks after administration of the drug is stopped. Terbinafine is extensively biotransformed by cytochrome P450 to at least 15 metabolites. Dosage of terbinafine should be altered when it is given with other drugs that either induce or inhibit cytochrome P450, and also in the presence of renal failure.

### Therapeutic Applications

The allylamines promise to be very effective for the treatment of difficult dermatophyte infections, especially those involving the nails.

## SUGGESTED READINGS

Como JA, Dismukes WE. Oral azole drugs as systemic antifungal therapy. *N Engl J Med.* 1994;330:263-272.

DeMuri GP, Hostetter MK. Resistance to antifungal agents. *Pediatr Clin North Am.* 1995;42:665-686.

Dismukes WE, Bradsher RW Jr, Cloud GC, et al. Itraconazole therapy for blastomycosis and histoplasmosis. NIAID Mycoses Study Group. *Am J Med.* 1992;93:489-497.

Elewski BE. Mechanisms of action of systemic antifungal agents. *J Am Acad Dermatol.* 1993;28:S28-S34.

Ernest JM. Topical antifungal agents. *Obstet Gynecol Clin North Am.* 1992;19:587-607.

Fielding RM. Liposomal drug delivery. Advantages and limitations from a clinical pharmacokinetic and therapeutic perspective. *Clin Pharmacokinet.* 1993;21:1155-1164.

Pearson MM, Rogers PD, Cleary JD, Chapman SW. Voriconazole: a new triazole antifungal agent. *Ann Pharmacother.* 2003;37:420-432.

Perfect JR. Use of newer antifungal therapies in clinical practice: what do the data tell us? *Oncology (Huntington).* 2004;13(suppl 7):15-23.

Sharkey PK, Rinaldi MG, Dunn JF, et al. High dose itraconazole in the treatment of severe mycoses. *Antimicrob Agents Chemother.* 1991;36:707-713.

Terrell C, Hermans PE. Antifungal agents used for deep-seated mycotic infections. *Mayo Clin Proc.* 1987;62:1116-1128.

# 52

# Antimicrobial Agents That Affect the Synthesis of Cellular Proteins

## J UETRECHT, EJ PHILLIPS, AND SL WALMSLEY

### CASE HISTORY

A 30-year-old man presented to the Sexually Transmitted Infections Clinic with a 4-day history of dysuria and purulent urethral discharge. He had a new sexual partner, a woman he had met in a bar about 1 week before the onset of the symptoms, and knew little about her health. Contrary to his usual practice, he had decided not to wear a condom.

A Gram stain of the urethral swab showed Gram-negative intracellular diplococci, and a diagnosis of gonorrhea was made. As the incidence of β-lactamase-producing gonorrhea in the area served by this clinic was more than 10%, and because of the patient's history of penicillin allergy, he was treated with a single intramuscular injection of 1 g spectinomycin. As was the policy of the clinic, it was also recommended that he receive treatment against *Chlamydia trachomatis*, and oral doxycycline, 100 mg twice a day for 7 days, was prescribed for him. When the patient went to get this prescription, he mentioned to the pharmacist that he had been under considerable stress recently and that he was taking antacids. The pharmacist was concerned about the potential for diminished absorption of doxycycline by antacids and called the physician. The doxycycline prescription was changed to azithromycin, 1 g orally. The patient returned to the clinic 1 week after treatment. All symptoms had resolved, and follow-up cultures were negative. He remained well.

About 2 years later, while on a camping trip, he developed periumbilical abdominal pain and fever. The pain became more intense and radiated into the right lower quadrant over the next few hours. He returned to the city for medical attention. On the trip back, the pain became even more intense, he was diaphoretic, and he complained of lightheadedness. On arrival in the emergency room, a diagnosis of acute appendicitis was made, and he was operated on within the hour.

Before surgery, he was given 500 mg metronidazole and 80 mg gentamicin intravenously as antibiotic prophylaxis. During surgery it was found that the appendix had ruptured and that there was fecal soiling of the abdominal cavity. He was treated post-operatively with intravenous clindamycin, 600 mg every 8 hours, and with intravenous gentamicin, 400 mg once per day, to cover bowel organisms. He made a successful and uneventful recovery.

## BACTERIAL PROTEIN SYNTHESIS

Protein synthesis occurs through translation of the genetic information coded in messenger RNA (mRNA). This process takes place on the ribonucleoprotein particles, the ribosomes, with the help of transfer RNA (tRNA), and it consists of three stages: initiation, elongation, and termination (shown schematically in Fig. 52-1).

In general, the functional unit of bacterial protein synthesis is the 70S ribosome, which consists of two subunits: 30S and 50S. The mRNA attaches to the 30S subunit, and the anticodon of aminoacyl-tRNA is matched to the codon on the mRNA. The aminoacyl group attached to the tRNA is bound to the 50S subunit, where peptide bond formation occurs. One of the proteins making up the 50S subunit is peptidyl transferase, which catalyzes peptide bond formation.

Initiation (i.e., formation of the 70S ribosome) involves various initiation factors by means of which a 30S subunit combines with mRNA and tRNA, and then with a 50S subunit, to complete the 70S ribosome. The tRNA, initially bound to the "A" (aminoacyl) site of the ribosome, is translocated to the "P" (peptidyl) site, freeing the "A" site for additional tRNA.

The elongation stage is essentially a response to a "request" by the codons of mRNA for additional aminoacyl-tRNA, which is first bound to the "A" site and then

**FIGURE 52-1** Schematic representation of the basic elements and steps of bacterial protein synthesis and the sites of action of antibiotics that inhibit synthesis. Principal mechanisms of action: (1) Aminoglycosides bind to 30S subunit, block initiation, block tRNA binding, distort codons of mRNA, and cause misreading of the genetic code. (2) Tetracyclines block "A" site binding (tRNA to mRNA); they also chelate essential cations. (3) Chloramphenicol inhibits peptidyl transferase and prevents peptide bond formation. (4) Macrolides block translocation and prevent peptide chain extension. (See text for additional details.)

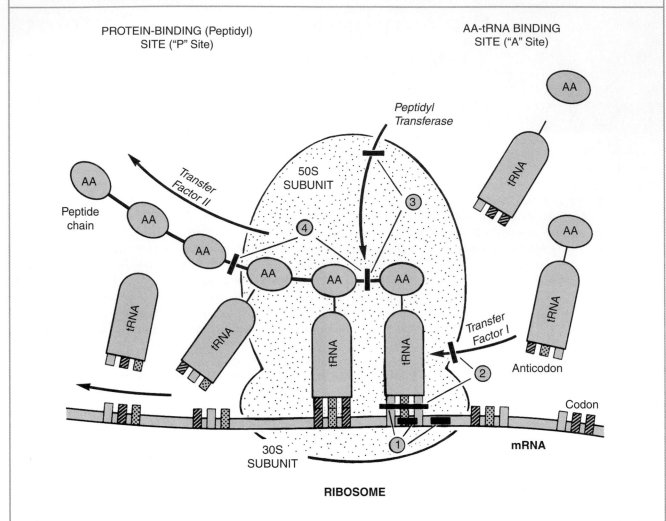

## MECHANISMS OF ACTION

Several antibiotics inhibit protein synthesis by interfering with translation. They bind to ribosomes and prevent normal peptide chain formation at one or more stages, which translocated to the "P" site. Various elongation factors are involved in this process, which is repeated until the entire message is read and the peptide is completed.

Termination of the peptide chain occurs when a terminating codon is reached and the completed chain is discharged from the ribosome. Various termination factors are involved in the release of completed peptides. The 50S and 30S subunits dissociate and join a pool of free subunits.

include peptide bond formation, translocation, and movement of the ribosomes along the mRNA. The basis for selective toxicity to bacteria with relatively low toxicity to mammalian cells is that, with the exception of the tetracyclines and chloramphenicol, these agents do not bind to mammalian ribosomes. (Chloramphenicol inhibits mammalian mitochondrial protein synthesis in bone marrow precursor cells.) The structure of the mammalian ribosome is different from that of bacteria. Mammalian ribosomes are 80S and are not easily split into subunits.

**Aminoglycosides** bind tightly to the 30S subunit of the bacterial ribosome and inhibit protein synthesis at several points by blocking the normal activity of the initiation complex, interfering with tRNA attachment, and distorting the triplet codon of mRNA so that the message is misread and faulty peptides are formed. **Spectinomycin,** like the aminoglycosides, binds to the 30S ribosomal subunit, thereby inhibiting protein synthesis. It does not, however, cause misreading of the genetic code.

**Tetracyclines** also bind to the 30S subunit and block the binding of tRNA to mRNA. They also bind to mammalian ribosomes, but susceptible bacteria concentrate the tetracyclines, and therefore the drugs can be used at a concentration that will kill bacteria but have little toxicity to mammalian cells. In addition, these agents chelate cations that are essential for protein synthesis, especially magnesium.

**Chloramphenicol,** lincosamides such as **clindamycin,** and macrolides such as **erythromycin** all bind to the 50S subunit. Chloramphenicol prevents peptide bond formation by inhibiting the responsible enzyme, peptidyl transferase, which is also located on the 50S subunit. Clindamycin and erythromycin prevent the extension of growing peptides on the ribosomes and also block translocation or progression to the next codon on mRNA.

It would be expected that agents that inhibit protein synthesis would inhibit bacterial growth and therefore be bacteriostatic rather than bactericidal. However, this is largely dependent on the bacterial organism as well as on the drug. Aminoglycosides display concentration-dependent bacterial killing and are generally bactericidal in clinical use.

# AMINOGLYCOSIDES

The aminoglycoside group of antibiotics includes a large number of structurally related compounds all derived from different species of *Streptomyces.* **Streptomycin** was the first of this group to be discovered (1943), by means of a systematic examination of soil fungi. Subsequently, **neomycin** (1949), **kanamycin** (1957), **gentamicin** (1964), and **tobramycin** (1971) were discovered. Semi-synthetic derivatives of these agents, including **amikacin** (1975) and **netilmicin** (1976), were then produced. The main impetus for the original search for these compounds was the lack of significant activity of the penicillins against Gram-negative organisms. The aminoglycoside class of antibiotics today remains one of the most important weapons against Gram-negative pathogens.

## Chemistry

The members of this group of antibiotics are characterized by the presence of amino sugars glycosidically linked to aminocyclitols (hence the name "aminoglycoside"; Fig. 52-2).

The pharmacokinetics, adverse reactions, and drug interactions of all systemically used aminoglycosides are very similar, mainly because of their common physicochemical characteristics. The dosages, regimens, routes of administration, and therapeutic applications do differ somewhat, and these aspects must therefore be considered separately for each agent.

## Bacterial Susceptibility

The aminoglycosides are active primarily against the Gram-negative aerobes and a limited number of Gram-positive aerobes (e.g., staphylococci). Just as their structure precludes adequate oral absorption or distribution into the central nervous system (CNS), it also makes simple diffusion of the aminoglycosides into bacteria insufficient for antibacterial activity. However, the aminoglycosides are taken up very efficiently by aerobic bacteria through an active transport mechanism linked to the oxidative phosphorylation system of these organisms. For this reason, the aminoglycosides are inactive against anaerobic bacteria, which do not possess this system, and are less active in anaerobic environments, which inhibit oxidative phosphorylation. Acidic environments protonate the basic aminoglycosides and decrease their uptake.

Streptomycin is also quite active against bovine and human mycobacteria (MIC ~0.5 µg/mL). Streptomycin, neomycin, and kanamycin are not active against *Pseudomonas aeruginosa,* but the other four aminoglycoside agents (gentamicin, tobramycin, amikacin, and netilmicin) have varying degrees of activity against this organism (Table 52-1). Of these four, tobramycin is the most active against the majority of *P. aeruginosa* isolates, and netilmicin is the least active. Other differences in the activity of the four most commonly used aminoglycosides against a variety of microorganisms can be seen in Table 52-1. For instance, gentamicin is the most active against *Serratia marcescens.*

An important aspect of activity against Gram-negative aerobes is that increasing resistance has developed in some hospitals and other enclosed environments after extensive use of aminoglycosides. However, problems with resistance to these agents are far less frequent than those observed with the new cephalosporins and quinolones. Resistance results from either chromosomal mutations or R plasmid–mediated factors that induce the bacteria to produce enzymes that can inactivate some or all of the aminoglycosides. These enzymes cause aminoglycoside inactivation by acetylation, adenylation, or phosphorylation of specific amino or alcohol groups that are necessary for activity (see Fig. 52-2). Of the aminoglycosides represented in Table 52-1, gentamicin is susceptible to the largest number of these enzymes (9 of 12), and amikacin, to the smallest number (1 of 12). It is thus not surprising that the development of resistance appears to be most common with gentamicin and least common with amikacin. When widespread resistance develops to one of the aminoglycosides being used in a particular hospital, it is often beneficial to change to another aminoglycoside (to which the bacteria are still sensitive) for some period of time.

**FIGURE 52-2** Structural formula of tobramycin, a representative aminoglycoside.

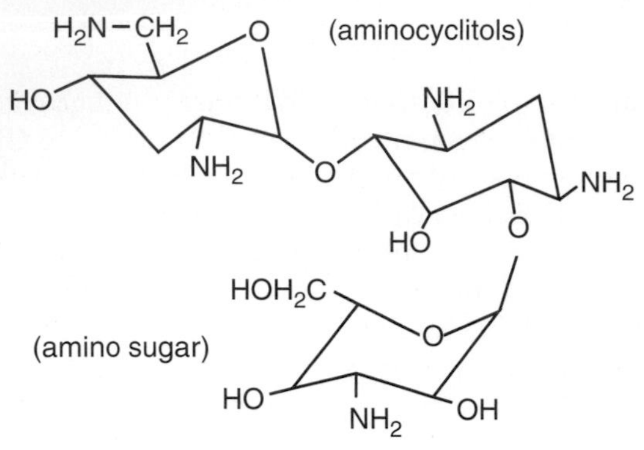

There are well-documented cases of endocarditis due to enterococci with a high level of resistance to aminoglycosides. Resistance results from disruption of the synergistic bactericidal interaction of cell wall–disrupting antibiotics and the aminoglycosides. Enterococci are intrinsically resistant to low concentrations of aminoglycoside (4 to 250 µg/mL) because of their anaerobic metabolism. Strains with MICs of 2000 µg/mL or more are defined as showing high-level resistance (HLR). HLR is mediated by modifying enzymes.

## Pharmacokinetics

Very little of an oral dose of any aminoglycoside is absorbed from the gastrointestinal tract, even after administration of large doses. Aminoglycosides are, however, rapidly absorbed after intramuscular injection, and they can also be given intravenously. The concentrations of aminoglycosides obtained after specified doses are outlined in Table 52-2. Neomycin is not included in this table as it is too toxic to use systemically.

The apparent volume of distribution of the aminoglycosides ranges from 0.25 to 0.7 L/kg. In general, it is lower in adults and higher in infants. The drugs are not highly protein-bound (less than 30%). They are distributed in all the extracellular fluids but do not generally attain sufficiently high concentrations in the cerebrospinal fluid (CSF) after parenteral administration to be of therapeutic benefit to patients with meningitis. The main site of uptake is the kidney, which accounts for approximately 40% of the total antibiotic in the body. The cortex accumulates approximately 85% of this load, and the resulting concentrations are more than 100 times greater than serum concentrations.

The aminoglycosides are not significantly biotransformed by body tissues but are eliminated unchanged, primarily by glomerular filtration in the kidneys. The complete dose is usually not excreted during the first 1 to 2 days of therapy, but thereafter, over a prolonged period, nearly 100% elimination occurs by this route. The serum elimination half-life of these agents in normal adults ranges from 1.5 to 2.5 hours.

## Adverse Reactions

The most important toxicities of the aminoglycosides are those affecting the inner ear and the kidneys.

**Ototoxicity** may be primarily vestibular or cochlear (in both cases, associated with ablation of hair cells). The agents most likely to cause **vestibular toxicity** are streptomycin and gentamicin. The most severe vestibular reactions are noted when streptomycin is used in high doses. Nearly 75% of patients who were given 2 g of streptomycin

| TABLE 52-1 | Median MICs (in µg/mL) of Aminoglycosides | | | | |
|---|---|---|---|---|---|
| **Bacterium** | **Gentamicin** | **Tobramycin** | **Amikacin** | **Netilmicin** |
| Gram-positive | | | | |
| *Staphylococcus aureus* | 0.39 | 0.5 | 1.8 | 0.5 |
| *Streptococcus* group A | 6.3 | >25.0 | >200 | 4.0 |
| *Streptococcus viridans* | 4.0 | – | >40 | – |
| *Enterococcus faecalis* | 25.0 | 25.0 | >80 | 16.0 |
| Gram-negative | | | | |
| *Haemophilus influenzae* | 1.0 | 0.8 | 5.0 | 1.0 |
| *Salmonella* | 0.78 | 0.4 | 0.8 | 0.4 |
| *Shigella* | 0.78 | 0.8 | 4.0 | 0.8 |
| *Klebsiella* | 1.0 | 1.5 | 3.0 | 1.0 |
| *Escherichia coli* | 3.2 | 2.0 | 2.0 | 0.7 |
| *Pseudomonas aeruginosa* | 4.0 | 1.6 | 6.0 | 8.0 |
| *Proteus mirabilis* | 1.0 | 1.0 | 2.0 | 1.0 |
| *Serratia marcescens* | 1.0 | 3.0 | 4.0 | 3.0 |

| TABLE 52-2 | Pharmacokinetics of Aminoglycosides | | |
| --- | --- | --- | --- |
| Agent | Unit Dose | Usual Serum Concentration (µg/mL) | Half-Life (hours) |
| Streptomycin | 500 mg | 15–20 | 2.5 |
| Kanamycin | 7.5 mg/kg | 25 | 2.0 |
| Gentamicin | 1.5 mg/kg | 5–7 | 2.4 |
| Tobramycin | 2.0 mg/kg | 6–8 | 2.0 |
| Amikacin | 7.5 mg/kg | 15–30 | 1.5–2.0 |
| Netilmicin | 1.0 mg/kg | 3.5–5.0 | 2.0–2.5 |

daily for 60 to 120 days manifested some vestibular disturbance, whereas reduction of the dose to 1 g daily decreased this incidence to approximately 25%. Inflammation of the meninges also appeared to predispose to ototoxicity, and repeated intrathecal injections of the drug caused earlier and more severe damage than did administration by other routes. The incidence of vestibular symptoms with gentamicin therapy is approximately 2%. This ranges from slight vertigo to an acute Ménière's syndrome. Damage is usually permanent, but patients may diminish their symptoms through adaptation.

The agents most likely to cause **cochlear toxicity** are neomycin, kanamycin, amikacin, and tobramycin. The cochlear toxicity of neomycin is so severe that the systemic use of this agent is precluded. Irreversible deafness will occur from just 1 to 2 weeks of daily intramuscular therapy using 0.5 to 1 g. The frequency of hearing loss with tobramycin and amikacin is low, but it may occur without any warning and may be irreversible.

Risk factors that seem to predispose to ototoxicity include increased serum concentrations, prolonged use, advanced age, pre-existing renal disease or hearing loss, and the concomitant administration of other ototoxic drugs (e.g., furosemide, ethacrynic acid; see Chapter 37).

The accumulation of aminoglycosides in the proximal tubules of the renal cortex predisposes to the development of **nephrotoxicity**. Early manifestations of nephrotoxicity include proteinuria, hypokalemia, glycosuria, alkalosis, hypomagnesemia, and hypocalcemia. The usual course is a non-oliguric renal failure that progresses gradually. This nephrotoxicity is dose-related and generally reversible. Its incidence may increase with the concomitant administration of cisplatin, furosemide, ethacrynic acid, or cephalothin, and it is potentiated by volume depletion.

Another adverse reaction to the aminoglycosides is a competitive type of **neuromuscular blockade** (blocking potency of the aminoglycosides is less than 1% that of d-tubocurarine), which occurs most frequently after intraperitoneal administration. Hypersensitivity reactions to the aminoglycosides are infrequent, although a contact dermatitis is the most common side effect of topically applied neomycin. This usually occurs after prolonged use and is unlikely to be noted with short-term treatment.

Over the years, considerable research has led to a better understanding of the pharmacokinetics and pharmacodynamics of aminoglycosides, ensuring the achievement of therapeutic concentrations to optimize antibacterial activity and lessen toxicity. Consequently, many hospitals have now adopted once-daily dosing schedules for administration of aminoglycosides.

The aminoglycosides demonstrate a property known as concentration-dependent killing. Clinical studies have demonstrated that achievement of high peak serum concentrations relative to the MIC of the infecting microorganism is a major determinant of the clinical response. This can best be obtained by once-daily administration. In addition, aminoglycosides demonstrate a property known as the post-antibiotic effect. This is defined as a period of time after complete removal of the antibiotic during which there is no growth of the organism. Therefore, despite the 12-hour period after which there are no detectable serum concentrations when aminoglycosides are given once daily, this post-antibiotic effect ensures that therapeutic efficacy is not compromised. The once-daily dosage schedule is also theoretically associated with lesser toxicity. The uptake and accumulation of aminoglycosides into renal cortical tissue demonstrate saturable kinetics, making peak concentrations irrelevant. Less frequent dosing does allow for serum concentrations to fall below the threshold for binding to tissue receptors and allows back-diffusion of the aminoglycosides from the renal cortex and inner ear. Numerous published studies have shown equivalent outcomes between once-daily and multiple-daily dosing of aminoglycosides with no excess toxicity of once-daily dosing, but with considerable cost savings and elimination of the need for therapeutic drug-level monitoring.

## Drug Interactions

The β-lactam ring of penicillins and cephalosporins reacts with the amino group of aminoglycosides and inactivates them; therefore, penicillins and cephalosporins should not be mixed in the same bottle with aminoglycosides. Inactivation can also occur in vivo, but this is of little clinical significance with the possible exception of patients with renal failure, in whom the concentration of penicillin can be very high. In such instances, the administration of the β-lactam and the aminoglycoside on a staggered schedule will minimize this interaction.

There is also a positive interaction (synergy) that can occur between aminoglycosides and β-lactams as well as other agents, such as vancomycin, which inhibit cell wall synthesis, because these agents increase the uptake of aminoglycosides into bacteria, especially Gram-positive bacteria. This helps the aminoglycoside to reach an effective concentration at its site of action, the ribosome. This is especially important for the treatment of bacterial endocarditis and *P. aeruginosa* infections.

Other nephrotoxic agents used in conjunction with aminoglycosides, such as amphotericin B, may increase the risk of renal toxicity.

## Dosage Regimens, Routes of Administration, and Therapeutic Applications

### Streptomycin

Adults are usually treated with 15 mg/kg/day intramuscularly, in one or two doses. The drug may be given only once or twice weekly in the initial treatment of tuberculosis. Streptomycin is not commonly used today as first-line treatment of tuberculosis, except in multidrug-resistant strains, because of its toxicity by this route and the availability of more acceptable therapeutic alternatives.

### Gentamicin (Cidomycin, Garamycin), tobramycin (Nebcin, Tobrex), amikacin (Amikin), and netilmicin (Netromycin)

The usual dosages and regimens of these four aminoglycosides are outlined in Table 52-3. (As stated earlier, however, there may be a move to once-a-day administration rather than the fractional doses described in this table.) They are administered intravenously and, rarely, intramuscularly. Occasionally, in the treatment of cephalosporin-resistant, Gram-negative meningitis and other CNS infections, these aminoglycosides are also administered by the intrathecal or intraventricular route. Topical formulations (e.g., ointments, ear drops, eye drops) are also available.

The most important indications for using one of these aminoglycosides are Gram-negative infections, including infections of blood, bones and joints, intra-abdominal and pelvic cavities, soft tissue and wounds, and the urinary tract. These drugs are also invaluable in the empirical treatment of neutropenic febrile hosts who are at great risk of Gram-negative septicemia. They also act in synergy with the penicillins or cephalosporins against numerous bacteria (see "Drug Interactions" above). This is particularly important in the treatment of serious enterococcal infections. The choice among the four aminoglycosides is influenced by several factors, including the resistance pattern of organisms within the institution, the familiarity of the clinicians with the individual antibiotics, and the cost of each agent to the patient.

## SPECTINOMYCIN

Spectinomycin (Trobicin) is an antibiotic produced by *Streptomyces spectabilis.* The drug is an aminocyclitol. It is active against a number of Gram-negative bacterial species but is inferior to other drugs. Its most important activity is

| TABLE 52-3 | Dosages and Regimens of Aminoglycosides | |
|---|---|---|
| Agent | Usual Daily Total Dose (mg/kg) | Usual Number of Fractional Doses per Day |
| Gentamicin | 4.5–5.0 | 3 |
| Tobramycin | 5.0–7.5 | 3 |
| Amikacin | 15–20 | 2–3 |
| Netilmicin | 4.5–6.0 | 3 |

that against *Neisseria gonorrhoeae,* which it inhibits at concentrations of 7 to 20 μg/mL.

Absorption, distribution, and excretion of spectinomycin are similar to those of the aminoglycosides. A single dose of 2 g produces peak plasma concentrations of 100 μg/mL at 1 hour.

Local discomfort after intramuscular injection is the most common adverse reaction. The risk of oto- and nephrotoxicity is low because the drug is administered as a single injection in a dose of 35 mg/kg (up to 2 g total). It is used exclusively for the treatment of gonorrhea suspected or proven to be due to a penicillin-resistant strain, when ceftriaxone or quinolones cannot be used, and is ineffective in oropharyngeal disease.

## TETRACYCLINES

The development of tetracycline antibiotics was the result of systematic screening of soil samples from many parts of the world. The first tetracycline, chlortetracycline, was introduced in 1948. The most recent tetracycline congener is minocycline (introduced in 1972).

## Chemistry

The tetracyclines are all derivatives of the polycyclic substance naphthacenecarboxamide (Fig. 52-3). There are a number of these agents, including **tetracycline** (Achromycin, Tetracyn), **chlortetracycline** (Aureomycin), **oxytetracycline** (Terramycin), **demeclocycline** (Declomycin), **rolitetracycline** (Reverin), **methacycline** (Rondomycin), **doxycycline** (Vibramycin), and **minocycline** (Minocin). Of these, the three most commonly used are tetracycline, doxycycline, and minocycline.

## Bacterial Susceptibility

The tetracyclines are active against a broad spectrum of bacteria. Susceptible strains include a wide range of Gram-positive and Gram-negative bacteria, *Mycoplasma, Rickettsia,* and *Chlamydia.* They are also very active against *Tre-*

| FIGURE 52-3 | Structural formulae of tetracyclines. |

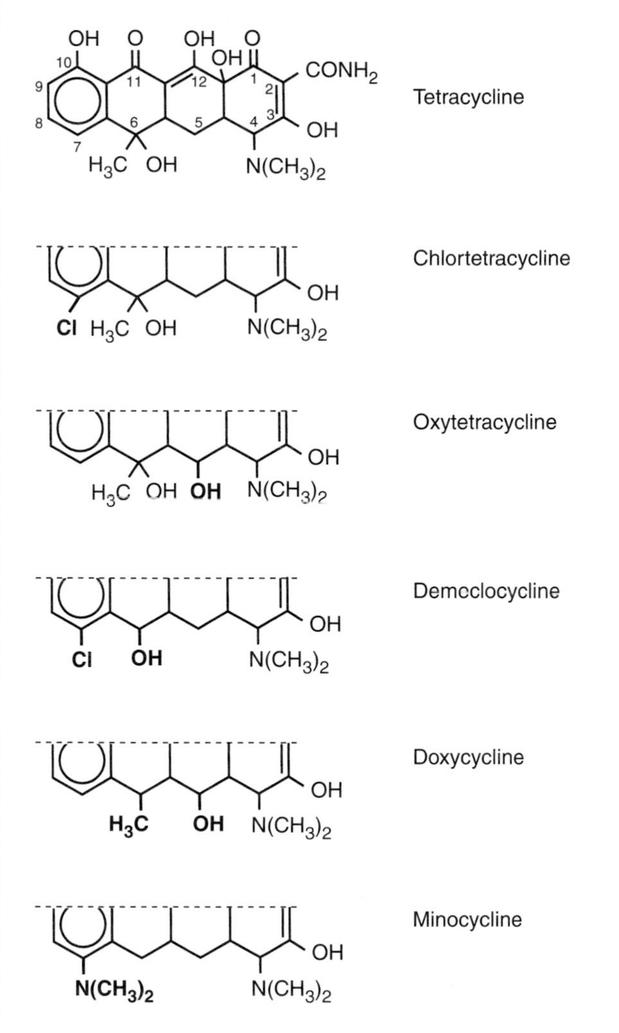

doxycycline, which do not have a hydroxyl group in the 6 position (see Fig. 52-3), the tetracyclines are unstable in the acidic environment of the stomach, and this contributes to their incomplete oral bioavailability.

Tetracyclines are effective chelating agents against various cations, with which they form poorly soluble complexes. Accordingly, absorption from the intestinal tract is impaired by milk and milk products, which contain $Ca^{2+}$, and by the co-administration of aluminum hydroxide gels or calcium, magnesium, or iron salts. After a 250-mg oral dose of tetracycline to an average-sized adult, the serum concentrations are 2 to 3 µg/mL. After a 100-mg oral dose of doxycycline or minocycline, serum concentrations are 1 to 2 µg/mL.

The volumes of distribution of the tetracyclines range from 0.4 L/kg for minocycline to 1 to 2 L/kg for doxycycline and tetracycline. Their protein binding ranges from 60% (tetracycline) to 80 to 95% (doxycycline). Tetracyclines are widely distributed, especially the highly lipid-soluble compounds minocycline and doxycycline. They enter the CSF quite freely, attaining concentrations 10 to 50% of those in the serum, but they are seldom used for meningitis because of better alternative agents. Because of chelation of tissue calcium deposits, the drugs become markedly bound to bones, teeth, and neoplasms, in which they cause yellow fluorescence; hence, these drugs should not be used in children less than 9 years of age or in pregnant women.

The main mode of elimination of most of the tetracyclines is renal glomerular filtration, but they are also eliminated to a greater or lesser extent via the biliary route. For most of the tetracyclines, 20 to 60% of the administered dose is found in the urine in unchanged form. Minocycline is recoverable in the urine and feces in significantly lower amounts than the other tetracyclines, and it appears to be biotransformed to a considerable degree. Doxycycline is excreted primarily in the feces (90%) as an inactive metabolite or perhaps as a chelate. The half-lives of these drugs range from 6 hours (tetracycline) to 24 hours (doxycycline).

## Adverse Reactions

Hypersensitivity reactions to the tetracyclines are rare. **Gastrointestinal disturbances** (nausea, vomiting, and diarrhea) are common, and pseudomembranous colitis has been described.

**Photosensitivity** reactions may be caused by any of the tetracyclines but are most frequent with doxycycline.

Tooth and bone deposition of these agents represents the most important side effect in pediatrics and is the reason these agents are **contraindicated in children less than 9 years old** and, because they cross the placenta, during fetal development. The depositions are in the calcifying areas of teeth and bones, and they may discolour both deciduous and permanent teeth. Tetracycline deposition in bone may result in temporary cessa-

*ponema pallidum*. The median MICs for three commonly used tetracyclines against representative organisms are shown in Table 52-4. Minocycline is generally the most active of the tetracyclines, especially against *Staphylococcus aureus*. When resistance develops, it is usually due to bacterial membrane transport proteins that prevent the accumulation of tetracyclines by decreasing the influx and increasing the ability of the bacteria to export antibiotics. Such proteins are coded for by plasmids, which can be transferred between bacteria and usually result in resistance to all tetracyclines.

## Pharmacokinetics

All tetracyclines are absorbed adequately but incompletely after an oral dose. Absorption is most active in the stomach and upper small intestine and is greater in the fasting state. With the exception of minocycline and

| TABLE 52-4 | Median MICs (in µg/mL) of Tetracyclines | | |
| --- | --- | --- | --- |
| Bacterium | Tetracycline | Doxycycline | Minocycline |
| Gram-positive | | | |
| Staphylococcus aureus | 3.19 | 1.6 | 0.78 |
| Streptococcus group A | 0.78 | 0.39 | 0.39 |
| Streptococcus viridans | 3.1 | 0.39 | 0.39 |
| Enterococcus faecalis | >100 | >100 | >100 |
| Streptococcus pneumoniae | 0.8 | 0.2 | 0.2 |
| Gram-negative | | | |
| Neisseria meningitidis | 0.8 | 1.6 | 1.6 |
| Neisseria gonorrhoeae | 0.78 | 0.39 | 0.39 |
| Haemophilus influenzae | 1.6 | 1.6 | 1.6 |
| Shigella | 100.0 | 100.0 | 100.0 |
| Klebsiella | 50.0 | 50.0 | 25.0 |
| Escherichia coli | 12.5 | 12.5 | 6.3 |
| Pseudomonas aeruginosa | 200.0 | 100.0 | 200.0 |
| Proteus mirabilis | >100 | >100 | >100 |
| Serratia | 200.0 | 50.0 | 25.0 |
| Bacteroides fragilis | 12.5 | – | – |
| Other Bacteroides | 0.25 | – | – |
| Others | | | |
| Mycoplasma pneumoniae | 1.6 | 1.6 | 1.6 |
| Treponema pallidum | 0.4 | 0.1 | – |
| Chlamydia | 2.0 | 2.0 | 2.0 |

tion of bone growth. This latter effect is reversible when the drug is discontinued.

Hepatotoxicity is an uncommon but serious adverse reaction, which has been described primarily after the intravenous administration of large doses of tetracycline to pregnant women. This reaction has usually been fatal. The liver shows extensive fatty infiltration at autopsy.

Outdated tetracycline products have resulted in a "Fanconi-like" syndrome (renal tubular abnormalities), with acidosis, nephrosis, and aminoaciduria. Tetracyclines may also cause further increases in blood urea nitrogen (BUN) and serum creatinine in patients with renal failure. These biochemical changes, as well as tetracycline-induced azotemia, have been attributed to an anti-anabolic effect of the drugs.

Benign increase of the intracranial pressure (i.e., pseudotumour cerebri) has been observed as a side effect of tetracycline therapy. It is reversible upon discontinuation of the medication.

Manifestations of neurotoxicity are observed frequently, and almost exclusively, with minocycline. Dizziness, weakness, ataxia, and vertigo appear within the first few days of therapy.

## Drug Interactions

Antacids containing the divalent cations $Ca^{2+}$, $Al^{3+}$, or $Mg^{2+}$, and iron salts used in the treatment of anemia, can bind these antibiotics and may result in diminished absorption of the tetracyclines from the intestinal tract when administered concomitantly.

Diuretics, presumably acting by plasma volume depletion, may aggravate the increases in BUN observed with the tetracyclines.

## Dosage Regimens and Routes of Administration

Tetracycline is usually administered orally at a daily dose of 25 to 50 mg/kg, divided into four equal doses. Minocycline is usually administered orally in a daily dose of 4 mg/kg, divided into two equal doses. The daily dose of doxycycline is 5 mg/kg, administered orally in two doses.

## Therapeutic Applications

Possible clinical indications for the tetracyclines include acute exacerbations of chronic bronchitis, Mycoplasma pneumonia, gonorrhea and syphilis in penicillin-allergic patients, early Lyme disease, Q fever, psittacosis, brucellosis, rickettsial infections, and lymphogranuloma venereum. Minocycline has a therapeutic advantage over the other tetracyclines in the treatment of Nocardia infections. Doxycycline and minocycline are unique among the tetracyclines in that they do not accumulate in renal insufficiency. Doxycycline can therefore be used in the rare situation in which a tetracycline is the drug of choice in a patient with renal insufficiency. It may also be the drug of choice for genital tract infection with *Chlamydia* or *Mycoplasma*.

# CHLORAMPHENICOL

Chloramphenicol (Chloromycetin) was first isolated in 1947 from *Streptomyces venezuelae,* an organism found in a soil sample from Venezuela. After the structural formula of this antimicrobial agent was determined, it was prepared synthetically.

## Chemistry

Chloramphenicol is a lipid-soluble compound lacking acidic and basic groups that could form salts. It is unique among natural compounds in that it contains a nitrobenzene moiety, which can be *reduced* by cytochrome P450 (see Chapter 4). Of the four stereoisomers of the propanediol moiety, only the D-threo isomer has antibacterial activity (Fig. 52-4).

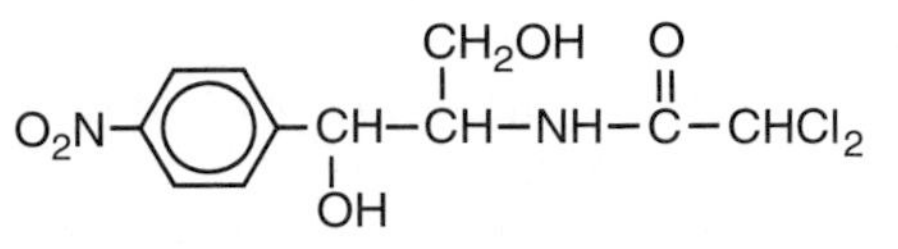

## Bacterial Susceptibility

Most aerobic bacteria (except *P. aeruginosa),* practically all anaerobes, and the majority of clinically important types of *Mycoplasma, Chlamydia,* and *Rickettsia* are susceptible to chloramphenicol at concentrations achievable in the serum. MICs of chloramphenicol against representative bacteria are outlined in Table 52-5.

Although chloramphenicol is bacteriostatic against most organisms, it is bactericidal in vitro against most strains of *Haemophilus influenzae, Streptococcus pneumoniae,* and *Neisseria meningitidis.* The mechanism of this bacterial killing action is not known.

The principal mechanisms of acquired resistance to chloramphenicol are the production of a bacterial acetyltransferase that inactivates the drug and the loss of permeability of the bacterial cell wall to chloramphenicol.

## Pharmacokinetics

Chloramphenicol is rapidly and completely absorbed from the intestinal tract. It is generally administered as

| TABLE 52-5 | MIC Ranges (in µg/mL) of Chloramphenicol |
|---|---|
| Bacterium | MIC |
| **Gram-positive** | |
| *Staphylococcus aureus* | 1.0–5.0 |
| *Streptococcus* group A | 0.3–6.0 |
| *Streptococcus viridans* | 0.6–2.5 |
| *Enterococcus faecalis* | 6.3 to >100 |
| *Streptococcus pneumoniae* | 0.06–12.5 |
| **Gram-negative** | |
| *Neisseria meningitidis* | 0.78–6.25 |
| *Neisseria gonorrhoeae* | 0.78–6.3 |
| *Haemophilus influenzae* | 0.2–3.5 |
| *Salmonella* | 0.75–5.0 |
| *Shigella* | 2.5–6.0 |
| *Klebsiella* | 0.5–25.0 |
| *Escherichia coli* | 3.0–50.0 |
| *Pseudomonas aeruginosa* | 8.0–1000 |
| *Proteus mirabilis* | 3.0–25.0 |
| *Serratia marcescens* | 2.5–5.0 |
| *Bacteroides fragilis* | 0.5–16.0 |
| Other *Bacteroides* | 0.1–16.0 |

the tasteless palmitate, which must be hydrolyzed to free active base in the intestinal lumen before absorption can occur. The peak serum concentration is approximately the same as that attained after a similar dose given intravenously, but the peak is not reached until 2 hours after an oral dose.

After administration of an intravenous dose of 500 mg of the succinate form to an adult, rapid hydrolysis to the free drug results in serum concentrations of 6 to 10 µg/mL.

The apparent volume of distribution of chloramphenicol is approximately 0.9 L/kg. It is 50 to 60% protein-bound. It diffuses into most body fluids and tissues, and, unlike many other antibiotics, chloramphenicol penetrates well into the CSF even in the absence of meningitis. In the presence of meningitis, CSF concentrations often reach 70 to 80% of serum levels; brain tissue concentrations exceed those in the serum.

Chloramphenicol is converted in the liver to a highly water-soluble monoglucuronide that has no biological activity. Impaired liver function might reduce the rate of conjugation to glucuronic acid (see Chapter 4) and correspondingly increase serum concentrations of active drug.

About 90% of chloramphenicol is excreted in the urine, but only 5 to 10% of this is in the unchanged active form. Active chloramphenicol is excreted only by glomerular filtration, but the inactive derivatives (glucuronic acid conjugates) are also eliminated by tubular secretion. Only a small amount of chloramphenicol (2 to 3%) is excreted in bile, mostly in the inactive form, and less than 1% appears in the feces. The serum half-life of chloramphenicol is approximately 3 hours.

---

| FIGURE 52-4 | Structural formula of chloramphenicol. |
|---|---|

$$O_2N - C_6H_4 - \underset{\underset{OH}{|}}{CH} - \underset{\underset{CH_2OH}{|}}{CH} - NH - \underset{\underset{O}{\|}}{C} - CHCl_2$$

## Adverse Reactions

The most feared complication of chloramphenicol therapy is **aplastic anemia**. It occurs in approximately one in 40 000 patients treated with this drug. The mechanism is unclear but appears to be related to the presence of the nitro group, because the analogue in which the nitro group is replaced with a methylsulfone group has not been associated with aplastic anemia.

A second type of hematopoietic depression is dose-related. Serum concentrations in excess of 20 to 25 µg/mL invariably result in reduced iron utilization by the bone marrow and vacuolization of erythroblasts, megakaryocytes, and leukocyte precursors. Anemia, thrombocytopenia, and leukopenia result. This type of **marrow toxicity,** apparently due to inhibition of mitochondrial protein synthesis in bone marrow precursor cells, is reversible and responds to discontinuation of the drug.

A toxic reaction to chloramphenicol observed almost exclusively in neonates is the **grey baby syndrome** (see Chapter 4). This is a form of circulatory collapse associated with excessive serum concentrations of unconjugated chloramphenicol that are maintained for several days because of immaturity of the glucuronyl transferase system in the liver of the neonate.

## Drug Interactions

Chloramphenicol may inhibit cytochrome P450–mediated metabolism of phenytoin, oral hypoglycemic agents, and oral anticoagulants, with resultant phenytoin toxicity, hypoglycemia, or hemorrhage, respectively.

Some drugs, such as phenobarbital, can induce liver microsomal enzymes and hence increase the total body clearance of chloramphenicol, resulting in reduced serum concentrations of the drug. Acetaminophen, on the contrary, can prolong the half-life of chloramphenicol and lead to drug accumulation, perhaps because of a reduction in its rate of biotransformation by glucuronidation.

## Dosage Regimens and Routes of Administration

The drug can be administered by the oral or intravenous route. The recommended dose by either route is the same, 50 to 100 mg/kg/day, divided into four doses. Significant dose reductions are necessary in neonates (see "Adverse Reactions" above). Marked variations in individual patient kinetics necessitate the monitoring of serum concentrations and appropriate adjustments in dosage.

## Therapeutic Applications

Chloramphenicol is active against most strains of bacteria that commonly cause meningitis, including *H. influenzae, N. meningitidis,* and *S. pneumoniae.* It is also active against *Salmonella,* including *S. typhi, Rickettsiae,* and almost all anaerobic bacteria that would be found in abscesses. However, the risk of aplastic anemia and the availability of new, safer alternatives have resulted in the replacement of chloramphenicol by other drugs for most indications, so it is now rarely used in the developed world. Some remaining indications are bacterial meningitis or brain abscesses in patients with a history of a severe hypersensitivity reaction to penicillins and cephalosporins, cases of penicillin-resistant pneumococcal meningitis, and rickettsial infections, such as Rocky Mountain spotted fever, typhus, and Q fever in children or pregnant women for whom tetracyclines would be contraindicated.

# CLINDAMYCIN

Lincomycin, the parent compound of clindamycin, was isolated from the fermentation products of a soil streptomycete found in Lincoln, Nebraska, which was named *Streptomyces lincolnensis.* Clindamycin is the 7-chloro-7-deoxy derivative of lincomycin. This family of agents is referred to as the **lincosamides.**

## Bacterial Susceptibility

The antibacterial activity of the lincosamides is very similar to that of erythromycin (see "Macrolides and Ketolides" below). Clindamycin is generally more active than lincomycin. These agents generally show activity against Gram-positive organisms, except the enterococci, but they are inactive against Gram-negative aerobes, with the exception of *H. influenzae.* They are also active against anaerobic bacteria, notably the cocci and Gram-negative rods. MICs against representative bacteria are given in Table 52-6.

## Pharmacokinetics

Clindamycin hydrochloride (Dalacin C) is well absorbed from the gastrointestinal tract; a dose of 300 mg produces peak serum concentrations of 4 to 5 µg/mL, 1 to 2 hours after administration. The ester, clindamycin palmitate hydrochloride, is available as a suspension. This compound must be hydrolyzed in vivo to the active base, but serum levels attained with it are nearly the same as those with clindamycin capsules.

The intramuscular and intravenous preparation is a 2-phosphate derivative. It, too, must be converted in vivo to its active form. Peak serum concentrations are considerably higher after intravenous administration. After a 300-mg intramuscular dose, the mean peak concentration is 4 to 5 µg/mL. After a similar intravenous dose, the mean peak concentration is 14 to 15 µg/mL.

The apparent volume of distribution of clindamycin is 0.6 to 0.75 L/kg. It is 90 to 95% protein-bound. It is widely distributed in the body and does not appear to be concentrated in any particular organ. Penetration into bone and across the inflamed meninges into the CSF is moderate, the concentrations reaching approximately 40% of those in serum.

After the administered compound is converted to active drug in the serum, biotransformation takes place primarily in the liver. Two metabolic derivatives are a dimethyl and a sulfoxide form. The former is more active, and the latter less active, than the base.

The main organ of clindamycin elimination is the liver, and only 8 to 28% of the drug is excreted in the urine. Thus, hepatic insufficiency has a more profound effect on clindamycin kinetics than does renal insufficiency. The half-life of clindamycin is normally 2 to 4 hours.

## Adverse Reactions

**Gastrointestinal disturbances** represent the most important group of adverse reactions to clindamycin. Diarrhea occurs in up to 30% of cases but is self-limited and subsides with discontinuation of therapy. It may be associated with nausea, vomiting, and/or abdominal cramps. A more significant gastrointestinal side effect is pseudomembranous colitis. This was first described in association with clindamycin, but almost every antibiotic has now given rise to cases of it. It is caused by the overgrowth of toxin-producing *Clostridium difficile* in the feces. The observed variation in incidence reflects the inconsistent presence of *C. difficile* in stools of patients in different locations and institutions.

Minor abnormalities of liver function tests occur with clindamycin use. No significant drug interactions have been reported.

## Dosage Regimens and Routes of Administration

The usual recommended oral dose of clindamycin is 10 to 25 mg/kg/day, administered in four equal doses. The intravenous or intramuscular daily dose is 10 to 40 mg/kg, divided into two to four equal doses.

## Therapeutic Applications

Clindamycin is primarily useful in the treatment of a variety of anaerobic infections, including those caused by *Bacteroides fragilis*. Lincomycin is rarely used clinically today. Some examples of anaerobic infections that have been successfully treated with clindamycin, either alone or in combination with other antimicrobial agents, include intra-abdominal and pelvic infections, aspiration pneumonia, anaerobic pleuropulmonary infections, infected decubitus ulcers, diabetic foot infections, and periodontal disease. Unfortunately, the incidence of resistance among *B. fragilis* is increasing; estimates as high as 19% have been reported recently.

| TABLE 52-6 | Median MICs (in μg/mL) of Clindamycin and Erythromycin | |
|---|---|---|
| Bacterium | Clindamycin | Erythromycin |
| Gram-positive | | |
| *Staphylococcus aureus* | 0.1 | 0.5 |
| *Streptococcus* group A | 0.04 | 0.04 |
| *Streptococcus viridans* | 0.02 | 0.5 |
| *Enterococcus faecalis* | 100.0 | 1.5 |
| *Streptococcus pneumoniae* | 0.01 | 0.1 |
| Gram-negative | | |
| *Neisseria meningitidis* | 12.5 | 0.78 |
| *Neisseria gonorrhoeae* | 3.1 | 0.94 |
| *Haemophilus influenzae* | 12.5 | 2.5 |
| *Salmonella* | >100 | >100 |
| *Shigella* | >100 | >100 |
| *Klebsiella* | >100 | >100 |
| *Escherichia coli* | >100 | >100 |
| *Pseudomonas aeruginosa* | >100 | >100 |
| *Proteus mirabilis* | >100 | >100 |
| *Serratia marcescens* | >100 | >100 |
| *Bacteroides fragilis* | 0.1 | 1.6 |
| Other Bacteroides | 0.1 | 1.0 |

Clindamycin is useful as an alternative to penicillin in a variety of staphylococcal and streptococcal infections, and it has recently been recommended for patients with structural heart defects who require prophylactic antibiotic therapy but are allergic to penicillin and intolerant to erythromycin. It is also used topically as an effective treatment for acne vulgaris.

Other uses that are being explored include combination with primaquine for the treatment of *Pneumocystis* pneumonia, combination with pyrimethamine for the treatment of toxoplasmosis, and combination with quinine for the treatment of chloroquine-resistant *Plasmodium falciparum* malaria (see Chapter 54).

## MACROLIDES AND KETOLIDES

**Erythromycin** (E-Mycin, Erythromid) was discovered in 1952 in the metabolic products of a strain of *Streptomyces erythreus,* originally obtained from a soil sample collected in the Philippine Archipelago. It is a macrolide antibiotic, so named because it contains a many-membered lactone ring to which deoxy sugars are attached.

New macrolides are being developed. One such erythromycin analogue, **clarithromycin** (Biaxin), is 6-methoxy-erythromycin. Clarithromycin and **azithromycin** (Zithromax) have recently been marketed, and others, such as **roxithromycin,** are under investigation. They have significant advantages over erythromycin, including less frequent dosing, less gastrointestinal toxicity, and higher tissue levels, but they are also much more expensive. They

**FIGURE 52-5** Structual formulae of representative macrolides and a ketolide (telithromycin).

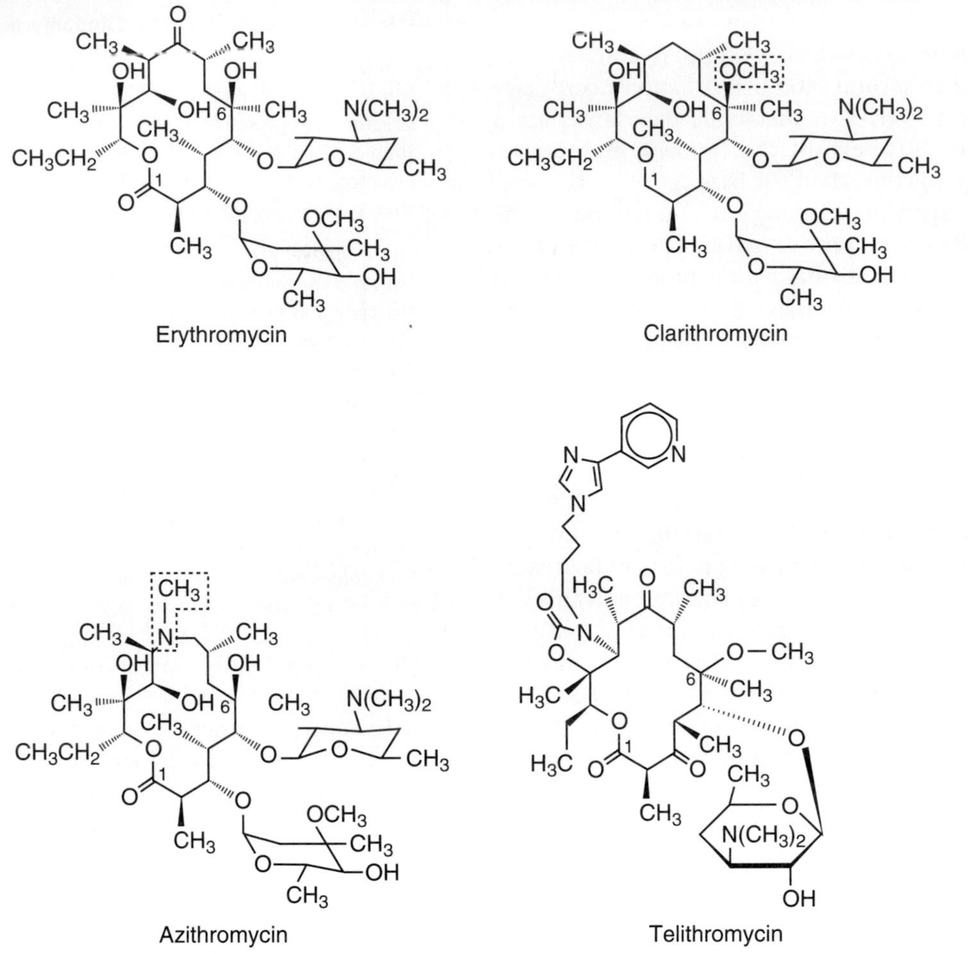

Erythromycin

Clarithromycin

Azithromycin

Telithromycin

have greater in vitro activity against many of the respiratory pathogens, including *H. influenzae, Legionella, Chlamydia pneumoniae,* and *Moraxella.* The structures of several macrolides and a ketolide are shown in Figure 52-5.

The **ketolides** are a newer group of macrolide-type antibiotics within the macrolide–lincosamide–streptogramin B family. Ketolides have a mechanism of action similar to that of macrolides, by binding to the 23S subunit of ribosomal RNA (rRNA). **Telithromycin** is the first drug in this class to be available. It is thought that, in the case of telithromycin, a stronger interaction with a specific portion of the 23S rRNA (domain II) confers activity against *Streptococcus pneumoniae* even when resistance occurs to erythromycin and the other macrolides. Telithromycin is given at a dose of 800 mg once daily. Aside from having activity against macrolide- and penicillin-resistant *S. pneumoniae,* its spectrum of activity is similar to that of the other macrolides, including respiratory tract pathogens such as *Moraxella catarrhalis, H.*

*influenzae, Streptococcus pyogenes, Mycoplasma pneumoniae, C. pneumoniae,* and *Legionella pneumoniae.*

## Bacterial Susceptibility

The antibacterial activity of **erythromycin** is very similar to that of clindamycin (see above). The agent is mainly active against Gram-positive aerobes. It is generally inactive against Gram-negative aerobes with the exceptions of *Neisseria* species, *Haemophilus, Bordetella, Campylobacter,* and *Legionella.* The Gram-negative anaerobes are not reliably sensitive. Erythromycin is also active against *Rickettsia, M. pneumoniae, Ureaplasma,* and *Chlamydia.* MICs against representative bacteria are shown in Table 52-6.

**Clarithromycin** is two to four times more active than erythromycin against most strains of *Staphylococcus* and *Streptococcus,* but cross-resistance with erythromycin has been observed. Clarithromycin also appears to have increased activity against *H. influenzae* and good activity in vitro against *Branhamella, Legionella, Mycoplasma,* and *Chlamydia.*

Development of resistance against the macrolides is uncommon, but it may develop by the following:

- Alteration in the single 50S ribosomal protein of the receptor
- Plasmid-mediated alteration (i.e., methylation of adenine moiety) in the 50S rRNA
- Enzymatic inactivation
- Decreased cell envelope permeability

## Pharmacokinetics

Erythromycin base is adequately absorbed from the gastrointestinal tract, although its activity is destroyed by gastric juice, and its absorption is delayed by food in the stomach. These problems are overcome by enclosing the drug in acid-resistant capsules or by administering a stearate derivative. Another derivative, erythromycin estolate, is less susceptible to acid, and food does not appreciably alter its absorption. Peak serum concentrations of erythromycin range from 0.5 to 1 µg/mL after a 500-mg oral dose of erythromycin base or stearate. Peak serum concentrations are two to four times higher when an equivalent dose of the estolate preparation is given. After intravenous administration of 500 mg of erythromycin, serum concentrations are approximately 5 µg/mL.

The volume of distribution of erythromycin is approximately 0.7 L/kg, and it is 70 to 75% protein-bound. It is distributed throughout the body water and tends to be retained longer in the liver and spleen than in the blood. Only very low levels are attained in the CSF even in the presence of inflamed meninges.

Only a small amount of erythromycin is excreted in its original form. It is presumed that the remainder is demethylated or otherwise degraded. Excretion occurs in both the urine and the bile, but only a fraction of the dose can be accounted for in this way. The half-life of erythromycin is approximately 1.5 hours.

## Adverse Reactions

**Gastrointestinal side effects,** including nausea, vomiting, diarrhea, and abdominal cramps, are frequent after oral erythromycin and represent a major limitation to its use. The incidence of gastrointestinal side effects associated with clarithromycin or azithromycin is significantly lower than with erythromycin, and patients who are unable to tolerate erythromycin can often tolerate the newer macrolides.

Hepatotoxicity, which has been documented with the estolate and other erythromycin preparations (although considerably less frequently), is felt to be due to the propionyl ester linkage. Manifestations may include jaundice,

fever, pruritus, rash, increased liver size, and eosinophilia. Liver histology reveals a hypersensitivity cholestasis with or without necrosis. This adverse reaction generally resolves when the antibiotic is discontinued.

Thrombophlebitis is a common side effect after intravenous administration. Ototoxicity, manifested as tinnitus and transient deafness, is a rare adverse reaction that has occurred more frequently after intravenous than after oral administration. Rashes are not uncommon in association with erythromycin use, but significant allergic reactions are rare.

## Drug Interactions

Erythromycin and clarithromycin have been found to inhibit some isozymes of cytochrome P450, especially CYP3A4. Thus, the use of erythromycin has led to increases in theophylline and cyclosporine concentrations when these drugs are administered concurrently with it. It was recently shown that the concomitant use of erythromycin and terfenadine or astemizole leads to elevated levels of their active metabolites. In some patients, this appears to be associated with a prolongation of the QT interval and cardiac arrhythmias. Inhibition of the metabolism of other drugs is likely, but evidence for other interactions will require further trials.

## Dosage Regimens and Routes of Administration

The usual recommended oral dose of erythromycin ranges from 20 to 50 mg/kg/day, divided into two to four equal doses. The daily intravenous dose is the same, usually administered in two doses.

## Therapeutic Applications

Erythromycin is useful in the treatment of staphylococcal, streptococcal, and pneumococcal infections in patients who cannot tolerate penicillins. Additional indications for erythromycin therapy include the treatment of *Mycoplasma* infections *(M. pneumoniae* and *Ureaplasma),* the eradication of *Bordetella pertussis* and *Corynebacterium diphtheriae* from the nasopharynx, the treatment of *Chlamydia* infections, the treatment of Legionnaire's disease, the treatment of gonorrhea or syphilis during pregnancy, and the eradication of *Campylobacter* from the stools of patients with *Campylobacter* gastroenteritis.

Clarithromycin and azithromycin are useful as alternatives to erythromycin in patients who have a gastrointestinal intolerance to erythromycin, or in serious infections where they are more active. They may be particularly useful in community-acquired pneumonia. Clarithromycin and azithromycin are also being used (in combination with other drugs) in the treatment and prevention of disseminated *Mycobacterium avium* infections in patients with AIDS. Telithromycin may be used in cases where macrolide- or penicillin-resistant *S. pneumoniae* is suspected.

## NEWER PROTEIN SYNTHESIS INHIBITORS

More recently, a new class of drugs, the **oxazolidinones**, has been developed particularly to target infections caused by multi-resistant, Gram-positive bacteria such as methicillin-resistant *Staphylococcus aureus* (MRSA) and vancomycin-resistant *Enterococcus* (VRE). **Linezolid** is the prototypical drug representing this class (Fig. 52-6). Like many other protein synthesis inhibitors, linezolid binds to the 50S subunit of the bacterial ribosome and prevents bacterial protein synthesis. Most other protein synthesis inhibitors allow mRNA translation to begin but then inhibit peptide elongation. Oxazolidinones, however, block the initiation complex for protein synthesis and prevent translation of the mRNA. The significance of this mechanistic difference is that the activity of linezolid against Gram-positive cocci is unaffected by rRNA methylases that modify the 23S rRNA, and therefore activity is maintained when resistance has developed to other drugs such as the lincosamides and macrolides. Furthermore, linezolid is equally active against MRSA, methicillin-sensitive *S. aureus* (MSSA), and VRE.

Linezolid also has favourable pharmacokinetic properties. Adverse reactions are few, but reversible thrombocytopenia and leukopenia have been described. Linezolid is a reversible inhibitor of monoamine oxidase B, and although food restrictions are not advised, caution should be used when administering it together with psychotropic drugs, since there have been case reports of a serotonin-type syndrome. More recently, peripheral neuropathy and optic neuritis have been described.

Another group of drugs active against multi-resistant, Gram-positive organisms is the **streptogramins**. The clinically available example is **quinupristin–dalfopristin** (Synercid; Fig. 52-7), so named because it is a combination of two different streptogramins that work at slightly different sites of bacterial cell wall synthesis and hence have synergistic activity. Dalfopristin is derived from a group A

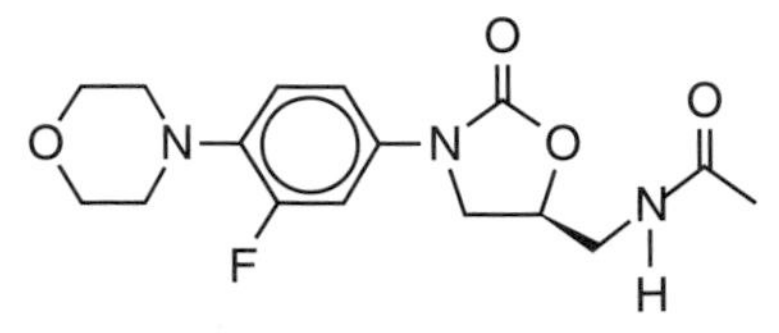

FIGURE 52-7 Structural formulae of quinupristin and dalfopristin.

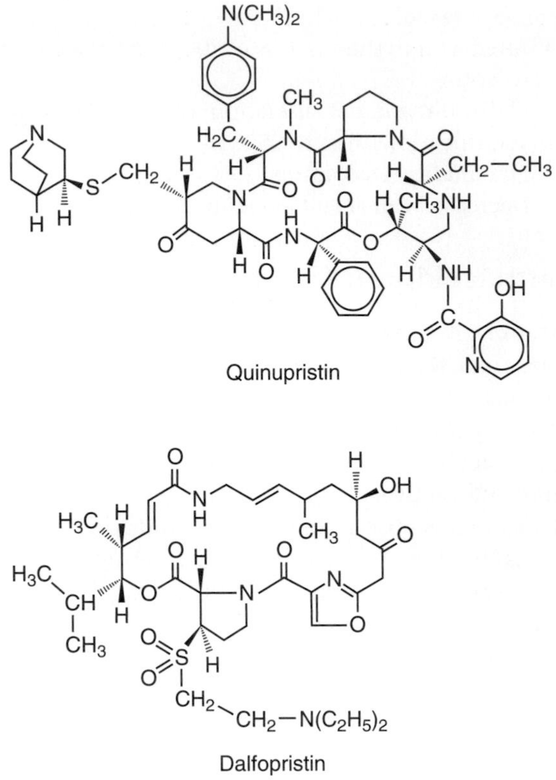

streptogramin, and quinupristin is a group B streptogramin. Each of these drugs has bacteriostatic activity when used individually, but when combined, they are bactericidal. The microbial spectrum of quinupristin–dalfopristin includes *Enterococcus faecium* (but not *E. faecalis*), MRSA, coagulase-negative staphylococci, and penicillin-resistant *S. pneumoniae*.

Quinupristin-dalfopristin is used only by intravenous infusion, and it has a short plasma half-life (less than 1 hour). Both components are metabolized in the liver, and dose reduction may be required in patients with hepatic insufficiency. The major side effects include myalgia associated with the infusion and non-specific infusion site reactions. The drug is also an inhibitor of CYP3A4 and therefore may cause adverse drug interactions.

## SUGGESTED READINGS

Alvarez-Elcoro S, Enzler MJ. The macrolides: erythromycin, clarithromycin and azithromycin. *Mayo Clin Proc.* 1999;74:613-634.

Barradell LB, Plosker GL, McTavish D. Clarithromycin: a review of its pharmacological properties and therapeutic use in *Mycobacterium avium*-intracellulare complex infection in

FIGURE 52-6 Structural formula of linezolid.

patients with acquired immune deficiency syndrome. *Drugs.* 1993;46:289-312.

Brittain DC. Erythromycin. *Med Clin North Am.* 1987;71:1147-1154.

Clark JP, Langston E. Ketolides: a new class of antibacterial agents for treatment of community-acquired respiratory tract infections in a primary care setting. *Mayo Clin Proc.* 2003;78: 1113-1124.

Davey P. Clinical use of the aminoglycosides in the 1990s. *Rev Med Microbiol.* 1991;2:22-30.

Eliopoulos GM. Quinupristin-dalfopristin and linezolid: evidence and opinion. *Clin Infect Dis.* 2003;36:473-481.

Gilbert DW. Once daily aminoglycoside therapy. *Antimicrob Agents Chemother.* 1991;35:399-405.

Klein NC, Cunha BA. Tetracyclines. *Med Clin North Am.* 1995;79: 789-802.

Leclercq R, Dutka-Malen S, Brisson-Noel A, et al. Resistance of enterococci to aminoglycosides and glycopeptides. *Clin Infect Dis.* 1992;15:495-501.

Lortholary O, Tod M, Cohen Y, Petitjean O. Aminoglycosides. *Med Clin North Am.* 1995;79:761-788.

Schlossberg D. Azithromycin and clarithromycin. *Med Clin North Am.* 1995;79:803-815.

Shaw KJ, Rather PN, Hare RS, Miller GH. Molecular genetics of aminoglycoside resistance genes and familial relationships of the aminoglycoside-modifying enzymes. *Microbiol Rev.* 1993; 57:138-163.

Smilack JD, Wilson WR, Cockerill FR. Tetracyclines, chloramphenicol, erythromycin, clindamycin, and metronidazole. *Mayo Clin Proc.* 1991;66:1270-1280.

Whitman MS, Tunkil AR. Azithromycin and clarithromycin: overview and comparison with erythromycin. *Infect Control Hosp Epidemiol.* 1992;12:357-368.

# 53

# Drugs That Affect Cellular Nucleic Acid Synthesis

## EJ PHILLIPS, J UETRECHT, AND SL WALMSLEY

### CASE HISTORY

A 36-year-old male immigrant from Sri Lanka saw his physician after a 3-week history of cough, hemoptysis, fever, and weight loss of about 5 kg (11 lb.). A chest X-ray revealed a right upper lobe infiltrate with cavity. A sputum smear was positive for acid-fast bacilli, and *Mycobacterium tuberculosis* was later confirmed on culture. The patient was started on treatment with isoniazid 300 mg/day, rifampin 600 mg/day, ethambutol 25 mg/kg/day, and pyrazinamide 25 mg/kg/day. His wife and children were also seen by the physician and were given isoniazid prophylaxis at a dose of 300 mg/day (wife) and 10 mg/kg/day (children) when their skin tests were found to be positive. On culture, the patient's infecting microorganisms were found to be sensitive to all first-line anti-tuberculous drugs.

Ethambutol and pyrazinamide were discontinued after 2 months of treatment. Isoniazid and rifampin were continued for another 4 months. His signs and symptoms resolved completely and his chest X-ray improved.

After full recovery from this bout of tuberculosis, he visited his homeland for a period of 1 month. Three days before his return to North America, he developed fever and bloody diarrhea, which was quite severe during the flight home. He immediately saw his family physician, who requested a stool specimen. Because he had a fever of 39°C and continued bloody diarrhea, the physician empirically started him on oral ciprofloxacin at a dose of 500 mg twice daily. The physician received a report that *Shigella* was isolated from the stool sample, whereupon ciprofloxacin was continued for a period of 7 days. All signs and symptoms of the disease resolved.

Bacterial replication, like that of all living cells, requires replication of the DNA and RNA that contain and transfer the genetic codes for the synthesis of all constituents of the cell. Compounds that inhibit the replication of bacterial nucleic acids but are sufficiently selective to have little or no effect on mammalian nucleic acids are potentially useful in treating infectious diseases. Inhibition of nucleic acid replication by these compounds may be either direct or indirect.

## DIRECT INHIBITORS OF NUCLEIC ACID REPLICATION

Rifampin (an antibiotic), and perhaps griseofulvin (an antifungal), directly inhibit the replication of nucleic acids. **Rifampin** acts by inhibiting bacterial RNA polymerase, which is concerned with RNA replication. Human DNA-dependent RNA polymerase, however, is resistant to rifampin. **Nalidixic acid** and the newer **fluoroquinolones** inhibit the enzymatic activities of bacterial DNA gyrase (DNA topoisomerase), which is responsible for introduc-

ing superhelical twists into closed double-stranded DNA. The DNA gyrase produces breaks in the DNA strands; supercoiling occurs by the passage of another strand of DNA through the break, and then the break is resealed. DNA topoisomerase is necessary in DNA replication, repair, and genetic recombination. Binding of a quinolone to the DNA gyrase results in inhibition of the rejoining reaction after a break in the strand has occurred.

It has been proposed that **griseofulvin** exerts its antifungal activity by inhibiting fungal DNA production. Griseofulvin also binds to microtubular protein and inhibits mitosis. It is also toxic to mammalian cells, and the basis for useful selective toxicity appears to involve the selective distribution of the drug to keratinized cells, especially those that are diseased.

**Flucytosine (5-fluorocytosine)** is also thought to inhibit the replication of nucleic acids directly, by acting as a fluorine analogue of the normal body constituent cytosine. It appears that this drug enters susceptible yeast cells and is deaminated by cytosine deaminase to the antimetabolite 5-fluorouracil. 5-Fluorouracil is converted through several steps to 5-fluorodeoxyuridylic acid monophosphate, a non-competitive inhibitor of thymidylate synthetase. This interferes with DNA synthesis. Conversion of flucytosine to 5-fluorouracil within the body occurs to a sufficient degree to be a possible explanation for its toxicity to bone marrow and the gastrointestinal tract (i.e., mucositis).

## INDIRECT INHIBITORS OF NUCLEIC ACID REPLICATION

**Sulfonamides, sulfones,** probably **para-aminosalicylic acid (PAS),** and the diaminopyrimidines (**trimethoprim** and **pyrimethamine**) inhibit the replication of nucleic acids more remotely by interfering with the synthesis of folic acid by microbial cells. Folic acid functions as a coenzyme for the transfer of one-carbon units from one molecule to another, a step necessary for the synthesis of thymidine and the other nucleosides. Mammals require preformed folic acid (it is a vitamin for them; see Chapters 39 and 63). In contrast, bacteria cannot use preformed

folic acid, which cannot enter the bacterial cell; instead, they must synthesize it intracellularly from para-aminobenzoic acid (PABA). Sulfonamides act by competitively inhibiting the incorporation of PABA into folic acid. The presence of an extraneous source of PABA (e.g., pus, blood, tissue exudates) can decrease the competitive effectiveness of the sulfonamides. Trimethoprim is a dihydrofolate reductase inhibitor. It potentiates the activity of sulfonamides by sequential inhibition of folinic acid synthesis (Fig. 53-1). The resulting depletion of folic or tetrahydrofolic acid within the bacterial or parasitic cells inhibits the formation of coenzymes necessary for the synthesis of purines, pyrimidines, and other substances required for growth and reproduction. Although this does not usually result in cell death, the sulfonamides and related compounds are selectively toxic to bacteria.

Pyrimethamine is more active than trimethoprim in inhibiting the dihydrofolate reductases of *Plasmodium* species and *Toxoplasma gondii,* whereas trimethoprim is more active against bacteria. Both drugs can inhibit mammalian dihydrofolate reductase at high concentrations.

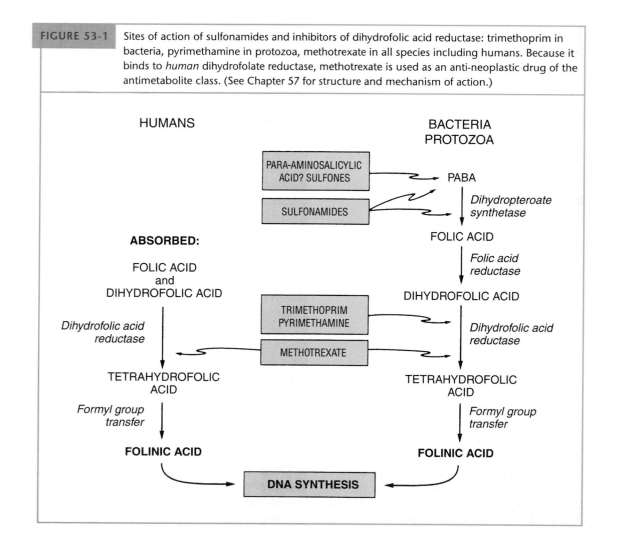

**FIGURE 53-1**   Sites of action of sulfonamides and inhibitors of dihydrofolic acid reductase: trimethoprim in bacteria, pyrimethamine in protozoa, methotrexate in all species including humans. Because it binds to *human* dihydrofolate reductase, methotrexate is used as an anti-neoplastic drug of the antimetabolite class. (See Chapter 57 for structure and mechanism of action.)

Trimetrexate is a lipid-soluble dihydrofolate reductase inhibitor with activity against *T. gondii* and *Pneumocystis carinii*. Methotrexate, which binds to *human* as well as microbial dihydrofolate reductase, is used as an antimetabolite in the treatment of severe psoriasis, rheumatoid arthritis, and some neoplastic diseases. (See Chapter 57.)

# ANTIFUNGAL AGENTS

## Griseofulvin (Fulvicin, Grisovin)

Griseofulvin was isolated from *Penicillium griseofulvum* in 1939, but it was not used clinically as an antifungal agent until nearly 20 years later.

It inhibits the growth in vitro of various species of *Microsporum, Epidermophyton,* and *Trichophyton*. Minimum inhibitory concentrations against sensitive fungi range from 0.18 to 0.42 µg/mL.

### Pharmacokinetics

Griseofulvin is reasonably well absorbed from the intestinal tract, although there is considerable variability and fluctuation in serum concentrations in the same subject and in different individuals receiving the same dose. A serum concentration of 1 to 2 µg/mL is attained about 4 hours after a 1-g dose. Concentrations are enhanced approximately twofold if the drug is taken after a fatty meal rather than in the fasting state.

The volume of distribution and degree of protein binding of this drug are unknown, but some of it is carried in the circulation to the skin, hair, and nails, where it is concentrated by selective binding to keratin.

Most of the absorbed drug is inactivated in the liver by dealkylation. This inactivation may be enhanced by barbiturates through induction of drug-biotransforming enzymes. The inactive metabolite of griseofulvin is excreted in the urine. A considerable proportion of an oral dose, which is unabsorbed, appears unchanged in the feces. The plasma half-life is 10 to 20 hours.

### Adverse reactions

Nausea, vomiting, diarrhea, headache, fatigue, and mental confusion may all occur with griseofulvin therapy but are uncommon.

### Drug interactions

The co-administration of barbiturates may increase the rate of biotransformation of griseofulvin, resulting in reduced serum concentrations.

Griseofulvin itself may induce liver microsomal enzymes and may increase the biotransformation of warfarin, thus diminishing the anticoagulant effect of the latter. It has also been found to increase the metabolism of contraceptive steroids and reduce their efficacy.

### Therapeutic applications

Griseofulvin is effective in the systemic treatment of dermatophyte infections caused by *Microsporum, Trichophyton,* and *Epidermophyton*. It is primarily useful in infections of the scalp, hands, feet, and nails that are refractory to topical therapy.

## 5-Fluorocytosine (5-FC, Flucytosine) (Ancobon)

5-Fluorocytosine (5-FC) was synthesized in 1957 as a cytosine antimetabolite for the treatment of leukemia but was ineffective for this purpose. However, in 1964, it was noted to possess selective antifungal activity.

### Fungal susceptibility

The drug inhibits *Cryptococcus neoformans* and *Candida albicans* in concentrations of 0.46 to 3.9 µg/mL and kills them at concentrations of 3.9 to 15.6 µg/mL. Other fungi that are sensitive to this drug include the non-*albicans* species of *Candida* and *Torulopsis glabrata*. *Aspergillus* species are variably sensitive, with minimum inhibitory concentration (MIC) ranges of 0.48 to 500 µg/mL.

Drug resistance arising during therapy is frequent, rapid, usually profound, and accompanied by clinical deterioration. Fungal mechanisms for resistance include loss of deaminase (for conversion of 5-FC to 5-fluorouracil) and decreased permeability. Because of this problem, 5-FC is usually used in combination with amphotericin B.

### Pharmacokinetics

5-Fluorocytosine is well absorbed following oral administration. Peak serum concentrations of approximately 45 µg/mL are attained 2 to 6 hours after a 2-g dose.

The volume of distribution of 5-FC is 0.6 to 0.7 L/kg. It is approximately 10% protein-bound. It is well distributed in body fluids and tissues, and during the treatment of fungal meningitis it attains concentrations in the cerebrospinal fluid (CSF) that are 50 to 100% of those in the serum.

A small amount of 5-FC is converted to 5-fluorouracil, and approximately 90% of 5-FC is excreted unchanged via the kidney by glomerular filtration. It must be used cautiously in patients with impaired renal function. Its plasma half-life is 3 to 4 hours, which may increase to more than 100 hours in the presence of renal disease. Unabsorbed 5-FC, usually less than 10%, is excreted unchanged in the feces.

### Adverse reactions

Dose-dependent hematological toxicity with thrombocytopenia and/or granulocytopenia is common and is dose-limiting. Agranulocytosis and aplastic anemia have also been reported. Nausea and vomiting are frequent. Given the high incidence of adverse reactions, it is imperative that the dosage recommendations be followed carefully, especially in patients receiving concurrent amphotericin B, and serum drug levels should be monitored.

## Dosage, route of administration, and therapeutic applications

5-Fluorocytosine is administered orally every 6 hours to provide a total daily dose of 50 to 150 mg/kg. It is most useful in the treatment of cutaneous and mucocutaneous candidiasis, *Candida* urinary tract infections, and in combination with amphotericin B in the treatment of cryptococcal meningitis. It may also play a therapeutic role as a synergistic agent in other systemic fungal infections caused by sensitive organisms.

# ANTI-TUBERCULOUS DRUGS

See also Chapter 50: "Cycloserine," "Isoniazid," and "Ethambutol."

## Rifampin (Rifadin, Rimactane)

Rifampin is a complex macrocyclic antibiotic produced by *Streptomyces mediterranei,* which was first isolated in 1959.

### Bacterial susceptibility

The drug is active against a wide range of Gram-positive and Gram-negative organisms (Table 53-1). However, resistance, which may emerge rapidly when rifampin is used alone, limits its widespread use. Its strongest antibacterial attribute is its activity against the majority of *M. tuberculosis* strains (MIC 0.5 µg/mL or less).

| TABLE 53-1 | Median MICs (in µg/mL) of Rifampin |
|---|---|
| **Bacterium** | **MIC** |
| Gram-positive | |
| *Staphylococcus aureus* | 0.001 |
| *Streptococcus* group A | 0.04 |
| *Streptococcus viridans* | 0.05 |
| *Enterococcus faecalis* | 4.0 |
| *Streptococcus pneumoniae* | 0.05 |
| Gram-negative | |
| *Neisseria meningitidis* | 0.016 |
| *Neisseria gonorrhoeae* | 0.2 |
| *Haemophilus influenzae* | 0.5 |
| *Klebsiella* | 10.0 |
| *Escherichia coli* | 5.3 |
| *Pseudomonas aeruginosa* | 20.0 |
| *Proteus mirabilis* | 3.9 |
| *Serratia* | 64.0 |
| *Bacteroides fragilis* | 0.26 |
| Other *Bacteroides* | 0.1 |
| *Mycobacterium tuberculosis* | 0.5 |

## Pharmacokinetics

Rifampin is well absorbed from the intestinal tract. The peak concentration of 8 µg/mL is reached approximately 2 hours after a 600-mg oral dose. Serum concentrations are lower if the drug is taken immediately after food.

The volume of distribution of rifampin is approximately 1.6 L/kg. It is 60 to 90% protein-bound. Rifampin penetrates well into most tissues and fluids, including lungs, liver, pleural and ascitic fluid, bone, tears, and saliva; it also enters the CSF, whether or not the meninges are inflamed. Concentrations in the CSF during therapy for tuberculous meningitis usually exceed 50% of serum concentrations.

Rifampin is deacetylated in the liver, and it must also be inactivated elsewhere in the body to some extent, because a proportion of the dose remains undetected in excretion studies.

## Adverse reactions

The major serious adverse reaction associated with the use of rifampin is liver disease. The type of injury is usually obstructive, and jaundice occurs in 0.6% of treated patients; however, hepatocellular disease with an increase in transaminases can also occur. The use of high doses, or the interruption and reinstatement of therapy, can lead to what appear to be immune-mediated reactions. Such reactions can consist of hemolytic anemia and thrombocytopenia, acute renal failure, a syndrome of fever, chills, myalgia, and arthralgia, and even hepatorenal syndrome. Rifampin has been reported to cause immune suppression, but the significance of this effect is unknown. Patients should be warned that rifampin leads to an orange–pink coloration of tears, urine, and sweat and can stain soft contact lenses.

## Drug interactions

Rifampin is a potent inducer of cytochrome P450, specifically the 3A4 and 2C9/19 isoforms, and thus can decrease the levels of many other drugs. This can lead to breakthrough bleeding and pregnancy in women using birth control pills.

## Therapeutic applications

The major indication for rifampin is the treatment of mycobacterial infections, especially tuberculosis. Despite its high activity, it should always be used in combination with at least one other agent for the treatment of active tuberculosis to decrease the emergence of resistant strains (see "Isoniazid," Chapter 50). Rifampin is also used for the chemoprophylaxis of contacts of patients with meningococcal or *Haemophilus influenzae* meningitis. It is effective against intracellular organisms. Its penetration into nasopharyngeal secretions also allows its use in combination with other drugs in the eradication of *Staphylococcus aureus* nasal carriage.

## Pyrazinamide (Tebrazid)

Pyrazinamide is a synthetic analogue of nicotinamide. Its mode of action on tubercle bacilli is not known. The drug is bactericidal at acidic pH, like that existing intracellularly in phagolysosomes, but replicating microorganisms become rapidly resistant to it when it is used alone. Metabolically inactive tubercle bacilli are resistant, rendering the drug inappropriate for long-term therapy. It may be used as an anti-tuberculous drug only together with other agents in multiple-drug treatment schedules.

### Pharmacokinetics

Pyrazinamide is well absorbed after oral administration. It is widely distributed, readily penetrates cells and diffuses into cavities, and enters the CSF when the meninges are inflamed. The drug is biotransformed in the liver to pyrazinoic acid and then to 5-hydroxypyrazinoic acid, which is excreted by renal glomerular filtration. The half-life is about 6 hours.

### Adverse reactions

Pyrazinamide at high doses (40 to 50 mg/kg/day) causes hepatotoxicity, which has resulted in fatal hepatic necrosis in some instances. Therefore, the drug is currently used at much lower dosage, but it still requires monitoring for hepatotoxicity during the entire period of therapy. Since pyrazinamide inhibits urate excretion, episodes of hyperuricemia are frequently observed, as well as occasional nausea, vomiting, fever, polymyalgia, and malaise. The hyperuricemic episodes may precipitate gouty arthritis.

### Dosage regimens and therapeutic application

Pyrazinamide is an important drug for short-term, multiple-drug therapy, primarily in areas with high primary resistance to anti-tubercular agents. In view of its rapid bactericidal action, it is typically used in combination with other first-line anti-tuberculous drugs for the first 2 months of treatment. The daily dosage is 20 to 35 mg/kg orally, divided into three or four equally spaced doses, not to exceed 3 g per day regardless of the patient's weight.

## Para-Aminosalicylic Acid (PAS) (Nemasol)

Over 50 years ago, it was determined that benzoic and salicylic acids increased the oxygen consumption of tubercle bacilli. It was speculated that similar compounds played a role in the normal metabolism of *M. tuberculosis,* and it was theorized that structurally altered analogues might have an opposite effect. This led to the discovery of para-aminosalicylic acid (PAS), a drug that is chemically closely related to salicylic acid and that probably acts as a competitive antagonist of para-aminobenzoic acid.

Thus, PAS inhibits folate synthesis, but also mycobactin synthesis. Mycobactin is a "siderophore," and its inhibition reduces the uptake of iron by mycobacteria.

### Pharmacokinetics

PAS is well absorbed from the intestinal tract. Maximum serum concentrations of 50 to 150 μg/mL are attained 1 to 2 hours after a 2-g dose. The drug is 50 to 60% protein-bound. It is distributed throughout the total body water and reaches concentrations in the pleural fluid and in caseous tissues approximately equal to those in the circulation. It does not yield effective CSF concentrations, possibly because it is actively transported out of the CSF.

PAS is biotransformed in the liver, mainly by acetylation. Over 80% of the drug is excreted in the urine by glomerular filtration and tubular secretion. Only 14 to 33% of the total dose is excreted in the urine as the active unchanged drug. The remainder is excreted as metabolites such as acetyl-*p*-aminosalicylic acid, para-aminosalicyluric acid, and other conjugated amines. The half-life of PAS is less than 1 hour.

### Adverse reactions

Nausea, vomiting, anorexia, abdominal cramps, and diarrhea occur to some extent in nearly all patients. These may be reduced by taking the drug with meals or by the concomitant administration of antacids.

### Drug interactions

PAS may enhance the effect of anticoagulants and inhibit the biotransformation of acetylsalicylic acid, thereby allowing toxic amounts to accumulate. Probenecid may inhibit tubular secretion of PAS, and PAS may impair the absorption of rifampin.

### Dosage regimen, route of administration, and therapeutic applications

The usual daily dose of PAS is 200 to 300 mg/kg administered orally, divided into two or three doses. This drug has largely been displaced by newer or first-line agents and is currently used as a second or third agent, in combination with other more effective agents, in the treatment of infections caused by *M. tuberculosis*. More recently, it has been used in combination with second-line, anti-tuberculous drugs in the treatment of multidrug-resistant tuberculosis.

# QUINOLONE ANTIBACTERIAL AGENTS

The prototype drug in this group is **nalidixic acid** (NegGram), an old drug with limited use as a urinary antiseptic. The development of **fluoroquinolones** has greatly extended the antibacterial spectrum and usefulness of these agents. Three examples of the early fluoroquinolones are **norfloxacin** (Noroxin), **ciprofloxacin** (Cipro), and **ofloxacin** (Floxin). More recently, newer drugs such as **moxifloxacin** (Avelox) and **gatifloxacin** (Tequin) have been developed (Fig. 53-2).

**FIGURE 53-2** Structural formulae of nalidixic acid and the fluoroquinolones.

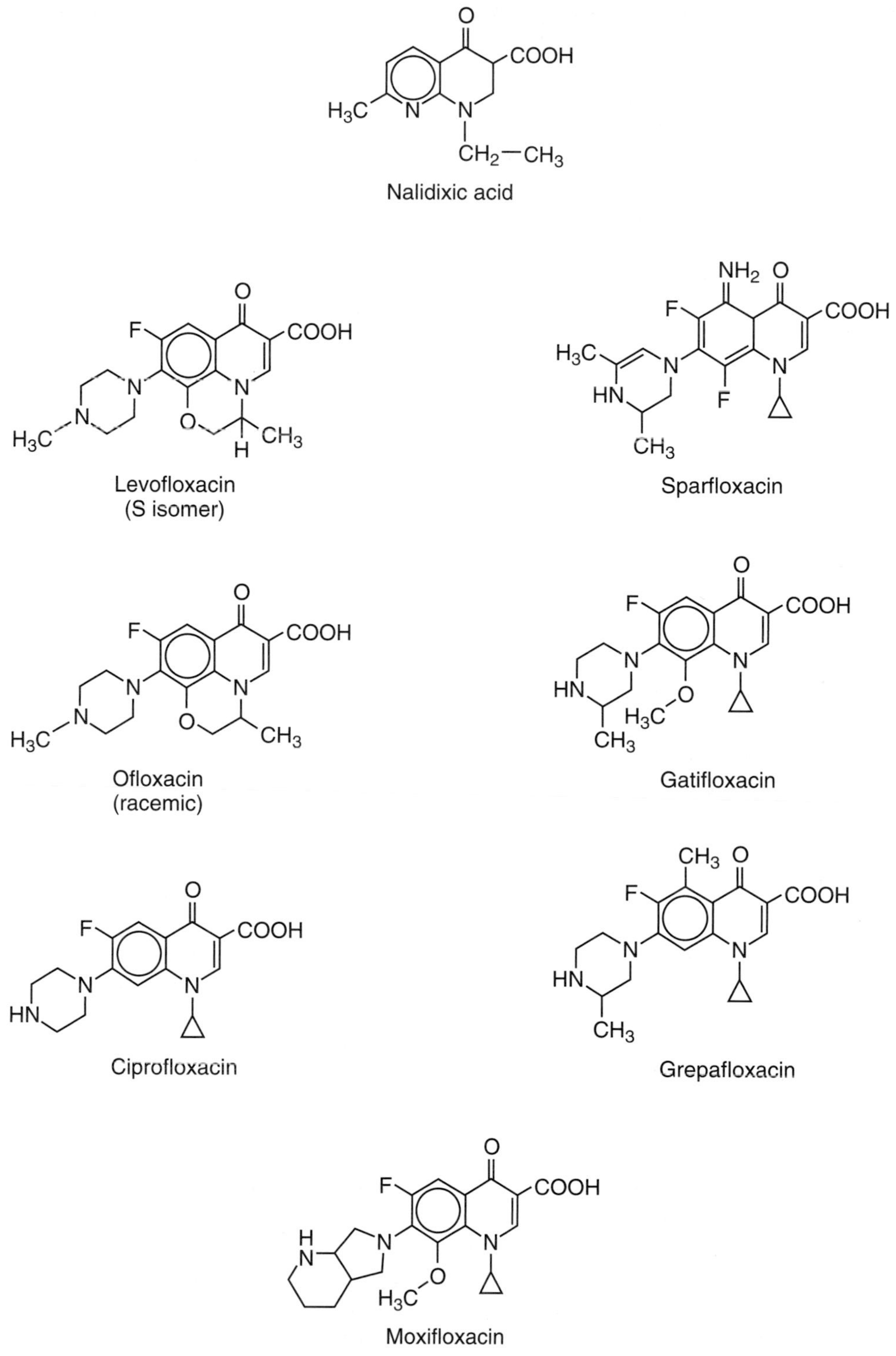

## Bacterial Susceptibility

Although nalidixic acid has a broad spectrum of activity against Gram-negative organisms, its activity is weak, resistance emerges rapidly, and it is inactive against all Gram-positive organisms.

Nalidixic acid is bacteriostatic. Addition of a fluorine and removal of the ethyl side group yields norfloxacin. The fluoroquinolones show activity against Gram-positive organisms and greater activity than nalidixic acid against Gram-negative organisms. The fluoroquinolones also are bactericidal. Their spectrum of activity includes *S. aureus* (including methicillin-resistant strains), most streptococci, enterococci, and most other Gram-negative enteric organisms, *H. influenzae,* and *Neisseria gonorrhoeae.* Addition of a piperazine ring, as in ciprofloxacin, increases fluoroquinolone activity against *Pseudomonas.* Importantly, ciprofloxacin is the only fluoroquinolone with reliable activity against *Pseudomonas aeruginosa.* Therefore, it is worrisome that increasing resistance of *P. aeruginosa* to ciprofloxacin (now in the range of 25 to 40% of isolates) has recently been reported from many centres.

More recently, newer fluoroquinolones have been developed in attempts to improve the activity against Gram-positive and anaerobic organisms. Levofloxacin is the *l*-isomer of ofloxacin and has improved activity against *Streptococcus pneumoniae;* its main target in clinical use is community-acquired respiratory tract infections such as community-acquired pneumonia. Newer examples of fluoroquinolones with Gram-positive and anaerobic coverage include moxifloxacin and gatifloxacin, which are available in both oral and intravenous preparations. Another drug called **trovafloxacin** also was developed for its enhanced activity against Gram- positives and anaerobes; its use is currently limited because of an idiosyncratic hepatic toxicity associated with the drug.

There has been a rapid emergence of resistant strains in a short period of time since the introduction of these drugs, which may seriously limit their continued usefulness. For example, in one prospective study, the incidence of resistance of methicillin-resistant strains of *S. aureus* to ciprofloxacin increased from 0 to 79% in just 1 year. The rate of development of resistance among *P. aeruginosa* and mycobacteria is also about 1000 times faster than that of most other bacteria. The development of such resistance is probably due to alteration of DNA gyrase and/or changes in the outer membrane proteins that lead to decreased permeability to the drug.

## Pharmacokinetics

The fluoroquinolones are well absorbed when given orally; most are available for both oral and parenteral administration. They penetrate well into most body fluids. However, the activity of norfloxacin is relatively low, and it does not achieve adequate concentrations in serum or tissues to treat most systemic infections; its use is limited to infections of the urinary tract. The half-lives of norfloxacin and ciprofloxacin are about 4 hours, and these agents need to be administered only every 8 to 12 hours. Elimination is about half by renal excretion and half by biotransformation, and the dose may need to be adjusted in renal and hepatic failure. Newer drugs, such as levofloxacin, moxifloxacin, and gatifloxacin, are administered once daily.

## Adverse Reactions

Severe adverse reactions are uncommon with the fluoroquinolones. The most common side effects are gastrointestinal symptoms. Central nervous system (CNS) symptoms, including headache, confusion, and hallucinations, are infrequent, and seizures have been reported but are rare. Rashes and other allergic reactions, including anaphylaxis, have also been observed. The fluoroquinolones cause damage to developing cartilage in animals, but there is no evidence that this also occurs in humans. Long-term follow-up of children who have received these agents has shown only transient reversible arthralgias; however, use of these agents in children and pregnant or nursing women is still controversial and should only be considered when the benefit clearly outweighs the risk or when alternative agents are not available. Although laboratory abnormalities such as increased transaminases and leukopenia have been reported, these abnormalities appear to be reversible.

Recently, Health Canada issued a warning that gatifloxacin may produce rare but severe, and even fatal, hypo- or hyperglycemia in patients with diabetes or other predisposing conditions. The mechanism is unknown. Hypoglycemia tends to occur in the first three days of therapy, and hyperglycemia between the fourth and tenth days.

## Drug Interactions

When co-administered with aluminum-, magnesium-, and, to a lesser degree, calcium-containing antacids, the quinolones have markedly reduced bioavailability, presumably due to the formation of cation–quinolone complexes. Some quinolones inhibit hepatic microsomal enzymes involved in theophylline and caffeine metabolism. This can result in decreased theophylline clearance and toxicity. This is a greater problem with ciprofloxacin than with ofloxacin and is not a problem with the newer fluoroquinolones.

## Therapeutic Applications

A major indication for the fluoroquinolones is the treatment of urinary tract infections and chronic prostatitis involving organisms, such as *P. aeruginosa,* that are resistant to other oral agents. They are also used as second-line therapy in complicated urinary tract infections or in patients who are allergic to sulfonamides. Another important indication is the treatment of chronic osteomyelitis and diabetic foot infections caused by Gram-negative organisms, and these agents have allowed many such infections to be treated at home rather than in hospital. In contrast, the only other antibiotics effective for this indication require frequent intravenous administration. Likewise, the use of fluoroquinolones for the treatment of pneumonia in patients with cystic fibrosis, commonly caused by *P. aeruginosa,* has allowed many patients to be treated at home. However, given their poor activity against *S. pneumoniae,* ciprofloxacin and ofloxacin should not be used in the treatment of most community-acquired pneumonia. Newer fluoroquinolones, such as levofloxacin, gatifloxacin, and moxifloxacin, have been recommended in guidelines for the treatment of community-acquired pneumonia.

Other uses for the fluoroquinolones include the empirical treatment of bacterial diarrhea, including traveller's diarrhea; treatment of invasive external otitis; treatment of gonorrhea, including penicillin-resistant strains; treatment, in combination with other agents, of disseminated *Mycobacterium avium* complex infections (*M. avium* and *Mycobacterium intracellulare*) in AIDS patients; prophylaxis in some patients at high risk of Gram-negative infections, such as cancer patients receiving chemotherapy; and the outpatient management of diabetic foot infections. Given their activity against Gram-negative organisms, fluoroquinolones are frequently used as "step-down therapy" (i.e., therapy that begins with intravenous administration for rapid effect and then changes to oral therapy with the same drug and dose) for patients with nosocomial pneumonia. As with imipenem, it is important to avoid the indiscriminate use of these agents in order to slow the development of resistant strains of bacteria.

## Dosage and Routes of Administration

Norfloxacin and ofloxacin are given orally, while ciprofloxacin is available in both oral and intravenous dosage forms. The recommended daily dose of ciprofloxacin for urinary tract infections is 500 mg divided into two doses, but for more severe infections, doses of up to 1.5 g/day are given. The recommended daily dose of norfloxacin for urinary tract infections is 800 mg, while that of ofloxacin is 400 to 800 mg, both divided into two doses. For community-acquired pneumonia, levofloxacin is given in a dose of 500 mg daily and gatifloxacin and moxifloxacin, 400 mg daily.

## Newer Developments

A new group of derivatives related to moxifloxacin and gatifloxacin, called **diarylquinolines**, is now starting to undergo clinical trials for the treatment of tuberculosis. They appear to act by a different mechanism from the currently available fluoroquinolones: they inhibit an enzyme involved in the synthesis of adenosine triphosphate (ATP). They are reported to have a bactericidal action on *M. tuberculosis* in a much shorter time than the anti-tuberculous agents currently in use. These compounds represent a possible future development in the treatment of tuberculosis in humans.

# ANTIFOLS

## Sulfonamides

Sulfonamides were the first group of synthetic antibacterial compounds for systemic use, based on Ehrlich's concepts of selective toxicity as outlined in Chapter 49. The original studies of the clinical effectiveness of Prontosil were reported by Domagk in 1935. At first, the claims pertained only to infections caused by hemolytic streptococci, but soon, with modifications of the molecule, activity against a wider range of bacteria was demonstrated.

### Chemistry

All sulfonamides are amides of para-aminobenzene–sulfonic acid (sulfanilamide, Fig. 53-3). Three basic features necessary for antibacterial action are (1) a benzene ring with a sulfonic acid group, (2) an amide nitrogen on the sulfonic acid, and (3) a free amino group in the para position of the benzene ring. The activity of the sulfonamides is also dependent on a negative charge on the amide nitrogen, which mimics the carboxylate anion of para-aminobenzoic acid (PABA). The free amino group in the para position represents the primary site of sulfonamide degradation.

### Bacterial susceptibility

The sulfonamides originally had a wide range of activity, but this range has been seriously reduced by acquired bacterial resistance. Resistance is usually due to either microbial overproduction of PABA or structural changes in the dihydropteroate synthase enzyme. Resistance may also be mediated by plasmids. This form of resistance has increased in recent years, often in combination with trimethoprim resistance.

Gram-positive bacteria that are usually sensitive to sulfonamides include group A streptococci, *Streptococcus viridans,* some *S. pneumoniae,* and *Nocardia.* Staphylococci are variably sensitive and *Enterococcus faecalis* is resistant. The most sensitive Gram-negative species are the *Neisseria,* many enterobacteria, *H. influenzae,* and *Bordetella pertussis.* Some representative bacteria and their median MICs are outlined in Table 53-2. Sulfonamides are also active against *Chlamydia, Toxoplasma,* and some *Plasmodium* species.

| FIGURE 53-3 | Structural formulae of para-aminobenzoic acid, some sulfonamides, trimethoprim, pyrimethamine, and dapsone. |
|---|---|

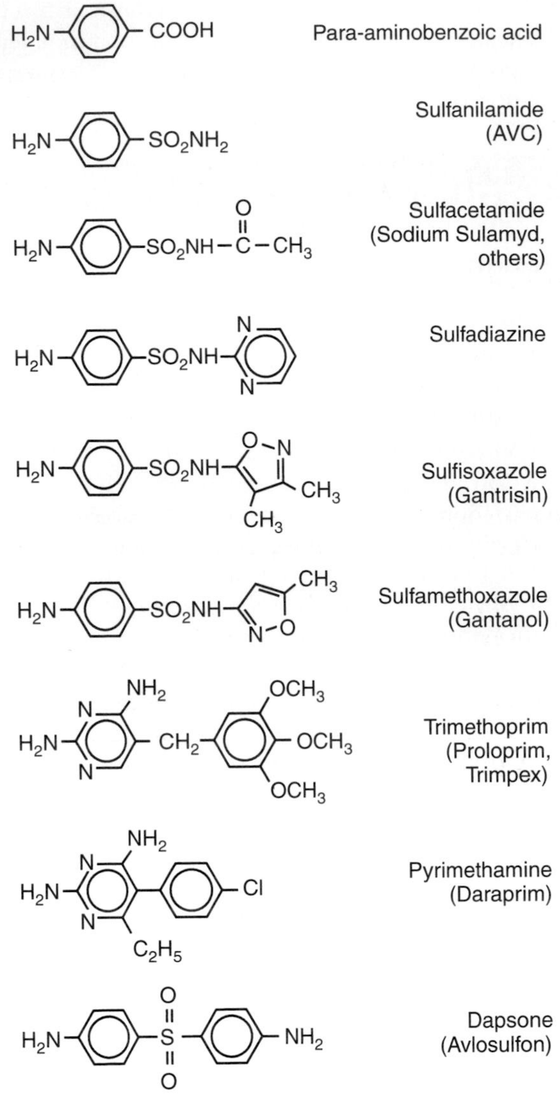

All sulfonamides (except sulfaguanidine and the other derivatives designed for use within the intestinal lumen) are well absorbed after oral administration. Serum concentrations vary somewhat among the sulfonamides. The peak concentration of sulfisoxazole after a 1-g dose ranges from 50 to 100 µg/mL. Intravenously injectable sulfonamides attain high plasma concentrations extremely well.

The sulfonamides are generally well distributed throughout the body, including the CSF. There is some variation in this distribution between individual agents. For instance, CSF concentrations of sulfisoxazole are approximately 30% of those in the serum, whereas the CSF concentrations of sulfadiazine are about 50% of serum concentrations. The volume of distribution of the sulfonamides is small, that of sulfisoxazole being 0.16 to 0.2 L/kg. Protein binding is quite variable among these agents, ranging from 20% for some of the short-acting forms to over 90% for the long-acting drugs.

A percentage of the absorbed sulfonamide is acetylated (at the para-amino group) in the liver, forming inactive conjugates. Individual acetylating capacity is variable in a manner analogous to that for isoniazid. Some sulfonamides also undergo glucuronide conjugation to inactive metabolites in the liver.

Free and conjugated sulfonamides are excreted via the kidneys by both glomerular filtration and tubular secretion. The long-acting forms, which are more extensively protein-bound, undergo more complete tubular reabsorption and hence have prolonged half-lives. Since the sulfonamides and their metabolites are weak acids, their clearance is increased in alkaline urine. Minimal amounts of sulfonamides are excreted in the bile. Half-lives of the

| TABLE 53-2 | Median MICs (in µg/mL) of Sulfonamides and Trimethoprim | |
|---|---|---|
| Bacterium | Sulfonamides* | Trimethoprim |
| **Gram-positive** | | |
| Staphylococcus aureus | 50.0 | 0.2 |
| Streptococcus group A | 12.5 | 0.4 |
| Streptococcus viridans | 8.0 | 0.25 |
| Enterococcus faecalis | 100.0 | 1.0 |
| Streptococcus pneumoniae | 32.0 | 1.0 |
| **Gram-negative** | | |
| Neisseria meningitidis | 5.0 | 8.0 |
| Neisseria gonorrhoeae | 4.0 | 12.0 |
| Haemophilus influenzae | 0.5 | 0.12 |
| Salmonella | 10.0 | 0.4 |
| Shigella | 4.0 | 0.4 |
| Klebsiella | 16.0 | 0.5 |
| Escherichia coli | 8.0 | 0.2 |
| Pseudomonas aeruginosa | 25.0 | >100 |
| Nocardia | 12.5 | >100 |

*Variations among individual sulfonamides occur.

## Pharmacokinetics

The sulfonamides are often classified on the basis of their pharmacokinetics, specifically on the basis of their half-lives. Hence, there are short-acting, medium-acting, long-acting, and ultra-long-acting forms. There are also those that are poorly absorbed from the intestinal tract. Only a few sulfonamides remain in use today, notably sulfadiazine, sulfisoxazole, and sulfamethoxazole. These drugs are described below as a group, using sulfisoxazole (a widely used, short-acting sulfonamide) as a representative. Where important differences exist between various agents, they are specifically noted below.

sulfonamides range from 2 hours to as long as 200 hours, depending on the individual agent. The half-life of sulfisoxazole is 5 to 6 hours.

### Adverse reactions

**Hypersensitivity reactions** ranging from a mild rash to severe Stevens-Johnson syndrome may occur. The latter reaction is an extreme form of erythema multiforme, characterized by bulla formation in the mouth, pharynx, anogenital region, and conjunctivae. Though rare, it produces serious morbidity when it does occur. It is more common in children, especially with long-acting sulfonamides. The incidence of adverse reactions in patients with AIDS who receive sulfonamides, usually co-trimoxazole for the treatment of *P. carinii* pneumonitis (PCP), is about 50% (or about 100 times higher than in other patients). The basis for this increased risk in AIDS patients is unknown. These reactions usually consist of a rash and fever with variable involvement of other organs such as the liver, kidneys, or bone marrow.

**Hematological toxicity** may also occur with sulfonamide use. Reactions include agranulocytosis, which is usually reversible on discontinuation of the drug, and hemolytic anemia in patients with glucose-6-phosphate dehydrogenase (G-6-PD) deficiency. Aplastic anemia has also been described as a rare complication.

In the neonate, sulfonamides are contraindicated because they may displace bilirubin from protein binding sites and hence predispose these patients to the development of jaundice and even kernicterus (see Chapter 61).

**Renal damage** was common with older forms of sulfonamides that were poorly water-soluble. Patients developed crystalluria, which led to obstruction and hematuria. However, this reaction is rare with the more soluble congeners in use today. Nevertheless, renal damage on the basis of hypersensitivity may still be observed.

### Drug interactions

Sulfonamides may accentuate the action of oral hypoglycemic agents and the degree of hypoprothrombinemia produced by oral anticoagulants by displacing these drugs from plasma protein binding sites and also, perhaps, by inhibition of their biotransformation. Sulfonamides may also interfere with the biotransformation of phenytoin, with resultant increase in serum concentrations of that drug.

### Dosage regimens and routes of administration

The usual daily dose of sulfisoxazole is 120 to 150 mg/kg orally, divided into four to six doses, and that of sulfamethoxazole is 50 to 60 mg/kg orally, divided into two equal doses.

### Therapeutic applications

Common clinical uses of the sulfonamides include the treatment of acute, uncomplicated urinary tract infections, either alone or in combination with trimethoprim (co-trimoxazole, co-trimazine); *Nocardia* infections, including those in the lung and CNS; *Toxoplasma* infections (in combination with pyrimethamine); and chloroquine-resistant *Plasmodium falciparum* malaria (in combination with pyrimethamine).

## Trimethoprim (Proloprim)

This drug, a 2,4-diaminopyrimidine, was first synthesized in 1956 as a result of a planned systematic study. It was designed at first as an antibacterial agent, but it was subsequently found to have valuable antiparasitic activity also.

### Bacterial susceptibility

Trimethoprim has an antibacterial spectrum similar to that of the sulfonamides, although it is more active than the sulfonamides against most bacterial species, with the exception of *Neisseria, Brucella,* and *Nocardia.* The enterococci, which are resistant to the sulfonamides, are sensitive to trimethoprim, as are malaria parasites (see Chapter 54). The comparative activities of trimethoprim and the sulfonamides are shown in Table 53-2. As may be expected from its mechanism of action (see Fig. 53-1), trimethoprim is synergistic with sulfonamides against many bacterial species.

### Pharmacokinetics

Trimethoprim is well absorbed from the gastrointestinal tract. A peak serum concentration of about 2 µg/mL is attained 1 to 2 hours after a 160-mg oral dose.

After absorption, trimethoprim is rapidly distributed in the body, and tissue concentrations often exceed serum concentrations except in the brain, skin, and fat. Its apparent volume of distribution is thus greater than total body water. Trimethoprim is 42 to 46% protein-bound.

A substantial proportion of trimethoprim is converted in the liver to at least five inactive metabolites, all of which are excreted in the urine. The amount of active (unchanged) drug excreted by this route during a 24-hour period ranges from 42 to 75% of an administered dose. A small amount of trimethoprim is excreted via the bile. The serum half-life is about 13 hours.

### Adverse reactions

Trimethoprim may cause nausea and diarrhea, especially at high doses. On rare occasions, trimethoprim may also be associated with various blood dyscrasias, including agranulocytosis, thrombocytopenia, and anemia. Inhibition of folate synthesis leading to anemia is a problem only in patients who are already folate-deficient and who are receiving large doses of the drug. This anemia is reversible with the administration of folates, preferably folinic acid, and this measure does not interfere with the antibacterial and antiparasitic effects of the drug. Trimethoprim may inhibit creatinine secretion and thus increase the serum creatinine concentration. Adverse reactions are more common when trimethoprim is administered in combination with a sulfonamide (e.g., sulfamethoxazole). The incidence of serious toxicity from this combination is especially high (about 50%) in patients with AIDS (see "Sulfonamides" above). The mechanism of this interaction is unknown.

### Dosage regimens and routes of administration

Trimethoprim is most commonly administered in a **fixed 1:5 ratio with sulfamethoxazole (co-trimoxazole,** Bactrim, Septra) **or sulfadiazine (co-trimazine,** Coptin). The usual dose of the trimethoprim contained in these combinations ranges from 5 to 20 mg/kg/day, with the specific dose determined by the infecting organism and the severity of the infection. The combinations may be administered orally or intravenously, divided into two to four equal doses. An oral preparation of trimethoprim alone is also available. Its usual daily dose is 4 mg/kg, divided into two equal doses.

### Therapeutic applications

The combination of trimethoprim with a sulfonamide (e.g., co-trimoxazole) is used extensively for the treatment of a variety of infections, including urinary tract infections, prostatitis, exacerbations of chronic bronchitis and pneumonia, sinusitis, otitis media, traveller's diarrhea *(Shigella, Salmonella,* enterotoxic *Escherichia coli),* brucellosis, nocardiasis, and *P. carinii* pneumonitis (PCP). Septicemia, pneumonia, and meningitis caused by multiresistant, Gram-negative aerobes (e.g., *Serratia marcescens, Pseudomonas cepacia, Stenotrophomonas maltophilia*) have also been treated successfully with this combination, as are some atypical mycobacterial species *(M. marinum, M. kansasi).* In addition, the combination of agents is often used prophylactically in patients with recurrent urinary tract infections, in immunocompromised patients at risk for PCP, and in neutropenic hosts to reduce the incidence of serious bacterial infections.

Trimethoprim alone may be used for the treatment and prevention of urinary tract infections. Trimethoprim (15 mg/kg divided into four equal doses) is used in combination with dapsone (100 mg/day) for the treatment of mild to moderate PCP in patients with HIV who are allergic to co-trimoxazole.

## Pyrimethamine (Daraprim)

This drug, which was first synthesized in 1951, is very similar to trimethoprim, also being a 2,4-diaminopyrimidine (see Fig. 53-3). It is more specific than trimethoprim in its activity against protozoan dihydrofolate reductase and is therefore useful in the treatment of protozoan infections (see Chapter 54). It is primarily active against *P. falciparum* and *T. gondii,* with lesser activity against other *Plasmodium species.*

### Pharmacokinetics

Pyrimethamine is completely and regularly absorbed from the intestinal tract. Blood concentrations are prolonged, and urinary excretion may persist for 30 days or more after ingestion of the last dose. Between 20 and 30% is excreted unchanged in the urine. The half-life is approximately 36 hours.

### Adverse reactions

Pyrimethamine can inhibit mammalian dihydrofolate reductase more strongly than trimethoprim does; it is therefore more toxic. **Gastrointestinal** disturbances are common, and **hematological** toxic effects such as megaloblastic anemia, leukopenia, and thrombocytopenia may occur if daily doses are administered without the concomitant administration of folinic acid.

### Dosage regimens, route of administration, and therapeutic applications

The drug is administered orally in one daily dose or divided into two equal doses. The total daily dose is 0.5 to 1 mg/kg, up to a maximum of 25 mg/day. The drug is given daily for the treatment of toxoplasmosis or malaria and every second week for the prophylaxis of malaria. See Chapter 54 for its specific use (also in combination with a sulfonamide) in *P. falciparum* malaria.

## Sulfones

The major sulfones used clinically are **dapsone (DDS)** (Avlosulfon) and its water-soluble derivative **sulfoxone sodium** (Diasone). Their mechanism of action is probably identical to that of the sulfonamides. Dapsone was first used against streptococcal infections but is now used for the treatment of leprosy, dermatitis herpetiformis, malaria, and *P. carinii* pneumonitis.

### Pharmacokinetics

Dapsone is slowly but almost completely absorbed from the gastrointestinal tract. Absorption of sulfoxone is not as great, but it causes less gastric distress. Sulfoxone is hydrolyzed to dapsone, which is the active agent. Distribution to most tissues is very good, and the drug can accumulate in the skin, muscle, liver, and kidneys. The major pathways of biotransformation involve *N*-acetylation and *N*-oxidation, which are reversible, and *N*-glucuronidation and *N*-sulfation, which lead to urinary excretion.

### Adverse reactions

The sulfones are aromatic amines, and their most common untoward effect, which occurs in most patients (especially those with erythrocytic G-6-PD deficiency) who are treated with 200 to 300 mg/day, is hemolysis of varying degree. Methemoglobinemia is also common but is not affected by G-6-PD deficiency. Anorexia, nausea, and vomiting can limit the use of dapsone, and sulfoxone is often better tolerated. An infectious mononucleosis-like syndrome occurs occasionally and can be fatal.

## Therapeutic applications

Dapsone is the primary drug used in the treatment of **leprosy.** The emergence of resistant strains has forced the search for alternate drugs. As mentioned earlier, dapsone can also be used in the treatment of chloroquine-resistant malaria and dermatitis herpetiformis. Dapsone is also used in combination with trimethoprim for treatment and prophylaxis of *P. carinii* infection.

## SUGGESTED READINGS

Andries K, Verhasselt P, Guillemont J, et al. A diarylquinoline drug active on the ATP synthesis of *Mycobacterium tuberculosis. Science.* 2005;307:223-227.

Buescher ES. Community-acquired methicillin-resistant Staphylococcus aureus in pediatrics. *Curr Opin Pediatr.* 2005;17:67-70.

Cockerill FR, Edson FS. Trimethoprim-sulfamethoxazole. *Mayo Clin Proc.* 1991;66:1260-1269.

Emmerson AM, Jones AM. The quinolones: decades of development and use. *J Antimicrob Chemother.* 2003;51(suppl 1):13-20.

Grim SA, Rapp RP, Martin CA, Evans ME. Trimethoprim-sulfamethoxazole as a viable treatment option for infections caused by methicillin-resistant Staphylococcus aureus. *Pharmacotherapy.* 2005;25:253-264.

Hooper DC, Wolfson JS. Fluoroquinolone antimicrobial agents. *N Engl J Med.* 1991;324:384-394.

Sanders EW. Oral ofloxacin: a critical review of the new drug applications. *Clin Infect Dis.* 1992;14:539-554.

Suh B, Lorber B. Quinolones. *Med Clin North Am.* 1995;79:869-894.

Van Scoy RE, Willowske CJ. Antimycobacterial therapy. *Mayo Clin Proc.* 1999;74:1038-1048.

Walker RC, Wright AJ. The fluoroquinolones. *Mayo Clin Proc.* 1991;66:1249-1259.

# 54

# Chemotherapy of Common Parasitic Infections

## JS KEYSTONE

A 30-year-old African-Canadian woman visited her physician because of fever, chills, aching muscles, and headache 2 weeks after having returned from a 3-month visit to her birthplace in Nigeria. She had taken no precautions against insect bites while in Africa, nor had she taken malaria chemoprophylaxis. At the time of the office visit, her blood films showed many ring forms of *Plasmodium falciparum* malaria and a moderately high (5%) parasitemia.

Believing it to be the correct action, the physician prescribed chloroquine for treatment, but the patient refused, explaining that she was allergic to the drug. She said that, during her childhood in Africa, she had developed marked itching whenever chloroquine was given to her.

The physician consulted a tropical disease expert, who explained that chloroquine was inappropriate therapy because chloroquine-resistant *P. falciparum* malaria is widespread in Africa. In addition, up to 45% of Black Africans develop pruritus with chloroquine treatment as a result of a drug metabolite that is deposited in the skin; in other words, the patient had, in fact, suffered no "allergy" to the drug. Since the reaction does not seem to occur with quinine, the expert recommended quinine as the drug of choice for this patient. When asked why she had not recommended atovaquone plus proguanil, the consultant indicated that this drug combination was not appropriate for the treatment of complicated malaria as evidenced by the patient's high parasitemia. A discussion of drug dosage ensued, and the consultant recommended an oral loading dose (twice the maintenance dose of 600 mg) of quinine sulfate because of the high parasitemia. She explained that, by administering a loading dose, steady-state plasma levels of the drug would be reached within hours, whereas initiating therapy with a maintenance dose would delay the attainment of steady-state levels for 2 to 3 days (half-life of quinine is 16 hours).

Twenty-four hours after the start of treatment, the patient complained of headache, severe ringing in the ears, mild hearing loss, and diarrhea. In a panic, the attending physician called the consultant, who explained that these symptoms, known as "cinchonism," are to be expected with quinine, a cinchona alkaloid, that they will occur in most patients, and that they will resolve after the drug is discontinued. However, when the attending physician mentioned that the patient was somewhat confused, diaphoretic, and had tachycardia, the consultant suggested that the patient's blood sugar be assessed immediately by a glucometer. The patient's blood sugar was 2.1 mmol/L. After the patient's condition was stabilized with an intravenous bolus of glucose, the consultant noted that hypoglycemia is an important and frequent complication of severe malaria, particularly when quinine is used for treatment since the drug is known to cause insulin to be released from the pancreas.

Three months later, the patient had a recurrence of fever and headache, at which time a diagnosis of *Plasmodium ovale* malaria was made. This bout of malaria occurred because the previous therapy for *P. falciparum* malaria did not eradicate the dormant hepatic forms (hypnozoites) of *P. ovale*. Quinine and adjuvant drugs such as tetracycline and clindamycin are blood schizonticides that act on developing parasites within red blood cells. They have little effect on the liver (exoerythrocytic) phase of the plasmodial life cycle.

The patient was treated with quinine again (because of her unwillingness to take chloroquine), followed by a 14-day course of primaquine. Four days into this latter therapy, she complained of fatigue and noticed reddish-coloured urine. A clinical diagnosis of drug-induced hemolysis was made, presumably due to the oxidant effects of primaquine. The diagnosis was confirmed when the patient's glucose-6-phosphate dehydrogenase (G-6-PD) level was found to be very low.

*For organisms not covered in this chapter, the reader is referred to standard parasitology textbooks and the Medical Letter monograph "Drugs for parasitic infections" at www.medletter.com.*

On a global basis, parasitic infections are the leading cause of chronic illness and contribute directly or indirectly to the deaths of millions of children annually in the developing world. However, it is important to understand that the majority of infected individuals are asymptomatic, either because the parasite has a low degree of virulence, the parasitic load is too low to cause tissue damage, or the host has the ability to control the infection. Consequently, the clinician must first decide whether or not a parasitic infection requires treatment before a therapeutic agent is even considered.

Antiparasitic drugs (Table 54-1) are directed against two major groups of parasites: (1) protozoa, which constitute the single-celled organisms, and (2) metazoa, the multi-celled organisms, or worms. Metazoa include the flatworms (cestodes and trematodes) and roundworms (nematodes). With a few notable exceptions, drugs that act against intestinal parasites are usually ineffective against tissue-dwelling or blood parasites and vice versa.

## INTESTINAL AND VAGINAL PROTOZOAN INFECTIONS

### Amoebiasis

Strictly speaking, amoebiasis refers to an infection by the intestinal protozoan *Entamoeba histolytica,* which has the ability to invade tissue. Since stool microscopy cannot distinguish *E. histolytica* from the identical-appearing non-pathogen, *Entamoeba dispar,* additional testing (serology, stool antigen, or polymerase chain reaction) should be carried out before a decision to treat is made. There are many other amoebae that are harmless commensals not requiring treatment. These include *Endolimax nana, Entamoeba coli, Entamoeba hartmanni,* and *Iodamoeba bütschlii.*

In the large bowel, *E. histolytica* is found in two forms: cyst and trophozoite. The motile trophozoite is the vegetative form that maintains the infection by replication. Under an unknown stimulus, trophozoites, which normally live as commensals, may invade the intestinal mucosa and give rise to amoebic colitis. Hematogenous spread to liver, lungs, or brain may result in the formation of an amoebic abscess. Under adverse conditions, bowel trophozoites develop a protective covering and transform themselves into cysts. Cysts are transmitted by the fecal–oral route via flies, fingers, food (and water), and fornication.

Amoebicides can be divided clinically into two groups: those acting in the intestinal lumen and those acting in the tissue.

### Agents acting in the lumen

These agents act directly on organisms in the lumen of the bowel. They are often poorly absorbed from the intestine and are used primarily for eradicating the infection at this site. These drugs cannot eradicate trophozoites that have invaded the intestinal wall and beyond. They include halogenated quinolines, diloxanide furoate, and antibiotics. In asymptomatic (or minimally symptomatic) persons passing cysts or trophozoites, in whom tissue invasion presumably has not occurred, a lumen-active agent is all that is required. For symptomatic invasive amoebiasis (intestinal or extra-intestinal), a tissue-active drug *plus* one that acts in the lumen are needed.

*Iodoquinol (Yodoxin).* This iodinated hydroxyquinoline compound is the only lumen-active agent of this group marketed in Canada and the United States. In addition to eradicating *E. histolytica,* iodoquinol is effective in some patients with *Dientamoeba fragilis, Balantidium coli,* and *Blastocystis hominis.* It functions by inactivating enzymes or halogenating proteins of the protozoan. The drug is absorbed moderately well from the intestine and is extensively biotransformed. Less than 10% of an oral dose is recovered in the urine, largely as glucuronides and ethanol sulfates.

Occasional adverse reactions include gastrointestinal (GI) upset, rash, and thyroid gland enlargement. Rarely, iodoquinol produces subacute myelo-optic neuropathy when larger-than-recommended doses are given. The drug is contraindicated in patients who are allergic to iodine.

*Diloxanide furoate (Furamide).* This non-absorbable amide is a safe and highly effective lumen-active agent for treatment of asymptomatic amoebiasis. Diloxanide furoate is classified as an emergency drug in the United States and Canada, available from the Centers for Disease Control Drug Service, Atlanta, Georgia, and by authorization of the Bureau of Human Prescription Drugs, Health Canada, Ottawa. Diloxanide is rapidly absorbed, and its ester linkage is largely hydrolyzed in the intestine. Peak blood levels are reached in 1 hour. The elimination half-life is approximately 6 hours; the major portion is excreted in the urine as glucuronide. The mechanism of action of diloxanide is unknown.

Toxicity is rare. Excessive flatulence is the most frequent side effect. GI upset and allergic reactions are uncommon.

*Paromomycin (Humatin).* Antibiotic amoebicides are transiently effective for invasive amoebiasis. When they are used alone, relapses are frequent. Antibiotics such as paromomycin and the tetracyclines are adjunct therapy, especially useful for symptomatic relief of severe amoebic dysentery. Although its primary role is as a luminal amoebicide, paromomycin has some tissue activity. Therefore, it is an alternative to metronidazole in mild-to-moderate

**TABLE 54-1**     Antiparasitic Drug Doses

| Infection | Drug | Adult Dosage | Pediatric Dosage |
|---|---|---|---|
| Amoebiasis (*Entamoeba histolytica*) | | | |
| 1. Asymptomatic or minimal symptoms | Lumen-active agents: Iodoquinol* | 650 mg tid × 20 days | 30–40 mg/kg/day in 3 doses × 20 days |
| | **or** | | |
| | Diloxanide furoate | 500 mg tid × 10 days | 20 mg/kg/day in 3 doses × 10 days |
| | **or** | | |
| | Paromomycin | 25–30 mg/kg/day × 10 days | Same as adult |
| 2. Moderate to severe disease or amoebic abscess | Metronidazole **plus** lumen-active agent | 750 mg tid × 5–10 days <br> Same as for 1 above | 35–50 mg/kg/day in 3 doses × 5–10 days <br> Same as for 1 above |
| Ascariasis (*Ascaris lumbricoides*, roundworm) | Mebendazole | 100 mg bid × 3 days | Same as adult |
| | **or** | | |
| | Pyrantel pamoate* | 11 mg/kg once (max 1 g) | Same as adult |
| | **or** | | |
| | Albendazole | 400 mg once | Same as adult |
| Clonorchiasis (*Clonorchis sinensis*) | Praziquantel | 25 mg/kg tid × 1 day | Same as adult |
| Cyclosporiasis (*Cyclospora cayetanensis*) | Co-trimoxazole (trimethoprim [TMP] / sulfamethoxazole [SMX]) | TMP 160 mg and SMX 800 mg bid × 7 days | TMP 5 mg/kg and SMX 25 mg/kg bid × 7 days |
| | Ciprofloxacin | 500 mg bid × 7 days | |
| Cysticercosis (*Cysticercus cellulosae*) | Albendazole* | 15 mg/kg/day in 2 doses × 15–30 days | Same as adult |
| | **or** | | |
| | Praziquantel | 50 mg/kg/day in 3 doses × 14 days | Same as adult |
| Dientamoebiasis (*Dientamoeba fragilis*) | Iodoquinol* | 650 mg tid × 20 days | 30–40 mg/kg/day in 3 doses × 20 days |
| | **or** | | |
| | Tetracycline | 500 mg qid × 10 days | 40 mg/kg/day in 4 doses × 10 days (max 2 g/day) |
| | **or** | | |
| | Paromomycin | 25–30 mg/kg/day × 10 days | Same as adult |
| *Diphyllobothrium latum* (fish tapeworm) | Praziquantel | 10–20 mg/kg once | Same as adult |
| Echinococcosis (*Echinococcus granulosus*, hydatid disease) | Albendazole | 400 mg bid × 3–6 months | 15 mg/kg/day × 3–6 months |
| Enterobiasis (*Enterobius vermicularis*, pinworm) | Pyrantel pamoate* | 11 mg/kg once (max 1 g); repeat after 2 wks | Same as adult |
| | **or** | | |
| | Mebendazole* | 100 mg once; repeat after 2 wks | Same as adult |
| | **or** | | |
| | Pyrvinium pamoate | 5 mg/kg once (max 250 mg); repeat after 2 wks | Same as adult |
| | **or** | | |
| | Piperazine citrate | 65 mg/kg (max 2.5 g) × 7 days; repeat after 2 wks | Same as adult |
| Fascioliasis (*Fasciola hepatica*, sheep liver fluke) | Triclabendazole | 11 mg/kg once | Same as adult |

*continued*

| TABLE 54-1 | continued | | |
|---|---|---|---|
| **Infection** | **Drug** | **Adult Dosage** | **Pediatric Dosage** |
| Giardiasis (*Giardia intestinalis*) | Metronidazole* | 2 g once × 3 days **or** 250 mg tid × 5–7 days | <25 kg: 35 mg/kg/day once × 3 days >25 kg: 50 mg/kg/day once × 3 days **or** 15 mg/kg/day in 3 doses × 5–7 days |
| | **or** Quinacrine | 100 mg tid × 7 days | 6 mg/kg/day in 3 doses × 7 days |
| | **or** Furazolidone | 100 mg qid × 10 days | 6 mg/kg/day in 4 doses × 10 days |
| Hookworm (*Ancylostoma duodenale, Necator americanus*) | Mebendazole* **or** Pyrantel pamoate **or** Albendazole | 100 mg bid × 3 days 11 mg/kg (max 1 g) × 3 days 400 mg once | Same as adult Same as adult Same as adult |
| Hymenolepiasis (*Hymenolepis nana,* dwarf tapeworm) | Praziquantel* | 25 mg/kg once | Same as adult |
| Isosporiasis (*Isospora belli*) | Co-trimoxazole (trimethoprim [TMP] / sulfamethoxazole [SMX]) | TMP 160 mg and SMX 800 mg bid × 10 days then bid × 3 wks | TMP 5 mg/kg and SMX 25 mg/kg |
| **Malaria** | | | |
| 1. Chloroquine-sensitive *P. falciparum* and *P. malariae* | Chloroquine phosphate | 1 g (salt) stat; 500 mg in in 6 h; then 500 mg/day × 2 days | 10 mg/kg (max 500 mg); then 5 mg/kg in 6 h; then 5 mg/kg/day × 2 days |
| 2. *P. vivax* and *P. ovale* | Chloroquine phosphate **plus** Primaquine | Same as for 1 above 30 mg/day (base) × 14 days | Same as for 1 above 0.6 mg/kg/day (base) × 14 days |
| 3. Chloroquine-resistant *P. falciparum* | Atovaquone/proguanil | 4 tabs once daily × 3 days | 11–20 kg; 1 adult tab 21–30 kg: 2 adult tabs 31–40 kg: 3 adult tabs >40 kg: adult dose once daily × 3 days |
| | **or** Quinine sulfate* **plus** (a) Tetracycline* | 600 mg tid × 3 days 250 mg qid × 7 days | 25 mg/kg/day in 3 doses × 3 days 20 mg/kg/day in 4 doses × 7 days |
| | **or** (b) Clindamycin | 900 mg tid × 3 days | 20–40 mg/kg/d in 3 doses × 3 days |
| | **or** Mefloquine | 15–25 mg/kg: 2/3 of dose stat and 1/3 in 12 h | Same as adult dose |
| | **or** Parenteral Quinidine gluconate | 10 mg/kg (salt) (max 600 mg) in normal saline over 1 h; then infusion of 0.02 mg/kg/min × 3 days max | Same as adult |
| | **or** Parenteral Quinine dihydrochloride | 20 mg/kg (salt) in 10 mL/kg 5% D/W over 4 h; then 10 mg/kg over 2–4 h q8h (max 1800 mg/day) until oral therapy can be given | Same as adult |

*continued*

| TABLE 54-1 | continued | | |
|---|---|---|---|
| **Infection** | **Drug** | **Adult Dosage** | **Pediatric Dosage** |
| Malaria prevention<br>1. Chloroquine-sensitive areas | Chloroquine | 500 mg/wk (salt); start 1 wk before and continue for 4 wks after last exposure | 8.3 mg/kg (salt) once/wk as for adults (max 500 mg/day) |
| 2. Chloroquine-resistant areas | Mefloquine* | 250 mg/wk; start 2–4 wks before and continue for 4 wks after last exposure | 15–19 kg: 1/4 tab; 20–30 kg: 1/2 tab; 31–45 kg: 3/4 tab; >45 kg: 1 tab |
| | **or**<br>Doxycycline | 100 mg daily and for 4 wks after last exposure | >8 years: 1 mg/kg/day (max 100 mg) |
| | **or**<br>Atovaquone/proguanil | 1 tablet daily & for 1 wk after last exposure | 11–20 kg: 1 pediat. tab<br>21–30 kg: 2 pediat. tabs<br>31–40 kg: 3 pediat. tabs<br>>40 kg: adult dose daily and for 1 wk after last exposure |
| Paragonimiasis (*Paragonimus westermanni*, lung fluke) | Praziquantel | 25 mg/kg tid × 2 days | Same as adult |
| Schistosomiasis (*Schistosoma haematobium*) | Praziquantel | 40 mg/kg/day in 2 doses × 1 day | Same as adult |
| (*S. japonicum*) | Praziquantel | 60 mg/kg/day in 3 doses × 1 day | Same as adult |
| (*S. mansoni*) | Praziquantel | 40 mg/kg/day in 2 doses × 1 day | Same as adult |
| Strongyloidiasis (*Strongyloides stercoralis*) | Ivermectin | 200 μg/kg/day × 1–2 days | Same as adult |
| | **or**<br>Albendazole | 400 mg bid × 7 days | Same as adult |
| Toxoplasmosis (*Toxoplasma gondii*) | Pyrimethamine*<br>**plus**<br>Sulfadiazine<br>**or**<br>Spiramycin | 25–100 mg/day × 3–4 wks<br><br>1–2 g qid × 3–4 wks<br><br>3–4 g/day × 3–4 wks | 2 mg/kg/day × 3 days, then 1 mg/kg/day (max 25 mg/day) × 4 wks<br>100–200 mg/kg/day × 3–4 wks<br><br>50–100 mg/kg/day × 3–4 wks |
| Trichomoniasis (*Trichomonas vaginalis*) | Metronidazole | 2 g once<br>**or**<br>250 mg tid orally × 7 days | 15 mg/kg/day orally in 3 doses × 7 days |
| Trichuriasis (*Trichuris trichiura*, whipworm) | Mebendazole*<br>**or**<br>Albendazole | 100 mg bid × 3 days<br><br>400 mg once | Same as adult<br><br>Same as adult |

*Drug of choice
IV = intravenously; 5% D/W = 5% dextrose in water.

intestinal amoebiasis and can be used to eliminate cyst passage. Paromomycin also has variable efficacy in giardiasis and cryptosporidiosis (see below). Some of the therapeutic action of paromomycin in intestinal amoebiasis occurs by modifying the intestinal bacterial flora, thereby depriving amoebae of nutrients and rendering the intestinal medium less favourable to parasite multiplication and invasion. It has greater amoebicidal activity than tetracycline. Paromomycin is poorly absorbed from the intact GI tract.

GI upset is the most frequently reported adverse reaction. Rash, headache, and vertigo occur occasionally.

## Agents acting in the tissues

These substances act directly on organisms that have invaded tissues. Therefore, unlike those acting in the lumen, they must be well absorbed, reach high concentrations in tissue, and be sufficiently non-toxic to permit systemic use. Metronidazole has now replaced emetine, its less toxic analogue dehydroemetine, and chloroquine as treatment for invasive amoebiasis.

*Metronidazole (Flagyl).* This agent has been considered the drug of choice for the treatment of vaginitis caused by *Trichomonas vaginalis,* and it is also effective against the protozoa *Giardia intestinalis, Blastocystis hominis, Dientamoeba fragilis,* and some anaerobic bacteria such as *Bacteroides fragilis.* Although metronidazole has been promoted as being efficacious against all stages of amoebiasis *(E. histolytica),* it appears to be a poor agent in the lumen but an excellent agent in tissues. Metronidazole is currently the drug of choice for the treatment of invasive amoebiasis, but it should be followed by a lumen-active agent. A parenteral form of metronidazole is available. **Tinidazole**, a metronidazole derivative, enjoys worldwide popularity because of its ease of administration (single dose for giardiasis, three once-daily doses for amoebiasis) and greater efficacy than metronidazole, with reduced side effects. It is available in the United States, but not in Canada.

Metronidazole is a nitroimidazole compound with a mode of action that is common to all nitroaromatics. The drug is reduced by enzymes present in susceptible anaerobic microorganisms, giving rise to reactive metabolites. These intermediates are oxidized by molecular $O_2$ to generate superoxide anions that, in turn, damage the parasite by producing toxic ionizing OH radicals that cause peroxidation of lipids and DNA in the parasite.

Absorption of metronidazole is rapid and complete. After a single oral dose, peak plasma concentrations are reached within 0.5 to 3 hours; the serum half-life is 7 hours. The drug is poorly protein-bound and therefore penetrates tissue readily, including the brain and cerebrospinal fluid (CSF); it also crosses the placenta. Most of the drug is excreted by the kidney, about 20% unchanged and the remainder as a variety of metabolites formed by side-chain oxidation and glucuronide conjugation.

Common adverse effects include dark urine (probably due to a drug metabolite), nausea, vomiting, diarrhea, headache, and a metallic taste in the mouth. Rarely, seizures and reversible peripheral neuropathy have been reported. Alcohol should not be consumed during treatment with metronidazole because of a possible disulfiram-like reaction (see Chapter 22).

Concern has been expressed about the ability of metronidazole to cause cancer and birth defects in experimental animals as well as gene mutations in bacteria. In high and prolonged dosage, the drug is carcinogenic in mice. Although it has been regarded by some clinicians as potentially dangerous in humans, there are no data to support this claim; retrospective studies have shown the drug to be safe in pregnancy. However, in this situation, metronidazole should not be used for trivial indications.

## Giardiasis

This is an infection of the small bowel with the flagellated protozoan *Giardia intestinalis* (previously known as *Giardia lamblia).*The parasite resides in the upper part of the small intestine and exists in two forms, trophozoite and cyst. The latter is the infective stage of the parasite. The trophozoite, with its ventral sucking disk, is responsible for the damage to the upper small bowel. Water-borne epidemics have occurred as well as person-to-person transmission by the fecal–oral route. Invasion beyond the bowel lumen does not occur. Only symptomatic infections or asymptomatic food handlers require treatment.

*Metronidazole.* This is the drug of choice for the treatment of giardiasis (see "Amoebiasis" above).

*Quinacrine (mepacrine HCl; Atabrine).* Quinacrine is less effective than metronidazole for the treatment of giardiasis and potentially has more adverse effects. Thus, in giardiasis, quinacrine is used primarily as an alternative for patients who have failed metronidazole therapy or who should not receive or do not tolerate metronidazole. It is available from several compounding pharmacies in the United States and Canada; in Canada, the drug may be requested through the Special Access Program of the Bureau of Human Prescription Drugs, Health Protection Branch, Health Canada.

Quinacrine is well absorbed and widely distributed in tissues, where it is largely bound and, therefore, excreted slowly for prolonged periods. Nausea and vomiting are the most common adverse effects. Prolonged administration stains the skin yellow. Up to 2% of adults receiving quinacrine have developed drug-induced psychosis. Aplastic anemia, exfoliative dermatitis, and acute hepatic necrosis are rare.

*Furazolidone (Furoxone) and nitazoxanide (Alinia).* These are liquid preparations that are easy to administer and are well tolerated by children. They are marketed in the United States but are available in Canada only through the Special Access Program, Bureau of Human Prescription Drugs, Health Canada.

*Paromomycin.* This drug has limited efficacy, approximately a 50% cure rate, against *G. intestinalis.* It is poorly absorbed and therefore is safe in pregnancy (see "Amoebiasis"). Recent studies suggest that it has limited efficacy against cryptosporidiosis in AIDS patients.

## Trichomoniasis

Vaginal infections with *Trichomonas vaginalis* are common during the reproductive years. Trichomonads may persist in the urethra and periurethral glands of both sexes. Therefore, both partners should be treated to prevent recurrence of infection.

**Metronidazole,** the drug of choice, may be administered orally or vaginally.

## Dientamoebiasis

*Dientamoeba fragilis* is a large-bowel flagellate that has been shown to be a potential human pathogen. It is likely transmitted in pinworm eggs and therefore is frequently seen in daycare children and institutionalized persons. For symptomatic individuals, the treatment of choice is **iodoquinol.** Alternatively, **tetracycline** and **paromomycin** have been shown to be effective. Asymptomatic infections do not require treatment.

## Blastocystosis

It is not yet clear whether *Blastocystis hominis,* a large-bowel protozoan, has the ability to produce gastrointestinal symptoms in infected humans. Limited clinical experience suggests that therapy with **iodoquinol,** high-dose **metronidazole,** or **paromomycin** results in a 60 to 70% cure rate. Treatment should be reserved for symptomatic individuals.

## Isosporiasis

Isosporiasis, caused by the coccidian parasite *Isospora belli,* is endemic in developing countries and has been seen in institutionalized patients. It is now recognized as an important opportunistic infection of the small bowel, causing chronic diarrhea in AIDS patients.

**Trimethoprim–sulfamethoxazole** (co-trimoxazole) or **pyrimethamine plus sulfadiazine** (see "Cyclosporiasis" and "Toxoplasmosis") are recommended therapy for this infection. High-dose pyrimethamine alone and the fluoroquinolone **ciprofloxacin** have also been shown to be effective. Although metronidazole and furazolidone have been reported to be effective, they should be relegated to second-line therapy because of limited efficacy data.

## Cyclosporiasis

*Cyclospora cayetanensis* is a relatively recently described coccidian protozoan of the small intestine that has been responsible for endemic diarrhea in the developing world and food-borne outbreaks in North America. Contaminated raspberries from Guatemala and fresh basil have caused self-limited diarrheal disease in hundreds of individuals. In patients with AIDS, the organism spreads beyond the intestine, causing disease in other organs, notably the liver, gallbladder, thyroid, eye, and lungs. Standard therapy for persistent or severe disease includes trimethoprim–sulfamethoxazole, but ciprofloxacin has been shown to be effective as well.

*Co-trimoxazole (trimethoprim–sulfamethoxazole; TMP-SMX; see also Chapter 53).* This drug combination is a broad-spectrum antimicrobial agent that (like pyrimethamine–sulfadiazine) acts by interfering with the synthesis of tetrahydrofolic acid. Trimethoprim, a diaminopyrimidine, inhibits dihydrofolate reductase, while sulfamethoxazole, a sulfonamide, inhibits the incorporation of para-aminobenzoic acid into dihydrofolate. The optimal ratio of concentrations of trimethoprim to sulfamethoxazole for antimicrobial synergy is 1:20. This ratio is achieved in the serum by using a combination of 1:5 (TMP to SMX).

Co-trimoxazole may be administered orally or intravenously. In healthy individuals, absorption from the GI tract is excellent. TMP and SMX are predominantly excreted in the urine and have an elimination half-life of 10 to 11 hours. Most of the TMP is excreted as unchanged drug, but about 80% of the SMX is excreted as the *N*-acetylated compound.

For those allergic to sulphonamides, ciprofloxacin has also been shown to be effective.

## Cryptosporidiosis

*Cryptosporidium parvum* is an important ubiquitous coccidian protozoan pathogen in both immunocompetent and immunosuppressed patients. In AIDS patients, the organism produces a chronic, unrelenting, watery diarrhea associated with weight loss and malabsorption. In hosts with normal immunity, *Cryptosporidium* causes self-limited watery diarrhea, particularly in children. No effective therapy has been found. Paromomycin (see "Amoebiasis"), alone or in combination with azithromycin, has been effective in some patients, but the clinical response to this drug has been generally disappointing. Recent studies with **nitazoxanide** are promising.

## Microsporidiosis

*Enterocytozoon bieneusi* and *Septata intestinalis* are two intestinal microsporidia—small intracellular protozoa that have recently been shown to be a common cause of diarrhea in AIDS patients. Other species may cause hepatitis, myositis, peritonitis, and keratopathy. At this time, there is no known treatment for the parasite, although **albendazole** (see "Intestinal Helminth Infections" below) appears to be beneficial against *S. intestinalis* only. For eye disease, the addition of **fumagillin** has been shown to be helpful.

# BLOOD AND TISSUE PROTOZOAN INFECTIONS

## Toxoplasmosis

*Toxoplasma gondii,* an obligate intracellular protozoan, causes a ubiquitous infection that is transmitted congenitally or orally through ingestion of tissue cysts in poorly cooked meat or through oocysts in cat feces. Clinical disease includes congenital toxoplasmosis, ocular toxoplasmosis, a mononucleosis-like picture in immunocompetent hosts, and central nervous system (CNS) disease in immunocompromised hosts, especially AIDS patients. Agents used for the treatment of toxoplasmic diseases include pyrimethamine–sulfadiazine, dapsone, atovaquone, and clindamycin. Spiramycin has been used in pregnancy. Therapy is generally not given for the lymphadenopathic form in immunocompetent hosts unless symptoms are particularly severe or persistent.

*Pyrimethamine–sulfadiazine.* The effect of this drug combination is synergistic; it acts by sequential blockage of two consecutive steps in the formation of folinic acid from para-aminobenzoic acid (PABA) by the parasite. Sulfadiazine prevents the parasite from utilizing PABA to synthesize folic acid; pyrimethamine inhibits dihydrofolate reductase, thereby preventing formation of tetrahydrofolic acid (folinic acid) (see also Chapter 53). This combination is the most effective therapy presently available for the treatment of toxoplasmosis. Unfortunately, sulfadiazine is no longer readily available.

Both drugs are well absorbed. Peak plasma concentrations are reached in 1.5 to 8 hours for pyrimethamine and in 2 to 4 hours for sulfadiazine. The elimination half-life for pyrimethamine and sulfadiazine is 50 to 100 hours and 10 to 12 hours, respectively. Both drugs are excreted primarily by the kidney.

Frequent adverse reactions include myelosuppression and thrombocytopenia, headache, GI upset, bad taste in the mouth, and rash (especially in AIDS patients). Convulsions and shock have been reported rarely. In order to minimize the marrow-suppressant effects of these antifols, folinic acid is administered concurrently. Since the parasite cannot utilize exogenous folinic acid, but must synthesize its own, the addition of folinic acid (as citrovorum factor) does not reduce the antiparasitic efficacy of the pyrimethamine–sulfadiazine combination.

In patients with AIDS, toxoplasmosis is one of the most important opportunistic infections causing CNS disease. Since the cyst form of the parasite is not susceptible to drug therapy, relapses after treatment occur in 80% or more of patients unless maintenance therapy with lower doses of the above drug combination is carried on indefinitely.

*Spiramycin (Rovamycine).* This macrolide antibiotic has been used successfully for the therapy of acutely infected pregnant women in the first trimester to prevent congenital infection. For other indications, it is less effective than the pyrimethamine–sulfadiazine combination. It is stable in gastric acid and is well absorbed from the intestine.

Adverse effects include GI disturbances and occasional allergic cutaneous reactions.

*Clindamycin (Dalacin, Cleocin).* Clindamycin is a lincosamide antibiotic (see Chapter 52) with a spectrum of antibiotic activity very similar to that of the macrolides. It is active against *T. gondii.* The drug is concentrated in the choroid of the eye and has been used for treatment of ocular toxoplasmosis with favourable results. Clindamycin has also been used with pyrimethamine for the treatment of toxoplasmic encephalitis in AIDS patients who have sulfonamide sensitivity. However, the response in this clinical setting may be due to pyrimethamine alone.

Adverse reactions include diarrhea (especially *Clostridium difficile* colitis), hepatotoxicity, hypersensitivity reactions, and myelosuppression.

*Systemic corticosteroids.* Corticosteroids are used as adjunct therapy for chorioretinitis and occasionally for cerebral toxoplasmosis to reduce cerebral edema. They should be administered with antiparasitic agents and preferably in brief courses.

## Malaria

Malaria parasites are blood protozoa of the genus *Plasmodium.* Four species infect humans: *Plasmodium falciparum* (malignant tertian malaria), *Plasmodium vivax* (benign tertian malaria), *Plasmodium malariae* (quartan malaria), and *Plasmodium ovale* (ovale tertian malaria).

The **plasmodial life cycle** begins when sporozoites are inoculated into humans from the salivary glands of a feeding female *Anopheles* mosquito. The organisms multiply in the liver and form tissue schizonts (**exoerythrocytic stage**). When liver schizonts rupture, merozoites are released into the bloodstream. In *P. vivax* and *P. ovale* malaria only, some merozoites, now called hypnozoites, may lie dormant in the liver and later cause a relapse of malaria. This stage is not present in *P. falciparum* and *P. malariae,* which have a single passage through the liver. In all species, merozoites released from the liver invade red blood cells and develop through a trophozoite stage into a schizont stage (**erythrocytic stage**). When the red cell schizont ruptures, most of the released merozoites invade new red cells. Some merozoites develop into male and female gametocytes that do not multiply; subsequently, they are ingested by a feeding mosquito. Mating of these gametocytes in the mosquito gut leads to sporozoite production and completion of the malaria cycle (Fig. 54-1).

The modern classification of anti-malarial drugs is based on the stage of the *Plasmodium* life cycle upon which the drugs act:

**Tissue schizonticides:** Primaquine acts in the liver on hypnozoites of *P. vivax* and *P. ovale* and has some activity against red cell schizonts. In addition to acting as

---

**FIGURE 54-1** Life cycle of malaria parasites in humans and sites of action of anti-malarial drugs. Omitted for simplicity is the phase of sporozoite development in *Anopheles* mosquitoes, which consists of the ingestion of gametocytes in a blood meal, their fusion and production of motile zygotes in the mosquito stomach, formation of oocysts on the outer stomach wall, and release of sporozoites from oocysts into salivary glands, from which they are injected into the bloodstream of humans during a mosquito bite.

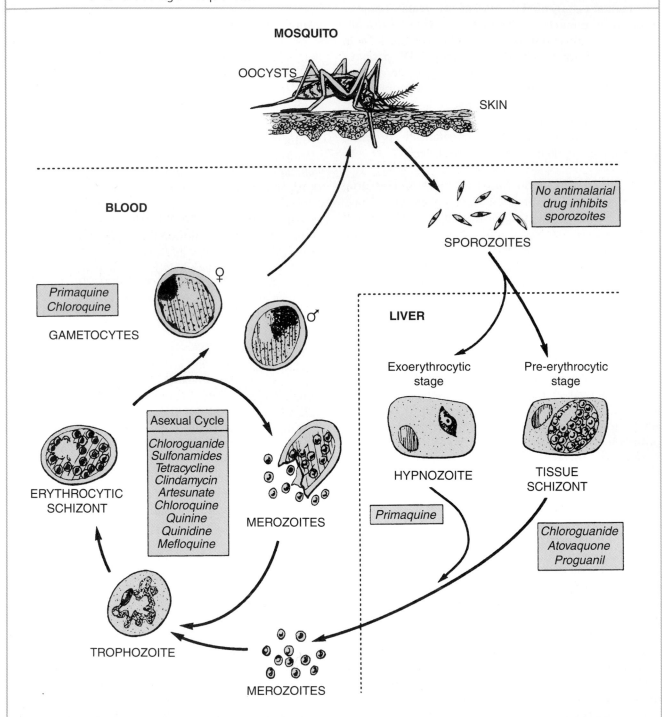

blood schizonticides, atovaquone, proguanil, and pyrimethamine act on the liver phase of *P. falciparum* only. These latter two drugs are known as "causal" prophylactics since they prevent symptoms of malaria from occurring by inhibiting the exoerythrocytic (liver) phase.

**Blood schizonticides:** Quinine, quinidine, chloroquine, mefloquine, proguanil, pyrimethamine, primaquine, sulfonamides, sulfones, clindamycin, tetracycline, atovaquone, and artemisinin derivatives (artesunate, artemether) act in the blood on the erythrocytic phase of all four species of malaria. When one of these drugs is used to prevent malaria, it is known as a "suppressive" agent because it suppresses the symptoms of malaria by eradicating parasites in the circulation.

## Tissue schizonticides

*Primaquine.* This drug is an 8-aminoquinoline that destroys the exoerythrocytic (hepatic) forms of malaria. Also, it is highly gametocytocidal and has some schizonticidal activity. Primaquine is not usually used as a prophylactic agent but rather to eradicate dormant hypnozoites of *P. vivax* and *P. ovale* after a blood schizonticide (such as chloroquine) has been used to arrest the clinical attack of malaria. However, the drug may be used prophylactically against all malaria species and as "terminal prophylaxis" when it is used to prevent late relapses of *P. vivax* in those who return from areas where the infection is highly endemic. *Plasmodium ovale* is sufficiently rare to make prophylactic use of primaquine unnecessary. When used for chemoprophylaxis, daily doses are administered one day before exposure, during exposure, and for 3 days afterwards. The mechanism of action of primaquine is unknown, but it appears to exert its effects through a metabolite. Partial resistance ("tolerance") of *P. vivax* to primaquine occurs in about one-third of those infected with the Chesson strain in Southeast Asia and Oceania. Recently, it has been described in Guyana and Somalia as well.

Primaquine is rapidly and completely absorbed, extensively distributed, and converted to carboxyprimaquine. Less than 5% of the administered dose is found in the urine.

The most serious adverse effect of primaquine is intravascular hemolysis manifested as acute hemolytic anemia in those with glucose-6-phosphate dehydrogenase (G-6-PD) deficiency. Ethnic groups in which G-6-PD deficiency is found include Mediterraneans, people of Black African descent, Asians, and Orientals (see also Chapter 10). Primaquine may cause GI upset, headache, and, rarely, leukopenia and agranulocytosis. Primaquine may also induce hemolysis in individuals with other defects of glucose metabolism and certain hemoglobinopathies.

A long-acting derivative of primaquine, **tafenoquine**, has been shown to be very effective in the prevention of malaria. The drug is not yet marketed but may revolutionize malaria chemosuppression when it becomes available. In a recent study of semi-immune patients in Africa, three daily doses of the drug administered at the beginning of the study provided effective protection against *P. falciparum* malaria for almost 3 months.

*Chloroguanide (Proguanil; Paludrine).* This biguanide breaks down to its active metabolite, cycloguanil. The latter is a dihydrofolate reductase inhibitor that prevents the conversion of dihydrofolic acid to tetrahydrofolic acid (folinic acid). Because of widespread resistance to the drug, it is always combined with another anti-malarial such as chloroquine, dapsone, or sulfamethoxazole. In combination with atovaquone (Malarone), it is highly synergistic against *P. falciparum* and other malaria species. In parts of Europe, the combination of weekly chloroquine with daily chloroguanide is often used to prevent malaria in chloroquine-resistant *P. falciparum* areas. However, because of the low efficacy of this combination (70%), it is not recommended in North America. Chloroguanide should not be given with primaquine as it inhibits the metabolic degradation of the latter.

Absorption of chloroguanide is slow; peak plasma levels are reached within 3 hours. Approximately half of the drug is excreted in the urine, about 60% as unchanged drug and the rest as a metabolite.

Chloroguanide is well tolerated and safe in pregnant women. Gastrointestinal upset and mouth ulcers are common but mild side effects.

## Blood schizonticides

*Quinine and Quinidine.* These cinchona alkaloids are rapidly acting blood schizonticides. They are optical isomers with qualitatively but not quantitatively identical pharmacological actions. Although quinidine appears to have greater efficacy against malaria, it is potentially more toxic. Both drugs are quinoline-containing anti-malarials (as are chloroquine and amodiaquine), which are weak bases that accumulate within the digestive vacuole of the malarial parasite. Current evidence suggests that these drugs specifically inhibit the malarial parasite enzyme heme polymerase, which converts the breakdown products of hemoglobin into a non-toxic malarial pigment, hemozoin. Inhibition of this enzyme leads to the accumulation of soluble ferric heme, which is highly toxic to the parasite membrane.

Because of their short half-lives and side effects, these drugs are used only for *treatment* of malaria, not for *prophylaxis,* and they are rarely employed alone because of drug resistance. Quinine is given orally or intravenously, while quinidine is administered only intravenously.

Quinine is well absorbed, widely distributed, and metabolized primarily in the liver. The elimination half-life is approximately 11 hours. In anti-malarial doses, quinine sulfate frequently causes mild to moderate cinchonism (tinnitus, headache, decreased hearing, blurred vision, nausea, and vomiting), but symptoms seldom necessitate cessation of treatment. Less common problems with both drugs include allergic reactions, hemolysis, thrombocytopenia, and agranulocytosis. Hypoglycemia has been well documented with treatment of severe malaria because these drugs cause insulin to be released from the pancreas. When used intravenously, they must be administered slowly to prevent arrhythmias and hypotension. Electrocardiographic monitoring should accompany parenteral quinidine use (see Chapter 33), and glucose monitoring is mandatory for both drugs, especially when the parenteral forms are used.

*Chloroquine (Aralen).* Chloroquine phosphate (sulfate or hydrochloride salt) is a 4-aminoquinoline that is effective against the erythrocytic phase of *P. malariae* and *P. ovale,* and, except for some strains in Southeast Asia and Latin America, it is very effective for *P. vivax.* However, chloroquine-resistant *P. falciparum* malaria is present everywhere in the world except in Central America, Haiti, the Dominican Republic, parts of the Middle East, and Central China. Therefore, the use of chloroquine for treatment and prevention of malaria has diminished considerably. The mechanism of chloroquine resistance involves active efflux of the drug from the parasite, by an energy-dependent drug transporter (see Chapter 2) that is inhibited by calcium-channel blockers.

The mechanism of action of chloroquine in malaria is inhibition of heme polymerase, leading to a build up of heme, a hemoglobin product that is toxic to the parasite. Chloroquine can be administered orally, intramuscularly, subcutaneously, and intravenously. Chloroquine is rapidly and completely absorbed and has a very large volume of distribution. The drug is concentrated in the liver and in the cornea and retina of the eye. The plasma half-life is 6 to 12 days. About 30% of the drug is metabolized in the liver; excretion is primarily by renal pathways.

Adverse reactions are dose-related and include GI upset, pruritus, headache, and CNS stimulation. Pruritus, seen primarily in Blacks of African origin, is not an allergic reaction. Permanent retinopathy is associated with prolonged daily use of chloroquine (such as in rheumatic diseases), but not when the drug is used weekly for malaria suppression. Acute overdosage (with as few as 10 tablets in adults) can lead to circulatory failure, respiratory and cardiac arrest, and death. Chloroquine can safely be used during pregnancy for treatment and prevention of malaria.

*Mefloquine (Lariam).* This is a quinoline methanol derivative that is used primarily for the *prevention* of chloroquine-resistant *P. falciparum* malaria. Mefloquine appears to act in the same way as chloroquine. It is less often used for *treatment* of malaria because of the increased frequency of serious neuropsychiatric reactions associated with higher dosage. The drug is well absorbed, partly biotransformed in the liver, and excreted mainly in feces. It has a long (1 to 4 weeks) terminal half-life.

Adverse events such as gastrointestinal upset, dizziness, headache, and sleep disturbances occur with the same frequency as when chloroquine is used for chemosuppression. However, dizziness, irritability, nightmares, depression, and anxiety occur more often with mefloquine than with other anti-malarials. Clinically significant neuropsychological side effects, severe enough to lead to drug discontinuation, occur in 1 to 5% of users. Although confusion, psychosis, and convulsions have been reported rarely with both chemosuppression (1 in 10 000 to 1 in 13 000) and treatment, these side effects are much more likely to occur with treatment (1 in 150 to 1 in 1700) and in those with a previous history of such problems. The drug is contraindicated for use by those with a recent history of anxiety reactions or depression as well as by those with any history of seizures or psychosis.

Mefloquine-resistant *P. falciparum* malaria has, for many years, been documented by in vitro studies in many countries, but it is not yet clinically significant except along the borders of Thailand, where the drug is no longer effective.

## Artemisinin derivatives

These drugs are new oral and intravenous derivatives of artemisinin (also known as ginghaosu), an anti-malarial derived from the ancient Chinese herb *Artemisia annua.* They are very short- and rapid-acting schizonticides that clear parasitemia and symptoms of malaria considerably faster than any other compound. They also inhibit the development of parasites in the mosquito, a property that makes them important in the control of malaria. **Artemether, artesunate,** and **arteether** are derivatives of artemisinin that are quickly converted to their active plasma metabolite, dihydroartemisinin, the chemical responsible for the anti-malarial activity. They produce ultra-structural changes to the growing trophozoite parasite; current evidence suggests that an endoperoxide bridge is essential for anti-malarial activity.

Recrudescence of *P. falciparum* malaria is common when these drugs are used alone; therefore, they are often combined with other longer-acting anti-malarials such as mefloquine, doxycycline, or lumefantrine. In many published clinical studies, artemisinins appear to be very well tolerated. Animal studies using fat-soluble derivatives (artemisinin, artemether, and arteether) have demonstrated midbrain toxicity, but this problem has not been documented to occur in humans. Their rapid action on the early blood-stage trophozoite makes them ideal drugs for the treatment of severe *P. falciparum* infections.

*Atovaquone–Proguanil (Malarone).* A new hydroxynaphthoquinone derivative, atovaquone is a rapid-acting blood schizonticide. Malarone is a drug combination containing 250 mg of atovaquone and 100 mg of proguanil per adult tablet. A pediatric preparation is available that contains 62.5 mg of atovaquone and 25 mg of proguanil per tablet. The site and mode of action of this drug combination are distinct from those of other anti-malarial blood schizonticides. The atovaquone and proguanil interfere with two different pathways involved in the biosynthesis of pyrimidines required for nucleic acid synthesis. Atovaquone is a selective inhibitor of parasite mitochondrial electron transport. The drug acts synergistically with proguanil (a dihydrofolate reductase inhibitor) during parasite development both in the liver and in red blood cells, leading to inhibition of cell replication. This drug combination is effective against multidrug-resistant *P. falciparum* as well as other species of malaria. However, atovaquone–proguanil does not eradicate hepatic hypnozoites found in relapsing malarias (*P. vivax* and *P. ovale*).

The elimination half-life of atovaquone is 2 to 3 days, whereas that of proguanil is 12 to 21 hours. Atovaquone is excreted mostly unchanged in the stool, whereas 40 to 60% of proguanil is excreted by the kidneys. The latter is metabolized by the liver to cycloguanil and other metabolites. The drug combination is best absorbed with a fatty meal.

Atovaquone–proguanil has been shown to be very safe, with gastrointestinal side effects similar to those of mefloquine but only half as many neuropsychiatric problems when used for prophylaxis. In several studies, side effects from atovaquone–proguanil were no different from those reported in controls. In a head-to-head comparison with mefloquine among non-immune travellers, fewer than 1% of atovaquone–proguanil users discontinued the drug due to side effects compared with 5% of mefloquine users. Because of its renal excretion, this drug combination is contraindicated in those with severe renal insufficiency.

*Antibiotics.* Tetracycline, doxycycline, and clindamycin are slow-acting blood schizonticides that are combined with quinine to treat drug-resistant *P. falciparum* malaria. In addition, like the atovaquone–proguanil combination, doxycycline is an effective chemosuppressant, even along the Thai–Myanmar and Thai–Cambodian borders, where multidrug-resistant strains of *P. falciparum* are endemic.

## Malaria treatment

Chloroquine is the drug of choice for treatment of *P. malariae, P. ovale,* most strains of *P. vivax,* and a few strains of *P. falciparum*. In the management of *P. vivax* and *P. ovale,* chloroquine or other blood schizonticides must be followed by a course of primaquine that will eradicate hepatic hypnozoites, thereby ensuring that relapse will not occur. Chloroquine-resistant *P. falciparum* malaria is widespread globally, whereas chloroquine-resistant *P. vivax* malaria and, more recently, *P. malariae* are well established in Indonesia.

Mefloquine, quinine in combination with tetracycline or clindamycin, halofantrine alone, artesunate followed by mefloquine, and atovaquone plus proguanil are all effective treatments of drug-resistant *P. falciparum* malaria. However, mefloquine alone is not generally recommended for treatment of malaria because of the relatively high incidence of severe neuropsychiatric reactions associated with treatment doses of this drug.

Artemisinin derivatives, in combination with another drug, enjoy widespread use in Africa and Southeast Asia. In Europe, the combination of artemisinin plus lumefantrine is now available. However, in North America, where artemisinin derivatives are not yet available, the current treatment of choice for uncomplicated *P. falciparum* malaria is atovaquone–proguanil because of its efficacy, side-effect profile, and ease of administration.

## Malaria chemosuppression (chemoprophylaxis)

Since no drug kills sporozoites, the traditional term "malaria chemoprophylaxis" is a misnomer. A better term is "malaria chemosuppression." Most anti-malarials act beyond the liver phase within erythrocytes, thereby suppressing the parasitemia and hence the symptoms of malaria. If chemosuppression with chloroquine, mefloquine, or doxycycline is continued after the liver stages of *P. falciparum* and *P. malariae* have been completed (i.e., for 4 weeks after exposure to malaria), a "suppressive cure" of these species will result and no late recrudescence will occur. The additional weeks of prophylaxis will not cure *P. ovale* and *P. vivax* malaria because these parasites may lie dormant in the liver and relapse at a later date. Only a tissue schizonticide, such as primaquine, will provide a "radical cure" of these latter infections. The recent introduction of atovaquone–proguanil and prophylactic studies with primaquine have added two additional drugs to the armamentarium for malaria chemoprophylaxis. Since both the atovaquone–proguanil combination and primaquine act on the primary exoerythrocytic cycle in the liver, they may be initiated the day before exposure and discontinued a mere 3 to 7 days afterwards.

Chloroquine is the drug of choice for suppression of all species of malaria, except in areas where resistant *P. falciparum* and *P. vivax* strains occur.

Choice of agents for malaria chemosuppression in chloroquine-resistant areas of the world has become a very complex and controversial subject among those responsible for making recommendations. At present, there is no uniformity of opinion concerning optimal regimens for this purpose. To make matters worse, the World Health Organization recently declared that **"no available chemoprophylaxis regimen will guarantee protection against malaria."**

In North America, mefloquine, doxycycline, and atovaquone–proguanil are regarded as the three drugs of choice for prevention of chloroquine-resistant *P. falciparum* malaria throughout the world. Along the Thai–Myanmar and Thai–Cambodian borders, where multidrug resistance is found, daily doxycycline or atovaquone–proguanil are the chemosuppressants of choice. Primaquine is considered to be a second-line drug when the others cannot be used. Regardless of which chemosuppressive regimen is used, travellers must take personal protection measures against mosquito bites (e.g., insect repellents, bed nets, screened accommodation) and seek medical attention at the first sign of fever while in a malarious area or within 1 year of departure from one. Pregnant women are advised not to travel to areas where mefloquine-resistant malaria is found because of the lack of safe and effective alternatives to mefloquine.

## INTESTINAL HELMINTH INFECTIONS

Intestinal helminths (Table 54-2) are metazoan worms found in the lumen of the large or small bowel, where they frequently attach themselves to the intestinal mucosa. Unlike protozoa, helminths do not usually multiply in the human host. This means that the worm burden (i.e., the total number of worms in the individual's gastrointestinal tract) may increase only when the patient is re-exposed to infective eggs or larvae. Since human morbidity from helminth infections is directly proportional to worm burden, it follows that reduction in worm burden, even without a parasitological cure, may produce an acceptable therapeutic result.

Disease outside of the intestine can occur from the systemic dissemination of eggs or larvae of certain worm species. **Hydatid disease** arises from the ingestion of tapeworm eggs (*Echinococcus granulosus* and *Echinococcus multilocularis*) from feces of dogs and related species. In the infected individual, larvae migrate from the intestine into the portal circulation and travel mostly to the liver or lungs (occasionally to kidneys, bone, and brain), where they form hydatid cysts of increasing size that can rupture and become the source of new cysts. **Cysticercosis** arises from the ingestion of eggs of the pork tapeworm (*Taenia solium*). These eggs develop into larval cysticercus forms in the brain, eye, and muscles, producing inflammation and cystic lesions.

### Mebendazole (Vermox)

This drug is a broad-spectrum benzimidazole anthelmintic. It is the drug of choice for trichuriasis and is effective

| TABLE 54-2 | Drugs Used in the Treatment of Selected Helminth Infections | | | | | | | |
|---|---|---|---|---|---|---|---|---|
| Worm | Species | Albendazole | Mebendazole | Piperazine citrate | Praziquantel | Pyrantel pamoate | Pyrvinium pamoate | Ivermectin |
| Roundworm | *Ascaris lumbricoides* | + | + | + | | + | | |
| Hookworm | *Ancylostoma duodenale, Necator americanus* | + | + | | | + | | |
| Pinworm | *Enterobius (Oxyuris) vermicularis* | + | + | + | | + | + | |
| Whipworm | *Trichuris trichiura* | + | + | | | | | |
| Threadworm | *Strongyloides stercoralis* | + | | | | | | + |
| Tapeworm | *Taenia saginata, Taenia solium, Diphyllobothrium latum, Hymenolepis nana* | + | + | | + | | | |
| Flukes | *Schistosoma* species, *Fasciolopsis buski*, *Paragonimus* species, *Clonorchis sinensis* | | | | + | | | |

Note: The symbol (+) means the drug is effective for that specific helminth infection.

for ascariasis, hookworm, and enterobiasis. For the management of invasive parasites (such as trichinosis, toxocariasis, and hydatid disease), it has been replaced by **albendazole,** since the latter is better absorbed and gives higher tissue levels.

By inhibiting glucose uptake into susceptible parasites, mebendazole causes a decrease in adenosine triphosphate (ATP) production and death of the organism. The drug is poorly absorbed (<10%) from the gastrointestinal tract. Bioavailability is very low (<5%) because of very high first-pass elimination. The elimination half-life of mebendazole ranges from 3 to 9 hours. Unchanged drug and its major metabolites are excreted in the urine.

Mebendazole is an extremely safe drug that only rarely causes mild GI upset, pruritus, and skin rash. Since it has been shown to be teratogenic in rats, mebendazole should not be used during pregnancy.

## Pyrantel Pamoate (Combantrin, Antiminth)

This is a drug of choice for ascariasis, hookworm, and enterobiasis; it is ineffective in trichuriasis and strongyloidiasis. Pyrantel acts as a depolarizing neuromuscular blocking agent that paralyzes worms, which subsequently "lose their grip" on the bowel mucosa and are expelled in the feces.

Pyrantel is poorly and incompletely absorbed from the GI tract; most of an oral dose is excreted unchanged in the feces. The drug is well tolerated except for infrequent, mild, GI upset.

## Piperazine Citrate (Entacyl)

Piperazine is an alternative drug for the treatment of ascariasis and enterobiasis, frequently used in the developing world. (Pyrantel and mebendazole are preferred for both infections.) The drug exerts its action by inducing flaccid paralysis of the worm, thereby causing it to detach from the intestinal mucosa.

Piperazine is well absorbed from the small intestine. Approximately two-thirds of a dose is eliminated unchanged in the urine within 24 hours. It is a relatively safe drug that occasionally produces GI upset, urticaria, and dizziness. It may reduce seizure threshold and is therefore contraindicated in patients with epilepsy.

## Pyrvinium Pamoate (Vanquin)

This salt of a cyanine dye has largely been replaced by pyrantel and mebendazole for the treatment of enterobiasis. The drug acts by inhibiting glucose uptake by the parasite.

Pyrvinium is poorly and incompletely absorbed from the GI tract and, hence, is one of the few anthelmintics considered to be safe in pregnancy. Mild GI upset is uncommon. Because it is a dye, it colours the stool orange and may stain the patient's underwear and bed sheets.

## Albendazole (Zentel)

This is one of the most potent and broad-spectrum benzimidazole anthelmintics. It is effective against adult and larval forms of many nematodes and cestodes. Like mebendazole, the drug acts by interfering with the parasite's uptake of glucose, with subsequent depletion of glycogen and ATP stores.

At present, albendazole is available in Canada only by emergency drug release but is available in the United States. Albendazole is highly effective as a single oral dose against ascarids, hookworms (including those that cause cutaneous larva migrans), pinworms, whipworms, and the threadworm *Strongyloides stercoralis*. It is somewhat less effective for adult tapeworm infections. However, because it is much better absorbed than mebendazole, it is effective for the treatment of larval cestode infections such as hydatid disease and cysticercosis. Recent data suggest that it is effective against filaria larvae (microfilaria), *Loa loa* adults, and against *G. intestinalis* and the microsporidium *Septata intestinalis*.

Approximately 50% of a dose of albendazole is absorbed, compared with less than 10% for mebendazole. The drug is rapidly converted to its active metabolite, albendazole sulfoxide, and then excreted in the urine. The elimination half-life of the metabolite is approximately 8 hours.

Short, 1- to 3-day courses are well tolerated; GI upset and dizziness occur infrequently. Prolonged courses of therapy used for larval cestode infections have occasionally caused reversible hepatotoxicity, neutropenia, and alopecia.

## Praziquantel (Biltricide)

This pyrazinoisoquinoline compound has a broad spectrum of activity against trematodes (flukes) and cestodes (tapeworms). It is the drug of choice for all species of schistosomiasis, and for clonorchiasis, opisthorchiasis, paragonimiasis, and fasciolopsiasis (*Fasciolopsis buski*) but not fascioliasis *(Fasciola hepatica)*. Praziquantel is effective for the treatment of taeniasis (*Taenia saginata, T. solium*), diphyllobothriasis (*Diphyllobothrium latum*), and hymenolepiasis (*Hymenolepis nana*). It is also very effective in the treatment of cysticercosis and in the eradication of echinococcal protoscolices that have leaked from a ruptured cyst. Recent studies suggest that the combination of albendazole and praziquantel may be more effective against cystic hydatid disease than either drug alone.

Praziquantel is readily absorbed, rapidly biotransformed in the liver by first-pass hydroxylation, and largely excreted in the urine. The unchanged drug has a serum half-life of approximately 1 hour with a terminal elimination half-life of 3 to 10 hours. Although the clinical significance is uncertain, corticosteroids and anticonvulsants have been shown to markedly decrease serum levels of the drug.

Praziquantel increases the permeability of the worm's cell membrane to calcium ions, causing spastic paralysis of its musculature and dislodgement from sites of attachment. Subsequently, disintegration of the worm tegument takes place, resulting in lysis of the parasite.

Dizziness, headache, malaise, drowsiness, abdominal pain, and nausea are common side effects, particularly when larger doses are used. Vomiting, urticaria, and mild to moderate increases in hepatic transaminases occur less frequently.

## Ivermectin (Mectizan)

Ivermectin is effective against the larvae of filarial worms, notably onchocerciasis, as well as Bancroftian filariasis and *L. loa*; it has little effect against adult worms. The drug is also effective against *S. stercoralis* and against ectoparasitic infections such as **head lice** and **scabies** when the arthropod parasite takes up ivermectin during a blood meal. The drug binds to glutamate-gated chloride channels in the parasite's nervous system, causing them to open and thereby leading to paralysis and death of the parasite.

Ivermectin is highly protein-bound and has a half-life of 22 to 28 hours. It does not cross the blood–brain barrier in humans. Rapidly absorbed from the gut, ivermectin is metabolized by the liver and excreted in the feces; less than 1% of the dose is excreted in the urine. The drug is usually administered as a single dose. Most individuals tolerate it remarkably well.

## SUGGESTED READINGS

Ali SA, Hill DR. Giardia intestinalis. *Curr Opin Infect Dis.* 2003;16: 453-460.

del Giudice P, Chosidow O, Caumes E. Ivermectin in dermatology. *J Drugs Dermatol.* 2003;2:13-21.

Derouin F. Anti-toxoplasmosis drugs. *Curr Opin Investig Drugs.* 2001;2:1368-1374.

Drugs for parasitic infections. *Med Lett Drugs Ther* 2004:1-12. Available at: http://www.medletter.com/freedocs/parasitic.pdf. Accessed October 13, 2005.

Garcia HH, Gonzalez AE, Evans CA, Gilman RH for the Cysticercosis Working Group in Peru. Taenia solium cysticercosis. *Lancet.* 2003;362:547-556.

Haque R, Huston CD, Hughes M, et al. Amebiasis. *N Engl J Med.* 2003;348:1565-1573.

Horton J. Albendazole: a broad spectrum anthelminthic for treatment of individuals and populations. *Curr Opin Infect Dis.* 2002;15:599-608.

Horton J. Albendazole for the treatment of echinococcosis. *Fundam Clin Pharmacol.* 2003;17:205-212.

Jong E. Intestinal parasites. *Prim Care.* 2002;29:857-877.

Kain KC, Shanks GD, Keystone JS. Malaria chemoprophylaxis in the age of drug resistance. I. Currently recommended drug regimens. *Clin Infect Dis.* 2001;33:226-234.

Katz DE, Taylor DN. Parasitic infections of the gastrointestinal tract. *Gastroenterol Clin North Am.* 2001;30:797-815.

Maitland K, Bejon P, Newton CR. Malaria. *Curr Opin Infect Dis.* 2003;16:389-395.

Minenoa T, Avery MA. Giardiasis: recent progress in chemotherapy and drug development. *Curr Pharm Des.* 2003;9:841-855.

Potts J. Eradication of ectoparasites in children. How to treat infestations of lice, scabies, and chiggers. *Postgrad Med.* 2001; 110:57-59, 63-64.

Shanks GD, Kain KC, Keystone JS. Malaria chemoprophylaxis in the age of drug resistance. II. Drugs that may be available in the future. *Clin Infect Dis.* 2001;33:381-385.

Shields JM, Olson BH. Cyclospora cayetanensis: a review of an emerging parasitic coccidian. *Int J Parasitol.* 2003;33:371-391.

Sibley LD. Intracellular parasite invasion strategies. *Science.* 2004;304:248-253.

Singh K, Wester WC, Trenholme GM. Problems in the therapy for imported malaria in the United States. *Arch Intern Med.* 2003; 163:2027-2030.

Stanley SL Jr. Amoebiasis. *Lancet.* 2003;361:1025-1034.

Stauffer W, Fischer PR. Diagnosis and treatment of malaria in children. *Clin Infect Dis.* 2003;37:1340-1348.

Wendel K, Rompalo A. Scabies and pediculosis pubis: an update of treatment regimens and general review. *Clin Infect Dis.* 2002;35(suppl 2):S146-S151.

White NJ. The treatment of malaria. *N Engl J Med.* 1996;335: 800-806.

# Antiviral Agents

## SL WALMSLEY

A 38-year-old gay man known to be HIV-infected had been treated with oral acyclovir 200 mg three times daily as suppressive treatment for recurrent perianal herpes simplex infections. He was well in all other respects. When he developed oral thrush (candidiasis), he approached his physician about treatment. This opportunistic candidal infection was treated with nystatin, 500 000 IU three times daily, using the "swish and swallow" technique. A blood test showed a low CD4 count of $200 \times 106/L$ and a moderately elevated viral load (35 000 copies of HIV RNA/mL). It was decided that the patient should initiate antiretroviral therapy, and the combination of combivir 1 tablet twice daily—this is a combination antiretroviral tablet containing zidovudine (AZT) at a dose of 300 mg and lamivudine (3TC) at a dose of 150 mg—together with nelfinavir (Viracept) at a dose of 1250 mg twice daily was chosen. This caused an initial increase in his CD4 count and suppression of HIV RNA to <50 copies/mL.

On screening laboratory evaluations, he was found to be co-infected with the hepatitis C virus. Given that his HIV was well controlled, it was decided to assess the status of his liver disease. A liver biopsy showed grade 2 inflammation and grade 2 fibrosis, and it was felt, in consultation with the hepatologist, that therapy should be considered. The patient was started on oral ribavirin 800 mg daily and weekly subcutaneous injections of 180 μg of pegylated interferon. This therapy, however, had to be discontinued after 2 weeks because of side effects characterized by flu-like symptoms, malaise, and myalgia, which occurred with each injection and interfered significantly with his quality of life and worsened his chronic anemia.

He remained well over the next 2 years, but then he started to develop some changes in his body appearance, with a loss of fat in the face and limbs and a gain of fat in the abdominal area (lipodystrophy). He felt that everyone around him saw these changes and thus knew that he had HIV, and he became quite depressed. Consequently, he started to be inconsistent with his antiretroviral drugs and eventually stopped them altogether.

One year later, his CD4 count had decreased to $30 \times 106/L$, his viral load had increased to 150 000/mL, and he complained of floaters in his visual field. A diagnosis of cytomegalovirus (CMV) retinitis in one of his eyes was made, and he was started on induction therapy with oral valganciclovir, 900 mg twice daily. It was felt that he should restart on HAART (highly active antiretroviral therapy). AZT therapy was not thought to be useful because of the patient's low hemoglobin (85 g/L) and neutrophil count ($1200 \times 106/L$); it was felt that the combined marrow-suppressant effects of AZT and valganciclovir would be too great. Further, because of his earlier inconsistencies with his antiretroviral therapy, it was thought that he might have developed resistance to all three components of his combination. Therefore, his new combination consisted of abacavir 300 mg twice daily, nevirapine 200 mg once daily for a week and then twice daily, and lopinavir/ritonavir (Kaletra) 400 mg/100 mg, three pills twice daily. Acyclovir was discontinued because valganciclovir at a maintenance dose of 900 mg/day provided adequate control of the herpes simplex infections.

Unlike bacteria, viruses are incomplete infectious organisms; the infectious particles, or *virions,* consist essentially of DNA or RNA surrounded by a protein capsule and sometimes by an additional outer covering of lipoprotein that may have glycoprotein or other inclusions. Viruses are obligatory parasites because they lack the enzymatic machinery for reproducing their own constituents; therefore, they must invade living cells of higher organisms and use the host cell's biosynthetic machinery, under the direction of the viral nucleic acid, to produce and release new viral particles. The sequence of steps in the invasion of the host cell by the virus and the intracellular reproduction and release of new viral particles are illustrated in Figure 55-1. Antiviral chemotherapy is aimed at blocking or disrupting one or more of these steps in viral replication.

The history of human antiviral chemotherapy is relatively short; the first agent was licensed for clinical use in North America within the past four decades. Despite drug developments, the major approach to the control of viral infections is through prevention. This includes prophylactic treatment in high-risk populations (e.g., recipients of organ transplants) and programs of vaccination.

A number of viral pathogens remain major therapeutic problems not only in the normal host but, more significantly, in those whose immunity has been compromised by underlying disease or its therapy. New viral pathogens continue to emerge.

The development of antiviral agents has been slow relative to that of other anti-infective agents because their effectiveness is closely related to cellular metabolism, and much had to be learned in this field before effective drugs could be devised. It was long believed that viral replication was so closely coupled with normal host cellular metabolism that antiviral therapy would not be possible without seriously compromising the host. Extensive research has increased our understanding of viral metabolism, especially those aspects of viral genome replication that are different from host cell replication. This has led to the development of antivirals that are selective for the virus and inhibit virus-specific events or, preferentially, inhibit virus-directed macromolecular synthesis. As these agents inhibit specific events in viral replication, most have a restricted spectrum of activity.

Despite these advances, few of the many antiviral drugs developed to date have had a sufficiently high ratio of therapeutic value to toxicity in animal models to warrant proceeding to clinical trials in humans. Even fewer have shown sufficient clinical benefit to achieve licensing.

The current epidemic of human immunodeficiency virus (HIV) infections has had an enormous impact on the field of virology. Infection with this virus has become a major public health problem worldwide since its recognition in 1981. It has posed a serious challenge to researchers concerned with developing viral vaccines and antiviral drugs. Many researchers have turned their efforts toward this problem, and although a solution to the epidemic is not yet in sight, remarkable advances have been made in our understanding of viruses, their replicative mechanisms, and the potential targets for antiviral drugs and vaccines. This knowledge was recently applied to the study of the putative coronavirus causing severe acute respiratory syndrome (SARS). The sequence of the virus was determined by polymerase chain reaction (PCR) technology within 1 month of the first clinical case and is now being used in the development of vaccines and antiviral agents.

## PRINCIPLES OF ANTIVIRAL CHEMOTHERAPY

Chemotherapeutic agents for viral infections can be classified into one of three major groups:

1. Agents that directly inactivate intact viruses (virucidal)
2. Agents that inhibit viral replication at the cellular level (antiviral)
3. Agents that augment or modify the host's response to infection (immunomodulating)

Virucidal drugs are usually too toxic for clinical use. The mechanisms of action of antivirals currently available for clinical use include (1) the prevention of viral fusion, penetration of the cell, and/or uncoating of the viral nucleic acid inside the cell, (2) the selective inhibition of enzymes specific for viral genome replication, (3) the shutting off of viral messenger RNA (mRNA) translation (e.g., interferon), (4) the inhibition of protein modification or cleavage, and (5) the prevention of release of newly synthesized virions from the infected cells. Immunomodulating agents are also available for some viral infections (see Chapter 40).

Many variables may influence the outcome of antiviral chemotherapy, including the following:

- Type of the underlying disease and immune competence of the host
- Age of the patient
- Stage of the illness at the time of initiation of treatment
- Dosage of the antiviral agent utilized
- Ability of the virus to remain latent within its host
- Ability of the virus to penetrate the central nervous system (CNS)
- Ability of the virus to change genetically over time
- Development of resistance by the virus to the inhibitory action of the drug

In clinical trials of antiviral agents, it is important that these variables be carefully considered during data analysis. It is also important to recognize that viral infections often follow an unpredictable course; some viral infections may improve even if the patient is treated with a placebo. For these reasons, it is imperative that any trial of antiviral chemotherapy be double blind and placebo-controlled until an agent with clinical efficacy is identified. This then becomes the standard against which newer agents are tested. As most agents are inhibitory rather than virucidal in their activity, viral infections may relapse when the compound is removed, especially when the host's immune function remains compromised, as in HIV infections and transplants.

Antiviral drugs act at various points in the viral replication cycle shown in Figure 55-1. Given these various steps in viral replication, it is possible to search for new drugs that will block some point in the replication cycle. Thus, there are agents that do the following:

- Interfere with virus attachment to host cell receptors, cell penetration, and viral uncoating
- Inhibit virion-associated enzymes such as reverse transcriptase
- Inhibit transcription of the parental genome
- Inhibit translation processes of viral mRNA
- Interfere with viral regulatory proteins
- Interfere with viral protein glycosylation or cleavage
- Interfere with viral assembly
- Interfere with release of virus through the membranes of infected cells

The agents discussed in this chapter are limited to those that are currently, or will soon be, available for clinical use (Table 55-1).

The use of combinations of antiviral agents with different mechanisms or sites of action is an active area of research. This is being investigated as a means to increase the antiviral activity, decrease drug toxicity, and prevent the development of resistant viruses.

## DRUGS THAT BLOCK VIRAL PENETRATION OR UNCOATING

The receptors to which viruses attach themselves before penetrating the cell are not unique viral receptors; they can be receptors for endogenous substances. For example, the human polyoma virus JCV can bind to serotonin

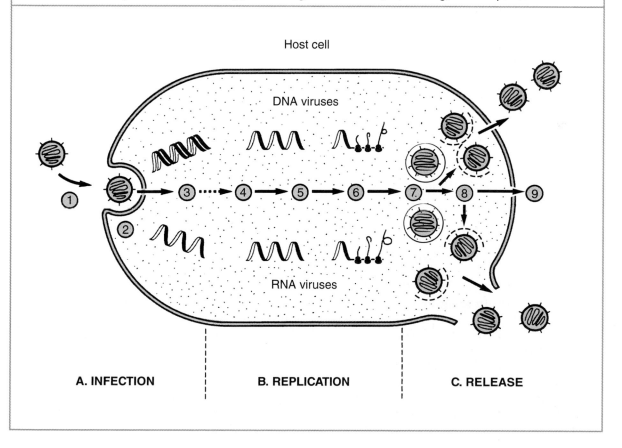

**FIGURE 55-1** Basic strategy (key steps) of viral replication. (A) Infection: (1) Adsorption of virion to host cell plasma membrane receptors. (2) Entry of virion into host cell (akin to phagocytosis). (3) Uncoating of virion (i.e., removal of protein capsid, exposure of viral nucleic acids to initiate replication). (B) Replication: (4) Viral DNA-dependent RNA polymerases (for DNA viruses) and RNA-dependent RNA polymerases or reverse transcriptases (for RNA viruses) catalyze the synthesis of mRNA for production of structural and non-structural viral proteins. (5) Viral genome may integrate into host chromosome. (6) Modification of viral proteins by glycosylation and cleavage. (C) Release: (7) Assembly of virions. (8) Removal of sialic acid by viral neuraminidase. (9) Slow leakage from host cell (i.e., budding) or cell rupture.

Host cell

DNA viruses

RNA viruses

**A. INFECTION**          **B. REPLICATION**          **C. RELEASE**

| TABLE 55-1 | Characteristics of Antiviral Agents | | |
|---|---|---|---|
| **Drug** | **Mechanism of Action** | **Clinical Indications** | **Main Adverse Effects** |
| Amantadine and Rimantadine | Interfere with uncoating of the virus | Prophylaxis and treatment of influenza A | Confusion; insomnia; anxiety |
| Zanamivir and Oseltamivir | Inhibit neuraminidase of influenza virus | Prophylaxis and treatment of influenza A and B | Bronchospasm by zanamivir; nausea by oseltamivir |
| Trifluorothymidine (Trifluridine) | Competitively inhibits the incorporation of natural nucleotide into viral DNA | Topical treatment of herpetic keratitis and herpetic skin ulcerations | Burning and irritation upon instillation |
| Pleconaril | Interferes with virus attachment and uncoating | Enterovirus meningitis | Gastrointestinal effects |
| Acycloguanosine (Acyclovir) | Inhibition of viral DNA polymerase | Herpes simplex encephalitis; herpes of the newborn; herpes in immuno-compromised hosts; genital herpes; varicella zoster in immuno-compromised hosts; herpes keratitis | Transient increases in blood urea nitrogen (BUN) and creatinine; thrombophlebitis |
| Ribavirin | Suppression of biosynthesis of guanosine-5'-monophosphate; blocks capping of viral mRNA | Influenza A and B; respiratory syncytial virus and paramyxovirus bronchiolitis and pneumonia; hepatitis C (in combination with interferon) | Macrocytic anemia; hemolytic anemia; conjunctival injection; lethal to embryo in some animal species |
| Ganciclovir (DHPG) | Inhibits DNA polymerase, thereby inhibiting DNA synthesis and terminating chain elongation | Serious cytomegalovirus (CMV) infections in compromised hosts | Bone marrow suppression; liver toxicity; psychosis |
| Foscarnet (PFA) | Inhibits DNA polymerase | CMV retinitis in compromised hosts | Transient increases in creatinine; anemia; nausea; tremor; genital ulcers |
| Zidovudine (AZT) | Inhibits reverse transcriptase; blocks DNA chain lengthening | HIV | Anemia; leukopenia; neutropenia; decreased vitamin $B_{12}$; myositis |
| Didanosine (ddI) | Inhibits reverse transcriptase | HIV | Peripheral neuropathy; pancreatitis; diarrhea |
| Zalcitabine (ddC) | Inhibits reverse transcriptase | HIV | Peripheral neuropathy; pancreatitis; aphthous stomatitis |
| Stavudine (d4T) | Inhibits reverse transcriptase | HIV | Peripheral neuropathy; pancreatitis; lipoatrophy; mitochondrial toxicity |
| Lamivudine (3TC) | Inhibits reverse transcriptase | HIV | Nausea |
| Abacavir | Inhibits reverse transcriptase | HIV | Hypersensitivity reaction; rash |
| Tenofovir | Inhibits reverse transcriptase | HIV | Nausea; renal abnormalities |
| Efavirenz | Inhibits reverse transcriptase | HIV | CNS symptoms; rash |
| Nevirapine | Inhibits reverse transcriptase | HIV | Hypersensitivity reaction; rash; increased liver transaminases |
| Delavirdine | Inhibits reverse transcriptase | HIV | Rash |
| Saquinavir/Invirase/Fortovase | Inhibits HIV protease | HIV | Diarrhea |

*continued*

| TABLE 55-1 | continued | | |
|---|---|---|---|
| Drug | Mechanism of Action | Clinical Indications | Main Adverse Effects |
| Indinavir | Inhibits HIV protease | HIV | Renal stones; dry skin, mouth; paronychia; "Crix" belly |
| Nelfinavir | Inhibits HIV protease | HIV | Diarrhea |
| Ritonavir | Inhibits HIV protease | HIV | Nausea; vomiting; diarrhea; circumoral paresthesia |
| Amprenavir | Inhibits HIV protease | HIV | Nausea; diarrhea; rash |
| Lopinavir/Ritonavir | Inhibits HIV protease | HIV | Nausea; diarrhea; increased cholesterol and triglycerides |
| Atazanavir | Inhibits HIV protease | HIV | Indirect hyper-bilirubinemia; nausea; diarrhea |
| Tipranavir and tipranavir/r | Inhibits HIV protease | HIV | Increased triglycerides and liver transaminases; diarrhea |
| Enfuvirtide | Inhibits membrane fusion | HIV, advanced disease | Injection site reactions |
| Imiquimod | Immunomodulator | Genital and cutaneous warts | Local skin reactions |
| Interferons | Activation of an endoribonuclease and phosphorylation of a peptide initiation factor | Herpes keratitis; rhinovirus prophylaxis and treatment; varicella zoster infection in immunocompromised hosts; chronic hepatitis C (in combination with ribavirin) | Headache; somnolence; gastrointestinal upset |

5-HT$_{2A}$ receptors, and its penetration into cells can be prevented by serotonin receptor blockers. However, blockade of viral binding to specific receptors has not yet become a practical therapeutic approach. Available drugs all act at other stages of the penetration process.

## Amantadine

This antiviral agent is a stable tricyclic amine that has been chemically synthesized and has a peculiar cage-like structure (Fig. 55-2). It increases the dopaminergic activity in the striatum and was initially used in the treatment of Parkinson's disease (see Chapter 17).

### Mode of antiviral action

The mode of action is not fully known, but amantadine is thought to interfere with the uncoating and nucleic acid release of certain RNA viruses. In vitro, it is active against certain myxoviruses (e.g., type A influenza), a paramyxovirus (Sendai virus), and a toga virus (rubella).

### Pharmacokinetics

Amantadine (as the hydrochloride, Symmetrel) is slowly but probably completely absorbed by the oral route, crosses the blood–brain barrier, and appears in the saliva and nasal secretions. It is available in capsule, tablet, and syrup forms. It has a long half-life of approximately 15 hours and is almost entirely recoverable unmetabolized in the urine. Plasma half-life increases in the elderly and in patients with impaired renal function, and doses are adjusted accordingly.

### Resistance

Resistance to amantadine is readily achieved in the laboratory. It develops from mutations in the matrix proteins of the virus. Drug-resistant strains have been isolated from treated and untreated patients, but more studies are needed to assess the clinical importance of such strains.

### Adverse reactions and toxicity

These include difficulty thinking, confusion, lightheadedness, hallucinations, anxiety, insomnia, and a reduced seizure threshold. The approximate incidence of these primarily CNS manifestations is 3 to 7%. Very often they may occur within 48 hours of initiating therapy, but they are usually reversible despite continuation of the drug. The side effects are related to CNS levels of the drug and are exacerbated by the concomitant use of other CNS-active agents, by renal insufficiency, and in those with a history of seizures. The other major side effects are gastrointestinal, including nausea and lack of appetite. Amantadine has been found to be embryotoxic and teratogenic in animals.

## Clinical indications

Amantadine at a dose of 200 mg/day is currently used in chemoprophylaxis and therapy of influenza A virus infections. In persons 65 years of age or older, the dose is decreased to 100 mg/day. It is compatible with influenza vaccine and may be used in combination therapy under epidemic conditions. As a chemoprophylactic agent, the drug has been found to reduce the incidence of clinical ill-

---

**FIGURE 55-2** Structural formulae of some antiviral agents.

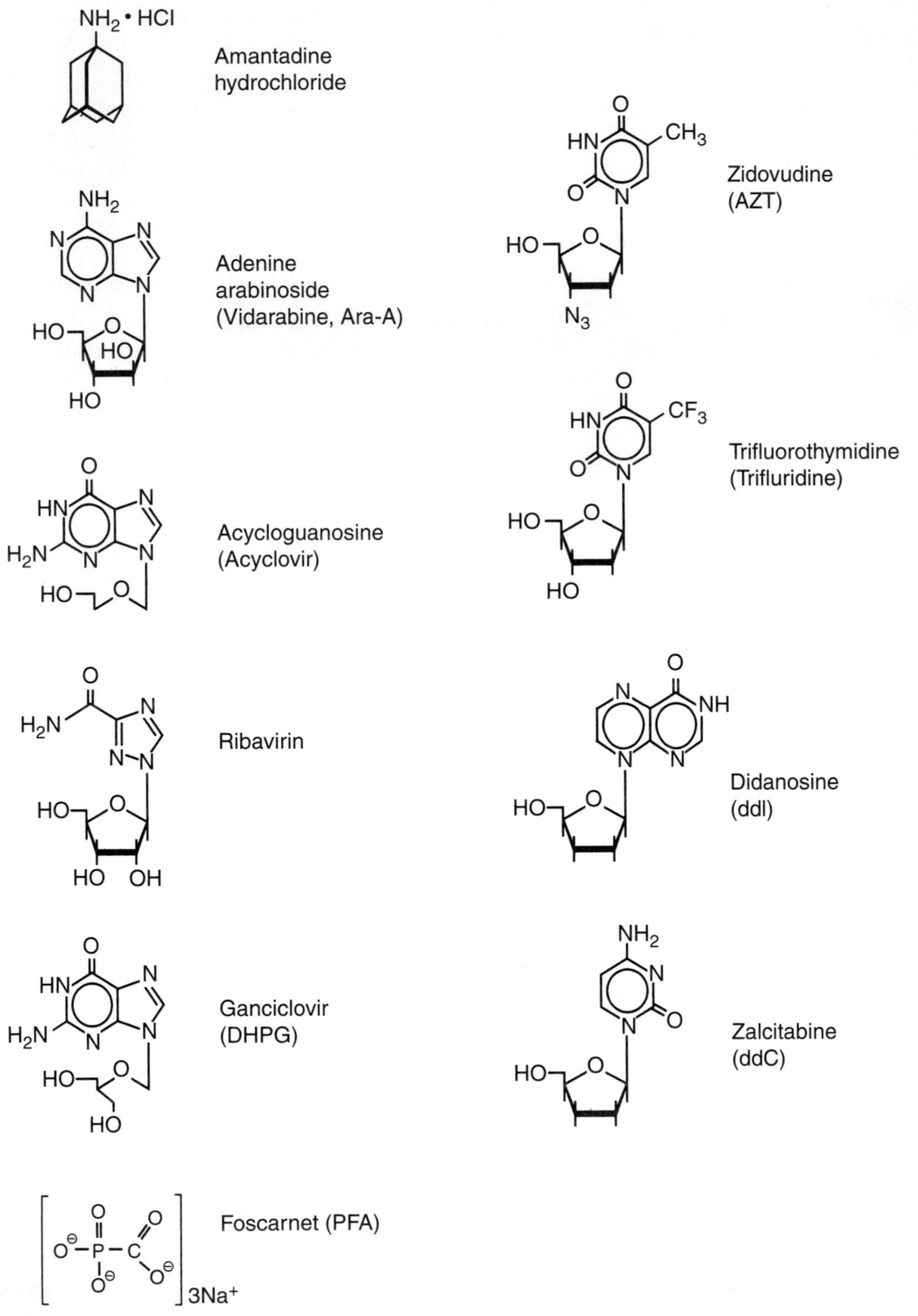

Amantadine hydrochloride

Adenine arabinoside (Vidarabine, Ara-A)

Acycloguanosine (Acyclovir)

Ribavirin

Ganciclovir (DHPG)

Foscarnet (PFA)

Zidovudine (AZT)

Trifluorothymidine (Trifluridine)

Didanosine (ddI)

Zalcitabine (ddC)

ness by 50 to 100% in persons at high risk (e.g., patients with chronic respiratory or cardiovascular disease). As a chemotherapeutic agent against influenza A virus infections, amantadine decreases fever in 50% of patients and reduces illness duration by 1 to 2 days if it is administered within the first 2 to 3 days of the illness. It also reduces viral shedding. It does not appear to be useful in the treatment or prophylaxis of influenza B.

## Rimantadine

This antiviral agent is a structural analogue of amantadine with an identical mechanism of action. Its activity against influenza A virus in vitro is four to eight times that of amantadine. It is also more efficacious against influenza A virus infections in animals. Until recently, it had been used primarily in the former Soviet Union. A clinical trial of its usefulness as a prophylactic agent against influenza A infections in humans, conducted in the United States, revealed that it is *not* more efficacious than amantadine but that it produces considerably fewer CNS side effects. This quality of rimantadine may soon make it the preferred agent. Gastrointestinal effects, however, are reported frequently. In contrast to amantadine, rimantadine is extensively metabolized, with less than 15% excreted unchanged in the urine and approximately 20% excreted as a hydroxylated metabolite. Its half-life averages 24 to 36 hours.

## Pleconaril

### Mechanism of action
Pleconaril inhibits picornavirus replication by binding to a specific hydrophobic pocket within the viral capsid and preventing viral attachment to the cell and/or uncoating of the viral genome.

### Pharmacokinetics
After oral administration, maximum plasma concentrations are reached in 1.5 to 5 hours. Peak plasma concentration averages 1.1 µg/mL and 2.4 µg/mL after doses of 200 mg and 400 mg, respectively, and is increased if the drug is taken with food. The half-life averages 25 hours.

### Adverse events
Pleconaril is generally well tolerated. The most common adverse events are headache, nausea, stomach upset, diarrhea, and discomfort. No serious organ damage has been reported.

### Clinical indication
The only current indication is enteroviral meningitis in adults. Pleconaril therapy results in significant shortening of the duration of illness, faster resolution of headache, and decreased use of analgesics. Studies of its

possible beneficial effects in other enteroviral infections are in progress.

## VIRAL NEURAMINIDASE INHIBITORS

The influenza virus, both type A and type B, is coated with a neuraminic acid derivative that must be acted on by a viral surface neuraminidase, which splits off sialic acid residues and enables the newly synthesized intracellular virus particles to pass through the cell membrane and exit the infected cell. There are now several drugs available that inhibit the viral neuraminidase and thus prevent release of the virus from the cell.

## Zanamivir (Relenza)

Zanamivir is a sialic acid analogue that is a potent and selective inhibitor of the influenza virus neuraminidase. It is active against both influenza A and B viruses by altering virus particle aggregation and inhibiting the release of infectious virions from the epithelial cells of the respiratory tract.

### Pharmacokinetics
The drug is available for inhalation from a "diskhaler" device using "rotadisks" containing the medication in powder form, in blisters delivering 5 mg of drug per inhalation. The recommended dosage is two inhalations (total dose 10 mg) twice daily for 5 days. In human pharmacokinetic studies, approximately 10 to 20% of the dose was systemically absorbed, yielding peak serum concentrations of 17 to 142 ng/mL within 1 to 2 hours. The serum half-life ranges from 2.6 to 5 hours, and the drug is entirely excreted unchanged in the urine. After inhalation, zanamivir is widely deposited at high concentrations throughout the respiratory tract and is thus delivered directly to the site of the influenza infection.

### Clinical indications
Zanamivir is used to treat uncomplicated acute illness due to influenza in patients more than 12 years of age who have been symptomatic for no more than 2 days. Some studies have shown that it may also be useful for prophylaxis in household contacts of acute cases.

### Adverse events and toxicity
Some patients being treated with zanamivir for influenza have experienced bronchospasm and decreased respiratory function. Many (but not all) of these patients had underlying airway disease such as asthma or chronic obstructive pulmonary disease. Therefore, zanamivir is not recommended for the treatment of influenza in patients with such underlying diseases because of the risk of serious adverse events and because efficacy has not been demonstrated in this group. Allergic or allergic-like

reactions, including facial and oropharyngeal edema, have been reported. Some elderly patients, and those with chronic musculoskeletal or neurological disorders affecting the function of the hands, may have difficulty using the inhaler device.

## Oseltamivir (Tamiflu)

Oseltamivir is available as a prodrug, the ethyl ester of oseltamivir carboxylate. It requires hydrolysis by hepatic esterases to convert it to the active metabolite, which is a selective inhibitor of the viral neuraminidase. It is readily absorbed (bioavailability about 80%) after oral administration. After activation in the liver, it is carried largely in unbound form in the plasma and excreted unchanged in the urine by both glomerular filtration and tubular secretion, so its plasma concentration is increased by probenecid (see Chapter 30). Renal clearance is reduced in patients with decreased creatinine clearance. The half-life of elimination of the parent drug is about 2 hours, but that of the active metabolite is 6 to 10 hours, and it is not altered by acetaminophen, which is frequently used for symptomatic relief in patients with influenza. Oseltamivir does not interact with either cytochrome P450 or glucuronyl transferases.

Like zanamivir, oseltamivir is used for treatment of uncomplicated infection with influenza virus, both type A and type B, in adults and children over 1 year of age. In vitro it is also active against the avian influenza virus. These agents can also be used for influenza prophylaxis in high-risk patients, but they should not affect the evaluation of individuals for annual influenza vaccination. Treatment of acute influenza with these drugs has been shown to alleviate symptoms and shorten duration. It may also decrease complications in previously healthy adults. Oseltamivir is available both as capsules and as a suspension in liquid. The recommended dosage is 75 mg twice daily for 5 days, beginning no more than 2 days after the onset of influenza symptoms.

The most frequently reported adverse events with oseltamivir are nausea and vomiting, which are transient, generally appearing with the first dose but disappearing despite continued administration. There are insufficient data in pregnant women to permit an evaluation of the potential for fetal toxicity.

## INHIBITORS OF VIRAL NUCLEIC ACID REPLICATION

## Trifluorothymidine (Trifluridine)

### Mechanism of action

Trifluridine (Viroptic) is a thymidine analogue (see Fig. 55-2). It is phosphorylated by cellular thymidine kinase to a monophosphate, which is further phosphory-lated by other cellular enzymes. The triphosphate is incorporated into DNA, competitively inhibiting the incorporation of the natural thymidine nucleotide. Viral DNA polymerase has a higher affinity for trifluridine triphosphate than does the DNA polymerase of uninfected host cells. Trifluridine is active against herpes simplex viruses, including some acyclovir-resistant strains.

### Clinical indications

Trifluridine is used primarily for the treatment of primary keratoconjunctivitis and recurrent epithelial keratitis due to herpes simplex virus. It has also been shown to be effective in the management of some chronic cutaneous ulcerations secondary to herpes simplex virus in HIV-infected patients with acyclovir-resistant strains.

The drug is given by drops onto the cornea and is continued for 7 days after re-epithelialization has occurred. It should not be given for more than 3 weeks.

Resistance of herpes simplex virus type II to trifluridine has been produced in vitro, and these strains are able to produce infection in vivo.

### Adverse reactions and toxicity

The drug is limited to topical usage, primarily ocular. Patients may experience burning on instillation, eyelid edema or irritation, and blurring of vision. Allergic reactions occur infrequently.

## Adenine Arabinoside (Ara-A, Vidarabine)

This agent (see Fig. 55-2) was first introduced as an anticancer drug in 1960. Its antiviral activity was noted in 1964.

### Mechanism of action

Vidarabine is a nucleoside derivative of adenine deoxyriboside that inhibits DNA synthesis by competitive inhibition of DNA polymerase. Vidarabine is phosphorylated by cellular enzymes to the triphosphate derivative. The principal metabolite is hypoxanthine arabinoside, a compound with 30 to 50 times less antiviral activity. It is primarily active against the DNA viruses, including members of the herpes group and pox viruses.

### Pharmacokinetics

When vidarabine (Vira-A) is administered by intravenous infusion, it is very rapidly deaminated to a hypoxanthine derivative. It may also be converted by phosphorylation to various phosphate nucleotides. The drug requires large administration volumes because of poor solubility (<0.5 mg/mL). When it is given intravenously at a dose of 1 mg/kg, plasma levels of 1 to 2 µg/mL have been achieved. The plasma half-life is 1.5 to 3 hours. After an intramuscular injection of 1 mg/kg, the peak serum concentration is only 0.2 to 0.3 µg/mL, but the half-life is prolonged to 10 to 16 hours. The difference in half-life is probably caused by protracted absorption from the intramuscular site. Most of the drug is excreted in the urine as an arahypoxanthine derivative. A dosage reduction of 25% has been recommended for patients with severe renal insufficiency.

## Adverse reactions and toxicity

The most important side effect is gastrointestinal upset consisting of anorexia, nausea, vomiting, weight loss, and diarrhea. Less commonly, but more importantly, CNS toxicities, including tremors, ataxia, paresthesias, dizziness, hallucinations, confusion, and even psychosis, may occur. These CNS side effects are most common in patients with reduced renal function. Another problem with vidarabine therapy relates to its poor solubility, which necessitates a large fluid volume for administration of the drug. In patients being treated for encephalitis, this large fluid volume is relatively contraindicated. Other adverse reactions include skin rashes, leukopenia, thrombocytopenia, anemia, megaloblastosis, and increased levels of aspartate aminotransferase (AST, formerly SGOT). This drug has been shown to be mutagenic, teratogenic, and oncogenic in animal models.

## Clinical indications

The only current use of vidarabine is in the form of an ophthalmic ointment for the topical treatment of keratoconjunctivitis caused by herpes simplex virus. For other indications, it has been replaced by more efficacious and less toxic agents such as acyclovir.

## Acycloguanosine (Acyclovir)

### Mechanism of action

This antiviral agent is a guanine derivative with an acyclic side chain (see Fig. 55-2). As a nucleoside derivative, it has a mechanism of action similar to that of vidarabine, but it displays a unique selectivity in action. It appears to be selectively taken up by virus-infected cells and converted to its monophosphate form by a virus-specific thymidine kinase. This monophosphate form is then converted by cellular enzymes to the active triphosphate form that interferes with viral replication by inhibiting viral DNA polymerase. Acyclovir is much more active against the viral DNA polymerase than it is against cellular DNA polymerase. It may also be incorporated into the viral DNA and act as a chain terminator for viral DNA synthesis. The spectrum of activity in vitro includes members of the herpes group of DNA viruses. It is most active against herpes simplex viruses and the varicella zoster virus, and it is less active against cytomegalovirus (CMV) and Epstein-Barr virus.

### Resistance

Alterations or deficiency in the viral thymidine kinase or alterations in viral DNA polymerase can cause acyclovir resistance in vitro. Most clinically significant viral isolates have been thymidine kinase–deficient mutants, usually isolated from immunocompromised patients on long-term or multiple treatment courses. These viruses have led to progressive mucocutaneous infections in these patients, particularly those infected with HIV.

### Pharmacokinetics

Acyclovir (Zovirax) is available in topical, oral, and intravenous preparations. The topical preparation consists of 5% acyclovir in polyethylene glycol ointment; there are no strong indications for its use. Oral acyclovir is slowly and incompletely absorbed from the gastrointestinal tract, with only 15 to 30% oral bioavailability. With multidose administration, steady-state concentrations (0.6 to 1.6 µg/mL, depending on the dose) are reached within 24 to 48 hours. Peak serum concentrations of 20 µmol/L to more than 100 µmol/L are achieved following a 1-hour infusion of acyclovir of 2.5 to 15 mg/kg. The terminal half-life is 2 to 3 hours in adults with normal renal function. Acyclovir prodrugs with increased absorption provide total exposures of acyclovir comparable to those following intravenous dosing, although peak serum concentrations are somewhat lower. Available newer derivatives include **famciclovir**, **valacyclovir**, and **pencyclovir**. After oral administration, they are rapidly and almost completely converted to acyclovir by first-pass enzymatic hydrolysis by hydrolases in the liver and intestine. They are of greatest benefit in the treatment of herpes zoster infection in which higher drug concentrations are required.

The excretion of acyclovir is primarily via the kidneys by both glomerular filtration and tubular secretion. There is minimal transformation of the drug in vivo. Dosage must be reduced in patients with renal insufficiency.

### Adverse reactions and toxicity

The topical and oral formulations of acyclovir are relatively free of side effects. The intravenous formulation can result in transient and reversible increases in blood urea nitrogen (BUN) and creatinine in approximately 5 to 10% of treatments, and local reactions consisting of thrombophlebitis or bullae formation have been noted in approximately 3% of patients.

Neurological symptoms, including lethargy, agitation, tremor, disorientation, and paresthesia, have been noted after intravenous infusion in approximately 1% of patients, especially after bone marrow transplantation or in those with renal failure. Psychiatric symptoms, including depersonalization, hallucinations, and hyperactivity, have also been observed. Complicating illnesses and concomitant drug use may be contributing factors. These adverse reactions are reversible when acyclovir is discontinued.

### Clinical indications

Extensive clinical evaluation has established acyclovir as the treatment of choice in many types of herpes simplex and varicella zoster viral infections.

**Oral acyclovir** at a dose of 200 mg five times a day is effective in the treatment of first-episode genital herpes simplex infection. Effects include decreased duration of viral shedding, decreased time to healing, and decreased duration of constitutional symptoms. Use of the drug does not alter the time to first recurrence. Oral acyclovir is associated with antiviral activity and, in some trials, with statistically significant but modest clinical effects in recurrent genital herpes simplex infection. Several placebo-controlled studies have shown that chronic suppressive treatment with oral acyclovir (200 mg three times per day) will reduce recurrences of genital herpes by up to 80%. Treatment should be interrupted every 12 months to reassess the need for continued suppression.

Similarly, long-term suppressive oral acyclovir may decrease recurrences of mucocutaneous herpes simplex infections in immunocompromised hosts, such as transplant recipients and patients with acquired immunodeficiency syndrome (AIDS).

Oral administration of acyclovir in high dose (800 mg five times per day) accelerates the rate of cutaneous healing from varicella zoster (shingles) if given within 72 hours of the onset of the rash. Early treatment of acute herpes zoster may also decrease the duration of post-herpetic neuralgia. For this purpose, the oral prodrugs valacyclovir or famciclovir, 500 mg three times a day, may be preferred as a means of achieving better patient adherence to the prescribed regimen.

Clinical trials have also shown that high-dose acyclovir can lead to more rapid healing of varicella (chickenpox) in children if given less than 24 hours after onset. Although the results were statistically significant, the clinical benefits are limited, and the role of acyclovir in immunocompetent (i.e., not compromised) children is controversial.

**Intravenous acyclovir** (like the oral formulation) is effective in the treatment of first-episode genital herpes simplex infections in immunocompetent patients. Effects are less dramatic in recurrent episodes. It is also effective in the prevention and treatment of mucocutaneous herpes simplex infections in the compromised host. The usual dose is 5 mg/kg three times per day.

Localized and disseminated infections due to varicella zoster in immunocompetent as well as immunocompromised hosts respond to intravenous therapy. In the compromised host, visceral dissemination of varicella zoster herpes is decreased by treatment with acyclovir.

Two large randomized trials of acyclovir and vidarabine in the treatment of herpes simplex encephalitis demonstrated increased survival and decreased morbidity in patients treated with acyclovir. Acyclovir is now considered the drug of choice in the treatment of herpes simplex encephalitis. The dose is 12.4 mg/kg every 8 hours.

Studies comparing vidarabine and acyclovir in the treatment of neonatal herpes simplex infection show the two drugs to be equally efficacious.

Acyclovir is of no benefit in the treatment of severe CMV infections in transplant recipients. The drug has been found to be useful as a prophylactic agent when used in high dose in renal and bone marrow transplant patients to decrease the frequency of symptomatic CMV infections.

## Ribavirin

This agent, 1-β-D-ribofuranosyl-1,2,4-triazole-3-carboxamide (Virazole; see Fig. 55-2), a guanosine analogue, was synthesized in 1972 as part of a major program to search for a compound with broad-spectrum antiviral activity. In vitro, it inhibits a wide range of DNA and RNA viruses, including myxoviruses, paramyxoviruses, arena, corona, bunya, RNA tumour, herpes, and pox viruses. In contrast, rotavirus, poliomyelitis, hepatitis B virus, and CMV seem relatively insensitive to inhibition by the drug.

### Mechanism of action

The mechanism of action is uncertain but relates to the alteration of cellular nucleotide pools and viral mRNA formation. Proposed mechanisms include (1) a decrease in intracellular guanosine 5'-triphosphate (GTP), (2) inhibition of 5'-cap formation of mRNA, and (3) inhibition of the initiation and elongation of viral mRNA through effects on RNA polymerase.

### Pharmacokinetics

After oral administration in humans, bioavailability averages 60% and is increased with a high-fat meal. The estimated serum half-life is 30 hours. Peak plasma levels of 1 to 3 μg/mL occur at 1 to 2 hours. Tenfold higher peak plasma levels occur following intravenous administration. Aerosol administration of the lyophilized agent by means of a small-particle aerosol generator delivering an estimated 0.8 mg/kg/hr achieves drug levels in respiratory secretions of 50 to 200 μg/mL, the actual concentration depending on ventilation and lung pathology. The half-life in tracheal secretions is 1 to 2 hours. The drug is biotransformed and secreted in the urine.

### Adverse reactions and toxicity

Aerosolized ribavirin is well tolerated except for mild conjunctival irritation, rash, and transient wheezing in some patients. When it is used in conjunction with mechanical ventilation, in-line filters, modified circuits, and frequent monitoring are required to prevent plugging of the valves or tubing with precipitates.

After oral administration, hemolytic anemia occurs in approximately 10% of patients, usually appearing in the first 1 to 2 weeks of therapy and stabilizing by the fourth week. Reversible increases in leukocytes, serum bilirubin, iron, and uric acid have been observed. The drug was found to be teratogenic and embryotoxic in small mammals during the first trimester. Adequate birth control is mandatory when the drug is used in human females of reproductive age. Prolonged use in animals has also caused macrocytic anemia.

## Clinical indications

Ribavirin by aerosol is effective in the treatment of lower respiratory tract infections (bronchiolitis and pneumonia) by the respiratory syncytial virus (RSV) in infants and young children with congenital heart disease, pulmonary disease, or immune deficiency. Infants treated with ribavirin showed a significantly faster improvement in their illness severity score. However, no differences were noted in viral shedding. Opinion varies about the overall clinical value, indications for use, and optimal length of treatment in RSV infections.

Other indications for ribavirin aerosols are respiratory infections secondary to influenza A and influenza B. Treated groups improve statistically more rapidly than controls; however, the clinical improvements are minimal. The drug cannot be used prophylactically for these infections.

In Sierra Leone, intravenous ribavirin was used for the treatment of Lassa fever. Mortality rates decreased significantly when treatment was initiated within the first 6 days of illness. Oral ribavirin was less effective.

The most common indication is in combination with interferon for the treatment of chronic hepatitis C in persons with compensated liver disease.

## Ganciclovir (DHPG)

This acyclic nucleoside analogue of guanine (Cytovene; see Fig. 55-2) has in vitro activity against all herpes virus strains, but its unique characteristic is its potent inhibition of CMV replication.

### Mechanism of action

The drug is an inhibitor of viral DNA synthesis. Intracellular ganciclovir is phosphorylated to its monophosphate derivative by infection-induced kinases. Ganciclovir diphosphate and triphosphate are formed by cellular enzymes. Ganciclovir triphosphate is a competitive inhibitor of deoxyguanosine 5′-triphosphate (dGTP) incorporation into DNA and preferentially inhibits viral DNA polymerase. The drug is incorporated into growing viral DNA and inhibits chain elongation.

### Resistance

Herpes simplex virus strains resistant to ganciclovir because of DNA polymerase mutations have been demonstrated in the laboratory. Ganciclovir-resistant strains of herpes and CMV have also been isolated from immune-compromised hosts.

### Pharmacokinetics

The oral bioavailability is very low (less than 5%), and therefore ganciclovir is usually given intravenously. Peak plasma concentrations average 8 to 11 µg/mL. Cerebrospinal fluid (CSF) levels average 25 to 70% of those in plasma. The elimination half-life averages 3 to 4 hours in patients with normal renal function. The drug is excreted unchanged in the urine, and dose reduction is necessary in patients with renal insufficiency. **Valganciclovir**, a prodrug that is converted to ganciclovir in the body, has greater bioavailability (60%) than oral ganciclovir and is currently considered the drug of choice for patients who can adequately take and absorb oral formulations. It is rapidly absorbed, reaching peak levels within 30 minutes, and is rapidly hydrolyzed to ganciclovir, which reaches its peak concentrations within 90 minutes. The plasma profile is similar to that of intravenous ganciclovir, with a similar elimination half-life of about 4 hours. The bioavailability is increased when the drug is taken with food.

## Adverse reactions and toxicity

The most common (and typically dose-limiting) adverse events have been anemia, neutropenia, and thrombocytopenia, occurring in up to 40% of treated patients. Central nervous system side effects, including headache, behavioural changes, psychosis, convulsions, and coma, have been described in 5 to 15% of patients. Rash, fever, abnormal liver function tests, nausea, and vomiting have also been reported. Ganciclovir is teratogenic in rabbits and mutagenic in a number of different systems.

## Clinical indications

The drug is used in the treatment and prophylaxis of serious CMV infections in immunocompromised hosts. In patients with AIDS, ganciclovir has been used successfully in the suppression of CMV retinitis. Approximately 80 to 90% of patients will respond to treatment. The dose used for induction of therapy is oral valganciclovir 900 mg twice daily or intravenous ganciclovir 5 mg/kg twice daily, usually for 2 to 3 weeks. Long-term maintenance therapy (900 mg of oral valganciclovir or 5 mg/kg of intravenous ganciclovir once daily) is required as relapse will occur after 1 to 2 months off the drug. For HIV patients who subsequently respond to HAART, long-term maintenance therapy may be safely discontinued. Intraocular drug administration by intravitreal injection and slow-release intraocular implants is also available but needs to be combined with systemic agents to prevent systemic dissemination of the disease.

Ganciclovir has also been found useful (clinical response up to 65%) in the management of other CMV syndromes in patients with HIV, including esophagitis, colitis, cholangitis, and pneumonia. The role of long-term maintenance therapy is controversial for these infections. In these situations, the intravenous formulation is preferred, given the uncertain absorption by mouth.

A randomized, placebo-controlled study has demonstrated efficacy of oral ganciclovir as prophylaxis against CMV infection in HIV patients at risk. However, given the declining incidence of CMV disease in the HAART era, it is generally not used.

In bone marrow transplant patients undergoing treatment with ganciclovir for CMV pneumonia, decreases in viral levels have been observed but there was no decrease in mortality. Increased survival has been reported when ganciclovir is used in combination with anti-CMV immunoglobulin.

Ganciclovir has been found useful in the prophylaxis and pre-emptive therapy of CMV infections and disease in bone marrow and solid organ transplant recipients. The optimal dose, duration, and appropriate selection of patients continue to be subjects of active research. Such therapy is usually considered in those at highest risk, such as CMV antibody–negative recipients of transplants from CMV antibody–positive donors, those receiving anti-lymphocyte globulin for transplant procedures, and lung and heart–lung recipients.

A recent, randomized, placebo-controlled study has demonstrated efficacy of oral ganciclovir as prophylaxis against CMV infection in HIV patients at risk.

## Foscarnet (PFA)

Trisodium phosphoformate hexahydrate (see Fig. 55-2) is an inorganic pyrophosphate analogue that inhibits herpes virus DNA polymerase and retroviral reverse transcriptase. It is active in vitro against most herpes viruses, including CMV and herpes simplex virus.

### Pharmacokinetics

Foscarnet is usually given by the intravenous route as a bolus followed by either continuous or intermittent infusions of 90 mg/kg. The plasma half-life averages 3 to 6 hours. It penetrates the CSF and the eye. The drug is excreted by the kidneys, and dosages must be adjusted in renal failure.

### Adverse reactions and toxicity

The major toxicity is renal insufficiency. The drug has been associated with malaise, nausea, vomiting, fatigue, and headache. Tremors, seizures, irritability, and hallucinations have been associated with increased serum concentrations. Local phlebitis, hypo- or hypercalcemia, hyperphosphatemia, and abnormal liver function tests may develop. Neutropenia has been reported infrequently. In a small number of patients, painful oral and genital ulcers have been described following the intravenous infusion of this drug. Nephrogenic diabetes insipidus is an uncommon complication.

### Clinical indications

Foscarnet (Foscavir) has been used primarily to treat CMV infections in HIV-infected patients or transplant recipients, especially those who are intolerant or resistant to ganciclovir. In CMV retinitis, clinical responses appear to be similar in frequency to those observed with ganciclovir and may be associated with a small survival benefit, given its additional anti-HIV activity. The problem of relapse after discontinuation of therapy is similar to that observed with ganciclovir, so long-term maintenance therapy is required in those patients not receiving, or unresponsive to, HAART. In transplant recipients, caution must be exercised because of the potential for renal toxicity and alterations in levels of immunosuppressive agents. Resistant strains have been described, probably resulting from mutations in the viral polymerase gene.

Foscarnet also appears to be a useful agent in the treatment of acyclovir- and ganciclovir-resistant strains of herpes simplex virus and CMV.

## Future Directions

The drugs described above act on known enzymes at various stages of viral DNA or RNA synthesis. Recently, it has been discovered that certain human microRNAs (21 to 24 nucleotides long) that play a regulatory role by silencing the expression of host genes can also block expression of viral genes that contain similar nucleotide sequences. This knowledge may give rise to new antiviral agents in the future.

# ANTIRETROVIRAL DRUGS

HIV infects the CD4 T lymphocytes, resulting in progressive deterioration of the cell-mediated immune system. As the CD4 count declines, patients are at increasing risk of opportunistic infections and malignancies, complicating their viral infection and resulting in AIDS. HIV is a chronic disease; patients survive an average of 8 to 10 years. No cure is presently available. However, numerous antiretroviral drugs have been developed to slow the progressive immunological deterioration, increase CD4 cell counts, decrease viral loads, and eventually delay complications and prolong survival. Unfortunately, resistance can develop to all of these drugs as a result of mutations at different points in the reverse transcriptase enzyme or in other enzymes involved in viral replication.

Antiretroviral therapy is currently prescribed as combination therapy with at least three agents from two or three different classes of drugs—the so-called "HIV cocktails." The use of combination therapy has resulted in much more profound effects on viral replication and immune function recovery, while minimizing the risk of emergence of drug resistance. However, the use of more agents can result in increased toxicity and can threaten the patient's adherence to the prescribed regimen. In addition, controversy remains as to when to start antiretroviral therapy, and it is unlikely that a clinical trial will ever be able to answer the question. Therefore, current management is guided by treatment guidelines written and regularly updated by experts in the field, based on the available data at the time. The most current recommendations are to start therapy in any HIV-infected patient who has symptoms, who is pregnant (to prevent transmission from mother to fetus), and who has more advanced disease characterized by a CD4 count less than 200 to 350/mm³. Some guidelines also recommend therapy for those with viral loads greater than 30 000 to 50 000 copies of HIV RNA/mL. Combination therapy is also used for post-exposure prophylaxis within 72 hours of needle use or sexual contact, in an attempt to minimize transmission.

Currently available antiretroviral therapy is carried out with drugs of four different classes:

1. Nucleoside and nucleotide reverse transcriptase inhibitors
2. Non-nucleoside reverse transcriptase inhibitors
3. Protcase inhibitors
4. Viral fusion inhibitors

Some representative drugs in these classes are illustrated in Figure 55-3.

## Nucleoside and Nucleotide Reverse Transcriptase Inhibitors

### Mechanisms of action and resistance

These agents are analogues that mimic the natural nucleosides or nucleotides. They are prodrugs that must be activated intracellularly by phosphorylation by host cell enzymes. The triphosphate derivatives are the active drugs, which are selective competitive inhibitors of the reverse transcriptase of HIV-1 and HIV-2. When the triphosphate metabolites of the analogues are incorporated into newly forming viral nucleic acid, they terminate nucleic acid chain elongation. This event interrupts the viral replication cycle.

However, viral resistance to the drugs can occur as a result of mutations of the reverse transcriptase enzyme. The thymidine-associated mutations were first found with AZT use, but are also selected for by stavudine (d4T). A total of three to six mutations can significantly decrease susceptibility to either drug, as well as to other members of the class. There is some level of cross-resistance between drugs of this class because some of the same mutations can arise during treatment with different agents of the class. Some mutations can confer high-level cross-resistance to all members of the class. Therefore, in antiretroviral combination therapy for HIV infection, in general, two nucleoside reverse transcriptase inhibitors are combined with either a protease inhibitor or a non-nucleoside reverse transcriptase inhibitor.

### Class-specific adverse events

Mitochondrial toxicity mediated by the nucleoside analogues results from inhibition of the mitochondrial gamma DNA polymerase, resulting in depletion of mitochondrial DNA. All agents in this class can inhibit this enzyme, but

they differ in their inhibitory potency. The inhibition is associated with a wide range of clinical toxicities, including myopathy, peripheral neuropathy, cardiomyopathy, pancreatitis, lactic acidosis, and peripheral lipoatrophy.

Lactic acidosis and severe hepatomegaly with hepatic steatosis should be considered in patients treated with these drugs who complain of fatigue, abdominal pain, nausea, vomiting, and dyspnea. This complication is life-threatening, and all nucleoside reverse transcriptase inhibitors should be stopped if an elevated serum lactate level occurs in combination with the typical symptoms. All members of this drug class can cause the complication,

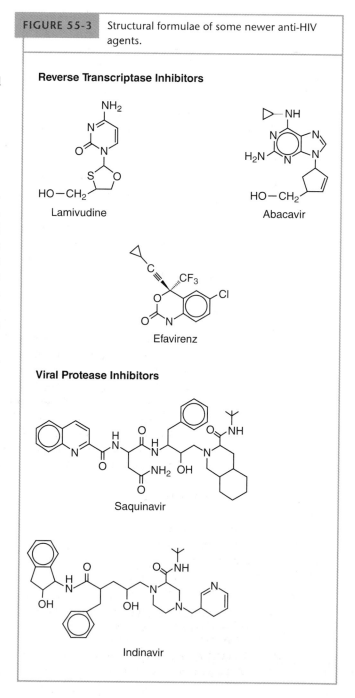

**FIGURE 55-3** Structural formulae of some newer anti-HIV agents.

but it occurs most commonly with a combination of didanosine and stavudine, which are described in the following sections.

## Zidovudine (AZT)

A deoxynucleoside analogue structurally related to thymidine, this drug, 3'-azido-3'-dideoxythymidine (see Fig. 55-2), was synthesized more than 25 years ago; however, no therapeutic application was found until recently. This was the first agent shown to be effective in the management of HIV-1 infections and was approved for use in 1987.

### Pharmacokinetics

The drug is well absorbed orally with 65% bioavailability, and it penetrates the CNS. Plasma protein binding is only 30%. Peak plasma concentrations of 5 µmol/L are achieved with intravenous doses of 2.5 mg/kg or oral doses of 5 mg/kg. Its half-life is approximately 1 to 1.5 hours. The determination of intracellular levels is difficult, but they are probably a more reliable indicator of the drug's antiviral activity.

Biotransformation is primarily hepatic (via glucuronidation) with subsequent renal excretion. The drug undergoes extensive first-pass metabolism to an inactive metabolite. After oral administration, 65 to 75% of the drug is recovered as a metabolite in the urine, and 8 to 15% as the parent compound; the remaining 15 to 20% is excreted by extra-renal mechanisms.

The dose needs to be decreased in patients with severe hepatic or renal dysfunction.

### Adverse reactions and toxicity

The major adverse effects include reversible anemia and leukopenia. Macrocytosis is a common finding but does not usually require treatment. Significant frequencies of nausea, headache, insomnia, and myalgia are reported. These symptoms occasionally require dosage adjustment, but they may resolve spontaneously despite continuation of the drug. Myositis with elevation of creatine phosphokinase (CPK) and proximal muscle weakness has been reported and may be a manifestation of mitochondrial toxicity. Nail pigmentation may occur in dark-skinned patients.

### Clinical indications

AZT in high dose was found to be effective in the treatment of HIV-associated neurological disease; it is also the preferred treatment for HIV-related thrombocytopenia.

AZT, when given orally to pregnant women (14 to 34 weeks) with CD4 counts more than $200 \times 10^6$/L during their pregnancy, when given intravenously during delivery, and when given as an oral suspension to newborns for the first 6 weeks, can lower the rate of maternal–fetal transmission from 25 to 8%. It is now used in combination therapy in these patients.

The recommended dose for long-term treatment is 500 to 600 mg/day, given as two or three fractional doses. AZT is also given as a constituent of combination tablets, such as Combivir (AZT plus 3TC) or Trizivir (AZT plus 3TC plus abacavir), to improve adherence to the therapy regimen.

## Didanosine (ddI) (Videx)

### Pharmacokinetics

This purine nucleoside analogue (2'3'-dideoxyinosine; see Fig. 55-2) has a plasma half-life of approximately 1 hour. The active metabolite has a longer intracellular half-life (25 to 40 hours), thereby allowing less frequent administration. It is acid-labile and therefore must be buffered for oral use. The drug is currently available as a chewable tablet, with average bioavailability of 43%. Unfortunately, many patients find the taste unpleasant. The dosage is 300 to 400 mg once a day based on body weight. It is taken on an empty stomach, thus improving bioavailability by 45%. A newer formulation of delayed-release enteric-coated capsules (Videx EC) is now available. This capsule can be swallowed whole rather than chewed, has improved palatability, and avoids buffer-related drug interactions and related side effects such as diarrhea. It is given at a dose of 250 to 400 mg once daily based on body weight and also should be taken on an empty stomach.

### Adverse reactions and toxicity

The main dose-limiting toxicity includes peripheral neuropathy and pancreatitis. Peripheral neuropathy occurs in 5 to 12% of cases and typically resolves or improves in 3 to 5 weeks when the drug is discontinued. Pancreatitis is reported in 1 to 9% of patients treated and is fatal in 6% of those affected. Other symptoms include diarrhea, dry mouth, headache, insomnia, irritability, and seizures. Hyperuricemia is commonly seen but is rarely clinically important. Hypokalemia, hypomagnesemia, and hypocalcemia have been described. There is a U.S. Food and Drug Administration (FDA) warning about the combination of ddI and ribavirin, which has given rise to 23 reported cases of pancreatitis, alone or combined with lactic acidosis, and so must be avoided or used with caution. Combination of ddI with the nucleotide reverse transcriptase inhibitor tenofovir results in increased levels of ddI, and dose reduction to 250 mg/day should therefore be considered. The combination of ddI and stavudine is contraindicated in pregnant women because it has caused cases of fatal lactic acidosis and hepatic steatosis.

## Zalcitabine (ddC) (Hivid)

The drug is a pyrimidine nucleoside analogue (2'3'-dideoxycytidine; see Fig. 55-2).

## Pharmacokinetics

The oral bioavailability of the drug is 87%. The plasma half-life is 0.34 hours and the intracellular half-life is 2.6 hours.

## Adverse reactions and toxicity

The major dose-limiting toxicity is peripheral neuropathy, especially in patients on higher doses and with more advanced infection. Pancreatitis has also been reported. Aphthous stomatitis with fever, malaise, and esophageal ulcerations can occur.

## Clinical indications

Zalcitabine (Hivid) is used infrequently now because of the availability of a large number of less toxic members of the same drug class and because of overlapping resistance patterns.

## Lamivudine (3TC)

This drug, 2′-deoxy-3′-thiacytidine, is a dideoxypyrimidine analogue that inhibits the HIV reverse transcriptase (see Fig. 55-3). The (–) enantiomer has greater activity and less toxicity than the (+) enantiomer and was selected for clinical testing and use. Lamivudine has activity against a wide range of retroviruses, including strains of HIV that are resistant to AZT. It is also synergistic with AZT in vitro and in vivo. Lamivudine is also a potent inhibitor of hepatitis B virus (HBV) replication, causing loss of HBV DNA, elimination of hepatitis B e antigen (HbeAg), improved levels of alanine transaminase (ALT) in the blood, and improved liver histology. Mutations in the YMDD (Tyr-Met-Asp-Asp) region of the viral polymerase gene confer lamivudine resistance at a rate of 20 to 25% per year during chronic treatment.

## Pharmacokinetics

The mean oral bioavailability of lamivudine is 86%, and the mean plasma half-life is approximately 2 to 4 hours, with a mean intracellular half-life of 12 hours. Renal excretion accounts for 71% of the administered dose. Studies have shown similar efficacy at dosages of 300 mg once daily and 150 mg twice daily. The recommended dosage for hepatitis B is 100 mg/day for a full year, but patients who are co-infected with HBV and HIV should receive the standard doses.

## Adverse reactions

The drug is generally well tolerated. Neutropenia and mild and transient episodes of diarrhea, headache, fatigue, nausea, and abdominal pain are the most frequent adverse events reported. Rare cases of pancreatitis have occurred.

## Stavudine (d4T)

This drug, 2′,3′-didehydro-2′,3′-dideoxythymidine, is a nucleoside reverse transcriptase inhibitor closely related to AZT. There is pharmacologic antagonism between stavudine and AZT, arising from the fact that AZT inhibits the intracellular phosphorylation of stavudine, and the two drugs should not be given together.

## Pharmacokinetics

Stavudine is rapidly absorbed with an overall mean bioavailability of 91%, which is not influenced by food. It is given at a dosage of 30 to 40 mg twice daily depending on body weight. At peak plasma concentrations of 1.2 to 4.2 mg/L, CSF concentrations range from 0.08 to 0.4 mg/L. The mean plasma half-life is 1 to 1.6 hours. Approximately 40% is excreted unchanged in the urine. Because of the prolonged half-life of the triphosphate metabolite, fewer daily doses are required than for the other reverse transcriptase inhibitors. An extended-release formulation (d4T XR) was shown to have similar efficacy and toxicity as the standard formulation, and it is given once daily at a dose of 75 to 100 mg depending on body weight.

## Adverse reactions

The major limiting toxicities are peripheral neuropathy (5 to 15%) and pancreatitis, for which the risks are dose-related. Other adverse events reported include headache, asthenia, gastrointestinal disturbance, and raised liver enzyme levels. A syndrome of ascending motor weakness resembling Guillain-Barré syndrome has been described in a small number of patients taking stavudine.

## Abacavir (Ziagen)

### Pharmacokinetics

This nucleoside analogue (see Fig. 55-3) is given orally at a dose of 300 mg twice daily. The bioavailability is 83%. The plasma half-life is 1.5 hours, and the intracellular half-life is more than 12 hours. CSF levels are about one-third of the corresponding plasma levels. About 81% of the dose is metabolized by alcohol dehydrogenase and glucuronyl transferase, and the metabolites are excreted in the urine. Dose modification is not required in patients with renal failure.

### Adverse events

A hypersensitivity reaction is seen in 3 to 9% of patients, usually within the first 2 weeks of administration. The clinical features include fever, skin rash, fatigue, malaise, nausea, vomiting, diarrhea, abdominal pain, arthralgias, and cough or dyspnea. If the drug administration is stopped and then restarted, an anaphylactic-like reaction may occur in 20% of cases, with hypotension, bronchoconstriction, and/or renal failure. Death has occurred in some cases. Treatment is supportive, consisting of drug discontinuation, intravenous fluids, and symptomatic medication. Steroids and antihistamines are usually not effective.

### Clinical use

The triple nucleoside combination of AZT, 3TC, and abacavir, available as trizivir (dose of one tablet twice daily), has been studied in clinical trials. It has the advantages of convenient dosing, a well-tolerated regimen, and delaying the use of protease inhibitors and non-nucleoside inhibitors until later in the course of HIV disease. The disadvantages include the risk of hypersensitivity reaction and possible reduced potency, especially in those with baseline viral loads greater than 100 000 copies/mL. Abacavir is also available in a fixed-dose combination tablet with 3-TC (Kivexa).

## Tenofovir (Viread)

### Mechanism of action

Tenofovir is a nucleotide analogue and has a mechanism of action similar to that of the nucleoside reverse transcriptase inhibitors. However, since it is a nucleotide analogue, it needs to have only two rather than three phosphates added in order to be converted to the active compound.

### Pharmacokinetics

It is given as a dose of 300 mg once daily, with food. The bioavailability is about 25% in the fasting state, rising to about 40% with food. The plasma half-life is 12 to 18 hours, and the intracellular half-life is 10 to 50 hours. The drug undergoes glomerular filtration as well as active secretion in the kidney tubules, and dose reductions are therefore required in patients with renal insufficiency. Tenofovir also interacts with ddI to increase the plasma AUC (area under the curve) of ddI by 40 to 60% when the drugs are co-administered. This increases the risk of peripheral neuropathy, pancreatitis, and lactic acidosis caused by the ddI. Ganciclovir and valganciclovir compete with tenofovir for active secretion in the renal tubule, thus increasing plasma levels of tenofovir.

### Adverse events

The major untoward effect of tenofovir is gastrointestinal intolerance, but it occurs infrequently. Elevation of serum creatinine and acute renal failure have also been reported in patients receiving tenofovir.

## NON-NUCLEOSIDE REVERSE TRANSCRIPTASE INHIBITORS

## Mechanism of Action

Unlike the nucleoside and nucleotide analogues, the non-nucleoside reverse transcriptase inhibitors (NNRTIs) do not require intracellular phosphorylation to become active. They bind directly to the viral reverse transcriptase at a different site from the nucleoside and nucleotide analogue triphosphates, and they function as non-competitive rather than competitive inhibitors. Resistance to this action arises through mutations of the reverse transcriptase; two different single-step mutations give rise to high-level cross-resistance to all drugs within this class.

## Clinical Indications

The NNRTIs are combined with two nucleoside or nucleotide reverse transcriptase inhibitors as first-line therapy for HIV infection. They can also be used in combination with a nucleoside or nucleotide inhibitor plus a protease inhibitor as part of second- or third-line antiretroviral therapy in those who have developed resistance to their first-line therapy. More recently, they have been used in "switch therapy" for patients well controlled on combinations containing protease inhibitors but who have become concerned about long-term adverse events or about having to take large numbers of pills.

## Efavirenz (Sustiva)

### Pharmacokinetics

This drug (see Fig. 55-3) is administered by mouth, at a dose of 600 mg once daily, at bedtime. The oral bioavailability is 40 to 45%, with or without food. The plasma half-life is 40 to 55 hours. Efavirenz is metabolized by cytochrome CYP 3A4 and is excreted both in the urine and the feces. No dose modification is required in the presence of impaired liver or kidney function. The drug both induces and inhibits the CYP 3A4, exerting a variable effect on the concentrations of other concurrently administered drugs that are metabolized by the same pathway. Dose adjustments are frequently required when efavirenz is used in combination with protease inhibitors.

### Adverse events

Approximately 15 to 30% of patients treated with this drug develop a self-limited morbilliform rash. More serious rashes requiring drug discontinuation occur in 1 to 2% of patients. CNS side effects occur in most users but result in drug discontinuation in only about 5% of cases. The symptoms occur with the first dose but usually resolve spontaneously after 2 to 4 weeks; they include confusion, abnormal thinking, impaired concentration, depression, depersonalization, abnormal dreams, and dizziness. Other side effects noted include somnolence, insomnia, hallucinations, and euphoria. Patients must be warned of these effects before starting therapy. Increased serum levels of liver transaminases are noted in 2 to 8%, more frequently in those co-infected with hepatitis B or C.

This drug has caused birth defects (anencephaly, anophthalmia, and microphthalmia) in offspring when given to pregnant monkeys. The current recommendation for humans is to avoid its use during the first trimester of pregnancy. There are two case reports in the literature of myelomeningocele in the newborn child of a woman taking efavirenz during conception and early pregnancy. The FDA now classifies efavirenz as a "D" agent in pregnancy.

## Nevirapine (Viramune)

### Pharmacokinetics

Nevirapine is given by mouth at a dose of 200 mg once daily for two weeks, and then 200 mg twice daily. The pharmacokinetic features of this drug also permit once-daily administration of 400 mg, but the higher peak level achieved this way has been associated with a higher incidence of adverse events. The bioavailability of the drug is 93% and is not affected by food or fasting. The plasma half-life is 25 to 30 hours. The drug is converted by CYP3A4 to hydroxylated metabolites that are excreted primarily in the urine. Nevirapine autoinduces hepatic cytochrome P450 enzymes, thus reducing its own half-life from 45 hours to about 25 hours over 2 to 4 weeks. Since it induces CYP3A4 enzymes, the possibility of drug interactions with other agents metabolized by the same isoform must be considered.

### Adverse events

Life-threatening cutaneous reactions and hepatotoxicity have been reported, usually during the first 8 weeks of treatment, and they are part of a hypersensitivity reaction that is characterized by fever, rash, arthralgias, and myalgias. Liver transaminases should be monitored closely, especially in the first 8 weeks. A maculopapular rash is seen in about 15 to 30% of users, and 7% will require discontinuation of the drug. NNRTIs should be discontinued if a severe rash occurs, or if the patient develops a rash accompanied by fever, blisters, mucous membrane involvement, conjunctivitis, or edema. Stevens-Johnson syndrome has been reported.

Hepatotoxicity occurring in the first 8 weeks of treatment is usually part of a hypersensitivity reaction and may be accompanied by rash, eosinophilia, and systemic features. It is more common in Black women and in those with higher CD4 cell counts. Overall increases in liver transaminases are seen in 5 to 20% of patients and are more common in those with chronic hepatitis B or C infection. They are also more common in women with CD4 counts >400/mm$^3$, for whom there is a warning in the product monograph.

### Clinical uses

In addition to the general indications for NNRTI use listed above, nevirapine has been used in protocols to prevent maternal–fetal transmission of HIV in the developing world. Given its prolonged half-life and pharmacokinetics in pregnancy (half-life increased to 66 hours), clinical studies have been conducted on the use of a single 200-mg oral dose to the mother at the onset of labour, plus a single dose of 2 mg/kg to the infant within 72 hours of birth. Although this decreases the risk of transmission to about 10 to 15%, drug resistance emerges in the women, some offspring are nevertheless infected with HIV, and the impact of the treatment protocol is diminished by breastfeeding.

## Delavirdine (Rescriptor)

### Pharmacokinetics

This agent is given orally as four 100-mg tablets three times daily. Absorption is 85% and is unaffected by food, but it is decreased by antacids, achlorhydria, or simultaneous administration of buffered ddI. The half-life of delavirdine is 5.8 hours. The drug is metabolized primarily by cytochrome P450 enzymes. It also inhibits CYP3A4, thus inhibiting its own metabolism, as well as that of other agents.

### Adverse events

Rash is noted in about 18% of cases, but it is usually self-limited and requires drug discontinuation in only about 4% of patients. Hepatotoxicity is less frequent and less severe than with nevirapine or efavirenz.

### Clinical use

In view of the similarity of efficacy of delavirdine to that of the other drugs in this class, the occurrence of complete cross-resistance, and the large number of pills that must be taken, delavirdine has largely been replaced by efavirenz and nevirapine.

## HIV PROTEASE INHIBITORS

This class of antiretroviral drugs has potent activity against HIV. The major enzymatic and structural proteins of the virus are synthesized as a polyprotein that must be cleaved into the individual proteins by a viral aspartic protease that is essential for the release of infectious virus. The protease inhibitors are selective inhibitors of this enzyme.

## Class-Specific Adverse Events

Lipodystrophy is a syndrome characterized by body fat redistribution and metabolic abnormalities. There is a peripheral loss of subcutaneous fat in the face and limbs, and accumulation of fat in the abdominal cavity, upper back, and breasts. Associated metabolic changes include elevations of blood triglycerides and cholesterol, increased fasting glucose level, and insulin resistance. The syndrome is reported in 20 to 80% of patients receiving antiretroviral therapy. Fat accumulation is more closely linked to the use of protease inhibitors, whereas lipoatrophy is more likely to occur with the nucleoside analogues. However, the exact cause and mechanism of the syndrome remain uncertain. Insulin resistance occurs in 30 to 90% of patients treated with protease inhibitors, and 1 to 10% develop overt diabetes. These changes start to occur usually within the first few months of therapy. Significant increases in triglycerides and cholesterol have been noted with HAART based on protease inhibitors (except atazanavir), but they are also observed in HAART based on efavirenz. There is concern that these changes may lead to increased cardiovascular risk in affected patients.

## Resistance

Resistance is a consequence of mutations in the gene for the HIV protease enzyme. Although there are unique "signature mutations" associated with the individual agents, a significant degree of cross-resistance occurs.

## Clinical Use

The protease inhibitors are combined with the NNRTIs as part of initial antiretroviral therapy. They are also combined with all other classes of antiretroviral agents as part of second- or third-line antiretroviral therapy in patients who have developed resistance. Given the low serum concentrations attained with most protease inhibitors, and their short half-lives, they are now frequently "boosted" with low-dose ritonavir. Ritonavir blocks the cytochrome P450 enzyme that metabolizes the protease inhibitors, thus increasing their concentrations over the dosing interval, increasing the half-life, decreasing the total daily dose required, and often increasing the dosing interval. Ritonavir boosting is used with saquinavir, indinavir, amprenavir, lopinavir, tipranavir, and atazanavir. The risk is that the lipid abnormalities are most closely linked with the use of ritonavir and are dose-dependent.

## Saquinavir (Invirase)

### Pharmacokinetics

This compound (see Fig. 55-3) has a low oral bioavailability of about 4% due to a combination of incomplete absorption (30%) and extensive first-pass metabolism. The extent of absorption is substantially increased following food. A gel capsule with increased bioavailability (Fortovase) is also available and is the formulation of choice if used without ritonavir boosting. In this setting, it is given at a dosage of 1200 mg (six 200-mg capsules) three times daily. The half-life of the drug is 1.1 to 1.9 hours. Protein binding is approximately 98%, and therefore, CSF penetration is low. There is extensive hepatic clearance, but only 4% is cleared by the kidney. Invirase is now re-emerging as the preferred formulation because of the favourable pharmacokinetics when combined with ritonavir and better gastrointestinal tolerability. The preferred dosage is 1000 mg of saquinavir plus 100 mg of ritonavir twice daily. A 500-mg film-coated tablet is now approved in many countries.

### Drug interactions

Saquinavir is metabolized by CYP3A4. Drugs that inhibit this isoenzyme (such as ketoconazole) cause an increase in the plasma concentrations of saquinavir. In contrast, drugs that induce the CYP3A4 isoenzyme (such as rifampin) can significantly decrease saquinavir plasma concentrations by up to 80%. Saquinavir itself can inhibit the biotransformation of other drug substrates of CYP3A4, such as the antihistamines terfenadine and astemizole (see Chapter 30).

### Adverse reactions

The majority of adverse reactions are mild. The most frequently reported reactions involve the gastrointestinal tract. They include diarrhea, abdominal discomfort, and nausea.

## Ritonavir (Norvir)

### Pharmacokinetics

The oral bioavailability of this drug is approximately 60 to 80%, and the half-life is 3 to 5 hours. These two factors allow for twice-daily dosing schedules. The drug is available in either 100-mg capsule or liquid formulation. Ritonavir is 99% protein-bound and does not penetrate well into the CNS. The drug induces its own metabolism, so plasma levels (and adverse events) are greatest during the first few days of treatment. To decrease the toxic effects, the drug dose is initially low (300 mg twice daily) and is increased gradually to 600 mg twice daily.

### Drug interactions

Ritonavir is metabolized by cytochrome P450 isoenzymes and therefore interacts with other medications that either inhibit or induce these isoenzymes. It is the most potent inhibitor of cytochrome P450 CYP3A4, and therefore, drug interactions are common and significant with other medications metabolized by this pathway. Amiodarone, astemizole, terfenadine, cisapride, lovastatin, simvastatin, midazolam, triazolam, ergot alkaloids, propafenone, quinidine, and St. John's wort are therefore contraindicated in patients receiving ritonavir.

### Adverse events

Adverse events are very common (85 to 100% of patients), especially during the first weeks of treatment, and include nausea, vomiting, diarrhea, headaches, asthenia, circumoral paresthesia, and increased plasma transaminase levels. In view of the problems with tolerability, the drug is rarely used as a single protease inhibitor; its use is largely restricted to "boosting" other protease inhibitors that are better tolerated.

## Indinavir (Crixivan)

### Pharmacokinetics

Indinavir (see Fig. 55-3) is well absorbed orally and is administered at a dose of 800 mg (two 400-mg tablets) three times daily, on an empty stomach. When it is boosted with ritonavir, the dose is reduced to 800 mg indinavir plus 100 mg ritonavir twice daily. Absorption can be reduced to 78% when the drug is administered with a standard meal high in calories, fat, and protein. It has a relatively short half-life of 1.8 hours. It is approximately 60% protein-bound. Less than 20% of indinavir is excreted in the urine. Patients should drink more than 1.4 L (48 ounces) of fluids daily to prevent indinavir-associated renal calculi.

## Adverse reactions

Indinavir is usually well tolerated. Nephrolithiasis has been reported in 4% of patients receiving this drug, but the frequency increases to 10% when indinavir is boosted with ritonavir. In general, these stones are not associated with renal dysfunction and resolve with hydration and temporary interruption of therapy. Asymptomatic elevation of the indirect bilirubin level is found in about 10 to 15% of patients. In less than 1%, this is associated with elevations of ALT or aspartate transaminase (AST). A number of patients develop rash, dry skin, taste disturbances, and paronychia. Indinavir should not be administered concurrently with terfenadine, triazolam, cisapride, astemizole, midazolam, or other substrates of CYP3A4. Less common adverse events include headache, nausea, diarrhea, and metallic taste.

## Nelfinavir (Viracept)

### Pharmacokinetics

This agent is administered orally at a dose of 1250 mg (two 650-mg tablets) twice daily with food. Absorption with meals varies from 20 to 80%; fatty meals increase absorption significantly. The half-life is 3.5 to 5 hours. The drug is metabolized by CYP3A4. Only 1 to 2% appears in the urine, but up to 90% appears in the feces, primarily as the hydroxylated metabolite designated M8, which also has anti-HIV activity.

### Adverse events

Nelfinavir is usually well tolerated. About 10 to 30% of patients report diarrhea or loose stools, which is rarely dose-limiting but can interfere with quality of life. Elevations of liver transaminases are reported in about 4 to 5% of patients, usually less than with other protease inhibitors.

## Amprenavir (Agenerase)

### Pharmacokinetics

This drug is given by mouth at a dose of 1200 mg (eight 150-mg capsules) twice daily, with or without food. When it is boosted with ritonavir, the dosage is either 600 mg amprenavir/100 mg ritonavir twice daily or 1200 mg amprenavir/200 mg ritonavir once daily. The bioavailability is estimated at 89%, but high-fat meals can decrease the AUC by 20%. The half-life is 7.1 to 10.6 hours. It is metabolized in the liver, and most of the administered dose appears in the feces. A prodrug, **fosamprenavir** (Telzir) decreases the required drug burden to 700 mg with 100 mg ritonavir twice daily.

### Adverse events

The major side effects are nausea, vomiting, diarrhea, rash, and headache. The large capsule size and drug burden can compromise adherence. The capsules contain large amounts of vitamin E, so further supplementation is to be avoided. Inhibition of CYP3A4 by amprenavir is less than that by ritonavir, indinavir, or nelfinavir, but drug interactions still need to be taken into consideration.

## Lopinavir/Ritonavir (Kaletra)

### Pharmacokinetics

This is the first co-formulated protease inhibitor. Three capsules, each containing 133 mg of lopinavir and 33 mg of ritonavir, are taken twice daily with food. A liquid formulation is also available. A new tablet formulation (200/50mg per tablet) is under review. Once-daily therapy with 800 mg lopinavir/200 mg ritonavir is now also approved. Bioavailability is about 48% on an empty stomach but increases to 80% with food. The mean lopinavir plasma concentrations are 15 to 20 times higher than after the same dose without ritonavir. The half-life is 5 to 6 hours. The drug is primarily metabolized by CYP3A4, and the drug also inhibits these enzymes. Less than 3% is excreted unchanged in the urine.

### Adverse events

The drug is generally well tolerated. The most common adverse reactions, leading to drug discontinuation in 2 to 4% of patients, are nausea and diarrhea. Increases in liver transaminases are noted in 10%. Drug precautions are the same as for ritonavir.

### Resistance

There is no known primary mutation that confers resistance, and, to date, no patient in whom a first-line therapy containing lopinavir/ritonavir has failed has demonstrated resistance to protease inhibitors. In experienced patients, resistance usually results from multiple resistance mutations.

## Atazanavir

### Pharmacokinetics

Atazanavir specifically inhibits HIV protease. It is formulated as a bisulfate salt that ranges from very to freely soluble in organic solvents, but only slightly soluble in water. It is administered once daily in a dose of 400 mg (300 mg if boosted with ritonavir) and is rapidly absorbed. It undergoes biliary secretion, the kidney playing only a minor role in its elimination. The half-life of atazanavir is 6.4 hours, increasing to 12 hours in those with impaired hepatic function. CYP3A4 is the major enzyme responsible for its metabolism, and the possibility of drug interactions needs to be considered when concomitant medications are used. Its absorption is impaired by tenofovir, and the two should not be used together unless the atazanavir is boosted by ritonavir. Concomitant administration of efavirenz decreases the AUC for atazanavir by 75%.

### Adverse events

The most commonly reported side effects include nausea, diarrhea, abdominal pain, and dizziness. Approximately 20% of subjects develop increased levels of unconjugated bilirubin and/or clinical jaundice, but this is typically not associated with increases in liver transaminases. Unlike other protease inhibitors, atazanavir has not been associated with clinically important changes in blood lipids.

## Tipranavir

This is the newest of the HIV protease inhibitors. It is a sulfonamide-containing dihydropyrone that binds strongly and selectively to the active site of the HIV-1 protease. Tipranavir is metabolized by CYP3A4 and it also induces this enzyme. It must be given boosted with ritonavir, in a combination (TPV/R) containing 500 mg/200 mg, twice daily.

### Pharmacokinetics

The median $C_{min}$ is 29–32 µmol/L, which is well above the 90% inhibitory concentration (0.16 µmol/L) for a susceptible strain of HIV. The absorption of tipranavir increases when it is given with food. It is excreted mainly in the feces. The median elimination half-life is 4 hours. The TPV/R combination inhibits CYP3A and induces P-glycoprotein, thus leading to the potential for many drug interactions.

### Adverse events

The most common adverse events are gastrointestinal upset (nausea and vomiting), occurring in about 10% of patients, and increases in liver transaminases (in about 6% of patients) and triglycerides (in about 20% of patients).

### Clinical use

Tipranavir has recently been approved as part of combination antiretroviral therapy for adults with high degrees of treatment experience or who have multiple protease inhibitor–resistant viruses. Two large controlled trials have demonstrated efficacy in this population.

## FUSION INHIBITORS

The newest class of antiretroviral drugs is the fusion inhibitors, which interfere with the entry of HIV into the CD4 lymphocytes. The only member of the class licensed so far is enfuvirtide, which interferes with viral entry mediated by the viral transmembrane glycoprotein gp41. Other compounds in development act at the site of the co-receptors, the chemokines.

## Enfuvirtide (T20) (Fuzeon)

### Mechanism of action

Enfuvirtide is derived from a naturally occurring sequence, amino acid residues 643 to 678 within the gp41 of HIV. It interferes with the entry of HIV into cells by inhibiting the fusion of the viral and cellular membranes. Enfuvirtide binds to the first heptad repeat (HR1) in the gp41 subunit of the viral envelope glycoprotein and prevents the conformational changes required for the membrane fusion.

### Pharmacokinetics

The drug is administered as a subcutaneous injection twice daily. A single 90-mg dose resulted in a mean $C_{max}$ of 4.6 µg/mL and an AUC of 55.8 µg·hr/mL, with an absolute bioavailability of 84%. Absorption from the subcutaneous injection site is comparable for abdominal, thigh, or arm sites. The steady-state trough concentration in plasma ranges from 2.6 to 3.4 µg/mL. As a peptide, enfuvirtide is expected to undergo catabolism to its constituent amino acids. The mean elimination half-life is 3.8 hours.

### Clinical use

Enfuvirtide is used in combination with other antiretroviral agents as salvage therapy, that is, in the management of treatment-experienced patients who present evidence of HIV replication despite ongoing therapy.

### Adverse events

Hypersensitivity reactions to enfuvirtide have developed during therapy and may occur upon re-challenge with the drug. These reactions have included rash, fever, nausea and vomiting, chills, rigor, hypotension, and increased liver transaminase levels in plasma. An increased incidence of bacterial pneumonia was observed in patients treated in clinical trials, but the exact relationship to the use of the drug is unclear. Local injection site infections were the most common adverse events (98%). Manifestations include pain and discomfort, induration, erythema, nodules and cysts, pruritus, and ecchymoses. Analgesics are required in approximately 10% of cases.

## MEDIATORS OF IMMUNE RESPONSE

Some viral infections can be treated by modification of the body's natural immune responses. The organization and functions of the immune system are described in detail in Chapter 40. Readers who are not familiar with this topic are advised to review Chapter 40 before reading the following sections.

## Interferon (IFN)

The interferons are a family of **host range–specific** glycoproteins (e.g., bovine IFN is not cross-protective for humans). These agents have become recognized as potent cytokines that are associated with complex antiviral, immunomodulatory, and anti-proliferative activity. They are synthesized by host cells in response to various inducers. The human interferons are divided into three classes:

1. **Leukocyte IFN (IFN-α;** Alferon, Intron, Roferon, Wellferon) is produced when null lymphocytes, B lymphocytes, and macrophages are stimulated by viruses, bacteria, foreign cells, and mitogens for B lymphocytes.
2. **Fibroblast IFN (IFN-β)** is produced in fibroblasts, epithelial cells, myeloblasts, lymphoblasts, and T lymphocytes when stimulated by viruses, polynucleotides, and inhibitors of RNA and protein synthesis.
3. **Immune IFN (IFN-γ;** Actimmune) is produced in T lymphocytes when stimulated by foreign antigens, mitogens for T lymphocytes, galactose oxidase, and calcium ionophores.

More recently, interferons have been produced by means of recombinant DNA technology, thereby providing adequate quantities of pure interferon for clinical trials.

The interferons have a range of biological and biochemical effects, including the following:

- Antiviral action
- Immunoregulatory action
- Anti-tumour action
- Cell growth inhibition
- Macrophage activation
- Enhancement of cytotoxicity of lymphocytes
- Induction of new cellular proteins
- Alteration of initiation factor eIF-2
- Induction of 2,5-oligoadenylic synthetase and activation of endonuclease activated by 2′,5′-oligoadenylic acid

The interferon system is the earliest appearing host defence against viral infection, coming into operation within a few hours of infection. As the viral infection subsides and the titre of virus declines, there is a corresponding drop in the level of interferon. Several other lines of evidence strongly suggest a causal relationship between the interferon system and natural recovery from many viral infections of humans and animals. In addition, there is increasing evidence that interferon may inhibit the growth of some tumours. Numerous trials are currently being carried out to determine the effects of the various interferons in the treatment of a variety of neoplasms, and as immunosuppressants.

## Mechanisms of action

Interferons can be induced by active and inactive viruses, double-stranded RNA, and a number of other compounds. They tend to be species-specific.

A wide range of viruses are sensitive to the antiviral effects of interferon, although considerable differences exist for different viruses and assay systems. Interferons are not directly antiviral but cause biochemical changes in exposed cells that lead to resistance to viruses. Depending upon the virus and cell type, interferon antiviral effects are mediated through inhibition of viral penetration or uncoating, synthesis or processing of mRNA, translation of viral proteins, or viral assembly and release. For most viruses, the primary step inhibited by interferon is protein synthesis. The interferon produced is released into the extracellular fluid and binds to specific cell receptors. This initiates a series of events leading to the production of two enzymes, protein kinase and 2,5-oligoadenylate synthetase. Protein kinase inhibits the formation of the initiation complex for protein synthesis, and 2,5-oligoadenylate synthetase activates a cellular endonuclease that degrades viral mRNA. Consequently, viral protein synthesis is inhibited at two stages.

## Pharmacokinetics

The pharmacokinetics of interferons are not well characterized. Orally administered doses do not result in detectable serum levels and are not used clinically. After intramuscular or subcutaneous injection, plasma levels are dose-related. Doses of interferon given every 12 hours provide relatively steady serum levels. Maximum levels in blood following intramuscular injection are achieved in 5 to 8 hours. Interferon does not penetrate well into the CSF.

Peginterferon alpha-2a (Pegasys) and peginterferon alpha-2b (PegIntron) are interferons conjugated with polyethylene glycol (PEG), which decreases their clearance rate and results in sustained concentrations, permitting less frequent dosing. The side effect profiles of pegylated and non-pegylated interferons appear to be similar.

## Adverse reactions and toxicity

Both purified natural and recombinant interferons cause dose-related toxicity that limits their clinical use. A systemic dose of $1 \times 10^6$ IU/day is generally well tolerated, but with prolonged systemic administration, an influenza-like syndrome of fever, chills, headaches, myalgias, nausea, vomiting, and diarrhea frequently occurs. Major toxicities that limit parenteral use are bone marrow suppression, mental confusion, behavioural changes, fatigue, myalgias, and cardiotoxicity. Local reactions consist of tenderness and erythema at the injection site. Intranasal administration is associated with mucosal friability, ulceration, and dryness.

## Clinical use

Extensive testing has been done with various formulations and routes of administration to assess the possible value of interferons in the prevention and treatment of various viral infections. Clinical use has been limited by the lack of potency and the high incidence of adverse reactions.

Topical administration (i.e., nasal sprays) has been studied most extensively in the prophylaxis and treatment of rhinovirus infections. Although trials have shown some response, the clinical significance is debatable.

Condyloma acuminatum has responded to various interferon preparations administered topically, subcutaneously, or directly into the lesion. Efficacy has been demonstrated in patients in whom previous conventional therapies had failed, but side effects frequently preclude long-term use.

Chronic hepatitis B viral infections have shown responsiveness to the parenteral administration of recombinant IFN-$\alpha$, which is associated with a loss of DNA polymerase activity. This therapy has been largely replaced by lamivudine and tenofovir.

The primary use is in combination with ribavirin, in the treatment of compensated chronic hepatitis C. The recommended doses are peginterferon alpha-2a 180 $\mu$g subcutaneously every week and ribavirin 1000 to 1200 mg daily, or peginterferon alpha-2b 1.5 $\mu$g/kg subcutaneously every week and ribavirin 800 mg daily. In place of the pegylated interferons, standard interferon can be used at a dosage of $3 \times 10^6$ IU intramuscularly or subcutaneously, three times a week. Response rates are higher for viral genotypes 2 and 3 than for 1 and 4, and they are decreased in patients co-infected with HIV and in those with higher hepatitis C viral loads. Overall, about 50% of hepatitis C patients treated with this combination show an effective long-term response; the reason for poor response in the other 50% is not yet known.

## Aldara (Imiquimod)

This is an immune response modifier. In vitro, it induces the release of IFN-$\alpha$ and other cytokines from human monocytes or macrocytes, and from keratinocytes. It is used for the treatment of external genital and perianal warts (condyloma acumionatum). It is applied as a topical cream three times a week and is left on the skin for 6 to 10 hours. Percutaneous absorption is minimal.

Local skin reactions such as erythema, erosion, excoriation, and flaking are common. In the event of a severe skin reaction, the cream should be removed with soap and water. These reactions are more frequent and more intense with daily application and may require a rest period.

## SUGGESTED READINGS

Atkinson WL, Arden NH, Patriarca PA, et al. Amantadine during an institutional outbreak of type A (H1N1) influenza. *Arch Intern Med.* 1986;146:1751-1756.

Baker DA. Valacyclovir in the treatment of genital herpes and herpes zoster. *Expert Opin Pharmacother.* 2002;3:51-58.

Burdge DR, Money DM, Forbes JC, et al. The Canadian consensus guidelines for the management of pregnancy, labour and postpartum care in HIV-positive pregnancy women and their offspring. *CMAJ.* 2003;168:1671-1674.

Clive D, Corey L, Reichman RC, et al. A double blind, placebo-controlled cytogenetic study of oral acyclovir in patients with recurrent genital herpes. *J Infect Dis.* 1991;164:753-757.

Crumpacker CS. Ganciclovir. *N Engl J Med.* 1996;335:721-729.

Davis GL, Esteban-Mur R, Rustgi V, et al. Interferon alfa-2b alone or in combination with ribavirin for the treatment of relapse of chronic hepatitis C. International Hepatitis Interventional Therapy Group. *N Engl J Med.* 1998;339:1493-1499.

Elphick GF, Querbes W, Jordan JA, et al. The human polyomavirus, JCV, uses serotonin receptors to infect cells. *Science.* 2004;306:1380-1383.

Englund JA, Piedra PA, Jefferson LS, et al. High-dose, short-duration ribavirin aerosol therapy in children with suspected respiratory syncytial virus infection. *J Pediatr.* 1990;117:313-320.

Hayden FG, Osterhaus ADME, Treanor JJ, et al. Efficacy and safety of the neuraminidase inhibitor zanamivir in the treatment of influenza virus infections. *N Engl J Med.* 1997;337:874-880.

Hirsch MS, Brun-Vézinet F, Clotet B, et al. Antiretroviral drug resistance testing in adults infected with HIV-1: 2003 recommendations of an international AIDS Society USA panel. *Clin Infect Dis.* 2003;37:113-128.

HIV Lipodystrophy Case Definition Study Group. An objective case definition of lipodystrophy in HIV infected adults: a case control study. *Lancet.* 2003;361:726-735.

Jacobson MA, Drew WL, Feinberg J, et al. Foscarnet therapy for ganciclovir resistance in the treatment of cytomegalovirus retinitis in patients with AIDS. *J Infect Dis.* 1991;163:1348-1351.

Lai CL, Chien RN, Leung N, et al. A one-year trial of lamivudine for chronic hepatitis B. *N Engl J Med.* 1998;339:61-68.

Lalezari J, Henry K, O'Hearn M, et al. Efficacy of enfuvirtide plus an optimized background of antiretrovirals in treatment experienced HIV-1 positive patients in North America and Brazil (TORO 1). *N Engl J Med.* 2003;348:2175-2185.

Lalezari J, Lindley J, Walmsley S, et al. A safety study of oral valganciclovir maintenance treatment of CMV retinitis. *J Acq Immun Def Synd.* 2002;30:392-400.

Lecellier CH, Dunoyer P, Arar K, et al. A cellular microRNA mediates antiviral defense in human cells. *Science.* 2005;308:557-560.

Martin D, Stempien MJ, Sierra-Madero J, et al. A controlled trial of valganciclovir as induction therapy for cytomegalovirus retinitis. *N Engl J Med.* 2002;346:1119-1126.

McHutchison JG, Gordon SC, Schiff ER, et al. Interferon alfa-2b alone or in combination with ribavirin as initial treatment for chronic hepatitis C. *N Engl J Med.* 1998;339:1485-1492.

Nicholson KG, Aoki FY, Osterhaus AD, et al. Efficacy and safety of oseltamivir in treatment of acute influenza: a randomized controlled trial. Neuraminidase Inhibitor Flu Treatment Investigator Group. *Lancet.* 2000;355:1845-1850.

Panel on Clinical Practices for Treatment of HIV Infection Convened by the Department of Health and Human Services (DHHS). *Guidelines for the Use of Antiretroviral Agents in HIV-1 Infected Adults and Adolescents.* Washington, DC: DHHS; 2003:1-78.

Rothbart HA, Webster AD, for the Pleconaril Treatment Registry Group. Treatment of potentially life-threatening enterovirus infections with pleconaril. *Clin Infect Dis.* 2001;32:228-235.

Sauder DN, Skinner RB, Fox TL, et al. Topical imiquimod 5% cream as an effective treatment for external genital and peri-anal warts in different patient populations. *Sex Transm Dis.* 2003;30:124-128.

Simmons A. Clinical manifestations and treatment considerations of herpes simplex virus infections. *J Infect Dis.* 2002;182(suppl 1):S71-S77.

Smith AE, Helenius A. How viruses enter animal cells. *Science.* 2004;304:237-242.

Walmsley S, Bernstein B, King M, et al. Lopinavir-ritonavir versus nelfinavir for the initial treatment of HIV infection. *N Engl J Med.* 2002;346:2039-2046.

# Antiseptics, Disinfectants, and Sterilization

## S LIM, K IVERSON, AND MA GARDAM

### CASE HISTORY

Mr. X is a 53-year-old man in good health. His father died at 57 years of age from colon cancer. On the advice of his family doctor, Mr. X had a screening colonoscopy performed for early detection of cancer, in view of his family history. He had no gastrointestinal symptoms upon entering the hospital for this procedure, and the colonoscopy itself was performed with no immediate complications. The following day, however, Mr. X developed fever, abdominal cramping, and bloody diarrhea. Laboratory testing of his stool samples revealed *Salmonella enterica* serotype Typhimurium. The gastroenterologist who performed the procedure became very concerned upon learning this result, as he knew that another patient who had a colonoscopy performed several hours prior to Mr. X was suffering from *Salmonella* diarrhea at the time of the procedure. Microbiological sampling from the implicated colonoscope used on both patients confirmed the presence of *Salmonella*. Further investigation revealed that the colonoscope had been cleaned with an enzymatic cleaner, but rather than undergoing high-level disinfection with glutaraldehyde as an intended second step, the scope was washed a second time with enzymatic cleaner only. Improper disinfection of the colonoscope was implicated as the cause of *Salmonella* transmission from patient to patient.

## HISTORY AND INTRODUCTION

Hospital-acquired infections were first recognized in the 1840s by the observations of Oliver Wendell Holmes and Ignaz Semmelweis. These individuals independently hypothesized that the high rates of maternal infections and mortality observed on obstetrical units were related to infectious agents passed on to pregnant women by the unwashed hands of physicians. Semmelweis ordered physicians to wash their hands with a chlorinated solution before examining their patients, and this subsequently reduced the mortality rate from about 12% to less than 2%. Following this, Louis Pasteur's landmark formulation of the germ theory of disease led Joseph Lister to use the antiseptic phenol to disinfect wounds and surgical instruments in his hospital, allowing his wards to remain clear of sepsis for 9 months.

These concepts remained unpopular and were met with indifference and even hostility until shortly before the 1900s, when appreciation of the roles of microorganisms in the transmission of infectious diseases and acceptance of aseptic surgical technique finally took hold. It is now recognized that approximately 5 to 10% of adults admitted to hospital acquire an infection that was neither present nor incubating prior to admission and that is, by definition, considered a nosocomial infection (from the Latin *nosocomium,* meaning hospital). Prevention of nosocomial infections depends on a number of factors, including the effective use of antiseptics, disinfectants, and sterilization procedures, along with other infection control measures to limit transmission of infection to patients and healthcare workers.

This chapter is divided into two major sections with respect to the prevention and control of nosocomial infections within the healthcare setting. The first, "Handwashing and Antisepsis," addresses the issue of preventing secondary disease transmission from the contaminated hands of healthcare workers or environmental surfaces to patients. "Cleaning, Sterilization and Disinfection" focuses on the role of cleaning and decontamination of reusable patient-care equipment.

## HANDWASHING AND ANTISEPSIS

The surface flora of human skin consist of "normal" resident microorganisms (colonizers) but, on occasion, can include transient contaminating microorganisms. Normal resident organisms, such as coagulase-negative staphylococci and *Corynebacterium* species, do not usually cause complicated nosocomial skin infections in patients with normal immune systems, but they may be implicated in minor infections if introduced into body tissues by trauma or by medical devices such as intravenous catheters. Transient microorganisms on the skin acquired from contaminated environments, equipment, or hands pose a more serious problem as these microorganisms are more frequently implicated as the source of nosocomial infections. The most common transient flora acquired in hospitals includes *Staphylococcus aureus* and Gram-negative coliforms such as *Escherichia coli*.

It is well recognized that hand carriage of bacteria is an important route of transmission of infection between healthcare workers and patients. It is estimated that at least one-third of all nosocomial infections are preventable, with a significant proportion of these due to cross-contamination and transmission of microorganisms by the hands of healthcare workers. Handwashing is considered the single most important intervention for preventing infections, with multiple studies demonstrating that appropriate handwashing results in a decreased incidence of nosocomial infections. This being said, motivating healthcare workers to wash their hands appropriately has been shown to be surprisingly difficult, and improvements in compliance are often not sustainable.

Handwashing limits the transmission of microorganisms by removing soil, organic material, and transient microorganisms from the skin. The different classes of agents for handwashing are defined below, while Table 56-1 provides further details.

## Detergents

These are cleansing agents that have no antimicrobial activity (e.g., soap).

## Antiseptic Agents

Antiseptics are substances that inhibit the growth of or destroy microorganisms. Antiseptics are used on living skin or mucous membranes, in contrast to disinfectants, which are used on inanimate objects. Table 56-2 lists the common antiseptic agents used in hospitals. Waterless hand scrubs are one form of antiseptic agent.

### Waterless hand scrubs

Barriers to handwashing among healthcare workers are numerous and include the time required, the inconvenience of finding a washbasin, and general disruption of busy workflow. One possible solution has been the introduction of alcohol-based hand washes for skin antisepsis. The alcohol in these preparations rapidly reduces microbial counts on the skin, and a 1-minute vigorous hand rub with enough of the preparation has been shown to be as effective as traditional soap and water for handwashing. Advantages to these products include their efficacy, which includes both immediate and delayed antimicrobial action, absence of the need for a sink and running water; and the convenience of pump-dispensed bottles of the hand wash placed outside patient rooms and throughout patient care areas. The major disadvantage is the drying effect of alcohol on the skin with repeated use;

| TABLE 56-1 | Agents for Handwashing | |
|---|---|---|
| **Product** | **Indications** | **Comments** |
| Plain soap (bar, liquid, granules) | • For routine care of patients<br>• For washing hands soiled with dirt, blood, or other organic material | • May contain very low concentrations of antimicrobial agents to prevent microbial contamination growth in the product |
| Waterless hand scrubs (rinses, foams, wipes, towelettes) | • Equivalent alternative to conventional soap<br>• Advantageous where handwashing facilities are inadequate, impractical, or inaccessible | • Not effective if hands are soiled with dirt or heavily contaminated with blood or other organic material<br>• Efficacy dependent upon alcohol concentration in product |
| Antiseptic agents | May be preferable for the following:<br>• Heavy microbial soiling<br>• Prior to performing invasive procedures<br>• Before contact with patients who have immune deficiencies, non-intact skin, or percutaneous implanted devices<br>• Before and after direct contact with patients who harbour antimicrobial-resistant organisms<br>• Critical care areas<br>• Operating room scrub | • For situations/conditions where reduction in the number of resident flora is important and/or level of microbial contamination is high<br>• Agents differ in activity (see Table 56-2) |

**TABLE 56-2** Antiseptic Agents

| Group and Examples | Advantages | Disadvantages | Comments |
|---|---|---|---|
| Alcohols<br>• alcohol-based waterless hand scrubs<br>• ethanol<br>• n-propanol<br>• isopropanol | Good for hand antisepsis, with rapid attainment of maximum reduction of bacterial counts; continued antimicrobial activity persists after use; activity not affected by small amounts of blood | Drying effect; not recommended in the presence of physical dirt and other organic material; may be toxic (rare) | Optimum alcohol concentration 70–90%; good activity against both Gram-positive and -negative organisms, mycobacteria, and various fungi and viruses |
| Chlorhexidine gluconate (CHG)<br>• 2% aqueous + 70% isopropyl alcohol<br>• 4% detergent<br>• 0.5% aqueous + 70% isopropyl alcohol<br>• other preparations available +/− isopropyl alcohol | Recommended for handwashing and surgical site skin preparation; activity not affected by blood or organic material | Toxicity associated with direct inoculation into mucous membranes, middle ear, and eyes | Persistent activity of CHG for 6 hours; addition of CHG to alcohol-based preparations more effective than alcohol alone; good activity against Gram-positive organisms, less against Gram-negative and some viruses, and minimal against mycobacteria |
| Hexachlorophene<br>• 3% aqueous | Handwashing; persistent activity | Can be toxic; not recommended for surgical site preparation; limited antimicrobial activity; slow to intermediate rate of action | Bacteriostatic for Gram-positive cocci; little activity against all other microorganisms |
| Iodine compounds | Surgical site preparation; safe; fast-acting | Too irritating for handwashing | Staining; good activity against Gram-positive and Gram-negative organisms, mycobacteria, viruses, and fungi |
| Iodophors<br>• povidone-iodine (varying concentrations from 0.05 to 10%) | Handwashing and surgical site preparation | Neutralized in the presence of organic materials; skin irritation; can have allergic/toxic effects | |
| Para-chloro-meta-xylenol (PCMX)<br>• varying concentrations of 0.5 to 3.75% | Hand washing; intermediate rate of action; persistent effect over few hours; activity minimally affected by organic matter | Neutralized by non-ionic surfactants | Good activity against Gram-positive organisms, less against Gram-negatives |
| Triclosan<br>• varying concentrations from 0.3 to 2% | Intermediate rate of action; excellent persistent activity; minimally affected by organic material | | Good activity against Gram-positive organisms and most Gram-negatives (but bacteriostatic); persistent activity on skin |

however, this can be ameliorated with skin lotion and other emollients.

Traditional handwashing, using friction generated by rubbing the hands together, along with an adequate amount of soap (detergent), followed by rinsing under running water and drying, removes most transient bacteria on hands. While several studies have not been able to demonstrate a significant decrease in infection rates with use of an antiseptic agent compared with soap for routine handwashing in the healthcare setting, some studies have suggested that antiseptic agents may be preferred in certain situations. These include (1) areas of the hospital that are at high risk of having antimicrobial-resistant organisms present, such as critical care settings, (2) the presence of known antimicrobial-resistant organisms, and (3) conditions of heavy microbial soiling.

## Selection of an antiseptic agent

If the decision is made to choose an antiseptic agent over a detergent, selection of an antiseptic agent is a three-step process. First, one must determine what agent characteristics are important for that particular use and setting (i.e., absence of absorption across skin or mucous membranes, persistence, rapid reduction in flora, spectrum of activity). Next, efficacy and safety evidence should be objectively evaluated. The final step is a consideration of workplace acceptance and use of the product (which will determine compliance) and cost issues.

## Handwashing Technique

Handwashing must be performed correctly to effectively reduce microbial counts. This involves first wetting the hands with water, applying enough of the product, rubbing hands together vigorously for at least 15 seconds to cover all surfaces of the hands and fingers, rinsing, and thorough drying. The faucets should be turned off with a towel to avoid re-contaminating the hands. Washing for 15 seconds reduces bacterial counts by 0.6 to 1.1 $log_{10}$, whereas washing for 30 seconds reduces counts by 1.8 to 2.8 $log_{10}$. The frequency of handwashing by the healthcare worker obviously depends upon a number of factors, including the type and duration of activity with the patient, the degree of contamination involved with the contact, and the patient's susceptibility to infection. However, Health Canada's recommendations for handwashing include the following:

1. Between direct contact with individual patients/residents/clients
2. Before performing invasive procedures
3. Before caring for patients in intensive care units and immunocompromised patients
4. Before preparing, handling, serving, or eating food, and before feeding a patient
5. When hands are visibly soiled
6. After situations or procedures in which microbial or blood contamination of hands is likely
7. After removing gloves
8. After personal body function, such as using the toilet or blowing one's nose

Despite guidelines from multiple international infection control organizations that have repeatedly emphasized the importance and significance of handwashing, compliance by healthcare workers remains poor. This is a complicated and multifactorial problem, including lack of motivation and inadequate understanding of the role of cross-transmission of infection by contaminated hands, and real or perceived obstacles such as inconveniently located handwashing basins, disruption of workflow, and dermatitis caused or aggravated by repeated handwashing. Strategies to improve handwashing include education, accessible and conveniently located handwashing facilities, and waterless antiseptic agents and other acceptable handwashing products.

## CLEANING, STERILIZATION, AND DISINFECTION

Cleaning, sterilization, and disinfection of certain types of medical equipment are essential to ensure that patient-care equipment does not transmit infectious pathogens from patient to patient. In the past, appropriate cleaning, disinfection, and sterilization procedures within the healthcare environment were primarily of interest to those involved in infection control. However, infectious complications and outbreaks related to improper cleaning and/or decontamination of reusable patient-care equipment have stirred both public and legal interest. Similarly, prion diseases such as Creutzfeldt-Jakob disease have also raised questions regarding the elimination of agents that exhibit resistance to conventional chemical and physical decontamination methods. There has been a gradual increase in public awareness of cleaning practices within healthcare settings, followed justifiably by a demand that hospitals and healthcare centres be held accountable for the safety of patients undergoing medical procedures that involve reusable equipment. It is now considered not only standard but overall good practice for all individuals involved in delivering patient care to have a general understanding of the principles of proper cleaning and decontamination within the workplace.

Numerous agents with different mechanisms of action can be used for cleaning, disinfection, and sterilization in the healthcare setting (Table 56-3).

**Cleaning** is the single most important step in making a medical device safe for handling. This is defined as the physical removal of foreign material (e.g., dust, soil, microorganisms, and organic material such as blood, secretions, and excretions), usually through wiping and/or using water with detergents or enzymatic products. Cleaning in itself does not kill microorganisms; however, reducing the microbial bioburden is an essential step prior to any subsequent processing, since both inorganic and organic materials that are not physically removed from the equipment's surfaces interfere with the subsequent disinfection processes.

Studies demonstrate that appropriate cleaning of flexible endoscopes can reduce bioburden by 4 $log_{10}$ units (i.e., to 0.0001 of the original value, or a 99.99% reduction). An item that has not been cleaned cannot be assuredly disinfected or sterilized. Unless the item can be cleaned immediately, it should be submerged in water and/or detergent to prevent organic matter from drying onto the surface, since this makes removal more difficult and again affects the subsequent disinfection or sterilization process. In addition, complete disassembly of each item is required, which can often be difficult for intricate devices with multiple components. The friction generated with either manual cleaning (scrubbing with a brush) or

| TABLE 56-3 | Susceptibility of Microorganisms to Chemical Disinfectants and the Level of Decontamination Achieved | |
| --- | --- | --- |
| Susceptibility | Microorganism | Level of Decontamination |
| Least susceptible | Prions | Disposal of instrument |
| | Bacterial spores (*Bacillus subtilis, Clostridium tetani, difficile,* and *botulinum*) Protozoa with cysts (*Giardia lamblia, Cryptosporidium parvum*) | Sterilization |
| | Mycobacteria (*Mycobacterium tuberculosis, Mycobacterium avium* complex) | High- or intermediate-level disinfection |
| | Non-enveloped viruses (coxsackieviruses, polioviruses, rhinoviruses, rotaviruses, noroviruses, hepatitis A virus) | Intermediate-level disinfection |
| | Fungi (*Candida, Cryptococcus,* and *Aspergillus* species, dermatophytes) | Low-level disinfection |
| Most susceptible | Vegetative bacteria (*Staphylococcus aureus, Pseudomonas aeruginosa,* coliforms) Enveloped viruses (human immunodeficiency virus, hepatitis B and C viruses, herpes simplex, influenza virus) | Low-level disinfection |

the use of a mechanical unit (ultrasonic cleaner, or combined washer-decontaminator or washer-sterilizer systems) is the key component of this process.

**Detergent solutions** or **enzymatic cleansers** are used to remove soil, with the latter also able to inactivate the proteinaceous enzymes in organic material. These agents must be compatible with the material undergoing cleaning in order to maintain equipment integrity. Following cleaning with detergents or enzymatic cleansers, rinsing with distilled or deionized water is required to remove both the organic material and detergent from the item, which could interfere with the subsequent disinfectant. Adequate rinsing of enzymatic cleaners is particularly important because these agents typically contain proteinaceous material, which can cause severe reactions in patients when the device is used. The final step involves drying the item as bacterial biofilms may form on surfaces left moist.

Unlike the quality assurance indicators available to validate sterilization (see later section on "Sterilization"), there is no practical way to confirm that adequate cleaning has been achieved.

**Sterilization** is the destruction and complete elimination of all forms of microbial life, including bacteria, viruses, spores, and fungi. In hospitals, this is achieved by either physical (steam under pressure, dry heat) or chemical (ethylene oxide gas, hydrogen peroxide gas plasma, peracetic acid) processes.

**Disinfection** is the elimination of many disease-producing microorganisms, with the exception of bacterial spores. Disinfectants are used on inanimate objects, as distinct from antiseptics, which are used on living tissue. In the healthcare setting, disinfection is accomplished through the use of liquid chemicals, wet pasteurization, or ultraviolet radiation. Disinfection can be divided into three levels—high, intermediate, and low—based on the type of microorganisms eliminated:

- **High-level disinfection** destroys vegetative bacteria, fungi, mycobacteria, enveloped and non-enveloped viruses, and some but not all bacterial spores.
- **Intermediate-level disinfection** destroys vegetative bacteria, mycobacteria, most fungi and enveloped viruses, and some non-enveloped viruses, but not bacterial spores.
- **Low-level disinfection** destroys most vegetative bacteria and some fungi and enveloped viruses. Most non-enveloped viruses, mycobacteria, and bacterial spores are not eliminated.

It should be kept in mind that many factors affect these categories. For example, high-level disinfectants are capable of sterilization when the contact or exposure time is prolonged. Similarly, concentration of the agent, temperature, pH, the extent of soilage, and nature of the microorganism bioburden all play a role in the level of disinfection achieved. See Table 56-4 for factors affecting the efficacy of disinfection and sterilization.

From a patient risk perspective, preferably all patient-care equipment would be single-use and discarded. In reality, however, not only is it unnecessary to sterilize all patient-care equipment and items, but rising healthcare costs and environmental concerns make this option next to impossible. Although cleaning alone often does not make an item safe for patient use, it is self-evident that the degree of disinfection required for neurosurgical instruments is greater than that of a blood pressure cuff that touches a patient's intact skin.

In the 1970s, Earle H. Spaulding developed an approach to disinfection and sterilization of patient-care equipment based upon the intended use of the item. His system classifies the cleaning, disinfection, and sterilization requirements for equipment into three categories based on the risk of infection involved in the use of the items. These

| TABLE 56-4 | Factors Affecting the Efficacy of Disinfection and Sterilization |
| --- | --- |
| **Factor** | **Effect** |
| Microorganism number (bioburden) | The larger the number of organisms, the longer it takes to destroy them all; cleaning helps to reduce the number prior to disinfection or sterilization. |
| Microorganism type | Spores are the most resistant form of pathogen; they are used as test organisms for FDA clearance to obtain a large safety margin, although most contaminating microorganisms on medical devices are vegetative bacteria. |
| Microorganism location | Surfaces must be in direct contact with the disinfectant/sterilant; equipment with multiple pieces, crevices, joints, and other difficult-to-access components requires prolonged exposure time (see "Duration of exposure" at bottom of table). Equipment with longer lumen lengths and smaller diameters has similar requirements. |
| Organic and inorganic matter | Persistent bioburden, inorganic, and organic matter reduce disinfection efficacy through chemical reactions between the disinfectant and matter or by providing the microorganism with a physical barrier against direct contact with the disinfectant. |
| Biofilm | This impairs exposure of the microorganism to the disinfectant/sterilizing agent. |
| Concentration and potency of disinfectants | More concentrated disinfectants generally have greater efficacy and shorter time to microbial elimination; concentration has an effect on the length of disinfection time. |
| Physical and chemical factors | Increased temperature improves efficacy; pH is variable; humidity affects gaseous disinfectants like ethylene oxide; and increased water hardness reduces the rate of microbial elimination. |
| Duration of exposure | Longer contact time increases efficacy; the microorganism location needs to be considered (see above). |
| FDA = U.S. Food and Drug Administration. | |

categories (critical, semi-critical, and non-critical) form the basis of guidelines produced by Health Canada and the U.S. Centers for Disease Control and Prevention (CDC) for cleaning, disinfecting, and sterilizing patient-care equipment in healthcare institutions.

**Critical items** are those that have contact with sterile tissue, non-intact mucous membranes, or normally sterile body sites. There is a high risk of infection and disease transmission if such an item is contaminated with any type of microorganism, including bacterial spores. Therefore, these items must be sterile prior to use. Items in this category include surgical instruments, implantable devices (e.g., cardiac pacemakers), needles, and any devices used to biopsy tissue. Further examples, and the common products or methods used to achieve sterilization, are shown in Table 56-5. In general, items that can undergo steam sterilization are processed in this manner; if the item is heat-labile, it may be treated with ethylene oxide gas, hydrogen peroxide gas plasma, or peracetic acid.

**Semi-critical items** are those that come in contact with mucous membranes or non-intact skin but do not enter sterile sites. Although these items must be free of all microorganisms, small numbers of bacterial spores may be present without posing a risk to the patient. Examples include most flexible endoscopes, laryngoscopes, and ultrasound probes. These devices require high-level disinfection as a minimum, usually with chemical disinfec-

tants and occasionally through wet pasteurization (see Table 56-5).

**Non-critical items** are those that come in contact with intact skin, which is an effective barrier against most infectious organisms. Examples of non-critical items include bedpans, blood pressure cuffs, bed rails, and patient furniture. Although there is virtually no risk of transmitting infectious agents from patient to patient through non-critical items provided that they have been appropriately cleaned, these items can cause secondary transmission through healthcare workers who do not wash their hands after touching contaminated items.

Although the Spaulding scheme provides a useful and rational framework for cleaning, disinfection, and sterilization, logistical difficulties arise when this approach is implemented. For example, many medical devices that require sterilization are heat-labile, yet the lengthy time associated with ethylene oxide sterilization is impractical for routine use in between patients. Similarly, optimal contact time to achieve the required degree of disinfection can be difficult to determine, particularly with intricate medical devices with difficult-to-access surfaces.

## Sterilization

Sterilization is required for all critical items. One major disadvantage of biologic indicators of sterilization is a required incubation time of 24 hours. Table 56-6 outlines

| TABLE 56-5 | Common Processes, Products, and/or Methods for Processing Reusable Medical Equipment | | |
|---|---|---|---|
| Process* | Category | Examples | Products or Methods† |
| Sterilization | Critical items | • All items contacting sterile tissue<br>• Surgical instruments<br>• All implantable devices:<br>  – Needles and syringes<br>  – Cardiac and urinary catheters<br>  – All intravascular devices<br>• Biopsy equipment<br>• Bronchoscopes<br>• Arthroscopes<br>• Cystoscopes<br>• Acupuncture needles and body piercing objects<br>• Neurologic test needles<br>• All instruments used for foot care | • Steam<br>• Dry heat<br>• Ethylene oxide gas<br>• 2% glutaraldehyde<br>• Hydrogen peroxide gas plasma<br>• 6–25% hydrogen peroxide<br>• Peracetic acid<br>• Ortho-phthalaldehyde |
| High-level disinfection | Semi-critical items | • Flexible endoscopes<br>• Laryngoscopes<br>• Respiratory therapy equipment<br>• Anaesthesia equipment<br>• Endotracheal tubes<br>• Vaginal specula<br>• Vaginal probes used in sonographic scanning | • 2% glutaraldehyde<br>• 6% hydrogen peroxide<br>• Peracetic acid<br>• Chlorine or chlorine compounds (5.25% sodium hypochlorite [household bleach] diluted to 100 ppm chlorine)<br>• Ortho-phthalaldehyde<br>• Pasteurization |
| Intermediate-level disinfection | Some semi-critical items | • Glass thermometers<br>• Electronic thermometers<br>• Hydrotherapy tanks (non-intact patient skin) | • 70–90% ethyl or isopropyl alcohol<br>• Sodium hypochlorite<br>• Iodophors<br>• Phenolics (not for use in nurseries) |
| Cleaning +/– low-level disinfection | All reusable equipment | • All reusable equipment after patient use<br>• Bedpans, urinals, commodes<br>• Stethoscopes<br>• Blood pressure cuffs<br>• Ear specula | Cleaning:<br>• Detergents<br>• Enzymatic agents<br>Low-level disinfection:<br>• 70–90% ethyl or isopropyl alcohol<br>• Sodium hypochlorite<br>• Quaternary ammonium compounds<br>• Some iodophors<br>• 3% hydrogen peroxide |

*All processes must be preceded by cleaning.

†For products or methods that appear in two categories, the manufacturers' directions differ for length of exposure time and concentration.

the major methods of sterilization, along with their advantages and disadvantages. In broad categories, sterilization is achieved through either physical (steam under pressure, dry heat, radiation) or chemical (ethylene oxide gas, hydrogen peroxide gas plasma, peracetic acid, ozone) processes. To meet sterility standards as advocated by the Association for the Advancement of Medical Instrumentation, a 12 $\log_{10}$ reduction in microorganisms is required for surgical instruments and implantable devices.

In the past, medical and surgical instruments used in the healthcare setting were primarily made of materials that were heat stable, and thus steam sterilization was the traditional method employed. It is still the recommended sterilization process if items are heat resistant, such as sur-

gical devices made of stainless steel, as it has the largest margin of safety. However, endoscopes and other medical instruments made of plastics cannot tolerate the temperatures required to achieve steam sterilization, and, therefore, ethylene oxide gas has been used since the 1950s for heat- and moisture-sensitive items. Since that time, hydrogen peroxide gas plasma and peracetic acid immersion systems have been introduced, which are also low-temperature processes that offer certain advantages over ethylene oxide gas sterilization.

Other sterilization methods sometimes employed, including boiling, microwave ovens, and glass bead sterilizers, are not recommended by Health Canada as accepted sterilization methods.

| TABLE 56-6 | Commonly Used Sterilization Methods* | |
|---|---|---|
| **Sterilization Method** | **Advantages** | **Disadvantages** |
| Steam<br>• gravity displacement sterilizers<br>• vacuum sterilizers | • Non-toxic to humans and environment<br>• Simple to control and monitor cycles<br>• Rapid and efficient<br>• Least affected by organic/inorganic substances<br>• Penetrates medical packing, devices with lumens<br>• Can be used to sterilize liquids, linens<br>• Inexpensive | • Unable to use for heat- or moisture-sensitive items<br>• Unable to use for anhydrous oils, powders, and lensed instruments<br>• Some instruments damaged by repeated exposure<br>• May leave instruments wet and prone to rust |
| Dry heat<br>• gravity convection<br>• mechanical convection | • Useful for anhydrous oils, powders, glass<br>• No corrosive or rusting effect on instruments<br>• Reaches surfaces of instruments that cannot be disassembled<br>• Inexpensive | • Lengthy cycle due to slowness of heating and penetration<br>• Unsuitable for temperature-sensitive items<br>• Limited choice of materials suitable for packing items to be sterilized |
| Ethylene oxide gas (ETO) | • For temperature-sensitive items<br>• Easily penetrates packaging and devices with lumens<br>• Systems in place to minimize gas leak and ETO exposure<br>• Simple to operate and monitor<br>• Compatible with most medical devices | • Lengthy cycle time<br>• Requires lengthy aeration time to remove ETO residue prior to use<br>• ETO is toxic, flammable, and a probable carcinogen<br>• Monitoring of residual gas levels in environment required<br>• ETO cartridges require storage in flammable liquid storage cabinet<br>• Highly reactive with other chemicals<br>• Small sterilization chamber<br>• Expensive<br>• Causes structural damage to some devices |
| Hydrogen peroxide gas plasma | • For temperature-sensitive items<br>• Safe for humans and the environment<br>• No toxic residues<br>• Cycle time rapid with no aeration needed<br>• Suitable for heat- and moisture-sensitive items<br>• Simple to operate, install, and monitor<br>• Compatible with most medical devices | • Cannot be used to process paper, linen, or liquids (inactivates hydrogen peroxide)<br>• Small sterilization chamber<br>• Limitations on length and lumen diameter of devices<br>• Requires synthetic packaging and special container tray |
| Peracetic acid | • For temperature-sensitive immersible items<br>• Rapid cycle time<br>• Safe for environment<br>• Liquid immersion suitable for small endoscope lumens<br>• Effective in presence of organic matter | • Point-of-use system (items unwrapped); therefore cannot have sterile storage<br>• Efficacy monitoring with biological indicator is questionable<br>• Can be used for immersible instruments only<br>• Some material incompatibility<br>• Cycle cannot process many devices at once |
| Glutaraldehyde | • Appropriate for temperature-sensitive items | • Unable to monitor sterilization<br>• Copious rinsing with sterile water required<br>• Toxic to humans and environment<br>• Lengthy process to achieve sterility |

*For methods that appear in both Tables 56-6 and 56-7, the level of decontamination achieved depends upon length of exposure time and concentration according to manufacturers' instructions.

## Steam sterilization

The underlying principle of steam sterilization is the exposure of an item to direct steam contact at a specified temperature and pressure for a specified length of time. Moist heat eliminates microorganisms through the irreversible coagulation and denaturation of enzymes and structural proteins. Pressure permits the attainment of the high temperatures required—either 121°C (250°F) for 30 minutes in a gravity displacement sterilizer or 132°C (270°F) for 4 minutes in a pre-vacuum sterilizer. As stated previously, steam sterilization should be used whenever possible on critical items that are resistant to heat and moisture.

## Flash sterilization

Flash sterilization is a modification of conventional steam sterilization and was originally defined as sterilization of an unwrapped object at 132°C (270°F) for 3 minutes at 27 to 28 lbs. of pressure in a gravity displacement sterilizer. Items are placed unwrapped in an open tray and are exposed to steam for 3 to 10 minutes at 132°C (270°F). Duration of sterilization depends upon the item being sterilized and the type of sterilizer: porous instruments with lumens and vacuum sterilizers (as opposed to gravity displacement) require longer settings. Until recently, lack of timely biological indicators (discussed below), absence of protective packaging following sterilization, and risk of contamination during transportation to operating rooms were major disadvantages. Although some of these issues have been addressed through new biological indicators that provide results in 1 to 3 hours, new packaging that allows steam penetration, and constructional changes to minimize the physical distance between operating rooms and the flash sterilizer, flashing is still not recommended as a routine method of sterilization. Its most appropriate setting for use is when there is insufficient time to sterilize an item by the preferred method, such as intra-operatively when a surgical instrument has been accidentally contaminated and the surgery must proceed without a lengthy time delay. Therefore, flash sterilization of equipment should not be performed out of convenience, to save time, or to minimize purchasing costs of equipment by shortening turnover time between uses. Flash sterilization of implantable devices should not be performed (unless indicated by the manufacturer's instructions), and, in cases where this is unavoidable, documentation of the biological indicator result and careful follow-up for the development of a surgical site infection are warranted.

## Ethylene oxide

Since the 1950s, ethylene oxide has been used as a low-temperature sterilant for processing items that are temperature- and moisture-sensitive. Its mode of action is through the alkylation of protein, DNA, and RNA to prevent normal cellular metabolism and replication. However, its major disadvantages include the lengthy cycle time (1 to 6 hours processing time, plus aeration time of 8 to 12 hours at 50 to 60°C), cost, and occupational hazards (skin and mucous membrane irritation, teratogenesis, mutagenesis, and carcinogenesis). To limit employee exposure, institutions are required to monitor and document ethylene oxide emissions in areas of use, and Environment Canada will be requiring hospitals to prevent or control the release of ethylene oxide into the atmosphere by 2007.

## Hydrogen peroxide gas plasma

Gas plasmas, considered a fourth state of matter, are generated when gas molecules are excited by radio frequency or microwave energy under deep vacuum conditions in a closed chamber. This produces charged particles and free radicals that disrupt cellular metabolism. Introduced in the late 1980s, hydrogen peroxide gas plasma is used for items that cannot undergo steam sterilization, and it is compatible with the materials of most medical devices.

## Peracetic acid

Like the hydrogen peroxide gas plasma system, peracetic acid sterilization is another low-temperature-process alternative. Peracetic acid is an oxidizing agent that denatures proteins and disrupts cell wall permeability. One limitation for use is that the item to be sterilized must be able to be submerged in liquid without sustaining damage.

## Other sterilization methods

Ozone sterilization has recently been approved by the United States Food and Drug Administration (FDA) as another low-temperature alternative to ethylene oxide. Preliminary reports on this new technology suggest it is safer, faster, and potentially more cost-effective than ethylene oxide. This technology has not yet been widely adopted, and the instability of ozone and difficulties in generating ozone in pure form remain barriers to its use. Other less employed or less common methods of sterilization are discussed in Table 56-6.

## Sterilization process

As sterilization is a process and not a single event, appropriate procedures must be in place to achieve and maintain sterility. The ability to validate the efficacy of sterilization is one important component of this process. Quality assurance monitoring can be achieved through three distinct methods:

1. **Mechanical monitoring:** temperature (and duration of temperature) and pressure graphs, charts, or printouts
2. **Chemical monitoring:** temperature and/or humidity sensitive tape, strips, or pellets that change colour when at least one parameter is met and can be located inside or outside each sterilized pack
3. **Biological monitoring:** spore-laden strips or vials

Mechanical and chemical indicators provide visual confirmation that the conditions required to achieve sterilization—such as time duration, temperature, and pressure—have been met. It is assumed that because these physical endpoints have been achieved, sterilization has occurred. However, only biological indicators demonstrate the actual effectiveness of the sterilization process, since the elimination of all microbes, including microbial spores, is the true definition of sterility. *Bacillus stearothermophilus* spores are used for steam and liquid peracetic acid sterilization, while *Bacillus subtilis* is used for dry heat, ethylene oxide, and hydrogen peroxide gas plasma cycles. As *Bacillus* spores are more resistant and present in greater numbers than are the common microbial contaminants found on patient-care equipment, a negative result (i.e., no sign of growth) with a biological indicator strongly suggests that all other potential pathogens present have been destroyed. A combination of all three indicators must be used to routinely monitor sterilizing conditions, as each indicator provides a different yet complementary piece of information. Thus, one result alone should not be used to determine if sterilization has been achieved. The monitoring frequency of each sterilization load should be outlined by the manufacturer, and it is dependent upon the type of indicator (loads should be monitored at least weekly with biological indicators, but with each load for mechanical and chemical indicators), the number of loads per day, and the contents of each load (e.g., implantable devices should *always* be monitored).

One major disadvantage of biological indicators is a required incubation time of 24 to 48 hours prior to reading. This means that an instrument load that has been sterilized should not be used prior to the availability of this result. Nonetheless, many healthcare facilities do not have the financial resources to purchase the quantities of equipment required to allow patient flow to continue at its requisite pace while holding back instruments for 1 to 2 days. Therefore, increasing reliance has been placed on the mechanical and chemical indicators, which poses a serious problem should the biological indicator return positive (i.e., the spores have not been eliminated, suggesting that the sterilization cycle has failed). In these situations, it is difficult to determine if the biological indicator result is falsely positive, or if the physical indicators have failed. Fortunately, new rapid readout biological indicators with a turnaround time of 1 to 3 hours have been developed and are being brought into use.

Quality assurance is vital through the entire sterilization process. For example, testing with physical and biological indicators is only useful if the results themselves are dependable. This highlights the importance of thoroughly evaluating, validating, and routinely testing all sterilization processes and equipment at regular intervals. Many requirements are constructional in nature, such as performing sterilization within a central processing department by trained staff with good technique and practice. The physical layout of the department should allow workflow from dirty areas (cleaning, decontamination) to clean (sterilization, packing, storage). Airflow, acceptable materials for floors and walls, and climatic considerations (temperature, humidity) are also important factors, but will not be discussed further here. Similarly important is adherence to the manufacturers' recommendations for appropriate use of sterilization equipment and products.

Maintenance of sterility is another component of ensuring quality. If possible, items to be sterilized should be packaged in appropriate wraps before undergoing sterilization. One of the major disadvantages to liquid chemical (peracetic acid) and flash sterilization is the inability to maintain sterility since the items are not wrapped before undergoing sterilization. The sterilized instruments are often used immediately; however, these items must still be transported to the operating suite or storage area for packaging in a way that minimizes contamination.

Lastly, items either sterilized or purchased as sterile should be stored in a protected area where they are unlikely to be exposed to moisture, dirt, dust, and vermin. Location, temperature, and humidity of the storage area are important factors to consider. Expiration dates on purchased items should be noted. Once the packaging of items is opened, the items are no longer sterile (unless opened in a sterile environment).

## Disinfection

Disinfection is performed when cleaning alone is inadequate to make an item safe for patient use, yet sterilization is above and beyond what is required. As in the case of sterilization, a number of factors determine the level of disinfection achieved (see Table 56-4). Table 56-7 summarizes the major classes of chemical disinfectants and gives examples of use, advantages, and disadvantages.

Although high-level disinfection is, by definition, the elimination of all microorganisms with the exception of bacterial spores, in reality it is often difficult to ensure complete elimination of all microorganisms. Therefore, the FDA accepts a 6 $\log_{10}$ unit reduction of microorganisms as achieving the standard of high-level disinfection.

Just as with the process of sterilization, quality assurance at each step of disinfection is required. Upon disinfection, semi-critical items must be rinsed with sterile water to prevent re-contamination. If sterile water is unavailable, tap water followed by an alcohol rinse and forced air-drying can be considered. Storing items in a sterile package or in an area that is routinely disinfected is required once they are dried.

Some semi-critical items that come in contact with non-intact skin for brief periods of time can be disinfected with intermediate-level disinfectants, such as 70% isopropyl alcohol. Items in this category include glass and electronic thermometers and hydrotherapy tanks.

Although chemical agents play a necessary role in disinfection, many of these compounds pose occupational risks to healthcare workers and the environment. **Glu-**

| TABLE 56-7 | Commonly Used Chemical Disinfectants* | | | |
|---|---|---|---|---|
| **Disinfectant** | **Level of Disinfection** | **Uses** | **Advantages** | **Disadvantages** |
| Alcohols | Intermediate | Thermometers; external surfaces of stethoscopes; equipment used for home health care; skin antisepsis | • Rapid action<br>• No residue | • Volatile<br>• Evaporation reduces concentration<br>• Inactivated by organic material<br>• Contraindicated for use in the operating room |
| Chlorines | Intermediate | Hydrotherapy tanks; dialysis equipment; environmental surfaces; following blood spills | • Rapid action<br>• Inexpensive | • Corrosive to metals<br>• Inactivated by organic material<br>• Skin and mucous membrane irritant<br>• Must be diluted; can be unstable when diluted, with short shelf life<br>• Must be used in well-ventilated areas |
| Ethylene oxide gas | High | Heat-sensitive items | • Can be used for heat-sensitive items | • Lengthy cycle and aeration times<br>• Occupational health issues (toxic, flammable, and probably carcinogenic)<br>• Monitoring of residual gas levels in environment required<br>• ETO cartridges require storage in flammable liquid storage cabinet<br>• Highly reactive with other chemicals<br>• Small sterilization chamber<br>• Expensive<br>• Causes structural damage to some devices |
| Glutaraldehyde | 2% solution: High | Heat-sensitive items (e.g., endoscopes, respiratory therapy equipment, anaesthesia equipment) | • Non-corrosive to metal<br>• Active in presence of organic material<br>• Compatible with lensed instruments<br>• Relatively inexpensive | • Skin and mucous membrane irritant<br>• Shortened shelf life when diluted<br>• Expensive<br>• Concentration must be monitored<br>• Fixes organic material if not removed by cleaning |
| Hydrogen peroxide | 6% solution: High<br><br>3% solution: Low | Flexible endoscopes; foot care equipment; soft contact lenses<br><br>Home healthcare equipment; floors, walls, furnishings | • Rapid action<br>• Strong oxidant<br>• Safe for environment<br>• No activation required | • Can be corrosive to aluminum, copper, brass, and zinc |
| Iodophors<br>Note: antiseptic iodophors are not suitable for surface disinfection | Low<br><br><br><br>Intermediate | Hard surfaces and equipment (e.g., IV poles, wheelchairs, beds)<br><br>Thermometers; hydrotherapy tanks | • Rapid action<br>• Relatively free of toxicity and irritancy | • Corrosive to metal unless combined with inhibitors<br>• Disinfectant may burn tissue<br>• Inactivated by organic materials<br>• May stain fabrics and synthetic materials |
| Ortho-phthalaldehyde | High | Heat-sensitive items (e.g., endoscopes, respiratory therapy equipment, anaesthesia equipment) | • Rapid action<br>• No activation required<br>• Compatible with most materials | • Limited clinical use (stains skin, clothing, environmental surfaces) |

*continued*

| TABLE 56-7 | continued | | | |
|---|---|---|---|---|
| Disinfectant | Level of Disinfection | Uses | Advantages | Disadvantages |
| Peracetic acid | High | Heat-sensitive items | • Rapid action<br>• Safe for environment<br>• Active in presence of organic material<br>• No activation required<br>• Automated, standardized cycle | • Used for immersible instruments only<br>• Can be corrosive<br>• Unstable when diluted<br>• Point-of-use system with no long-term sterile storage<br>• Efficacy monitoring with biological indicator is questionable<br>• Some material incompatibility<br>• Cycle cannot process many devices at once |
| Phenolics | Low/ intermediate | Hard surfaces and equipment (e.g., floors, walls, furnishings, IV poles, wheelchairs, beds) | • Residual film | • Contraindicated for use in nurseries and food contact surfaces<br>• May be absorbed through skin or by rubber |
| Quaternary ammonium compounds | Low | Floors, walls, furnishings; blood spills | • Non-irritating to skin<br>• Non-corrosive | • Not for disinfecting instruments<br>• Limited use (narrow antimicrobial spectrum) |

*For products that appear in both Tables 56-6 and 56-7, the level of decontamination achieved depends upon length of exposure time and concentration according to manufacturers' instructions.

taraldehyde is one such example. It is widely used as a high-level disinfectant in the healthcare setting for medical devices such as endoscopes and for anaesthesia and respiratory therapy equipment because it is non-corrosive and relatively fast-acting. It has the ability to also act as a chemical sterilant if the contact time is prolonged. Glutaraldehyde is biocidal when activated by changing the pH of the solution from acidic to alkaline. A 2% aqueous solution is used for 20 minutes at room temperature to achieve high-level disinfection.

However, if equipment is processed with glutaraldehyde in a poorly ventilated room, its vapour can cause skin and mucous membrane irritation. Specific safety requirements, such as the installation of fume hoods, protective equipment for workers, and increased air exchanges in the work area, have been legislated in some Canadian provinces to minimize exposure and provide a safer work environment for employees.

## Pasteurization

This is a process of hot water disinfection, achieved when items are exposed to water above 75°C (158°F) for 30 minutes. Pasteurization is most commonly performed in the healthcare setting on anaesthesia and respiratory therapy equipment, which is typically plastic and immersible. As before, all equipment must be thoroughly cleaned prior to pasteurization. Major advantages of this method include lack of toxicity, rapid cycle, and moderate cost of both machinery and its upkeep. Disadvantages are that it is not sporicidal, it may cause splash burns, the equipment has not been standardized, and it is difficult to validate the effectiveness of the process. Although monitoring of temperature and time is performed, biological indicators are not used in this process.

## Ultraviolet radiation

Exposure to ultraviolet (UV) light with a wavelength range of 250 to 280 nm (UVc wavelength) can inactivate many microorganisms through the formation of thymine dimers in DNA. Although many potential applications exist, use of UV radiation in hospitals is limited to the elimination of airborne organisms or microorganisms on surfaces. This occurs primarily in operating rooms, isolation rooms, and biological safety cabinets within the laboratory setting. This is because the effectiveness of UV is affected by many factors—organic matter, wavelength, amount of turbidity, temperature, type of microorganism, and UV intensity, which is affected by distance from, and by dust or dirt on, the UV lamp. UV irradiation can be used as an adjunct in tuberculosis control through air cleaning of ventilation ducts or bronchoscopy suites. From an occupational hazard standpoint, UV light may cause skin and eye burns and has been theoretically linked to cataracts and skin cancer.

## Surface disinfection

Surfaces are considered non-critical items and pose little to no risk of transmission of infection. However, some bacteria such as *Clostridium difficile* and viruses such as the noroviruses can contaminate hospital floors and surfaces and significantly contribute to the spread of disease. Similarly, cross-transmission through unwashed hands of healthcare workers can also transmit infection. Low- or intermediate-level disinfectants are generally recommended over detergents since detergents themselves become contaminated with microorganisms and continued use can further contaminate the environment. Several guidelines (CDC, Health Canada) exist to direct both cleaning and disinfection of the hospital environment.

# MISCELLANEOUS ISSUES

## Creutzfeldt-Jakob Disease

Creutzfeldt-Jakob disease (CJD) is a degenerative and fatal neurological disease caused by a proteinaceous infection agent, or prion. CJD is one of several human transmissible spongiform encephalopathies of which the causal agent demonstrates an unusual resistance to conventional chemical and physical decontamination processes. The routine sterilization practices discussed in this chapter do not inactive prions. Iatrogenic CJD has been described primarily as a result of injection of pituitary hormones contaminated with the prion and after implantation of contaminated dura mater and corneal human grafts, but the use of contaminated medical equipment (stereotactic electrodes) has also been implicated. It is believed that the infrequent transmission of CJD via contaminated medical devices is likely a reflection of the inefficiency of transmission unless neural tissue transfer is involved.

Nonetheless, CJD protocols are being developed to ensure proper handling of equipment used in brain biopsies and other neurosurgical procedures on patients with known or suspected CJD. Disposal of instruments is the safest option, particularly if they are difficult or impossible to clean. If this choice is not available, three factors determine how the medical device is decontaminated: (1) risk of the patient having prion disease, (2) infectivity of the body tissue (brain, spinal cord, and eye versus all other tissues), and (3) the intended use of the medical device (critical or semi-critical).

## Reuse of Single-Use Medical Devices

Many Canadian hospitals reuse medical devices labelled as single-use by the manufacturer by developing in-house sterilization or disinfection procedures. This practice began in the late 1970s as a cost-saving measure. Labelling a device as "single-use" is at the discretion of the manufac-

turer. While this may mean, in some cases, that the device cannot be reprocessed because it becomes non-functional after single use, it may also mean that a validated reprocessing procedure has simply not been determined, and the manufacturer is unwilling to assume responsibilities for reuse of the device. This complex issue involves regulatory, ethical, medical, legal, and economic issues, and it remains both controversial and difficult to this day. Reuse committees consisting of experts in biomechanics, infection control, materials management, and sterilization have been formed to address many of these concerns.

However, a 2001 Health Canada survey found that only 38% of institutions with more than 250 beds had a reuse committee, and many hospitals practise reuse in the absence of protocols. In 2000, the FDA passed legislation stating that hospitals or companies that reprocess single-use devices must comply with the same standards that the original manufacturer would have needed to comply with in order to license the device as a reusable device. Thus, those wanting to reprocess a single-use device had to prove to the FDA that it was safe. There is no similar legislation in Canada; however, Manitoba has banned the reprocessing of critical single-use devices. Recently, the Ontario Hospital Association recommended that hospitals not reprocess critical and semi-critical devices.

# CONCLUSION

The concepts of antisepsis, disinfection, and sterilization are important ones that directly relate to patient safety. It is important that the right process be used for each setting and device and that appropriate quality assurance measures be taken. Because these processes can be complicated, it is important that national standards be accessible, understood, and followed.

# SUGGESTED READINGS

Association for the Advancement of Medical Instrumentation (AAMI). *Good Hospital Practice: Steam Sterilization and Sterility Assurance.* Arlington, Va: AAMI; 1993.

Block SS, ed. *Disinfection, Sterilization and Preservation.* 5th ed. Philadelphia, Pa: Lippincott Williams & Wilkins; 2001.

Boyce JM, Pittet D. Guideline for hand hygiene in health-care settings. Recommendations of the Healthcare Infection Control Practices Advisory Committee and the HICPAC/SHEA/APIC/IDSA Hand Hygiene Task Force. *Morb Mortal Wkly Rep.* 2002;51(RR16):1-44.

Garner JS. Guideline for isolation precautions in hospitals. The Hospital Infection Control Practices Advisory Committee. *Infect Control Hosp Epidemiol.* 1996;17:53-80.

Health Canada. Hand washing, cleaning, disinfection and sterilization in health care. *Can Commun Dis Rep.* 1998;24S8:1-55.

Health Canada. Routine practices and additional precautions for preventing the transmission of infection in health care. Revision of isolation and precaution techniques. *Can Commun Dis Rep.* 1999;25S4:1-142.

Larson EL. APIC Guideline for handwashing and hand antisepsis in health care settings. *Am J Infect Control.* 1995;23:251-69.

Sehulster L, Chinn RYW. Guidelines for environmental infection control in health-care facilities. Recommendations of CDC and the Healthcare Infection Control Practices Advisory Committee (HICPAC). *Morb Mortal Wkly Rep* 2003;52(RR10): 1-42.

# 57

# Anti-neoplastic Drugs

## EX CHEN AND MJ MOORE

### CASE HISTORY

In early June 1994, a 62-year-old man presented to his family physician with a 2-month history of intermittent bright red blood per rectum, and laboratory investigations showed hemoglobin of 110 g/L, with a MCV of 75, consistent with iron deficiency anemia. A colonoscopy revealed an ulcerative lesion in the sigmoid colon, 25 cm from the anal verge. Biopsies of this lesion were positive for adenocarcinoma. He underwent surgical resection in September 1994. Pathological examination of the surgical specimen showed a moderately differentiated adenocarcinoma, 4.2 cm in diameter, with clear resection margins, and involvement of 6 out of 15 removed lymph nodes.

A chest film, ultrasound examination of the liver, and routine laboratory investigations did not reveal any evidence of metastasis. The patient underwent adjuvant chemotherapy with 5-fluorouracil (5-FU) and leucovorin for 6 months, finishing in April 1995. He tolerated treatment well with mild mucositis. Afterwards, he was followed regularly by his surgeon and medical oncologist with physical examination, routine laboratory investigations, including serum level of carcinoembryogenic antigen (CEA), and ultrasound of the liver.

In June 1996, on routine follow-up, the serum CEA was found to be elevated at 12.5. Ultrasound of the liver showed two new lesions, measuring 2.0 cm and 3.2 cm in the right lobe. These lesions were confirmed with computer tomography (CT) of the abdomen. Metastatic workup, including CT of the chest and bone scan, was negative. The patient underwent surgical resection of liver lesions and pathological examination was consistent with metastatic colon cancer.

In April 1998, CT of the abdomen showed diffuse liver lesions consistent with metastatic disease. The patient was asymptomatic at the time. After discussion with his medical oncologist, he participated in a randomized phase III clinical trial evaluating a new drug, irinotecan (CPT-11), in combination with 5-FU and leucovorin. This combination chemotherapy was administered weekly for 4 consecutive weeks, and the cycle of chemotherapy was repeated every 6 weeks. During the infusion of the first irinotecan dose, the patient developed abdominal cramping and diarrhea. These symptoms were successfully treated with atropine 0.4 mg subcutaneously. Atropine was then administered prophylactically before each subsequent irinotecan infusion. After two cycles, CT showed improvement in his liver lesions, consistent with a partial response. CEA was also reduced to 4.5 from a pre-treatment value of 34.6. He was treated with four more cycles of chemotherapy, and after the sixth cycle of therapy, radiological imaging showed the disease to be stable.

He remained well until February 2000 when he developed nausea, vomiting, abdominal distension, and pain. Abdominal X-ray confirmed small bowel obstruction, and the patient was managed conservatively with a nasogastric tube. CT of the abdomen showed diffuse peritoneal carcinomatosis and progression of the liver lesions. After resolution of the small bowel obstruction, he was treated with oxaliplatin in combination with infusional 5-FU and leucovorin. This treatment was repeated every 2 weeks. Repeat CT of the abdomen after 2 months of therapy showed improvements in the liver lesions and peritoneal nodules. After eight cycles of treatment, he developed numbness and tingling sensations in his fingertips and toes immediately after drug administration. These symptoms, which gradually resolved after 4 days, were consistent with oxaliplatin-induced peripheral neuropathy. After discussion, it was decided to continue the chemotherapy with careful re-evaluation of his neurological symptoms. After a further four cycles of therapy, neurological symptoms persisted, and the patient began to have difficulty doing up buttons on his shirts. Oxaliplatin was discontinued.

The patient remained relatively well after the discontinuation of oxaliplatin for 5 months. He gradually developed fatigue, abdominal pain and distension, and peripheral edema. Therapy with oral capecitabine was initiated. However, the patient continued to deteriorate and died on June 17, 2001.

Malignant transformation of normal cells is characterized by uncontrolled proliferation of transformed cells at the expense of the host. Cancers spread by invasion of the surrounding tissues and by metastasizing to distant sites. Tumours may be very heterogeneous with respect to karyotype, morphology, immunogenicity, rate of growth, ability to metastasize, and responsiveness to anti-neoplastic drugs. Although surgery and radiation can often cure or control tumours locally, many patients eventually succumb because of distant metastases. Most present-day treatments for systemic disease employ cytotoxic or hormonal agents, or both. More recently, several agents that specifically target features of the malignant cell, but are not cytotoxic, have been introduced into clinical practice. In patients with cancer, anti-neoplastic drugs are used to control established metastases, to prevent disease recurrence after local treatment (adjuvant therapy), or to decrease tumour size prior to local treatment (neoadjuvant therapy).

## PRINCIPLES OF CANCER CHEMOTHERAPY

1. A "clonogenic" cell is one that has the potential for unlimited replication. A single clonogenic malignant cell can give rise to sufficient progeny to kill the host. The effectiveness of chemotherapy depends on its ability to eliminate *all* clonogenic cells.

2. The cell kill caused by anti-neoplastic drugs follows first-order kinetics; that is, in each successive time period, a constant percentage or fraction rather than a constant number of cells is killed by a given therapeutic intervention. For example, a patient with cancer might harbour $10^{12}$ malignant cells (about 1 kg). A drug treatment that kills 99.99% of these cells would reduce the tumour mass to about 100 mg (i.e., a complete clinical remission). However, $10^8$ malignant cells would survive, and any remaining clonogenic cells would cause a recurrence of the disease.

3. Most anti-neoplastic drugs have a low therapeutic index and are not specific for cancer cells. Many normal body tissues such as bone marrow, gonads, oral mucosa, and hair follicles may be damaged as well. Doses and schedules of drug administration that can be used to achieve tumour cell kill are limited by normal tissue tolerance. Therefore, most anti-neoplastic drugs are administered intermittently. These intermittent schedules allow time for recovery of normal host tissues between drug treatment cycles.

4. Tumour cells may grow in body compartments (e.g., the central nervous system) to which chemotherapeutic agents have limited or no access. Local drug administration (e.g., intrathecal) can be effective in eradicating malignant cells in such sites. Other examples of regional chemotherapy involve instillation of drugs into the bladder for treatment of superficial bladder cancer, injection of drugs into the peritoneal cavity in patients with peritoneal metastatic disease, or direct arterial infusion into limbs and liver.

5. Several drugs used together (combination chemotherapy) are more effective than drugs used individually. Ideally, each drug in the combination has a different mechanism of action, is effective as a single agent, and has qualitatively different toxicities, so all can be given at or near their individual maximum tolerated doses.

6. Theoretically, it would be best to start treatment early when the number of cancer cells is small, when the fraction of dividing cells is high, and when there is a low probability of resistant cells. This principle has led to the development of **adjuvant chemotherapy**, defined as the administration of drugs to patients who have no evidence of disease by currently available methods of study but who are at high risk of developing recurrent cancer according to current knowledge. It is assumed that such patients have small numbers of cancer cells and a low probability of resistant cells. This approach has been quite successful in the treatment of breast and colorectal cancers. In the case history described, the use of fluorouracil and leucovorin after surgery was adjuvant therapy, while the remaining therapies were used in the presence of metastatic disease.

7. Combined-modality treatments involving surgery, radiation, and chemotherapy are now used commonly. Such an approach is particularly successful in the treatment of childhood cancers and in breast, colorectal, and head and neck cancer in adults.

## CLASSIFICATION OF ANTI-NEOPLASTIC DRUGS

Anti-neoplastic drugs are classified on the basis of their mechanism of action (Fig. 57-1, Table 57-1).

In the following sections, representative drugs from each class are discussed, and properties of more commonly used agents are summarized. Practical considerations for drug administration are outlined in Table 57-2. Some indications of the therapeutic uses of anti-neoplastic drugs are given in each section.

## ALKYLATING AGENTS

Alkylating agents are chemically diverse drugs that act through the covalent bonding of alkyl groups (e.g., $CH_2Cl^-$) to intracellular macromolecules. These agents generate highly reactive, positively charged intermediates, which then combine with electron-rich "nucle-

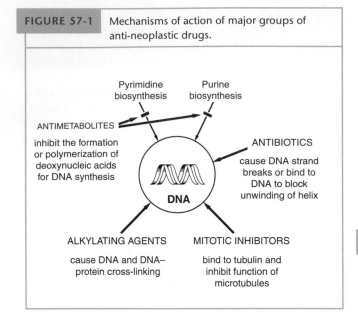

**FIGURE 57-1** Mechanisms of action of major groups of anti-neoplastic drugs.

ophilic" groups such as amino, phosphate, sulfhydryl, or hydroxyl moieties in intracellular macromolecules. Alkylating agents are classified as monofunctional (one reactive group) or bifunctional (two reactive groups). Bifunctional alkylating agents can react with one nucleophilic group on each of the two strands of DNA, thus preventing cell replication unless the DNA is repaired. The cytotoxicity of monofunctional alkylating agents is related to the recognition of the single-strand DNA lesion by the cell and the cellular response to this lesion.

Alkylating agents were the first agents used for treating malignant disease and are now used in many of the combination chemotherapy regimens. The prototypic alkylating agents are nitrogen mustard and its derivatives melphalan, chlorambucil, cyclophosphamide, and ifosfamide (Fig. 57-2). Structurally, they contain two chloroethyl groups ($CH_2CH_2Cl^-$), which, on separation of the chloride ions, form highly reactive carbonium ions crucial to the mechanism of action of these compounds. Therefore, these agents are bifunctional. Other alkylating agents include nitrosoureas, dacarbazine, and temozolomide.

Alkylating agents have many effects in common. The usual dose-limiting toxicity is myelosuppression (a reduction in the production of white blood cells and platelets). Neutropenia (a neutrophil count below 1500/µL) appears about 10 days after drug administration, and the lowest or nadir blood counts are seen at around 15 days. Recovery to baseline levels usually occurs by 21 to 28 days. However, nitrosoureas produce delayed myelosuppression with nadirs of both neutrophils and platelets occurring at 5 to 6 weeks after drug administration. Nausea and vomiting are common but short-lived (usually less than 24 hours after administration). Alopecia (loss of hair) is frequent with cyclophosphamide and ifosfamide and occurs after two to four courses of treatment.

Alkylating agents may cause significant gonadal toxicity in long-term survivors. These drugs can induce amenorrhea in women and oligospermia in men. The degree and duration of these side effects depend on the duration of drug treatment and the patient's age at the time of treatment. Second malignancies in patients receiving long-term treatment with alkylating agents and birth defects in infants of women inadvertently treated with these drugs during pregnancy reflect the **mutagenic effect** of these drugs.

Some alkylating agents, such as carmustine (BCNU), can cause severe skin and tissue damage if extravasation occurs

| **TABLE 57-1** | Classification of Anti-neoplastic Agents According to Mechanisms of Action or Derivation |
|---|---|

**Alkylating agents**
  Cyclophosphamide, ifosfamide, melphalan, chlorambucil
  Carmustine (BCNU), lomustine (CCNU)
  Dacarbazine (DTIC), temozolomide
  Busulphan, mitomycin C

**Platinating agents**
  Cisplatin, carboplatin, oxaliplatin

**Antimetabolites**
  Methotrexate, pemetrexed
  5-Fluorouracil, capecitabine
  Cytosine arabinoside (Ara-C), gemcitabine
  6-Mercaptopurine, 6-thioguanine
  Fludarabine, 2-chlorodeoxyadenosine (2-CdA)

**Topoisomerase inhibitors**
  Irinotecan (CPT-11), topotecan
  Doxorubicin, daunorubicin, epirubicin
  Etoposide (VP-16), teniposide (VM-26)

**Anti-microtubular agents**
  Vincristine, vinblastine, vinorelbine
  Paclitaxel, docetaxel

**Miscellaneous cytotoxic agents**
  L-Asparaginase
  Hydroxyurea
  Bleomycin

**Molecular targeted agents**
  Rituximab
  Imatinib
  Trastuzumab
  Bevacizumab
  Cetuximab, erlotinib, gefitinib
  Bortezomib

**Hormones**
  Glucocorticoids
  Tamoxifen, toremifen, anastrozole, letrozole, exemestane
  Progestational agents
  Leuprolide, buserelin, goserelin
  Flutamide, bicalutamide, nilutamide, cyproterone

**TABLE 57-2**  Doses, Routes of Administration, Schedules, Elimination, and Toxicities of Common Anti-neoplastic Agents

| Drug | Route of Administration | Dose* (mg/m²) | Frequency† | Major Route of Elimination‡ | Commonly Encountered Toxicities |
|---|---|---|---|---|---|
| Melphalan | Oral | 9 | Daily × 4 days every 4–6 weeks | Renal | Myelosuppression, mild nausea, vomiting |
| Cyclophosphamide | Intravenous Oral | 500–3500 100 | Every 3 weeks Daily × 14 days | Biotransformation | Myelosuppression, alopecia Nausea, vomiting, cystitis |
| Cisplatin | Intravenous | 50–100 | Every 3 weeks | Renal | Nausea, vomiting, mild myelosuppression, renal failure |
| Carboplatin | Intravenous | AUC 5-7* | Every 3 weeks | Renal | Myelosuppression, nausea, vomiting |
| Oxaliplatin | Intravenous | 85 | Every 2 weeks | Renal | Sensory neuropathy |
| Methotrexate | Intravenous | 30–60 | Every 2–4 weeks | Renal | Myelosuppression, mucositis |
| Pemetrexed | Intravenous | 500 | Every 3 weeks | Renal | Myelosuppression |
| 5-Fluorouracil | Intravenous | 200–600 | Daily × 5 days, weekly, or continuous infusion | Biotransformation | Myelosuppression, diarrhea, mucositis, skin rash |
| Capecitabine | Oral | 2500 mg | Daily × 14 days | Biotransformation | Mucositis, hand–foot syndrome |
| Ara-C | Intravenous infusion | 100 | 5–10 days | Biotransformation | Myelosuppression, mucositis, neurotoxicity |
| Gemcitabine | Intravenous | 1000 | Weekly | Biotransformation | Myelosuppression |
| 6-Mercaptopurine | Oral | 100 | Daily × 5 days | Biotransformation | Myelosuppression, cholestasis |
| Topotecan | Intravenous | 1.5 | Daily × 5 days | Renal | Myelosuppression |
| Irinotecan | Intravenous | 125–350 | Weekly or every 3 weeks | Biotransformation | Nausea, vomiting, myelosuppression, diarrhea |
| Doxorubicin | Intravenous | 75 | Every 3 weeks | Biotransformation | Myelosuppression, nausea, vomiting, alopecia, cardiomyopathy |
| Etoposide (VP-16) | Intravenous | 100–120 | Daily × 3 days | Biotransformation | Myelosuppression, neuropathy |
| Vincristine | Intravenous | 1.4 | Weekly | Biotransformation | Neuropathy, SIADH |
| Vinblastine | Intravenous | 6 | Every 1–2 weeks | Biotransformation | Mucositis, myelosuppression |
| Paclitaxel | Intravenous | 50–250 | Weekly or every 4 weeks | Biotransformation | Nausea, vomiting, myelo-suppression, allergic reactions |
| Docetaxel | Intravenous | 50–100 | Weekly or every 3 weeks | Biotransformation | Nausea, vomiting, myelo-suppression, allergic reactions |
| Bleomycin | Intravenous Intramuscular Subcutaneous | 10–15 | Weekly | Renal | Skin and pulmonary fibrosis, fever, allergic reactions |
| Rituximab | Intravenous | 375 | Weekly | Unknown | Infusion-related reactions, malaise |
| Imatinib | Oral | 400–800 mg | Daily | Biotransformation | Nausea, vomiting, diarrhea, edema |
| Trastuzumab | Intravenous | 2–4 mg/kg | Weekly | Unknown | Infusion-related reactions, heart failure |
| Bevacizumab | Intravenous | 5–10 mg/kg | Every 2 weeks | Unknown | Hypertension, proteinuria, hemorrhage, ↓ wound healing |

*continued*

| TABLE 57-2 | continued | | | | |
|---|---|---|---|---|---|
| Drug | Route of Administration | Dose* (mg/m²) | Frequency† | Major Route of Elimination‡ | Commonly Encountered Toxicities |
| Cetuximab | Intravenous | 250–400 | Weekly | Unknown | Skin rash, infusion-related reactions |
| Erlotinib | Oral | 150 mg | Daily | Biotransformation | Skin rash, diarrhea |
| Gefitinib | Oral | 250 mg | Daily | Biotransformation | Skin rash, diarrhea |
| Bortezomib | Intravenous | 1.3 | Twice weekly | Biotransformation | Nausea, vomiting, peripheral neuropathy |

*Dose as a single agent. AUC = area under the concentration–time curve, expressed in mg/mL × min.

†Frequency when given as a single agent.

‡"Renal" means renal excretion of unchanged drug. "Biotransformation" includes both hepatic and extrahepatic reactions: the metabolites may be excreted in the urine and bile.

SIADH = syndrome of inappropriate antidiuretic hormone secretion.

↓ = reduced or impaired.

at the time of drug administration. Patients often complain of severe pain, followed by erythema and edema at the site of catheter insertion. Supportive measures, such as cold compresses, local corticosteroids, and sling, are indicated.

## Nitrogen Mustard

Nitrogen mustard (mechlorethamine; Mustargen) was the first anti-cancer drug introduced into clinical practice. Its discovery was based on observations of reductions in white blood cells and lymph nodes seen in men exposed to mustard gas (sulfur mustard), a chemically similar compound, in World War I. Nitrogen mustard is useful in the treatment of Hodgkin's disease as part of the MOPP (Mustargen, vincristine [Oncovin], procarbazine, prednisone) regimen. It is unstable, reacting with water and other nucleophiles within a few minutes of preparation. It also can cause severe tissue necrosis if extravasation outside the intravenous injection site occurs. With addition of ring structures to the nitrogen mustard molecule, more active and chemically stable analogues of nitrogen mustard are created, and they have largely replaced nitrogen mustard in clinical use.

## Melphalan

Melphalan (L-phenylalanine mustard; Alkeran) is an alkylating agent that is taken up into the cell via active amino acid transport. It can be administered both orally and intravenously. About 50% of an orally administered dose is absorbed, but there is marked inter-individual variability in bioavailability. Some patients with no effect after oral administration could respond after intravenous administration of melphalan. The major clinical uses for this agent are in the treatment of multiple myeloma and

in some high-dose bone marrow transplant protocols. Common doses, frequency of administration, and route of elimination are summarized in Table 57-2.

## Cyclophosphamide

Cyclophosphamide (Cytoxan) is the most commonly used alkylating agent. It is inactive in vitro and is metabolized by P450 enzymes in the liver to active metabolites. Metabolites are excreted in the bile and urine and may irritate the bladder mucosa, resulting in a chemical cystitis. Acrolein has been identified as the metabolite most responsible for this effect. This complication can be limited by adequate hydration, which dilutes the concentration of acrolein in the urine. Cyclophosphamide can be given orally or intravenously in a wide range of doses ranging from 100 mg/day orally in treating autoimmune diseases and breast cancer, up to 3500 mg/day as part of marrow ablation regimens prior to allogeneic transplantations. It is also active against leukemia, lymphomas, lung cancer, and sarcomas. Cyclophosphamide dosages and schedule of administration are listed in Table 57-2.

**Ifosfamide** (Ifex) is a structurally related compound that also requires metabolic activation in the liver but by pathways different from that of cyclophosphamide. As a result, higher doses are required and the side-effect profile is somewhat different. Hemorrhagic cystitis due to acrolein is common with ifosfamide, and patients receiving ifosfamide should also be given **mesna (sodium 2-mercaptoethane sulfonate)**, which conjugates with acrolein in urine and renders it inactive. As mesna is inactive in plasma, and is converted to the active form only in urine, it does not affect the cytotoxicity of ifosfamide or cyclophosphamide at other sites. Ifosfamide is used in the treatment of soft-tissue sarcomas, testicular cancer, and lung cancer.

## FIGURE 57-2 · Structural formulae of mustard alkylating agents.

R—N(CH₂CH₂Cl)(CH₂CH₂Cl)

R = H₃C—  Nitrogen mustard

R = HOOC—CH—CH₂—⬡—  Melphalan
|
NH₂

R = (O=P—, NH₂, O)  Cyclophosphamide

R = HOOC—(CH₂)₃—⬡—  Chlorambucil

Ifosfamide

to function through formation of a metabolite with alkylating properties. The drug is used mainly for treatment of sarcomas, Hodgkin's disease, and melanoma. It causes nausea and vomiting in a high proportion of patients, and the dose-limiting toxicity is myelosuppression. **Temozolomide** (Temodar) is an oral agent that contains a triazene that is thought to be the active component of dacarbazine. It undergoes spontaneous decomposition to an alkylating intermediate and has a more predictable pharmacology than dacarbazine. Temozolomide has shown some activity against malignant glioma and melanoma.

**Busulfan** (Myleran) is an alkyl sulfonate that has a different mechanism of action from nitrogen mustards. It forms DNA cross-links by a direct displacement reaction. Busulfan causes marked myelosuppression and is used mainly in high-dose bone marrow transplantation regimens. Busulfan is eliminated via hepatic metabolism, and high doses of busulfan have been associated with veno-occlusive disease in patients who metabolize the drug slowly.

**Mitomycin C** (Mutamycin) is derived from a *Streptomyces* species and requires activation to an alkylating metabolite by reductive metabolism. The drug is more active against hypoxic than against aerobic cells in tissue culture, but it has not been shown to have preferential toxicity for hypoxic cells in vivo. It causes a delayed and rather unpredictable myelosuppression. More seriously, the drug can produce a hemolytic–uremic syndrome that is usually fatal and is probably due to small-vessel endothelial damage. Another potentially lethal effect is interstitial lung disease that progresses to pulmonary fibrosis. It has limited use in treating cancer of the anal canal, in combination

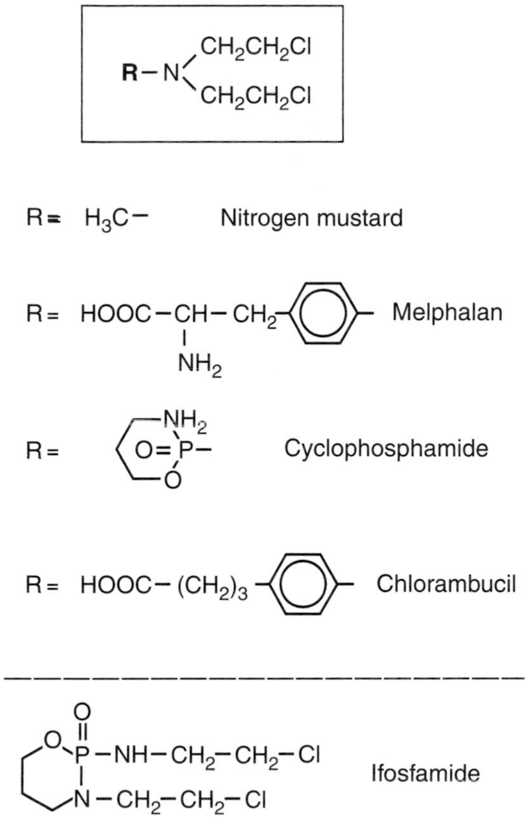

## Nitrosoureas

Nitrosoureas such as BCNU (**carmustine;** BiCNU) and CCNU (**lomustine;** CeeNU) are non-mustard alkylating agents (Fig. 57-3). One major difference between these drugs and other alkylating agents is their lipophilic character, which enables a significant fraction of these drugs to cross the blood–brain barrier and act against tumours in the central nervous system (CNS). Whereas most alkylating agents cause leukocyte nadirs about 10 days after administration, and recovery by day 21 to 28, the nitrosoureas cause two nadirs, one occurring at about day 10 and a second about day 28, with recovery by about day 42. Therefore, these agents are given at intervals of 6 to 8 weeks instead of 3 to 4 weeks as for other alkylating agents. These agents are also highly leukemogenic. Pulmonary toxicity (interstitial pneumonitis) can occur with chronic use. The nitrosoureas now have a very limited role in the treatment of cancers.

## Other Alkylating Agents

**Dacarbazine** (DTIC) was originally synthesized as an antimetabolite to inhibit purine biosynthesis. It is believed

## FIGURE 57-3 · Structural formulae of nitrosoureas.

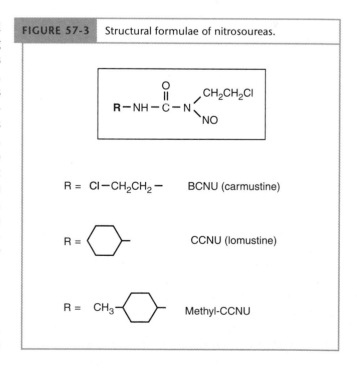

R—NH—C(=O)—N(CH₂CH₂Cl)(NO)

R = Cl—CH₂CH₂—  BCNU (carmustine)

R = ⬡—  CCNU (lomustine)

R = CH₃—⬡—  Methyl-CCNU

with radiation therapy, and sometimes it is used intravesically to treat superficial bladder cancer.

## PLATINATING AGENTS

The discovery of platinum drugs followed a series of experiments in which an electric current was delivered to bacterial cultures via platinum electrodes, and inhibition of bacterial growth was observed. The active compound was subsequently identified as cisplatin.

## Cisplatin

Cisplatin (*cis*-diamminedichloroplatinum; Platinol) is a platinum coordination complex with two chlorine leaving groups in the *cis* position (Fig. 57-4). While not a classical alkylating agent, its chlorine atoms are leaving groups that may be compared to those of nitrogen mustards. These chlorine atoms may be displaced directly by nucleophilic groups or indirectly after chloride ions are replaced by hydroxyl groups through reactions with water. These reactions occur spontaneously in environments where the chloride concentration is low, such as the intracellular environment. Cisplatin and its analogues react preferentially at the N-7 position of guanine and adenine bases to form DNA adducts, resulting in intra- and interstrand cross-linkages. The cytotoxic effects of platinum drugs correlate with their DNA cross-linking activity. However, the exact mechanism of cytotoxicity is not known. The presence of DNA adducts may cause faulty DNA repair, resulting in accumulation of DNA strand breaks and activation of apoptotic pathways. Cisplatin is given intravenously and binds avidly to proteins; a lesser proportion is excreted unchanged by the kidneys. Cisplatin causes severe and universal nausea and vomiting. 5-Hydroxytryptamine analogues such as **ondansetron**, together with glucocorticoids, are the most useful agents in controlling this problem. Nephrotoxicity with progressively declining creatinine clearance is dose-limiting but may be prevented in part by adequate hydration with a chloride-containing solution and mannitol-induced diuresis. Renal tubular damage may result in magnesium wasting with associated hypomagnesemia.

Multiple courses of cisplatin may cause irreversible ototoxicity, manifested initially by high-frequency hearing loss, and neurotoxicity manifested by a sensory peripheral neuropathy. The peripheral neuropathy is reversible, although the recovery is slow. There is no known strategy to circumvent these problems, and they are more common in patients with pre-existing hearing or neurological problems. These toxicities will limit the total number of cisplatin cycles that can be given. Cisplatin causes mild myelosuppression as a single agent but can add to myelosuppression caused by other drugs. Cisplatin is one of the most useful anti-neoplastic agents. It is the

FIGURE 57-4  Structural formulae of platinating agents.

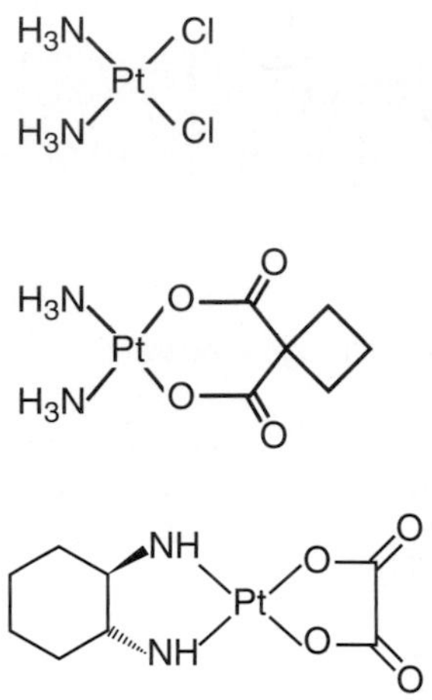

drug of choice for the treatment of testicular tumours, and cisplatin-based combinations can cure the majority of patients with advanced disease. It is also part of first-line therapy for lung, bladder, ovarian, gastric, cervical, and head and neck cancers and part of second-line therapy for malignant lymphomas. It is relatively inactive against colorectal cancer.

Because of the toxicities of cisplatin, there were major efforts to identify platinum analogues with less toxicity and broader activity. The two analogues in routine clinical use are carboplatin and oxaliplatin.

## Carboplatin

Carboplatin (*cis*-diammino [1,1-cyclobutanedicarboxylato] platinum [II]; Paraplatin) has a dicarboxylate chelate ligand replacing the two chlorine atoms in cisplatin (see Fig. 57-4). The presence of the dicarboxylate group renders carboplatin more stable and thus less reactive with proteins and DNA. The anti-tumour activity in vivo is comparable to that of cisplatin, but the spectrum of toxicity differs. Nausea and vomiting, neurotoxicity, nephrotoxicity, and ototoxicity are less severe, while myelosuppression, particularly low platelet count (thrombocytopenia), is dose-limiting. The severity of thrombocytopenia is related to the total exposure to the drug (area under the concentration–time curve; AUC), which is related to drug dose and renal function, as carboplatin is primarily excreted unchanged by the kidney. The clearance of carboplatin is determined by glomerular flow rate (GFR); therefore, the dose of carboplatin required to achieve a desired AUC can be calculated from the renal function. The Calvert formula is widely used clinically to individualize carboplatin dose:

$$\text{Carboplatin dose (mg)} = \text{target AUC (mg/mL} \times \text{min)} \times [\text{GFR (mL/min)} + 25]$$

Despite its more favourable toxicity profile, carboplatin has not replaced cisplatin in clinical practice, except perhaps in ovarian cancer. It is less active than cisplatin against testicular, bladder, and lung cancers. In addition, because its primary toxicity is myelosuppression, it can be a poor substitute for cisplatin in combination regimens with other myelosuppressive agents.

## Oxaliplatin

Oxaliplatin (Eloxatin) is one of a series of cisplatin analogues with substitution of a diaminocyclohexane for the main carrier group. Oxaliplatin has shown activity alone or in combination with 5-fluorouracil/leucovorin in metastatic colon cancer, which is resistant to cisplatin. In addition, it has a different toxicity profile. It has minimal nephrotoxicity, no ototoxicity, and causes only mild nausea and vomiting. Oxaliplatin causes a unique cumulative sensory neurotoxicity with marked sensitivity to cold (cold dysesthesia). In severe cases, patients may experience laryngopharyngeal spasm, which is not associated with significant respiratory symptoms and resolves with supportive care. The sensory neurotoxicity is cumulative, but reversible with drug discontinuation.

## ANTIMETABOLITES

Antimetabolites are synthetic drugs that act as inhibitors of critical biochemical pathways in the synthesis of DNA or as abnormal substitutes for naturally occurring nucleic acid bases, resulting in the formation of abnormal DNA. They are most active against rapidly dividing cells, and the most common toxicities are seen in the gastrointestinal mucosa (stomatitis and diarrhea) and the bone marrow (neutropenia and thrombocytopenia). Unlike the alkylating agents, the effects of these drugs are more dependent upon the schedule of administration than upon the total dose administered. Late-term toxicities such as infertility are not seen with the antimetabolites.

## Methotrexate

Methotrexate (4-amino-$N^{10}$-methylpteroylglutamic acid, also known as amethopterin; Rheumatrex, Folex) is a folic acid analogue (Fig. 57-5) that competes with dihydrofolate (a naturally occurring folate) for binding to the enzyme dihydrofolate reductase (DHFR). This leads to inhibition of tetrahydrofolate synthesis and a decrease in intracellular reduced folates. Reduced folates play a central role in methyl group transfer reactions that are necessary in purine biosynthesis and in the conversion of deoxyuridine monophosphate (dUMP) to thymidine phosphate (dTMP). Therefore, competitive inhibition of DHFR by methotrexate results in decreased purine biosynthesis, depletion of deoxythymidine triphosphate (dTTP),

a cessation of DNA synthesis, and cell death. Unfortunately, this action is exerted not only on malignant cells but also on rapidly reproducing normal cells such as those in bone marrow. The reduced folate leucovorin (folinic acid) may overcome the effect of inhibition of this pathway in normal tissues if given within 48 hours of methotrexate administration.

Methotrexate can be given orally, intravenously, or intrathecally (directly into the cerebrospinal fluid, or CSF). It can cross membranes slowly and accumulate in body cavities and spaces such as pleural effusions and ascites, from which it will slowly redistribute. This release from "third space" fluid collections can lead to excessive toxicity, and drainage of such collections prior to high-dose methotrexate administration should be considered. The kidney excretes the parent compound and metabolites; dose adjustment is necessary in the presence of renal dysfunction. Weak organic acids, such as acetylsalicylic acid and penicillins, can inhibit the renal excretion of methotrexate. Acetylsalicylic acid, non-steroidal anti-inflammatory agents, and sulfonamides can displace methotrexate from its binding sites on serum albumin and lead to increased toxicity.

"High-dose" methotrexate treatment, ranging from about 200 mg/m$^2$ to 20 g/m$^2$, has also been used. With this treatment, a high urine output must be maintained, and the urine must be kept alkaline in order to minimize the likelihood of drug precipitation in the renal tubules. Leucovorin must be given 24 to 48 hours after such doses of methotrexate to "rescue" normal tissues such as bone marrow and gastrointestinal mucosa from drug toxicity. Otherwise, such high doses of methotrexate would be lethal.

The major clinical uses of methotrexate are the systemic treatment of leukemia, lymphoma, choriocarcinoma, and bladder and breast cancers. Methotrexate is given intrathecally for meningeal leukemia or carcinomatosis. This will result in higher concentrations of methotrexate in the CSF than can be achieved by conventional doses given intravenously. The major forms of systemic toxicity are myelosuppression and mucositis. The use of prolonged low-dose oral methotrexate can cause hepatic fibrosis once a total dose of more than 3 g has been given.

## Pemetrexed

Pemetrexed (Alimta; see Fig. 57-5) is a novel antifolate agent. It is transported into cells through the reduced folate carrier system and converted to polyglutamate forms. These polyglutamate forms are retained in cells for long periods, and they inhibit folate-dependent enzymes involved in the *de novo* synthesis of thymidine and purine nucleotides, such as thymidylate synthase (TS), DHFR, and glycinamide ribonucleotide formyltransferase (GARFT).

Pemetrexed is administered intravenously and was recently approved for the treatment of malignant pleural

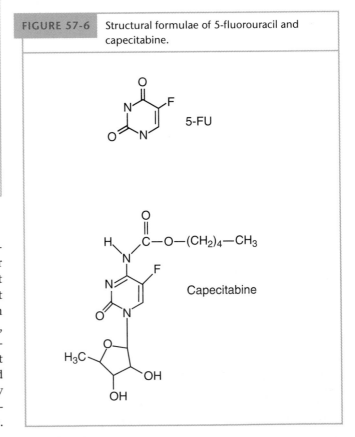

FIGURE 57-5  Structural formulae of folic acid, methotrexate, and pemetrexed.

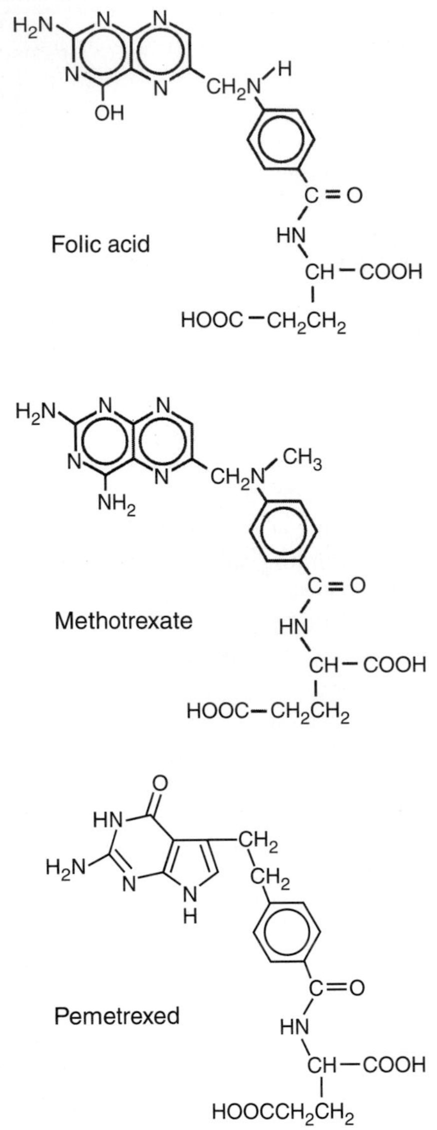

Folic acid

Methotrexate

Pemetrexed

In addition, patients should receive one intramuscular injection of vitamin $B_{12}$ during the week preceding the first dose of pemetrexed and every three cycles thereafter.

## 5-Fluorouracil

5-Fluorouracil (5-FU; Adrucil and others) is a fluorinated pyrimidine derivative, originally synthesized in 1957, that functions as an antimetabolite (Fig. 57-6). 5-FU remains today as one of the most widely used anti-cancer drugs with activity against gastrointestinal adenocarcinomas and cancers of the breast, esophagus, and head and neck.

The primary mechanism of 5-FU cytotoxicity is inhibition of TS through the generation of the intracellular nucleotide 5-fluorodeoxyuridine monophosphate (FdUMP), which binds to TS and prevents formation of dTMP. The ability of 5-FU to inhibit TS can be enhanced in the presence of reduced folates such as leucovorin that stabilize the binding of FdUMP to TS and allow for a more sustained inhibition of dTMP formation. In addition, 5-FU can be metabolized to FUTP intracellularly, thus interfering with RNA synthesis. 5-FU in combination with leucovorin is part of the standard treatment for patients with metastatic colorectal cancer. Toxic effects of 5-FU include stomatitis, diarrhea, skin rash, and myelosuppression. The toxicity profile depends upon whether 5-FU is given by repeated daily doses, weekly, or by continuous intra-

FIGURE 57-6  Structural formulae of 5-fluorouracil and capecitabine.

5-FU

Capecitabine

mesothelioma in combination with cisplatin and as a single agent for the treatment of non-small-cell lung cancer (NSCLC) in patients who received prior chemotherapy. It is mainly eliminated through renal excretion, and it is not recommended in patients with renal clearance less than 45 mL/min. Major toxicities include myelosuppression, gastrointestinal toxicities, and skin rash. Supplementation with folic acid and vitamin $B_{12}$ can reduce toxicity. It is recommended that patients start taking oral folic acid supplement daily for at least five doses during the 7-day period preceding the first dose of pemetrexed and continue through therapy and for 21 days after the last dose.

venous infusion. 5-FU is rapidly inactivated to dihydrofluorouracil by the enzyme dihydropyrimidine dehydrogenase (DPD). Approximately 3 to 5% of patients have a partial deficiency (autosomal recessive in inheritance) of this enzyme and are at risk of severe toxicity from 5-FU.

**Capecitabine** (Xeloda; see Fig. 57-6) is an oral fluoropyrimidine that is absorbed intact through the gastrointestinal tract. It is subsequently converted to 5-FU via a three-step process, the last step of which is mediated by the enzyme thymidine phosphorylase. Thymidine phosphorylase can be more concentrated in tumour tissues than in normal tissue, resulting in preferential conversion of capecitabine in tumour tissues. Capecitabine is usually given orally for 2 consecutive weeks on a three-week schedule, mimicking continuous infusion of 5-FU. It is commonly used in the treatment of metastatic colorectal cancer and breast cancer. Side effects are similar to those of prolonged 5-FU infusion with lower incidences of myelosuppression and stomatitis, but higher incidences of palmar–plantar erythrodysesthesia (hand–foot syndrome) and diarrhea than seen with intravenous bolus 5-FU.

## Cytosine Arabinoside (Ara-C, Cytarabine)

Ara-C (Cytosar) is an arabinose nucleoside that differs from the nucleoside deoxycytidine by the presence of a β-OH group in the C-2 position of the sugar (Fig. 57-7). It is phosphorylated to ara-cytosine triphosphate (ara-CTP) intracellularly, which is a competitive inhibitor of DNA polymerase. By binding to this enzyme, ara-CTP arrests DNA synthesis, and replicating cells die. Ara-C can also be incorporated into DNA directly, leading to DNA chain termination due to defective ligation or incomplete synthesis of the complementary DNA strand. Therefore, this agent is more effective against cycling cells.

The drug is given intravenously, either by frequent injections or by continuous infusion, since it is rapidly degraded (half-life of 7 to 20 minutes) by the enzyme cyti-

dine deaminase found in blood. The parent compound and its inactive metabolite, uracil arabinoside, are excreted in the urine. Myelosuppression is the major dose-limiting toxicity, but gastrointestinal toxicity is also common. CNS toxicity, with abnormal behaviour and mentation, occurs uncommonly. This agent is used primarily for the treatment of acute leukemia and may be given intrathecally for meningeal infiltration by leukemia.

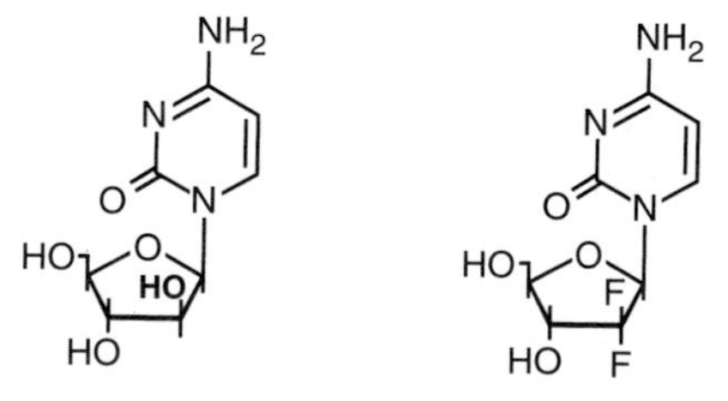

## Gemcitabine

Gemcitabine (2′,2′-difluorodeoxycytidine; Gemzar) is a cytosine analogue with structural similarities to cytosine arabinoside (see Fig. 57-7). Unlike ara-C, gemcitabine has significant activity against a variety of solid tumour cell lines, likely due to a longer intracellular retention. Similarly to ara-C, gemcitabine requires intracellular activation to its triphosphate derivative, which is incorporated into DNA and then inhibits DNA replication. Gemcitabine also has potent radiosensitizer properties, which may be associated with the depletion of deoxyadenosine triphosphate via the inhibition of ribonucleotide reductase. In clinical studies, gemcitabine is active against NSCLC and cancers of the pancreas, breast, head and neck (especially nasopharyngeal carcinoma), and bladder. The major toxicity is myelosuppression.

## Purine Antimetabolites

**6-Mercaptopurine** (6-MP; Purinethol) is a thiopurine analogue of hypoxanthine, a naturally occurring purine base. It is transformed intracellularly to ribonucleotide forms. These may be incorporated into RNA or DNA or act at several enzymatic steps in purine biosynthesis to inhibit purine formation. 6-MP is usually given orally, and its reported bioavailability is about 50%. The drug is degraded by xanthine oxidase to 6-thiouric acid, which is devoid of anti-tumour activity. Allopurinol, used for the treatment of hyperuricemia, may inhibit the degradation of 6-MP and thereby increase its toxicity. The major toxicity of 6-MP is myelosuppression. It is used clinically in the treatment of acute leukemia, particularly in children.

Analogues of adenine and adenosine are the DNA base analogues most recently introduced into clinical practice. **Fludarabine** (Fludara) is an adenosine derivative that is resistant to deamination by adenosine deaminase (ADA). It is rapidly dephosphorylated to 2-fluoro-ara-A, which is then transported into cells and converted to the active triphosphate derivative. Its mechanism of cytotoxicity includes inhibition of DNA polymerase, leading to termination of DNA and RNA replication. Fludarabine is active mainly against hematological tumours with low proportions of actively cycling cells (low-grade lymphomas, chronic lymphocytic leukemia, hairy cell leukemia, and Waldenstrom's macroglobulinemia). The major toxicities

---

**FIGURE 57-7** Structural formulae of cytosine arabinoside and gemcitabine.

Cytosine arabinoside

Gemcitabine

are myelosuppression and immunosuppression; other toxic effects are mild or infrequent.

**2-Chlorodeoxyadenosine** (2CdA; Cladribine) is a more potent fluorinated adenosine derivative. Its spectrum of activity and toxicity profile are similar to those of fludarabine.

**Deoxycoformycin** (Nipent) is an inhibitor of ADA that has demonstrated activity against hairy cell leukemia and some indolent lymphomas. It is not clear why an accumulation of normal adenine nucleosides would be cytotoxic, but it may lead to a secondary inhibition of DNA synthesis. The dosages required to maximally inhibit ADA lead to significant toxicity. However, "hairy cell" leukemias have low ADA activity, and the dose of deoxycoformycin required to treat this disease is therefore lower and has minimal toxicity.

# TOPOISOMERASE INHIBITORS

DNA topoisomerases I and II are ubiquitous nuclear enzymes that regulate the torsional strain of supercoiled DNA double helices during critical cellular processes such as replication, transcription, recombination, and repair. Torsional strain is relieved via the formation of a single-strand nick (topoisomerase I) or a double-strand nick (topoisomerase II), followed by swivelling of the DNA at the nick(s) and subsequent re-ligation. Topoisomerase inhibitors bind to and stabilize the DNA/topoisomerase "cleavable complex," thus preventing the re-ligation of DNA strands. Irreversible damage results when an advancing DNA replication fork encounters the drug-stabilized cleavable complex, ultimately leading to lethal double-stranded breaks and cell death.

## Topoisomerase I Inhibitors

### Camptothecin derivatives

The camptothecin derivatives are the only topoisomerase I inhibitors currently in clinical usage. Camptothecin was isolated from the stem wood of *Camptotheca acuminata*, a tree indigenous to northern China. Although the drug had demonstrable anti-tumour activity, clinical development in the early 1970s was terminated because of severe and unpredictable toxicity, namely hemorrhagic cystitis and severe diarrhea. Interest in developing camptothecins was renewed only when the mechanism of camptothecin anti-tumour activity was found to be inhibition of just topoisomerase I. Structure–activity studies established that several structural analogues, such as topotecan and irinotecan, had increased anti-tumour activity and better safety profiles.

The basic structure of camptothecin is a pentacyclic alkaloid (Fig. 57-8). Although the closed-ring lactone form is essential for its cytotoxic activity, all camptothecins can undergo a rapid, reversible, pH-dependent, non-enzymatic hydrolysis of the closed lactone ring to yield an open-ring carboxylate form. Human serum albumin preferentially binds to the carboxylate form, thereby shifting the equilibrium in favour of the inactive carboxylate. As a result, the carboxylate form predominates at physiological pH in vivo.

**Irinotecan** (CPT-11; Camptosar; see Fig. 57-8) is mainly degraded by the liver to inactive metabolites, with approximately 10% converted to an active metabolite SN-38 by carboxylesterase. SN-38 is conjugated to SN-38 glucuronide, which is then excreted via the biliary tract. Pharmacokinetic studies of CPT-11 demonstrate a triphasic plasma clearance curve with a half-life of 9 to 14 hours.

| FIGURE 57-8 | Structural formulae of camptothecins. |
| --- | --- |

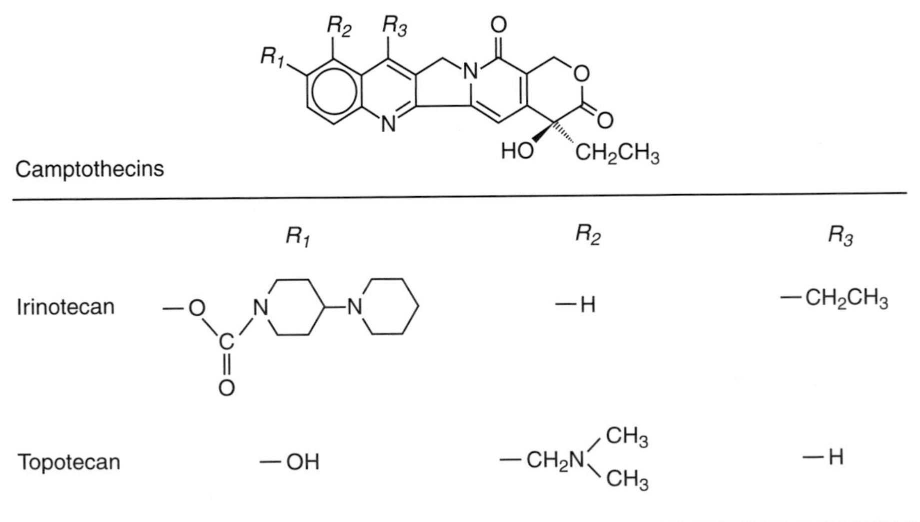

| Camptothecins | $R_1$ | $R_2$ | $R_3$ |
| --- | --- | --- | --- |
| Irinotecan | | —H | —$CH_2CH_3$ |
| Topotecan | —OH | —$CH_2N$ $\begin{smallmatrix}CH_3\\CH_3\end{smallmatrix}$ | —H |

The major side effects are myelosuppression and diarrhea. Irinotecan can produce a cholinergic syndrome consisting of abdominal cramps, diarrhea, and diaphoresis. This syndrome often occurs during or immediately after irinotecan infusion and can be effectively treated with subcutaneous or intravenous atropine. Prophylactic atropine prior to subsequent irinotecan infusions may prevent further episodes. A second distinct type of diarrhea, more severe and protracted, tends to have a delayed onset. This type of diarrhea is related to damage to the gastrointestinal mucosa caused by unconjugated SN-38. It requires aggressive pharmacological and supportive measures, such as loperamide, intravenous hydration, and hospitalization if persistent. Irinotecan is a useful drug for treating colorectal cancer, and it also has activity against small-cell lung cancer, other gastrointestinal cancers, and gynecological cancers.

**Topotecan** (Hycamtin; see Fig. 57-8) is administered intravenously or orally. It is primarily eliminated unchanged via renal excretion; therefore, dose reduction is required in patients with renal dysfunction. The drug has been used in the treatment of patients with NSCLC and ovarian cancer. Unlike irinotecan, it is not active against colorectal cancer. The major toxic effect is myelosuppression; other side effects include alopecia, mild diarrhea, and elevation of liver enzymes.

## Topoisomerase II Inhibitors

### Epipodophyllotoxins
**VP-16** (etoposide; VePesid) and **VM-26** (teniposide; Vumon) are semi-synthetic glycosidic derivatives of podophyllotoxin, which is an anti-mitotic agent derived from the mandrake plant. Although podophyllotoxins bind to tubulin, their cytotoxic activity is mainly mediated through inhibition of DNA topoisomerase II. Resistance to these drugs is correlated with decreased activity of DNA topoisomerase II, as well as over-expression of P-glycoprotein that promotes increased drug efflux from the tumour cells.

VP-16 is usually given intravenously, although it can be given orally with approximately 50% bioavailability and considerable inter-individual variability. After intravenous administration, the elimination of VP-16 from plasma follows a two-compartment model with initial and terminal elimination half-lives of approximately 3 and 15 hours. About 45% of administered drug is excreted unchanged in the urine and an additional 15% in the feces. Its dose-limiting toxicity is myelosuppression. VP-16 is used in treating small-cell lung cancer, testicular cancer, pediatric cancers, and lymphomas. Because of its lack of other toxicity, VP-16 is also commonly used in higher-dose chemotherapy regimens given prior to bone marrow transplantation. VM-26 is mainly used in childhood hematological malignancies.

## Anthracyclines

**Doxorubicin** (Adriamycin) and **daunorubicin** (Cerubidine) are antibiotics produced by the fungus *Streptomyces peucetius*. These drugs have a tetracyclic ring structure with an unusual sugar, daunosamine, attached by a glycosidic linkage (Fig. 57-9); their chemical structures differ by a single hydroxyl group at position C-14. Their mechanism of cytotoxicity is complex. A major effect involves binding with DNA topoisomerase II and inhibiting the re-ligating activity of this enzyme, thereby causing DNA double-stranded breaks and cell death. Other actions include DNA intercalation leading to partial unwinding of the DNA helix, and free radical formation by oxidation–reduction of the quinone-hydroquinone group.

**Doxorubicin** is administered intravenously and has an initial plasma half-life of 10 to 15 minutes and a terminal half-life of 25 to 30 hours. It is distributed widely in body tissues and is approximately 75 to 80% protein-bound in plasma. Doxorubicin is metabolized in the liver to doxorubicinol, which has some cytotoxic activity, and to several other inactive metabolites. Doxorubicin and its metabolites are then excreted via the biliary tract. Therefore, patients with hepatic dysfunction require dosage adjustment.

Doxorubicin is one of the most useful anti-neoplastic drugs available for the treatment of lymphoma, breast cancer, lung cancer, and sarcomas. Major acute adverse effects include myelosuppression, alopecia, local tissue necrosis (if extravasation occurs during intravenous administration), and mucositis. A major long-term toxicity is cardiomyopathy, which occurs with increasing frequency once the accumulative dose is over 500 mg/m². Patients with pre-existing cardiac diseases or those who have received mediastinal radiation are more likely to develop

FIGURE 57-9    Structural formulae of two anthracyclines.

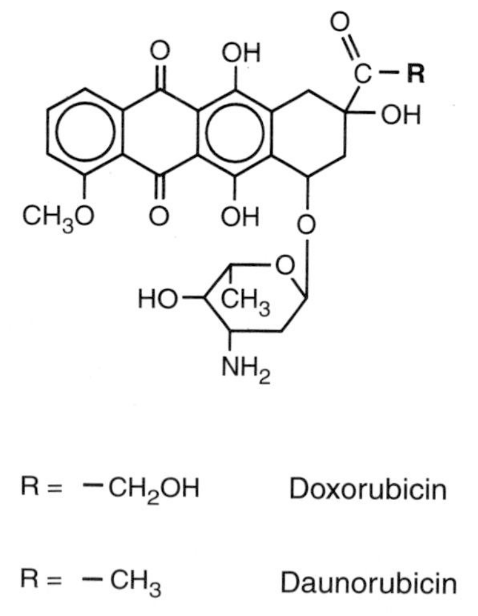

cardiomyopathy. The mechanism of cardiomyopathy is probably related to damage to sarcoplasmic reticulum of cardiac muscle by doxorubicin-induced free radicals. **Dexrazoxane**, an iron-chelating agent, has been shown to reduce cardiac toxicity without compromising efficacy when administered concurrently with doxorubicin.

**Epirubicin** (Pharmorubicin) differs from doxorubicin only in the position of the hydroxyl group on the daunosamine sugar. The clinical activity and toxicity are similar to those of doxorubicin, but the drug may be somewhat less cardiotoxic.

**Daunorubicin** is used in the treatment of acute leukemia in children and adults. Its toxic effects are similar to those of doxorubicin, except that it is less cardiotoxic.

**Mitoxantrone** (Novantrone) is a synthetic drug with a tricyclic structure; it intercalates between DNA bases and inhibits DNA topoisomerase II, thereby causing DNA double-stranded breaks and cell death. It lacks the ability to produce quinine-associated free radicals and therefore produces less cardiomyopathy. Mitoxantrone is used clinically in the treatment of breast and prostate cancer and in acute myeloblastic leukemia as an alternative to daunorubicin. Mitoxantrone causes fewer acute toxicities such as nausea, vomiting, and alopecia than are seen with doxorubicin.

## Actinomycin D

Actinomycin D (dactinomycin; Cosmegen) is produced by a fungus of the genus *Streptomyces*. It acts by intercalating between base pairs of DNA; it thus inhibits synthesis of RNA at low drug concentrations and synthesis of both RNA and DNA at higher drug concentrations. Like doxorubicin and daunorubicin, it also interacts with DNA topoisomerase II to produce DNA strand breaks. Dose-limiting toxicity is myelosuppression; other side effects include ulceration of the oral mucosa and gastrointestinal tract. Actinomycin D is used primarily in pediatric oncology in the treatment of Wilms' tumour, Ewing's sarcoma, and embryonal rhabdomyosarcoma.

## ANTI-MICROTUBULAR AGENTS

### Vinca Alkaloids

Vinca alkaloids are structurally similar compounds consisting of two multi-ringed subunits, vindoline and catharanthine (Fig. 57-10). The commonly used vinca alkaloids are **vincristine** (Oncovin, Vincasar), **vinblastine** (Velban), and **vinorelbine** (Navelbine). Vincristine and vinblastine are derived from the periwinkle plant, *Vinca rosea*.

The vinca alkaloids bind to tubulin and inhibit its polymerization to form microtubules. Microtubules have several important cellular functions, including formation of the mitotic spindle responsible for separation of chromosomes and structural and transport functions in axons of nerves. Microtubules are in a state of dynamic equilibrium, with continuous formation and degradation from cytoplasmic tubulin. This process is interrupted by treatment with vinca alkaloids, and lethally damaged cells may be observed to enter an abortive metaphase and then lyse.

The pharmacokinetics of vincristine and vinblastine are somewhat different because of their side-chain substitutions. Both drugs are given intravenously. Vincristine clearance is rapid, with a terminal half-life of 2 to 3 hours, while vinblastine is eliminated more slowly (terminal half-life of 20 hours). Both drugs are eliminated by hepatic biotransformation.

Vinblastine is used in the treatment of Hodgkin's disease and as a second-line drug in testicular cancer; vincristine is commonly used in treating non-Hodgkin's lymphoma and childhood leukemias. Their major toxicities are also different: neuropathy is the main dose-limiting toxicity for vincristine, and myelosuppression for vinblastine. Vincristine can also cause a syndrome of inappropriate antidiuretic hormone secretion (SIADH).

Vinorelbine (Navelbine) is a novel vinca alkaloid that differs structurally from the other vinca alkaloids in having a modified catharanthine subunit. Vinorelbine is administered intravenously. Its plasma clearance consists of a rapid distribution to peripheral tissues, an intermediate component representing drug metabolism, and a slow tertiary phase of drug efflux from those tissues. Clinically, the drug has been used to treat patients with advanced NSCLC and patients with metastatic breast cancer who have not responded to other chemotherapy.

### Taxanes

**Paclitaxel** (Taxol) and **docetaxel** (Taxotere) are plant alkaloids derived from the bark of the Pacific yew tree (*Taxus*

**FIGURE 57-10** Structural formulae of vinca alkaloids.

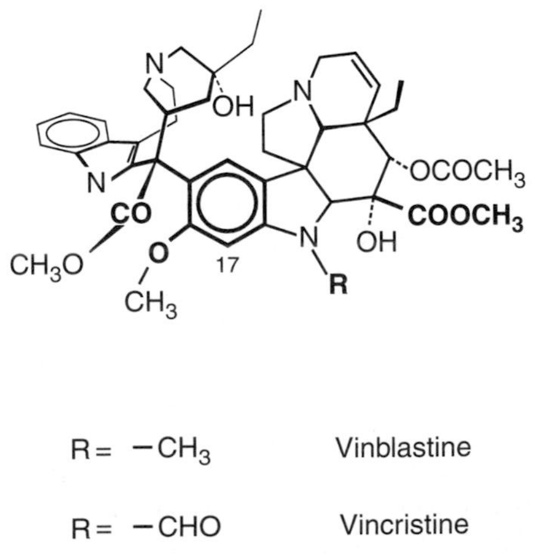

R = —CH₃      Vinblastine

R = —CHO      Vincristine

*brevifolia)* and the needles of European yew tree *(Taxus baccuta),* respectively. They consist of a 15-member taxane ring with an ester side chain attached to the C-13 position (Fig. 57-11). The ester side chain is essential for taxane anti-tumour activity. Taxanes bind to microtubules, but at sites different from those of vinca alkaloids. In contrast to vinca alkaloids, taxanes inhibit microtubule depolymerization and disrupt the normal growth and breakdown of microtubules essential for cell division.

Paclitaxel and docetaxel are administered intravenously and have large apparent volumes of distribution with extensive tissue binding. Both are mainly metabolized in the liver by cytochrome P450 enzymes. Therefore, agents that affect these enzymes can influence clearance and toxicity of taxanes. For example, patients on anticonvulsants have increased clearance and reduced toxicity. In addition, doses of both paclitaxel and docetaxel need to be adjusted in patients with hepatic dysfunction.

Taxanes can cause hypersensitivity reactions with bronchial constriction, urticaria, and hypotension. This problem can be prevented by prophylactic treatment with corticosteroids and histamine antagonists. Vehicles (Cremophor EL and polysorbate 80) in which taxanes are formulated to increase their water solubility have been implicated as possible causes of the hypersensitivity reaction. Paclitaxel and docetaxel share many other common toxicities, and for both of them the dose-limiting toxicity is myelosuppression. A peripheral sensory neuropathy can occur after repeated administration. Docetaxel can cause fluid retention and skin and nail changes.

Paclitaxel has activity against ovarian, breast, bladder, stomach, and non-small-cell lung cancers. It has also been used in combination with carboplatin for treating cancers of unknown origins. Docetaxel is used in treating breast, prostate, and non-small-cell lung cancers (NSCLC).

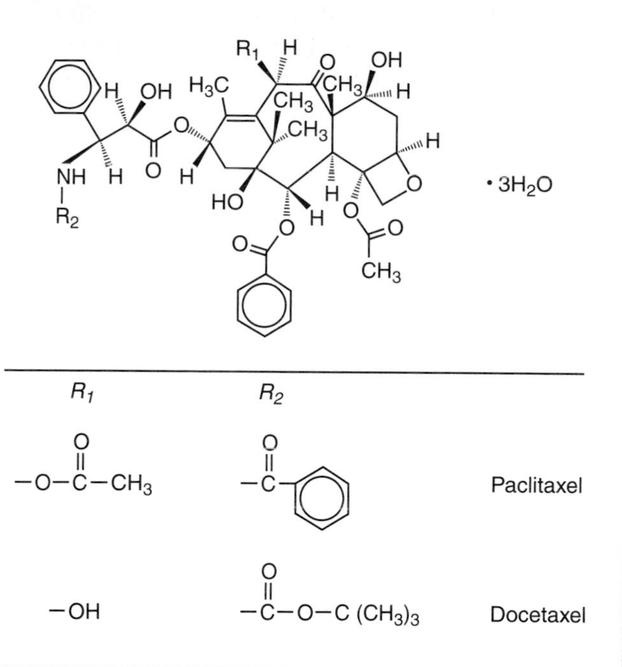

## MISCELLANEOUS CYTOTOXIC AGENTS

### L-Asparaginase

L-Asparaginase degrades L-asparagine to aspartic acid and ammonia. L-Asparagine is a non-essential amino acid synthesized by transamination of L-aspartic acid, catalyzed by the enzyme L-asparagine synthetase. Certain leukemic cells are deficient in this enzyme and therefore are dependent upon an extracellular supply of L-asparagine. If this supply is depleted by administration of L-asparaginase, cells lacking L-asparagine synthetase suffer marked inhibition of protein synthesis and cannot survive. In contrast, most normal cells can synthesize asparagines from aspartic acid by induction of L-asparagine synthetase. This treatment has proven useful in approximately 50% of cases of childhood acute lymphoblastic leukemia (ALL). Resistance occurs as a result of up-regulation of the expression of the gene for L-asparagine synthetase in cells exposed to L-asparaginase.

**FIGURE 57-11** Structural formulae of taxanes.

L-Asparaginase is usually administered intravenously. Two major side effects are hypersensitivity reactions and protein depletion. The enzyme is derived from *Escherichia coli* or *Erwinia carotovora* and is thus a foreign protein in humans; after repeated courses of treatment, hypersensitivity reactions such as urticaria, angioneurotic edema, bronchospasm, and hypotension may be observed. Inhibition of protein synthesis leads to depletion of anticoagulant and thrombolytic factors such as protein C, protein S, antithrombin III, and plasminogen and may result in thrombosis of major vessels. Other toxic effects that have been observed are nausea, vomiting, chills, and acute pancreatitis.

### Hydroxyurea

Hydroxyurea is a derivative of urea that is used primarily to rapidly reduce high white blood cell counts in patients with chronic myelogenous leukemia (CML). Its mechanism of action is inhibition of the enzyme ribonucleotide reductase, thereby depleting intracellular nucleotide pools and causing an accumulation of cells in late $G_1$ and early S phase of the cell cycle. Hydroxyurea is rapidly absorbed after oral administration. The drug has also been used to maintain patients with CML in remission, especially those who have developed resistance to the alkylating agent busulfan.

### Bleomycin

Bleomycin (Blenoxane) consists of a mixture of antibiotic peptides derived from fungal cultures with the predominant component being the bleomycin A2 peptide. Bleomycin produces DNA strand breaks through a complex sequence of reactions involving the binding of a bleomycin–ferrous iron complex to DNA, leading to DNA intercalation. In addition, the bleomycin–ferrous ion complex may catalyze formation of superoxide or hydroxyl radicals. Bleomycin is administered intravenously and is mainly eliminated unchanged in the urine. It is useful in combination chemotherapy for treating testicular cancer and lymphomas. It has little myelosuppressive activity but may cause fever, chills, hyperpigmentation, and skin thickening. Its dose-limiting toxicity is interstitial pulmonary fibrosis, the incidence of which is related to cumulative dose, age, renal function, and concurrent use of other agents that may cause lung damage, such as high-concentration oxygen therapy or radiation therapy.

## MOLECULAR TARGETED AGENTS

Cancer cells are characterized by self-sufficiency in growth signals, insensitivity to anti-growth signals, evasion of apoptosis, unlimited replicative potential, sustained angiogenesis, and tissue invasion and metastasis. With advances in molecular biology, many agents have been designed to specifically target certain steps in these processes. The majority of these agents are still in various stages of clinical development. Four currently approved agents are discussed briefly below.

### Rituximab

Rituximab (Rituxan) is a humanized monoclonal antibody against CD20, a protein present on the surface of almost all normal and malignant B cells. Although its exact mechanism remains unknown, rituximab can lyse CD20 cells in vitro through antibody-dependent cell-mediated cytotoxicity (ADCC), activation of the complement cascade, and induction of apoptosis. Rituximab was the first monoclonal antibody approved for therapeutic use against cancers, and it is indicated for treating B-cell lymphomas, either alone or in combination with chemotherapy. Infusion-related side effects are common and include fever, chills, hypotension, and nausea. These side effects are related to cytokine release after rituximab infusion and are more severe with the initial infusion. 5-HT$_3$ antagonists are used to manage these reactions.

### Imatinib

Most patients with CML carry the Philadelphia chromosome, which results from a reciprocal exchange of genetic material between the long arms of chromosomes 9 and 22. As a result of this translocation, a fusion gene, *bcr-abl* is formed. The BCR-ABL protein has tyrosine kinase activity and is constitutively active. It is thought to be the main cause of CML. Imatinib mesylate (STI-571; Gleevec) is a 2-phenylaminopyrimidine (Fig. 57-12) that specifically inhibits the BCR-ABL protein kinase activity, and it is active in chronic and blast phases of CML. In addition, imatinib can inhibit the tyrosine kinase activity of *c-kit*, which is commonly over-expressed in patients with gastrointestinal stromal tumours (GISTs). Recent studies show that imatinib can induce sustained responses in patients with advanced unresectable or metastatic GISTs. Imatinib is absorbed rapidly after oral administration and is mainly metabolized in the liver. The half-life of imatinib ranges from 13 to 16 hours. Imatinib is well tolerated. Common side effects include mild superficial edema, nausea, musculoskeletal pain, fatigue, and diarrhea. In addition, imatinib could cause elevation of liver enzymes and neutropenia in some patients.

### Trastuzumab

Trastuzumab (Herceptin) is a humanized monoclonal antibody against the human epidermal growth factor receptor 2 (HER2). HER2 is over-expressed in 25 to 30% of human breast cancers and is associated with a poorer prognosis. Trastuzumab is administered intravenously, once weekly, either alone or in combination with chemotherapy for metastatic breast cancer that over-expresses HER2. Common side effects include chills, asthenia, fever, and nausea. Rarely, trastuzumab can cause cardiac dysfunction. However, the risk of cardiac dysfunction increases significantly if trastuzumab is given together with other cardiotoxic agents such as anthracyclines.

### Bevacizumab

Bevacizumab (Avastin) is a humanized monoclonal antibody that binds and inhibits the human vascular endothelial growth factor (VEGF). VEGF is a soluble protein that plays an important role in inducing blood vessel formation, thereby allowing tumours to grow beyond a few millimetres in size. Bevacizumab is administered in combination with intravenous 5-FU-based chemotherapy for the treat-

**FIGURE 57-12** Structural formula of imatinib.

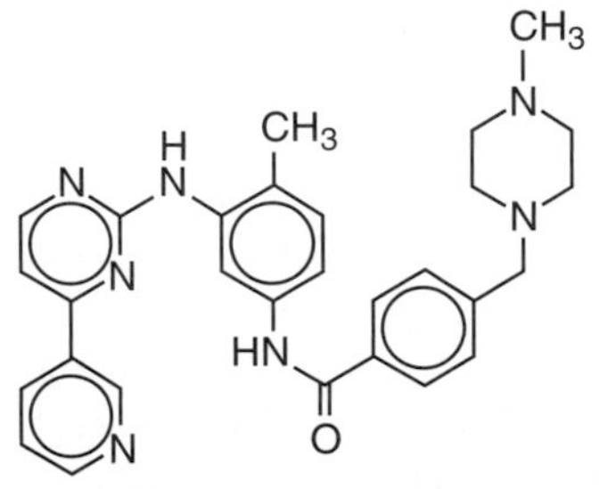

ment of metastatic colorectal cancer. Recent studies indicate that bevacizumab is also active in advanced NSCLC and breast cancer. Due to its anti-angiogenic action, bevacizumab can interfere with wound healing and increase the risk of bleeding or gastrointestinal perforation. Other side effects include hypertension and proteinuria.

## Inhibitors of Epidermal Growth Factor (EGFR)

The epidermal growth factor receptor (EGFR) is a transmembrane glycoprotein composed of an extracellular ligand-binding domain, a short transmembrane domain, and an intracellular domain that has tyrosine kinase activity. Binding of a specific ligand, such as epidermal growth factor, to the extracellular domain of EGFR induces conformational changes within the receptor and increases the activity of associated tyrosine kinases. This activity results in autophosphorylation and increased biological activity, which may include cell proliferation and/or differentiation. Abnormal EGFR expression, either through a mutation or over-expression, has been demonstrated in many malignancies. Inhibition of EGFR can be achieved by preventing ligand binding with an anti-EGFR antibody or by inhibiting EGFR-associated tyrosine kinases.

**Cetuximab** (Erbitux) is a human/mouse chimeric monoclonal antibody that binds to the extracellular domain of EGFR. Cetuximab reverses the resistance of colorectal cancer to irinotecan and is used in combination with irinotecan in the treatment of EGFR over-expressing metastatic colorectal cancer in patients who are refractory to irinotecan. The most common side effect of cetuximab is an acne-like rash. It is interesting to note that the development of the rash is associated with a higher likelihood of tumour control.

**Erlotinib** (OSI-774; Tarceva; Fig. 57-13) is an orally active, potent, and selective inhibitor of EGFR tyrosine kinases. Growth inhibition and tumour regression have been seen in human xenograft models in lung, prostate, breast, and colorectal cancers. Erlotinib is approved for the treatment of refractory advanced NSCLC. However, recent studies have shown promising results in advanced pancreatic cancer and as an adjuvant therapy for NSCLC. Toxicity is mainly skin rash and diarrhea. **Gefitinib** (Iressa; see Fig. 57-13) is another orally administered quinazoline-based molecule that inhibits EGFR tyrosine kinases. Gefitinib is also indicated for the treatment of refractory NSCLC.

## Bortezomib

Bortezomib (PS-341; Velcade) is a boronic acid dipeptide which binds to the 26S proteasome and inhibits the proteasome pathway. The ubiquitin–proteasome pathway plays an important role in regulating intracellular concentrations of proteins and maintaining intracellular homeostasis. Although bortezomib is currently indicated

for the treatment of multiple myeloma, it has also shown activity in other cancers, such as lymphoma and NSCLC. Common side effects include myelosuppression, peripheral neuropathy, and gastrointestinal toxicities.

## HORMONES

## Glucocorticoids

These agents have useful roles in the treatment of many cancers, either for their anti-tumour effect or for treatment of complications related to malignancy. **Dexamethasone** in combination with a 5-HT$_3$ antagonist is effective in treating chemotherapy-induced nausea and vomiting. **Prednisone** is often combined with other drugs in the treatment of leukemia, myeloma, lymphomas, and prostate cancer. Glucocorticoids are also useful for treating patients with brain edema and hypercalcemia.

## Hormones for the Treatment of Breast Cancer

Many breast cancers grow more rapidly in the presence of female hormones. Whether a breast cancer will respond to hormonal therapy can often be predicted by the amounts of estrogen and progesterone receptors in the tumour tissue. The hormonal treatments for breast cancer include anti-estrogens (tamoxifen), aromatase inhibitors (anastrozole, letrozole, exemestane), or progestational agents (megestrol acetate). For tumours that are positive for hormone receptors, a hormonal treatment would generally be

**FIGURE 57-13** Structural formulae of erlotinib and gefitinib.

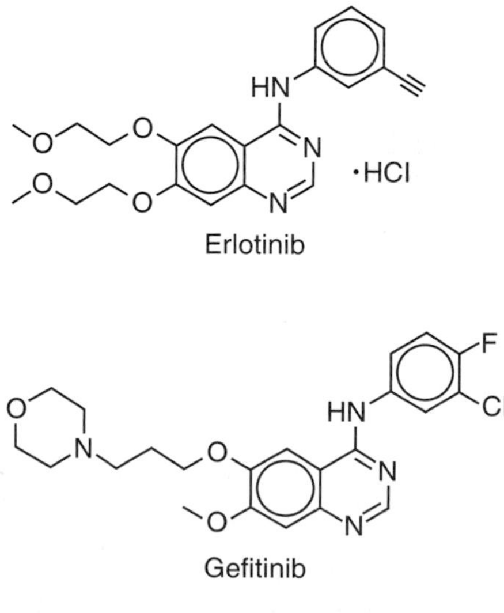

used before any chemotherapy because there is a higher chance of success and the toxicities are generally less severe.

## Selective estrogen receptor modulators (SERMs)

**Tamoxifen** (Nolvadex and others; see Fig. 46-7) is a non-steroidal analogue of clomiphene (see Chapter 46). It competitively binds to the estrogen receptor, but with a lower affinity than that of estrogen. When this tamoxifen–estrogen receptor complex is translocated to the nucleus, transcription of estrogen-responsive genes involved in the development and growth of breast cancer is attenuated. However, tamoxifen may exert estrogen agonist effects in other tissues, such as bone and uterus.

Approximately 70% of breast cancers are positive for estrogen and progesterone receptors and may respond to tamoxifen. The drug is given orally and undergoes extensive hepatic biotransformation. The two major metabolites, 4-hydroxytamoxifen and desmethyltamoxifen, have long half-lives and also have anti-estrogen activity. Conjugates are excreted in the bile and undergo extensive enterohepatic recirculation. Toxicity is generally mild, consisting chiefly of nausea and menopausal symptoms, but the drug can produce a transient flare-up of pain and other symptoms arising from the breast cancer and metastases. In addition, long-term use of tamoxifen is associated with increased risks of thromboembolic disorders and endometrial cancer. The incidence of endometrial cancer is approximately four times greater in women receiving 5 years of tamoxifen compared with that of the general population. Tamoxifen is indicated for the prevention of breast cancer in high-risk women; for adjuvant therapy after surgery, chemotherapy, and radiation in women with early-stage breast cancer; or for treating metastatic breast cancer.

**Toremifene** (Fareston) was developed as a result of efforts to find tamoxifen analogues without estrogen agonist properties. It is as effective as tamoxifen in treating metastatic breast cancer in post-menopausal women, but the risk of endometrial cancer is also similar to that of tamoxifen.

## Aromatase inhibitors

Aromatase is the enzyme that catalyzes the final and rate-limiting step in the synthesis of estrogens. In post-menopausal women, estrogen synthesized in tissues such as muscle and fat becomes the dominant source of estrogen. Enzymes related to aromatase also catalyze the conversion of cholesterol to pregnenolone, an important step in the synthesis of steroid hormones.

The first aromatase inhibitor introduced clinically, **aminoglutethimide** (Cytadren), is a non-specific inhibitor of aromatase and other related enzymes. Thus, patients treated with aminoglutethimide require co-administration of corticosteroids. More specific aromatase inhibitors with better toxicity profiles have replaced it in clinical practice. Currently available aromatase inhibitors fall into two classes: class I inhibitors have a steroidal structure and bind to aromatase irreversibly, while class II inhibitors are non-steroidal and bind to aromatase reversibly.

**Anastrozole** (Arimidex) and **letrozole** (Femara) are class II aromatase inhibitors (see Fig. 46-8). Blood levels of estrogens can be suppressed 85% or more from baseline with chronic administration of anastrozole or letrozole. Both agents are administered orally, with rapid absorption and extensive hepatic metabolism. Half-lives of anastrozole and letrozole are approximately 2 days. Both agents are generally well tolerated, although about 20% of patients using them do initially experience mild menopausal-like symptoms or nausea.

**Exemestane** (Aromasin) is a class I aromatase inhibitor. It is rapidly absorbed after oral administration with a bioavailability of approximately 40%. Exemestane is extensively distributed and mainly converted to inactive metabolites in the liver. Like anastrozole and letrozole, exemestane is generally well tolerated.

These three agents have similar activity, and they have not been compared with one another in randomized trials. Anastrozole and letrozole are used for treating advanced breast cancer in post-menopausal women. Exemestane is currently used as second-line treatment after tamoxifen failure. It has also demonstrated activity in patients whose diseases are refractory to non-steroidal aromatase inhibitors. Recently, letrozole has been shown to be effective as adjuvant therapy in patients who have completed 5 years of tamoxifen.

## Progestational agents

It is not clear how these drugs act to suppress breast cancer, but **medroxyprogesterone** and **megestrol** are both known to be active against hormone-sensitive cancers. Aromatase inhibitors have largely replaced them.

# Hormones for the Treatment of Prostate Cancer

Most prostate cancer cells are stimulated by androgens. It was discovered over 50 years ago that the removal of male hormones by surgical castration could lead to regression of advanced prostate cancer. More recently, a variety of pharmacological approaches have been developed, based either on inhibition of androgen production or on blockade of androgen action (anti-androgens). Androgen synthesis occurs mainly in the testis, but a small proportion (5 to 10%) occurs in the adrenal gland. To achieve nearly complete androgen blockade, an inhibitor of testicular androgen production is combined with an anti-androgen. The agents used are described below.

## Gonadotropin-releasing hormone agonists

Gonadotropin-releasing hormone (GnRH) is a hypothalamic polypeptide that binds to receptors in the pituitary gland and stimulates the production of luteinizing hormone (LH) and follicle-stimulating hormone (FSH). In the male, LH stimulates testosterone production and secretion. Normal secretion is pulsatile; with continuous GnRH secretion, there is an immediate increase in LH and FSH secretion followed by complete inhibition of their release. Various synthetic GnRH analogues cause a biochemical castration by binding very strongly to the receptor and suppressing the pituitary–gonadal axis. These analogues are given parenterally or intranasally; monthly and three-monthly depot formulations are also available. The commercial preparations include **leuprolide** (Lupron), **buserelin** (Suprefact), and **goserelin** (Zoladex); all provide results equivalent to an orchiectomy and differ mainly in the route of administration. These agents have similar side effects related to the ablation of androgens, such as hot flashes, sweating, and nausea.

## Estrogens

High doses of estrogens will also inhibit androgen production by feedback inhibition of LH release. The preparation most commonly used has been **diethylstilbestrol**. The use of estrogens has fallen out of favour because of excessive cardiovascular side effects with the higher doses.

## Anti-androgens

**Flutamide** (Euflex, Eulexin), **bicalutamide** (Casodex), and **nilutamide** (Anandron) are non-steroidal agents that block effects of dihydrotestosterone (DHT) at the androgen receptor. The side effects are primarily related to androgen deficiency. A compensatory increase in testosterone secretion may partially overcome the effects of these drugs. Anti-androgens are not appropriate as single agents in the therapy of prostate cancer but are most effective in combination with an inhibitor of androgen production.

**Cyproterone** (Androcur) is a steroidal anti-androgen that also blocks DHT at the androgen receptor. It does have anti-gonadotrophic effects as well; it produces feedback inhibition of GnRH release so that no compensatory increase in testosterone secretion occurs. It is thus suitable for single-agent therapy of prostate cancer.

## DEVELOPMENT OF NEW CANCER TREATMENTS

Currently available chemotherapy can cure testicular cancer, Hodgkin's disease, non-Hodgkin's lymphoma, choriocarcinoma, and many childhood cancers. Although some of the common solid tumours can be cured by adjuvant chemotherapy, most are relatively resistant. The development of new drugs and strategies to improve the results of cancer chemotherapy is a priority.

The screening of naturally occurring and synthetic compounds is one strategy of drug development. New compounds are screened for activity against human and animal tumour cell lines in vitro. The most promising agents are tested further to identify the maximally tolerated dose in mice and other species. Other new agents are developed as specific inhibitors of pathways known to be important in cancer growth and metastasis. As our understanding of cancer biology continues to grow, more drugs are being developed on the basis of known pathways involved in cancer progression and unique activity in preclinical models, rather than through large-scale screening of naturally occurring compounds.

Initial testing of new anti-cancer drugs in humans is often performed in cancer patients when no other treatment is available or when conventional therapy has been unsuccessful. In analogy to universal drug development and testing rules, these studies are referred to as phase I or dose-finding trials. The starting dose, based on the patient's body surface area, is usually equivalent to one-tenth of the maximally tolerated dose in the mouse. If this produces no major toxicity, the dose may be escalated by 25 to 100% in the next group of patients. This process continues until the maximally tolerated dose (MTD) is determined. Once the MTD has been ascertained, phase II studies are conducted. These studies involve patients with cancer of a specific type or site who meet defined eligibility criteria. A drug dose slightly less than the MTD is used. Assessment of anti-tumour efficacy is the major purpose. If the drug shows promising activity (usually defined as reduction in the size of measurable lesions), then further studies are performed. These might include studies of combination therapy with other active drugs or comparisons with the best available current therapy in randomized phase III trials.

## SUGGESTED READINGS

Chabner BA, Longo DL, eds. *Cancer Chemotherapy and Biotherapy: Principles and Practice.* 3rd ed. Philadelphia, Pa: Lippincott Williams & Wilkins; 2001.

Chu E, DeVita VT Jr. Principles of cancer management: chemotherapy. In: DeVita VT Jr, Hellman S, Rosenberg SA, eds. *Cancer: Principles and Practice of Oncology.* 6th ed. Philadelphia, Pa: Lippincott Williams & Wilkins; 2001:289-306.

Perry MC, Anderson CM, Donehower RD. Chemotherapy. In: Abeloff MD, Armitage JO, Lichter AS, Niederhuber JE, eds. *Clinical Oncology.* 2nd ed. New York, NY: Churchill Livingstone; 2000:378-422.

Pharmacology of cancer chemotherapy. In: DeVita VT Jr, Hellman S, Rosenberg SA, eds. *Cancer: Principles and Practice of Oncology.* 6th ed. Philadelphia, Pa: Lippincott Williams & Wilkins; 2001:335-460.

Siu LL, Moore MJ. Pharmacology of anticancer drugs. In: Tannock I, Hill R, eds. *The Basic Science of Oncology.* New York, NY: McGraw-Hill; 2004:317-337.

# Part X

Special Topics of Pharmacology

# 58

# Sources of Individual Variation in Drug Response

## H KALANT

In all textbooks of pharmacology, medicine, and therapeutics, recommended dosages of drugs are given in absolute amounts (e.g., 10 mg three times daily) or, less frequently, in amounts relative to body weight (e.g., 1 mg/kg). Such dosages represent a combination of statistical statement and value judgement because they are based on extensive clinical observations indicating that the recommended dosage will, in *most* patients, on *most* occasions, produce the desired therapeutic effect with an *acceptably low* risk of toxicity.

Like all statistical statements, dosage recommendations represent mean values and imply that some individuals will require more than the mean and some will require less. This chapter deals with the following basic question: If an accepted normal dosage of a drug is prescribed, why do some patients show either too much or too little response? The answer to this question is really a composite of the answers to four subsidiary questions:

1. Was the prescribed dosage (both amount and frequency) actually taken by the patient? This is dealt with below under the heading "**Compliance.**"
2. If it was taken as prescribed, was it properly absorbed and delivered to the systemic circulation? This is considered under "**Bioavailability.**"
3. If absorbed and delivered to the circulation, was the drug distributed normally in the body, in such a way as to achieve the intended concentration and duration at the site(s) of action? This is examined under sources of "**Pharmacokinetic Variation.**"
4. If the drug was distributed in the expected way, did the target tissue(s) respond to it in the usual manner? This is considered under sources of "**Pharmacodynamic Variation.**"

## COMPLIANCE (ADHERENCE)

Most patients probably do intend to comply with (adhere to) their physicians' instructions concerning prescribed medication because most prescriptions are filled promptly. One study showed that 97% of the prescriptions written by physicians were filled within 5 days. If the patients did not intend to take the drugs, it is unlikely that they would go to the trouble and expense of having the prescriptions filled at a pharmacy. However, other studies have found that actual compliance with the physician's instructions is quite variable: for *short-term preventive* medication (i.e., medication intended to prevent the development of symptoms rather than to treat existing ones), the compliance rate was found to be about 80%; for *long-term preventive* medication (e.g., for the treatment of asymptomatic hypertension), compliance was only 40%.

## Methods of Studying Compliance

There are two basic types of method used for studying drug compliance: self-report and independent (non-self) measures. Self-report methods include the use of drug diaries, in which the patient is required to mark down the date, time, drug name, and amount of each dose taken; questionnaires; and patient interviews by a physician or nurse. Independent measures include a variety of quite different methods, such as pill counts or weighing the container when the patient brings the medication vials to the physician's office at periodic visits, electronic microprocessors built into the vial cap that record every opening of the container, measurement of drug levels in plasma or blood, and administrative records of claims submitted to insuring agencies for reimbursement of drug costs.

The degree of concordance between self-report and independent measures varies widely with the different methods used. Interview data have a significantly poorer agreement with independent measures than questionnaire or diary data do. This means that if the physician suspects non-compliance with the prescribed regimen, it will be necessary to do more than simply ask the patients if they have been taking their medications as prescribed.

## Factors Affecting Degree of Compliance

Investigators have assessed the possible contributions of many individual factors that might conceivably affect the patient's understanding of the physician's instructions and the willingness or determination to follow them.

A variety of **demographic factors** such as sex, socio-economic status, educational level, and ethnic background do not appear to exert any significant effect on the degree of compliance. Age per se also does not appear to be a significant factor, but it does have an important indirect role. With increasing age, there is a higher probability of having more than one illness at the same time and, therefore, of having more than one prescribed medication to be used concurrently. This introduces an element of increased complexity in the treatment schedule, which increases the likelihood of forgetting some of the doses or confusing the amounts to be taken (see Chapter 62). In addition, some elderly persons have memory problems that can interfere with their ability to adhere to dosage regimens even though they intend to do so.

There is also no significant correlation with any **specific disease** for which the medication is prescribed. Non-compliance is a frequent problem in conditions as diverse as grand mal epilepsy, diabetes mellitus, arterial hypertension, chronic affective disorder, HIV infection, and even immunosuppression therapy after organ transplants. Recent meta-analyses have shown non-compliance rates as high as 70% in hypertension, 50% in type 2 diabetes mellitus, and 45% in depression. The pathophysiology in these various diseases is obviously quite unrelated, but they have in common the fact that they are chronic diseases that require prolonged or lifetime drug therapy, in many cases, with more than one drug concurrently.

It is possible that in the cases of some psychiatric illnesses, such as schizophrenia, the disease itself may interfere with the patient's attention to, or comprehension of, the physician's explanations or may give rise to negative responses, apathy, or inertia. In such cases, responsibility for ensuring that the prescribed dosage schedule is followed should probably be assigned to a family member, friend, or guardian of the patient.

The degree of **complexity** and **inconvenience** of the treatment schedule can have an important effect in decreasing compliance. The larger the number of different drugs the patient must take, the poorer the compliance, especially if the drugs are to be taken at varying times of day and for different numbers of times each day. In general, compliance is better with drugs that have a long half-life or come in special formulations that permit once-daily dosage than with drugs or preparations requiring multiple daily doses. This may be one reason for the marketing of pharmaceutical mixtures, in which a single tablet or capsule contains fixed proportions of two or more drugs that are frequently prescribed together for patients with certain illnesses. Among the very numerous examples are combinations of a thiazide diuretic with a hypotensive agent (for hypertension), an atropine-like anticholinergic agent with a sedative (for peptic ulcer), a non-steroidal anti-inflammatory agent with an $H_2$ receptor blocker or prostaglandin $E_1$ (for rheumatoid arthritis), and a glucocorticoid with a β-adrenergic agonist (for bronchial asthma). It is possible that compliance is improved by such mixtures as the patient has to remember only a single dosage instruction. However, the serious disadvantage is the loss of therapeutic flexibility since the dosages of the individual constituents of the mixture cannot be separately adjusted according to the patient's needs and responses.

In contrast, several factors contribute significantly to improved compliance. One is the **continuity and ease of contact with the physician.** The longer the patient has known and trusted the physician and the more convenient and prompt the follow-up visits are, the better the physician's opportunity to remind the patient about the importance of the drugs and to strengthen the patient's motivation to use them. Closely related to this factor is the **patient's perception of the seriousness of the disease and the importance and efficacy of the drug therapy.** Compliance tends to improve if the patient believes that the disease is serious or that the drug is effective. In contrast, medications or treatment schedules with a high incidence of unpleasant side effects generally give rise to poor compliance.

**An illustrative case:** High blood pressure per se does not cause obvious and troublesome symptoms in the majority of patients. On the other hand, the adverse effects of antihypertensive drugs may cause some patients to feel miserable. It is not surprising, therefore, that patients who are not feeling ill frequently fail to comply with their physician's recommendations to take drugs that are intended to prevent the occurrence of cerebral, cardiac, or renal consequences of hypertension at some unknown time in the future.

A study carried out by the employee medical service of a large steel factory yielded interesting results on improvement of compliance in hypertension. Of 230 hypertensive employees, 38 were identified as non-compliant with instructions on medication. Twenty of these employees were placed on an experimental protocol for 6 months. Even when these men were given better opportunities to see the doctor, for instance during working hours, or received instruction about the nature of hypertension, most of them remained non-compliant, and their blood pressure remained elevated. However, when the patients were taught to measure their own blood pressure, were asked to chart their own pressure readings and record the taking of their medication, and were taught how to fit drug-taking into their daily routines, and when these behaviours were reinforced with supervision every 2 weeks, the compliance increased by 21%, and the control of their blood pressure improved significantly (Fig. 58-1). This study demonstrated that compliance with medication instructions can be improved in hypertensive patients by the use of proper methods.

Important measures to assure compliance in long-term therapy include simplified dosage schedules, use of long-acting rather than short-acting drugs, choosing drugs with minimal side effects, giving written instructions about the medications, and assuring continuous supervision of the patient. In addition, patients should be thoroughly familiarized with the importance of taking prescribed drugs regularly in order to prevent the serious consequences of high blood pressure. The physician can help to monitor compliance by asking patients to bring their medication bottles with them when they come for checkups. Comparison of the number of tablets or capsules prescribed and the number remaining will help to identify patients who are not taking the drugs regularly. *Such principles are not specific for antihypertensive therapy, but apply equally to medications used in long-term treatment of other diseases.*

# BIOAVAILABILITY

The concept of bioavailability, methods of measuring it, and its clinical significance are all covered in detail in Chapters 5 and 6. Therefore, the topic is mentioned only briefly here as one potentially important source of variation in drug response.

As described in Chapter 5, the term "bioavailability" refers to the fraction of an administered dose (by any route other than intravenous) that is absorbed and reaches the systemic circulation in its original (i.e., unmetabolized) form. Bioavailability is most commonly measured by determining the area under the concentration–time curve after an administered dose and expressing it as a percentage of

the corresponding area after intravenous injection of the same dose. This percentage can be reduced, for the same preparation of the same drug, by a variety of physiological and pathological factors in the gastrointestinal tract and liver. For example, the rate of gastric emptying has a marked influence on the apparent bioavailability of drugs that are absorbed primarily in the upper small intestine. The presence of food in the stomach and the resulting delay in gastric emptying can result in an apparent decrease in bioavailability; unusually rapid emptying can result in an apparent increase. Intestinal hypermotility, diarrhea, steatorrhea, biliary obstruction, reduced gastrointestinal blood flow, and induction of hepatic or intestinal drug uptake and biotransformation (see Chapter 4) can all reduce the fraction of an oral dose that finally reaches the systemic circulation and hence reduce the drug effect. In contrast, liver disease, especially in cases that produce intrahepatic or extrahepatic shunts (see Chapter 43), may result in an unusually large fraction of the dose reaching the circulation and producing an unexpectedly large effect. Inhibition of hepatic or intestinal drug-metabolizing enzymes can also increase systemic drug levels and drug effects.

Some drugs are administered as prodrugs that must be acted on by intestinal enzymes before the active drug can be absorbed. For example, flavonoids such as quercetin exist in the diet as glycosides, and rutin (quercetin rutinoside) is administered as a vasoprotective agent. These glycosides must be split by intestinal mucosal β-glucosidases before the aglycone can be absorbed. Marked variability in the activity of these enzymes results in substantial interindividual variability in the bioavailability of quercetin.

The factors affecting drug bioavailability differ according to the route of administration, but the effect is not the same for all drugs. For example, inter-individual variation in bioavailability is greater for rectal administration than for oral administration of the anti-malarial agent artemisinin, but it is greater for oral than for rectal administration of tetrahydrocannabinol.

Independently of the patient, however, bioavailability may vary because of differences in the formulation of the preparation, leading to differences in the rate and completeness of release of the active drug into solution in the gastrointestinal fluid. Dissolution is a necessary first step before the drug can be absorbed. If it does not occur rapidly enough, the undissolved part of the dose may be lost in the feces. For this reason, an overly compacted tablet may exhibit lower bioavailability than the same dose of the drug given as a solution (Fig. 58-2). Different companies marketing the same drug may use different tablet formulations, which may differ significantly in disintegration rate and uniformity. Some preparations may be better formulated than others, giving better and more uniform bioavailability (Fig. 58-3), and the physician must be aware of potential differences of this type when evaluating different products in clinical practice.

FIGURE 58-1 | The effect on blood pressure of improved compliance with dosage recommendations due to combined strategies. (From Haynes et al., 1976. Reprinted with permission.)

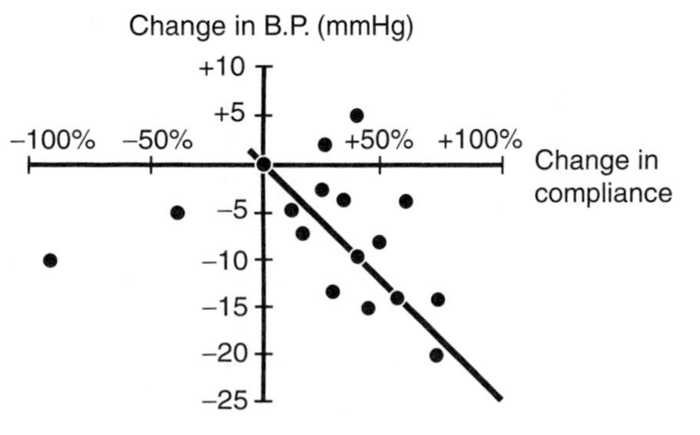

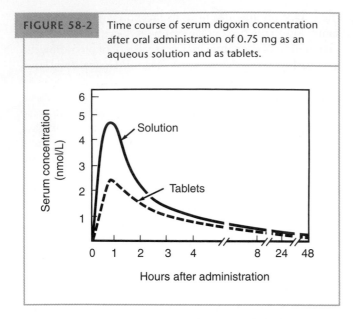

FIGURE 58-2  Time course of serum digoxin concentration after oral administration of 0.75 mg as an aqueous solution and as tablets.

## PHARMACOKINETIC VARIATION

Apart from variations in drug absorption and bioavailability mentioned above, other important pharmacokinetic factors contributing to variation in drug response are differences in drug distribution, biotransformation, and elimination. Some of the main sources of **variation in drug biotransformation** are reviewed in Chapter 4. Genetically determined alterations in biotransformation are discussed in Chapter 10. The effects of liver disease on drug biotransformation and elimination are covered in some detail in Chapter 43.

The potential magnitude of these variations is illustrated by the following examples:

- In a group of geriatric inpatients, the mean plasma half-life of antipyrine was 45% greater and that of phenylbutazone was 29% greater than in young controls (i.e., impaired hepatic biotransformation).
- Absorption of a 400-mg oral dose of mecillinam was only slightly reduced in a group of elderly subjects (aged 65 years or more) compared with a group of young adults, but the elimination half-life was markedly prolonged (4 versus 0.9 hours), and the urinary drug levels were correspondingly lower in the elderly (i.e., impaired renal excretion).
- The plasma levels of phenacetin after a standard dose were markedly lower in regular smokers than in non-smokers (i.e., induction of biotransforming enzymes) (Table 58-1).

The main causes of variation in **drug distribution** are those associated with early infancy (see Chapter 61) and

advanced age (see Chapter 62). However, drug distribution may be affected at any age by differences in **body composition.** It is generally recognized that dosage for adults should take account of body size and body build. Obviously, a large person will need more drug than a small person to achieve the same desired drug concentration in the blood or tissues. This is the basis for giving dosages in relative values (such as mg/kg). However, the modifying factor of the percentage of body fat must be taken into account. Many differences in drug response between men and women (e.g., to ethanol; see Chapter 22) are due to differences in body composition, especially in the percentage of body fat. An obese person will require a lower dose of a highly water-soluble drug than a lean person *of the same total body weight* in order to avoid excessively high drug concentration in the body water, including the plasma water. Conversely, the obese person will probably require more of a lipid-soluble drug than the lean person to achieve the same plasma level, but the large store of drug in body fat may result in greatly prolonged drug action.

Drug distribution may also be modified by disease processes. For example, normally the blood–brain barrier hinders the passage of penicillin and various other antibiotics into the central nervous system; however, in the presence of inflammatory conditions (meningitis), the permeability of the blood–brain barrier is increased, and these antibiotics pass much more readily and attain a higher concentration in the central nervous system (CNS). This improves their therapeutic value but may also increase the risk of seizures or other toxic effects in the brain. In contrast, when an inflammatory process gives rise to a localized abscess or other walled-off infection (e.g., empyema), systemic antibiotic therapy may be ineffective because the drug will not be distributed into the abscess or other cavity in which the bacteria are growing. For this reason, surgical

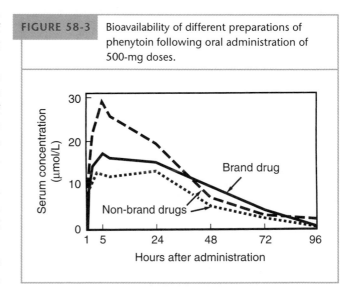

FIGURE 58-3  Bioavailability of different preparations of phenytoin following oral administration of 500-mg doses.

| TABLE 58-1 | Plasma Levels of Phenacetin (µg/mL) in Cigarette Smokers and Non-smokers at Various Times after Oral Administration of 900 mg of Phenacetin | | | |
|---|---|---|---|---|
| | **Hours after Phenacetin Administration** | | | |
| | 1 | 2 | 3.5 | 5 |
| Non-smokers | 0.81 | 2.24 | 0.39 | 0.12 |
| Smokers | 0.33 | 0.48 | 0.09 | 0.02 |

(Data from Kuntzman R et al. Phenacetin metabolism: Effect of hydrocarbons and cigarette smoking. *Clin Pharmacol Ther.* 1977;22:757-764.)

drainage may be required, together with local application of the antibiotic directly into the affected site.

## VARIATION IN REQUIRED DOSAGE IN CHILDREN

A special case of pharmacokinetic variation as a source of variation in drug response is encountered in relation to dosage in children of different ages. As noted above, body composition can account for substantial differences in the drug concentration produced by a given dose. However, the required dose for a given individual is usually more strictly proportional to **body surface area** than to body weight. The discrepancy is not large for adults but is important for babies and small children, whose surface-to-mass ratio is considerably higher than that of adults. The relationship is described by the equation $S$ (cm$^2$) = $W^{0.425}$ (kg) $\times$ $H^{0.725}$ (cm) $\times$ 71.8, but this is obviously impractical for calculating dosages in a physician's office or a patient's home. Therefore, simplified approximations have been made for calculating **children's doses** on the basis of age or surface area.

### Calculation of children's dose by age (Young's rule):

Age/(age + 12) = fraction of adult dose to be given to child

### Calculation of children's dose by body surface area:

(1.5 $\times$ weight in kg) + 10 = percentage of adult dose to be given to child

Each of these calculations is based on some standard of comparison. Young's rule makes the assumption that a 12-year-old, weighing 35 to 40 kg, should receive one-half of an adult dose. The surface area rule is based on the assumption that the average adult has about 65 kg of metabolically active mass and a corresponding surface area of about 1.7 m$^2$. Table 58-2 illustrates the relative doses calculated by these two methods. The younger the child, the more clearly superior is the surface area method of calculation.

## PHARMACODYNAMIC VARIATION

Variations in drug response are probably less frequently attributable to changes in responsiveness of the target tissue than to the causes discussed in the preceding sections. Nevertheless, there are some important instances. Examples of **genetically determined abnormalities** of tissue response to drugs, such as malignant hyperthermia and β-adrenergic receptor polymorphisms, are described in Chapter 10.

Other changes in tissue response can be caused by **disease processes.** For example, hyperthyroidism is frequently associated with an increased number of β-adrenoceptors, leading to increased sensitivity to the cardiovascular and other effects of noradrenaline and related catecholamines.

Sometimes **drug interactions** will alter pharmacodynamic sensitivity to one or more of the drugs concerned (Chapter 60). Patients with chronic left ventricular failure, for example, may be given a diuretic as well as a cardiac glycoside. Improvement in cardiac output by the cardiac glycoside increases renal blood flow and may therefore improve the urinary response to the diuretic. Conversely, if the diuretic then causes excessive loss of K$^+$ in the urine, the hypokalemia will increase myocardial sensitivity to the digitalis glycoside and increase the risk of arrhythmia (see Chapter 32).

Previous drug history can also affect target tissue sensitivity. This is perhaps seen most clearly in relation to central nervous system depressants such as alcohol (Chapter 22), benzodiazepines and other sedatives and anxiolytics (Chapter 23), and opioid analgesics (Chapter 19). Prolonged or high-dose use of these drugs usually leads to changes in receptor number or sensitivity or to other compensatory functional changes that offset the drug effects and give rise to **tolerance** (Chapter 70). This not only decreases the response to the drug itself, but it may also lead to **cross-tolerance,** that is, decreased response to other drugs with similar effects. A well-recognized example is the decreased sensitivity to general anaesthetics that is frequently encountered in alcoholics.

## CONCLUSIONS

Every aspect of drug absorption, distribution, action, and elimination is subject to greater or lesser degrees of variability, from an infinite range of causes. It is impossible to catalogue all the sources of variation in this chapter. The physician prescribing drugs must be aware of the importance of these variations and be prepared to modify the dosage in individual patients in light of the most probable factors operating in any given case.

| TABLE 58-2 | Comparisons of Age, Weight, Surface Area, and Relative Doses for Children | | | | |
|---|---|---|---|---|---|
| | | | | Relative Drug Dose as Percent of Adult Dose* | |
| Age | Weight (kg) | Surface Area (m²) | Percent of Adult Area | By Young's Rule | By Body Surface Rule |
| Newborn | 3 | 0.2 | 12 | 0 | 15 |
| 3 months | 6 | 0.3 | 18 | 2 | 19 |
| 1 year | 10 | 0.45 | 26 | 8 | 25 |
| 6 years | 20 | 0.8 | 47 | 33 | 40 |
| 9 years | 30 | 1.0 | 59 | 43 | 55 |
| 12 years | 40 | 1.3 | 76 | 50 | 70 |
| 14 years | 50 | 1.5 | 88 | 54 | 85 |
| 24 years (adult) | 65–70 | 1.7 | 100 | 100 | 100 |

*For this purpose, the adult dose referred to is the average dose (in mg) for a 65- to 70-kg person of normal body build.

# SUGGESTED READINGS

Bangsberg DR, Moss AR, Deeks SG. Paradoxes of adherence and drug resistance to HIV antiretroviral therapy. *J Antimicrob Chemother.* 2004;53:696-699.

Cramer JA, A systematic review of adherence with medications for diabetes. *Diabetes Care.* 2004;27:1218-1224.

Elliott WJ. Optimizing medication adherence in older persons with hypertension. *Int Urol Nephrol.* 2003;35:557-562.

Erlund I, Kosonen T, Alfthan G, et al. Pharmacokinetics of quercitin from quercitin aglycone and rutin in healthy volunteers. *Eur J Clin Pharmacol.* 2000;56:545-553.

Garber MC, Nau DP, Erickson SR, et al. The concordance of self-report with other measures of medication adherence: a summary of the literature. *Med Care.* 2004;42:649-652.

Haynes RB, Sackett DL, Gibson ES, et al. Improvement of medication compliance in uncontrolled hypertension. *Lancet.* 1976;I:1265-1268.

Sackett DL, Haynes RB, Gibson ES, et al. Randomized clinical trial of strategies for improving medication compliance in primary hypertension. *Lancet.* 1975;1:1205-1207.

Schmidt D, Leppik IE, eds. *Compliance in Epilepsy.* New York, NY: Elsevier; 1988.

Stillings M, Havlik I, Chetty M, et al. Comparison of the pharmacokinetic profiles of soluble aspirin and paracetamol tablets in fed and fasted volunteers. *Curr Med Res Opin.* 2000;16:115-124.

# 59

# Adverse Drug Reactions

## NH SHEAR

### CASE HISTORY

A 48-year-old woman developed a urinary tract infection with an organism that is known to be sensitive to ciprofloxacin. Her physician initiated treatment, and the patient seemed to tolerate the medication well. Later that week while playing tennis, she ruptured her Achilles tendon. When her physician examined her, she asked if the tendon rupture could be related to her treatment. Her physician thought this very unlikely but agreed to investigate. After a simple Google search using "ciprofloxacin tendon rupture," he found that there is a well-established link. He informed his patient of his findings and agreed to report the case to the national regulatory body.

## IDENTIFYING ADVERSE REACTIONS TO DRUGS

### Epidemiological Approach

All drugs have the potential to cause deleterious effects. Before a drug can be approved for general use, it must be carefully studied in several thousand patients. While some adverse effects are detected in such pre-marketing studies, some serious but relatively infrequent types of toxicity may become apparent only when the drug is used in a large population of patients over long periods of time. Consequently, the early detection and assessment of adverse drug reactions has become increasingly important.

### History

From the time humans first used different substances as medicines, toxic effects were observed. Reference to the toxicity of drugs is found in the writings of several famous physicians of ancient times. For example, Hippocrates (460–377 B.C.) instructed his students and fellow physicians that they should "above all, do no harm"; this was obviously a reference to the potential hazards associated with remedies of that time. The balance between the beneficial and toxic effects of drugs has been a continuing concern as medicine has progressed. Occasionally, wise laymen, such as Voltaire in his work *Le Médecin Malgré Lui,* have expressed doubts about the proper use of drugs by physicians: "They poured drugs of which they knew little into bodies of which they knew less." However, interest in the detection and prevention of serious drug toxicity reached a peak after the occurrence of the thalidomide disaster in 1961.

In that year, there was a sudden outbreak of births of babies suffering from deformities known as phocomelia or micromelia. Astute physicians suspected that the development of these abnormalities was associated with a new and presumably safe hypnotic, thalidomide, which was used by the mothers of these babies to control nausea and vomiting during the first trimester of pregnancy when the forelimb buds were forming and developing (see also Chapters 61 and 68). Case–control studies established that thalidomide was indeed the factor responsible for the malformations. All these events led to a reassessment of the methodology and regulations applied to the testing of drug safety. As a consequence, more stringent legislation was implemented in several countries in order to improve the possibility of detecting serious toxicity before drugs were administered to humans.

In recent years, new knowledge has been acquired concerning the diagnosis, assessment, mechanism, treatment, and prevention of adverse drug reactions. This chapter is a brief review of the most relevant knowledge and procedures.

### Clinical Approach

Patients may develop unwanted symptoms during drug therapy. This is called an adverse drug event (ADE). If the ADE is believed to be caused by the drug therapy, then the reaction is called an adverse drug reaction (ADR). The clinical management of a patient with an ADE includes four steps:

1. Diagnosis of the reaction
2. Differential diagnosis of the reaction
3. Drug history
4. Determination of the probability that the drug caused the reaction

Each of these steps is critical for the optimal management of an ADR, and each will be discussed in greater detail.

## DEFINITIONS, MECHANISMS, AND CLASSIFICATION

An adverse drug reaction is any noxious, unintended, or undesired effect of a drug that is observed at usual therapeutic doses administered in humans. This definition excludes cases of drug overdose, drug abuse, or therapeutic errors.

The severity of an ADR is usually classified as mild, moderate, severe, or lethal, as follows:

- **Mild:** No antidote, therapy, or prolongation of hospitalization
- **Moderate:** Requires a change in drug therapy, although not necessarily discontinuation of the offending drug; may prolong hospitalization and require specific treatment
- **Severe:** Potentially life-threatening; requires discontinuation of the drug and specific treatment of the adverse reaction
- **Lethal:** Directly or indirectly contributes to the death of the patient

The adequate assessment and classification of ADRs requires knowledge of the mechanisms by which they are produced. ADRs are the result of an interaction between the characteristics of the administered drug and some inherent or acquired characteristics of the patient that determine the individual pattern of drug response. Thus, there are some reactions that are determined principally by the drug (physicochemical and pharmacokinetic characteristics, formulation, dose, rate and route of administration), others that are determined chiefly by the patient's characteristics (genetic, physiological, or pathological), and others in which both drug and patient variables are important.

ADRs are usually referred to as **dose-related** and **not dose-related,** and this practice is followed in the present chapter simply because of its wide currency. However, it should be understood that all drug effects are dependent on dose. What is true is that some ADRs will not occur in most patients at any dose, and some patients may have an

ADR at a subtherapeutic dose, but a dose can always be found that will not cause an ADR in any patient. In fact, one way to deal with a severe allergy to penicillin, an ADR which is considered not dose-related, is to give the patient very small doses of penicillin (starting at about 1/1000 of a normal dose), and, in most cases, this will permit desensitization that leads to tolerance to normal doses.

**Dose-related** ADRs (e.g., central nervous system depression by sedative hypnotics) are the most common (about 95% of cases). In these cases, the frequency and severity of the ADR are directly proportional to the administered dose and, therefore, can be prevented and/or treated by adjusting the dosage to the patient's needs and tolerance. In some patients, impairment of drug elimination by renal disease (for drugs such as digoxin, predominantly excreted by the kidney) or liver dysfunction (for drugs eliminated after biotransformation in the liver) can contribute to the development of toxicity. The ADR can represent an extension of the usual pharmacological effects of the drugs or an unusual toxicity caused by the drug and/or its metabolites. These reactions are usually predictable from animal toxicity studies.

So-called **not dose-related** ADRs are less common (about 5% of cases) and are due to an increased susceptibility of the patient. The ADR is usually manifested as a qualitative change in the patient's response to drugs, and it may be caused by a pharmacogenetic variant (see Chapter 10) or an acquired drug allergy. Most reactions with a pharmacogenetic basis are detected only after the patient is exposed to the drug and are therefore difficult to prevent on first administration. An example of toxicity that is, in part, genetically determined is the hypersensitivity reaction caused by abacavir. This ADR is much more common in patients with certain human leukocyte antigen (HLA) genotypes.

The identification of a reaction as dose-related or not dose-related sometimes allows practical decisions concerning the treatment of an individual patient and/or the prevention of ADRs. The main features of these reactions are summarized in Table 59-1.

The mechanisms of most ADRs that are classed as not dose-related are very poorly defined. There is a large amount of circumstantial evidence to suggest that most such reactions are due to reactive metabolites of drugs rather than to the drugs themselves, but this has not been proven. Penicillin is chemically reactive without metabolism, and there is very good evidence that this reactivity is responsible for most penicillin-induced ADRs.

The characteristics of these reactions suggest that they are immune-mediated. These characteristics include a delay between starting a drug and the onset of the ADR. For drug rashes, this delay is usually 1 to 2 weeks; for idiosyncratic drug-induced liver failure and agranulocytosis, the delay is usually 1 to 6 months; and for generalized autoimmunity, the delay can be more than a year. In con-

| TABLE 59-1 | Adverse Drug Reactions (ADRs) | |
|---|---|---|
| | **Dose-Related** | **Not Dose-Related** |
| Nature of abnormality | Quantitative | Qualitative |
| Incidence | High | Low |
| Is ADR predictable? | Yes | No |
| In the presence of liver and/or kidney dysfunction | Increased toxicity, depending on the main route(s) of elimination of the drug in question | Not affected, unless the excretion of toxic metabolites is impaired (e.g., allopurinol) |
| Prevention | Adjustment of dose | Avoid drug administration |
| Treatment | Adjustment of dose | Discontinue drug administration |
| Mortality | Usually low | Usually high |

trast, if a sensitized patient is re-exposed to the offending drug, the onset of the ADR is usually very rapid, sometimes within minutes. However, with the exception of a few examples, such as penicillin-induced anaphylaxis, the evidence for an immune-mediated mechanism is far from conclusive. It is also unclear how reactive metabolites lead to an immune response. The dominant theory is the "hapten hypothesis," in which the reactive metabolite (acting as a hapten) binds to proteins, making them "foreign"; in some patients, this can lead to an immune response that is manifested as an ADR. However, it is likely that reactive metabolites also cause other types of cell damage that help to stimulate an immune response.

**Allergic or hypersensitivity** immunological reactions have been classified into four main clinical types: (1) anaphylactic, (2) cytotoxic, (3) immune complex–mediated, and (4) cell-mediated.

**Type 1 anaphylactic,** or immediate hypersensitivity, reactions involve interaction of the allergen (the drug) with IgE antibody on the surface of basophils and mast cells, resulting in the release of chemical mediators such as histamine, slow-reacting substances of anaphylaxis, kinins, and prostaglandins that lead to capillary dilatation, contraction of smooth muscle, and edema. A type 1 reaction may be limited to cutaneous weals and flares, but it can also result in life-threatening systemic anaphylaxis (characterized by shock and bronchoconstriction), asthma, or laryngeal angioneurotic edema. Anaphylactic reactions may occur after the injection of penicillin and other antimicrobials. For example, many drugs and biological response modifiers can cause urticaria and angioedema. For most, the mechanism is unknown but is not related to IgE. Up to 25% of asthmatic patients may demonstrate intolerance to acetylsalicylic acid (ASA) and other non-steroidal anti-inflammatory drugs (NSAIDs), which may cause severe bronchospasms, a pharmacological reaction that is not due to IgE but presumably is due to a shift in arachidonic acid metabolism away from prostaglandins toward leukotrienes.

**Type 2** cytotoxic reactions are complement-fixing reactions between antigen and antibody on a cell surface (e.g., RBC, WBC, platelets) that lead to lysis of the cell. Drugs are usually haptens, binding to a protein on the cell surface to constitute a complete antigen against which a specific antibody is formed. Subsequent antigen–antibody reactions with complement fixation may lead to hemolytic anemia (e.g., methyldopa, chlorpromazine), agranulocytosis (e.g., amidopyrine, cephalothin, sulfonamides), or thrombocytopenic purpura (e.g., ASA, quinidine, phenytoin).

**Type 3** hypersensitivity reactions (toxic immune-complex reactions) occur when antigen–antibody complexes deposit on target tissue cells. Complement is then activated and causes tissue destruction by releasing lysosomal enzymes. This mechanism may cause glomerulonephritis, collagen diseases, and vasculitic skin eruptions. The classic adverse reaction associated with immune complex formation is the serum sickness reaction. This is a syndrome of fever, arthralgia/arthritis, rash consisting of an exanthem and purpura, and nephritis. It is due to foreign proteins used in therapy, such as anti-thymocyte globulin for immune suppression. Drugs may cause a reaction that has been confused with serum sickness but is very different. The serum sickness–like reaction (SSLR) is defined as the triad of fever, arthralgia/arthritis, and an exanthematous or urticarial rash, but this is not associated with immune complexes, and renal disease is very rare. The drug most commonly associated with this reaction is the antibiotic cefaclor. Other drugs commonly implicated in these reactions are penicillins, sulfonamides, erythromycin, hydralazine, and nitrofurantoin.

Cell-mediated **type 4** allergic reactions arise from a direct interaction between an allergen (the drug) and sensitized lymphocytes, resulting in the release of cytokines (see Chapter 40). Most cases of eczematous and contact dermatitis are cell-mediated allergic reactions. Common causes are topical antihistamines, para-aminobenzoic acid compounds, and mercury derivatives. A delayed hypersensitivity reaction (HSR) syndrome is believed to be initiated by the formation of reactive metabolites of the drug, which act as haptens and evoke a type 4 response. HSR is a syndrome of fever, rash (exanthema, erythema multiforme, Stevens-Johnson syndrome, or toxic epidermal necrolysis), and internal organ involvement. The most common internal manifestations are hepatitis, nephritis, agranulocytosis, and thrombocytopenia. Drugs that are commonly implicated are aromatic anticonvulsants (phenytoin, phenobarbital, carbamazepine, and lamotrigine; see Chapter 18) sulfonamides, allopurinol, and NSAIDs.

However, as indicated earlier, the mechanisms of most "not dose-dependent" ADRs are not well defined, and most of the above designations are only our best guess. Furthermore, it is often difficult to fit a hypersensitivity ADR into any of these four categories.

## EPIDEMIOLOGY OF ADVERSE DRUG REACTIONS

### Pre-approval Clinical Trials

Adverse reactions are carefully collected and analyzed during the drug approval process. The prevalence of reactions is noted and reported in contrast to comparative drugs or placebo in the study population. These data will become a key part of the drug monograph and package insert and will be used to inform healthcare professionals and patients after the drug is approved. Specific warnings in susceptible or unstudied populations will also become part of the same documentation. Although such clinical trials are valuable to determine the incidence of frequent ADRs, they typically only involve about 3000 patients and therefore are not able to detect uncommon ADRs. If 1 in 10 000 patients develops a life-threatening ADR, such as liver failure, it will not be detected in clinical trials but will appear only in post-marketing surveillance after many patients have been given the drug, and it is usually sufficient to lead to withdrawal of the drug.

### Drug Monitoring Methods

Drug monitoring is the systematic collection, recording, and assessment of information on ADRs. This information is collected to allow the early identification of severe ADRs, to determine the possible causal association of drugs and adverse events, to establish the frequency of ADRs, and to identify the factors predisposing to their development.

Estimation of the frequency of adverse reactions to a drug depends on the reliable identification of the number of subjects presenting the adverse event (numerator) and the accurate estimate of the number of subjects exposed to the drug (denominator). The determination of these two numbers is generally difficult because the denominator is usually unavailable, and the numerator can be over- or underestimated. Information on ADRs is collected using several methods that are briefly described below.

### Spontaneous communication to national drug monitoring centres

After the thalidomide disaster of the 1960s, several countries established national drug monitoring centres to collect information on ADRs. These agencies encourage physicians and other health personnel to report any clinical event suspected of being an ADR. The system has met with varying success. The most active drug monitoring centres are located in the United Kingdom and Sweden, and they periodically report their findings. This system mostly collects information on the number of cases of ADRs, but it is not designed to yield information on the number of prescriptions for various drugs. Another disadvantage is that the collection of information is highly dependent on the motivation of physicians to report the events. Therefore, under-reporting is common. However, these systems have obviously contributed to an early recognition of severe reactions, and thus they are still operative in various countries. In the United States, the Food and Drug Administration (FDA) has an Adverse Event Reporting System (AERS) to which physicians can report information on suspected ADRs. The corresponding monitoring agency in Canada is Health Canada's Canadian Adverse Drug Reaction Monitoring Program (CADRMP) and its associated Canadian Adverse Drug Reaction Information System (CADRIS) computerized database (see "Online Resources" at end of chapter). The monitoring agencies in many countries are united in an international network, reporting data regularly to a World Health Organization Collaborating Centre in Uppsala, Sweden.

### Cohort studies

Another procedure frequently used has been the systematic collection of prospective information on drug therapy and adverse events in subjects with a particular characteristic (patient-oriented) or receiving a particular drug (drug-oriented). This system allows the collection of information on both the number of subjects with ADRs and the number of subjects receiving the drug. This procedure has been applied mostly to medical patients in teaching hospitals. The best-known example is the Boston Collaborative Drug Surveillance Program. In this and similar programs, information on the demographic and clinical characteristics of patients, the drugs administered to them, and the suspected ADRs is collected by trained nurse or pharmacist monitors. The data are subsequently analyzed to establish the drugs most commonly inducing ADRs, the frequency of different types of ADR, and the factors predisposing to them. These procedures have provided information about the clinical use of, and adverse reactions to, the most commonly prescribed drugs. They have also been used to determine the clinical toxicity of drugs in subjects with special characteristics, for example, those suffering from renal or liver dysfunction. However, these data have obvious shortcomings, the most important being that the information has been collected exclusively on medical inpatients in university hospital centres, making extrapolation of results to other populations difficult.

More recently, the post-marketing surveillance of a cohort of subjects receiving a new drug has gained popularity. These studies begin immediately after a new drug has been marketed, and the drug's performance is closely monitored during months or years when widespread use may result in the discovery of rare side effects or previously unknown drug interactions. Cohort studies are expensive and difficult to perform because large populations must be studied if the incidence of uncommon but severe ADRs is to be determined.

## Case–control studies

These studies are retrospective but useful for suggesting cause–effect relationships between drugs and adverse events. In the case of a suspected ADR, the relative use of the suspected drug is compared in subjects with the presumed drug-induced illness and in a matched control group without the illness. If the illness really is associated with the drug, those showing the adverse event will have had a greater exposure to the drug. This procedure was employed to discover the link between thalidomide and phocomelia. In his classic letter to the *Lancet,* McBride (1961) reported that "congenital abnormalities are present in approximately 1.5% of babies. I have observed that the incidence of severe abnormalities in babies of women who were given the drug thalidomide ... during pregnancy ... [was] almost 20%." This method is very efficient when the undesirable event is clinically unique. However, when the adverse event is a common clinical occurrence such as jaundice, ulcer, or depression, it may not be suspected as an ADR, and the event may be attributed to causes other than the drug. This is why so many adverse effects (e.g., ASA-induced bleeding) remained unrecognized for a long time. The most obvious limitation of this procedure is that it is retrospective; therefore, it is difficult to confirm the validity of the history of drug exposure. However, in spite of this problem, it is a very useful method for generating hypotheses about possible drug-induced illness.

## Frequency of ADRs

The reported overall incidence of ADRs in different studies varies widely from 1% or less to approximately 30%. This disparity is a reflection of the different methodologies used to detect and report the ADRs, the different populations surveyed, the different prescribing habits in various countries, and the inclusion or exclusion of mild reactions. However, most prospective studies show that the incidence of ADRs (excluding the mild ones) in hospitalized patients is between 10% and 20%. Admission to hospital due to an ADR is relatively common; a recent review of published studies indicated that in highly developed industrialized countries, 0.2 to 21% (median, 5%) of patients are admitted to a hospital because of an ADR (e.g., digitalis intoxication). About 10 to 20% of ADRs occurring in hospitalized patients are severe. Drug-induced deaths occur in 0.5 to 0.9% of medical inpatients.

The drugs most commonly causing ADRs vary from one study to another. This reflects the differences in the populations surveyed and in the methods employed for collecting the data. Most studies have been conducted in hospitalized medical patients. In such patients, most reactions are caused by cardiac glycosides, diuretics, antimicrobials, anticoagulants, and NSAIDs.

## Risk Factors Associated with ADRs

There are few well-conducted studies of the factors that predispose to ADRs. However, epidemiological studies in hospitalized patients have identified some of these factors, and laboratory-based investigations of systemic HSRs due to pharmacogenetic defects have helped to identify individual differences in drug metabolism.

### Age

Most studies show that older subjects (over 60 years of age) are more susceptible to ADRs. For example, it has been consistently shown that, compared with younger subjects, older patients are more likely to bleed during heparin treatment, are more sensitive to potent analgesics, are at higher risk of developing digitalis toxicity, and are more likely to develop potassium depletion during diuretic therapy. Impaired drug elimination and increased receptor sensitivity to drugs have been proposed as likely mechanisms responsible for this increased susceptibility to ADRs. However, older patients usually have concomitant diseases and receive more drugs than younger patients; both of these factors are associated with higher incidence of ADRs. The newborn, particularly when premature, is also more sensitive to some ADRs, probably as a consequence of incomplete development of enzymes involved in the biotransformation of drugs. The increased toxicity of chloramphenicol in the newborn may be explained by this mechanism (see also Chapters 4, 52, and 61).

### Sex

Women are more likely than men to develop ADRs, especially drug-induced gastrointestinal symptoms. Women also appear to be more susceptible to the toxic effects of digoxin. In the over-60 age group, women are more likely than men to show bleeding induced by heparin.

**Other factors**

Patients on multiple-drug therapy have an increased probability of developing ADRs. This may be due merely to the additive risk of ADRs when receiving several drugs or to the increased opportunity for drug–drug interactions.

A patient history of "allergic disorders" is a good predictor of ADRs, including those that are *not* allergic in nature. The predisposition to HSRs may be inherited, and close relatives may be at an increased risk (e.g., for idiosyncratic reactions to sulfonamides and anticonvulsants). Patients who have previously presented with an ADR are also more likely to develop a new adverse reaction. The disease state of the patient can also influence the susceptibility to ADRs. For example, impaired renal function predisposes patients to adverse reactions of those drugs that are mainly excreted by the kidneys. Hepatic dysfunction has a similar effect in relation to drugs that are inactivated in the liver. However, few drug monitoring studies have conclusively documented these relationships.

## Important Adverse Reactions Detected since the Thalidomide Reports

A summary of the most important ADRs identified since the occurrence of the thalidomide-induced congenital abnormalities, together with the drug monitoring methods that contributed to their discovery, is presented in Table 59-2. A similar summary of important recent drug withdrawals due to ADRs is provided in Table 59-3. It is of interest to note that a simple and relatively inexpensive procedure, the spontaneous reporting system (case reports), has allowed the identification of the majority of these reactions.

## CLINICAL ASSESSMENT OF INDIVIDUAL CASES OF ADRs

A major problem in the evaluation of an adverse event in a particular patient is to establish whether there is a causal association between the untoward clinical event and the suspected drug. This can be particularly difficult because the manifestations of ADRs are not unique to that drug. The suspected drug is often administered together with other drugs, and frequently, the features of the adverse clinical event cannot be distinguished from the symptoms of the underlying disease.

The four-step approach described at the beginning of this chapter helps in the evaluation of adverse events. The correct *diagnosis* is essential before further assessment should be done. If the diagnosis is an entity that is never caused by a drug, obviously the drug is unlikely to be the cause of this specific event. The diagnostic possibilities for drug reactions include almost every known disease and some specific drug-related syndromes, including SSLR, delayed HSR syndrome, and many rare conditions, such as the dermatological fixed drug eruption. The *differential diagnosis* is important to give a perspective on all the possible causes of the reaction. Thus, an exanthematous rash could be due to an infection as well as to the drug. This diagnostic list is vital to ensure that important causes are looked at in a comprehensive manner. The list of *drugs* that the patient has been exposed to is not always easy to obtain. The list should include non-prescription medication, herbal and traditional treatments, as well as the prescribed drugs.

Conventionally, the **degree of probability** that an adverse event is associated with the administration of a

| TABLE 59-2 | Ten Important Adverse Drug Reactions Detected after the Occurrence of Thalidomide-Induced Reactions | |
|---|---|---|
| **Adverse Drug Reaction** | **Drug** | **Method of Discovery** |
| Oculomucocutaneous syndrome | Practolol | Case reports |
| Thromboembolism | Oral contraceptives | Case–control study |
| Nephropathy | Analgesics (especially phenacetin) | Case reports |
| Lactic acidosis | Phenformin | Cohort study |
| Deaths from asthma | Sympathomimetic aerosols | Case–control study |
| Subacute myelo-optic neuropathy | Clioquinol | Case reports |
| Vaginal cancer (in daughters) | Diethylstilbestrol (maternal) | Case–control study |
| Aplastic anemia | Chloramphenicol | Case reports |
| Jaundice | Halothane | Case reports |
| Retroperitoneal fibrosis | Methysergide | Cohort study |
| (Data from Venning, 1983.) | | |

| TABLE 59-3 | Ten Important Recent Drug Withdrawals from the Market due to Adverse Drug Reactions | |
|---|---|---|
| Drug | Adverse Drug Reaction | Method of Discovery |
| Cisapride | Cardiac arrhythmias | Case reports |
| Nefazodone | Hepatotoxicity | Case reports |
| Cerivastatin | Rhabdomyolysis | Case reports |
| Fenfluramine | Cardiac valvular disease | Case reports |
| Terfenadine | Cardiac arrhythmias | Case reports |
| Troglitazone | Hepatotoxicity | Case reports |
| Tolcapone | Hepatotoxicity | Case reports |
| Trovofloxacin | Hepatotoxicity | Case reports |
| Rofecoxib | Cardiac mortality | Case–control studies |
| Valdecoxib | Toxic epidermal necrolysis | Case reports |
| (Data adapted from Lexchin, 2005.) | | |

particular drug has been classified as definite, probable, possible, or doubtful, as follows.

- **Definite:** The reaction (1) either follows a reasonable temporal sequence after administration of the drug, or is one for which the drug level has been measured in body fluids or tissues; (2) follows a known pattern of response to the suspected drug; (3) is confirmed by improvement upon removal of the drug and by reappearance on re-challenge; and (4) cannot be explained by the known characteristics of the patient's disease.
- **Probable:** The reaction (1) follows a reasonable temporal sequence after drug administration; (2) follows a known response pattern; (3) is confirmed on suspension of the drug ("de-challenge") but not on re-challenge; and (4) cannot be explained by the known characteristics of the patient's disease.
- **Possible:** The reaction (1) follows a reasonable temporal sequence; (2) may or may not follow a known response pattern; but (3) *could* be explained by the known characteristics of the patient's clinical state.
- **Doubtful:** The event is more likely related to factors other than the suspected drug.

However, physicians often disagree on their assessment of the probability of ADRs. In an attempt to standardize the assessment of causality of ADRs, several algorithms of varying complexity have been developed. A simple method, the Adverse Drug Reaction Probability Scale (APS), is valid and reliable in a variety of clinical situ-

ations. The APS is a short questionnaire (Table 59-4) that systematically analyzes the various components described here that must be assessed to establish a causal association between drug(s) and adverse events. Each question can be answered positive (yes), negative (no), or unknown/inapplicable (do not know) and is scored accordingly. The probability of the ADR is given by the total score, which can range from –4 (a drug-unrelated event) to +13 (a definitely drug-related event). The use of such procedures for assessing cases of ADRs observed in daily practice, as well as those reported in medical journals, should be encouraged.

Recently, a Bayesian Adverse Reaction Diagnostic Instrument (BARDI) has been developed. This method considers the assessment of the causality of ADRs as a special case of conditional probability. The application of this methodology to clinical practice has been simplified by the development of a computer program.

## DISCOVERY OF ADVERSE EVENTS INDUCED BY NEW DRUGS IN HUMANS

The toxicity of new drugs is assessed in animal and human studies as prescribed by law. Nevertheless, toxicological studies in animals do not always predict the toxicity in humans. In addition, the possibility of discovering ADRs in clinical trials that are designed primarily to assess the efficacy and safety of new drugs depends on a variety of factors, of which the most important are (1) the relative frequency of drug-related and drug-unrelated events, (2) the mechanism of the drug toxicity (i.e., dose-related or not dose-related reactions), (3) the number of subjects exposed to the drug, and (4) the methodology used for detecting ADRs. Since the contribution and limitations generated by these various factors are often ignored, it is appropriate to briefly analyze how they may influence the discovery of drug-induced illness.

### Relative Frequency of Drug-Related and Drug-Unrelated Events

The manifestations of ADRs are usually non-specific, and the contribution of the drug must be distinguished from other possible etiologies. Accordingly, the discovery of an ADR depends on the relative magnitudes of two risks: the added risk of illness experienced by the users of a drug and the baseline risk in the absence of the drug. In the event that the drug-induced illness is frequent and severe, it is usually recognized very early during clinical use of the drug, and the identification is mostly based on well-documented case reports in medical journals and/or from national drug monitoring centres. In contrast, when the drug-induced illness is less common, prospective investigations of cohorts of patients receiving the drug and retrospective case–control studies are indicated.

| TABLE 59-4 | Adverse Drug Reaction Probability Scale (APS)* | | | | |
|---|---|---|---|---|---|
| | | Yes | No | Do Not Know | Score |
| Are there previous conclusive reports on this reaction? | | +1 | −0 | 0 | |
| Did the adverse event appear after the suspected drug was administered? | | +2 | −1 | 0 | |
| Did the adverse reaction improve when the drug was discontinued, or a specific antagonist was administered? | | +1 | −0 | 0 | |
| Did the adverse reaction reappear when the drug was re-administered? | | +2 | −1 | 0 | |
| Are there alternative causes (other than the drug) that could on their own have caused the reaction? | | −1 | +2 | 0 | |
| Did the reaction appear when a placebo was given? | | −1 | +1 | 0 | |
| Was the drug detected in the blood (or other fluids) in concentrations known to be toxic? | | +1 | −0 | 0 | |
| Was the reaction more severe when the dose was increased, or less severe when the dose was decreased? | | +1 | −0 | 0 | |
| Did the patient have a similar reaction to the same or similar drugs in any previous exposure? | | +1 | −0 | 0 | |
| Was the adverse event confirmed by any objective evidence? | | +1 | −0 | 0 | |
| Total score: | | | | | |

*To assess the ADR, the questions are answered by inserting the pertinent score for each. The total score (which can range from −4 to +13) indicates the increasing probability of an observed event being drug-related.

(From Naranjo et al., 1981. Reprinted with permission.)

## Mechanism of Drug-Induced Toxicity

The probability of discovery of an ADR may be determined by its mechanism. As described before, ADRs can be dose-related and dose-unrelated. Since dose-related ADRs are the most common, they are easier to detect in the early phases of human studies. In addition, animal studies are usually good predictors of the toxicity that must be ascertained in humans. In contrast, dose-unrelated ADRs (drug allergy and pharmacogenetically based reactions) are peculiar to a group of subjects with very discrete genetic or immunological characteristics. Therefore, these reactions are detected only when the new drug is administered to individuals with such characteristics. These reactions are rarely detected in early clinical trials and generally are not predictable from toxicological studies in animals.

## Sample Size Required for Detecting Drug-Induced Disease

Clinical trials are usually short-term studies conducted in a few hundred patients before the drug is marketed. Therefore, only the most common, acute, dose-related ADRs are detected in the pre-marketing phase. A dramatic example of the limitation imposed by this factor is the case of the antipsychotic drug clozapine. Clozapine was introduced in Finland in 1975 when only about 200 subjects had been previously treated. Within the first 6 months of use, 17 cases of serious hematological reactions (10 cases of agranulocytosis and 7 of neutropenia) were reported to the Finnish national drug monitoring centre from among about 3200 users, indicating that the risk of developing agranulocytosis or severe granulocytopenia during clozapine treatment was at least 0.6 to 0.7% in Finland. (For unexplained reasons, this frequency was 21 times higher than in other countries.) Because of these reactions, the drug was withdrawn from the market. Interestingly, clozapine has been reintroduced for the treatment of schizophrenia resistant to other medications. Recently, other drugs have been discontinued because of inadequate safety (e.g., benoxaprofen). A new quinolone antibacterial agent, temafloxacin, was withdrawn from the market only 15 weeks after being made available for clinical use in the United States because post-marketing monitoring showed it to have much more frequent and serious ADRs than the related drugs ciprofloxacin, norfloxacin, and ofloxacin. These examples illustrate the importance of the close post-marketing monitoring of any new drug, irrespective of the safety shown in clinical trials, and the important role of physicians in evaluating the toxicity of newly introduced drugs by voluntarily reporting ADRs to national drug monitoring agencies. No currently available method for detecting ADRs could have predicted such reactions; only the administration of the drug to a sufficient number of subjects resulted in the discoveries.

## Methods for Assessing ADRs

Methods for collecting information on ADRs in clinical trials are varied and consist of unstructured and structured interviews, physiological and physical examinations, and laboratory tests. The procedures most commonly used are the unstructured interview, designed to eliminate the risk of suggestion of reactions to the patient, and a standardized list of symptoms (checklist). The frequency of symptoms elicited by these scales during treatment with the test drug is compared with symptoms observed during treatment with a placebo. Those symptoms most commonly observed with the test drug are suspected of being ADRs. However, since the clinical manifestations of ADRs are usually non-specific, the detected associations may be difficult to interpret. Therefore, despite the above-mentioned scales, a more definite assessment of individual cases of suspected ADRs is possible only by using the procedures for assessing causality mentioned above.

The discovery of ADRs also depends on the frequency of assessments and the validity, reliability, and sensitivity of the tests employed. Theoretically, if frequent assessments are performed with a sensitive method, all ADRs should be detected. In practice, no such procedure exists. However, the systematic recording of all adverse events occurring during a drug trial greatly improves the chances of detecting ADRs.

## CONCLUSIONS

The discovery and evaluation of ADRs depends on information collected in the pre-clinical and clinical studies. The most common dose-related acute ADRs are usually detected before a drug is marketed. However, uncommon ADRs or manifestations of chronic toxicity may become apparent only after the drug has been used in a large number of subjects for long periods of time. A more definite assessment of individual cases of ADRs should include the use of the APS or similar methods. Because knowledge about the clinical toxicity of a new drug will always be incomplete at the time of marketing, further investigation of the frequency and determinants of ADRs must be pursued in the post-marketing phase.

## SUGGESTED READINGS

Bernstein JA. Nonimmunologic adverse drug reactions. How to recognize and categorize some common reactions. *Postgrad Med.* 1995;98:120-122, 125-126.

Davey P, McDonald T. Postmarketing surveillance of quinolones, 1990 to 1992. *Drugs.* 1993;45(suppl 3):46-53.

Davies DM. *Textbook of Adverse Drug Reactions.* 3rd ed. London, United Kingdom: Oxford University Press; 1985.

Einarson TR. Drug-related hospital admissions. *Ann Pharmacother.* 1993;27:832-840.

Jankel CA, Fitterman LK. Epidemiology of drug-drug interactions as a cause of hospital admissions. *Drug Saf.* 1993;9:51-59.

Ju C, Uetrecht J. Mechanism of idiosyncratic drug reactions: reactive metabolite formation, protein binding and the regulation of the immune system. *Curr Drug Metab.* 2002;3:367-377.

Lexchin J. Drug withdrawals from the Canadian market for safety reasons, 1959–2004. *CMAJ.* 2005;172:765-767.

Liebler DC, Guengerich FP. Elucidating mechanisms of drug-induced toxicity. *Nat Rev Drug Discov.* 2005;4:410-420.

McBride WG. Thalidomide and congenital abnormalities. *Lancet* 1961;2:1358.

Naranjo CA. A clinical pharmacologic perspective on the detection and assessment of adverse drug reactions. *Drug Inf J.* 1986;20:387-393.

Naranjo CA, Busto U, Sellers EM, et al. A method for estimating the probability of adverse drug reactions. *Clin Pharmacol Ther.* 1981;30:239-245.

Naranjo CA, Shear NH, Lanctôt KL. Advances in the diagnosis of adverse drug reactions. *J Clin Pharmacol.* 1992;32:897-904.

Park BK, Kitteringham NR, Powell H, Pirmohamed M. Advances in molecular toxicology—towards understanding idiosyncratic drug toxicity. *Toxicology.* 2002;153:39-60.

Recchia A, Shear NH. Organization and functioning of an adverse drug reaction clinic. *J Clin Pharmacol.* 1994;34:68-79.

Rieder MJ. Mechanisms of unpredictable adverse drug reactions. *Drug Saf.* 1994;11:196-212.

Shear NH, Spielberg SP. Anticonvulsant hypersensitivity syndrome: in vitro assessment of risk. *J Clin Invest.* 1988;82:1826-1832.

Stricker BH, Psaty BM. Detection, verification and quantification of adverse drug reactions. *BMJ.* 2004;329:44-47.

Uetrecht J. Screening for the potential of a drug candidate to cause idiosyncratic drug reactions. *Drug Discov Today.* 2003;8:832-837.

Venning GR. Identification of adverse reactions to new drugs. I. What have been the important adverse reactions since thalidomide? *BMJ.* 1983;286:199-202.

## ONLINE RESOURCES

Canadian Adverse Drug Reaction Information System (CADRIS) computerized database:

http://www.hc-sc.gc.ca/hpfb-dgpsa/tpd-dpt/fact_cadris_e.html

# 60

# Drug Interactions

## EM SELLERS, K SCHOEDEL, AND MK ROMACH

## CASE HISTORY

A 63-year-old man who had been receiving medication for major depression boarded Air Canada flight #007, which departed Toronto at 1930 hours and arrived at London's Heathrow Airport at 0730 hours. Upon arrival, the cabin crew were shocked to discover an unrousable passenger in seat 83A. His passport indicated that he was 63 years old. A search of his carry-on bag revealed three prescription containers. One was nefazodone for depression; the prescription label indicated that the patient had been taking the medication regularly for 1 month. The second was a 6-month supply of ketoconazole for a fungal infection. The label of the third container indicated that it had contained three tablets of triazolam 0.125 mg for "transient insomnia," and it was dated the day of departure. One tablet of triazolam remained.

## INTRODUCTION

The simultaneous use of several therapeutic agents has become commonplace. Concomitant prescription of multiple drugs for ambulatory patients occurs with many diseases. Furthermore, patients commonly consume analgesics, cold remedies, herbal remedies, and other drugs that are available without prescription. In the United States, 40% of the adult population takes more than one prescription daily, 20% take three or more, and 7% take five or more. The median number of drugs administered to patients during one hospitalization is 10 to 13, and many patients receive 20 or more drugs. The number of drugs prescribed increases with age, the number of physicians seen by patients, certain chronic conditions (e.g., pain, major depression), in-patient treatment settings, healthcare delivery systems, and the presence of more than one chronic condition. In addition, the number of drugs prescribed is higher for females than for males. As a consequence, a number of drugs have been withdrawn from the market due to the high risk of clinically important drug interactions. For instance, terfenadine, astemizole, grepafloxacin, cisapride, and mibefradil have been associated with the occurrence of torsades de pointes, a cardiac conduction abnormality linked with increased ventricular arrhythmia risk.

One drug may change the effect of another either by altering its metabolic fate or by enhancing or opposing its activity at the site of action. The latter type of interaction is more predictable and more generally understood, particularly when it is related to the expected pharmacological actions of the drugs. It is not surprising that β blockers can alter the actions of drugs that increase heart rate, or that there are interactions between insulin and glucagon. Metabolic interactions between drugs are generally more subtle and are fully predictable only when the processes of absorption, distribution, binding, biotransformation, and excretion of each drug are thoroughly understood. Since this is seldom the case among practising physicians, the frequency of unexpected, adverse, and sometimes serious drug interactions has grown with the increasing use of potent drugs.

## CLASSIFICATION OF DRUG INTERACTIONS

The classification of drug interactions is summarized in Table 60-1.

### Consequence

The consequence of drug interactions can be either of the following:

- Beneficial (enhancement of therapeutic effectiveness, diminution of toxicity)
- Adverse (diminution of therapeutic effectiveness, enhancement of toxicity)

| TABLE 60-1 | Classification of Drug Interactions |
|---|---|
| Consequence<br>   Beneficial or adverse | |
| Site<br>   External or internal | |
| Mechanism<br>   Pharmacodynamic<br>   Pharmacokinetic<br>   Physiological | |

The tactics of optimal modern drug therapy often rely on the wise combination of drugs with complementary modes of action in order to reduce toxicity or enhance therapeutic efficacy. A few examples are shown in Table 60-2.

## Site of Interaction

### External

Not surprisingly, there are many physicochemical incompatibilities when drugs are mixed in intravenous infusion vials or syringes. Precipitation or inactivation may occur. In general, it is better not to mix drugs together in the same solution. Hospital pharmacies can usually provide a full listing of intravenous incompatibilities when this information is needed.

### Internal

This can be a body site or system (e.g., gastrointestinal tract, liver) or the site of drug action (e.g., cell membrane, receptor site, enzyme). With respect to interactions at drug receptors, much of pharmacology is in fact the study of drug interactions:

- **Cholinergic receptors:** Some antibiotics (e.g., gentamicin) potentiate the depolarizing block produced by succinylcholine at the neuromuscular junction;

atropine competitively blocks pilocarpine at muscarinic receptors (see Chapters 12, 15, and 52).
- **Adrenergic receptors:** Phentolamine, phenothiazines, and phenoxybenzamine block noradrenaline action on $\alpha$-adrenoceptors in blood vessels. Metoprolol blocks $\beta_1$-adrenoceptor agonists such as isoproterenol (see Chapters 13 and 24).
- **Opioid receptors:** Morphine-induced respiratory depression is reversed by the opioid antagonist naloxone (see Chapter 19).

## Magnitude

With respect to quantitating the magnitude of pharmacodynamic drug interactions, several descriptive terms are encountered.

- **Additive:** The consequence *(C)* of an interaction is the simple sum of the separate effects of each drug *(A* and *B): C = A + B*
- **Supra-additive:** $C > A + B$
- **Infra-additive:** $C < A + B$

These terms have very limited usefulness because they are only correct for a particular drug effect at a specified dose (or more accurately, at a specified drug concentration in plasma or at the site of action), at a specified point in time, under specified conditions. These terms say nothing about mechanisms of interaction.

## Mechanism

### Pharmacodynamic interaction

This term refers to drug-induced changes in the effects of other drugs and needs to be distinguished from interactions based on changes in disposition (i.e., "pharmacokinetic" or metabolic interaction).

The barbiturate–ethanol interaction shown in Table 60-3 is a pharmacodynamic interaction. The term **pharmacological interaction**, which may be encountered in some publications, refers to drug actions that are exerted at or on different sites or systems but have the net effect of augmenting or offsetting each other, for example,

| TABLE 60-2 | Examples of Drug–Drug Interactions and Their Consequences | |
|---|---|---|
| **Therapeutic Efficacy** | | **Toxicity** |
| Enhanced<br>   Combination drug therapy in cancer, hypertension, angina pectoris, infection, etc. | | CNS depressants + ethanol (see Table 60-3) |
| Diminished<br>   Quinidine decreases codeine analgesia by inhibiting the metabolism of codeine to morphine | | Naloxone + opiates<br>Carbidopa + L-dopa |

| TABLE 60-3 | Blood Concentrations of Barbiturate and Ethanol Associated with Death in Various Groups of Overdose Patients | |
|---|---|---|
| Mean **barbiturate** concentration in blood | | (mg/L) |
|    Death from barbiturate alone | | 3.67 |
|    Death from barbiturate + ethanol | | 2.55 |
| Mean **ethanol** concentration in blood | | |
|    Death from ethanol alone | | 6500 |
|    Death from ethanol + barbiturate | | 1750 |

combining an angiotensin-converting enzyme (ACE) inhibitor with a thiazide diuretic to treat hypertension or administering a muscle relaxant or anxiolytic to offset the agitation caused by a selective serotonin reuptake inhibitor (SSRI) while treating major depression.

### Pharmacokinetic interaction

Pharmacokinetic interactions are changes in the pharmacokinetics of one drug that are produced by the presence of another drug. Table 60-4 classifies pharmacokinetic interactions, which are taken up in detail in the remainder of this chapter.

## PHARMACOKINETIC INTERACTIONS

## Gastrointestinal Absorption

### Physicochemical interactions

The following five examples illustrate physicochemical interactions that may affect the absorption of a drug from the stomach or small intestine (Fig. 60-1).

1. **Changes in gastrointestinal pH:** A proton pump inhibitor, such as omeprazole, can affect the ionization of another drug (see Chapter 41).
2. **Chelation:** Tetracycline chelates $Ca^{2+}$ and $Fe^{3+}$ (see Chapter 52).
3. **Exchange resin binding:** Cholestyramine binds warfarin and other drugs (see Chapter 35).
4. **Adsorption:** Activated charcoal adsorbs many drugs. This observation is used therapeutically in drug poisonings by giving patients activated charcoal to adsorb the ingested drug (see Chapter 72).

5. **Dissolution:** The therapeutic agent may dissolve in non-absorbable material present in the gastrointestinal tract (e.g., fat-soluble vitamins that become dissolved in mineral oil taken as a laxative).

### Changes in gastrointestinal motility

Changes in gastrointestinal (GI) motility affect the rate and/or the completeness of drug absorption (i.e., the absolute bioavailability). It is important to realize that absorption may be complete in spite of being slowed, since absorption of some substances occurs along the whole GI tract. The clinical importance of interactions brought about through changes in GI motility depends on the rate of onset of action of the affected drug and its therapeutic index.

*Increased gastric emptying and intestinal motility.* Administration of metoclopramide increases the rate of gastric emptying and hence might result in earlier and higher peak concentrations for drugs that are rapidly absorbed from the upper small intestine (see Chapter 12). Cathartics increase intestinal motility and might decrease the completeness of drug absorption by moving the medication to the colon, where absorption for some drugs is poor (see Chapter 42).

*Decreased gastric emptying and intestinal motility.* All opioid analgesics and drugs with anticholinergic activity decrease the rate of gastric emptying and intestinal motility (e.g., codeine, morphine, atropine, loperamide; see

| TABLE 60-4 | Pharmacokinetic Interactions |
|---|---|
| Absorption | |
| Physicochemical interaction | |
| Altered gastrointestinal motility | |
| Change in bacterial flora | |
| Mucosal damage | |
| Distribution | |
| Blood flow | |
| Serum binding | |
| Tissue binding | |
| Active transport to/from site of action | |
| Biotransformation | |
| Hepatic | |
| Other sites (e.g., lung, kidney, brain) | |
| Excretion | |
| Renal | |
| Biliary | |
| Other sites | |

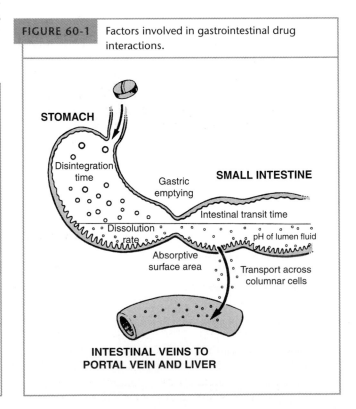

**FIGURE 60-1** Factors involved in gastrointestinal drug interactions.

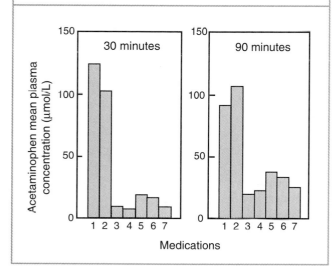

Mean plasma acetaminophen concentrations (standard error omitted for clarity) in 46 women in labour and 10 women postpartum at 30 and 90 minutes after a single oral dose of 1.5 g, with and without administration of opioid analgesics alone or in combination with metoclopramide. Condition: 1 = no opioids; 2 = postpartum; 3 = pentazocine; 4 = meperidine; 5 = meperidine/metoclopramide; 6 = heroin; 7 = heroin/metoclopramide. (Modified from Prescott LF, et al. Drug absorption interactions. In: Grahame-Smith DG, ed. *Drug Interactions*. Baltimore, Md: University Park Press; 1977:45-51, by permission of Dr. Grahame-Smith.)

tions with other drugs. For example, cytotoxic drugs used to treat cancer (see Chapter 57) can damage intestinal mucosa, leading to impaired absorption of drugs.

## Distribution

### Blood flow

Since organ uptake and clearance of drugs are dependent on organ blood flow, it is not surprising that some drug interactions involve alterations in blood flow. For example, β blockers and some anti-arrhythmics may produce an important decrease in cardiac output. This in turn can reduce hepatic blood flow and hepatic clearance of drugs with high extraction ratios, such as lidocaine (see Chapter 6).

### Tissue uptake, extraction, or binding

Drug localization in tissues is both specific (at sites of action) and non-specific (largely determined by physicochemical properties). Many drugs localize in tissues at sites that have nothing to do with the desired therapeutic action of the drug (e.g., digoxin in skeletal muscle). Tissue binding of these drugs serves as a potentially large store from which they can be displaced by other drugs.

The strategic placement of the liver between the small intestine and the systemic circulation can result in important drug interactions. Recall that $F$ (bioavailability) = $1 - E$ (extraction ratio). A drug that interferes with hepatic uptake, biotransformation, intracellular binding, or bil-

Chapters 12 and 19). A decreased rate of gastric emptying is associated with slower absorption, lower peak drug concentrations, and later times of peak concentration.

Figure 60-2 summarizes the results of a study that determined the effects of opioids (pentazocine, meperidine, heroin) on drug absorption. The analgesic acetaminophen was used as the test drug. Note that metoclopramide, acting as a dopaminergic direct prokinetic agent, did not reverse the decreased gastric emptying caused by the opioids.

### Changes in bacterial flora

Bowel bacteria may play an important role in synthesizing the vitamin K that is essential for normal clotting function or may reactivate some inactive drug metabolites that are excreted via the bile by deconjugating them. Hence, chronically administered broad-spectrum antibiotics may interact indirectly with these drugs by modifying or eliminating intestinal flora (see Chapters 52 and 53).

### Drug-induced changes in mucosal function

Drugs with specific GI toxicity may damage the GI mucosa or block active transport. This action can result in interac-

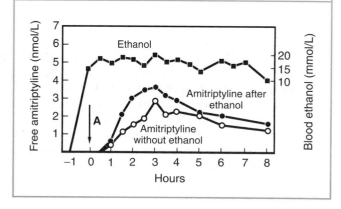

Mean plasma concentrations of free amitriptyline (nmol/L) and ethanol (mmol/L) for five subjects. Ethanol was administered as an oral loading dose of 0.9 g/kg lean body weight, followed by approximately 0.1 g/kg every half-hour to maintain blood ethanol levels at 15 to 20 mmol/L. Amitriptyline 25 mg (A) was administered at time zero, with or without a preceding dose of ethanol. (Modified from Dorian P, et al. Amitriptyline and ethanol: pharmacokinetic and pharmacodynamic interaction. *Eur J Clin Pharmacol*. 1983;25:325-331, with permission.)

iary excretion of other drugs may markedly increase systemic bioavailability during the absorptive phase if the drugs are subject to high first-pass effects. For example, ethanol, administered 1 hour before amitriptyline, causes a doubling of amitriptyline concentrations during the absorptive phase of this antidepressant (Fig. 60-3). Cimetidine has similar effects on the uptake of propranolol.

### Serum protein binding interactions

Many drugs are highly bound to serum proteins, especially to albumin. The literature often points out that other highly bound drugs that are administered concurrently may displace the initially administered highly bound drugs. For example, warfarin is displaced by trichloroacetic acid (a metabolite of chloral hydrate), and thus increased anticoagulation may occur. Bilirubin is displaced by some sulfonamides, and kernicterus may result (see Chapter 53).

When a displacing drug is added to therapy, it can, in theory, cause the immediate appearance of toxicity or otherwise altered response by causing a large relative increase in the free active fraction of the drug in the serum (Table 60-5). However, the displaced drug does not remain confined in the circulation but redistributes throughout the body. After such redistribution, the increase in free drug concentration in serum and extracellular fluid depends mainly on the apparent volume of distribution of the free drug. If the distribution volume of the free drug is large, the increase in free drug concentration will be small and probably pharmacologically unimportant.

Other processes also act to buffer the consequences of the acute changes in free concentration after partial displacement of the drug from albumin. An increase in the concentration of unbound drug in the serum also makes more drug available for glomerular filtration or hepatic biotransformation. For drugs exclusively eliminated by the liver, this displacement results in a greater elimination of the free drug (via first-order Michaelis–Menten kinetics), which may be reflected temporarily as a slight shortening of the serum half-life of total drug. At the new steady state, the total drug concentration in the serum is lower than before displacement, the serum half-life of total drug is the same, and the free drug concentration in the serum is a higher fraction of the total. Clearance of free drug will be the same as before displacement, but clearance calculated on the basis of total drug will appear to be greater.

For drugs that are removed from the circulation by high-capacity or high-affinity uptake mechanisms in the kidney or liver, displacement from albumin may decrease the rate at which drug is delivered to these sites of elimination. Thus, displacement of such drugs from albumin can, in theory, increase both their total and free concentrations (see Chapter 6).

Clinically important pharmacokinetic interaction due to displacement from plasma proteins will occur only when (1) administration of the displacing drug is started in high doses during chronic therapy with the displaced drug; (2) the volume of distribution of the displaced drug is small; and (3) the response to the drug occurs faster than redistribution or enhanced elimination. Maximum potentiation occurs shortly after addition of the displacing drug; however, the potentiation is usually transient.

Because the free drug level is the determinant of the pharmacological effect, changes in *total* steady-state levels may not predict a clinically important change in pharmacological effect during concurrent therapy with an interacting drug. For example, inhibition of warfarin biotransformation, coupled with its displacement from plasma proteins, could result in "normal" steady-state *total* drug concentration in the plasma, yet free concentrations would be markedly elevated and result in a prolonged prothrombin time (see Chapter 38).

| TABLE 60-5 | Potential Consequences of Drug Displacement from Plasma Proteins | | |
|---|---|---|---|
| | | Immediately after Displacement* | At Steady State |
| Free drug fraction in serum | | Increased | Increased |
| Free drug concentration in serum | | Increased | Unchanged |
| Total drug concentration in serum | | Unchanged | Decreased |
| Pharmacological activity | | Increased | Unchanged |
| Glomerular filtration | | Increased | Unchanged |
| Tubular secretion | | Variable | Unchanged |
| Diffusion into liver cells | | Increased | Unchanged |
| Active hepatic uptake | | Variable | Unchanged |

*All changes are compared with those concentrations and effects immediately prior to displacement. This phase may last only a short time because redistribution starts to occur immediately.

## Drug transporters

Active drug transport through cell membranes is another important site of potential interactions. For instance, P-glycoprotein is an ATP-dependent drug efflux pump expressed in human liver, kidney, colon, adrenal gland, placenta, and blood capillaries in the brain, predominately in the cells surrounding the luminal space or exterior. P-glycoprotein plays an important role as a detoxifying transporter by actively extruding drugs and xenobiotics and preventing their entrance to the body. In the case of some drugs (Table 60-6), this can markedly diminish the absorption or prevent the entry of the drug into the organ. Since P-glycoprotein is located in the intestinal mucosa and the liver, it can markedly affect the systemic bioavailability of its substrates. Drugs and chemicals that inhibit P-glycoprotein will remove its "protective" function, resulting in large and clinically important increases in the systemic bioavailability of P-glycoprotein–transported drugs.

## Biotransformation

Many drugs are metabolized by cytochrome P450 (CYP) enzymes, principally in the liver. These enzymes exist in specific isoforms that display catalytic selectivity for particular drugs (see Chapter 4 for classification and nomenclature). Table 60-7 summarizes drugs that are known substrates, inhibitors, and inducers for particular CYP enzymes. This table includes only common examples of drugs with a narrow margin of safety. For more detailed information, see the Online Resources at the end of the chapter. The utility of this type of summary is that one can anticipate that cytochrome-selective inhibitors will result in inhibition of the biotransformation of a substrate

metabolized by the same CYP. The fact that inhibition can be demonstrated in vitro does not necessarily mean that clinically important interactions will occur. However, the possibility of such an interaction should raise one's index of clinical caution. The likelihood of clinically significant interactions depends on the potency of the inhibitor, the proportion of the metabolism of the affected drug that is catalyzed by a particular CYP, the relative concentrations of the substrate drug and inhibitor drug, and the therapeutic index of the drug.

## Enzyme induction

Stimulation of microsomal enzyme activity by drugs and other chemicals is an important clinical problem. Hundreds of drugs, including analgesics, anticonvulsants, oral hypoglycemics, sedatives, and tranquillizers, stimulate their own biotransformation or that of other drugs (see Chapter 4). Enzyme induction does the following:

- Increases the rate of hepatic biotransformation of drug
- Increases the rate of production of metabolites
- Increases hepatic drug clearance
- Decreases serum drug half-life
- Decreases serum total and free drug concentrations
- Decreases pharmacological effects if the metabolites are inactive

Drugs and xenobiotics that induce major increases in drug-biotransforming enzymes in humans include phenobarbital (and other barbiturates), rifampin, polycyclic aromatic hydrocarbon (PAH) constituents of tobacco smoke, and ethanol (chronic).

With barbiturates, approximately 4 to 7 days is required before any clinically significant effect occurs, but enzyme induction may take 2 to 4 weeks to disappear after barbiturate administration ends. This period of offset of induction can be important. For example, phenobarbital enhances the biotransformation of the anticoagulant warfarin, and higher doses of warfarin will be needed to achieve satisfactory anticoagulation if phenobarbital is given concurrently. If the phenobarbital is discontinued and the warfarin dose is not adjusted, bleeding may result (Fig. 60-4).

The antibiotic rifampin is another potent enzyme inducer. Concurrent administration of rifampin with oral contraceptives can result in contraceptive failure because of increased biotransformation of the steroids. Similar increases in biotransformation during rifampin therapy have been shown with midazolam, simvastatin, verapamil, most dihydropyridine calcium-channel antagonists, prednisone, oral anticoagulants, and some hypoglycemics.

Herbal remedies, such as St. John's wort, can also induce cytochrome P450 enzymes. Cases of organ transplant rejection have been observed in patients taking St. John's wort because of increased biotransformation of the transplant anti-rejection drug cyclosporin A.

| TABLE 60-6 | P-Glycoprotein Drug Interactions | |
|---|---|---|
| **P-Glycoprotein** | | |
| Substrate | Inhibitor | Inducer |
| Paclitaxel | Grapefruit juice | Rifampin |
| Erythromycin | Saquinavir | |
| Simvastatin | Quinidine | |
| Ritonavir | Ketaconazole | |
| Phenytoin | Verapamil | |
| Saquinavir | | |
| Digoxin* | | |
| Tacrolimus | | |
| Cyclosporin | | |
| *Not CYP3A substrate. | | |

## Enzyme inhibition

Inhibition of microsomal enzymes does the following:

- Decreases the rate of hepatic biotransformation of drug
- Decreases the rate of production of metabolites
- Decreases total clearance
- Increases serum drug half-life
- Increases serum total and free drug concentrations
- Increases pharmacological effects if the metabolites are inactive

Clinically important inhibitors of drug biotransformation include acute ethanol exposure, macrolide anti-biotics, cimetidine, ketoconazole, ritonavir, and some anti-arrhythmics such as amiodarone and quinidine (see Table 60-7).

Some clinically important drug interactions that are usually attributed to altered albumin binding of one or both drugs can actually involve other mechanisms as well. For example, phenylbutazone can displace both warfarin isomers from plasma albumin in vivo and in vitro and can importantly enhance prothrombin international normalized ratios (PT-INR) in patients on anticoagulant therapy with warfarin. However, phenylbutazone also inhibits the biotransformation of the *S*-isomer of warfarin (by inhibiting CYP2C9) while stimulating the elimination of

| TABLE 60-7 | Selected Substrates, Inhibitors, and Inducers of Specific Cytochromes P450* (CYPs) | | |
|---|---|---|---|
| CYP Isoform | Substrate | Inhibitor | Inducer |
| 1A2 | Clozapine<br>Imipramine | Cimetidine<br>Fluoroquinolones<br>Fluvoxamine<br>Ticlopidine | Tobacco |
| 2C19 | Diazepam<br>Phenytoin<br>Amitriptyline<br>Clomipramine<br>Cyclophosphamide | Fluvoxamine<br>Ketoconazole<br>Lansoprazole<br>Omeprazole<br>Ticlopidine | |
| 2C9 | Tolbutamide<br>Glyburide<br>Irbesartan<br>Losartan<br>Phenytoin<br>Tamoxifen<br>Tolbutamide<br>Warfarin | Amiodarone<br>Fluconazole<br>Isoniazid<br>Ticlopidine | Rifampin |
| 2D6 | *S*-Metoprolol<br>Propafenone<br>Timolol<br>Amitriptylline<br>Clomipramine<br>Desipramine<br>Imipramine<br>Haloperidol<br>Risperidone<br>Thioridazine<br>Codeine<br>Dextromethorphan<br>Flecainide<br>Mexiletine<br>Ondansetron<br>Tamoxifen<br>Tramadol<br>Venlafaxine | Amiodarone<br>Chlorpheniramine<br>Cimetidine<br>Clomipramine<br>Fluoxetine<br>Haloperidol<br>Methadone<br>Paroxetine<br>Quinidine<br>Ritonavir | |
| 2E1 | Acetaminophen<br>Chlorzoxazone<br>Ethanol | Disulfiram | Ethanol |

*continued*

| TABLE 60-7 | continued | | |
|---|---|---|---|
| **CYP Isoform** | **Substrate** | **Inhibitor** | **Inducer** |
| 3A4/5 | Clarithromycin | Indinavir | Carbamazepine |
| | Erythromycin | Nelfinavir | Phenobarbital |
| | Quinidine | Ritonavir | Phenytoin |
| | Alprazolam | Saquinavir | Rifabutin |
| | Diazepam | Amiodarone | Rifampin |
| | Midazolam | Cimetidine | St. John's wort |
| | Triazolam | Clarithromycin | Troglitazone |
| | Cyclosporin | Diltiazem | |
| | Tacrolimus | Erythromycin | |
| | Indinavir | Fluvoxamine | |
| | Ritonavir | Grapefruit juice | |
| | Saquinavir | Itraconazole | |
| | Amlodipine | Ketoconazole | |
| | Diltiazem | Mibefradil | |
| | Felodipine | Nefazodone | |
| | Nifedipine | Troleandomycin | |
| | Nisoldipine | Verapamil | |
| | Verapamil | | |
| | Atorvastatin | | |
| | Cerivastatin | | |
| | Lovastatin | | |
| | Simvastatin | | |
| | Methadone | | |
| | Pimozide | | |
| | Tamoxifen | | |
| | Trazodone | | |
| | Vincristine | | |

*This table can be used to anticipate some potential interactions between drugs that are substrates and those that are inhibitors or inducers.

the *R*-isomer. Since the *S*-isomer is five times more potent than the *R*-isomer, potentiation of warfarin-induced anticoagulation occurs. *In general, inhibition of drug biotransformation is the clinically most prevalent mechanism of pharmacokinetic interaction.*

An interesting association of CYP3A and P-glycoprotein exists in terms of localization and substrate overlap. Many drugs that are substrates of CYP3A are also P-glycoprotein substrates, and many drugs that inhibit or induce CYP3A also inhibit P-glycoprotein. The consequence of this is that P-glycoprotein, when active, can work in concert with CYP3A to alter disposition. However, the extent of independent modulation of P-glycoprotein and CYP3A expression in the intestine is affected by hormones, age and concurrent drug therapy, making the prediction of effects difficult. In addition, in the intestine, the situation is further complicated by the differing substrate and inhibitor selectivities of P-glycoprotein and CYP3A, making prediction of the clinical importance even more difficult.

Drug interactions are most likely to be clinically important when (1) the therapeutic index of the affected drug is narrow, and (2) the changes in either the peak drug concentration ($C_{max}$) or the area under the concentration curve (AUC) are large. For enzyme inducers or inhibitors to importantly affect the target drug's plasma concentrations, the target drug typically needs to be metabolized predominately (e.g., ≥50%) by a single cytochrome P450. Examples of drugs with narrow margins of safety include warfarin, digoxin, theophylline, phenytoin, cyclosporin A, and numerous anti-arrhythmics.

Two examples are described below:

1. **Grapefruit juice interaction:** An interesting interaction, based on inhibition of specific cytochrome P450 enzymes, occurs when *grapefruit juice* is drunk by patients undergoing treatment with certain medications. Grapefruit juice, whether fresh or frozen, contains bioflavonoids (such as naringin, which is biotransformed in human liver to naringenin) and furanocoumarins (such as 6′,7′-dihydroxybergamottin). These compounds appear to be potent inhibitors of CYP3A4 and thus reduce the hepatic metabolism of a number of drugs that are substrates for this enzyme, including several calcium-channel blockers (felodipine, nifedipine, nimodipine, and verapamil), cyclosporine, terfenadine, midazolam, and caffeine. As a result, the

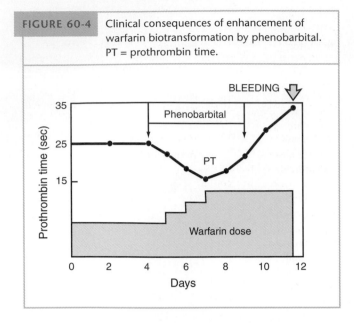

**FIGURE 60-4** Clinical consequences of enhancement of warfarin biotransformation by phenobarbital. PT = prothrombin time.

oral bioavailability of these drugs, as reflected by their plasma levels and AUC values, is increased when the drugs are taken after drinking grapefruit juice.

2. **Inhibition of CYP3A increases triazolam plasma concentrations and effects:** Triazolam, a sedative–hypnotic benzodiazepine, is extensively metabolized by CYP3A isoforms. As determined by in vitro studies, many macrolide antibiotics (e.g., erythromycin, clarithromycin, and troleandomycin) are potent inhibitors of CYP3A. On the other hand, azithromycin has a high $IC_{50}$ for CYP3A ($>250\,\mu M$), predicting that much higher concentrations of this drug would be needed to inhibit triazolam biotransformation by CYP3A in vivo than the previously mentioned macrolide antibiotics. Clinical studies have verified this prediction, as illustrated in Figure 60-5. When erythromycin (E) and clarithromycin (C) are given in typical oral doses concurrently with triazolam in healthy normal volunteers, triazolam plasma $C_{max}$, AUC, and terminal elimination half-life are all significantly increased. These changes indicate a decrease in triazolam biotransformation during both the absorption and post-absorption phases of the drug. These changes were accompanied by a 40 to 60% decrease in performance on a digit symbol substitution test and a 25 to 30% increase in electroencephalogram (EEG) beta wave amplitude, indicating that the changes were large enough in magnitude to produce an observable pharmacodynamic effect. On the other hand, concurrent azithromycin (A) administration does not alter triazolam plasma pharmacokinetics.

## Excretion

Drug interactions may alter the rates of elimination of drugs by any of the excretory routes (urine, feces, bile, sweat, tears, and lungs). However, the only drug interactions of this type that have received careful study are those involving renal excretion. The following major types have been observed:

1. Glomerular filtration of drugs is increased by displacement from albumin.
2. Tubular reabsorption of filtered drugs is decreased by
   • Diuretics (in some instances),
   • Urine alkalinizers (e.g., $NaHCO_3$) for weakly acidic drugs such as salicylates, and
   • Urine acidifiers (e.g., ascorbic acid, $NH_4Cl$) for weak amines such as amphetamines, methadone, and quinidine.
3. Tubular secretion of drugs is decreased by competition for active transport systems so that their half-life in the body is prolonged (e.g., the ability of probenecid to block tubular secretion of penicillin G was important when penicillin G was in short supply during World War II).

Digoxin (a cardiac glycoside used to treat heart failure; see Chapter 32) provides an example of an interaction involving the renal excretion of drugs. Digoxin concentrations rise almost twofold when the anti-arrhythmic drug quinidine is given concurrently, and this increase is associated with clinically important toxicity. Similar effects occur with verapamil and amiodarone. Studies suggest that the basis of this interaction is a fall in the renal clearance of digoxin without a change in glomerular filtration, a decrease in the apparent volume of distribution, and a decrease in total body clearance, while elimination half-life is not greatly altered. Other studies suggest that quinidine may also displace digoxin from tissue binding sites.

## CONCLUDING EXERCISES

### 1. Predicting Drug Interactions

Clinically important interactions frequently arise because of the presence of multiple concurrent risk factors. Adverse drug–drug interactions are often predictable based on knowledge of the mechanisms of action and pharmacological principles.

As illustrations, consider the interactions of the following (see Table 60-8):

• Sulfonylurea agents (e.g., glyburide) used to treat diabetes interacting with sulfonamide antibiotics that can inhibit CYP2C9 (which biotransforms glyburide)
• Digoxin toxicity occurring when the antibiotic clarithromycin, a P-glycoprotein inhibitor, is given
• Angiotensin-converting enzyme (ACE) inhibitors interacting with potassium-sparing diuretics to produce hyperkalemia

We can address these interactions by considering the dangerous clinical outcome of concern and the antecedent

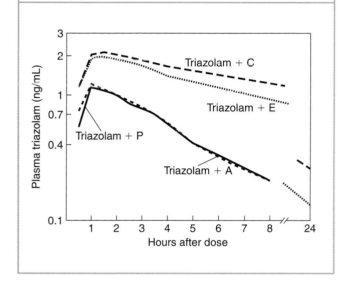

**FIGURE 60-5** Mean plasma concentrations of triazolam following single-dose administration of triazolam (0.125 mg) and co-administration with azithromycin (A), erythromycin (E), clarithromycin (C), or placebo (P). Co-administration of triazolam and azithromycin resulted in triazolam plasma levels similar to those observed with triazolam and placebo. Co-administration with clarithromycin and erythromycin produced large increases in triazolam concentrations. (Adapted in part from Greenblatt, et al., 1998, with permission.)

predictors and conditions that might contribute to the interaction. In individual patients, any or a combination of these risk factors could result in the particular outcome (see Table 60-8).

A case–control survey of hospital admissions among individuals over the age of 66 indicated that patients admitted to hospital with hypoglycemia were significantly more likely to have received glyburide in combination with co-trimoxazole (sulfisoxazole plus trimethoprim) in the week before admission than those receiving glyburide alone. Digoxin toxicity was strongly associated with clarithromycin co-administration. In addition, hyperkalemia was much more common in patients receiving an ACE inhibitor plus a potassium-sparing diuretic (see Suggested Readings).

Knowledge of the risk factors associated with drug interactions can make many of them preventable. When they do occur, prompt recognition that the adverse clinical effect is due to the interaction, and not another disease process, expedites management of the problem.

## 2. Predict an Interaction

From Table 60-7, select one clinically used drug that is a substrate for CYP3A4/5 and one inhibitor of the same enzyme, and see if any clinically important interactions have been reported. Many potential interactions can be demonstrated in vitro. The clinical importance of such *potential* interactions must be shown in vivo. Carefully controlled studies, incorporating both pharmacokinetic and pharmacodynamic measures, are an important way to establish the potential clinical importance of drug interactions. However, determining overall clinical importance in general populations of patients requires prospective epidemiological studies to assess the frequency and severity of the interactions in clinical practice settings.

## 3. Case History

The case history at the beginning of this chapter is an example of the type of interaction one may find reported.

| TABLE 60-8 | Predicting Drug Interactions | | |
|---|---|---|---|
| Outcome | Drug | Potential Risk Factors | Specific Drugs |
| Hypoglycemia | Glyburide | Other oral hypoglycemic agents<br>Insulin preparation<br>Agents causing hyperglycemia<br>CYP2C9 inducer<br>CYP2C9 inhibitor | Other hypoglycemic agents<br>Insulins<br>Thiazides, β-adrenergic antagonists, corticosteroids<br>Rifampin, barbiturates, dexamethasone |
| Digoxin toxicity | Digoxin | P-glycoprotein inhibitor<br>Agents decreasing digoxin concentration<br>Agents causing hypokalemia | Verapamil, amiodarone, cyclosporine, propafenone<br>Cholestyramine<br><br>Thiazides and loop diuretics |
| Hyperkalemia | ACE inhibitors | Potassium supplements<br>Inhibitors of kaliuresis<br>Promoters of kaliuresis | Potassium chloride/glucuronate<br>Trimethoprim and others<br>Thiazides and loop diuretics |
| | | Agents altering transmembrane potassium distribution | β-Adrenergic antagonists |

Ketoconazole and nefazodone are CYP3A inhibitors that can increase the AUC of triazolam. Often, the duration, timing, and order of dose ingestion are important. Could the circumstances in the described case be changed so that the medications implicated could be taken safely together? Propose an alternative, less risky treatment regimen for the patient in the case history.

## SUGGESTED READINGS

Bernard SA, Bruera E. Drug interactions in palliative care. *J Clin Oncol.* 2000;18:1780-1799.

Doering W. Quinidine-digoxin interaction. *N Engl J Med.* 1979; 301:400-404.

Ernst E. St John's wort supplements endanger the success of organ transplantation. *Arch Surg.* 2002;137:316-319.

Greenblatt DJ, von Moltke LL, Harmatz JS, et al. Inhibition of triazolam clearance by macrolide antimicrobial agents: in vitro correlates and dynamic consequences. *Clin Pharmacol Ther.* 1998;64(3):278-285.

Juurlink DN, Mamdani M, Kopp A, Laupacis A, Redelmeier DA. Drug-drug interactions among elderly patients hospitalized for drug toxicity. *JAMA.* 2003;289:1652-1658.

Juurlink DN, Mamdani MM, Lee DS, et al. Rates of hyperkalemia after publication of the Randomized Aldactone Evaluation Study. *N Engl J Med.* 2004;351:543-551.

Newton DJ, Wang RW, Lu AYH. Cytochrome P450 inhibitors: evaluation of specificities in the in vitro metabolism of therapeutic agents by human liver microsomes. *Drug Metab Dispos.* 1995;23:154-158.

Rizack MA, ed. *The Medical Letter on Drugs and Therapeutics Handbook on Adverse Drug Interactions.* New Rochelle, NY: The Medical Letter; 2004.

Ross EM, Kenakin TP. Pharmacodynamics: mechanisms of drug action and the relationship between drug concentration and effect. In: Hardman JG, Limbird LE, Goodman Gilman A, eds. *Goodman & Gilman's the Pharmacological Basis of Therapeutics.* 10th ed. New York, NY: McGraw-Hill; 2001:31-44.

Somogyi A, McLean A, Heinzow B. Cimetidine-procainamide pharmacokinetic interaction in man: evidence of competition for tubular secretion of basic drugs. *Eur J Clin Pharmacol.* 1983;25:339-345.

## ONLINE RESOURCES

Cytochrome P450 Drug Interaction Table, Indiana University School of Medicine:
http://medicine.iupui.edu/flockhart/table.htm

# 61

# Perinatal Pharmacology

## LA MAGEE AND G KOREN

### CASE HISTORY

Mrs. M. is a 25-year-old woman with a history of epilepsy since childhood who has come for pre-pregnancy counselling. Her only medication is phenytoin 300 mg daily. Her last plasma phenytoin concentration was 45 µmol/L (normal 40 to 80 µmol/L), and her last seizure was 2 years ago.

The patient has been told by another physician that carbamazepine is considered by many to be the drug of choice for epilepsy in pregnancy given the evidence that phenytoin may have neurotoxic effects on the developing central nervous system. However, she is also aware that changing from one anticonvulsant to another puts her at risk of seizure recurrence. She does not want to lose her driver's licence, and she wishes to remain on phenytoin throughout pregnancy. Mrs. M.'s only other medication is a prenatal vitamin preparation that contains 0.8 mg/day of folic acid. She is otherwise well.

If she remains on phenytoin throughout pregnancy, what are the implications of such a decision with respect to maternal pharmacokinetics, risk of teratogenicity, and the feasibility of breastfeeding while on therapy?

Throughout pregnancy, progressive maternal physiological changes occur that affect maternal pharmacokinetics and pharmacodynamics. At the same time, there are many developmental changes in pharmacokinetics and pharmacodynamics that take place in the fetus and the newborn. These changes occur along a continuum and are inextricably linked to maternal pharmacology by the uteroplacental circulation (for the fetus) and the breast milk (for the neonate). Perinatal pharmacology and toxicology therefore involve consideration of all the interactions among mother, fetus, and newborn, as illustrated in part in Figure 61-1. An understanding of the general principles and their application to the individual mother–child pair is a prerequisite for safe and appropriate drug therapy during this unique time in human life.

## RISK ASSESSMENT

Maternal drug ingestion occurs in 40 to 90% of pregnancies. While some agents are unnecessary or avoidable, others are critical to the physical and psychological well-being of the mother, upon which the fetus, and subsequently the neonate, relies. It is often not appropriate to deny beneficial drug therapy to the pregnant woman since the vast majority of drugs used in pregnancy are not known to be harmful to the fetus or neonate.

The potential fetal risks of drugs used in gestational pharmacotherapy are assessed by mandatory reproductive toxicology studies in animals during the pre-marketing phase of drug development. However, interspecies differences in genetics, drug disposition, and embryology, as well as the large doses of drugs administered to animals, give these studies limited positive predictive value with respect to possible harm to the human fetus. In contrast, the negative predictive value is quite high. As it is obviously unethical to administer agents to pregnant women solely to assess fetal effects, post-marketing surveillance of inadvertent or unavoidable drug exposures during human pregnancy is a critical step in information gathering.

Post-marketing research on gestational pharmacotherapeutic agents is voluntarily conducted by drug manufacturers in North America. However, such information is often incomplete and potentially biased; women whose babies have malformations are more likely to report drug exposures than are women whose babies are normal. In addition, the data are not readily accessible and are not usually included in product monographs. The product monographs generally contain disclaimers advising that therapy with the drug in question is not recom-

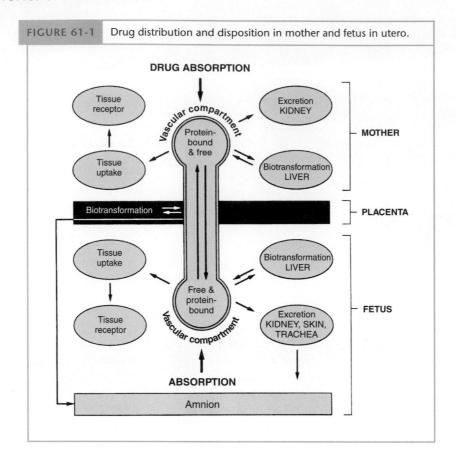

**FIGURE 61-1** Drug distribution and disposition in mother and fetus in utero.

mended during pregnancy or that the risks have not been assessed, but that, if the drug is used, the "potential benefits must outweigh the potential risks." Such vague statements may be made even when a significant body of literature exists about a drug's *safety,* and they do nothing to dispel the misconception that all drug exposures during pregnancy are teratogenic or fetotoxic. The situation is made worse by the frequent failure to recognize or acknowledge that (1) other factors, such as maternal disease, can adversely affect pregnancy outcome and thereby confound the interpretation of adverse drug effects, and (2) all women, regardless of illness or drug therapy, have a baseline risk for spontaneous abortion (in excess of 10 to 15%), major birth defects (1 to 5%), and other adverse pregnancy outcomes.

There is currently somewhat sparse evidence for pregnancy-induced alterations in maternal receptor sensitivity, but some changes do occur, such as alterations in uterine contractile responses and an increase in the hepatotoxicity of some agents (e.g., tetracyclines). Physiologically induced modifications in pharmacokinetics are thought to be responsible for other changes in maternal drug effects and in control of maternal disease that may indirectly affect fetal well-being. For example, a decrease in free levels of anticonvulsant medication may precipitate a maternal seizure, which (particularly if prolonged)

may cause fetal hypoxemia. Drug action on uterine muscle or uteroplacental vasculature may also indirectly affect the fetus.

Direct fetal effects occur only when agents reach the fetal circulation, and the extent to which they do so depends on maternal drug disposition, placental drug transfer, and fetal drug disposition. Given that fetal exposure occurs, the nature of the agent and the timing of exposure relative to conception will determine the potential adverse outcomes. If the drug is administered at term, the infant may be born with drug in its systemic circulation, and neonatal pharmacodynamics and pharmacokinetics will contribute to the risk of neonatal health problems. This chapter collectively considers all of the aforementioned factors as part of an integrated approach to gestational pharmacotherapy.

## MATERNAL PHARMACOKINETICS

Drugs known to have low systemic absorption (e.g., some topical preparations that are not administered for systemic disease) do not reach the maternal systemic circulation and cannot directly or indirectly affect the fetus. There are no known clinically important changes in absorption of orally administered drugs during pregnancy, despite decreases in gastric emptying rate and gut motility. However, in hyperemesis gravidarum with persistent severe vomiting, or in active labour, oral administration may be unreliable and parenteral drug administration may be required.

The substantial increases in total body water (by as much as 8 L) and plasma volume (by 50%) that occur during the average normal pregnancy may increase the distribution of drugs into water compartments. Decreases in plasma albumin (by 5 to 10 g/L) and reduced binding to plasma albumin (through competition with endogenous ligands such as free fatty acids) may increase the free drug fraction; the same may occur for basic drugs that bind to $\alpha_1$-acid glycoprotein. This reduction in protein binding may increase the amount of free drug available for maternal clearance, but also for placental transfer to the fetus (e.g., **salicylates**).

Metabolizing systems may be altered by changes in hormone levels in pregnancy. Although wide inter-patient variability in metabolic rate makes it sometimes difficult to discern pregnancy-induced changes in bio-transformation, drugs such as **phenytoin** and **metoprolol,** for which clearance is limited by intrinsic hepatic metabolism (see Chapter 6), have been found to exhibit shorter elimination half-lives during pregnancy. On the other hand, the clearance of **caffeine** is impaired during pregnancy, presumably due to the down-regulation of the cytochrome P450 isoform (CYP1A2) primarily responsible for its biotransformation. However, the hepatic clearance of many agents is not modified as their transformation is often limited primarily by hepatic blood flow, which is unchanged in pregnancy. Agents cleared primarily or exclusively by the kidney may also exhibit shorter elimination half-lives due to increases of up to 50% in renal blood flow and glomerular filtration rate. This does not necessarily lead to a change in dosing recommendations, as discussed below for β-lactam antibiotics.

Pregnancy-induced changes in maternal pharmacokinetics are likely to be of greatest importance for drugs with small volumes of distribution or high protein binding. If serum drug concentrations are closely correlated with maternal drug effects, and if the therapeutic index is low, the problem can be magnified. Anticonvulsants such as **phenytoin** and **carbamazepine** are excellent examples. Serum concentrations of both drugs decrease during pregnancy because of increases in plasma volume, free fraction, and intrinsic hepatic clearance. As a result, there may be increased seizure activity. **Ampicillin** is another drug exhibiting lower serum concentrations in pregnancy, due to increases in distribution volume, free fraction, and renal clearance. However, because of its high therapeutic index, this drug is usually administered to patients in high doses that produce plasma and tissue concentrations well above the minimum therapeutic levels. Therefore, a good therapeutic effect can usually still be achieved in pregnant women, despite the reduced serum concentrations. **Aminoglycosides** are an example of drugs that are eliminated by glomerular filtration; increased renal clearance during pregnancy may cause reductions in serum concentration and a resulting decrease in therapeutic effect. Cefoxitin may be a better choice for treatment of postpartum fever given that cefoxitin (like ampicillin) has both good coverage of Gram-negative and anaerobic organisms and a high therapeutic index, which allows it to be given in high doses likely to achieve adequate tissue levels.

In the end, what is important is the knowledge that pregnancy-induced alterations in drug disposition *may* occur and the application of this knowledge to the clinical status of the *individual patient.* As with all drug therapy, changes in drug concentration should be interpreted in light of the patient's clinical status.

## PLACENTAL DRUG TRANSFER

Most drugs cross the placenta. However, the degree of transfer is dependent upon characteristics of the placenta, the drug, and fetal blood pH (Table 61-1).

### The Placenta

Aside from the thickness and surface area of the placental epithelial layer, the most important determinant of the rate of drug transfer may be uteroplacental blood flow. Transit may be very rapid, especially for highly lipid-soluble agents. For example, nitrous oxide attains concentrations in the fetus that are 80% of maternal levels within 3 minutes of induction of maternal anesthesia. The mechanisms by which placental perfusion is regulated are complex and poorly understood. It is known that the placenta is not innervated and that local production of autacoids may be important for regulation of blood flow. It is also

| TABLE 61-1 | Factors Promoting Placental Drug Transfer |
|---|---|
| Placental characteristics |
|   High placental blood flow |
|   Active placental transport mechanisms |
|   No/minimal placental metabolism |
| Drug characteristics (favouring transfer) |
|   Not bound to plasma proteins |
|   High lipid solubility |
|   Low molecular weight |
|   Weakly basic |
| Fetal characteristics |
|   Lower fetal blood pH |
|   (lower than maternal by 0.1–0.15 pH units) |

known that the uteroplacental vasculature may be directly affected by drugs that exhibit effects on the cardiovascular system (such as antihypertensive agents or vasoconstrictors such as cocaine), even if the agents themselves do not cross the placenta.

The most important mode of placental transport is passive diffusion along a concentration gradient, although some agents also cross by means of specialized transport mechanisms. Some drugs may assert their influence on the fetus by affecting these transport systems. For example, cocaine and nicotine may increase the risk of intrauterine fetal growth restriction by interfering with the activity of amino acid transporters that are necessary to maintain the nutrient gradients needed for the fetus to achieve its growth potential. The placenta also has drug biotransformation systems capable of oxidation, reduction, hydrolysis, and conjugation. For most agents at steady state, the contribution of placental biotransformation is thought to be small relative to maternal metabolism; however, placental enzymatic activity may theoretically be of clinical importance when a drug is administered rapidly (e.g., a bolus of cocaine). Even so, twin studies have shown that despite the equivalent maternal systemic exposure to cocaine, there can be large disparities in the fetal exposure of the twins. As another example, placental metabolism of most corticosteroids is known to decrease their transfer to the fetus; it is the lower degree of placental metabolism of betamethasone that has led to its use for promotion of fetal lung maturity.

## The Drug

It is free (unbound) drug that equilibrates across the placenta. The fetal to maternal ratio of free drug is usually close to unity, even if the ratio of total drug is not. Exceptions may occur in the case of drugs that are subject to ion trapping in the fetus (see "Fetal Blood pH" below). As the placenta, like other biological membranes, contains lipid barriers to drug diffusion, it follows that lipid-soluble, non-ionized drugs generally cross most readily. The placenta is impermeable to drugs with molecular weights of more than 1000 Da. Most drugs have molecular weights less than 600 Da and cross easily (e.g., penicillins, aminoglycosides). Within the range of 100 to 1000 Da, both molecular weight and lipid solubility are important factors in placental transfer. Many drugs are relatively unbound, non-ionized, lipid-soluble molecules of rather low molecular weight and can therefore cross the placenta readily. This fact has enabled physicians to administer drugs to the mother in order to treat fetuses suffering from such conditions as cardiac arrhythmia and heart failure.

Standard heparin and low-molecular-weight heparins are notable exceptions, having mean molecular weights of 15 000 and 5000 Da, respectively; consequently, these agents do not cross the placenta. From the fetal point of view, they represent superior alternatives to the known ter-atogenicity of warfarin when the mother requires anticoagulant therapy. However, even low-dose heparin given for a few months may, in some cases, cause maternal osteoporosis and vertebral crush fractures. This fact illustrates the weighing of risks and benefits that must be done when pharmacotherapy is prescribed for pregnant patients.

## Fetal Blood pH

Fetal blood is slightly more acidic (by 0.1 to 0.15 pH units) than maternal blood; as a result, ionization and ultimate trapping of weakly basic drugs (e.g., lidocaine or procainamide) in the fetal circulation may occur. Fetal acidosis, such as that associated with maternal cardiac arrhythmia and hypotension, will magnify such pH differences and result in more ion trapping. Intracellular accumulation of weak acids may also occur because of the greater pH gradient between the intracellular and extracellular compartments in the fetus. Such accumulation, especially in the central nervous system (CNS), is an important factor in the fetal toxicity of **salicylates.**

## FETAL DRUG DEPOSITION

The fetus is not simply a passive bystander during maternal drug therapy. Rather, drugs delivered into the fetal bloodstream are subject to fetal pharmacokinetics that may be altered by peculiarities of the fetal circulation.

Amniotic fluid is a potential source of drugs that can act on the fetus, in addition to that delivered through the uteroplacental circulation. Agents that are excreted by the fetal kidney into the amniotic fluid may be swallowed by the fetus and reabsorbed from the gastrointestinal tract, thus creating what is termed the "enterorenal cycle." This also provides a route for fetal therapy, such as the injection of thyroid hormone into the amniotic fluid for the in utero treatment of fetal hypothyroidism. Drug absorption may also occur directly across the fetal respiratory epithelium or through unkeratinized fetal skin. After keratinization has taken place at 24 to 26 weeks, the skin is an unlikely transfer site other than for very lipid-soluble, low-molecular-weight compounds (e.g., carbon dioxide).

The affinity of fetal plasma albumin and other proteins for drugs may sometimes be higher (e.g., salicylates) but is usually lower (e.g., phenytoin) than that of maternal proteins. Protein binding may also change as a function of the gestational age.

Although the placenta is the main organ involved in fetal drug clearance, both fetal renal clearance (glomerular filtration and tubular secretion) and fetal hepatic biotransformation do occur. Drugs that are cleared by the liver may show increased bioavailability and decreased clearance in the fetus, because a substantial proportion (15 to 40%) of portal venous blood bypasses the fetal liver via the ductus venosus for up to 20 weeks of gestation. Biotransformation (at least at steady state) occurs primarily in the mother, although enzymatic systems necessary for drug transformation are present and functional to varying degrees early in gestation. In general, parent drugs are metabolized in the fetus to more polar compounds, just as they are after birth, and the polar metabolites are less likely than non-polar compounds to transfer back into the maternal circulation.

One of the proposed mechanisms for **thalidomide**-induced birth defects (see Chapters 59 and 68) was the fetal production of a toxic intermediate metabolite. Fetal biotransformation may play a particularly important role in the metabolism of parent compounds to reactive intermediates and the clearance of drugs in non-steady-state conditions, such as in maternal **acetaminophen overdose.** *Acetaminophen overdose is the most common poisoning in pregnancy.* Hepatic toxicity results from the formation, by hepatic cytochrome P450 activity, of the highly reactive intermediate *N*-acetyl-benzoquinoneimine, which is normally excreted as a urinary sulfate or glucuronide. In an overdose, detoxification occurs by conjugation with glutathione, which becomes depleted when stores fall below 70% of normal. The specific antidote is *N*-acetylcysteine (NAC), which acts as a glutathione precursor (see also Chapters 4, 43, and 72).

Acetaminophen is known to cross the placenta. Metabolic studies using human fetal hepatocytes at 18 to 23 weeks of gestation demonstrated low levels of cytochrome P450 activity (about 10% of normal adult levels). This would be protective for the fetus because only low levels of the toxic metabolite are produced. However, cytochrome P450 activity was found to increase linearly with advancing gestational age, suggesting that fetal risk may be higher when maternal acetaminophen overdose occurs later in pregnancy. These findings give rise to concern because the same metabolic studies failed to demonstrate the presence in fetal hepatocytes of the glucuronidation mechanism necessary to conjugate the harmful acetaminophen metabolite. There are several reports of stillbirth attributed to fetal hepatic necrosis following acetaminophen overdose in the third trimester. However, NAC has recently been shown to cross the human placenta and achieve fetal levels in the range of those present in maternal blood; therefore, NAC may protect the fetus when given to the mother.

## TIMING OF EXPOSURE

### Early Exposures: Teratogenicity

Maternal drug therapy during pregnancy must be understood in the context of the development of the embryo. From conception until day 14, damage to the embryo may result in its death (in which case the woman may not even know that she was pregnant) or in complete repair and recovery. For obvious reasons, this is termed the "all-or-none" phenomenon.

Drug exposure during days 14 through 60 after conception (i.e., the time of major organogenesis) may result in fetal death (i.e., spontaneous abortion) or in structural malformations or functional changes. The compounds that produce these fetal abnormalities are called teratogens. With the exception of the brain and eye, both of which develop throughout gestation, organogenesis is complete by the end of the first trimester. Each organ exhibits a sensitive period during which major malformations are more likely to occur, although exposures prior to complete organ formation can potentially affect tissue development. This must be considered when interpreting the link between a drug exposure and an associated adverse effect. If a causal relationship seems feasible on the basis of embryological principles, one then looks at the consistency of defects described in the available case reports. Most teratogens produce not one particular abnormality, but, rather, constellations of abnormalities (termed syndromes), particularly after exposure during a specific (critical) period of gestation (see also Chapter 68). Well-known examples include the fetal warfarin syndrome, following exposure during the 6 to 9 weeks post-LMP (last menstrual period, based on a 28-day cycle), and the fetal hydantoin syndrome following exposure to phenytoin.

In contrast, exposures after day 60 following conception do not result in major structural malformations unless there is a substantial disruption of vascular supply. For example, it is thought that in pregnancies exposed to warfarin, CNS malformations (despite ultrasonographic demonstration of normal CNS anatomy at 18 to 20 weeks' gestation) may have resulted from anticoagulation of the fetus and CNS bleeding. Instead, such exposures have the potential to impair fetal growth or function, especially that of the CNS. Such effects may extend into infancy and childhood and are discussed below under "Later Exposures: Fetotoxicity."

It is remarkable that, given the rapidly expanding number of therapeutic agents, relatively few drugs have been found to be human teratogens (Table 61-2). In fact, various authors have estimated that only 1% of malformations can be attributed to drug, chemical, or physical exposures during pregnancy, whereas 65 to 70% remain completely unexplained and are thought to have multifactorial causes (which *may* include some drug effect).

**Isotretinoin** (Accutane), a vitamin A congener, is the drug with the highest human teratogenic potential. It has most of the characteristics that have been described as factors in the development and expression of teratogenicity and fetotoxicity. Isotretinoin crosses the human placenta, and in pre-marketing animal studies, it produced malformations in 38% of exposed fetuses. The knowledge gained from these studies helped to avoid a catastrophe on the scale of that caused by thalidomide. However, case reports of inadvertent exposures during human pregnancy have

| TABLE 61-2 | Recognized Human Teratogens/Fetotoxins* |
|---|---|

**Drugs**
- Alcohol
- Angiotensin-converting enzyme (ACE) inhibitors
- Anticonvulsants
- Carbon monoxide
- Chemotherapeutic (anti-neoplastic) agents
- Coumarins
- Diethylstilbestrol (DES)
- Lithium
- Misoprostol
- Organic solvents
- Retinoids
- Streptomycin
- Tetracyclines
- Thalidomide
- Thionamides

**Physical exposure**
- Heat
- High-dose radiation

**Infections**
- Cytomegalovirus
- Parvovirus B19
- Rubella
- Syphilis
- Toxoplasmosis
- Varicella

*In addition to various maternal diseases and maternal nutrition.

## Later Exposures: Fetotoxicity

The principles of teratogenicity apply equally to exposures later in pregnancy, which have the capacity to produce non-specific fetal effects, such as the growth restriction associated with antihypertensive therapy (with β blockers or other medications) and with cigarette smoking. However, effects may also be specific to a particular target organ, depending on the pharmacodynamics of the drug as well as the sensitivity and maturity of the fetal organ in question. For example, **angiotensin-converting enzyme (ACE) inhibitors** are contraindicated in pregnancy because they have been associated with fetal renal failure; the fetal kidney appears to be more dependent on angiotensin II–mediated renal perfusion than the adult kidney, which is usually adversely affected only in the presence of bilateral renal artery stenosis. **Propylthiouracil** may produce fetal hypothyroidism in up to 15% of exposed fetuses, but this will occur only after exposures that occur at a gestational age of more than 12 to 14 weeks, when the fetal thyroid begins to concentrate iodide. **Tetracyclines** chelate calcium ions and are deposited in developing teeth, producing discoloration; this occurs only with exposures after 16 to 20 weeks gestation, when the deciduous teeth begin to calcify.

It must be remembered that fetotoxic effects may not become manifest until later in life. There are far fewer examples of such effects, as adequate long-term follow-up has been conducted for few medications. Transplacental carcinogenesis has been described in animals, although development of vaginal carcinoma in young women exposed in utero to **diethylstilbestrol (DES)** represents the only established example in humans.

Behavioural teratogenesis has also been well described in animals. Of particular concern are the effects of psychotropic or other agents that affect neurotransmitter activity, since this may be important for regulating cell proliferation. Conflicting reports have appeared in the literature concerning the possible adverse effects of in utero exposure to phenytoin, carbamazepine, tricyclic antidepressants, selective serotonin reuptake inhibitors, and even of maternal depression itself, on fetal and postnatal neurobehavioural development. This is a good example of how developmental effects can be confounded by other factors, such as maternal epilepsy, socio-economic factors, and parenting skills.

## NEONATAL PHARMACOLOGY

The neonate may carry a drug burden from three potential sources: in utero exposure, direct administration after birth, and ingested breast milk. The half-life of drugs may be very prolonged because renal function is immature at birth; renal plasma flow and glomerular filtration rate (GFR) are only 30 to 40% of adult values (especially in pre-

confirmed that the drug has powerful teratogenic effects on the human embryo similar to those seen in the animal studies. The interaction between the drug and the unique genetic makeup of the fetus is probably responsible for the fact that about 38% rather than 100% of exposed fetuses have had major birth defects. Isotretinoin and its major metabolite, 4-oxo-isotretinoin, produce a classic retinoid embryopathy characterized particularly by CNS and craniofacial abnormalities and agenesis and/or stenosis of the external ear canal.

The drug is thought to act by binding to a nuclear receptor, thereby affecting transcription of developmental control genes that play a role in the differentiation and migration of cranial neural crest cells. The critical period for birth defects to occur is 2 to 5 weeks post-conception (4 to 6 weeks post-LMP, based on a 28-day cycle), although there is also a high rate of spontaneous abortions. Exposure later in pregnancy presents a significant risk for neurobehavioural deficits given the fact that the brain develops throughout gestation. Vitamin A consumption during pregnancy is encouraged at the recommended daily allowance of 1 mg; however, isotretinoin is prescribed at a much higher dose, about 40 mg/day, which clearly contributes to its dose-dependent, teratogenic–fetotoxic potential (see also Chapter 63).

term babies born before 34 weeks' gestation). Although GFR increases rapidly thereafter, the development of tubular secretion lags behind, and functional maturity is not achieved until 1 year of age. Hepatic biotransformation can be quite variable in terms of the pathways involved and their enzymatic activity. The best-known example of this is the neonatal jaundice due to immaturity of the hepatic mechanism for glucuronidation of bilirubin. It should be noted, however, that more active pathways may compensate for deficiencies in an enzymatic pathway by which a drug is commonly metabolized—a good example is the increased sulfation of the intermediate metabolite of acetaminophen in neonates as compared with adults. The potential problems created by low drug clearance rate are magnified if the drug has a long elimination half-life to begin with and if the neonate is more sensitive to the known pharmacological and toxicological effects of the drug.

## Drug Burden at Birth

After birth, the neonate must eliminate drugs entirely on its own, without the aid of maternal or placental clearance. Neonates may be forced to clear drugs that they would not normally receive. Psychotropic drugs are examples. Tricyclic antidepressants administered to the mother during late pregnancy are slowly biotransformed by the newborn and may produce irritability, tremor, muscle spasms, seizures, and urinary retention within a few hours after birth. Neonatal sedation may follow administration of high doses (>30 mg) of **diazepam** during labour because the drug has a long half-life and an active metabolite (desmethyldiazepam). Use of shorter-acting benzodiazepines (e.g., lorazepam) having inactive metabolites may pose less of a risk, although sedation of the neonate has still been described.

Drug-withdrawal reactions after birth may also be a problem following long-term drug exposure in utero. The opioid withdrawal syndrome (manifested by irritability, tremor, increased tonus, tachypnea, convulsions, and high-pitched cry) usually occurs within 24 hours of delivery, although signs may be delayed if **methadone,** which has a considerably longer half-life than **morphine** or **heroin,** is used. High doses of other opioids, such as **codeine** at more than 50 mg/day, may also be associated with this reversible neonatal syndrome.

## Drug Exposure through Breastfeeding

The health benefits of breastfeeding have been recognized to include decreased neonatal morbidity and mortality. Given that over 90% of infants worldwide are breastfed at birth, and that a high percentage of women receive at least one drug in the postpartum period, it follows that nursing infants have a high chance of being exposed to medications through ingestion of breast milk.

Whether a drug is excreted in milk depends on its movement from the maternal circulation into the alveolar acini of the mammary glands and then into the breast milk. Only free drug will pass into milk, and drugs with high protein binding (e.g., warfarin) are therefore less likely candidates for transfer. Given the relatively high fat content of milk, transfer is also facilitated by high lipid solubility (e.g., amiodarone) and low molecular weight. High $pK_a$ (i.e., basic drugs) also increases the likelihood of transfer because the lower pH of breast milk (pH 6.9 to 7.2) compared with maternal plasma (pH 7.4) increases ionization of basic drugs in the milk, and they cannot then easily transfer back into maternal plasma.

The estimated drug dose received by a nursing infant, as a fraction of the maternal dose, can be calculated from the following formula:

$$\text{Dose per feed} = \frac{C_{max} \times 30 \text{ mL/kg/feed}}{\text{Maternal (dose/weight)}}$$

$C_{max}$ is the maximum drug concentration in the breast milk, and 30 mL/kg/feed is the estimated infant milk consumption per feed. Other formulae are also available, based on the milk to plasma ratio of drug. However, isolated ratios of drug concentration can be misleading because the average daily amount of drug ingested by the infant may be small and of no potential harm.

To determine drug safety during lactation, the dose per feed (there are usually five feedings per day in a newborn) is related to a therapeutic dose of that drug for an infant. By convention, it is assumed that if the neonate receives less than 10% of the therapeutic dose (expressed in mg/kg), then dose-dependent adverse effects are unlikely. For most drugs, the amount consumed by nursing infants is less than 5% of the maternal dose (in mg/kg) and has no appreciable effect on the infant. A number of good reference sources are available from which one may estimate drug excretion into breast milk.

Even if the estimated dose of drug ingested by the nursing infant is small, it is still important to monitor the breastfed infant for unwanted drug effects. Many factors other than dose can come into play. For example, neonates may be more sensitive to the CNS effects of narcotics and sedatives because of immaturity of the blood–brain barrier. Drug-induced idiosyncratic adverse reactions may also occur. Also, the neonate may fail to clear the drug adequately, a point that is well illustrated by atenolol. **Atenolol** is renally excreted, and there have been reports of adverse reactions, which are predictable from the known pharmacology of the drug and are based on prolonged drug half-life in the neonate. Drug effects may also be potentially harmful to the infant during the early period of growth and development for reasons that are not yet known. For example, the American Academy of Pediatrics lists a group of agents "whose effect on nursing infants is unknown but may be of concern." This statement was based mostly on psychotropic drugs, for which clinically demonstrable short-term adverse effects have not been reported in nursing infants.

## BIOLOGICAL MARKERS OF DRUG EXPOSURE

Biological markers of fetal drug exposure can be tested in amniotic fluid, meconium, neonatal urine, and neonatal hair. Each provides different information and is therefore of different clinical usefulness.

Least useful are amniotic fluid and neonatal urine. Amniotic fluid may be obtained before delivery by amniocentesis, or it may be collected at the time of delivery. Not only is collection often complicated, but the measured drug levels may not reflect drug originating in the fetal circulation. Agents may be present due to fetal urine production, as well as from diffusion across the chorioallantoic membranes. Neonatal urine reflects only very recent drug exposure at term, which may be useful if neonatal drug withdrawal is a concern, as with opioids. However, meconium and hair offer distinct advantages because they act as stable matrices for drugs and their metabolites, and they are easy to obtain.

Meconium is fetal stool formed from the 12th to 16th week of gestation onward that is passed within the first few days of life. It contains drug from both swallowed amniotic fluid and biliary excretion. Positive assays may reflect early or late fetal drug exposure. In contrast, terminal fetal hair grows during the third trimester and, therefore, reflects drug exposure only late in gestation. Hair growth occurs at a rate of approximately 1 cm per month, and drugs are incorporated into the shaft of the hair, from which they can be extracted and assayed. Fetal hair with which the infant is born is not lost until 5 to 6 months after birth, so there is a large window during which fetal drug exposure can be assessed; in contrast, meconium is only available for 1 or 2 days after birth. Concomitant maternal hair analysis also affords the opportunity to more exactly ascertain the timing of exposure, given that maternal hair also grows at a fairly constant rate of 1.0 to 1.5 cm per month. Therefore, hair analysis offers distinct advantages over other biological markers of fetal drug exposure.

Biological markers have been used for over a decade, primarily to investigate fetal exposure to drugs of abuse. Cocaine (and its active metabolite benzoylecgonine) and nicotine (and its major metabolite cotinine) are notable examples. Maternal reports of exposure (or cessation) have been validated using hair analysis. Importantly, these biological markers reflect the amount of drug that reached the fetus, which is the key. Twin studies have demonstrated the important role that the placenta plays; the same exposure to maternal cocaine may result in exposure of one fetus but not the other. Clearly, sorting out the potential fetal impact of a maternal ingestion is a complex process about which much is to be learned.

## ANSWER TO QUESTION IN CASE HISTORY

During pregnancy, particularly in late pregnancy, the phenytoin concentrations in the mother's serum are likely to decrease because of increased body weight, distribution volume, and clearance rate. She may need more drug. However, most laboratories report total, and not free, drug concentrations, which may not change much, if at all, in pregnancy. Therefore, a small decrease in total levels in a woman who is well may not require a dosage adjustment. The mother should be made aware of the risk of fetal hydantoin syndrome, including facial and bony changes, and of an increased risk of developmental delay. Vitamin $K_1$ (10 to 20 mg/day orally) should be taken during the last month of pregnancy to decrease the risk of early neonatal bleeding. Excretion of phenytoin into breast milk is minimal, and the infant can be safely breastfed.

## SUGGESTED READINGS

American Academy of Pediatrics. WIC Program. Provisional section on breastfeeding. *Pediatrics.* 2001;108:1216-1217.

Bar-Oz B, Nulman I, Koren G, Ito S. Anticonvulsants and breast feeding: a critical review. *Paediatr Drugs.* 2000;2:113-126.

Brent RL. The complexities of solving the problem of human malformations. *Clin Perinatol.* 1986;13:491-503.

Briggs GG, Freeman RK, Yaffe SJ. *Drugs in Pregnancy and Lactation: A Reference Guide to Fetal and Neonatal Risk.* 6th ed. Baltimore, Md: Lippincott Williams & Wilkins; 2002.

Cunningham AS, Jelliffe DB, Jelliffe EFP. Breast-feeding and health in the 1980s. A global epidemiologic review. *J Pediatr.* 1991;118:659-666.

Jelovsek FR, Mattison DR, Chen JJ. Prediction of risk for human developmental toxicity: how important are animal studies for hazard identification? *Obstet Gynecol.* 1989;74:624-636.

Johnson D, Schwartz H, Forman R, et al. Assessment of in utero exposure to cocaine: radioimmunoassay testing for benzoylecgonine in meconium, neonatal hair and maternal hair. *Can J Clin Pharmacol.* 1994;1:83-86.

Kearns GL, Abdel-Rahman SM, Alander SW, et al. Developmental pharmacology–drug disposition, action, and therapy in infants and children. *N Engl J Med.* 2003;349:1157-1167.

Koren G, ed. *Maternal-Fetal Toxicology: A Clinician's Guide.* 3rd ed. New York, NY: Marcel Dekker; 2001.

Koren G, Chan D, Klein J, Karaskov T. Estimation of fetal exposure to drugs of abuse, environmental tobacco smoke, and ethanol. *Ther Drug Monit.* 2002;24:23-25.

Koren G, Pastuszak A, Ito S. Drugs in pregnancy. *N Engl J Med.* 1998;338:1128-1137.

Magee LA. Antihypertensives. *Best Pract Res Clinl Obstet Gynaecol.* 2001;15:827-845.

Morselli PL. Clinical pharmacology of the perinatal period and early infancy. *Clin Pharmacokinet.* 1989;17(suppl 1):13-28.

Nulman I, Rovet J, Stewart DE, et al. Child development following exposure to tricyclic antidepressants or fluoxetine throughout fetal life: a prospective, controlled study. *Am J Psychiatry.* 2002;159:1889-1895.

Schimmel MS, Eidelman AJ, Wilschanski MA, et al. Toxic effects of atenolol consumed during breast feeding. *J Pediatr.* 1989; 114:476-478.

Whitelaw AGL, Cummings AJ, McFadyen IR. Effect of maternal lorazepam on the neonate. *BMJ.* 1981;282:1106.

Zahn CA, Morrell MJ, Collins SD, et al. Management issues for women with epilepsy: a review of the literature. *Neurology.* 1998;51:949-956.

# 62

# Geriatric Clinical Pharmacology

## DS SITAR

### CASE HISTORY

A community-dwelling, 75-year-old woman with mild congestive heart failure is controlled with a single daily dose of furosemide (40 mg). Recently she has had trouble sleeping, and her physician prescribed diazepam (5 mg) to treat this condition. On the second evening after starting to take the diazepam, she awoke with urinary urgency and fell on her way to the bathroom. The patient self-medicated with ibuprofen (400 mg every 6 hours) for relief of the pain resulting from the fall. She became confused, her heart failure worsened, and she now appears in the emergency room of her community hospital for assessment.

*Pharmacological Issues in This Case*
- Benzodiazepines in the elderly
- Self-medication
- Choice of analgesic
- Drug interactions
- Prostaglandins and renal function

The United Nations Report of 2002 indicated that 10% of the world's population was older than 60 years, with 12% of these persons older than 80 years. In the more developed areas of the world, 20% of the population was older than 60 years, with 17% of these persons older than 80 years. This cohort of the population probably will increase more rapidly than any other age group over the next several years. In fact, the largest increase in population over the next 20 years is projected to be of persons older than 85 years. Operating definitions of the elderly have divided them arbitrarily into two groups, the "young-old," 65 to 84 years, and the "old-old," 85 years and older. Much of our most recent knowledge with respect to pharmacological issues in aging is based on studies in the young-old cohort.

## DISEASE AND DRUG USE PREVALENCE IN THE ELDERLY

The prevalence of disease increases substantially as people age, and they utilize a greater fraction of their own resources and those of society in an effort to maintain acceptable health status. Drug therapy is an important tool in this effort. Most often, diseases of the elderly are chronic and multiple, and polypharmacy is a major factor in the high incidence of adverse drug reactions, which increase with patient age (Table 62-1; see also Chapter 59).

Together with the increase in disease prevalence, the elderly have less effective and more variable homeostatic responses to the multitude of functional disturbances they suffer. As we age, physiological responses become more heterogeneous, reflecting the variable rate of declining organ and tissue function. Thus, the predictability of patient response to drug therapy becomes less certain. Suboptimal drug therapy often stems from disease progression, increased adverse drug reactions, defective adherence to prescribed regimens due to the complication of timing the doses of many drugs with differing dose schedules, and the inevitable attempt by the patient to self-medicate with over-the-counter drugs and herbal remedies purchased without prior consultation with physicians or other healthcare professionals.

The problem of drug-related adverse patient events (DRAPEs) has been known for many years, but its preva-

| TABLE 62-1 | Age and Adverse Drug Reactions |
|---|---|
| Age of Patient (years) | Incidence (%) |
| 10–19 | 3.1 |
| 20–29 | 3.0 |
| 30–39 | 5.7 |
| 40–49 | 7.5 |
| 50–59 | 8.1 |
| 60–69 | 10.7 |
| 70–79 | 21.3 |
| 80–89 | 18.6 |

(From Hurwitz N. Predisposing factors in adverse reactions to drugs. *BMJ* 1969;1:536-539.)

lence remains the same despite the greater knowledge and educational efforts of the last 25 years. This finding has led to an increasing acceptance of the need to individualize drug doses for older patients.

In North America, the Boston Collaborative Drug Surveillance Program has provided valuable information, indicating a higher incidence of adverse drug reactions with increasing age. Although the observation has been attributed to increasing frailty with older age, most studies that have specifically examined the effect of age on the risk of DRAPEs have failed to demonstrate such an association. It must be remembered, moreover, that although this type of information is useful in alerting the physician to a potential problem with a particular drug or drug group in the elderly, it does not tell us the mechanism(s) underlying these observations. The mechanisms remain to be determined by more detailed examination of the problem in the affected patient group.

However, it is universally accepted that the number of drugs prescribed and the number of diseases diagnosed correlate much better with the incidence of observed adverse drug reactions than does age (Fig. 62-1). Since these two predictive factors are not independent variables, it is likely that the increased prevalence of chronic diseases in the older patient population is the most important determinant of the observed increase in adverse drug reactions (Fig. 62-2).

Both pharmacokinetic and pharmacodynamic explanations are possible for the apparently altered responses of older patients to drug therapy. It is most likely that both processes contribute. Without an understanding of the effects of aging on both of these processes, a rational approach to drug treatment of older patients is not possible. A more detailed examination of the evidence for potential and demonstrated contributions of aging to alterations in pharmacokinetics and pharmacodynamics is presented here.

## PHARMACOKINETIC CHANGES IN THE ELDERLY

For the following discussion, it is useful to recall some of the fundamental pharmacokinetic equations. For this short summary, only the model-independent relationships are presented:

$$Cl_p = \text{dose} / \text{AUC} = V_d \times \lambda$$

$$\lambda = Cl_p / V_d$$

$$t_{1/2} = 0.693 / \lambda = 0.693 \times V_d / Cl_p$$

In these equations, $Cl_p$ is plasma (serum) clearance, AUC is the area under the plasma (serum) concentration versus

| FIGURE 62-1 | (A) Relationship of DRAPE risk to the number of diseases ($r = 0.81$; $P < 0.026$) and (B) to the number of prescribed drugs used ($r = 0.77$; $P < 0.001$). (From Grymonpre et al., 1988. Reprinted with permission.) |
|---|---|

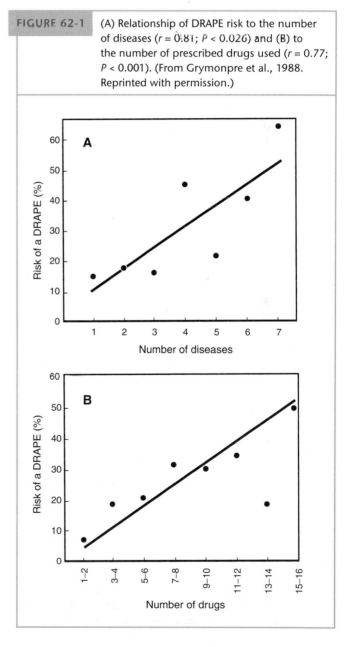

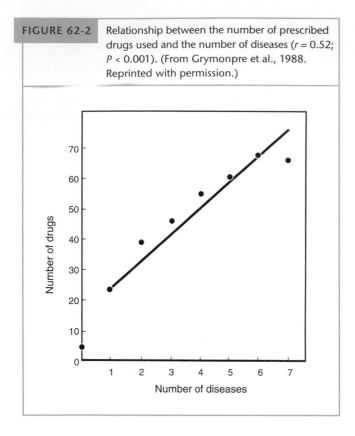

**FIGURE 62-2** Relationship between the number of prescribed drugs used and the number of diseases ($r = 0.52$; $P < 0.001$). (From Grymonpre et al., 1988. Reprinted with permission.)

time curve, $V_d$ is the apparent volume of distribution, $\lambda$ is the terminal disposition rate constant, and $t_{1/2}$ represents the half-life corresponding to the terminal disposition rate constant.

Earlier investigators inferred, from observed alterations of $t_{1/2}$, that the elderly handled drugs differently than the young. The problem with this simplistic approach is that $t_{1/2}$ is a hybrid of $V_d$ and $Cl_p$ (third equation above). Thus, if $V_d$ changes, then $t_{1/2}$ does not necessarily reflect the ability of the body to eliminate the drug ($Cl_p$). The mechanism could, in fact, be the inability of the drug to reach the clearance site. However, $Cl_p$ represents the ability of an elimination site to act on that fraction of the drug dose that does reach it, regardless of the concurrent presence of additional drug molecules at remote sites. Although the overall observed effect may be a decrease in the rate of drug elimination, without knowledge of the $V_d$ it is impossible to determine whether the observation is related to altered drug distribution, impaired elimination capability by the responsible organs, or a combination of both.

See Chapter 5 for a more detailed discussion of pharmacokinetic relationships.

## Physiological Changes with Increasing Age

### Body composition

The proportion of fat as a fraction of total body weight is a function of several variables, including height, weight, sex, age, diet, and physical activity. Generally, women have a higher proportion of total body weight as fat than men do. In both sexes, the proportion of total body weight as fat increases with age. The increment in fat content is generally localized to the middle and upper body regions. In women, there appears to be a post-menopausal acceleration of this trend. In the elderly, a considerable fraction of body fat tends to accumulate within organs rather than being localized as adipose tissue. Recent studies suggest a maximum age for fat accumulation around the sixth decade of life, with a plateau phase, and a subsequent reduction in the amount and proportion of body fat in the old-old population. It can be anticipated that distribution of drugs will be affected by this altered accumulation and distribution profile of body fat.

Body water content is closely related to the amount of fat-free mass. For all ages, the proportion of body weight attributed to water is less in women than in men. Body water as a percentage of total body weight generally declines with increasing age. In women, for example, it decreases from about 56% at age 20 to about 45% at age 70. This trend continues until approximately age 80, when the percentage of water begins to increase again. In men, this decline in body water begins with middle age. It is less rapid in women until about the sixth decade, when it accelerates. At the same time, the fraction of muscle per unit of body weight decreases with increasing age in both sexes.

If dosage is based on total body weight, drugs that are localized to lean tissue (i.e., hydrophilic drugs with lower lipid/water partition coefficients) will achieve a higher plasma concentration for the same dose per weight in older patients. As well, there will be increased tissue sequestration of more lipophilic drugs (i.e., those with higher lipid/water partition coefficients) and a lower circulating drug concentration.

The profile of plasma proteins in the circulation also changes with age. Serum albumin concentration decreases with increasing age, although it remains within the normal range unless it is affected by clinically important pathology. Reduced serum albumin concentration could result in an increased circulating free fraction of the acidic drugs that bind to albumin, such as non-steroidal anti-inflammatory drugs (NSAIDs). However, serum $\alpha_1$-acid glycoprotein concentration increases with age. The lability of this glycoprotein makes it difficult to determine whether its concentration contributes to the altered pharmacological response to basic drugs that bind to it (e.g., tricyclic antidepressants). This change in protein profile may have important consequences for drugs that are highly protein-bound, but studies of this issue have been restricted mostly to drugs that are highly bound to albumin.

### Organ function

Organ function tends to change with time, usually in the direction of decreased functional reserve with increasing age. Thus, the glomerular filtration rate of the kidney, as reflected by creatinine clearance, decreases in the majority of older patients. However, serum creatinine concentration may not be elevated even in the presence of clinically important renal impairment because of its decrease resulting from decreased muscle mass. In about one-third of apparently healthy community-dwelling elderly persons, renal function remains high and stable even in old age.

Liver size as a fraction of body weight decreases with increasing age. Although liver blood flow per unit of organ weight may not be significantly different in older persons, the decrease in mass results in decreased total hepatic blood flow and decreased rates of elimination of many drugs from the body, especially those that are lipophilic and have a high hepatic extraction ratio.

Cardiac output is also lower in older patients, but it is unclear to what degree this is due to a more sedentary lifestyle, to progressive tissue degeneration due to aging, or to disease. There is often a redistribution of cardiac output to maintain optimum blood flow to critical organs. Thus, perfusion of sites of drug elimination is often compromised in cardiac failure. Also, the baroreceptor reflex is decreased in older patients, resulting in their increased susceptibility to orthostatic hypotension.

Decline in the function of other organs is also more prevalent with increasing age and often forms the basis of the need for drug therapy (e.g., hypothyroidism and type 2 diabetes). Some representative changes in body composition and function are presented in Table 62-2.

| TABLE 62-2 | Average Changes in Body Composition and Function (Males and Females) |
|---|---|
| | Change from Age 20 to Age 80 (%) |
| Body fat/total body weight | +35 |
| Plasma volume | −8 |
| Plasma albumin | −10 |
| Plasma globulin | −10 |
| Total body water | −17 |
| Extracellular fluid (from age 20 to age 65) | −40 |
| Conduction velocity | −20 |
| Cardiac index | −40 |
| Cardiac output | −30 to −40 |
| Vital capacity | −60 |
| Glomerular filtration rate | −50 |
| Splanchnic and renal blood flow | −40 |

## Consequences for Drug Disposition

### Absorption

Various data indicate that gastric acid secretion decreases, gastric emptying time increases, and the surface area of the upper intestinal tract decreases with age. Also, cardiac output may be lower, and blood flow to the gastrointestinal tract may be reduced in the elderly patient. Although these observations provide a theoretical basis for predicting altered drug absorption in the aged, few examples exist to indicate that it is an important practical problem. Nevertheless, the possibility must be considered when multiple drugs are ingested concurrently, especially when their pharmacology includes modification of gastrointestinal physiological function (e.g., drugs with anticholinergic properties). Variation in drug absorption through the skin of older patients also has not been shown to be a clinically important problem related to the aging process.

The reductions in liver size and in surface area of the upper intestinal tract with advancing age are given as reasonable hypotheses to explain the reduced pre-systemic drug elimination and increased bioavailability of drugs that are normally subject to pre-systemic elimination, such as morphine and propranolol (Fig. 62-3). Although these postulated mechanisms seem reasonable, more research is required to confirm their contribution to the observed increase in drug bioavailability in some elderly patients.

### Tissue distribution

The changes in body composition with increasing age, described previously, have important clinical consequences with respect to the choice of drug and dose optimization in the elderly patient. Thus, relatively hydrophilic drugs (e.g., alcohol and morphine) will achieve higher concentrations in blood for the same weight-adjusted dose. The perception that the elderly are more sensitive to these central nervous system (CNS) depressants is likely to be explained, at least in part, by increased delivery to the brain due to the reduced $V_d$.

However, relatively lipophilic drugs (e.g., diazepam) will have a lower circulating concentration for an equivalent dose due to distribution into the increased fat of the older patient. Although the elderly are capable of biotransforming diazepam to an extent similar to that in younger patients (Fig. 62-4), delivery to the liver is decreased, and the drug persists longer in the body at levels that exert a CNS-depressant effect. Although the plasma half-life of diazepam approximates chronological age in adults (Fig. 62-5), this is not due to decreasing ability of the body to metabolize diazepam as much as to increased tissue sequestration (Fig. 62-6).

Another example of an important quantitative difference in tissue sequestration in the elderly is provided by digoxin. This drug is highly concentrated in muscle tissue. Since the proportion of muscle in the body invariably

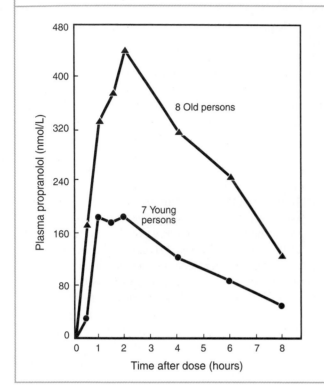

FIGURE 62-3 Mean plasma propranolol concentration in two different age groups, following a single oral dose of 40 mg. The difference between the age groups is statistically significant. (From Castleden CM, George, CF. The effect of aging on the hepatic clearance of propranolol. *Br J Clin Pharmacol.* 1979;7(1):49-54. Reprinted with permission.)

administered drugs with similar protein-binding properties, usually to the detriment of the patient. An informative example is provided by the interaction of tolbutamide and salicylates. In this instance, the salicylic acid displaces tolbutamide from its protein binding sites, thus increasing the hypoglycemic effect of tolbutamide. Although tolbutamide will also displace salicylate from its protein binding sites, the clinical consequences for the pharmacology of salicylate are not usually considered.

## Drug biotransformation

In vitro studies with human liver microsomes have failed to demonstrate a consistent decrement in intrinsic drug biotransformation capability with increasing age. However, results from in vivo studies are less clear. Most of the available evidence suggests that drug biotransformation decreases with increasing age, primarily in males, and this effect is seen with phase I reactions (oxidation, reduction, and hydrolysis). Interpretation of studies published to date is confounded by environmental influences that have a profound effect on inter-patient variability in drug biotransformation, such as exposure to drug-metabolizing enzyme inducers (see Chapter 4). Evidence for a decrease in phase II reactions (conjugation) with increasing age is much less compelling and is generally believed not to be an important consideration in altered drug biotransformation in geriatric patients.

Reduced liver blood flow due to reduced organ size remains an important confounding factor in interpreting the mechanisms contributing to observations of decreased drug clearance in the geriatric patient.

There is reasonable evidence that the inductive effect of some commonly prescribed drugs (e.g., rifampicin) on

declines with increasing age, the circulating concentration of digoxin will be higher than expected for a given dose per weight. Although this is not the sole determining factor in dose estimation for digoxin, it is an important one that is often overlooked.

## Protein binding

The decrease in plasma albumin and increase in $\alpha_1$-acid glycoprotein have implications for acidic and basic drugs that bind to them. Thus, the decrease in plasma albumin is implicated in the increased toxicity of acetylsalicylic acid in older patients at an equivalent total plasma concentration of salicylic acid. It is possible that increased binding of some basic drugs by $\alpha_1$-acid glycoprotein could cause the total drug concentration to be misleading, since only the free drug concentration is believed to determine the intensity of pharmacological activity. This might be an important contributing factor for variable responses to tricyclic antidepressant drugs in the elderly, but the possibility remains virtually unexplored. However, it can be reasonably assumed that drugs that have a small $V_d$ and that are extensively bound to plasma proteins are likely to alter the pharmacological response of concurrently

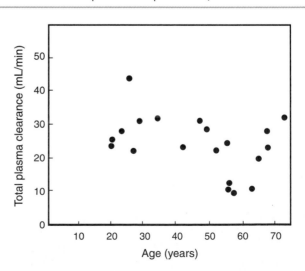

FIGURE 62-4 Relationship of total plasma clearance of diazepam to age. Each point represents a single normal individual. (From Klotz et al., 1975. Reprinted with permission.)

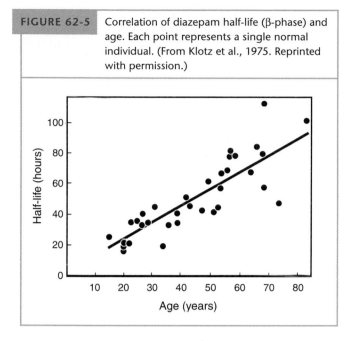

Correlation of diazepam half-life (β-phase) and age. Each point represents a single normal individual. (From Klotz et al., 1975. Reprinted with permission.)

procainamide) will have to be prescribed in smaller doses or at greater time intervals. It should also be remembered that a "normal" serum creatinine concentration in an older patient actually reflects impaired renal function, since creatinine production is reduced due to decreased muscle mass. If it is not possible to determine creatinine clearance directly, renal function may be estimated from the widely accepted algorithm of Cockroft and Gault

$$Cl_{\text{creatinine}} \text{ [mL/min]} = \frac{(140 - \text{age}) \times \text{weight [kg]}}{0.8145 \times C_{\text{p,creatinine}} \text{ [μmol/L]}}$$

in which $C_{\text{p,creatinine}}$ is the concentration of creatinine in the plasma. Values for creatinine clearance in women should be multiplied by 0.85. It cannot be overemphasized that this relationship provides only an approximation of renal function in the older patient and that direct determination of plasma concentrations for drugs with narrow therapeutic indices is recommended when available. Alternatively, consideration should be given to the possibility of drug therapy with an agent having a higher therapeutic index.

The increasing incidence of incontinence in the elderly often is addressed by decreasing their fluid intake. Together with the decreased homeostatic response to dehydration, there is decreased urine formation and an increased drug concentration in the bladder, which is able to diffuse back into the body down a concentration gradient. Both processes may contribute to a net decrease in the rate of drug excretion by the kidney. Also, this situation leads to an increased possibility of crystalluria due to precipitation of poorly soluble drugs and metabolites (e.g., acetylated sulfonamides) in the smaller urine volume.

the phase I reactions of other drugs is suppressed in older patients. However, there is also evidence that the multiple isoforms of tissue cytochrome P450 are not uniformly suppressed with increasing age. Thus, the induction effect of smoking on theophylline biotransformation is not blunted in elderly males. The alteration of dose in an older patient concurrently taking a known inducer of drug biotransformation often will differ from that required in younger patients.

In the older patient, multiple drug ingestion is more likely to result in toxicity due to inhibition of biotransformation. The increased frequency of this phenomenon in older patients is undoubtedly related, at least in part, to the competition for the available mechanisms of elimination among the drugs used concurrently to treat their chronic disease states. It is likely that influenza virus infection, which can produce a relatively non-specific depression of the cytochrome P450 enzymes, could also be an important contributing mechanism of increased drug toxicity in the elderly. Diet is also a potentially confounding factor in altering drug biotransformation. The rate of biotransformation is depressed with high-carbohydrate and stimulated with high-protein diets. Diminishing affluence in the older patient cohort makes it more likely that carbohydrates constitute an increasing fraction of their total caloric intake and contribute to the decrease of drug biotransformation rate.

### Excretion
Although renal function does not inevitably decline with increasing age, it is clear that most older patients have decreased renal function compared with younger patients. Thus, drugs that depend on renal elimination of a substantial fraction of the dose (e.g., amantadine, digoxin,

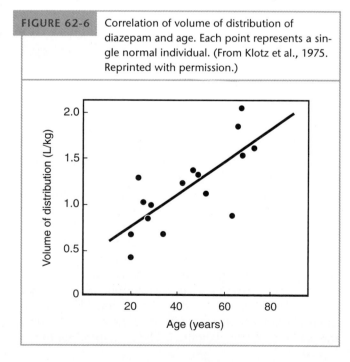

Correlation of volume of distribution of diazepam and age. Each point represents a single normal individual. (From Klotz et al., 1975. Reprinted with permission.)

## PHARMACODYNAMIC CHANGES IN THE ELDERLY

Much less is known about altered pharmacodynamics as a function of increasing age, but some important examples have become better appreciated recently.

There has been considerable controversy regarding the mechanisms contributing to the observed increase in the response to CNS-depressant drugs in the elderly. Alteration in pharmacokinetic disposition has been convincingly demonstrated for some drugs (e.g., ethanol and benzodiazepines), but pharmacodynamic changes have been more difficult to prove. The suggestion of increased neuronal sensitivity to drugs such as alfentanil, fentanyl, and nitrazepam is based on changes in the observed effect relative to concurrently measured drug concentrations in plasma. However, these data are based on the unproved assumption of an unchanged equilibrium between drug concentration in plasma and that in the brain.

There is more convincing evidence that older persons are less responsive to β-adrenergic receptor agonists, especially of the $\beta_1$ receptor type. This finding suggests the possibility of a blunted response to β blocker drug therapy in older patients. However, the therapeutic implications of this interaction have not yet been clearly outlined by definitive studies in the patient population at risk.

There is an increasing incidence of abnormal glucose tolerance tests in older persons. This is conventionally attributed to an altered insulin response rather than to a deficiency of the hormone. Recent studies implicate a post-receptor defect. Since exercise is known to improve tissue utilization of glucose, it may be that part of this observed insulin resistance could be explained by the increasingly sedentary lifestyle of older people.

## REPRESENTATIVE DRUG CLASSES FOR PHARMACOTHERAPY OF DISEASE IN ELDERLY PATIENTS

### Analgesics

Chronic pain occurs commonly in older patients, and it is often poorly managed. Recent studies have indicated that acetaminophen in analgesic doses is just as effective as equivalent analgesic or anti-inflammatory doses of NSAIDs in the treatment of osteoarthritis. Thus, the question arises as to whether acetaminophen might be a safer treatment in those patients with reduced creatinine clearance when renal prostaglandin synthesis is an important factor in maintaining residual tubular function.

In those patients with rheumatoid arthritis and impaired renal function, consideration may be given to the use of the NSAID sulindac, since the kidney converts the active sulfide metabolite back to the prodrug in the majority of patients. However, its use does not guarantee protection of renal prostaglandin synthesis. Concurrent use of diuretics increases the kidney's susceptibility to inhibitors of prostaglandin synthesis and to renal impairment by NSAIDs. However, the interaction is reversible on cessation of therapy with the offending analgesic if renal ischemia has not already induced acute tubular necrosis.

Recent studies, which have shown that acetaminophen but not acetylsalicylic acid raises pain threshold, suggest that use of these two analgesics together to improve pain control may eliminate the need to switch to an opioid analgesic. Also, there is evidence to show that caffeine improves the analgesic efficacy of non-opioid drugs. Thus, alternatives to opioid analgesics exist if the mechanism of pain is amenable to them.

For management of severe pain, morphine remains the opioid agent of choice. The relatively recent appreciation that morphine-6-glucuronide contributes substantially to the analgesic response raises the question of optimal dose schedules in older patients with decreased renal function. It must be emphasized that sufficient analgesic doses at regular intervals represent the optimal use of this drug class. Too low a starting dose may actually increase pain of gastrointestinal origin due to increased smooth muscle spasm that usually precedes the analgesic response. Rationing of doses until severe pain has returned will often result in the requirement for larger doses with concomitantly increased respiratory depression and decreased mental acuity. Meperidine should be used with extreme caution in these patients since the likelihood of accumulation of the proconvulsant metabolite normeperidine is substantially increased.

### Cardiovascular Drugs

Among all drug groups, cardiovascular drugs are the most commonly prescribed for older patients. Although the use of these drugs is often life-saving, many of them have a low therapeutic index, and large inter-patient variability in response is to be expected.

Most diuretics are prone to cause electrolyte disturbances in geriatric patients. Although hypokalemia is recalled more often as an undesirable side effect, the negative effect on body calcium stores is often forgotten. In the elderly female patient with osteoporosis, chronic use of diuretics may increase susceptibility to fractures. In this situation, use of hydrochlorothiazide is least likely to disturb calcium homeostasis. However, long-acting diuretics may increase the risk of episodes of incontinence and thus limit the social activities of geriatric patients. Although the benefit of treating hypertension with diuretics and other cardiovascular drugs has been demonstrated convincingly in elderly patients, their increased susceptibility to orthostatic hypotension usually will limit the choice and dose of drug that may be considered for this purpose.

Oral anticoagulants produce morbid events more often in elderly patients than in younger ones. Although some controversy exists about the proposed mechanisms contributing to the exaggerated responsiveness, the probable causes include concurrent ingestion of other drugs that impair coagulation (e.g., NSAIDs), reduced receptor sensitivity to and increased clearance of vitamin K, and decreased availability of other clotting factors. Thus, lower warfarin doses usually will suffice in this patient group. Dose should be guided by the plasma prothrombin time, conventionally reported as the international normalized ratio (INR; see Chapter 38).

Digoxin dose is commonly a problem in the older patient. By itself, dose adjustment must take into consideration the decreased muscle mass and renal function. Also, quinidine and calcium-channel blockers increase plasma digoxin concentration when added to the therapeutic regimen. Depletion of potassium body stores by diuretics is likely to increase digoxin toxicity.

## Psychotropic Drugs

Benzodiazepines are rather commonly prescribed for older patients. Lipophilic benzodiazepines persist for a much longer time in the elderly; thus, with chronic ingestion, the body burden is likely to be much greater than in younger patients. The susceptibility to cognitive impairment is substantial and may compromise the ability of the patient to maintain an independent lifestyle. Because of altered drug disposition in the elderly, there is an increasing belief that the more lipophilic benzodiazepines (e.g., diazepam and flurazepam) are contraindicated in older patients. If prescription of a benzodiazepine is deemed necessary, serious consideration should be given to the use of a congener with lower lipophilicity that is biotransformed primarily by conjugation (e.g., oxazepam).

Antidepressant drugs, particularly tricyclics (e.g., amitriptyline and imipramine), are much more likely to cause side effects in older patients. Prominent among the side effects are postural hypotension, anticholinergic activity that can cause or aggravate urinary retention and impair gastrointestinal motility, and sedation.

All CNS depressants increase the risk of cognitive impairment, falls, and hip fractures. The consequent morbidity and mortality from these side effects should weigh heavily in the decision to prescribe these drugs and in the expected benefit to risk ratio.

## ADVERSE DRUG REACTIONS AND PATIENT ADHERENCE

There is ample evidence that appropriately prescribed drug therapy for elderly patients can assist in maintaining an improved quality of life in an independent setting.

However, an older patient who has an undesirable experience with a prescribed drug may be reluctant to adhere to instructions to continue its use. Because the patient may not wish to offend the physician, this problem may not be communicated between them, and the result may be a misinterpretation of the outcome of the prescribed treatment. It has been estimated that up to half of elderly patients are non-adherent to prescribed drug therapy. Thus, it is incumbent on the prescriber to simplify dose regimens and communicate effectively the importance of adherence to prescribed therapy in order that outcome is correctly attributed.

Although there has been emphasis on consideration of the prescribing habits of the physician as a major contributing factor to DRAPEs, the confounding influence of concurrent ingestion of over-the-counter drugs and herbal remedies has been relatively ignored. Older patients commonly ingest multiple vitamins in order to maintain their health. Often, these vitamin preparations contain significant amounts of iron. Recently, it has been demonstrated that iron can interact with drugs containing phenolic groups and thus decrease their bioavailability. Important examples include the interaction of iron with thyroxine, with levodopa and carbidopa, and with quinolone antibiotics. In the case of thyroxine, there will be decreased hormone absorption with resultant elevation of serum thyroid-stimulating hormone. In the case of levodopa and carbidopa, the interaction is likely to be reflected by more erratic control of the rigidity and tremor of Parkinson's disease. In the case of quinolone antibiotics, interaction with iron is likely to be reflected by reduced antibiotic efficacy, especially against microorganisms with intermediate or low sensitivity to that particular drug.

## SUMMARY OF ISSUES FOR CONSIDERATION IN GERIATRIC DRUG THERAPY

1. Is drug therapy really necessary? Are alternate treatments with acceptable outcomes available to the patient?
2. What are the goals of drug therapy?
3. What other drugs or herbal remedies, both prescribed and over-the-counter, is the patient taking that might cause the symptoms or might alter the physician's choice of agent? Is the benefit to risk ratio in older patients better for an alternate drug in this pharmacological category (e.g., a short-acting diuretic in preference to a long-acting one)?
4. Is the dose schedule likely to confuse the patient with respect to concurrently ingested drugs? What about the drug formulation and its packaging? Is it convenient for the patient? Will the patient remember the instructions? Does the patient understand the consequences of non-adherence? Has the dose been modi-

fied to account for altered body composition and physiological response to the drug effects?

5. Has the physician waited long enough to ensure that the patient is at steady state before increasing the dose or changing the choice of drug therapy?

## SUGGESTED READINGS

Chandler F, ed. *Herbs: Everyday Reference for Health Professionals.* Ottawa, Ontario: Canadian Pharmacists Association and Canadian Medical Association; 2000:1-217.

Grymonpre RE, Mitenko PA, Sitar DS, et al. Drug-associated hospital admissions in older patients. *J Am Geriatr Soc.* 1988;36:1092-1098.

Klotz U, Avant GR, Hoyumpa A, et al. The effects of age and liver disease on the disposition and elimination of diazepam in adult man. *J Clin Invest.* 1975;55:347-359.

Montamat SC, Cusack BJ, Vestal RE. Management of drug therapy in the elderly. *N Engl J Med.* 1989;321:303-309.

Ray WA, Griffin MR, Schaffner W, et al. Psychotropic drug use and the risk of hip fracture. *N Engl J Med.* 1987;316:363-369.

Renton KW. Cytochrome P450 regulation and drug biotransformation during inflammation and infection. *Curr Drug Metab.* 2004;5:235-243.

Schmucker DL. Aging and drug disposition. An update. *Pharmacol Rev.* 1985;37:133-148.

Sitar DS, ed. Focus on drugs and aging. *Pharmaceutical News.* 2001;8(6):11-41.

# 63

# Vitamins and Other Micronutrients

## WE WARD

## GENERAL CONCEPTS

The term *micronutrient* collectively refers to vitamins and minerals that are present in foods and the body in much smaller quantities than macronutrients (e.g., protein, carbohydrate, and fats). Vitamins are a diverse group of organic chemicals that either cannot be synthesized in the body at all or not in sufficient amounts to maintain normal tissue function. Vitamins are essential coenzymes and are required for cell functions as diverse as energy metabolism, red blood cell synthesis, amino acid metabolism, nerve transmission, and gene expression. While some vitamins such as vitamins A and D can function as hormones, their vitamin designation has been retained since a food source is still required to obtain these vitamins. Similarly, minerals have a myriad of functions that include acting as critical cofactors for a multitude of enzymes, regulating gene expression, maintaining pH, regulating muscle contraction and nerve function, and producing energy. Many minerals are also major constituents of bone, making bone hard and resistant to fracture. All micronutrients must be supplied from exogenous sources such as foods or diet supplements.

In the past, much of what we knew about micronutrients arose from learning how micronutrient deficiencies were associated with various diseases. Overt micronutrient deficiencies are now rare in developed countries but remain commonplace in developing countries, particularly deficiencies of iron, iodine, and vitamin A. Most recently, the focus has switched to the role of optimal intakes of micronutrients in preventing chronic disease and maintaining overall health. Recent surveys suggest that up to 60% of North American adults consume vitamin and/or mineral supplements for health reasons. Perhaps not surprisingly, individuals at risk for specific diseases are more likely to take a micronutrient supplement. For example, individuals at risk of cardiovascular disease may take an antioxidant supplement, while women at risk of osteoporosis often take calcium and vitamin D supplements.

## Categories of Micronutrients

Traditionally, the **vitamins** have been categorized as water- or fat-soluble on the basis of their solubility in water or fat solvents:

| Water-Soluble | Fat-Soluble |
|---|---|
| B vitamins | Vitamins A, D, E, K |
| Vitamin C | |

A number of other compounds normally synthesized in the body become, under some circumstances (e.g., prematurity, total parenteral feeding, genetic aberrations) "conditionally" essential (e.g., choline, carnitine).

**Minerals** are classified as macrominerals, microminerals (or trace minerals), or ultra trace minerals. Due to the paucity of data available on the health effects of ultra trace minerals and the fact that there are no dietary recommended intakes at present (except that tolerable upper intake levels have been established for some of the ultra trace minerals, Table 63-4), these minerals will not be discussed. Moreover, some minerals such as arsenic are known to be toxic. Macrominerals are differentiated from microminerals on the basis of requirement: the daily requirement for all macrominerals is greater than 100 mg/day.

| Macrominerals | Microminerals | Ultra Trace Minerals |
|---|---|---|
| Calcium (Ca) | Iron (Fe) | Nickel (Ni) |
| Phosphorus (P) | Zinc (Zn) | Silicon (Si) |
| Magnesium (Mg) | Copper (Cu) | Vanadium (Vn) |
| Sodium (Na) | Fluoride (F) | Boron (B) |
| Chloride (Cl) | Selenium (Se) | Cobalt (Co) |
| Potassium (K) | Iodine (I) | Arsenic (Ar) |
| Sulfur (S) | Manganese (Mn) | |
| | Chromium (Cr) | |
| | Molybdenum (Mo) | |

## Nomenclature of Micronutrients

The familiar (or alpha) nomenclature of the vitamins designates (in general) the historical order in which the function or structure of the vitamins was elucidated. In some cases (e.g., vitamins E, K, A, B6), the familiar name is a generic descriptor of a family of chemically related compounds that have comparable biological functions; these members of the same vitamin family are termed "vitamers." Two vitamins, vitamin A and niacin, have precursor forms, β-carotene and tryptophan, respectively, which can be metabolized to the active form of the vitamin.

In nature, some minerals can exist in multiple oxidation states, but in biological systems, most minerals exist in only one or possibly two different states to regulate various aspects of mineral metabolism such as intestinal absorption, transport in blood, or storage in the body. Iron, Zn, and Cu are among the most common minerals that exist in multiple states. Minerals are capable of interacting with charged amino acid residues of proteins and peptides, and these interactions can be strong, moderate, or weak depending on the valence state of the mineral. Sulfur amino acids (e.g., cysteine, methionine) as well as histidine are commonly bound with minerals in biological systems to enhance intestinal absorption or facilitate transport in the blood.

## Dietary Reference Intakes (DRIs)

A significant portion of nutritional research is focused on determining the roles of micronutrients in preventing chronic disease, with the overall aim of determining optimal intakes. From these data, many countries, and scientific committees such as the Food and Nutrition Board of the Institute of Medicine, National Academy of Medicine in the United States (in collaboration with Health Canada), have established recommended intakes for essential nutrients. As new evidence of the physiological relevance of nutrients becomes available, guidelines are periodically revised by panels of expert scientists. Canada and the United States embarked on a joint effort to harmonize dietary recommendations in 1995 and, in 1997, published the first guidelines that included recommendations for intakes of Ca, P, Mg, F, and vitamin D (see Suggested Readings). Subsequent publications have documented the recommendations for other micronutrients. These dietary recommendations are collectively referred to as the dietary reference intakes (DRIs) and include four categories of reference values: estimated average requirement (EAR); recommended dietary allowance (RDA); adequate intake (AI); and tolerable upper intake level (UL). These DRIs are gender- and age-specific and also make specific recommendations for pregnant and lactating women. The DRIs replaced the recommended nutrient intakes (RNIs) established in 1991 for Canadians and the recommended daily allowances (RDAs) established in 1989 for Americans. They are defined as follows:

- **EAR:** This is the average daily nutrient intake level estimated to meet the requirement of half the healthy individuals in a specific life stage or gender group based on specific criteria of nutrient adequacy. The criteria for determining nutritional adequacy of a specific micronutrient may differ according to life stage or gender group, and these criteria are detailed in the respective reports of each scientific panel (see Suggested Readings). The EAR is used to calculate the RDA.

- **RDA:** This is the average daily nutrient intake level sufficient to meet the nutrient requirement of nearly all (97 to 98%) healthy individuals in a specific life stage or gender group. The RDA is calculated as the EAR plus 2 standard deviations (SD) if the requirement is normally distributed and the variation in requirements is well defined:

$$RDA = EAR + 2\ SD_{EAR}$$

If the variation (e.g., SD) is inconsistent among studies and/or limited data are available, a standard estimate of variance of 10% is used. The RDA is to be used as a goal for individual intake.

- **AI:** This is a recommended average daily nutrient intake level based on observed or experimentally determined estimates of nutrient intakes by a group or groups of healthy people. As identified in Tables 63-1 and 63-2, several vitamins (D, K, pantothenic acid, biotin, choline) and minerals (Ca, F, Cr, Mn) have an AI rather than a RDA for all life stage groups. The AI is to be used as a goal for individual intake of a specific nutrient *only when there are insufficient data to determine an RDA.*

- **UL:** This is the highest average daily nutrient intake level likely to pose no risk of adverse health effects to almost all individuals. With the widespread use of vitamin and mineral supplements among North Americans, establishing ULs is important for providing guidance in order to avoid toxicity to individuals consuming these supplements.

In formulating the DRIs, it is assumed that these amounts (RDA or AI) will prevent a nutrient deficiency in healthy individuals. The RDAs or AIs are not intended to be sufficient for individuals who are malnourished or who are suffering or recovering from an illness. Also, these recommendations do not allow for losses of nutrients during processing of food and commercial and shelf storage. The current DRIs (RDA or AI) for micronutrients, intended for use in Canada and the United States, are presented in Tables 63-1 (vitamins) and 63-2 (minerals). It is important to note that values are presented as either an RDA or AI depending on the quantity and quality of data available. The ULs for micronutrients are presented in Tables 63-3 (vitamins) and 63-4 (minerals).

## Micronutrient Deficiencies

A micronutrient deficiency may be classified as a primary deficiency (i.e., an inadequate dietary intake) or as a secondary deficiency due to malabsorption, drug–nutrient interactions, mineral–mineral interactions, or increased vitamin needs due to physiological stress or disease.

### Inadequate dietary intake

In developed countries, a micronutrient deficiency is likely to be observed only in individuals who are dieting vigorously to lose weight; among the poor who have insufficient incomes to purchase or prepare foods; in those who do not appreciate the need for, or who have lifestyles incompatible with, balanced diets (e.g., "bachelor's scurvy"); in those who respond to gastrointestinal or other symptoms by restricting their diet without medical advice; or in those who acquire restrictive or bizarre eating patterns based on religious or philosophical convictions. Loss of appetite, poor dentition, and inadequate cooking facilities are common causes among the elderly. In poorly industrialized and economically depressed areas, extreme poverty and unsatisfactory food production and/or distribution are major factors. In some cultures, weaning practices often do not provide sufficient nutrients to support optimal growth and health of the young child.

### Drug–nutrient interactions

A large number of therapeutic agents interfere with absorption and increase the rate of turnover of some vitamins. Addiction to, or excessive use of, common substances such as alcohol, caffeine, and nicotine also interfere with vitamin metabolism. Little is known about the specific effects of illicit drugs, as distinct from the effects of poor dietary habits of heavy users of illicit drugs.

### Mineral–mineral interactions

There are many examples of mineral–mineral interactions that can potentially lead to a deficiency of one or more minerals. Realistically, this interaction occurs only if individuals are consuming mineral supplements (containing one or multiple minerals). Most of these interactions occur in the intestine, affecting the absorption of minerals across the brush-border membrane and/or the transport of a specific mineral across the basolateral membrane of the mucosal cell. For example, consumption of high levels of Zn or Fe, attainable only through the use of supplements and not diet alone, results in reduced Cu or Zn absorption, respectively, and may lead to a deficiency.

### Increased micronutrient needs

Normal physiological processes such as growth, pregnancy, and lactation impose higher requirements for micronutrients. For this reason, the RDA or AI for micronutrients varies according to life stage group; in addition, specific requirements have been established for pregnancy and lactation (see Tables 63-1 and 63-2). Increased needs for some vitamins may also occur in post-surgical, burn, or trauma patients and in a number

of disease processes. There is now convincing evidence that intakes above the recommended levels of some micronutrients, especially folate, are effective in reducing the incidence of neural-tube defects in newborns if taken by the mother during the initial months of the pregnancy. Cohort studies have reported that folate and $B_6$ are associated with a lower risk of cardiovascular disease; large prospective clinical trials of folate, $B_6$, and $B_{12}$ in relation to cardiovascular disease are ongoing. There is some evidence of an inverse relationship between the intake of certain specific vitamins and the incidence of some types of cancer. The vitamins so implicated may act as antioxidants (vitamin E, β-carotene, vitamin C) or may alter DNA methylation (folate) and thereby have protective effects upon cells and tissues. However, these data are far from conclusive. Much of the uncertainty and controversy stems from differences in study designs (prospective vs. case–control studies) and the status of subjects studied (e.g., smokers vs. non-smokers, alcohol use, other lifestyle factors). Other micronutrient–disease relationships that are currently being investigated are selenium, vitamin D, and prostate cancer; and calcium, vitamin D, and colon cancer. A recent statement by the United States Preventive Services Task Force, which evaluated published studies on multivitamin supplement use and disease risk, concluded that there is currently insufficient evidence to recommend for or against the use of vitamins A, C, or E; multivitamins with folic acid; or antioxidants for the prevention of chronic diseases such as cancer or cardiovascular disease.

## FAT-SOLUBLE VITAMINS

## Vitamin A

### Structure, dietary sources, and recommended intake

Vitamin A, as the preformed vitamin, exists as all-*trans* retinol (the physiologically active form; Fig. 63-1), as long-chain fatty acyl esters of retinol (the main storage form in tissues), and as retinal (the active form in the retina). In the cells, retinol is converted to retinoic acid, also considered to be physiologically active. The *cis*-isomers have no significant vitamin activity. Vitamin A activity is also provided by β-carotene (provitamin A), which can be converted to retinol. Other members of the carotenoid group have marginal activity.

Preformed vitamin A, as retinyl esters, is found only in animal products, the major sources being liver, fish liver oils, milk and dairy products, egg yolk, and fortified margarine. β-Carotene occurs in plant foods such as green and yellow vegetables and yellow fruits. In humans with a mixed diet, the activity of β-carotene is approximately only one-twelfth that of retinal because of incomplete absorption and inefficient conversion to retinal.

1 RAE (retinal activity equivalent) = 1 µg of all-*trans*-retinal
= 12 µg of all-*trans*-β-carotene
= 24 µg of other dietary
provitamin A carotenoids

One-third to one-half of the daily intake of vitamin A in mixed diets is β-carotene. In strict vegetarian diets containing no animal foods, β-carotene is virtually the sole source of vitamin A. The recommended intakes for vitamin A are expressed as RDAs in micrograms (see Table 63-1).

## Pharmacokinetics

The preformed vitamin is well absorbed from the upper intestine by a carrier-mediated process at low intakes and by diffusion at higher doses. β-Carotene is cleaved to retinol mainly in the intestinal mucosal cells during absorption and to a lesser extent by liver and other tissues. Bile salts enhance retinol absorption and are required for the absorption of β-carotene. Both vitamin A and β-carotene are transported from the intestine in the chylomicrons via the lymph, in a manner identical to that seen in fat absorption.

The liver is the major storage organ, and it can sequester very large amounts of vitamin A as the ester. Smaller amounts are found in kidney, adipose tissue, and lung. Stored vitamin A is released from the liver into the plasma as retinol, bound to a specific retinol-binding protein, by a tightly regulated process to maintain a constant supply of retinol to the target tissues. Normal plasma retinol levels are maintained at 30 to 70 µg/dL (1.05 to 2.45 µmol/L) and are not significantly reduced even in vitamin A deficiency until depletion of liver stores is well advanced. When large amounts of vitamin A, in excess of the normal requirement, are taken in chronically, they are not excreted but are stored in the liver and can ultimately exceed the hepatic storage capacity.

| TABLE 63-1 | Vitamins: Dietary Reference Intakes (DRIs) for Healthy Individuals* | | | | | |
|---|---|---|---|---|---|---|
| Life Stage Group (years) | Vitamin A (µg/day) | Vitamin C (mg/day) | Vitamin D (µg/day) | Vitamin E (mg/day) | Vitamin K (µg/day) | Thiamin (mg/day) |
| Infants | | | | | | |
| 0–0.5 | 400 | 40 | 5 | 4 | 5 | 4 |
| 0.5–1 | 500 | 50 | 5 | 5 | 5 | 5 |
| Children | | | | | | |
| 1–3 | **300** | **15** | 5 | **6** | 30 | **0.5** |
| 4–8 | **400** | **25** | 5 | **7** | 55 | **0.6** |
| Males | | | | | | |
| 9–13 | **600** | **45** | 5 | **11** | 60 | **0.9** |
| 14–18 | **900** | **75** | 5 | **15** | 75 | **1.2** |
| 19–30 | **900** | **90** | 5 | **15** | 120 | **1.2** |
| 31–50 | **900** | **90** | 5 | **15** | 120 | **1.2** |
| 51–70 | **900** | **90** | 10 | **15** | 120 | **1.2** |
| >70 | **900** | **90** | 15 | **15** | 120 | **1.2** |
| Females | | | | | | |
| 9–13 | **600** | **45** | 5 | **11** | 60 | **0.9** |
| 14–18 | **700** | **65** | 5 | **15** | 75 | **1.0** |
| 19–30 | **700** | **75** | 5 | **15** | 90 | **1.1** |
| 31–50 | **700** | **75** | 5 | **15** | 90 | **1.1** |
| 51–70 | **700** | **75** | 10 | **15** | 90 | **1.1** |
| >70 | **700** | **75** | 15 | **15** | 90 | **1.1** |
| Pregnancy | | | | | | |
| ≤18 | **750** | **80** | 5 | **15** | 75 | **1.4** |
| 19–30 | **770** | **85** | 5 | **15** | 90 | **1.4** |
| 31–50 | **770** | **85** | 5 | **15** | 90 | **1.4** |
| Lactation | | | | | | |
| ≤18 | **1200** | **115** | 5 | **19** | 75 | **1.4** |
| 19–30 | **1300** | **120** | 5 | **19** | 90 | **1.4** |
| 31–50 | **1300** | **120** | 5 | **19** | 90 | **1.4** |

*Values are presented as either the RDA (bold type) or AI (roman) for a specific micronutrient.

(From Standing Committee on the Scientific Evaluation of Dietary Reference Intakes, 1997, 1998, 2000, 2001.)

## Physiology

In the retina of the eye, all-*trans* retinol is converted to the aldehyde and isomerized to 11-*cis* retinal, which then combines with the protein opsin in the rod cells of the retina to produce rhodopsin. This compound is responsible for vision in dim light. In the cone cells, iodopsin is similarly formed and is responsible for daylight vision.

Retinol and retinoic acid, a metabolite of retinol, are required for normal cell differentiation, particularly of the mucus-secreting epithelial cells. In the absence of retinol, mucus-secreting cells are replaced by keratin-producing cells in many body tissues. The action of retinol on cell differentiation may be exerted via its influence on gene expression in the nucleus. Retinol also serves as a carrier for mannose to effect its incorporation into cell-surface glycoproteins, which appear to serve a number of functions including that of regulation of cell differentiation. The requirement for vitamin A in normal reproduc-

tion, bone development, and growth, as well as its influence on the immune system, may be allied to the general function of cell differentiation.

## Deficiency

Vitamin A deficiency is most prevalent in preschool children in Southeast Asia and parts of Africa and South America because of poor intakes of both vitamin A and β-carotene. Also at risk is the newborn (especially the premature infant), since liver stores of vitamin A at birth are low. In the alcoholic individual, liver structure is affected (see Chapter 43) and storage of vitamin A is compromised. In the non-alcoholic adult, vitamin A deficiency occurs largely as a consequence of gastrointestinal abnormalities resulting in fat malabsorption. The major deficiency signs include night blindness (nyctalopia) and xerophthalmia, the latter characterized by a progressive drying (xerosis) of the conjunctiva and cornea of the eye,

| Riboflavin (mg/day) | Niacin (mg/day) | Vitamin $B_6$ (mg/day) | Folate (µg/day) | Vitamin $B_{12}$ (µg/day) | Pantothenic Acid (mg/day) | Biotin (µg/day) | Choline (mg/day) |
|---|---|---|---|---|---|---|---|
| 0.3 | 2 | 0.1 | 65 | 0.4 | 1.7 | 5 | 125 |
| 0.4 | 4 | 0.3 | 80 | 0.5 | 1.8 | 6 | 15 |
| 0.5 | 6 | 0.5 | 150 | 0.9 | 2 | 8 | 200 |
| 0.6 | 8 | 0.6 | 200 | 1.2 | 3 | 12 | 250 |
| 0.9 | 12 | 1.0 | 300 | 1.8 | 4 | 20 | 375 |
| 1.3 | 16 | 1.3 | 400 | 2.4 | 5 | 25 | 550 |
| 1.3 | 16 | 1.3 | 400 | 2.4 | 5 | 30 | 550 |
| 1.3 | 16 | 1.3 | 400 | 2.4 | 5 | 30 | 550 |
| 1.3 | 16 | 1.7 | 400 | 2.4 | 5 | 30 | 550 |
| 1.3 | 16 | 1.7 | 400 | 2.4 | 5 | 30 | 550 |
| 0.9 | 12 | 1.0 | 300 | 1.8 | 4 | 20 | 375 |
| 1.0 | 14 | 1.2 | 400 | 2.4 | 5 | 25 | 400 |
| 1.1 | 14 | 1.3 | 400 | 2.4 | 5 | 30 | 425 |
| 1.1 | 14 | 1.3 | 400 | 2.4 | 5 | 30 | 425 |
| 1.1 | 14 | 1.5 | 400 | 2.4 | 5 | 30 | 425 |
| 1.1 | 14 | 1.5 | 400 | 2.4 | 5 | 30 | 425 |
| 1.4 | 18 | 1.9 | 600 | 2.6 | 6 | 30 | 450 |
| 1.4 | 18 | 1.9 | 600 | 2.6 | 6 | 30 | 450 |
| 1.4 | 18 | 1.9 | 600 | 2.6 | 6 | 30 | 450 |
| 1.6 | 17 | 2.0 | 500 | 2.8 | 7 | 35 | 550 |
| 1.6 | 17 | 2.0 | 500 | 2.8 | 7 | 35 | 550 |
| 1.6 | 17 | 2.0 | 500 | 2.8 | 7 | 35 | 550 |

| TABLE 63-2 | Minerals: Dietary Reference Intakes (DRIs) for Healthy Individuals* | | | | |
|---|---|---|---|---|---|
| Life Stage Group (years) | Calcium (mg/day) | Chromium (µg/day) | Copper (µg/day) | Fluoride (mg/day) | Iodine (µg/day) |
| Infants | | | | | |
| 0–0.5 | 210 | 0.2 | 200 | 0.01 | 110 |
| 0.5–1 | 270 | 5.5 | 220 | 0.5 | 130 |
| Children | | | | | |
| 1–3 | 500 | 11 | **340** | 0.7 | **90** |
| 4–8 | 800 | 15 | **440** | 1 | **90** |
| Males | | | | | |
| 9–13 | 1300 | 25 | **700** | 2 | **120** |
| 14–18 | 1300 | 35 | **890** | 3 | **150** |
| 19–30 | 1000 | 35 | **900** | 4 | **150** |
| 31–50 | 1000 | 35 | **900** | 4 | **150** |
| 51–70 | 1200 | 30 | **900** | 4 | **150** |
| >70 | 1200 | 30 | **900** | 4 | **150** |
| Females | | | | | |
| 9–13 | 1300 | 21 | **700** | 2 | **120** |
| 14–18 | 1300 | 24 | **890** | 3 | **150** |
| 19–30 | 1000 | 25 | **900** | 3 | **150** |
| 31–50 | 1000 | 25 | **900** | 3 | **150** |
| 51–70 | 1200 | 20 | **900** | 3 | **150** |
| >70 | 1200 | 20 | **900** | 3 | **150** |
| Pregnancy | | | | | |
| ≤18 | 1300 | 29 | **1000** | 3 | **220** |
| 19–30 | 1000 | 30 | **1000** | 3 | **220** |
| 31–50 | 1000 | 30 | **1000** | 3 | **220** |
| Lactation | | | | | |
| ≤18 | 1300 | 44 | **1300** | 3 | **290** |
| 19–30 | 1000 | 45 | **1300** | 3 | **290** |
| 31–50 | 1000 | 45 | **1300** | 3 | **290** |

*Values are presented as either the RDA (bold type) or AI (roman) for a specific micronutrient.

(From Standing Committee on the Scientific Evaluation of Dietary Reference Intakes, 1997, 2000, 2001.)

culminating in disintegration of the cornea and extrusion of the lens, and hence irreparable blindness. There is also keratinization of other epithelial cells in the bronchorespiratory, genitourinary, and gastrointestinal tracts and in sweat glands, leading to an increased frequency of infections in these tissues.

### Therapeutic use

Supplementation is necessary only to treat frank deficiency or as a preventive measure in pregnancy, lactation, or infancy when dietary intakes are obviously inadequate. In the last case, the supplement plus usual dietary intake should not exceed the recommended intake. In areas where intake of vitamin A is chronically inadequate, prophylactic intramuscular injections of 30 to 120 mg retinol given every 3 to 6 months to infants and small children have proven effective in reducing blindness induced by vitamin A deficiency.

Vitamin A palmitate and, more recently, isomers of retinoic acid have proved effective in the treatment of various skin disorders, including acne vulgaris and psoriasis, albeit not without toxic side effects.

### Toxicity

The ULs for each life stage group and gender are shown in Table 63-3. Vitamin A is highly toxic when taken in large amounts well in excess of the ULs, either acutely or chronically. Hypervitaminosis A occurs most frequently as a result of overenthusiastic supplementation of children's diets or self-medication, but it may also result from the excessive consumption of retinol-rich foodstuffs (e.g., a single serving of polar bear liver or chronic intakes of large portions of chicken or beef liver).

Acute toxicity may result from a single dose of about 200 mg (666 000 IU) of vitamin A in adults or half of this amount in children. Toxicity signs include headache,

| Iron (mg/day) | Magnesium (mg/day) | Manganese (mg/day) | Molybdenum (μg/day) | Phosphorus (mg/day) | Selenium (μg/day) | Zinc (mg/day) |
|---|---|---|---|---|---|---|
| 0.27 | 30 | 0.003 | 2 | 100 | 15 | 2 |
| 11 | 75 | 0.6 | 3 | 275 | 20 | 3 |
| 7 | 80 | 1.2 | 17 | 460 | 20 | 3 |
| 10 | 130 | 1.5 | 22 | 500 | 30 | 5 |
| 8 | 240 | 1.9 | 34 | 1250 | 40 | 8 |
| 11 | 410 | 2.2 | 43 | 1250 | 55 | 11 |
| 8 | 400 | 2.3 | 45 | 700 | 55 | 11 |
| 8 | 420 | 2.3 | 45 | 700 | 55 | 11 |
| 8 | 420 | 2.3 | 45 | 700 | 55 | 11 |
| 8 | 420 | 2.3 | 45 | 700 | 55 | 11 |
| 8 | 240 | 1.6 | 34 | 1250 | 40 | 8 |
| 15 | 360 | 1.6 | 43 | 1250 | 55 | 9 |
| 18 | 310 | 1.8 | 45 | 700 | 55 | 8 |
| 18 | 320 | 1.8 | 45 | 700 | 55 | 8 |
| 8 | 320 | 1.8 | 45 | 700 | 55 | 8 |
| 8 | 320 | 1.8 | 45 | 700 | 55 | 8 |
| 27 | 400 | 2.0 | 50 | 1250 | 60 | 13 |
| 27 | 350 | 2.0 | 50 | 700 | 60 | 11 |
| 27 | 360 | 2.0 | 50 | 700 | 60 | 11 |
| 10 | 360 | 2.6 | 50 | 1250 | 70 | 14 |
| 9 | 310 | 2.6 | 50 | 700 | 70 | 12 |
| 9 | 320 | 2.6 | 50 | 700 | 70 | 12 |

nausea and vomiting, increased cerebrospinal fluid pressure, blurred vision, and bulging of the fontanelle in infants. Larger doses cause extensive peeling of the skin.

Chronic toxicity may follow repeated intakes of vitamin A over long periods of time (3 to 6 months or more) in amounts greater than 10 times the recommended intake. There is an extensive array of symptoms that vary with the individual, the more serious including hepatotoxicity (fibrosis, cirrhosis, central vein sclerosis, portal hypertension), hypercalcemia, hyperlipemia, spontaneous abortions, and fetal malformations. Although fatalities are not common, they have occurred; for example, a death from apparent vitamin A toxicity has been reported in a newborn receiving 25 mg/day for 11 days.

In both acute and chronic toxicity, the symptoms are transient and disappear after withdrawal of the supplement. Toxic dose levels also vary considerably because of marked variation in individual sensitivity to large intakes.

Retinoic acid isomers (e.g., etretinate and isotretinoin) used in the treatment of skin disorders cause minor side effects, including dryness of mucous membranes and conjunctivitis, but, more importantly, they are teratogenic if taken in early pregnancy.

Large intakes of β-carotene produce an orange coloration of the skin. Hypercarotenemia is a benign condition that does not result in vitamin A toxicity because of the slow conversion of β-carotene to retinol.

## Vitamin D

### Structure, dietary sources, and recommended intake

This vitamin exists in two major precursor forms, 7-dehydrocholesterol and ergosterol, which are converted to their vitamin forms cholecalciferol (vitamin $D_3$) and ergocalciferol (vitamin $D_2$), respectively, upon exposure to

| TABLE 63-3 | Vitamins: Tolerable Upper Intake Levels (ULs) for Healthy Individuals | | | | | | |
|---|---|---|---|---|---|---|---|
| Life Stage Group (years) | Vitamin A (µg/day) | Vitamin C (mg/day) | Vitamin D (µg/day) | Vitamin E (mg/day) | Vitamin K | Thiamin (mg/day) | Riboflavin |
| Infants | | | | | | | |
| 0–0.5 | 600 | ND | 25 | ND | ND | ND | ND |
| 0.5–1 | 600 | ND | 25 | ND | ND | ND | ND |
| Children | | | | | | | |
| 1–3 | 600 | 400 | 50 | 200 | ND | ND | ND |
| 4–8 | 900 | 650 | 50 | 300 | ND | ND | ND |
| Males/Females | | | | | | | |
| 9–13 | 1700 | 1200 | 50 | 600 | ND | ND | ND |
| 14–18 | 2800 | 1800 | 50 | 800 | ND | ND | ND |
| 19–70 | 3000 | 2000 | 50 | 1000 | ND | ND | ND |
| >70 | 3000 | 2000 | 50 | 1000 | ND | ND | ND |
| Pregnancy | | | | | | | |
| ≤18 | 2800 | 1800 | 50 | 800 | ND | ND | ND |
| 19–50 | 3000 | 2000 | 50 | 1000 | ND | ND | ND |
| Lactation | | | | | | | |
| ≤18 | 2800 | 1800 | 50 | 800 | ND | ND | ND |
| 19–50 | 3000 | 2000 | 50 | 1000 | ND | ND | ND |

ND = Not determinable due to lack of adverse effects in this age group and concern with regard to lack of ability to handle excess amounts.

(From Standing Committee on the Scientific Evaluation of Dietary Reference Intakes, 1997, 1998, 2000, 2001; and Trumbo et al., 2001.)

| TABLE 63-4 | Minerals: Tolerable Upper Intake Levels (ULs) for Healthy Individuals | | | | | | | |
|---|---|---|---|---|---|---|---|---|
| Life Stage Group (years) | Calcium (g/day) | Chromium | Copper (µg/day) | Fluoride (mg/day) | Iodine (µg/day) | Iron (mg/day) | Magnesium (mg/day) | Manganese (mg/day) |
| Infants | | | | | | | | |
| 0–0.5 | ND | ND | ND | 0.7 | ND | 40 | ND | ND |
| 0.5–1 | ND | ND | ND | 0.9 | ND | 40 | ND | ND |
| Children | | | | | | | | |
| 1–3 | 2.5 | ND | 1000 | 1.3 | 200 | 40 | 65 | 2 |
| 4–8 | 2.5 | ND | 3000 | 2.2 | 300 | 40 | 110 | 3 |
| Males/Females | | | | | | | | |
| 9–13 | 2.5 | ND | 5000 | 10 | 600 | 40 | 350 | 6 |
| 14–18 | 2.5 | ND | 8000 | 10 | 900 | 45 | 350 | 9 |
| 19–70 | 2.5 | ND | 10000 | 10 | 1100 | 45 | 350 | 11 |
| >70 | 2.5 | ND | 10000 | 10 | 1100 | 45 | 350 | 11 |
| Pregnancy | | | | | | | | |
| ≤18 | 2.5 | ND | 8000 | 10 | 900 | 45 | 350 | 9 |
| 19–50 | 2.5 | ND | 10000 | 10 | 1100 | 45 | 350 | 11 |
| Lactation | | | | | | | | |
| ≤18 | 2.5 | ND | 8000 | 10 | 900 | 45 | 350 | 9 |
| 19–50 | 2.5 | ND | 10000 | 10 | 1100 | 45 | 350 | 11 |

ND = Not determinable due to lack of adverse effects in this age group and concern with regard to lack of ability to handle excess amounts.

(From Standing Committee on the Scientific Evaluation of Dietary Reference Intakes, 1997, 2000, 2001; and Trumbo et al., 2001.)

| Niacin (mg/day) | Vitamin $B_6$ (mg/day) | Folate (µg/day) | Vitamin $B_{12}$ | Pantothenic Acid | Biotin | Choline (g/day) |
|---|---|---|---|---|---|---|
| ND | ND | ND | ND | ND | ND | ND |
| ND | ND | ND | ND | ND | ND | ND |
| 10 | 30 | 300 | ND | ND | ND | 1.0 |
| 15 | 40 | 400 | ND | ND | ND | 1.0 |
| 20 | 60 | 600 | ND | ND | ND | 2.0 |
| 30 | 80 | 800 | ND | ND | ND | 3.0 |
| 35 | 100 | 1000 | ND | ND | ND | 3.5 |
| 35 | 100 | 1000 | ND | ND | ND | 3.5 |
| 30 | 80 | 800 | ND | ND | ND | 3.0 |
| 35 | 100 | 1000 | ND | ND | ND | 3.5 |
| 30 | 80 | 800 | ND | ND | ND | 3.0 |
| 35 | 100 | 1000 | ND | ND | ND | 3.5 |

| Molybdenum (µg/day) | Phosphorus (g/day) | Selenium (µg/day) | Zinc (mg/day) | Nickel (mg/day) | Arsenic | Boron (mg/day) | Silicon | Vanadium (mg/day) |
|---|---|---|---|---|---|---|---|---|
| ND | ND | 45 | 4 | ND | ND | ND | ND | ND |
| ND | ND | 60 | 5 | ND | ND | ND | ND | ND |
| 300 | 3 | 90 | 7 | 0.2 | ND | 3 | ND | ND |
| 600 | 3 | 150 | 12 | 0.3 | ND | 6 | ND | ND |
| 1100 | 4 | 280 | 23 | 0.6 | ND | 11 | ND | ND |
| 1700 | 4 | 400 | 34 | 1.0 | ND | 17 | ND | ND |
| 2000 | 4 | 400 | 40 | 1.0 | ND | 20 | ND | 1.8 |
| 2000 | 3 | 400 | 40 | 1.0 | ND | 20 | ND | 1.8 |
| 1700 | 3.5 | 400 | 34 | 1.0 | ND | 17 | NS | ND |
| 2000 | 3.5 | 400 | 40 | 1.0 | ND | 20 | ND | ND |
| 1700 | 4 | 400 | 34 | 1.0 | ND | 17 | ND | ND |
| 200 | 4 | 400 | 40 | 1.0 | ND | 20 | ND | ND |

**FIGURE 63-1** Structural formulae of the fat-soluble vitamins A, E, and K.

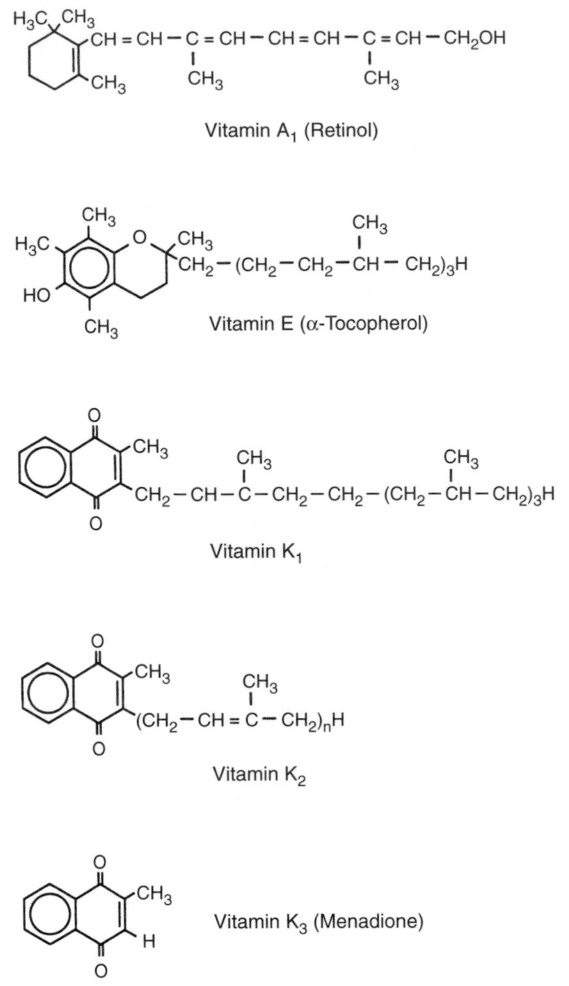

Vitamin A₁ (Retinol)

Vitamin E (α-Tocopherol)

Vitamin K₁

Vitamin K₂

Vitamin K₃ (Menadione)

ultraviolet radiation. This photobiosynthesis of vitamin D₃, occurring in the skin upon exposure to sunlight, is of major importance in humans. The physiologically active form appears to be 1,25-dihydroxycholecalciferol, or calcitriol (1,25(OH)₂D₃; Fig. 63-2). Vitamin D levels are particularly high in fish liver oils. Few other natural foods contain the vitamin in significant amounts, and it has therefore been necessary to add the vitamin to some foods in countries where the amount of sunlight is inadequate due to a northern climate or in areas with heavy air pollution that occludes ultraviolet penetration.

The policy governing the choice of foods that may be fortified varies in different countries. In North America, milk, margarine, butter, cheese, and infant foods are fortified with vitamin D₃.

The recommended intakes for vitamin D are expressed as AIs in micrograms (see Table 63-1). Vitamin D content is often expressed in international units (IU), and the conversion to micrograms is the following: 1 μg vitamin D = 40 IU vitamin D.

## Pharmacokinetics

Both vitamins D₂ and D₃ are absorbed from the intestine, the latter more completely. As with other fat-soluble vitamins, vitamin D absorption is dependent on normal fat absorption; it is thus dependent on hepatic and biliary function.

The first step in the activation of vitamin D₃ (now considered the prohormone form) occurs in the liver, where it is hydroxylated to 25(OH)D₃. From there it circulates to the kidney, where it is further hydroxylated to its active hormone form, 1,25(OH)₂D₃. This latter hydroxylation is tightly regulated and responds to changes in serum concentrations of calcium and phosphorus. Parathyroid hormone and calcitonin are also involved.

There is no significant storage of vitamin D in the liver (as occurs with vitamin A). It is distributed among various tissues in the body; adipose and muscle tissue are considered the major storage sites in humans. Excretion of vitamin D and its metabolites occurs primarily in the feces with the aid of bile salts. The details of the functional metabolism of vitamin D₃ are shown in Figure 63-2.

## Physiology

Vitamin D has a primary role in the homeostatic regulation of serum calcium and phosphate levels through the promotion of intestinal absorption and renal reabsorption of calcium and phosphorus and the resorption of calcium and phosphate from bone (see Chapter 65). Maintenance of serum calcium levels permits mineralization and remodelling of bone and the maintenance of normal excitability in the central autonomic and somatic nervous systems.

Because it is produced exclusively in the kidney in response to hypocalcemia and hypophosphatemia and exerts its function on specific target tissues, vitamin D is considered to be a hormone. The finding of high-affinity receptors for 1,25(OH)₂D₃ in a number of tissues (e.g., pancreas, skin, muscle, brain, and hematopoietic cells) not related to calcium homeostasis suggests additional roles for vitamin D (e.g., in cell growth and differentiation).

## Deficiency

Vitamin D deficiency occurs mainly as a consequence of inadequate exposure to sunlight and/or dietary deficiency. It can also occur as a result of an increased requirement (e.g., multiple pregnancies, lactation) or a deficit in the 1-hydroxylation pathway of 25(OH)D₃. Deficiency results in rickets in children and osteomalacia in adults, as a consequence of decreased mineralization of bone and teeth. The matrix is decalcified, so the bone is softened and may become grossly deformed. Rickets was formerly a major problem in Canada and northern regions of the

United States because of insufficient sunlight during the winter, but it has been largely eliminated by vitamin D fortification of milk.

## Therapeutic use

Rickets due to inadequate exposure to sunlight can be reversed by 10 µg vitamin D daily. Fully developed rickets

and osteomalacia may require dosages of 0.1 to 1.0 mg daily, depending on the etiology of the disease.

A form of vitamin D–dependent rickets that has a genetic rather than dietary etiology will respond to 1.25 to 2.50 mg (50 000 to 100 000 IU) of vitamin D daily. More recently, vitamin D supplements (17.5 µg/day, or 700 IU/day), in combination with Ca supplements

**FIGURE 63-2**    Current concepts of the functional metabolism of vitamin $D_3$.

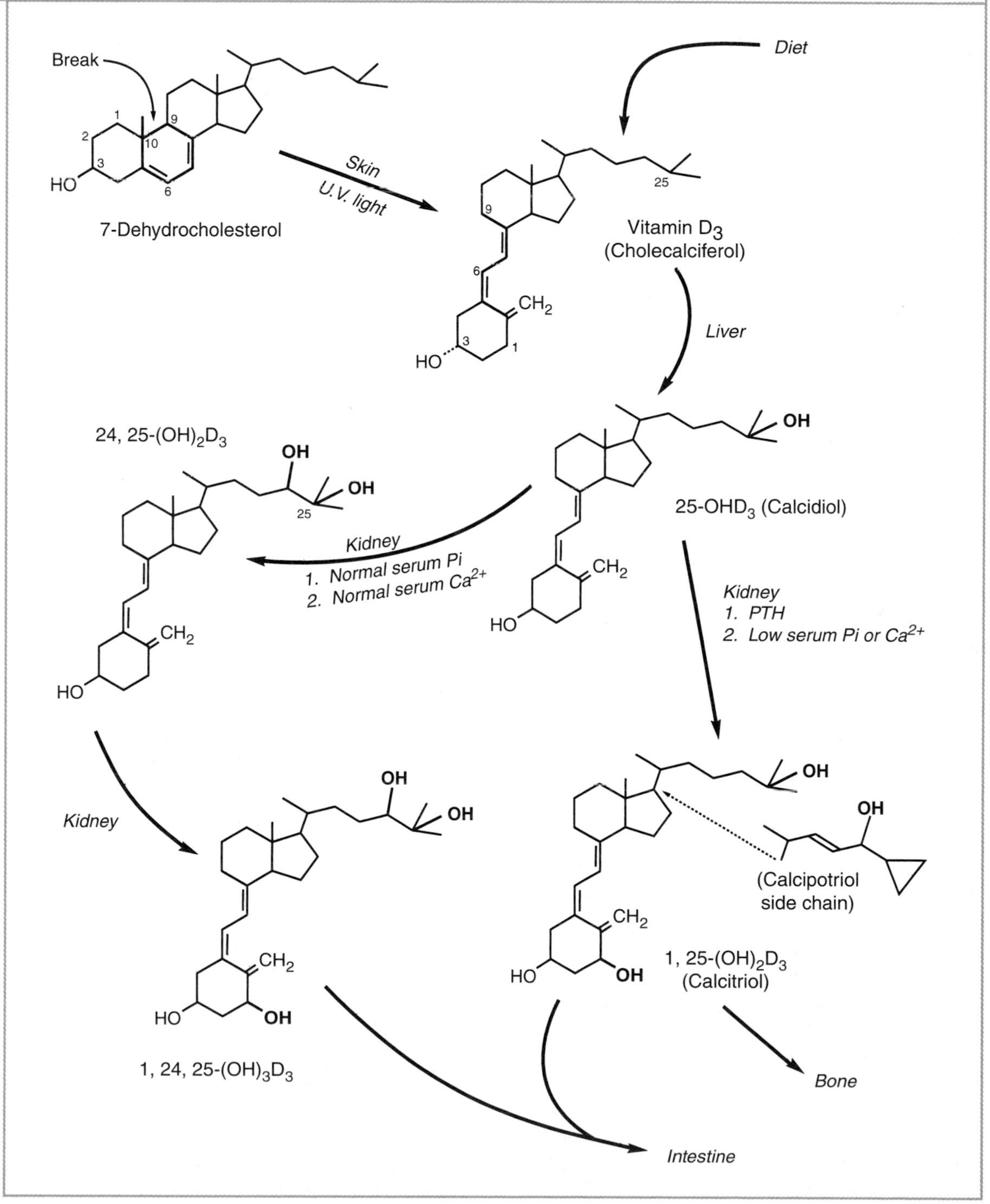

(500 mg/day), have been shown to be useful in slowing the loss of bone mass that occurs with aging among both men and women over age 65 (see "Calcium" below and Suggested Readings). A review published in 2005 suggests that vitamin D intakes of older men and women should be 20 to 25 µg (800 to 1000 IU) per day, higher than the current AI, to lower the risk of osteoporotic fracture. Optimal levels of vitamin D for maintance of overall health are still under active study.

### Toxicity

An excessive intake of vitamin D leading to toxicity is unlikely from natural food sources but can result from overzealous use of vitamin D supplements. For this reason, fortification of foods with vitamin D is regulated in most countries. The UL for vitamin D is 50 µg for individuals over the age of 1 year and 25 µg for infants under 1 year of age (see Table 63-3). However, data collected since the establishment of this UL suggest that intakes of 100 µg/day are safe for adults.

Symptoms of vitamin D toxicity include fatigue, headache, diarrhea, and hypercalcemia, which may lead to calcium deposition in kidneys, heart, lungs, blood vessels, and skin. Hypercalcemia may also lead to an arrest of growth that cannot be fully reversed. This may be associated with irreversible effects on calcitonin production (see Chapter 65).

## Vitamin E

### Structure, dietary sources, and recommended intake

Several tocopherols are known to have vitamin E activity. The highest biological activity is shown by $d$-α-tocopherol (RRR-α-tocopherol; see Fig. 63-1). Animal tissues contain primarily this form. The vitamin is found mainly in plant products; the richest sources are vegetable oils and wheat germ.

The RDA for vitamin E is expressed in milligrams (see Table 63-1). The older terminology for vitamin E activity is the IU: 1 IU = 1 mg $dl$-α-tocopheryl acetate (all-$rac$-α-tocopheryl acetate), the commercially synthesized form, or 1.49 mg $d$-α-tocopherol, the naturally occurring form.

### Pharmacokinetics

Absorption of vitamin E, like that of other fat-soluble vitamins, depends on the integrity of fat absorption processes in the intestine. At normal intakes, approximately 50% of dietary tocopherols are absorbed. Efficiency of absorption falls to less than 10% with pharmacological doses (e.g., 200 mg or more). Tocopherols are carried in the blood by plasma β-lipoproteins. Liver and muscle are the major storage sites. Although large amounts are also deposited in the adipose tissue, tocopherol is mobilized only very slowly from adipocytes.

### Physiology

Vitamin E is an antioxidant and probably acts as a free radical scavenger in cell membranes to protect membrane polyunsaturated fatty acids from peroxidation. It appears to act in concert with other antioxidant systems in the cell (e.g., selenium-dependent glutathione peroxidase, superoxide dismutase, catalase, and ascorbic acid).

Vitamin E not located in the membranes likely serves as a protective antioxidant for other easily oxidized lipid-soluble compounds such as vitamin A.

### Deficiency

Vitamin E is accepted as an essential nutrient for humans, but although deficiency states have been clearly defined in animals, this is a subject of much debate in human health and nutrition.

Adults rarely develop a vitamin E deficiency due to poor dietary intake. However, individuals with chronic fat malabsorption or a genetic deficiency of β-lipoprotein, the plasma carrier for vitamin E, are at risk. In these individuals, erythrocyte stability is diminished, resulting in decreased erythrocyte survival, although severe anemia does not usually ensue.

Premature newborns have limited tissue stores of vitamin E at birth and have intestinal malabsorption for the first few weeks of life. Decreased erythrocyte survival in these infants leads to a severe hemolytic anemia. In both children and adults, severe fat malabsorption results in a progressive neurological disorder that has been attributed to vitamin E deficiency.

### Therapeutic use

Correction of the deficiencies noted above may require up to 300 mg vitamin E. Vitamin E in high doses (about 300 mg) also appears to be effective in treating intermittent claudication in adults and in ameliorating oxygen-induced retrolental fibroplasia in premature infants. Claims for its efficacy in treating a myriad of other conditions (the effects of aging, cardiovascular disease, sexual dysfunction, etc.) are largely unfounded. A number of epidemiological studies indicate an inverse correlation between the mean intake of α-tocopherol and the incidence of coronary heart disease in a population. However, the results of large-scale, double-blind, placebo-controlled studies of the effect of vitamin E supplements on the risk of coronary heart disease are still controversial (see Suggested Readings).

### Toxicity

Vitamin E has extremely low toxicity, producing only mild gastrointestinal upsets or fatigue in some individuals, so not surprisingly, the ULs are relatively high compared with the RDA (see Table 63-3). However, high intakes of vitamin E may exacerbate a vitamin K deficiency, especially in those individuals on anticoagulant therapy with coumarin compounds.

# Vitamin K

## Structure, dietary sources, and recommended intake

Vitamin K (see Fig. 63-1) exists in two forms, one of plant origin (phylloquinone, or $K_1$) and the other of bacterial origin (a series of menaquinones, $K_2$). A number of synthetic quinones have vitamin K–like activity, of which the most important is menadione ($K_3$). Sources in the diet are green leafy vegetables, cheese, egg yolk, and liver.

One-half of the requirement for vitamin K is usually met by intestinal bacterial synthesis. The recommended intakes are expressed as AIs for all life stage groups and genders (see Table 63-1).

## Pharmacokinetics

Vitamin K is readily absorbed by the usual pathways of fat absorption, and it is therefore dependent on the presence of bile salts. There is only limited tissue storage of vitamin K, and the stores can be depleted in 10 to 20 days.

## Physiology

Vitamin K is required for the γ-carboxylation (activation) of glutamic acid residues in a number of inactive precursors of biologically important proteins. The best known of these are prothrombin and at least seven other factors involved in the coagulation of blood (see Chapter 38).

Other vitamin K–dependent proteins have been identified (e.g., osteocalcin in bone and proteins in plasma and kidney cortex). The common feature of these proteins is their capacity to bind calcium, presumably at the γ-carboxyglutamyl sites.

Oral anticoagulants of the coumarin class (including warfarin; see Chapter 38) are vitamin K antagonists and are useful in reducing thrombus formation in patients at risk of intravascular clotting, as in ischemic heart disease and non-hemorrhagic strokes. Paradoxically, vitamin K in megadose amounts has been reported to prolong the prothrombin time; a dose of 1200 IU may potentiate the anticoagulant effects of the coumarin drugs and cause bleeding.

## Deficiency

Requirements are easily met by the dietary content plus the synthesis by intestinal bacteria. In adults, deficiency is usually secondary to malabsorption or the administration of a vitamin K antagonist. In deficiency, there is an increased prothrombin time and a tendency to hemorrhage.

Newborn infants, particularly premature ones, are susceptible to a vitamin K deficiency, "hemorrhagic disease of the newborn." Little vitamin crosses the placenta to the fetus, and the gut is sterile for the first few days of life. Human breast milk is sterile and contains little vitamin K, placing the breastfed infant at further risk. Therefore, vitamin K is usually administered prophylactically to the newborn.

## Therapeutic use

The only rational uses of vitamin K are to increase the hepatic biosynthesis of clotting factors, especially as an antidotal agent in oral anticoagulant therapy (see Chapter 38) and in the prevention of hemorrhagic disease of the newborn.

## Toxicity

Excessive doses of menadione ($K_3$) produce a hemolytic tendency and kernicterus in infants. It irritates mucous membranes and may depress liver function. Vitamin $K_1$ does not have these effects, and, moreover, it is non-toxic in animals. In humans, flushing, dyspnea, and death have occurred, but these may have been due to other constituents in the pharmaceutical dosage forms of vitamin $K_1$ used in those cases.

# WATER-SOLUBLE VITAMINS

## B-Complex Vitamins

### Thiamin (vitamin $B_1$)

*Structure, dietary sources, and recommended intake.* Thiamin (Fig. 63-3) consists of a pyrimidine and a thiazole moiety. It is widely distributed in foods, but most contain low concentrations. The major dietary sources are yeasts (brewer's or baker's yeast), pork, beef, liver, wheat germ, whole or enriched cereals, and grains and legumes.

The vitamin is easily destroyed by heat (during cooking), in alkaline medium, and by oxidation or by sulfites added in food processing. Thiamin is also destroyed by agents occurring naturally in foods (e.g., heat-labile thiaminases in raw fish, or heat-stable thiamin antagonists such as polyphenols in tea, ferns, and betel nut).

Recommended intakes for thiamin are expressed as RDAs in milligrams for individuals aged 1 and older (see Table 63-1).

*Pharmacokinetics.* Thiamin is absorbed from the upper small intestine by a carrier-mediated active transport process when intakes are less than 5 mg/day (well above the recommended intake). At higher intakes, passive diffusion contributes. Absorption is significantly impaired in alcoholics and in patients with folate deficiency.

The body pool is small, about 30 mg in the adult, half of which is in skeletal muscle and the remainder in heart, liver, kidney, and brain. Excess thiamin is not stored but is excreted in the urine. In addition to free thiamin, the urine also contains a number of catabolites of thiamin that arise as a consequence of the coenzyme action of thiamin.

*Physiology.* Thiamin pyrophosphate functions as a coenzyme in the oxidative decarboxylation of pyruvic and

**FIGURE 63-3** Structural formulae of the water-soluble vitamins of the B complex.

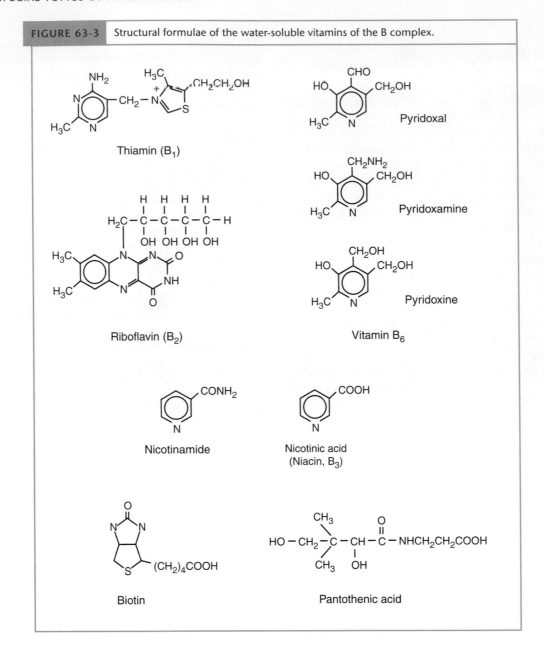

α-ketoglutaric acids and in the "transketolase" reactions of the triose phosphate pathway.

Thiamin is also required, likely as thiamin triphosphate, for nerve function in a reaction that is unrelated to its role as a coenzyme.

*Deficiency.* Beriberi is associated with white polished rice diets, as seen in Southeast Asia, and with highly milled wheat diets. The deficiency has become much less common because most countries now fortify foods with thiamin.

Acute deficiency (wet, or cardiovascular, beriberi) results from diets that are very low in thiamin and high in carbohydrates. Signs include edema, enlarged heart, elec-

trocardiogram (ECG) changes, and cardiac failure associated with increased cardiac output ("high-output failure").

Slightly higher, but still inadequate, intakes produce a chronic deficiency (dry, or neuritic, beriberi), the essential feature of which is polyneuropathy with depressed peripheral nerve function, sensory disturbance, loss of reflexes and motor control, and muscle wasting.

In populations whose diet is not based on rice, thiamin deficiency is frequently seen in alcoholics because of a combination of poor diet and inhibition of the thiamin uptake mechanism by alcohol. It is the causal factor in three conditions often seen in alcoholics: alcoholic polyneuritis indistinguishable from dry beriberi; a thiamin-responsive cardiomyopathy; and an encephalopathy, known as the Wernicke–Korsakoff syndrome, which is characterized by impairment of memory, apathy, irritability, nystagmus, and oculomotor paralysis.

*Therapeutic use.* Deficiency may be treated with 15 to 30 mg/day of thiamin hydrochloride. Pharmacological doses of 50 mg/day are required for a few rare and poorly described thiamin-responsive inborn errors of metabolism.

*Toxicity.* No marked toxicity has been observed, and there are no ULs for thiamin (see Table 63-3). The very small number of isolated reports of alleged toxicity may have been due to individual hypersensitivity in patients receiving large amounts of thiamin intramuscularly.

## Riboflavin (vitamin B₂)

*Structure, dietary sources, and recommended intake.* Riboflavin (see Fig. 63-3) is a heterocyclic flavin linked to ribose, analogous to the nucleosides in RNA. Green leafy vegetables contain significant amounts of riboflavin; however, milk and meats are the most important contributors of riboflavin to the North American diet. The vitamin is heat-stable but is easily destroyed when exposed to light. The recommended intakes for individuals aged 1 and older are RDAs and are expressed in milligrams (see Table 63-1).

*Pharmacokinetics.* Riboflavin is absorbed from the upper part of the ileum by a saturable active transport process. Bile salts facilitate absorption. The absorptive capacity is limited to 20 to 25 mg in a single dose. Riboflavin is distributed to all tissues; very little is stored.

Conversion of riboflavin to coenzymes occurs in most tissues. It is excreted in urine unchanged. Since there is little storage, urinary excretion reflects dietary intake. Excretion increases with conditions associated with tissue breakdown, such as weight loss, starvation, prolonged bed rest, and uncontrolled diabetes.

*Physiology.* Riboflavin phosphate (flavin mononucleotide, FMN) and flavin adenine dinucleotide (FAD) are involved as coenzymes in the metabolism of carbohydrates, fats, and proteins. In general, flavin dehydrogenases (e.g., NADH dehydrogenase and succinate dehydrogenase) function as hydrogen carriers from specific substrates to the respiratory chain, resulting in the production of ATP. Other riboflavin enzymes not involved in energy metabolism include the *d*- and *l*-amino acid oxidases, pyridoxine-5-phosphate oxidase, and glutathione reductase.

*Deficiency.* Deficiency symptoms, which are generally non-specific, include cheilosis (vertical fissures in the lips), angular stomatitis (cracks in the corners of the mouth), glossitis, corneal vascularization, photophobia, seborrheic

dermatitis, and a normochromic normocytic anemia. Peripheral neuropathy of the hands and feet may also develop. Overt clinical signs are seldom seen in industrialized societies; however, a "subclinical" deficiency, in which the activity of riboflavin-dependent enzymes is less than optimal, is common. This may result in subnormal growth in children. Deficiency is usually the result of an inadequate dietary intake, especially a low consumption of milk.

*Therapeutic use.* For the treatment of deficiency, 5 to 10 mg orally (or intravenously) is administered along with other B-complex vitamins, since ariboflavinosis is usually associated with other B-vitamin deficiencies.

*Toxicity.* There is no known toxicity of riboflavin and thus there are no ULs (see Table 63-3). Limited absorption, poor solubility, and urinary excretion of excess vitamin likely preclude the risk of toxicity even with megadoses.

## Niacin (nicotinic acid, vitamin B₃)

*Structure, dietary sources, and recommended intake.* Niacin is the generic descriptor of pyridine-3-carboxylic acid (nicotinic acid) and the physiologically active amide derivative nicotinamide (see Fig. 63-3). Nicotinamide is metabolically active as a constituent of the pyridine nucleotide coenzymes NADH and NADPH. Tryptophan, an essential amino acid, can be converted to nicotinamide adenine dinucleotide (NAD), but less than 2% of tryptophan metabolism follows this pathway. The conversion ratio of tryptophan to NAD is approximately 60:1. Therefore, dietary intake of niacin is essential.

Dietary sources are meats, enriched cereals, and enriched grains. In many cereal grains, particularly corn, most of the niacin is bound in an unabsorbable form. Milk and eggs contain little niacin but are good sources of tryptophan. Recommended intakes are expressed as RDAs in milligrams for individuals over 1 year of age (see Table 63-1).

*Pharmacokinetics.* At low intakes, niacin is readily absorbed from the intestine by a carrier-mediated facilitated diffusion. It is distributed to all tissues. The vitamin forms are converted to the coenzyme forms in tissues. Niacin released from the breakdown of NAD can be reused within the cells. Little niacin is excreted as such in the urine; most is transformed to methylated derivatives prior to urinary excretion.

*Physiology.* Niacin in its amide form is part of NAD and NAD phosphate (NADP). These coenzymes serve as hydrogen carriers for many reactions catalyzed by dehydrogenases. NAD is required in all of the major metabolic pathways involving the oxidative catabolism of carbohydrates, fats, proteins, and alcohol to energy. NADP systems are common to biosynthetic reactions, and NADPH is required as a hydrogen donor for the cytochrome P450 system (see Chapter 4).

*Deficiency.* In niacin deficiency (pellagra), the tissues most affected are the skin, the gastrointestinal tract, and the nervous system. Early signs are non-specific and include lassitude, anorexia, weakness, mild gastrointestinal disturbances, and emotional changes such as anxiety, irritability, and depression.

As the deficiency progresses, a bilateral, pigmented, scaly dermatitis develops on areas exposed to the sun. In the gastrointestinal tract, the mucosa becomes inflamed and atrophic, which may account for a profuse watery diarrhea. Glossitis, angular stomatitis, and cheilosis are frequent. Mental changes intensify to include confusion, hallucinations, memory loss, and frank psychosis. Peripheral motor and sensory disturbances may also occur. Anemias are frequent, but they are likely due to associated deficiencies.

*Therapeutic use.* In the treatment of pellagra, the recommended oral dose is 50 mg given up to 10 times a day or 25 mg intravenously at least twice a day. Additional therapy with riboflavin and pyridoxine is usually carried out.

Large doses of niacin (1 to 3 g/day) have been reported to lower serum cholesterol (see also Chapter 35). This appears to be a pharmacological effect unrelated to its role as a vitamin. Nicotinamide does not share this activity.

*Toxicity.* One gram or more of niacin per day produces marked peripheral vasodilatation (flushing), an effect that is not shared by nicotinamide. Doses over 3 g/day have been associated with activation of peptic ulcer, abnormal glucose tolerance, cardiac arrhythmias, and hepatotoxicity.

Nicotinamide is more toxic than nicotinic acid. Chronic administration of 3 g/day produces effects such as heartburn, nausea, headache, fatigue, sore throat, and an inability to focus the eyes. The ULs for niacin are shown in Table 63-3.

## Vitamin B6

*Structure, dietary sources, and recommended intake.* Vitamin B6 is the preferred descriptor of three naturally occurring pyridine derivatives: pyridoxal, pyridoxamine, and pyridoxine (see Fig. 63-3). They are present in low concentrations in virtually all plant and animal tissues. Recommended intakes for vitamin B6 are expressed in milligrams as RDAs for individuals aged 1 and older (see Table 63-1).

*Pharmacokinetics.* It is well absorbed from the small intestine, likely by passive diffusion, although the vitamin in plant foods is in a glycosylated form of very low bioavailability.

The adult body pool of B6 compounds is about 25 mg. The vitamin is excreted in the urine mainly as its major metabolite, 4-pyridoxic acid, along with small amounts of the three vitamin forms and their phosphates. Excretion reflects recent dietary intake.

*Physiology.* All three forms of vitamin B6 are physiologically active; they are interconvertible. The major coenzyme form is pyridoxal phosphate, which functions in amino acid metabolism in many pathways including decarboxylation, deamination, transamination, transsulfuration, heme synthesis, and the conversion of tryptophan to niacin.

*Deficiency.* A dietary deficiency of vitamin B6 is uncommon because of the diversity of foods containing the vitamin, although epileptiform convulsions have been observed in infants fed a milk formula in which vitamin B6 had been destroyed during processing. Deficiency symptoms include peripheral neuritis, seborrheic dermatitis and other skin lesions, and a B6-dependent sideroblastic anemia resembling iron deficiency anemia. Inborn errors of metabolism that respond to high doses of vitamin B6 have also been reported.

Vitamin B6 deficiency can occur also as a result of interaction with certain drugs. Pregnant women and those taking oral contraceptives have shown abnormalities in tryptophan metabolism suggestive of B6 depletion that responds to B6 supplementation. Hydralazine, isoniazid, and penicillamine have similar effects, all of which appear to be due to inhibition of pyridoxal kinase, one of the enzymes that convert B6 to its active form, pyridoxal phosphate.

*Therapeutic use.* Pyridoxine is included in all B-complex supplementation and is routinely used to prevent peripheral neuritis in patients receiving isoniazid. The efficacy of vitamin B6 in amounts up to 200 mg/day in the treatment of sickle-cell disease, asthma, premenstrual tension, and carpal tunnel syndrome has yet to be confirmed.

*Toxicity.* The ULs are set at 30 to 100 mg/day depending on the life stage group (see Table 63-3). Sensitivity to doses above 200 to 250 mg/day appears to vary among individuals. Instances of transient physiological dependence on vitamin B6 (i.e., the need for an increased daily dose) have been reported in adults receiving 200 mg/day for a month. Therapeutic doses of 2 to 3 g/day for periods ranging from several months to 2 to 3 years have caused incapacitating peripheral sensory neuropathy, which subsided slowly after withdrawal of the supplement.

## Vitamin B12 (cyanocobalamin)

*Structure, dietary sources, and recommended intake.* A number of forms of vitamin B12 have biological activity (Fig. 63-4). Naturally occurring cobalamins are hydroxycobalamin and the two coenzyme forms, 5′-deoxyadenosyl cobalamin (coenzyme B12) and methylcobalamin

**FIGURE 63-4** Structural formula of cobalamins.

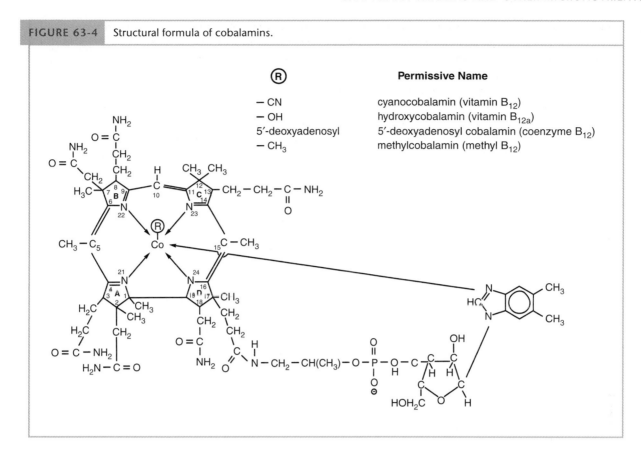

| ® | Permissive Name |
|---|---|
| — CN | cyanocobalamin (vitamin $B_{12}$) |
| — OH | hydroxycobalamin (vitamin $B_{12a}$) |
| 5′-deoxyadenosyl | 5′-deoxyadenosyl cobalamin (coenzyme $B_{12}$) |
| — $CH_3$ | methylcobalamin (methyl $B_{12}$) |

(methyl-$B_{12}$). Cyanocobalamin is an artifact of the isolation process of the vitamin but is used in clinical practice because of its greater availability and stability.

Vitamin $B_{12}$ is found only in tissues of animals that have obtained the vitamin from synthesis by their intestinal flora and in foods that have been fermented by vitamin $B_{12}$–producing bacteria. Liver, the major storage site for the vitamin, is the richest source. Muscle meats, dairy products, eggs, and fish are significant sources.

The RDA for individuals over the age of 1 is very small, in microgram quantities, and it is readily available in a mixed diet (see Table 63-1). However, strict vegetarians (vegans) are at risk of a deficiency, and individuals older than 51 years are advised to consume foods fortified with $B_{12}$ or to take a $B_{12}$ supplement, since malabsorption of food-derived $B_{12}$ is prevalent beyond this age.

*Absorption.* The absorption of vitamin $B_{12}$ is a multi-step process. Initially, $B_{12}$ is bound to R factors in gastric juices. The R–$B_{12}$ complex is non-absorbable, but pancreatic proteases release the vitamin from the R factor in the upper small intestine, where it then binds to the glycoprotein intrinsic factor (IF) secreted by the gastric parietal cells. IF protects the $B_{12}$ during passage down the intestine. The $B_{12}$–IF complex binds to specific receptor sites in the ileum (distal small bowel), where cobalamin is transported across the mucosal cell into the plasma. In the plasma, cobalamin is bound to its transport protein transcobalamin, which exists in different forms; transcobalamin II (TCII) is the most biologically active. The circulating TCII–$B_{12}$ complex attaches to its cell surface receptor, and $B_{12}$ enters the cell by endocytosis. Inside the cell, $B_{12}$ is converted to its coenzyme forms.

There is appreciable storage in the body; 60% of the total body pool is in the liver, and 30% is in the muscle. The large storage capacity and a very low turnover rate (0.1 to 0.2% of the body pool per day) mitigate against rapid depletion during dietary deprivation. An enterohepatic circulation further conserves body stores.

*Physiology.* Adenosylcobalamin functions in two mutase reactions that are instrumental in the degradative pathway of propionate and in the synthesis of leucine. Methylcobalamin serves as the methyl-group carrier between the donor, 5-methyl-$H_4$-PteGlu$_n$, and the acceptor, homocysteine, in the methylation of homocysteine to methionine. This reaction is important for the production of methionine, an important methyl-group donor, and the regeneration of $H_4$-PteGlu$_n$, the key functional form of folate (see "Folate" below).

*Deficiency.* A vitamin $B_{12}$ deficiency produces a failure of cell division in all replicating cells, most notably in the intestinal mucosa and hematopoietic tissue, due to the arrested synthesis of DNA precursors. This in turn is due to a lack of folate coenzymes (see "Folate" below). The hematological picture is described in detail in Chapter 39. Disturbed maturation of buccal and intestinal mucosal cells is often present. In addition, nerve demyelination eventually occurs, beginning with the peripheral nerves and progressing to the posterior and lateral columns of the spinal cord. Early peripheral demyelination responds to vitamin $B_{12}$ treatment; however, the later central nervous system demyelination is irreversible.

The most common cause of vitamin $B_{12}$ deficiency is malabsorption of the vitamin due to inadequate secretion of IF, probably a familial, immunologically based trait. The deficiency due to a lack of IF is termed "pernicious anemia" and normally affects individuals past middle age. Impaired absorption may, however, result from other causes such as pancreatic insufficiency, gastric atrophy, gastrectomy, resection of the ileum (the absorptive site for the vitamin), or diseases of the ileum (e.g., celiac or tropical sprue and ileitis). Deficiency from these causes may take 5 to 7 years to become evident because of the large stores of the vitamin in the body.

Absorption is also impaired by various drugs, including $p$-aminosalicylic acid (PAS), colchicine, neomycin, and the biguanides metformin and phenformin, which are used in the treatment of diabetes.

A nutritional deficiency is rare but is seen in individuals consuming a strict vegetarian (vegan) diet containing no animal products. Clinical signs take 10 to 20 years to develop in such cases. Several instances of a deficiency in breastfed infants of vegan mothers have been reported.

*Therapeutic use.* The only therapeutic use of vitamin $B_{12}$ (as cyanocobalamin) is the treatment of a vitamin $B_{12}$ deficiency. Although oral administration of large doses is effective in the treatment of pernicious anemia (150 µg/day, or a single weekly dose of 1000 µg), monthly intramuscular or subcutaneous injection of 60 to 100 µg is the preferred treatment.

*Toxicity.* Preparations of cyanocobalamin are non-toxic. There are no ULs established for vitamin $B_{12}$ (see Table 63-3).

## Folate

*Structure, dietary sources, and recommended intake.* Folate (Fig. 63-5) is the generic descriptor for folic acid (pteroylmonoglutamic acid, PteGlu) and related compounds that have biological activity. The naturally occurring and metabolically active compound is the reduced form of folic acid, 5,6,7,8-tetrahydrofolic acid ($H_4$-PteGlu), which is conjugated intracellularly with up to eight glutamyl residues ($H_4$-PteGlu$_n$).

The richest dietary sources of folates are green leafy vegetables, mushrooms, and liver. However, the bioavailability of folate is variable (30 to 80%) and is lower for folates from plant sources. Folates are easily oxidized and are unstable under cooking and storage conditions.

The recommended intakes of folate are RDAs (see Table 63-1). The increased requirement for folate in pregnancy makes the use of a folate supplement a necessity for most women. Because the neural tube closes very early in the first trimester, a time when many women are unaware they are pregnant, it is difficult to rely on a prenatal folate supplement for prevention of a neural tube defect in the fetus. Thus, while it is recommended that women take a prenatal supplement prior to conception, this is not an ideal and effective strategy. Therefore, mandatory folate fortification of flour (Canada) and cereal grains (United States) was introduced in the late 1990s and has dramatically improved the serum and red blood cell folate status of women in child-bearing years, and in all other segments of the population. The incidence of neural tube defects has been substantially reduced. The effects of these higher levels of folate on various health outcomes in the general population are under investigation.

*Pharmacokinetics.* Dietary folates in the polyglutamate form must be cleaved to the monoglutamate form by a zinc-dependent conjugase enzyme prior to absorption. The overall efficiency of absorption is about 50% (10 to 90%) but is sharply reduced by zinc depletion. Absorption is predominantly by active transport in the duodenum and jejunum. After uptake by tissue cells, the monoglutamate form is conjugated with up to eight glutamyl residues.

**FIGURE 63-5** Structural formulae of folic acid and tetrahydrofolic acid ($H_4$-PteGlu).

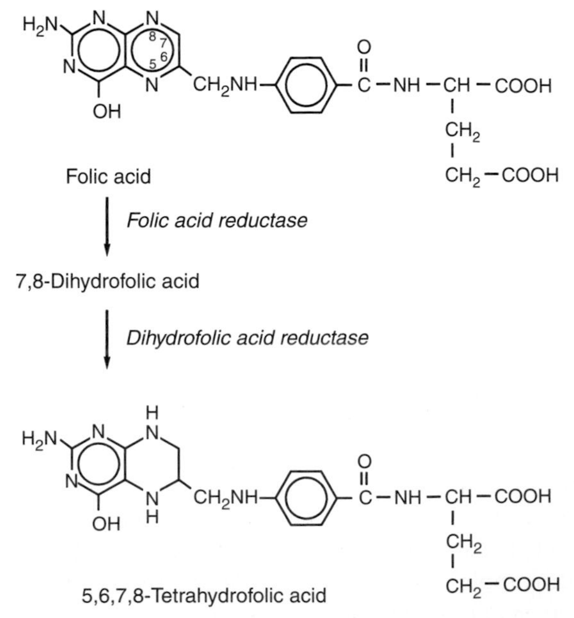

About 50% of the body pool of folate is in the liver. Small amounts of folate metabolites are excreted in the urine and bile (in feces). There is a significant degree of conservation of body folate by reutilization of folates released from senescent cells and by enterohepatic circulation of folate.

*Physiology.* Folate ($H_4$-PteGlu$_n$) functions as a coenzyme to transfer single carbon units (in the oxidation of methanol and formate, but not $CO_2$), for example, in the interconversions of some amino acids and in purine and pyrimidine nucleotide synthesis. This is of particular importance in the synthesis of DNA and, hence, in cell replication and maturation.

*Deficiency.* A poor intake of folate results in the failure of developing erythroid cells to mature past the megaloblast stage because of a suppression of DNA synthesis. Cells with rapid turnover rates (e.g., gastrointestinal mucosa) and red blood cells are most profoundly affected, resulting in malabsorption and a megaloblastic anemia, respectively. The anemia is indistinguishable from that caused by a vitamin $B_{12}$ deficiency. A striking clinical difference, however, is the absence of myelin degeneration and its neurological consequences in folate deficiency.

A vitamin $B_{12}$ deficiency may induce a secondary folate deficiency. Vitamin $B_{12}$ is required as an intermediate methyl-group acceptor in the conversion of homocysteine to methionine. In the absence of vitamin $B_{12}$, this transfer is blocked and $H_4$-PteGlu is "trapped" in the methyl derivative form, thus blocking its ability to transfer other single-carbon units.

Chronic alcoholism and intestinal malabsorption sharply reduce folate absorption. Chronic liver disease and vitamin C deficiency (diminished protection of folate in its reduced $H_4$-PteGlu form) also contribute to folate deficiency. The anticonvulsant phenytoin may produce folate deficiency in a small percentage of epileptics.

*Therapeutic use.* The main therapeutic use of pteroylglutamic acid is the treatment of folate deficiency. Folic acid supplements, usually 1 mg/day, are given to women with child-bearing potential in the periconceptual period to reduce the incidence of primary neural-tube defects in newborns. Larger doses (4 mg/day) are used against recurrences of such defects. Large "rescue doses" of 5-formyl-$H_4$-PteGlu (folinic acid, or leucovorin) are used as a specific antidote for the toxic effects of anti-neoplastic therapy with methotrexate (see Chapter 57).

Folate is also a cofactor in the conversion of homocysteine to methionine. Patients with hyperhomocysteinemia due to genetic deficiencies in the metabolism of homocysteine have an increased risk of premature atherosclerosis, leading to myocardial infarction and stroke. The possible value of folate supplements, to reduce homocysteine levels and prevent these complications, is currently being studied.

*Toxicity.* The ULs for folate range from 300 to 1000 µg/day for individuals beyond age 1 (see Table 63-3). Higher intakes (5 mg/day orally) correct the megaloblastic anemia of vitamin $B_{12}$ deficiency but may mask the concurrent development of neurological lesions. Thus, the indiscriminate use of large folate supplements is unwise. The sale of over-the-counter folic acid supplements is restricted to unit doses that will produce a response only to a folate deficiency.

## Biotin and pantothenic acid

These two vitamins are usually included in B-complex preparations. Other than the treatment of rarely occurring primary or induced deficiencies, they have no established therapeutic use. It is assumed that an adequate intake is provided in the diet. They are both virtually nontoxic. The structures are given in Figure 63-3.

*Biotin.* Biotin is widely distributed in the diet and may be synthesized by the bacterial flora. The recommended intakes for biotin are all expressed as AIs in microgram quantities (see Table 63-1).

A naturally occurring deficiency is an extreme rarity. In two reported cases, large quantities of raw eggs (6 to 12 eggs/day) were consumed over periods of months or years. Raw egg white contains avidin, which binds biotin and renders it biologically unavailable.

Experimental deficiencies are characterized by anorexia, nausea and vomiting, and a dry, scaly dermatitis.

Biotin is involved in fatty acid synthesis as the coenzyme for acetyl-CoA carboxylase and other carboxylation pathways. There are no established ULs for biotin (see Table 63-3).

*Pantothenic acid.* Pantothenic acid is present in almost all foods, and it is therefore very rare to observe a deficiency. All recommended intakes are expressed as AIs as for biotin, but in milligram quantities (see Table 63-1). Pantothenic acid is converted to coenzyme A, which is involved in the intermediary metabolism of carbohydrates, fats, and proteins, as well as the many synthetic reactions involving acetylation.

No naturally occurring deficiency has been reported in humans. There are no established ULs for pantothenic acid (see Table 63-3).

## Vitamin C

### Structure, dietary sources, and recommended intake

Vitamin C is the generic term for L-ascorbic acid and its oxidized form dehydroascorbic acid (Fig. 63-6), both of which have vitamin C activity. The two forms are readily interconvertible. The most important dietary sources of vitamin C are citrus fruits, vegetables, and fruit drinks supplemented with ascorbic acid. Organ meats (liver, kidney,

FIGURE 63-6  Structural formulae of ascorbic acid and its oxidation product, dehydroascorbic acid (both vitamin C).

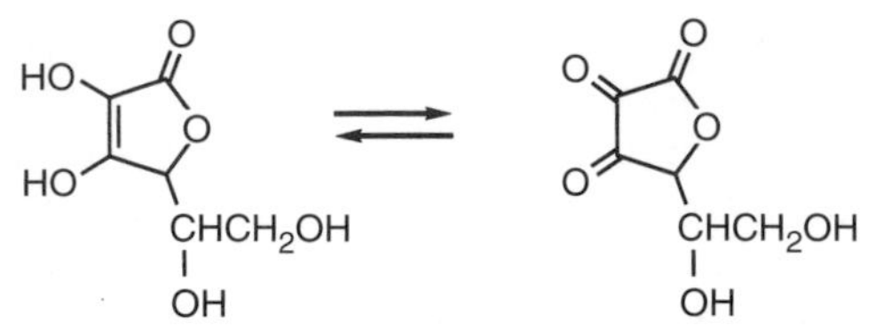

and brain) are also significant sources. However, muscle meats and milk contain very little ascorbic acid. Vitamin C is particularly labile and is easily destroyed by exposure to air, heat, or prolonged storage. The recommended intakes for individuals aged 1 and older are RDAs (see Table 63-1).

## Pharmacokinetics

Vitamin C is well absorbed from the small intestine by a saturable active transport process. The efficiency of absorption decreases with increasing intake. The vitamin is distributed in most tissues throughout the body, and levels in leukocytes are used to estimate tissue levels. The adult body pool is approximately 1500 mg. Excess vitamin C is not stored: at plasma concentrations below 1.4 mg/dL (80 μmol/L), ascorbic acid is reabsorbed by the kidney; above that level, it is actively excreted. A large number of metabolites also appear in the urine. Urinary excretion of ascorbic acid closely reflects recent dietary intake. Tissue saturation occurs when the plasma level is between 1 and 2 mg/dL (56.8 and 113.6 μmol/L). Cigarette smoking, as well as some types of stress, may drastically lower plasma ascorbate levels.

If ascorbic acid ingestion is reduced following long-term supplementation with 250 mg/day or more, the kidney continues to excrete ascorbic acid. This results in a rebound phenomenon in which plasma ascorbate may fall to scorbutic levels (especially if prior ingestion was 2 g/day or more). There is a report that after daily ingestion of 10 g of vitamin C for a week, withdrawal resulted in frank symptoms of scurvy.

## Physiology

The functions of vitamin C appear to reflect its redox capacity. Thus, it is involved in a number of hydroxylation reactions in which it maintains optimal enzyme activity by donating electrons; examples include collagen synthesis (and thus wound healing and bone matrix formation), synthesis of carnitine and the neurotransmitters serotonin and noradrenaline, the metabolism of histamine and cholesterol, and the activity of detoxifying enzymes in the liver. Vitamin C also enhances the absorption of non-heme iron and serves as an important mechanism to

inactivate highly reactive free radicals in the tissue cells. It retards the formation of nitrosamines, which are potential carcinogens. Mounting evidence links ascorbic acid to many elements of the immune system.

## Deficiency

Humans, monkeys, guinea pigs, and fruit bats have lost the ability to synthesize ascorbic acid from glucose (the terminal enzyme in the reaction sequence, L-gulonolactone oxidase, has been lost by these species). Dietary deficiency of ascorbic acid can therefore give rise, in these species, to the symptoms of scurvy, which include pathological lesions of bones, teeth, gums, skin, and blood vessels. These all appear to be due to depolymerization of connective tissue and disappearance of collagen. Death ensues if the scorbutic state is not corrected. In humans, infantile scurvy has been a problem, and Health Canada reports that there may be clinical vitamin C deficiency among the Inuit and the elderly.

## Therapeutic use

There is an increased requirement for ascorbic acid in tuberculosis, peptic ulcer, and other stress conditions (e.g., surgery). This can be met by ingestion of 100 to 200 mg/day. A transient tyrosinemia seen in some neonates has been treated with 100 mg/day. Scurvy is usually treated with 1 to 2 g/day until tissue saturation is attained.

## Toxicity

Normal dietary levels are without toxicity, but ULs have been established (see Table 63-3). High dietary intake (in excess of 1 g/day) may cause diarrhea, and in some sensitive individuals, it may promote the precipitation of cystine or oxalate stones in the urinary tract. At higher levels of ascorbate intake, the possibility of rebound effects on withdrawal should be considered. There is a danger of scurvy in the newborns of mothers who ingested large amounts of ascorbate during pregnancy.

# MACROMINERALS

While there are seven macrominerals, this section will focus on calcium, phosphorus, and magnesium. Three of the other four macrominerals (Na, Cl, and K) are discussed in Chapter 37.

## Calcium

### Structure, dietary sources, and recommended intake

The richest dietary sources of Ca are dairy foods (milk, cheese, ice cream, yogourt) and fish such as canned salmon and sardines if bones are consumed. While Ca is also present in broccoli, spinach, kale, and legumes, the bioavailability is highest from dairy foods. Spinach, in particular, contains oxalates that bind Ca so that it is largely unabsorbed and excreted in the feces. In North America, Ca is added to some breakfast cereals, orange juice, and soy milk (as well as vitamin D), making these foods good sources of Ca as well. Ca is predominantly present in foods as a relatively insoluble salt and must be converted to its ionized ($Ca^{2+}$) form in the intestine prior to absorption. Calcium requirements are expressed as AIs in milligrams for all life stage groups and both sexes (see Table 63-2).

## Pharmacokinetics

When Ca intakes are relatively low, absorption occurs by a saturable, active transport mechanism primarily in the duodenum or jejunum, but when Ca intakes are high, Ca absorption occurs via a non-saturable, paracellular transport mechanism in the jejunum and ileum. The former mechanism is regulated by the active form of vitamin D ($1,25(OH)_2D_3$), which stimulates production of the calcium-binding protein calbindin that facilitates the transport of Ca into the intestinal mucosal cell. Once inside the mucosal cell, Ca is released at the basolateral membrane via a vitamin D–dependent pump ($Ca^{2+}/Mg^{2+}$-ATPase). A number of dietary factors, such as fibre, free fatty acids, phytate, and oxalate, present in the intestine can bind or form complexes with Ca, inhibiting its absorption. Due to mineral–mineral interactions, divalent cations such as $Mg^{2+}$ can also compete for absorption, and the outcome of this competition is dependent on the concentrations of each mineral in the intestine.

In the blood, Ca circulates in its ionized form ($Ca^{2+}$), bound to proteins such as albumin or complexed with sulfate, phosphate, or citrate. Ca concentrations are tightly regulated by several hormones including parathyroid hormone (PTH), $1,25(OH)_2D_3$ (calcitriol), and calcitonin. When blood Ca concentrations decrease, PTH increases the production of active vitamin D ($1,25(OH)_2D_3$) from $25(OH)D_3$ (calcidiol) in the kidney. $1,25(OH)_2D_3$ then acts to increase blood Ca levels by stimulating resorption of Ca from bone and increasing intestinal absorption of Ca via increased production of calbindin, while PTH acts directly on the renal tubules to stimulate the reabsorption of Ca. Once blood Ca levels are restored, calcitonin counters the actions of PTH, preventing further loss of Ca from bones. Small quantities of Ca are located intracellularly in mitochondria, endoplasmic reticulum, and sarcoplasmic reticulum. Intracellular Ca levels are maintained by ATP-dependent Ca pumps that tightly regulate the movement of Ca within a cell.

## Physiology

Over 99% of the body's Ca is found in bones and teeth, and thus a major role of Ca is providing strength to these tissues. Calcium becomes incorporated with critical bone matrix proteins such as collagen, forming strong bone. Ca is commonly found incorporated into bone and bone matrix in a crystal form, termed hydroxyapatite ($Ca_{10}(PO_4)_6(OH)_2$). Ca

also has a number of other critical functions, including roles in muscle contraction, nerve transmission, blood pressure regulation, blood clotting, and the activation of a number of diverse enzymes. Some of these functions are regulated via fluctuations in intracellular Ca levels.

## Deficiency

Osteoporosis, characterized by a low bone mass that predisposes individuals to an increased risk of fracture, is a major consequence of Ca deficiency (see Chapter 65). Of note is the fact that most North Americans do not consume the recommended levels (AIs) for Ca. In children, Ca deficiency leads to rickets as a result of inadequate Ca relative to bone matrix, giving rise to soft bones that cannot support the weight of the child. Tetany can also result from low dietary Ca intakes; this involves increased excitability at the nerve–muscle junction and resulting alterations in muscle contractions and spasms. Chronic low Ca intakes may also have a role in hypertension and colon cancer, although these findings require confirmation.

## Therapeutic use

Large prospective clinical trials have shown that Ca supplementation slows the loss of bone mass (a surrogate measure of fracture risk) that occurs during aging in men and women (>65 years of age) (see Suggested Readings). The 2002 clinical practice guidelines for the diagnosis and management of osteoporosis in Canada recommend that post-menopausal women and men over age 50 should be consuming 1500 mg of Ca per day, slightly higher than the AI (see Table 63-2), to assist in preventing osteoporosis. Due to dietary preferences and/or lactose intolerance, it is difficult for some individuals to attain this level of Ca by diet alone. In such cases, Ca supplements are advised. Ca supplements are most effective when consumed at multiple times during the day and with meals to enhance absorption. While there are many different forms of Ca supplement available, small differences in absorption are unlikely to result in different biological effects.

## Toxicity

A UL of 2.5 g/day has been established for Ca (see Table 63-4). Individuals consuming higher amounts of Ca may be at risk of developing kidney stones due to excessive concentration of Ca in the tubular fluid. Because Ca can compete with other cations for absorption, chronic high intakes may lead to increased loss of Zn and/or Fe and, therefore, increased need.

# Phosphorus

## Structure, dietary sources, and recommended intake

Phosphorus in foods is present in both inorganic ($PO_4^{2-}$) and organic forms (phospholipids, phosphorylated sugars, phosphoproteins). Phosphorus is abundant in meats (chicken, beef), eggs, and dairy products with lesser quantities in breads, cereals, nuts, seeds, and legumes. The DRI for P is expressed as an RDA, except for infants up to 1 year of age, for which there are AIs (see Table 63-2).

## Pharmacokinetics

Organic P must first be cleaved by hydrolyzing enzymes (i.e., alkaline phosphatase, phospholipase C) in the intestinal lumen, and the resulting organic P is absorbed by either carrier-mediated active transport (at low dietary concentrations of P) or diffusion (at high dietary concentrations of P) across the brush-border membrane of the mucosal cell. Because some food sources such as cereals contain most of their P in the form of phytate, and humans lack the enzyme phytase that cleaves P from phytate, this form of P is largely unavailable for absorption. P absorption may also be reduced by the presence of competitive cations. Mg can form a complex with P ($Mg_3(PO_4)_2$) that is excreted in the feces. Ca can also form a complex with P and reduce its absorption. P is transported in the blood complexed with proteins, phospholipids, Ca, Mg, or as free P ($H_2PO_4^-$ or $HPO_4^{2-}$). Plasma P is usually in the range of 2.5 to 4.4 mg/dL. Phosphorus metabolism is largely regulated by the kidneys.

## Physiology

Like Ca, most phosphorus is in bone and teeth, and smaller amounts are present in blood and soft tissues such as muscle. In bone and teeth, P is incorporated into crystals such as hydroxyapatite, which are incorporated with bone matrix proteins such as collagen. P is also an integral component of cell membranes and nucleic acids, is directly involved with energy production and storage in the form of ADP and ATP, and serves to regulate pH within cells. Phosphorus also serves to activate or inactivate a number of enzymes through phosphorylation or dephosphorylation activity.

## Deficiency

Phosphorus deficiency is extremely rare, particularly since our diets tend to be high in P due to the high P content in soft drinks and the widespread use of preservatives in packaged foods. However, in conditions in which intake is low or absorption of P is poor, as occurs with anorexia or inflammatory bowel disease, respectively, P deficiency can result. P deficiency can also lead to osteoporosis in adults, rickets in children, and neuromuscular abnormalities.

## Therapeutic use

Because dietary P is rarely limiting, supplementation with phosphorus would only occur in extremely rare situations.

## Toxicity

Phosphorus toxicity is rare, mostly due to the fact that P metabolism is regulated by the kidneys in such a way that high intakes of P result in greater excretion in the urine. Accordingly, the ULs for P are relatively high compared with the RDA (see Table 63-4). Individuals with impaired kidney function may experience toxicity if the P content of their diet is not closely controlled. The ratio of calcium to phosphorus is considered to be important. A high level of P relative to Ca may result in increased stimulation of PTH, which in turn stimulates a loss of Ca from bone.

# Magnesium

## Structure, dietary sources, and recommended intake

A wide variety of foods are good sources of magnesium, including vegetables, legumes, meats, seafood, nuts, cereal grains, and soybeans. Because Mg is associated with chlorophyll, green leafy vegetables are an excellent source. RDAs are established for individuals aged 1 year and older (see Table 63-2).

## Pharmacokinetics

Mg is primarily absorbed in the jejunum and ileum by a carrier-mediated, saturable transport mechanism at low to normal dietary intakes of Mg. However, at higher dietary intakes, Mg is absorbed via passive diffusion. As with other divalent cations, $Mg^{2+}$ absorption can be reduced by the presence of other minerals ($Ca^{2+}$), and Mg may form complexes with free fatty acids, resulting in its loss in the feces. Mg is transported in the circulation bound to protein as a complex with phosphate or citrate, or in its free form.

## Physiology

Most Mg in the body is in bone and teeth; the rest is present in muscle and extracellular fluids. In addition to serving as a structural component of bone, Mg is essential for nerve impulse transmission and for several steps in protein synthesis including RNA and DNA transcription. Mg serves as an essential cofactor for more than 300 enzymes. Mg also acts to stabilize ATP by forming a $Mg^{2+}$–ATP complex and assists in the transfer of the high-energy phosphate group. In the membranes of organelles, such as the endoplasmic reticulum and mitochondria, Mg is associated with phospholipids, thereby stabilizing their structure.

## Deficiency

Although relatively rare, Mg deficiency resulting from kidney failure or malabsorption (i.e., gastrointestinal disorder) may result in growth failure, tetany, convulsions, impaired neuromuscular function, and/or changes in cardiovascular measures (pulse, blood pressure).

## Therapeutic use

Other than treatment of Mg deficiency, there are no confirmed conditions, at present, for which individuals would benefit from Mg supplementation.

## Toxicity

Mg toxicity is rare, as excessive Mg is excreted by the kidneys. However, if a patient with impaired kidney function takes Mg-containing laxatives or antacids, toxicity could potentially occur. Symptoms of toxicity include vomiting, low blood pressure, and cardiovascular changes. The UL is set at 350 mg/day for individuals aged 9 and older.

# MICROMINERALS

This section will focus on the microminerals for which we have the most information regarding human health: iron, zinc, copper, iodine, fluoride, and selenium.

## Iron

### Structure, dietary sources, and recommended intake

In biological systems, Fe exists in the ferrous ($Fe^{2+}$) or ferric ($Fe^{3+}$) form. Fe is present in red meats as heme Fe (derived from hemoglobin or myoglobin), which is more bioavailable (20 to 30% absorbed) than the non-heme Fe present in plant foods (1 to 5% absorbed). The recommended intakes are expressed as RDAs for infants older than 6 months of age (see Table 63-2). Dietary iron is mainly in the ferric form and must be converted to the ferrous form for absorption in the gastrointestinal tract. This is described in Chapter 39.

### Pharmacokinetics

When assessing Fe absorption, it is important to consider the fact that there are many different dietary factors that can enhance or inhibit the absorption of Fe (see Suggested Readings).

### Physiology

A primary function of Fe is oxygen transport via hemoglobin and myoglobin. In addition, Fe is critical for the function of many different heme-containing enzymes such as the cytochromes that are involved in electron transfer through the respiratory chain. In addition, many different monooxygenase and dioxygenase enzymes involved with a variety of pathways in the body are Fe-dependent. The role of Fe in human health is complicated in that Fe can have both antioxidant and pro-oxidant activity. Catalase, an Fe-dependent enzyme, protects against tissue damage by converting hydrogen peroxide to an inert form. In contrast, Fe in the form of $Fe^{3+}$ can react with hydrogen peroxide (called the Fenton reaction) to ultimately form a hydroxyl radical ($\cdot OH$) that can initiate tissue damage.

### Deficiency

Populations that are at greatest risk of Fe deficiency are infants and young children, adolescents undergoing the pubertal growth spurt (in which Fe demands are great), females who are menstruating (child-bearing years), pregnant women because of the increased demands by the fetus, vegans since non-heme iron is not as available for absorption as heme iron, and elite athletes due to iron losses during training (see Suggested Readings).

In Canada, multiple studies have demonstrated that infants and children are at particular risk of iron depletion and iron deficiency anemia. This is distressing as Fe deficiency is linked with impaired cognitive function. Breastfed infants who are born at term and healthy have sufficient Fe stores to meet their needs until 4 to 6 months of age. For formula-fed infants, an Fe-fortified infant formula is recommended until 12 months of age. To ensure adequate Fe intake in young infants and children, it is important that they consume Fe-fortified cereals, particularly as first foods. In addition, meat intake is an important determinant of Fe status. Fe deficiency anemia results in poor cognitive and motor development. In school-aged children, scholastic achievement is compromised. Fe supplements are commonly used to improve Fe status in individuals with low levels. Doses and duration of therapy vary widely depending on the individual situation. Ingestion of excessive amounts of iron can cause serious toxicity (see Chapter 39). The established ULs for Fe are shown in Table 63-4.

## Zinc

### Structure, dietary sources, and recommended intake

Zinc exists as a cation ($Zn^{2+}$) in the human body and is abundant in a wide variety of foods: seafood and meat, with lesser amounts in other foods including cereal grains, dairy products, and eggs, and the lowest amounts in vegetables and fruits. Recommended intakes for Zn are expressed as RDAs for individuals over 6 months of age (see Table 63-2).

### Pharmacokinetics

Many aspects of the pharmacokinetics of Zn are similar to those of Fe. To facilitate absorption, Zn must first be cleaved from proteins or other food components in the stomach and intestine by acid and proteases. Furthermore, there are many enhancers (citric acid, cysteine, histidine, glutathione) and inhibitors (tannins, polyphenols, oxalate, fibre, phytate) of Zn absorption. Zn absorption is highest when body stores of Zn are low. Inside the intestinal mucosal cell, Zn stimulates the production of metallothionein, a storage protein that binds Zn and Cu. Zn that is transported across the basolateral membrane is carried in the blood to target tissues bound to proteins (albumin, α2-macroglobulin, transferrin) or amino acids (histidine, cysteine).

### Physiology

Zn is essential for the normal functioning of more than 100 enzymes, including superoxide dismutase, which, like catalase (see "Iron"), protects against oxidant stress and free radical damage. Other major functions of Zn include a role in gene expression, where it is a structural component of "Zn-fingers," which facilitate the binding of key hormones and proteins to regulatory regions of genes. Zn is also involved with cell replication and cell membrane stability and is a structural component of bone.

## Deficiency

While not common, Zn deficiency can occur because Zn is not stored in appreciable quantities. However, Zn deficiency is likely to be observed only in malabsorptive or hypermetabolic conditions, including alcoholism, AIDS, and cancer, or as a result of trauma, including surgery. Because Zn is most abundant in seafood and meat, vegans can be at risk of Zn deficiency if adequate levels are not obtained through other food sources. In children, Zn deficiency is manifested as growth retardation and delayed sexual maturation. General symptoms of Zn deficiency include dermatitis, hair loss, and depressed immunity.

## Therapeutic use

The only known therapeutic use for Zn at this time is to correct a Zn deficiency. Zn supplements are available in many different forms: Zn acetate, gluconate, oxide, and sulfate. Research into the effect of Zn on immune status is ongoing.

## Toxicity

Zinc toxicity resulting from the use of Zn or multimineral supplements (a single dose of 1 to 2 g) results in headaches and gastrointestinal upset, including vomiting, cramping, loss of appetite, and diarrhea. Moreover, copper deficiency can result when Zn supplements are taken in doses of more than 50 mg/day (above the ULs for Zn) due to competition for absorption at the brush-border membrane, and also due to the fact that Zn induces the production of metallothionein in intestinal mucosal cells. Since Cu has a higher binding affinity for metallothionein, it binds to metallothionein and is thus trapped inside the intestinal cells, which are sloughed off every 3 to 5 days. The resulting Cu deficiency can in turn affect Fe metabolism as the ceruloplasmin level decreases and ceruloplasmin is not available to oxidize ferrous iron to ferric iron, an essential step that allows Fe to bind to transferrin. ULs have been established for all life stage groups (see Table 63-4).

# Copper

## Structure, dietary sources, and recommended intake

Similarly to Fe, Cu exists in two states ($Cu^{1+}$, $Cu^{2+}$) in biological systems. The richest sources of Cu are organ meats, particularly liver and kidney; smaller amounts are present in nuts, seeds, and legumes. The recommended intakes for Cu are RDAs for individuals aged 1 and over (see Table 63-2). Cu is required in much smaller quantities than Fe and Zn, measured in µg rather than mg.

## Pharmacokinetics

Prior to intestinal absorption, Cu is cleaved from food components by acid and proteases and can be absorbed by a saturable, active-transport mechanism at lower dietary levels and by passive diffusion at higher dietary levels. As with Fe and Zn, specific enhancers (ascorbic, citric, lactic and acetic acids; glutathione, methionine, cysteine) or inhibitors (high dietary Zn or high dietary Fe) of Cu absorption exist. Cu is transported in the blood bound to albumin, transcuprein, or specific amino acids such as cysteine or histidine. Only small amounts of Cu are stored in the body (approximately 100 mg), but a variety of tissues store it, including brain, muscle, hair, nails, and bone.

## Physiology

Cu has a number of critical functions in which it serves as an essential cofactor for enzymes. Ceruloplasmin is a Cu-dependent enzyme, also referred to as a ferroxidase, as it converts ferrous iron to ferric iron, a step necessary for the binding and transport of Fe by transferrin. Superoxide dismutase is both Cu- and Zn-dependent and is responsible for quenching superoxide radicals ($^-O_2$) that promote tissue damage. Cu is also involved with cytochrome C oxidase and thus with the transfer of electrons. Neurotransmitter synthesis is also Cu-dependent, as is the activity of lysyl oxidase, which is responsible for cross-linking collagen to stabilize bone matrix and facilitate mineralization of bone.

## Deficiency

Cu deficiency is very rare under normal dietary conditions. However, as discussed in previous sections (see "Iron" and "Zinc" above), it can be induced by mineral–mineral interactions between Zn and Cu, resulting in anemia. Cu deficiency can also be manifested as scurvy due to the involvement of the Cu-dependent enzyme lysyl oxidase in the cross-linking of collagen fibrils. Cu deficiency can result in changes in hair colour and texture and weakening of cardiac muscles. It can occur as a result of a genetic disorder, Menkes disease, in which the transport of Cu to tissues is impaired.

## Therapeutic use

Currently, there is no therapeutic use for Cu other than for correcting a Cu deficiency.

## Toxicity

Cu toxicity is rare and would only occur through use of supplements containing high quantities of Cu or as a result of a genetic disorder, Wilson's disease, in which Cu accumulates to a level that is damaging in critical organs (see Chapter 43). The ULs for copper are shown in Table 63-4 and are substantially higher than the RDAs.

## Iodine

### Structure, dietary sources, and recommended intake

Iodine is present in the food supply bound to amino acids or as iodide ($I^-$) or iodate ($IO_3^-$). The iodine content of foods varies according to the natural levels of iodine in the environment. Thus, salt-water fish have much higher concentrations of iodine than fresh-water fish, and fruits and vegetables grown in areas rich in iodine also contain higher levels. Meats with the highest levels of iodine are from animals grazing on plants and feed rich in iodine. Similarly, eggs are often a good source if chickens have consumed feed containing iodine. Because many countries have mandatory fortification programs involving the iodization of salt, table salt is often a major contributor to iodine intake. RDAs for iodine have been established for individuals aged 1 and older (see Table 63-2).

### Pharmacokinetics

Absorption of iodine in the intestine is extremely effective, and most ingested iodine appears in the circulation. The thyroid gland has the ability to sequester iodine for the production of thyroid hormones, thyroxine ($T_4$) and 3,5,3′ triiodothyronine ($T_3$), via a sodium-dependent, active transport mechanism (see Chapter 45). Consequently, the thyroid gland contains the highest concentration of iodine in the body (>70%). $T_3$ and $T_4$ are released from the thyroid gland and transported to target cells either bound to transport proteins (albumin, prealbumin, thyroid-binding globulin) or as free hormones. It is the free forms of $T_3$ and $T_4$ that are biologically active and available to target cells; however, $T_3$ is more biologically active than $T_4$.

### Physiology

The major role of iodine is the production of thyroid hormones ($T_3$ and $T_4$) that regulate a variety of enzymes and metabolic processes. Thyroid hormones, particularly thyroxine, regulate the basal rate of metabolism, oxygen consumption, and heat production. $T_4$ is less biologically active than $T_3$, and conversion of $T_4$ to $T_3$ by the enzyme 5′-deiodinase increases the availability of active thyroid hormone that can act on target tissues.

### Deficiency

Iodine deficiency is rare in developed countries due to mandatory iodization of table salt; however, it remains prevalent in some developing countries in which fortification programs do not reach entire populations. A common clinical sign of iodine deficiency is goiter due to hyperplasia of the thyroid gland. Hyperplasia results from the constant stimulation of the thyroid gland by thyroid-stimulating hormone, released by the anterior pituitary in response to low levels of thyroid hormones. Severe iodine deficiency in utero can result in cretinism, which is characterized by growth failure, deafness, and mental retardation. A "masked" iodine deficiency may also occur in states of selenium deficiency due to low activity of 5′-deiodinase, a selenium-dependent enzyme. A detailed discussion of thyroid hormones appears in Chapter 45.

### Therapeutic use

Supplementation with iodine in the form of fortified foods, injections, or iodized oil can eliminate goiter and improve iodine status. The duration and dose of administration depend on the severity of the iodine deficiency.

### Toxicity

In some individuals, chronic high intakes of iodine can result in a different type of goiter with hyperthyroidism. ULs for iodine have been established (see Table 63-4).

## Fluoride

### Structure, dietary sources, and recommended intake

A major source of fluoride is from fluoridated drinking water, which contains approximately 1 mg/L. Other sources include tea, meats, fish (if bones are consumed), legumes, and grains. If ingested, toothpaste can be a significant source of fluoride. The recommended intakes for fluoride are expressed as AIs (see Table 63-2).

### Pharmacokinetics

A unique feature of fluoride in comparison to other minerals is that it is predominantly and rapidly absorbed in the stomach and not the small intestine.

### Physiology

Fluoride is a critical component in bones and teeth, which, as for Ca, contain approximately 99% of fluoride in the body. In bones, it is essential for mineralization, providing strength to bones throughout life. Fluoride becomes incorporated into hydroxyapatite crystals (see "Calcium") by exchanging with a hydroxyl group. There is evidence that fluoride also acts directly on osteoblasts (bone-forming cells). In teeth, fluoride is also incorporated into apatite crystals, making teeth more resistant to acid and hence to the development of caries.

### Deficiency

Fluoride deficiency leads to an increased incidence of dental caries, or cavities. A classic study in the 1940s demonstrated that individuals living in areas without fluoridated water had the highest number of dental caries. Because the greatest benefits of fluoride to dental health occur during childhood, it is recommended that children living in areas where water is not fluoridated receive a fluoride supplement that is available by prescription.

### Therapeutic use

Fluoridation of public water systems has proven beneficial in reducing the incidence of dental caries. For many years, the use of fluoride supplements as a treatment for osteoporosis has been debated and remains controversial, particularly since other more established treatments such as bisphosphonate drugs are available and have proven to reduce fragility fractures (see Chapter 65). However, some fluoride intervention studies have shown improvements in bone mass with reductions in fractures. Studies are ongoing.

### Toxicity

ULs for fluoride have been established for all life stage groups (see Table 63-4). High intakes of fluoride during early development lead to fluorosis, a mottling of the teeth. Fluorosis is observed in children who ingest significant quantities of toothpaste containing fluoride, as 100% of the fluoride in toothpaste is absorbed, and this level can exceed the established ULs for children. With the wide variety of available toothpastes with appealing flavours, children are prone to consume them and should therefore be monitored closely. In the most severe cases of fluoride toxicity, individuals experience nausea and vomiting as well as abnormalities in bone structure, neuromuscular function, and kidneys.

## Selenium

### Structure, dietary sources, and recommended intake

A unique feature of Se is that it can substitute for sulfur in amino acids and thus create seleno-amino acids such as selenomethionine and selenocysteine. Se is most abundant in dietary sources in areas where the environment (soil and water) is high in it. Inorganic forms of Se such as selenate and selenite are present in commercial animal feed and thus appear in the human food supply. The recommended intake for Se is expressed as RDAs for individuals aged 1 and older (see Table 63-2).

### Pharmacokinetics

Se is efficiently absorbed across the intestinal mucosal cell, regardless of whether it is present in organic or inorganic form, and is subsequently transported in the blood bound to sulfhydryl groups in $\alpha$- or $\beta$-globulins (including the lipoproteins VLDL and LDL). Se is present in muscle, liver, kidney, and pancreas, with smaller amounts in other tissues. In the liver, Se may be stored as selenomethionine, be used for protein synthesis, or be metabolized to selenocysteine or selenocystine. In turn, selenocysteine may be incorporated into Se-dependent enzymes or metabolized

further to yield free Se. Many details regarding Se metabolism are still being elucidated.

### Physiology

The primary role of Se in human health is as an essential cofactor for two enzymes. Glutathione peroxidase converts hydrogen peroxide or other organic peroxides to an inert form, thereby protecting lipids, proteins, and nucleic acids against free radical damage. Se is also essential for the activity of 5′-iodinase, which produces triiodothyronine ($T_3$) from thyroxine (see "Iodine").

### Deficiency

Se deficiency is most prevalent in geographical regions that naturally contain low amounts of Se in the environment. These regions include areas in China, where Keshan disease, manifested as muscle weakness and cardiomyopathy, and Kashin–Beck disease, characterized by destruction of joints/cartilage, are observed. Provision of supplemental Se can attenuate the disease severity but does not necessarily completely reverse all effects, such as cardiomyopathy and joint abnormalities.

### Therapeutic use

The relationship between Se supplements and chronic diseases (i.e., cardiovascular disease, cancers) is currently under study.

### Toxicity

Selenium toxicity has been observed in miners exposed to high levels of Se in their working environment. Reported symptoms include extreme fatigue, nausea, and vomiting. Use of Se supplements can also result in toxicity, and ULs for Se have been established (see Table 63-4).

## SUGGESTED READINGS

Brown JP, Josse RG. 2002 clinical practice guidelines for the diagnosis and management of osteoporosis in Canada. *CMAJ.* 2002;167(10 suppl):S1-S34.

Dawson-Hughes B, Harris SS, Krall EA, et al. Effect of calcium and vitamin D supplementation on bone density in men and women 65 years of age or older. *N Engl J Med.* 1997;337:670-676.

Dawson-Hughes B, Heaney RP, Holick MF, et al. Estimates of optimal vitamin D status. *Osteoporosis Internat.* 2005;16:713-716.

Fairfield KM, Fletcher RH. Vitamins for chronic disease prevention in adults: scientific review. *JAMA.* 2002;287:3116-3126.

Lonn E, Yusuf S, Hoogwerf B, et al. Effects of vitamin E on cardiovascular and microvascular outcomes in high-risk patients with diabetes: results of the HOPE study and MICRO-HOPE substudy. *Diabetes Care.* 2002;25:1919-1927.

Pasut L. *Iron for All Ages: Iron for Health.* Ottawa, Ontario: National

Institute of Nutrition; 2002. Available at: http://epe.lac-bac. gc.ca/100/200/300/beef_info_centre/iron_for_all_ages-e/ iron.pdf. Accessed October 14, 2005.

Standing Committee on the Scientific Evaluation of Dietary Reference Intakes, Panel on Micronutrients, Subcommittees on Upper Reference Levels of Nutrients and of Interpretation and Uses of Dietary Reference Intakes, Food and Nutrition Board, Institute of Medicine. *Dietary Reference Intakes for Vitamin A, Vitamin K, Arsenic, Boron, Chromium, Copper, Iodine, Iron, Manganese, Molybdenum, Nickel, Silicon, Vanadium, and Zinc.* Washington, DC: National Academy Press; 2001. Available at: http://www.nap.edu/books/0309072794/html. Accessed October 14, 2005.

Standing Committee on the Scientific Evaluation of Dietary Reference Intakes, Panel on Dietary Antioxidants and Related Compounds, Subcommittees on Upper Reference Levels of Nutrients and Interpretation and Uses of Dietary Reference Intakes, Food and Nutrition Board, Institute of Medicine. *Dietary Reference Intakes for Vitamin C, Vitamin E, Selenium, and Carotenoids.* Washington, DC: National Academy Press; 2000. Available at: http://www.nap.edu/catalog/9810.html. Accessed October 14, 2005.

Standing Committee on the Scientific Evaluation of Dietary Reference Intakes and its Panel on Folate, Other B Vitamins, and Choline and Subcommittee on Upper Reference Levels of Nutrients, Food and Nutrition Board, Institute of Medicine. *Dietary Reference Intakes for Thiamin, Riboflavin, Niacin, Vitamin B6, Folate, Vitamin B12, Pantothenic Acid, Biotin, and Choline.* Washington, DC: National Academy Press; 1998. Available at: http:// books.nap.edu/catalog/6015.html. Accessed October 14, 2005.

Standing Committee on the Scientific Evaluation of Dietary Reference Intakes, Food and Nutrition Board, Institute of Medicine. *Dietary Reference Intakes for Calcium, Phosphorus, Magnesium, Vitamin D, and Fluoride.* Washington, DC: National Academy Press; 1997. Available at: http://www.nap.edu/catalog/5776.html. Accessed October 14, 2005.

Trumbo P, Schlicker S, Poos M. Dietary reference intakes: vitamin A, vitamin K, arsenic boron, chromium, copper, iodine, manganese, molybdenum, nickel, silicon, vanadium and zinc. *J Am Diet Assoc.* 2001;101:294-301.

Waters DD, Alderman EL, Hsia J, et al. Effects of hormone replacement therapy and antioxidant vitamin supplements on coronary atherosclerosis in postmenopausal women: a randomized controlled trial. *JAMA.* 2002;288:2432-2440.

# 64

# Herbal Preparations and Nutritional Supplements

## WE WARD

## INTRODUCTION

Herbal and nutritional supplements have become increasingly popular in North America over the last decades. While Native American, European, and Asian populations have used these various supplements for centuries, North Americans are now using them in significantly higher numbers than ever before as complementary medicine. In Canada, the prevalence of herbal and nutritional supplement use, classified as natural health products, is 46% and 33% among women and men, respectively. Moreover, estimates from the United States suggest that 15 million adults combine nutritional or herbal supplements with conventional drug therapy.

There are likely many reasons for the growing consumer interest in these supplements. One reason is that North Americans live in an aging society, in which individuals are increasingly searching for natural remedies to *prevent* chronic disease, rather than waiting to *treat* a condition once it develops. There also exists the mistaken belief that *natural* compounds, such as herbal preparations and nutritional supplements, have no adverse effects and no interactions with drugs. In addition, among some groups, there is a strongly held belief that *natural* is equated with *good,* and *synthetic* with *bad.*

Menopausal and post-menopausal women have become particularly interested in alternatives to traditional approaches, such as hormone replacement therapy (HRT), to manage menopausal symptoms and preserve bone health. In a Canadian survey, the highest prevalence of supplement use was among women aged 50 to 65 years, most of whom would be menopausal or post-menopausal. Women are often searching for alternative approaches to conventional drug therapies, such as HRT, particularly due to the findings from the Women's Health Initiative (WHI) trial. This trial, the largest multi-centre, randomized controlled trial of HRT to date, demonstrated that the risks of breast cancer, thromboembolism, and stroke were increased among women taking HRT.

Research over the past 20 years or so has provided a scientific basis for suggesting that some specific herbal preparations (Table 64-1) and novel foods, such as soy and flaxseed, or their unique food components (Table 64-2), which are often naturally part of a vegetarian diet, have health benefits. Both Canada and the United States have legislation in place to regulate dietary supplements. In 1994, the United States Congress defined a dietary supplement as a product that is intended to supplement the diet; contains one or more dietary ingredients, including vitamins, minerals, herbals or other botanicals, amino acids, or other substances or their constituents; is intended to be taken by mouth as a pill, capsule, tablet, or liquid; and is labelled as being a dietary supplement.

Using this definition, the Food and Drug Administration (FDA) controls dietary supplements in the United States by regulating label claims (including health claims, nutrient content claims, structure–function claims). A health claim identifies a relationship between a food, food component, or dietary supplement ingredient and a reduction in the risk of a specific disease or health-related condition. As an example, a health claim for soy was approved by the FDA in 1999 (see "Soy and Its Isoflavones" below for further details). The FDA also requires manufacturers to provide data on the safety of the supplement; other mandatory information includes identification of the product as a supplement, quantity of components of interest and compositional information, source of production, directions for use, serving size, and other general information.

Regulatory legislation for dietary supplements in Canada is more recent, starting in January 2004, and is anticipated to take up to 6 years to be fully implemented. Health Canada refers to supplements as natural health products, with the definition of a natural health product encompassing vitamins, minerals, herbal remedies, and homeopathic medicines. As stated by Health Canada, the natural health products regulations include provisions on definitions, product licensing, site licensing, good manufacturing practices, clinical trials, labelling and packaging requirements, and adverse reaction reporting. During the implementation of this legislation, natural health products will be given a natural product number (NPN) or, if they are currently or were previously classified as a drug, they will be given a drug information number for homeopathic medicine (DIN-HM). These regulations in the United States and Canada are important for encouraging quality and safety of dietary supplements. However, the potential for adverse interactions with drugs is a reality, and some examples are discussed in the last section of this chapter.

Given the multitude of herbal preparations and nutritional supplements available to consumers, this chapter is by no means exhaustive but rather focuses on the most commonly used supplements. The 10 top-selling herbal supplements in the United States for 2002 were the following:

1. garlic
2. ginkgo
3. echinacea
4. soy (which is often included as a nutritional supplement)
5. saw palmetto berry
6. ginseng
7. St. John's wort
8. black cohosh
9. cranberry
10. valerian

Other common supplements include glucosamine, chondroitin, and creatine. The herbal and nutritional supplements discussed in this chapter are summarized in Tables 64-1 and 64-2, respectively. The Suggested Reading list at the end of the chapter provides several comprehensive resources on the topic of herbal preparations and nutritional supplements.

## HERBAL PREPARATIONS

The compositions of the most commonly used herbal supplements have been extensively reported, but the effects of some of their specific bioactive components on human health are less certain. Furthermore, the scientific evi-

| TABLE 64-1 | Commonly Used Herbal Preparations | |
|---|---|---|
| **Common Name** | **Botanical Name** | **Potential Health Benefits In Humans*** |
| Black cohosh root | *Cimicifugae racemosae rhizoma* | ↓ Menopausal symptoms |
| Echinacea | *Echinacea purpurea herba* *Echinacea purpurea radix* | Improved immune function: ↑ Cellular immune function of peripheral blood monocytes ↑ Activation of natural killer cells ↓ Acute upper respiratory infections/common cold and their symptoms[†] |
| Garlic | *Allii sativi bulbus* | ↓ Low-density lipoprotein[‡] ↓ Triglycerides[‡] ↓ Total cholesterol[‡] ↓ Hypertension[§] ↓ Plaque formation[‖] ↓ Platelet aggregation |
| Ginkgo biloba leaf | *Ginkgo folium* | Improved cognition Delayed onset of cognitive impairments Improved activity among individuals with peripheral arterial disease[¶] |
| Ginseng root | *Ginseng radix* | ↓ Fatigue May aid in management of type 2 diabetes and ↓ risk of some cancers |
| Saw palmetto berry | *Sabal fructus* | ↓ Symptoms of benign prostatic hyperplasia |
| St. John's wort | *Hyperici herba* | Antidepressant for mild to moderate depression |
| Valerian root | *Valerianae radix* | Improved sleep quality |

*Potential health benefits for which there is some scientific evidence.
[†]Greatest effects observed for subjects with compromised immune function.
[‡]Most effective among individuals with hyperlipidemia.
[§]Most effective among individuals with hypertension.
[‖]Among individuals with significant plaque formation and hyperlipidemia.
[¶]As assessed by the distance subjects are able to walk on a treadmill.

**TABLE 64-2** Commonly Used Nutritional Supplements

| Nutritional Supplement | Main Components | Potential Health Benefits in Humans* |
|---|---|---|
| Soy | Protein<br>Isoflavones<br>Omega-6 fatty acids<br>Fibre<br>Micronutrients<br>Saponins | Improved blood lipids[†]: ↓ low-density lipoprotein (LDL), triglyceride (TG), and total cholesterol<br>↓, ↔ Menopausal symptoms<br>↓ Bone loss |
| Soy isoflavones (extract) | Genistein<br>Daidzein<br>Glycitein<br>Formononetin<br>Biochanin A<br>Equol | ↓, ↔ Menopausal symptoms<br>↓ Bone loss |
| Flaxseed (whole or ground seed) | Mammalian lignan precursor:<br>Secoisolariciresinol diglucoside (SDG, a mammalian lignan precursor)<br>α-Linolenic acid (ALA)<br>Micronutrients<br>Protein | Improved blood lipids[†]: ↓ LDL, TG, and total cholesterol<br>↓ Platelet aggregation<br>↓ Menopausal symptoms<br>↑ Laxation |
| Fish oil | Omega-3 long-chain polyunsaturated fatty acids (LCPUFAs):<br>• Docosahexaenoic acid (DHA)<br>• Eicosapentaenoic acid (EPA) | ↓ Serum TG<br>↓ Platelet adhesion and aggregation<br>↑ Endothelial function<br>↓ Mortality due to cardiovascular disease event[‡]<br>Mild and moderate regression of coronary artery atherosclerosis[§] |
| Glucosamine, chondroitin, or combination of the two | Glucosamine sulfate<br>Chondroitin sulfate | Attenuates osteoarthritis: ↓ joint pain, ↑ joint mobility, and ↑ quality of life |
| Creatine | Creatine monohydrate | May improve muscle mass, strength, and performance during short bouts of intense exercise<br>May improve muscle function in individuals with neuromuscular disorders |

*Potential health benefits for which there is some scientific evidence.

[†]Most effective among individuals with hyperlipidemia.

[‡]Among patients who had already experienced a non-fatal myocardial infarction prior to entry into the study.

[§]Patients with coronary artery atherosclerosis prior to entry into the study.

dence regarding the potential health benefits of herbal supplements is often sparse and inconclusive, owing to the fact that the studies in humans tend to be small, uncontrolled trials that are often of short duration. However, ongoing or planned studies include larger randomized controlled trials to provide stronger data regarding the relationship between herbals and specific disease outcomes or states.

Another difficulty in assessing the available data is that the purity and precise composition of herbal preparations were not regulated until recently (as discussed earlier), making it difficult to compare the findings of different studies. The data presented in the following sections are based on the strongest scientific evidence from human studies that exists to date. Because there is little known about the potential interactions of specific herbals with

medications, concurrent use may be harmful, and studies are urgently needed to fully assess the safety of such use. Users who combine prescribed pharmaceuticals and self-selected herbal supplements should be urged to consult with their caregiver. Some potential interactions between herbal preparations and drugs that could result in potential adverse effects are summarized in Table 64-3 and are discussed in the final section of the chapter.

## Black Cohosh

Black cohosh is a plant indigenous to North America. Dietary supplements are prepared from the roots and rhizomes of the plant. In general, black cohosh extracts are standardized to contain 1 mg of triterpene saponins per 20 mg of extract. Black cohosh has been most extensively

| TABLE 64-3 | Examples of Interactions of Herbals and Drugs with Potential Adverse Effects | |
|---|---|---|
| **Herbal Preparation** | **Drug** | **Potential Adverse Effect** |
| Ginseng root, garlic, or ginkgo biloba leaf | Aspirin | Antiplatelet activity, leading to excessive bleeding |
| Ginseng | Opioids | Decreased/impaired analgesic effect |
| Valerian root | Opioid analgesics | Enhanced depression of central nervous system |
| Garlic | Anti-cancer drugs (various), chlorzoxazone, ritonavir, saquinavir | Altered pharmacokinetics of drugs metabolized by cytochrome P450 enzymes |
| Ginkgo biloba leaf | Anti-cancer drugs, chlorzoxazone, dapsone, mephenytoin, nifedipine, omeprazole | Altered pharmacokinetics of drugs metabolized by cytochrome P450 enzymes |

studied with respect to relief of menopausal symptoms, as assessed by a variety of instruments such as Kupperman's Menopause Index, the Self-Evaluation Depression Scale, and the Clinical Global Impression Scale, as well as by vaginal cytology and measurement of sex hormone levels (i.e., luteinizing hormone, follicle-stimulating hormone). Common menopausal symptoms that are studied include hot flashes, profuse sweating, insomnia, depression, and anxiety. A commercially available black cohosh preparation, Remifemin, is the most widely studied form.

Several studies comparing black cohosh (Remifemin) with placebo and HRT (conjugated estrogens) have reported that black cohosh is as effective as HRT in attenuating menopausal symptoms. This suggests that black cohosh may be an appropriate therapy for women in whom HRT is contraindicated because of either the patient's medical history or concerns over the risks of long-term use of HRT, particularly in view of recent findings from the WHI trial (as discussed in the "Introduction"). Larger randomized controlled trials of longer duration are currently being conducted. The mechanism of action of black cohosh is currently unknown. It had been assumed that it interacted with the estrogen receptor and activated estrogen-dependent genes, but more recent data suggest non-estrogen-mediated mechanisms.

Based on the clinical data available, a dose of 40 to 80 mg of black cohosh per day is recommended to attenuate menopausal symptoms. There are currently no known interactions with any medications. Black cohosh may be contraindicated during pregnancy due to potential hormonal effects, and there is concern that liver problems may develop with long-term use.

## Echinacea

Echinacea, commonly known as purple coneflower, is native to North America. There are several different types of echinacea, but *Echinacea purpurea* has been the most extensively studied and, on the basis of current data, appears to have the strongest effect on the immune system. While the design of many of these studies is not opti-

mal, it has been concluded that echinacea stimulates the immune system, resulting in a decreased incidence of upper respiratory tract infections and common colds or a lessening of symptoms; however, the greatest effects were observed for subjects with compromised immune function. It is important to note that these findings are by no means consistent in all studies. The discrepancies are likely due to differences in the preparations (pure extract versus combination with other herbals), the part of the echinacea plant that was used (flowers and leaves versus root, or a mixture of both), the dose administered, and the duration of the intervention.

A careful placebo-controlled, double-blind study in which different doses were compared found that only the high dose (900 mg/day of echinacea root) and not the lower dose (450 mg/day) was effective at combating a cold. Among subjects who suffered three or more colds over a period of 1 year, 8 mL/day of echinacea (fresh pressed juice) for a duration of 8 weeks produced a reduction in the number of subjects who developed a cold compared with subjects receiving placebo. The duration of the cold and the severity of the symptoms were reduced, and the time between colds was increased.

There is some evidence that the mechanism by which echinacea acts is activation of natural killer cells and peripheral blood monocytes; elucidation of the precise mechanism of action remains an active area of research. Based on the doses of *Echinacea purpurea* used in clinical studies, the recommended dose is 6 to 9 mL of fresh juice from the plant, 0.9 g of cut root, or the equivalent quantity in an extract form. There are no known interactions between echinacea and any drugs, but it may affect the CYP3A4 enzyme and thus alter drug metabolism.

## Garlic

Garlic contains alliin, which is converted to a bioactive thiosulfinate, allicin, by the enzyme alliinase. Alliinase acts on alliin when the garlic bulb is destroyed by mincing, bruising, crushing, or chewing. Allicin is purported to be the active ingredient responsible for cardioprotective effects, including an improved blood lipid profile, reduced blood pressure, decreased platelet aggregation, and reduced plaque formation (see Table 64-1 for details on which subjects benefited most); however, other sulfur compounds in garlic may also have a role. The majority of clinical studies assessing the health benefits of garlic have investigated effects on the blood lipid profile. These studies have reported that both subjects with and without elevated levels of serum low-density lipoprotein (LDL), triglyceride (TG), and total cholesterol (TC) respond favourably to garlic supplementation.

Dietary supplementation with 900 mg/day of garlic powder for 4 years resulted in a significant reduction in plaque volume in femoral and carotid arteries, while patients receiving placebo experienced a significant increase in plaque volume, indicating the progression of cardiovascular disease. All of the patients studied had significant plaque formation and at least one other risk factor for cardiovascular disease prior to the start of the study. Epidemiological studies suggest that diets rich in garlic are associated with a lower risk of developing cancers, but prospective trials in humans have not yet been conducted.

Studies have used a variety of different forms of garlic (i.e., fresh, dried, oil, powdered, or aged garlic), but despite differences in form, the doses of garlic used are often attainable in the diet. The recommended dose to observe these effects, and the dose used in most studies to date, is between 2 and 5 g of fresh garlic per day (1 or 2 cloves) or the equivalent quantity in a supplement form, usually a powder (about 400 to 1200 mg of garlic powder).

Garlic has been shown to have anticoagulant properties, prolonging bleeding time, so patients taking warfarin are advised to be cautious in their use of garlic as an herbal preparation. Allicin-containing supplements may affect CYP3A4 enzymes and thereby have potential adverse effects on the metabolism of certain drugs (see Table 64-3).

## Ginkgo Biloba Leaf

*Ginkgo biloba* leaf comes from the ginkgo tree, indigenous to China. Ginkgo contains a variety of bioactive compounds that may mediate its effects: flavonoids (glycosides), sesquiterpenes, and terpenes. Findings from placebo-controlled studies reported that ginkgo delayed the onset of cognitive impairments among individuals with early signs of dementia or Alzheimer's disease. Further, among individuals with an existing dementia (mild to moderate), ginkgo improved their cognitive function or slowed the progression of their cognitive deterioration.

Ginkgo also appears to have favourable effects with respect to peripheral vascular disease. Several well-controlled studies have reported that after 6 months of treatment with ginkgo extract, patients with peripheral vascular disease walked greater distances, pain-free, than patients taking placebo. The mechanism of this effect is unclear, as blood flow was not improved in any of these studies.

The recommended dose of ginkgo is 40 to 80 mg of ginkgo extract, three times a day.

## Ginseng Root

Ginseng is an herb that has been used for centuries in Asia to treat stress in humans. Ginseng root is currently used with the goal of managing or treating a wide variety of ailments, including fatigue and type 2 diabetes, and reducing the risk of developing certain cancers. The active components in ginseng root are the saponins, called ginsenosides.

Some (but not all) studies have reported that ginseng reduces fatigue and symptoms of depression in women. A randomized controlled trial demonstrated that individuals with type 2 diabetes experience improved glucose control, while some other studies suggest that ginseng reduces the risk of certain cancers. To confirm these findings, newer studies are ongoing. It is well documented that the composition (i.e., level of ginsenoside) can vary significantly among preparations, thus making it impossible to directly compare the findings of different studies. With the newer regulations regarding dietary supplements (United States) and natural health products (Canada), more precise effects of ginseng and the effective dose ranges will be identifiable in future studies.

The recommended dose of ginseng depends on its form: 1 to 2 g of dried root per day or 100 to 300 mg of extract up to three times daily. Some supplements are standardized for the level of ginsenosides. Some side effects of ginseng include vaginal bleeding, mastalgia, agitation, and anxiety, possibly due to hormonal effects. For this reason, women are advised not to use ginseng during pregnancy. It is also recommended that ginseng not be used in combination with stimulants, including caffeine.

## Saw Palmetto Berry

Saw palmetto is a type of palm tree indigenous to North America, particularly common in the southeastern region of the United States. It is specifically the berries of the saw palmetto that have been reported to be effective in treating the symptoms of benign prostatic hyperplasia. Individual studies, and later a meta-analysis of these studies, concluded that extract from saw palmetto berries attenuated painful urination, reduced the frequency of nighttime urination, and reduced the retention of urine in the bladder by improving the peak flow of urine. The fat portion of the berries contains a variety of fatty acids, esters, and sterols, believed to be the components that act on the prostate.

However, the precise mechanisms of action have not yet been elucidated. Some studies have directly compared the effect of saw palmetto berry extract to finasteride, a testosterone 5-α reductase inhibitor (see Chapter 46), and have found that the extract is as effective as finasteride at reducing symptoms of benign prostatic hyperplasia. Therefore, it is hypothesized that saw palmetto berries may inhibit 5-α-reductase activity, but this awaits confirmation. Interestingly, the saw palmetto extract is reported to have fewer side effects than finasteride. Effective dosages are 1 to 2 g of cut fruit or 320 mg of lipophilic extract. Most clinical studies have administered 320 mg/day of lipophilic extract. There are no known interactions of saw palmetto berry with any drugs.

## St. John's Wort

St. John's wort is indigenous to Europe, Western Asia, and North Africa but is now also grown in Australia and North and South America. Like garlic preparations, it is available in a variety of forms: dried herb (extract or capsules), water-based infusion, or alcoholic tincture. The major health benefit of St. John's wort is purported to be its ability to treat mild to moderate depression. Many placebo-controlled trials have demonstrated that St. John's wort attenuates depression, but because it has not undergone the rigorous testing required of pharmacological agents, it is generally recommended only for use in mild to moderate depression. A criticism of many of the studies investigating St. John's wort for the treatment of depression is the fact that the length of the intervention is relatively short, often 6 weeks or less.

Hyperforin is currently hypothesized to be the bioactive agent in St. John's wort that acts as the antidepressant. In a study testing two different concentrations of hyperforin (0.5% and 5%), only the higher dose resulted in a reduction in depression scores, and patients with the most severe depression had a greater response to treatment. In addition to hyperforin, there are a number of other bioactive compounds in St. John's wort, such as proanthocyanidins, xanthones, phloroglucinol, and a number of flavonol derivatives, that may also mediate antidepressant effects.

The recommended dose, based on clinical studies, is 2 to 4 g of dried herb, consisting of the aerial portions of the plant that are collected during the flowering season, or 0.2 to 1 mg of hypericin if St. John's wort is taken in other forms (many extracts are standardized for their hypericin content).

There are currently no known interactions between St. John's wort and any drugs. However, a recent study in healthy volunteers showed that cytochrome P450 enzymes are altered after a 14-day course of St. John's wort (900 mg/day). Thus, long-term use of St. John's wort may alter the effectiveness of medications or may result in a higher dosage requirement. It may also increase the risk for phototoxicity.

## Valerian Root

Valerian root, from a perennial herb, is marketed for sleep disorders, with the claim of improving sleep quality and treating insomnia, likely through depression of the central nervous system (CNS). While the active ingredient has not been conclusively identified, supplements are often standardized according to the content of valerenic acid, a volatile oil. Other potential active components include valepotriates, but most supplements do not contain valepotriates. Valerian can be taken as tablets, capsules, teas, or tinctures.

Intervention trials have evaluated a variety of sleep outcomes, including movement during sleep, and have used pre- and post-sleep questionnaires regarding quality of sleep and morning drowsiness. Several randomized controlled trials have demonstrated that valerian root (400 to 600 mg/day) improved sleep quality and decreased sleep latency but did not result in greater total sleep time or alter the number of movements during sleep. Data suggest that a higher dose of valerian (900 mg/day) does not result in improved sleep outcomes compared with lower doses.

Recommended doses are highly variable, from 200 to 1500 mg, with randomized controlled trials primarily testing doses ranging from 400 to 600 mg/day. As discussed at the end of the chapter, valerian is not recommended for use in combination with drugs that depress the CNS.

# NUTRITIONAL SUPPLEMENTS

Among the most common nutritional supplements are soy and its isoflavones, flaxseed and its lignans, and fish oil, a rich source of omega-3 fatty acids. An important consideration when deciding how to increase the consumption of a novel food component is that there is a much greater risk of toxicity from consuming purified extracts (e.g., isoflavones or lignans) than from whole foods (e.g., soy or flaxseed). As noted with herbal preparations, the purity of extracts varies, and the differences in growing conditions can affect the isoflavone or lignan content of soy or flaxseed, respectively.

Glucosamine, although not naturally present in foods, is another popular substance that can be classified as a nutritional supplement; it is being used to treat osteoarthritis. In addition to discussing popular nutritional supplements with potential health benefits, such as soy, flaxseed, and fish oil, it is also important to consider creatine, a popular ergogenic aid used as a performance enhancer.

## Soy and Its Isoflavones

Soy is a complex food containing many components, such as a high-quality protein, isoflavones, micronutrients, fibre, and omega-6 fatty acids, all of which can have health benefits. Arguably, the strongest health benefit of soy to date is the effect of soy protein on elevated blood lipids, which are a risk factor for cardiovascular disease. A meta-analysis of 38 studies investigating the effect of eating soy protein on blood lipids showed significant reductions in the levels of LDL, serum cholesterol, and TG. The effects were greatest among individuals who were hyperlipidemic. The average amount of soy protein consumed was 47 g/day.

The overwhelming evidence from this meta-analysis, that soy protein has a favourable effect on the blood lipid profile, provided the rationale for the FDA in the United States to allow companies to make the following health claim on their products: "Diets low in saturated fat and cholesterol that include 25 grams of soy protein a day may reduce the risk of heart disease." The food must contain 6.25 g of soy protein per serving (assuming four servings of the food a day) and must also be low in total fat (<3 g), saturated fat (<1 g), cholesterol (<20 mg), and sodium (<480 mg for individual foods and <960 mg if the portion is the size of a meal). A similar health claim is currently under consideration in other countries.

Diets rich in soy protein have also been reported to improve cardiovascular disease risk by improving endothelial function, lowering blood pressure, and reducing oxidized LDL. To date, studies suggest that these effects are primarily due to the soy protein and not the isoflavones present in soy.

Studies of the effect of soy consumption in a variety of other diseases or conditions have focused not only on the effects of soy protein, but also on the isoflavones naturally present in soy. Isoflavones possess estrogen-like activity, albeit weaker than that of endogenous 17-β-estradiol. For this reason, isoflavones are also sometimes referred to as phytoestrogens ("plant estrogens") or dietary estrogens. Isoflavones are present in foods as glycosides, which are subsequently converted to aglycones by bacteria in the intestine or by an intestinal epithelial β-glycosidase. The aglycones are the biologically active forms: genistein, daidzein, and glycitein. Biochanin A and formononetin are precursors of genistein and daidzein, respectively. Daidzein can be further metabolized to equol, an isoflavone that has even greater estrogenic activity than daidzein itself or genistein.

The extent of the conversion of daidzein to equol varies among individuals according to the type and quantity of bacteria present in the intestine. The aglycones are absorbed across the intestine and travel to the liver, where they are conjugated with either glucuronic acid or sulfate and subsequently undergo enterohepatic circulation. Isoflavones are ultimately excreted in bile or urine.

Because it is possible to alter the level of isoflavones in soy, investigators have studied the effects of soy protein preparations with varying isoflavone content on hormone-sensitive tissues such as bone (osteoporosis) and on menopausal symptoms. The frequency of hot flushes is commonly used as a measure of menopausal symptoms. Some, but not all, studies have reported a reduction in the frequency of hot flushes among women who consume soy foods (containing isoflavones) or purified isoflavones. There are a number of reasons for the inconsistent findings.

The placebo effect has been shown to account for up to a 40% reduction in hot flushes. Moreover, it is almost impossible to conduct a crossover trial because (1) menopausal symptoms resolve spontaneously over time, and the duration that a woman experiences hot flushes is variable, and (2) the level of isoflavones consumed often varies among studies. Thus, there is a continuing challenge to design and conduct clinical trials in order properly to assess the effectiveness of nutritional supplements at alleviating or attenuating menopausal symptoms.

Several feeding trials have reported that bone loss (bone mineral content and bone mineral density) is attenuated with the consumption of 40 g/day of soy protein, but only if it contains a high level of isoflavones (>56 mg/day). Since most studies provide a mixture of isoflavones, it is uncertain whether all isoflavones have similar or equal biological effects. One randomized controlled trial reported that providing genistein extract (54 mg/day of genistein) to postmenopausal women improved bone mass by reducing bone resorption and increasing bone formation, as assessed by measurement of biochemical markers of bone turnover. Although positive effects on bone have been demonstrated, the effects are modest when compared with those of drug treatments such as HRT or bisphosphonates. To date, no studies have assessed fracture risk or have made direct comparisons of the effects of soy interventions on bone metabolism with those of HRT or bisphosphonate drugs.

While a high proportion of specific cancers such as breast and prostate cancer are known to be hormone-sensitive, there is currently no conclusive evidence as to whether soy and/or its isoflavones affect the risk of developing these specific cancers or alter their survival rate.

## Flaxseed and Its Lignans

Flaxseed, like soy, contains a variety of different components, including fibre, α-linolenic acid (ALA, an omega-3 fatty acid), and a mammalian lignan precursor, secoisolariciresinol diglucoside (SDG). Studies in humans have primarily investigated the effects of whole seed (either ground or unground) or ALA in various disease states. In humans, a proportion of ALA is converted to long-chain polyunsaturated fatty acids, such as eicosapentaenoic acid (EPA) and docosahexaenoic acid (DHA), which may at least partially mediate some of the reported positive health effects of ALA (see "Fish Oil" below). Although purified lignans are now available to consumers, studies in humans regarding these purified lignans are lacking, whereas studies using animal models are abundant. The mammalian lignan precursor SDG is converted to the mammalian lignan enterodiol by bacteria in the colon. Enterodiol can be further oxidized by colonic bacteria to form another mammalian lignan, enterolactone.

As with soy feeding, studies of the effects of flaxseed in humans have focused mainly on cardiovascular disease, with only a few investigating effects on menopausal symptoms. Trials in which individuals were fed 38 to 50 g/day of whole, ground flaxseed reported significant reductions in LDL and TG, thereby lowering the risk of cardiovascular disease. However, it is possible that the fibre in the flaxseed mediated the positive effects on blood lipids, as an inverse relationship between dietary fibre intake and risk of cardiovascular disease is well documented in the literature. Other studies have demonstrated that eating flaxseed reduces platelet aggregation. This effect is mediated by the ALA present in flaxseed.

Similar to isoflavones, lignans may also have some estrogenic activity, and the effects of flaxseed on bone metabolism and menopausal symptoms have therefore been studied. While flaxseed does not appear to protect against bone loss in post-menopausal women, the only study that has directly compared the effect of flaxseed with HRT, the gold standard for alleviation of menopausal symptoms, reported that 40 g/day of ground flaxseed was as effective as HRT (0.625 mg conjugated equine estrogens or combined with 100 mg progesterone, depending on the presence or absence of a uterus) in reducing the incidence and severity of the most common menopausal symptoms. Another potential health benefit of flaxseed is its proven ability to act as an effective laxative, resulting in a higher number of bowel movements.

## Fish Oil

Fish and fish oil supplements are an abundant source of the omega-3 long-chain polyunsaturated fatty acids EPA and DHA. Although all fish contain some EPA and DHA, salmon, herring, and mackerel are particularly rich sources. By weight, cod liver oil is an even richer source. Thus, the fattier the fish, the greater the polyunsaturated fatty acid content. Fish oil capsules, containing varying levels of EPA and DHA, are widely available to consumers. Upon consumption of fish or fish oils, EPA and DHA accumulate in cells and tissues. Because both EPA and DHA are precursors of eicosanoids, they can favourably alter the production of specific thromboxanes, leukotrienes, and prostaglandins (see Chapter 27). These actions are believed to mediate many of the positive effects of fish oil on human health.

Like eating soy and flaxseed, consumption of fish oil (and thus of EPA and DHA) has been shown to reduce the risk of cardiovascular disease or attenuate the disease progression in individuals with pre-existing cardiovascular disease. These favourable changes in risk factors include a reduction in serum TG level, improved endothelial function, and decreased platelet adhesion and aggregation. Some studies reported that elevations in serum LDL accompany the reduction in serum TG, and the mechanism of action is under investigation. The greatest reductions in serum TG are generally observed among individuals with elevated serum TG who are consuming high doses of fish oil through supplement use.

Among subjects who had previously had a myocardial infarction, 1 g/day of fish oil for 3.5 years resulted in a significant reduction in mortality due to cardiovascular disease events. Another study of patients with pre-existing cardiovascular disease (coronary artery atherosclerosis) demonstrated that 6 g/day of fish oil for 3 months followed by 3 g/day for 21 months resulted in a slowing of the narrowing of the coronary arteries compared with patients receiving placebo.

A common question is how much fish oil needs to be consumed to confer cardioprotective effects. Based on current knowledge, it is suggested that adults consume about 650 mg/day of long-chain polyunsaturated fatty acids (i.e., DHA and EPA), which can be achieved by consuming about 1 serving of fish per day or by taking a fish oil supplement. These guidelines are also supported by the American Heart Association, which advises individuals with cardiovascular disease to consume at least 1 serving of fatty fish each day to reduce mortality due to cardiovascular disease.

Fish oil supplements have also been studied in relation to specific inflammatory diseases such as inflammatory bowel disease (ulcerative colitis and Crohn's disease) and rheumatoid arthritis, but findings are somewhat inconclusive, likely because of problems with study design. However, because omega-3 long-chain polyunsaturated fatty acids suppress the conversion of arachidonic acid to proinflammatory and prothrombotic omega-6 eicosanoids, thereby stimulating the production of anti-inflammatory eicosanoids, there is a biological basis for using fish oil to manage or possibly prevent a wide variety of inflammatory diseases.

## Glucosamine and Chondroitin

Glucosamine and chondroitin are naturally present in articular cartilage and have been investigated for their efficacy in treating osteoarthritis. Glucosamine is an amino sugar, while chondroitin is a glycosaminoglycan that is endogenously synthesized by chondrocytes. Glucosamine supplements are derived from the chitinous exoskeleton of crustaceans, while shark cartilage or bovine trachea is a common source of chondroitin. Glucosamine and chondroitin sulfates are marketed as tablets, capsules, or powders. Glucosamine may produce favourable effects by stimulating the production of proteoglycans and glycosaminoglycans important for healthy joints. It has been claimed that chondroitin exerts beneficial effects by preventing the degradation of collagen.

A meta-analysis of 16 randomized controlled trials found that the majority of these studies demonstrated that glucosamine or chondroitin was effective at attenuating the symptoms of osteoarthritis, but not at regenerating the cartilage of affected joints. The majority of studies evaluated the knee joint using measurements of knee joint pain, inflammation, and mobility in addition to other indices, including measures of quality of life. It is uncertain whether the form of glucosamine or chondroitin results in differences in effectiveness, as most studies have tested these compounds as glucosamine sulfate and chondroitin sulfate. Most studies have provided glucosamine or chondroitin orally, but a few administered these compounds as intra-arterial or intramuscular injections. The duration of the studies has also varied considerably, from 1 month to 3 years for glucosamine and 90 days to 1 year for chondroitin.

Glucosamine trials have generally used doses of glucosamine sulfate of 750 to 1500 mg/day, with most trials being performed at the latter dose. Furthermore, 1500 mg of glucosamine is generally recommended as a daily dose. Chondroitin sulfate trials have used more variable doses, ranging from 800 to 2000 mg/day, and supplements are generally marketed as capsules containing 250 to 750 mg. There are many combined preparations of the two.

## Creatine

Creatine, in the form of creatine monohydrate, is popular among athletes and is marketed as a nutritional supplement to increase muscular strength and delay the onset of fatigue during intense, short bouts of exercise. Creatine is synthesized endogenously from glycine and arginine as a step in the urea cycle. About 95% of the total body creatine is present in skeletal muscle, where it is converted to phosphocreatine, which serves as an anaerobic source of ATP for energy utilization in intensive muscle activity. The richest sources of dietary creatine are meat and fish, providing approximately 1 g/day. More commonly, those wishing to *creatine load* will take creatine supplements in the form of powder, tablets, or beverages to achieve significantly higher levels of creatine in skeletal muscle than can be achieved by foods alone. In general, creatine is taken at a dose of 20 g/day for 5 days to ensure maximal levels in skeletal muscle and is then lowered to a maintenance dose of 2 to 5 g/day. Thus, to achieve these levels, modification of diet alone is insufficient.

A multitude of studies have investigated the effects of creatine supplementation on exercise performance, and mixed results have been reported. Combined with resistance or strength training, some studies report positive effects on performance while others report no effect. Differences in findings may be due to the type of outcome measured: endurance studies generally show no benefit with creatine supplementation, while intense exercise may be improved. However, this is not a consistent finding as elite swimmers experienced no significant improvement in their sprint times. Another reason for these discrepant findings may be the variation in initial levels of creatine stores in skeletal muscle. It is speculated that creatine supplementation may be most effective for patients with neuromuscular disorders in which muscle phospho-

creatine and ATP levels tend to be low, and this continues to be an active area of research. A side effect of creatine supplementation may be a rapid gain in body weight, likely due to an increase in body water.

## DRUG INTERACTIONS WITH POTENTIAL ADVERSE EFFECTS

It is essential from a safety perspective to acknowledge that *natural* compounds do have biological and chemical activity just as drugs do and thus can have potentially adverse interactions with drugs. Some of these known or postulated interactions are identified in Table 64-3. It is known that ginseng root, garlic, and ginkgo biloba leaf interact with aspirin and may enhance the prevention of platelet aggregation, which may result in excessive bleeding. Valerian root interacts with opioid analgesics and results in enhanced depression of the CNS.

Cancer patients often combine alternative therapies such as herbal preparations and dietary supplements with traditional anti-cancer drugs without being aware of potential adverse interactions. Most of the known interactions between herbal preparations and anti-cancer and other drugs relate to effects on cytochrome P450 enzymes (see Table 64-3). For example, garlic interacts with various drugs, such as anti-cancer agents, chlorzoxazone, ritonavir, and saquinavir. Similarly, ginkgo biloba can affect the activity of chlorzoxazone, dapsone, mephenytoin, nifedipine, and omeprazole. It is important to acknowledge that many other interactions exist, and future studies are needed to extensively identify these potential adverse interactions.

Due to the fact that herbal preparations may interact with medications used in relation to surgery, including anaesthetics, it is prudent for individuals who are scheduled for surgery to stop taking supplements at least 1 week prior. Moreover, there are reports of cardiac arrhythmias, poor wound healing, and excessive bleeding after surgery due to some herbal preparations.

## SUGGESTED READINGS

Anderson JW, Johnstone BM, Cook-Newell ME. Meta-analysis of the effects of soy protein intake on serum lipids. *N Engl J Med.* 1995;333:276-282.

Blumenthal M. Herbs continue slide in mainstream market. *Herbal Gram.* 2003;58:71.

Blumenthal M, Goldberg A, Brinckmann J, eds. *Herbal Medicine: Expanded Commission E Monographs.* Newton, Ma: Integrative Medicine Communications; 2000.

Ciocon JO, Ciocon DG, Galindo DJ. Dietary supplements in primary care. Botanicals can affect surgical outcomes and follow-up. *Geriatrics.* 2004;59:20-24.

Eisenberg DM, Davis RB, Ettner SL, et al. Trends in alternative medicine use in the United States, 1990-1997. *JAMA*. 1998; 280:1569-1575.

Holub BJ. Clinical nutrition: 4. Omega-3 fatty acids in cardiovascular care. *CMAJ*. 2002;166:608-615.

Hrastinger A, Dietz B, Bauer R, et al. Is there clinical evidence supporting the use of botanical dietary supplements in children? *J Pediatr*. 2005;146:311-317.

Mahady GB. Is black cohosh estrogenic? *Nutr Rev*. 2003;61:183-186.

Mahady GB, Parrot J, Lee C, et al. Botanical dietary supplement use in peri- and postmenopausal women. *Menopause*. 2003; 10:65-72.

Messina MJ, Loprinzi CL. Soy for breast cancer survivors: a critical review of the literature. *J Nutr*. 2001;131:3095S-3108S.

Persky AM, Brazeau GA. Clinical pharmacology of the dietary supplement creatine monohydrate. *Pharmacol Rev*. 2001;53: 161-176.

Richy F, Bruyere O, Ethgen O, et al. Structural and symptomatic efficacy of glucosamine and chondroitin in knee osteoarthritis. A comprehensive meta-analysis. *Arch Intern Med*. 2003; 163:1514-1522.

Rossouw JE, Anderson GL, Prentice RL, et al. Risks and benefits of estrogen plus progestin in healthy postmenopausal women: principal results from the Women's Health Initiative randomized controlled trial. *JAMA*. 2002;288:321-333.

Sparreboom A, Cox MC, Acharya MR, et al. Herbal remedies in the United States: potential adverse interactions with anticancer agents. *J Clin Oncol*. 2004;22:2489-2503.

Tesch BJ. Herbs commonly used by women: an evidence-based review. *Am J Obstet Gynecol*. 2003;188:S44-S55.

Thompson LU, Cunnane SC, eds. *Flaxseed in Human Nutrition*. 2nd ed. Champaign, Ill: American Oil Chemists Society Press; 2003.

Towheed TE, Maxwell L, Anastassiades TP, et al. Glucosamine therapy for treating osteoarthritis. *Cochrane Database Syst Rev*. 2005;(2):CD002946.

Troppmann L, Johns T, Gray-Donald K. Natural health product use in Canada. *Can J Public Health* 2002;93:426-430.

Ward WE. *Potential Health Benefits of Soy*. NIN Review No 34. Ottawa, Ontario: National Institute of Nutrition; 2002.

Williamson EM. Drug interactions between herbal and prescription medicines. *Drug Saf*. 2003;26:1075-1092.

Wilt TJ, Ishani A, Stark G, et al. Saw palmetto extracts for treatment of benign prostatic hyperplasia: a systematic review. *JAMA*. 1998;280:1604-1609.

World Health Organization. *WHO Monographs on Selected Medicinal Plants*. Vol 1. Geneva, Switzerland: World Health Organization; 1999.

## ONLINE RESOURCES

Center for Food Safety and Applied Nutrition, U.S. Food and Drug Administration:
http://www.cfsan.fda.gov/~dms/supplmnt.html

The Cochrane Collaboration:
http://www.cochrane.org/index0.htm

Drugs & Health Products, Health Canada:
http://www.hc-sc.gc.ca/hpfb-dgpsa/nhpd-dpsn/index_e.html

The European Scientific Cooperative on Phytotherapy:
http://www.escop.com/index.htm

HerbMed:
http://www.herbmed.org

Natural Standard:
http://www.naturalstandard.com

Office of Dietary Supplements, National Institutes of Health:
http://dietary-supplements.info.nih.gov/factsheets/dietarysupplements.asp

# 65

# Drugs That Alter Bone Metabolism for the Treatment of Osteoporosis

## JD ADACHI AND A PAPAIOANNOU

### CASE HISTORY

A 51-year-old white woman who was menopausal at age 49 was referred by her family physician to a specialist with an interest in bone diseases. The patient's medical history included polymyositis and lactose intolerance. Polymyositis had been diagnosed at age 32 and was initially treated with prednisone 40 mg daily for a period of approximately 6 months; the dose was then gradually tapered to a maintenance dose of 5 mg. The patient had two disease flare-ups and required higher doses of prednisone with early tapering to maintenance levels of 7.5 mg daily. At the time of presentation, she was also on weekly methotrexate. She gave no history of known fractures but spoke of two episodes of acute-onset back pain with slow resolution in each case and residual aching pain in the lower back. Because of chronic lactose intolerance, the patient had low dietary intake of calcium for many years, and only in the past 2 years had a supplement of calcium carbonate been prescribed, giving 500 mg of elemental calcium daily. She was not on any vitamin D supplement, and she received no other prescription medications.

Findings on physical examination were within normal limits, except for some tenderness on heavy percussion over the thoracolumbar spine. X-rays revealed anterior compression of the twelfth thoracic vertebra and first lumbar vertebra. The provisional diagnosis was osteoporosis secondary to the effects of long-term glucocorticoid treatment and low intake of calcium and vitamin D, with the menopause and immobilization contributing to bone loss.

Bone densitometry showed significant osteopenia in both the lumbar spine and femoral neck. Laboratory tests revealed ionized calcium levels just below the lower limit of normal, elevated alkaline phosphatase, low urinary calcium excretion, elevated intact parathyroid hormone (PTH), and 25-OH vitamin D near the lower limit of the reference range.

The patient had no contraindications to hormone replacement, and after normal gynecological and breast examinations, she was placed on conjugated equine estrogen (Premarin 0.625 mg) and medroxyprogesterone acetate (Provera 2.5 mg), both to be taken daily. She was changed from calcium carbonate to calcium citrate to give a daily calcium intake of approximately 1000 mg. Vitamin D, 1000 IU daily, was also begun, and she was urged to actively exercise as frequently as possible. The patient had some bothersome menstrual spotting for 3 months and read about the increased risk of side effects with hormone replacement. As a result, she elected to discontinue therapy. She had no side effects from calcium and vitamin D, and the plasma levels of ionized calcium and 25-OH vitamin D increased into the normal range. Intact PTH and alkaline phosphatase levels and urinary calcium excretion also became normal.

Recent studies reported the benefits of bisphosphonate therapy in preventing bone loss and reducing fracture risk. As a result, she was given alendronate 70 mg weekly.

During the next 3 years of follow-up, there was a progressive increase in bone density and a resulting reduction in the risk of fracture. Indeed, she has not had any fractures, and her long-term prognosis is good as long as she continues the present treatment and is able to minimize the dose of glucocorticoid used to treat her polymyositis.

## PHYSIOLOGY OF BONE

The histological structure, metabolism, and density of bone are closely related to serum calcium concentration. Close physiological control of serum calcium within a narrow range from 2.2 to 2.6 mmol/L is maintained by secretion of parathyroid hormone (PTH) and calcitonin (CT) and production of 1,25-dihydroxyvitamin $D_3$. These three hormonal substances act on (1) bone to control the transfer of calcium between extra- and intracellular fluid, as well as bone resorption, formation, and mineralization;

(2) the gastrointestinal tract to regulate the absorption of calcium and phosphorus; and (3) the renal tubule to regulate reabsorption of calcium and phosphate.

It has been estimated that a calcium intake of about 1 g/day is required to maintain calcium balance in the normal adult. Net calcium absorption is normally about 15 to 45% of the oral intake when measured by isotopic calcium absorption methods. The fraction of the total calcium absorption that occurs in any specific segment of the intestine depends on the length of that segment and the transit time along it, in addition to the calcium concentration in that part of the intestinal lumen. The duodenum has the greatest capacity for transport of calcium per unit length of intestine, but the largest fraction of the total calcium absorption occurs in the ileum.

Urinary excretion of calcium ranges up to 7.5 mmol/24 hours. Many factors affect total urinary calcium excretion, including age, sex (males absorb and excrete more calcium than do females), seasonal variations, exercise, and sodium and phosphorus intake. In adults, about 100 mL of plasma water is filtered by the kidneys every minute, but only about 1% of this filtered water and less than 2% of filtered calcium is excreted in the urine. The greatest part of the filtered load of calcium is reabsorbed by the renal tubules (Fig. 65-1).

If input of calcium from intestinal absorption and renal reabsorption is not sufficient to maintain extracellular fluid calcium concentration in the normal range, PTH is released from the parathyroid glands, and calcium can be rapidly mobilized from bone under the influence of PTH. This transfer is mediated by osteocytes and osteoblasts, and only if the deficiency is prolonged is there an increase in osteoclast-mediated bone resorption secondary to sustained increase in PTH secretion.

Ninety-nine percent of total body calcium is in the skeleton. Radioisotopic studies with $^{45}$Ca and $^{47}$Ca indicate that 1% of skeletal calcium is freely exchangeable with extracellular fluid. Bone metabolic activity ensures not only that bone is continuously undergoing remodelling or turnover but also that the readily exchangeable pool of calcium is maintained. The morphological unit of compact bone is the osteon, which has been defined as "an irregular, branching and anastomosing cylinder composed of a more or less centrally placed cell-containing neurovascular canal surrounded by concentric, cell-permeated lamellae of bone matrix." At one level of an osteon, the predominant cells may be osteoclasts, and bone resorption the prevailing process, while at another level of the same osteon, the predominant cell type may be osteoblasts, which are forming, depositing, and mineralizing the collagen matrix of bone.

Bone resorption and formation are normally closely coupled (Fig. 65-2). As matrix formation and mineralization continue, the active osteoblasts become encircled with mineralized matrix and become osteocytes lying within lacunae. Osteocytes are capable of active bone resorption (a process known as osteolysis) and transport of mineral ions to the osteoblasts via a cytoplasmic canalicular system. Osteolysis rather than osteoclast-mediated resorption is probably the primary metabolic activity of bone responsible

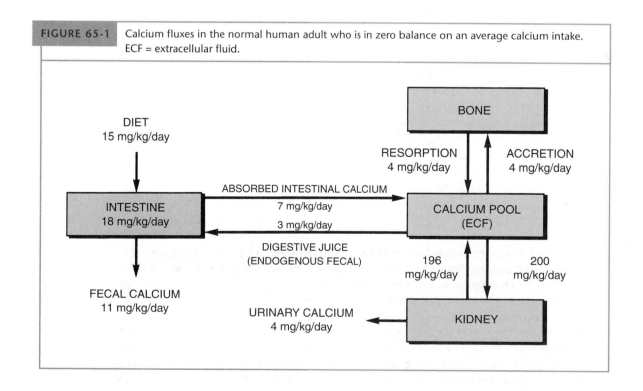

**FIGURE 65-1** Calcium fluxes in the normal human adult who is in zero balance on an average calcium intake. ECF = extracellular fluid.

FIGURE 65-2    Normal bone remodelling.

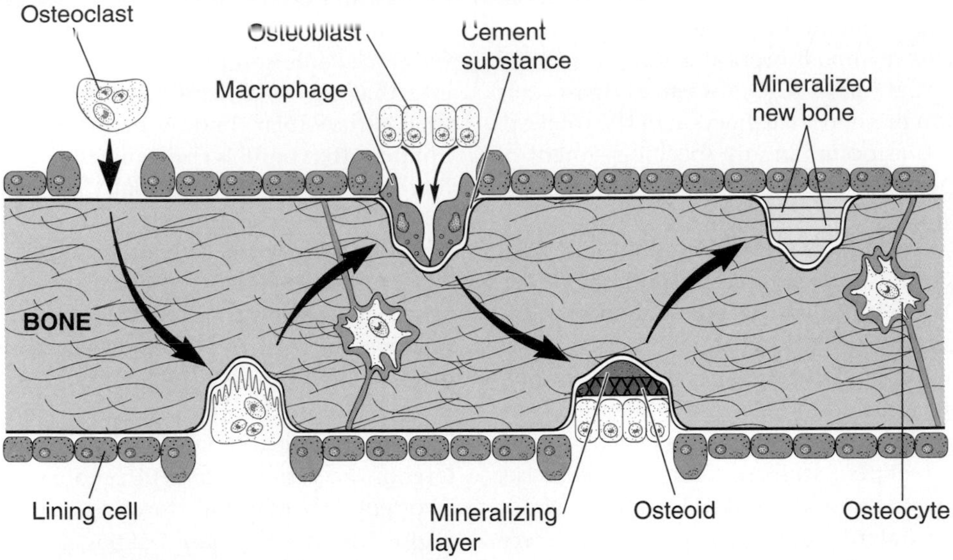

for maintaining normal extracellular fluid concentration of calcium. Osteoclasts are derived from the monocyte/macrophage system of cells of the hematopoietic system. They are important for the resorption of bone in the remodelling process, but their contribution to the normal control of calcium homeostasis is minimal.

In predominantly trabecular bone, the same cellular metabolic processes prevail; however, osteoclast-mediated resorption and osteoblast synthesis of bone occur on the surface of trabeculae rather than within osteons.

Studies of osteoblasts have indicated that the term "osteoblast" describes heterogeneous cells of a common mesenchymal origin, but with differentiated functions. There is increasing evidence that cells of osteoblast lineage serve a central function in bone matrix turnover, not only stimulating synthesis of new matrix but also controlling matrix resorption by osteoclasts as well. Several circulating hormones such as PTH, 1,25-dihydroxyvitamin D, and sex hormones control the formation of osteoclasts. The microenvironment of the bone marrow is an essential source of cytokines such as tumour necrosis factors and interleukins. These systemic and local factors exert their effect by acting first on cells of the osteoblastic lineage, which possess a cell surface molecule known as receptor activator of nuclear factor κB ligand (RANKL). This cell surface receptor, a member of the tumour necrosis factor (TNF) ligand family, then interacts with osteoclast precursors from the hemopoietic lineage by binding to RANK, an osteoclast precursor cell surface receptor, and promoting the differentiation, fusion, and, eventually, the formation of mature osteoclasts. Osteoprotegerin (OPG), a soluble

TNF receptor produced by cells of the osteoblast lineage, is an effective inhibitor of osteoclast formation. It performs this function by acting as a decoy receptor, binding to RANKL and blocking its interaction with RANK. The calciotropic hormones and cytokines appear to stimulate osteoclastogenesis in two ways: by inhibiting the production of OPG and by stimulating the production of RANKL and RANKL-stimulated osteoclastogenesis. Recent results of the first clinical trial with OPG have supported its potential as a therapeutic agent for osteoporosis.

## OSTEOPOROSIS

Osteoporosis is a skeletal disorder characterized by compromised bone strength that predisposes a person to an increased risk of fracture. Bone strength reflects the integration of two main features: bone density and bone quality. The major clinical consequences of osteoporosis are fractures. Major risk factors for fracturing include: age, previous fracture, low bone mineral density (BMD), and family history of osteoporosis. Major and minor risk factors are outlined in Table 65-1. Over the past decade, the treatment of osteoporosis has been the focus of much research. Advances in therapy and knowledge about the mechanisms of action of osteoporosis drugs have increased exponentially. Today, patients and physicians have a wide variety of available therapies to choose from. For the most part, anti-resorptive therapies have been the focus; however, more recently, anabolic therapies have offered new treatment alternatives.

| TABLE 65-1 | Factors Identifying the Need for Osteoporosis Assessment |
| --- | --- |
| **Major Risk Factors** | **Minor Risk Factors** |
| Age >65 years | Rheumatoid arthritis |
| Vertebral compression fracture | Past history of |
| Fragility fracture after age 40 | clinical hyperthyroidism |
| Family history of osteoporotic | Chronic anticonvulsant |
| fracture (especially maternal | therapy |
| hip fracture) | Low dietary intake |
| Systemic glucocorticoid | of calcium |
| therapy of >3 months | Smoker |
| Malabsorption syndrome | Excessive alcohol intake |
| Primary hyperparathyroidism | Excessive caffeine intake |
| Propensity to fall | Weight <57 kg |
| Osteopenia apparent on | Weight loss >10% of |
| X-ray film | weight at age 25 |
| Hypogonadism | Chronic heparin therapy |
| Early menopause | |
| (before age 45) | |

## ANTI-RESORPTIVE THERAPIES

## Calcium and Vitamin D

Calcium and vitamin D are important contributors to overall bone health. It is recommended that all individuals get adequate amounts of calcium and vitamin D and to supplement in those circumstances when dietary intake is inadequate. For post-menopausal women, the Osteoporosis Society of Canada recommends 1500 mg of calcium and 800 IU of vitamin D per day. A more detailed discussion of nutritional aspects of calcium is found in Chapter 63.

Various salts of calcium are available for medicinal use, such as calcium chloride, calcium citrate, calcium lactate, calcium gluconate, and calcium carbonate. Calcium chloride contains 27% elemental calcium, calcium citrate 21%, calcium lactate 13%, and calcium gluconate 9%; insoluble calcium carbonate, which is converted to soluble calcium salts in the body, contains 40% elemental calcium.

Vitamin D is either ingested in our diet, principally through fortified milk, or is converted from vitamin D precursors by sunlight exposure to the skin. From there, it is hydroxylated in the liver to 25-hydroxyvitamin D and is further hydroxylated in the kidney to its most active form, 1,25-dihydroxyvitamin D (see Chapter 63). Vitamin D is available for therapy as vitamin $D_3$, vitamin $D_2$, 1α-hydroxyvitamin D, D3 (1α-hydroxycholecalciferol), and 1,25-dihydroxyvitamin D (calcitriol) (Fig. 65-3).

### Pharmacokinetics
Calcium is best absorbed with a meal, particularly in the presence of achlorhydria. Gastrointestinal absorption of orally administered vitamin D is usually adequate. Since bile is essential for vitamin D absorption, hepatobiliary disease may be associated with decreased absorption of vitamin D. Also, fat malabsorption may impair the absorption of this fat-soluble vitamin.

### Adverse effects
A common adverse effect of intravenously administered calcium chloride is irritation of veins. Oral calcium supplements may cause gastric irritation, nausea, and constipation. Administration of excessive calcium can lead to hypercalcemic toxicity. Ingestion of large quantities of calcium salts, however, is unlikely to produce hypercalcemia unless large amounts of vitamin D are also administered.

The only adverse or toxic effects of vitamin D are those related to overtreatment and development of hypercalcemia and hyperphosphatemia. Impairment of renal function due to nephrolithiasis or nephrocalcinosis, localized or generalized decreases in bone density, and gastrointestinal complaints are the most common sequelae of vitamin D toxicity.

### Drug interactions
Calcium salts should not be taken orally at the same time as tetracycline because the absorption of tetracycline will be decreased by the formation of a calcium–tetracycline chelate. Similarly, the co-administration of fluoride or phosphates with calcium may be associated with decreased absorption due to formation of insoluble compounds in the gastrointestinal tract.

### Efficacy in the treatment of osteoporosis
A recent systematic review summarizes the controlled trials examining the effect of calcium on bone density and fractures in post-menopausal women. Calcium was more effective than placebo in reducing rates of bone loss. From this systematic review of calcium supplementation alone, it was concluded that calcium had a small positive effect on BMD. The data did show a trend toward reduction in vertebral fractures but did not meaningfully address the possible effect of calcium on reducing the incidence of non-vertebral fractures.

In another systematic review, vitamin D reduced the incidence of vertebral fractures and showed a trend toward reduced incidence of non-vertebral fractures. Most patients in the trials that evaluated vertebral fractures received hydroxylated vitamin D, and most patients in the trials that evaluated non-vertebral fractures received standard (non-hydroxylated) vitamin D. Hydroxylated vitamin D had a consistently greater impact on bone density than did standard vitamin D. Hydroxylated vitamin D at doses above 50 μg vitamin D resulted in an increased risk of discontinuing medication in comparison with control groups as a result of either symptomatic adverse effects or abnormal laboratory results, which were similar in trials of standard and hydroxylated vitamin D. Vitamin D decreases vertebral fractures and may decrease non-vertebral fractures.

**FIGURE 65-3** Structural formulae of clinically important vitamin D preparations and analogues.

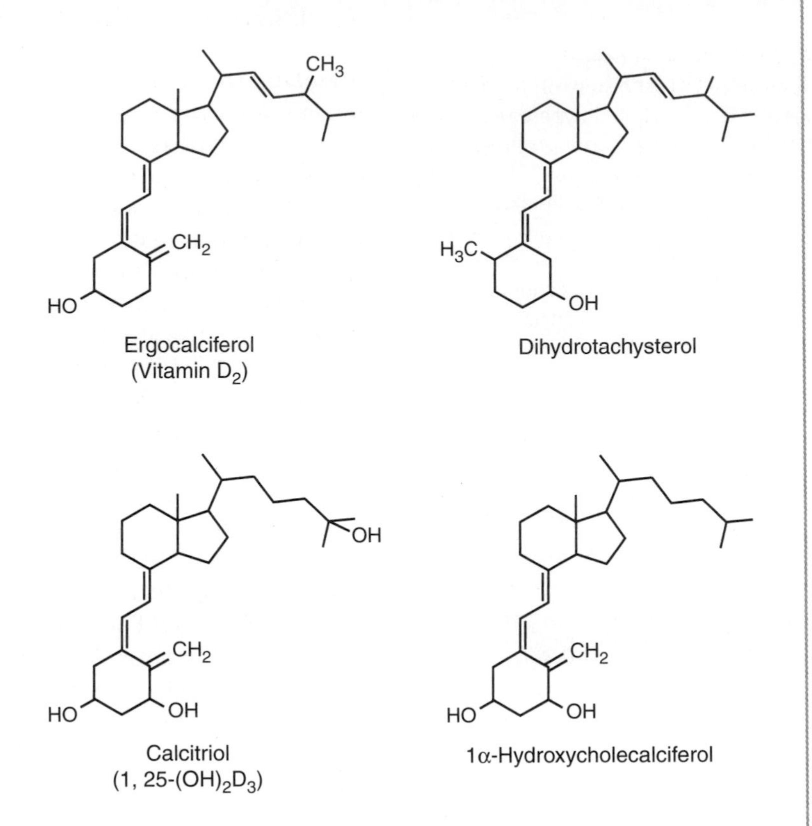

Ergocalciferol
(Vitamin $D_2$)

Dihydrotachysterol

Calcitriol
$(1, 25\text{-}(OH)_2D_3)$

$1\alpha$-Hydroxycholecalciferol

In the elderly, therapy with vitamin D may be particularly effective because vitamin D levels are often low in this population as a result of lack of exposure to sunlight.

# Calcitonin

Calcitonin is a 32-amino-acid polypeptide produced by the C cells of the thyroid gland. Calcitonin is available as a nasal spray and as subcutaneous and intramuscular injections.

## Cellular effects

Calcitonin receptors are present mainly on osteoclasts but are also present in the kidney, gastrointestinal (GI) tract, and the brain. Calcitonin decreases osteoclast size and motility and causes the osteoclasts to cease their bone resorbing activity. This hormone inhibits the increased rate of bone turnover that is induced by parathyroid hormone. It is also known to act on the central nervous system, having an analgesic effect. Calcitonin levels are affected by the GI tract, with gastrin and pancreozymin stimulating its secretion. In the kidney, calcitonin increases the excretion of sodium, potassium, phosphate, calcium, and magnesium. Post-menopausal women tend to have lower levels of plasma calcitonin compared with age-matched men or pre-menopausal women.

## Pharmacokinetics

Absorption of calcitonin from injection sites is rapid, although it is slowed by addition of gelatin to the vehicle. In the circulation, the half-life of calcitonin is on the order of 20 minutes. It is weakly and insignificantly bound to protein and is catabolized in the liver and kidney. Availability of calcitonin when administered as a nasal spray ranges from 3 to 50%, relative to intramuscular injection.

## Adverse effects

Adverse effects of calcitonin therapy are generally dose-related and consist of anorexia, nausea, and facial flushing. These side effects are more frequent with parenteral administration and are seldom seen with the nasal spray. Rhinitis, nasal dryness, and mild epistaxis are the most common adverse effects with the nasal spray. Urticaria or anaphylaxis is rare. A consequence of long-term calcitonin usage is the development of neutralizing antibodies and the potential for host resistance. The extent to which they may interfere with calcitonin action remains unresolved; however, long-term fracture efficacy data suggest that they are likely to be inconsequential.

Drug interactions are uncommon, but the concomitant administration of calcitonin and thiazide diuretics may be associated with potassium depletion.

### Efficacy in the treatment of osteoporosis

A systematic review of the efficacy of calcitonin in post-menopausal osteoporosis revealed that calcitonin reduced the incidence of vertebral fractures but did not clearly decrease non-vertebral fractures. Changes in BMD ranged from 3.0 to 3.8% depending on the site measured. Methodologically weaker studies tended to show greater treatment effects on BMD and vertebral fracture. It was concluded that calcitonin likely increases BMD in post-menopausal women when given in weekly doses greater than 250 IU and likely reduces the risk of vertebral fractures. Its effect on non-vertebral fractures remains uncertain.

## Hormone Replacement Therapy

The effects of hormone replacement therapy (HRT) on bone cannot be discussed in isolation, and the risks and benefits of therapy must be addressed. HRT has been shown to have a positive impact on BMD in all areas of the skeleton that have been studied, and it has been shown to reduce the risk of osteoporotic fractures. Positive effects of estrogen on the cardiovascular system have been reported; however, more recently, there is good evidence to the contrary. Indeed, the weight of the evidence shows that HRT should not be used either in primary or secondary prevention of cardiovascular disease. The association of unopposed estrogen therapy with increased incidence of uterine cancer is established, and the addition of a progestational agent reduces that risk. The association of estrogen therapy with an increased risk of breast cancer has now been confirmed. Venous thromboembolism is another known complication of HRT. HRT unequivocally aids menopausal symptoms and is the reason most women consider it. Recent suggestions that associate improved memory with HRT remain controversial. The amount of information that needs to be assimilated by both patient and physician is formidable, making the decision to commence HRT a difficult one.

### Cellular effects of estrogen deficiency

The cellular hallmark of bone loss caused by estrogen deficiency is increased bone remodelling, which is characterized by an imbalance of bone resorption over bone formation. The osteoclast plays a crucial role in the imbalance seen with estrogen deficiency. An increase in the proliferation and differentiation of hematopoietic osteoclast progenitors, an increase in stromal/osteoblastic cell number and support of osteoclast formation, and a decrease in the incidence of osteoclast apoptosis are seen with ovariectomy.

### The effects of estrogen on bone active cytokines

An increase in interleukin-1 (IL-1), interleukin-6 (IL-6), and tumour necrosis factor (TNF) occurs with the loss of estrogen. IL-1, IL-6, and TNF stimulate osteoclast progenitor replication and differentiation. An important characteristic of these cytokines that regulate osteoclast forma-tion is their ability to stimulate their own and each other's synthesis in an autocrine and synergistic fashion. Not only do IL-1, IL-6, and TNF induce their own synthesis, but TNF acts synergistically with IL-1 to stimulate both TNF and IL-6. PTH also acts synergistically with TNF to stimulate IL-6 production. Consistent with evidence that IL-6 mediates the increase in osteoclast formation caused by estrogen deficiency, estrogen suppresses production of IL-6 by inhibiting the IL-1- and TNF-stimulated biosynthesis of IL-6 in stromal/osteoblastic cells.

The differentiation of osteoclast precursors into functional osteoclasts depends on factors that are produced by stromal/osteoblastic cells. Physical contact between the progenitors and the support cells is thought to be required. It is likely that stromal/osteoblastic cells represent a subset of the marrow stromal cells that support hematopoiesis. They are in intimate contact with the endocortical and cancellous bone surfaces, as well as with marrow monocytes, hematopoietic progenitors, and the endothelial cells lining the blood vessels of the extravascular intersinusoidal space. Thus, they are ideally poised to respond to endocrine factors such as sex steroids and PTH that are present in the circulation, as well as to the cytokines and growth factors that are made in the bone marrow. Together with increased cytokine production, changes in the number and activity of stromal/osteoblastic cells appear to play a key role in the increased osteoclast formation caused by estrogen deficiency. Ovariectomy stimulates osteoblast formation. In view of the close relationship of stromal/osteoblastic cells to the osteoblast lineage, it is likely that the number of cells capable of supporting osteoclast formation is also increased in estrogen deficiency.

Recent findings indicate that apoptosis is stimulated by estrogen either directly or indirectly via the regulation of cytokines that influence osteoclast apoptosis. In vitro studies have demonstrated that TGFβ stimulates osteoclast apoptosis, while IL-1, TNF, and IL-6 inhibit it. Thus, it is highly likely that an ovariectomy-induced increase in the latter cytokines, together with decreased levels of TGFβ, prolongs the lifespan of osteoclasts.

### The effects of HRT on bone mineral density

HRT has a beneficial effect on BMD. In one representative three-year randomized clinical trial comparing estrogen treatment regimens, those assigned to the placebo group lost BMD by the third year of the study, while those assigned to active regimens gained BMD. Older women, women with low initial BMD, and those with no previous hormone use gained significantly more bone than younger women, women with higher initial BMD, and those who had used hormones previously. Long-term estrogen therapy is of benefit in the prevention of bone loss. A 10-year study showed that lumbar spine BMD was significantly higher in HRT-treated women than in those who remained untreated.

A dose–response relationship between the dose of estrogen and BMD has clearly been demonstrated. Studies have been performed examining the route of estrogen administration on BMD and have demonstrated that transdermal estradiol 0.05 mg/day and oral conjugated equine estrogens 0.625 mg/day prevented bone loss. However, 12% of women on either transdermal or oral treatment lost a significant amount of bone from the femoral neck in 3 years. Therefore, women taking therapy primarily for hip fracture prevention may require a follow-up BMD measurement to establish the efficacy of treatment.

### The effects of HRT on vertebral fractures and hip fractures

Most randomized clinical trials have been performed to demonstrate BMD benefit in both primary and secondary prevention. In a high-risk group of post-menopausal women with at least one vertebral fracture, treatment resulted in both an increase in BMD and a reduction in vertebral fractures. More recently, the Women's Health Initiative (WHI) published the results of the combination of conjugated equine estrogen and medroxyprogesterone on fractures as a secondary outcome measure. They found that there were fewer hip fractures, symptomatic vertebral fractures, and osteoporotic fractures.

The effect of HRT on reducing hip fractures has been documented in a number of cohort and case–control studies. Results from these trials suggest that for protection against fractures, estrogen should be initiated soon after menopause and continued indefinitely. The only prospective randomized clinical trial to demonstrate hip fracture efficacy came from the WHI, where a hip fracture benefit was seen.

### Summary of HRT

Hormone replacement therapy is beneficial in the prevention of vertebral and non-vertebral fractures. BMD actually increases in the first years following institution of therapy. There is a dose response, with higher doses being more effective than lower doses in increasing BMD. Both oral and transdermal routes of administration are effective. The beneficial effects of hormone therapy on bone may be abrogated by smoking. Other benefits of HRT include the control of menopausal and urogenital symptoms and a reduction in colon cancer. Risks include the increase in cardiovascular and cerebrovascular disease, gallbladder disease, deep venous thrombosis, pulmonary emboli, and risk of breast cancer.

## Raloxifene

Selective estrogen receptor modulators (SERMs) are non-hormonal agents that bind to estrogen receptors with an affinity equivalent to that of estradiol, but they produce estrogen agonist effects in some tissues while having antagonist effects in others. Raloxifene (Fig. 65-4), 60 mg/day, is

the only SERM that has been approved for the prevention and treatment of osteoporosis.

### Pharmacokinetics

Raloxifene is rapidly absorbed with 60% absorbed after an oral dose. It undergoes significant first-pass metabolism with extensive presystemic glucuronide conjugation. As a result, only 2% is bioavailable. Raloxifene is highly bound to plasma proteins.

### Drug interactions

Cholestyramine significantly reduces the absorption and enterohepatic cycling of raloxifene and should not be co-administered.

### Effects on fractures, BMD, and bone turnover

A large randomized clinical trial, the Multiple Outcomes of Raloxifene Evaluation (MORE), examined the anti-fracture efficacy of raloxifene in late post-menopausal women with osteoporosis with or without prior vertebral fractures. Raloxifene significantly reduced the incidence of new vertebral fractures in women with (30% reduction) and without (50% reduction) prior vertebral fracture and significantly reduced the incidence of multiple new vertebral fractures in both groups. Non-vertebral fracture risk was not significantly reduced in the a priori analysis. In a post-hoc analysis, non-vertebral fractures were reduced in a subset of those with severe vertebral fractures, a subset that is at greatest risk for fracturing. In another post-hoc analysis involving a small proportion of the study population, raloxifene decreased the risk for new clinical vertebral fractures at one year by 68% compared with placebo. Moreover, data from the fourth year of the MORE trial suggest a sustained vertebral anti-fracture efficacy. Com-

**FIGURE 65-4** Structures of estradiol and raloxifene.

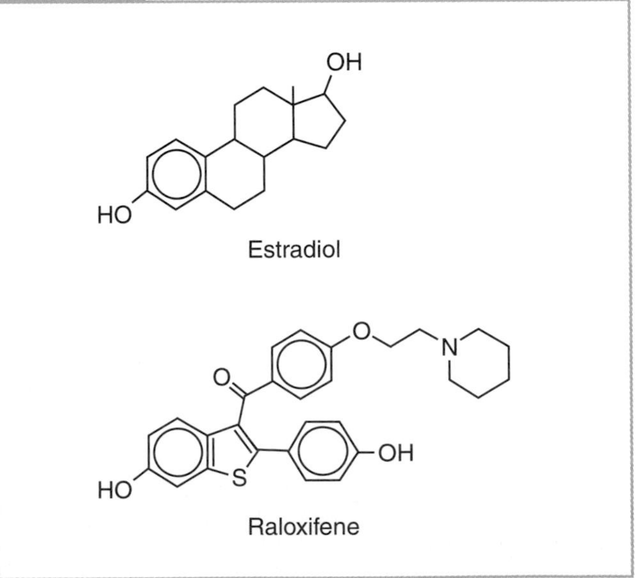

Estradiol

Raloxifene

pared with placebo, raloxifene significantly increased BMD at the lumbar spine and femoral neck and significantly reduced the bone turnover markers.

## Extra-skeletal effects

Raloxifene significantly reduces total and low-density lipoprotein cholesterol, but does not significantly change high-density lipoprotein cholesterol and triglyceride levels. Four-year results from the MORE trial showed similar effects on lipids. Raloxifene did not significantly affect the overall risk of cardiovascular events in the total population, but it did significantly reduce the risk of such events among women at high risk and among those with established cardiovascular disease.

Raloxifene reduced the incidence of estrogen receptor–positive invasive breast cancer by 84% in post-menopausal women with osteoporosis who were at low risk of breast cancer.

## Adverse effects

Raloxifene is generally safe and well tolerated. It increases hot flashes and leg cramps, which are usually mild to moderate in nature. There is no association between leg cramps and the risk of venous thromboembolism (VTE). VTE is a side effect associated with raloxifene, although it is reported infrequently. The magnitude of the relative risk is similar to that observed with HRT. Raloxifene is contraindicated in patients with past history of VTE. Raloxifene did not cause more vaginal bleeding or endometrial cancer than placebo.

## Summary of raloxifene

Raloxifene is efficacious in preventing vertebral fractures in post-menopausal women with osteoporosis. It increases BMD at the spine and femoral neck. Raloxifene has not yet been shown to be effective in preventing non-vertebral fractures, but a retrospective analysis suggests that it might well be of benefit. In post-menopausal women with osteoporosis, raloxifene decreases the incidence of estrogen receptor–positive invasive breast cancer, and in high-risk individuals it decreases the incidence of cardiovascular and cerebrovascular disease. Raloxifene does not increase the risk of endometrial hyperplasia or endometrial cancer. Raloxifene increases the risk of VTE from 0.5 to 1.1% over three years. Raloxifene has no beneficial effect on vasomotor symptoms and may increase their incidence.

## Bisphosphonates

Bisphosphonates (Fig. 65-5) are a novel class of drugs that have revolutionized the therapy of bone diseases. Several bisphosphonates have been registered for a wide variety of clinical applications, including the treatment of Paget's disease, hypercalcemia of malignancy, bone metastases, and osteoporosis.

## Pharmacokinetics

Bisphosphonates are poorly absorbed by the intestine, and their absorption is further reduced by food. Only up to 2% of any bisphosphonate may be absorbed when taken during fasting. They should, therefore, be administered in the fasting state 30 minutes to 1 hour before a meal, only with water.

The plasma half-life of bisphosphonates is 1 hour. The bisphosphonates are not metabolized, and after absorption they are excreted unchanged in the urine (50 to 80% within 24 hours) or removed from the circulation by binding to bone (20 to 50%), where they may persist for the lifetime of the patient.

## Mechanism of action

Bisphosphonates are stable analogues of naturally occurring pyrophosphate (see Fig. 65-5). They contain two phosphonate groups attached to a single carbon atom, to give a "P-C-P" structure. This renders them chemically stable and is responsible for the strong affinity of bisphosphonates for the skeleton.

Bisphosphonates inhibit bone resorption by cellular effects on osteoclasts. They interfere with osteoclast recruitment, differentiation, and action as well as osteoclast apoptosis. Bisphosphonates can be classified into at least two groups with different modes of action. Those that most closely resemble pyrophosphate, like etidronate, can be incorporated into cytotoxic ATP analogues. The more potent nitrogen-containing bisphosphonates affect cellular activity by interfering with protein prenylation through their effects on the mevalonate pathway, and, therefore, they impair the intracellular trafficking of key regulatory proteins (Fig. 65-6). The identification of these two mechanisms of action may help to explain some of the other pharmacological differences between the two classes of bisphosphonates.

Currently, the bisphosphonates approved for the treatment of osteoporosis in Canada include etidronate, alendronate, and risedronate. There are considerable differences between the bisphosphonates with respect to potency, ability to inhibit bone resorption, toxicity, and dosing regimens.

## Etidronate

Etidronate is given intermittently in a dose of 400 mg daily for 2 weeks followed by calcium 500 mg daily for 13 weeks. This regimen is then repeated. It is well tolerated, with diarrhea being an infrequent complaint, and it fits into the schedule of most patients.

Several studies have examined the anti-fracture efficacy of cyclical etidronate in women with severe osteoporosis. These studies indicate that treatment is effective in preventing new vertebral fractures in post-menopausal women with low bone mass and multiple previous vertebral fractures. However, randomized clinical trials have not shown intermittent etidronate to be effective in reducing hip fracture risk, and a recent meta-analysis confirmed the lack of efficacy against non-vertebral fracture. There is ample evidence that cyclical etidronate therapy maintains bone mass in patients undergoing treatment with corticosteroids, and it may also reduce the risk of vertebral fractures in glucocorticoid-treated post-menopausal women.

## Alendronate

Alendronate is given continuously in a dose of 5 mg/day for the prevention of osteoporosis and a dose of 10 mg daily or 70 mg weekly for the treatment of established osteoporosis. In the initial 3-year study, alendronate significantly reduced the incidence of new vertebral deformities. Its efficacy has since been examined in two large populations of post-menopausal women, one with and one without pre-existing vertebral fractures, in the Fracture Intervention Trial (FIT). In the vertebral fracture group, treatment with alendronate reduced the incidence of clinical fractures of the spine, hip, and wrist by about 50%. Alendronate also reduced the risk of multiple vertebral fractures and the incidence of new hip fractures.

The anti-fracture efficacy of alendronate was also examined in post-menopausal women with no prior vertebral fractures. Alendronate increased BMD at all measured sites. Treatment significantly reduced vertebral fractures by 44%, but it did not significantly reduce *all* clinical fractures. A pre-planned subset analysis of the clinical fracture data, however, revealed that the treatment significantly reduced fracture rates among women with osteoporosis but not among women with osteopenia. Alendronate prevents bone loss in normal post-menopausal women, but anti-fracture efficacy in this context has not been demonstrated. Alendronate also reduces the risk of fractures in glucocorticoid-treated post-menopausal women.

## Risedronate

Risedronate is given in a dose of 5 mg daily for the treatment of osteoporosis. More recently, it has become available as a 35-mg once-weekly tablet. Risedronate has been shown to have anti-fracture efficacy in osteoporotic women. In a randomized controlled trial of post-menopausal women with one or more vertebral fractures

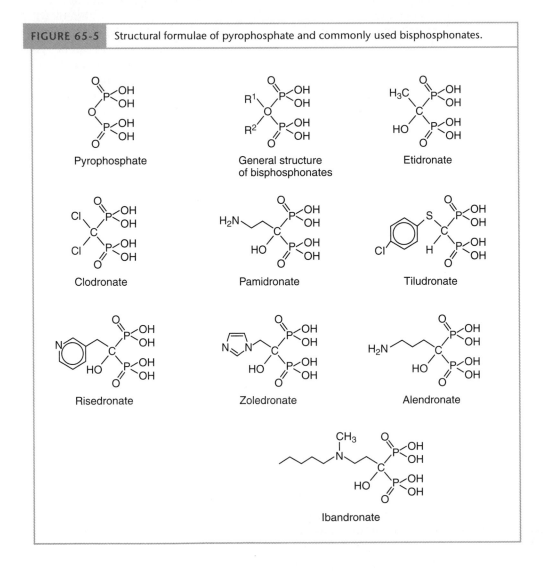

**FIGURE 65-5** Structural formulae of pyrophosphate and commonly used bisphosphonates.

at baseline, treatment with risedronate 5 mg daily decreased new vertebral fracture incidence by 65% in the first year and by 41% at the end of the third year. Risedronate also significantly lowered the incidence of nonvertebral fractures by 39%. In the European arm of the pivotal phase III trials, similar efficacy with respect to BMD and fractures was demonstrated. Very recently, risedronate has been shown to decrease the risk of hip fracture in elderly women with low BMD. However, in a stratum of the study, which recruited women with risk factors for falls, the effects of risedronate on hip fracture were not evident. Risedronate has also recently been reported to be of benefit in the prevention and treatment of glucocorticoid-induced bone loss and fracture.

## Adverse effects of bisphosphonates

High doses of etidronate can induce osteomalacia, but with the regimen used for osteoporosis, no clinically significant osteomalacia has been reported from the clinical trials. Diarrhea is an infrequent but reported problem with etidronate. Neither alendronate nor risedronate given to patients for up to 3 years impaired mineralization of newly formed bone. Alendronate can cause irritation of the esophageal and gastric mucosa, resulting in dyspepsia, heartburn, and nausea or vomiting. Although placebo-

and alendronate-treated patients in clinical trials did not differ significantly in frequency of adverse effects, a few cases of severe esophagitis have been reported in alendronate-treated patients. Like alendronate, risedronate also has a safe profile in clinical trials. Post-marketing safety data are not yet available. Oral administration of aminobisphosphonates is contraindicated in patients with esophageal pathology. Instructions for their use should be carefully followed. No drug interactions have been reported with the bisphosphonates.

## Summary of bisphosphonates

The evidence clearly demonstrates that, as a class, the nitrogen-containing bisphosphonates are the treatment of choice for the prevention of fractures in populations of patients at high risk for fracture.

# ANABOLIC THERAPIES

## Parathyroid Hormone (PTH)

PTH was reported as a clinical treatment for osteoporosis in 1980. The synthetic N-terminal fragment of PTH, recombinant hPTH(1-34), has been used in pharmaceuti-

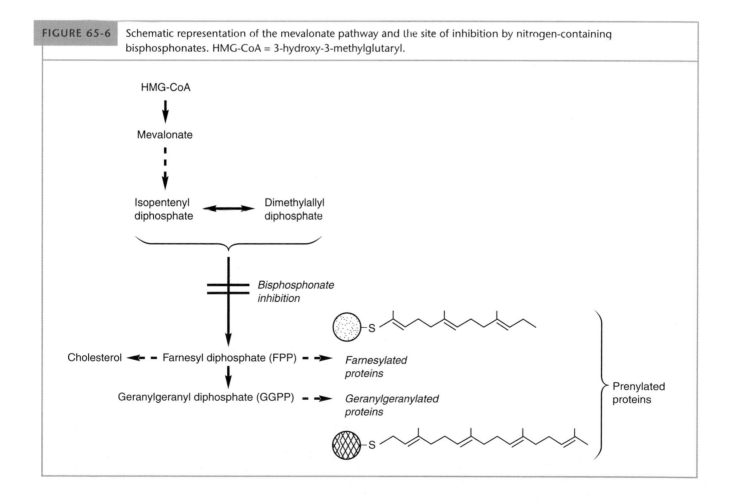

**FIGURE 65-6** Schematic representation of the mevalonate pathway and the site of inhibition by nitrogen-containing bisphosphonates. HMG-CoA = 3-hydroxy-3-methylglutaryl.

cal trials under the name **teriparatide**, and another PTH hormone, **recombinant hPTH(1-84)**, is currently undergoing phase III evaluation.

The pivotal randomized clinical trial evaluated the efficacy of teriparatide to reduce vertebral and non-vertebral fractures in post-menopausal women with at least one existing vertebral fracture. It was terminated prematurely because of the occurrence of osteosarcomas in a toxicology study in rats treated with large doses of teriparatide from infancy to senescence, which was subsequently felt to be of little significance in humans. There was a significant clinical fracture reduction in treated patients. For new vertebral fractures, the relative risk was 0.35 in the treated group, and for non-vertebral fractures the relative risk was 0.47. Teriparatide resulted in dose-dependent increments in measured BMD in both the lumbar spine (10 to 14%) and total/femoral neck (3 to 4%). Other smaller randomized clinical trials of recombinant hPTH(1-34) have shown similar consistent increments in spine and hip BMD observed over periods of 1 to 3 years of therapy.

Glucocorticoid-induced osteoporosis has been studied in a randomized clinical trial in post-menopausal women who had been on chronic estrogen therapy. Compared with the estrogen control group, treatment with PTH resulted in a significant 11.1% gain in BMD over the lumbar spine and an insignificant average gain of 2.9% over the femoral neck. The trial cohort was followed for an additional 12 months off therapy while the women continued chronic estrogen therapy. Further increments in BMD were observed.

### Adverse effects

Very few side effects occurred during PTH therapy. Nausea, headaches, dizziness, and leg cramps were observed infrequently as dose-dependent side effects during the teriparatide trials. PTH resulted in occasional episodes of hypercalcemia and/or hypercalciuria during the teriparatide trials, which were obviated by either cessation of concurrent calcium supplementation or minor dose reductions.

To date, the teriparatide toxicology data, documenting late-onset osteosarcomas in rats treated with large doses from infancy to senescence, have not been replicated in human studies. Current consensus is that limited exposure (1 to 2 years) to PTH therapy in older individuals with osteoporosis does not expose this population to the risk of osteosarcoma or any other neoplasm.

### Summary of PTH

Recombinant hPTH(1-34) is efficacious in preventing both vertebral and non-vertebral fractures in post-menopausal women with severe osteoporosis. It increases BMD at all skeletal sites with the exception of the radius. In men with severe osteoporosis and in post-menopausal women with glucocorticoid-induced osteoporosis, recombinant hPTH(1-34) increases BMD at the spine.

## Fluoride

Sodium fluoride is a potent stimulator of bone formation. It was initially investigated as a therapy for osteoporosis in 1964 and gained popularity through the 1970s and 1980s. The decade of the 1990s saw the introduction of randomized controlled trials into osteoporosis research and the use of precise vertebral fracture morphometry. Fluoride compounds had previously not been adequately investigated in accordance with modern evidence-based standards. Almost all of the studies were small and had limited analytical power. Furthermore, the clinical profile of fluoride treatments varied greatly with different pharmacological compounds and formulations in terms of bioavailability and side effect profile.

Fluoride is incorporated into bone as hydroxyfluoroapatite, which is resistant to resorption. More importantly, however, it appears to stimulate the synthesis of new bone matrix by osteoblasts. Precisely how or why this effect occurs is as yet unknown. At the same time, fluoride appears to retard the mineralization of the newly formed matrix.

### Pharmacokinetics

Soluble fluoride compounds such as sodium fluoride are almost completely absorbed. Fluoride is probably concentrated only in calcified tissues or sites of extra-skeletal calcification. The major route of fluoride excretion is the kidney.

### Efficacy

In an attempt to determine whether fluoride had any treatment effect, 11 studies were included in a meta-analysis. Increase in lumbar spine BMD was higher with treatment after 2 and 4 years, but the relative risk for new vertebral fractures was not significantly reduced at either 2 or 4 years.

### Adverse effects

New non-vertebral fractures are increased with fluoride therapy. Gastrointestinal side effects are also increased with fluoride. The only known pharmacological effects of fluoride other than on bone and teeth, where it inhibits dental caries, are toxic effects. Fluoride inhibits some enzyme systems, including enzymes involved in anaerobic glycolysis and tissue respiration, and it is an effective in vitro anticoagulant. It also inhibits glucose utilization by erythrocytes in vitro. However, these effects occur only at doses far in excess of those used therapeutically or prophylactically. The fluoride dose to cause death in an adult is approximately 2.5 to 5 g of sodium fluoride, taken in a single dose.

### Summary of fluoride

In light of more recent studies with sound methology, it has been concluded that although fluoride has an ability to increase BMD at the lumbar spine, it does not result in a reduction in vertebral fractures. Increasing the dose of fluoride increases the risk of non-vertebral fractures and gastrointestinal side effects without any effect on the vertebral fracture rate.

## CONCLUSION

Osteoporosis is a cause of significant morbidity and mortality. Recent research has shown that there are a number of efficacious treatments. Our challenge for the future is to recognize those patients who would benefit most from therapy. The Osteoporosis Society of Canada has recently published a comprehensive set of guidelines for the identification and treatment of those at risk for osteoporosis.

## SUGGESTED READINGS

Adachi JD, Bensen WG, Brown J, et al. Intermittent etidronate therapy to prevent corticosteroid-induced osteoporosis. *N Engl J Med.* 1997;337:382-387.

Barrett-Connor E, Grady D, Sashegyi A, et al. Raloxifene and cardiovascular events in osteoporotic postmenopausal women: four-year results from the MORE (Multiple Outcomes of Raloxifene Evaluation) randomized trial. *JAMA.* 2002;287: 847-857.

Brown JP, Josse RG, for the Scientific Advisory Council of the Osteoporosis Society of Canada. 2002 clinical practice guidelines for the diagnosis and management of osteoporosis in Canada. *CMAJ.* 2002;167(10 suppl):S1-S34.

Cauley JA, Norton L, Lippman ME, et al. Continued breast cancer risk reduction in postmenopausal women treated with raloxifene: 4-year results from the MORE trial. Multiple outcomes of raloxifene evaluation. *Breast Cancer Res Treat.* 2001;65:125-134.

Cauley JA, Robbins J, Chen Z, et al. Effects of estrogen plus progestin on risk of fracture and bone mineral density: the Women's Health Initiative randomized trial. *JAMA.* 2003;290:1729-1738.

Chesnut CH III, Silverman S, Andriano K, et al. A randomized trial of nasal spray salmon calcitonin in postmenopausal women with established osteoporosis: the prevent recurrence of osteoporotic fractures study. PROOF Study Group. *Am J Med.* 2000;109:267-276.

Cranney A, Guyatt G, Krolicki NL, et al. A meta-analysis of etidronate for the treatment of postmenopausal osteoporosis. *Osteoporos Int.* 2001;12:140-151.

Cranney A, Tugwell P, Zytaruk N, et al. Meta-analyses of therapies for postmenopausal osteoporosis. VI. Meta-analysis of calci-

tonin for the treatment of postmenopausal osteoporosis. *Endocr Rev.* 2002;23:540-551.

Delmas PD, Genant HK, Crans GG, et al. Severity of prevalent vertebral fractures and the risk of subsequent vertebral and non-vertebral fractures: results from the MORE trial. *Bone.* 2003;33:522-532.

Ettinger B, Black DM, Mitlak BH, et al. Reduction of vertebral fracture risk in postmenopausal women with osteoporosis treated with raloxifene: results from a 3-year randomized clinical trial. Multiple Outcomes of Raloxifene Evaluation (MORE) Investigators. *JAMA.* 1999;282:637-645.

Harris ST, Watts NB, Genant HK, et al. Effects of risedronate treatment on vertebral and nonvertebral fractures in women with postmenopausal osteoporosis: a randomized controlled trial. Vertebral Efficacy with Risedronate Therapy (VERT) Study Group. *JAMA.* 1999;282:1344-1352.

Jilka RL. Cytokines, bone remodeling, and estrogen deficiency: a 1998 update. *Bone.* 1998;23:75-81.

Liberman UA, Weiss SR, Broll J, et al. Effect of oral alendronate on bone mineral density and the incidence of fractures in postmenopausal osteoporosis. The Alendronate Phase III Osteoporosis Treatment Study Group. *N Engl J Med.* 1995;333: 1437-1443.

McClung MR, Geusens P, Miller PD, et al. Effect of risedronate on the risk of hip fracture in elderly women. Hip Intervention Program Study Group. *N Engl J Med.* 2001;344:333-340.

Neer RM, Arnaud CD, Zanchetta JR, et al. Effect of parathyroid hormone (1-34) on fractures and bone mineral density in postmenopausal women with osteoporosis. *N Engl J Med.* 2001;344:1434-1441.

Papadimitropoulos E, Wells G, Shea B, et al. Meta-analyses of therapies for postmenopausal osteoporosis. VIII: Meta-analysis of the efficacy of vitamin D treatment in preventing osteoporosis in postmenopausal women. *Endocr Rev.* 2002;23:560-569.

Rossouw JE, Anderson GL, Prentice RL, et al. Risks and benefits of estrogen plus progestin in healthy postmenopausal women: principal results from the Women's Health Initiative randomized controlled trial. *JAMA.* 2002;288:321-333.

Russell RG, Rogers MJ. Bisphosphonates: from the laboratory to the clinic and back again. *Bone.* 1999;25:97-106.

Saag KG, Emkey R, Schnitzer TJ, et al. Alendronate for the prevention and treatment of glucocorticoid-induced osteoporosis. Glucocorticoid-Induced Osteoporosis Intervention Study Group. *N Engl J Med.* 1998;339:292-299.

Shea B, Wells G, Cranney A, et al. Meta-analyses of therapies for postmenopausal osteoporosis. VII. Meta-analysis of calcium supplementation for the prevention of postmenopausal osteoporosis. *Endocr Rev.* 2002;23:552-559.

# 66

# Drugs Used in Dermatology

## GAE WONG AND NH SHEAR

### CASE HISTORY

A 47-year-old man presented with a 20-year history of chronic plaque psoriasis. On clinical examination, he had thick, scaly, red plaques of psoriasis widely distributed on his scalp, trunk, and limbs covering 30% of his body surface area. His past medical history included hypertension and hypercholesterolemia treated with atenolol and atorvastatin, respectively. He worked as a retail salesman. He stated that his psoriasis was extremely embarrassing at work and was also affecting his social life. He had tried many topical therapies a long time ago but had given up because "none of them work," but he had never had any form of phototherapy or systemic therapy for his psoriasis. Assessment of the severity of this patient's condition and a discussion of management options were undertaken.

Treatment was commenced with a combination of a topical vitamin D analogue and a corticosteroid, applied daily. After 1 month, the patient returned for review, stating that, although there had been some improvement in his skin condition, he was finding the treatment inconvenient to apply. He was also unable to make the time commitment required for phototherapy. In view of his history of hypertension and hyperlipidemia, cyclosporin and acitretin were considered to be relatively contraindicated. After appropriate screening blood tests, he was commenced on oral methotrexate. After 8 weeks of methotrexate 15 mg once weekly, his psoriasis was virtually clear, and he reported that his quality of life was considerably improved.

## PRINCIPLES OF DRUG THERAPY IN DERMATOLOGY

Skin diseases affect individuals both physically and psychologically. Treatment of many of these diseases can be extremely challenging; however, there are some potential advantages to the clinician: affected areas can be immediately assessed visually, they are readily accessible for diagnostic biopsy if necessary, and they are amenable to both topical and systemic therapy. Therapeutic success (or failure) can be assessed visually by both the patient and clinician. Common skin diseases include infections (bacterial, fungal, and viral), skin cancers (malignant melanoma, squamous cell carcinoma, basal cell carcinoma, cutaneous T- and B-cell lymphomas), atopic eczema, psoriasis, infestations, urticaria, acne, vasculitis, connective tissue diseases, and autoimmune conditions.

Depending on the severity of the disease, dermatologists may initially try to treat skin disorders with topical agents. Topical drug therapy allows direct application of a drug to the affected areas and minimizes the risk of systemic complications. The potential disadvantages include the time commitment required to apply the treatment and the messiness of some applications. Many variables affect the efficacy of topical drug therapy, and these include drug factors (e.g., molecular size, lipophilic properties, concentration), vehicle factors (e.g., ointment, cream, gel, lotion, solution), skin factors (e.g., stratum corneum thickness and integrity, degree of hydration, degree of vascularity), and application factors (e.g., frequency, dose applied, use of occlusion).

Phototherapy with ultraviolet B (UVB) and photochemotherapy with psoralen and UVA (PUVA) are useful in many inflammatory skin disorders, including atopic eczema and psoriasis. These modalities are also used to treat cutaneous T-cell lymphoma, and in some centres, vitiligo. Advantages include efficacy with limited systemic adverse effects. Disadvantages are the time commitment required to attend the treatment (usually 2 to 3 times per week for several weeks) and potential skin photoaging and skin cancers associated with long-term phototherapy.

Systemic drug therapy is indicated for severe skin disease or diseases failing to respond to topical treatment. Advantages of systemic treatment include efficacy and convenience of oral medication (compared with time-consuming topical applications). The risks of serious adverse effects are greater with drugs administered systemically than with drugs administered topically. Therefore, a careful assessment of the "risk-benefit ratio" of a particular treatment, whether topical or systemic, for a particular skin condition, in a particular patient, has to be made by the clinician. This information should then be discussed with the patient in a manner that will be understood.

This chapter briefly reviews some of the topical and systemic drugs used for common skin disorders. Drugs such as antihistamines, systemic corticosteroids, and drugs used for infectious diseases are discussed in other chapters and are not presented here.

# TOPICAL DRUG USE IN DERMATOLOGY

## Topical Corticosteroids

Topical corticosteroids were first used in the 1950s and have become some of the most effective and widely used drugs in dermatology. Hydrocortisone was the first topically active corticosteroid. Modifications or additions of functional groups to the basic hydrocortisone molecule result in effects on potency, lipophilicity, and relative glucocorticoid and mineralocorticoid properties. The vehicle in which the corticosteroid is incorporated, and the location and nature of the skin to which the compound is applied, also affect the efficacy and potential adverse effects of the treatment.

### Mechanism of action
Topical corticosteroids have a multitude of effects that can be summarized in the following categories: vasoconstriction, anti-inflammatory, immunosuppressive, and antiproliferative. Many of these effects are mediated by interaction of the corticosteroid with glucocorticoid receptors in the cell cytoplasm. The complex of glucocorticoid and its receptor then migrates to the nucleus, where it results in effects on gene transcription (see Chapter 48).

### Indications
Topical corticosteroids have a role in the treatment of many skin disorders. These include various types of dermatitis (e.g., atopic, contact, seborrheic), psoriasis, immunobullous disorders (e.g., bullous pemphigoid, pemphigus vulgaris), connective tissue diseases (e.g., lupus erythematosus), autoimmune diseases (e.g., alopecia areata, vitiligo), and a host of other miscellaneous skin diseases (e.g., lichen planus, cutaneous T-cell lymphoma).

### Adverse effects
Cutaneous atrophy is a potential adverse effect, particularly if high-potency corticosteroids are applied for pro-

longed periods of time in susceptible sites such as the face and body flexures. Tachyphylaxis, or tolerance to drug effects, can be minimized by using corticosteroids intermittently. Allergic contact dermatitis may develop to components of the vehicle or, less commonly, to the corticosteroid itself. Potential suppression of the hypothalamic–pituitary–adrenal axis due to significant percutaneous absorption of corticosteroids should be avoidable with judicious use of these agents.

## Topical Vitamin D Analogues

### Calcipotriol, tacalcitol, and calcitriol

*Mechanism of action.* Vitamin D is produced in the skin from 7-dehydrocholesterol. This biosynthetic pathway requires the action of ultraviolet irradiation on the skin. Vitamin D then enters the circulation and is sequentially hydroxylated to 25-hydroxyvitamin $D_3$ in the liver, and then to 1,25-dihydroxyvitamin $D_3$ (calcitriol; Silkis) in the kidneys (see Chapter 63). Calcipotriol (also known as calcipotriene in the United States; Dovonex) and tacalcitol (Curatoderm) are synthetic derivatives made by modifying the side chain of calcitriol (Fig. 66-1).

Vitamin D and its synthetic analogues interact with vitamin D receptors (VDRs). VDRs are nuclear receptors in the same family as corticosteroid and retinoic acid receptors. Activation of VDRs has effects on keratinocyte proliferation, epidermal differentiation, and the production of inflammatory cytokines.

*Indications.* Topical vitamin D analogues are effective for the treatment of psoriasis. Formulations in combination with topical corticosteroids are also effective treatments.

*Adverse effects.* Topical vitamin D analogues may cause local skin irritation. If used in large quantities (e.g., >100g/week of calcipotriol), there is a small risk that sufficient percutaneous absorption may occur to give rise to hypercalcemia and hypercalciuria.

## Topical Vitamin A Analogues (Retinoids)

The term retinoid describes compounds, either synthetic or naturally occurring, with similarities to vitamin A (retinol; see Chapter 63). The use of retinoids in skin disease has been of interest since the early twentieth century when low dietary levels of vitamin A were noted to be associated with epidermal changes.

Vitamin A (all-trans retinol) is an essential nutrient, with dietary intake in the form of its precursors, retinyl esters and beta-carotene. All-trans retinol is transported in the circulation by plasma retinol-binding proteins to target tissues, and within cells it interacts with cellular retinol-binding protein (CRBP). All-trans retinol is then

**FIGURE 66-1** Structural formulae of calcitriol, calcipotriol, and tacalcitol.

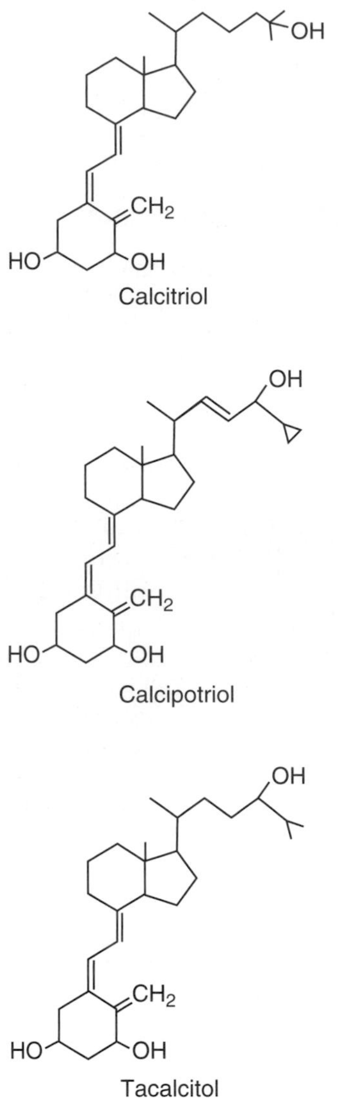

Calcitriol

Calcipotriol

Tacalcitol

either esterified to retinyl esters or sequentially oxidized to all-trans retinoic acid (ATRA), which then binds to cellular retinoic acid binding protein (CRABP). ATRA is the predominant biologically active form of retinoic acid and interacts with nuclear receptors.

Retinoids bind to nuclear retinoic acid receptors (RARs) and retinoid X receptors (RXRs). RARs and RXRs belong to a family of nuclear receptors that includes the steroid, vitamin D, and thyroid hormone receptors. RARs and RXRs act as transcription factors and bind to retinoic acid response elements in DNA. This interaction results in effects on gene transcription and modulation of cell growth and differentiation, and it may have immunomodulatory effects.

Synthetic retinoids have been developed to take advantage of their wide-ranging effects on skin disease. First-generation synthetic monoaromatic retinoids include **tretinoin** (ATRA) and **isotretinoin** (13-*cis* retinoic acid). Second-generation monoaromatic retinoids include **etretinate** and **acitretin**. Third-generation polyaromatic retinoids (arotinoids) include **bexarotene, adapalene,** and **tazarotene** (Fig. 66-2).

### Tretinoin, adapalene, and tazarotene

*Mechanism of action.* Topically applied tretinoin (ATRA) diffuses through skin and is taken up by keratinocytes. It binds to CRABP and then interacts with the nuclear receptors RAR and RXR to exert its effects on gene transcription, leading to effects on cell proliferation and differentiation. It also down-regulates skin androgen receptors.

Adapalene is a synthetic retinoid with affinity for RARs. It is thought to concentrate in sebum and act principally on hair follicle epithelium.

Tazarotene is a synthetic retinoid that is rapidly hydrolyzed to tazarotenic acid. Tazarotenic acid has affinity for RARs.

*Indications.* Tretinoin, adapalene, and tazarotene are all used in the treatment of acne. Their main effect in acne is to normalize follicular hyperkeratosis and thus reduce the accumulation of sebum within the sebaceous glands. Tretinoin is also used in the treatment of photoaged skin, for which its main beneficial effects are improvements in fine wrinkling and dyspigmentation.

Tazarotene is also used in treating psoriasis. Its effects in psoriasis are to normalize keratinocyte differentiation and proliferation and thus prevent the formation of psoriatic plaques.

*Adverse effects.* All topical retinoids can cause local irritation, erythema, and desquamation. Photosensitivity may occur, probably as a result of stratum corneum thinning. Teratogenicity is a theoretical risk, although significant systemic absorption is not thought to occur with topical retinoids.

## Topical Immuno-Inhibitory Drugs

### Tacrolimus and pimecrolimus

Tacrolimus and pimecrolimus are macrolide lactone antibiotics (see Chapters 40 and 52) derived from a soil fungus, *Streptomyces tsukubaensis*. They belong to the class of agents known as **calcineurin inhibitors**.

*Mechanism of action.* These drugs combine with specific cytoplasmic binding proteins to form complexes that inhibit calcineurin-mediated dephosphorylation of "nuclear factor of activated T cells." This action leads to

**FIGURE 66-2** Structural relationships among the three generations of retinoids.

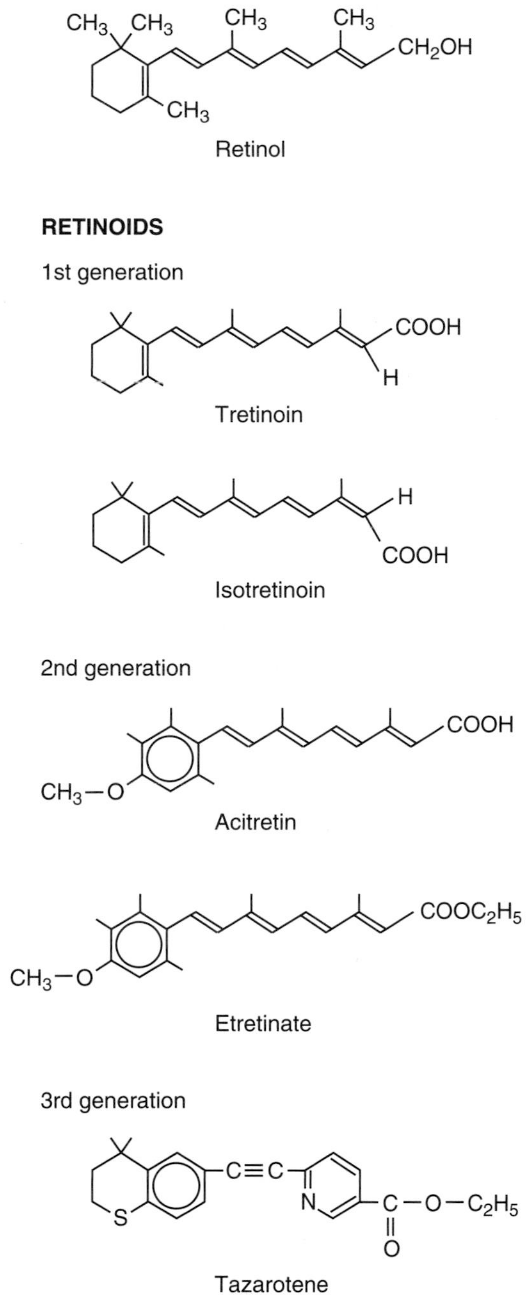

Retinol

**RETINOIDS**

1st generation

Tretinoin

Isotretinoin

2nd generation

Acitretin

Etretinate

3rd generation

Tazarotene

inhibition of the production of inflammatory cytokines, including interleukin-2 and interferon-γ (see Chapter 40).

*Indications.* Both tacrolimus (FK-506; Prograf, Protopic) and pimecrolimus (Elidel) are effective in the treatment of atopic dermatitis that has failed to respond well to steroid or other conventional therapy. Their main advantage over topical steroids is that they do not cause skin atrophy with long-term use.

*Adverse effects.* When used systemically as immunosuppressants to prevent organ graft rejection, they can give rise to a variety of side effects, of which the most important are renal damage, hypertension, and diabetes. However, when used topically, they carry relatively little risk. Their main side effect is a burning sensation at the site of application (more problematic with tacrolimus than with pimecrolimus). Sufficient transdermal absorption can occur to cause these drugs to appear in breast milk; however, there is little evidence so far concerning fetal effects in pregnant women. The U.S. Food and Drug Administration (FDA) has recently required the topical preparations to carry a warning on the label to indicate that excessive use of these agents may carry a risk of cancer.

## Topical Immuno-Enhancing Drugs

### Imiquimod and resiquimod
These agents are imidazoquinoline derivatives (Fig. 66-3) that can be applied to the skin to enhance immune reactions against certain viral infections.

*Mechanism of action.* Their mechanism of action has not been entirely elucidated; however, topical application of imiquimod has been shown to induce production of several cytokines through interaction with a toll-like receptor (TLR7), which is part of the innate immune system. This increases production of tumour necrosis factor alpha (TNFα), interferon-α, interferon-γ, and interleukin-1, -6, -8, and -12.

*Indications.* Imiquimod is FDA-approved for the treatment of genital and perianal warts caused by the herpes simplex virus. It is also used "off-label" for the treatment of resistant palmar and plantar viral warts and molluscum contagiosum (due to pox virus). The FDA has also approved imiquimod for the treatment of actinic keratosis, an early non-melanoma skin cancer that can progress to squamous cell carcinoma, and for the topical treatment of superficial basal cell carcinoma.

*Adverse effects.* Imiquimod is applied as a 5% cream that is usually well tolerated. The main adverse effect is an inflammatory reaction at the site of application.

### Diphencyprone

*Mechanism of action.* Diphencyprone (DPC) is a potent topical contact allergen. Patients are sensitized to a 2% DPC solution, and then more dilute preparations are applied at 1- to 4-week intervals to elicit a non-specific immune response.

FIGURE 66-3    Structural formulae of imiquimod and resiquimod.

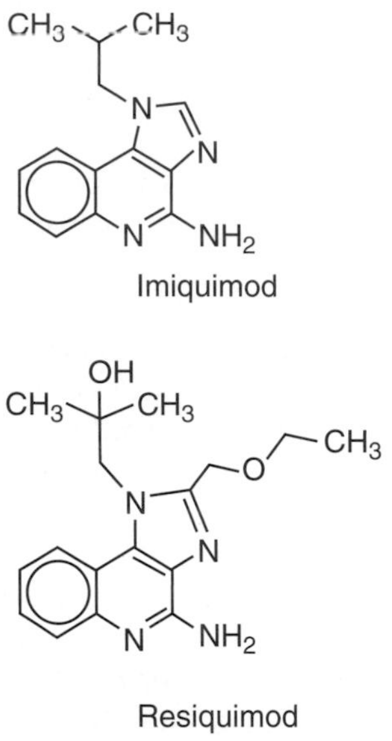

Imiquimod

Resiquimod

**Indications.** DPC can be used for the treatment of alopecia areata and viral warts.

**Adverse effects.** The main adverse effect of DPC is an acute eczematous reaction (redness, blistering) at the site of application.

## Topical Chemotherapeutic Agents

The various antibacterial, antiviral, and antifungal agents that are used both topically and systemically in dermatological treatment are described in Chapters 50 to 53 and 55 and will not be dealt with again in the present chapter. The agents briefly described below are anti-cancer chemotherapeutic agents that are occasionally used topically for skin diseases.

### 5-Fluorouracil

**Mechanism of action.** 5-Fluorouracil (5-FU) is a structural analogue of thymine and inhibits DNA formation by blocking thymidylate synthetase. Its systemic use is as an anti-cancer agent, and its pharmacology is covered in greater detail in Chapter 57.

**Indications.** The main use of topical 5-FU is for the treatment of precancerous skin conditions such as actinic keratosis, actinic cheilitis, and Bowen's disease (intraepidermal squamous cell carcinoma in situ). It can also be used to treat superficial basal cell carcinoma.

**Adverse effects.** Topical 5-FU causes a local inflammatory response, with pain and burning sensation at the application site.

### Nitrogen mustard (mechlorethamine)

**Mechanism of action.** Topical nitrogen mustard (mechlorethamine) acts as an alkylating agent, thereby inhibiting DNA replication (see Chapter 57).

**Indications.** Topical nitrogen mustard is predominantly used in the treatment of cutaneous T-cell lymphoma.

**Adverse effects.** Immediate contact sensitivity, presenting as urticarial skin lesions, occurs in about 8% of patients. Treatment should be discontinued if this occurs. A larger proportion of patients on long-term treatment develop a delayed eczematous reaction, similar to allergic contact dermatitis. In this case, treatment can be continued at a lower drug concentration. There is a possibility of increased risk of non-melanoma skin cancer in patients treated with topical nitrogen mustard.

# SYSTEMIC DRUG USE IN DERMATOLOGY

## Systemic Retinoids

### Isotretinoin, acitretin, and bexarotene

**Pharmacology and mechanism of action.** The mechanism of action of the retinoids after systemic administration is the same as described above for topical use.

**Pharmacokinetics.** Oral absorption of retinoids is enhanced when they are taken with food. Isotretinoin undergoes first-pass metabolism in the liver. Its major metabolite is 4-oxoisotretinoin, and its half-life is 20 hours.

Etretinate is more lipophilic, accumulates in adipose tissue, and therefore has a prolonged half-life of up to 120 days. This is a particular disadvantage in women of childbearing potential in view of the teratogenic effects of retinoids. Therefore, etretinate is no longer available.

Acitretin is formed from etretinate by the cleavage of an ester linkage. Its absorption is also increased when it is taken with food. Its major metabolite is its *cis* isomer. Unlike its parent drug etretinate, acitretin has a much shorter half-life of 2 days, and, therefore, it has replaced etretinate in clinical use. Acitretin can re-esterify to form etretinate, particularly in the presence of alcohol consumption.

Bexarotene is oxidized to 6- and 7-hydroxybexarotene, then to 6- and 7-oxobexarotene. The half-life of bexarotene is 7 to 9 hours. Excretion occurs via the hepatobiliary system. Bexarotene acts through RXRs.

*Indications.* Isotretinoin is extremely effective in the treatment of severe acne. It is usually given in daily doses of 0.5 to 1.0 mg/kg/day, aiming for a cumulative dosage of 120 mg/kg.

Acitretin is used to treat skin conditions such as psoriasis, ichthyoses, keratodermas, Darier's disease, and pityriasis rubra pilaris.

Bexarotene is used in the treatment of cutaneous T-cell lymphoma as part of combination therapy.

More recently, systemic retinoids have been used to reduce the risk of skin cancers in transplant recipients who are taking high-dose immunosuppressant medication.

Low-dose systemic retinoid regimens may offer efficacy with less risk of adverse effects, although further clinical studies are required to confirm this.

*Adverse effects.* Systemic retinoids cause drying and irritation of the skin and mucous membranes in almost all patients. Reversible changes in liver function tests and triglyceride levels may occur. Other adverse effects include myalgia, arthralgia, and hyperostosis (with long-term treatment). Systemic retinoids are teratogenic. Women of child-bearing potential should avoid getting pregnant for at least 2 months after discontinuing isotretinoin, and for at least 3 years after discontinuing acitretin. Effects of isotretinoin treatment on mood (depression) and an increased suicide risk in acne patients remain to be confirmed.

## Systemic Immunosuppressive Agents (Anti-metabolites and Cytotoxic Drugs)

### Azathioprine

*Mechanism of action.* Azathioprine (see Chapter 40) is a prodrug that is converted to 6-mercaptopurine (6-MP), which is then metabolized further by three enzyme pathways. Xanthine oxidase (XO) and thiopurine methyltransferase (TPMT) convert 6-MP to inactive metabolites. Hypoxanthine–guanine phosphoribosyl transferase (HGPRT) converts 6-MP to active purine analogues, such as 6-thioguanine and other monophosphate nucleotide analogues. These active purine analogues can be incorporated into DNA and RNA, resulting in inhibition of purine synthesis.

*Pharmacokinetics.* Variations in the activity of the three enzymes involved in azathioprine metabolism contribute to the variable efficacy and toxicity of the drug. TPMT activity is inherited in an autosomal co-dominant fashion. Most people (89%) have high TPMT activity, 11% have intermediate activity, and less than 1% (1 in 300) have low activity. Low TPMT activity results in more 6-MP undergoing conversion to active metabolites, with potentially greater adverse effects. XO inhibitors, such as allo-

purinol, cause accumulation of active metabolites in a similar way. Patients with **Lesch-Nyhan syndrome** (genetic HGPRT deficiency) are resistant to the effects (and side effects) of azathioprine.

*Indications.* Dermatologic use of azathioprine includes treatment of immunobullous diseases (e.g., pemphigus vulgaris), vasculitis, lupus erythematosus, photodermatoses, and atopic dermatitis. Azathioprine is often used in conjunction with corticosteroids and may allow a lower dose of corticosteroid to be used.

*Adverse effects.* Nausea, vomiting, and diarrhea may be problems with high azathioprine doses. Hepatitis and pancreatitis due to azathioprine use have been reported. Myelosuppression, with pancytopenia, is a potential adverse effect, particularly in patients with low TPMT activity. Azathioprine may increase the risk of malignancy (lymphoproliferative and skin cancer) and opportunistic infections. A drug hypersensitivity syndrome with fever, rash, and internal organ involvement has been described. Re-exposure can be fatal.

### Cyclophosphamide

*Mechanism of action.* Cyclophosphamide is converted by cytochrome P450 enzymes (2B, 2C) in the liver to active metabolites hydroxycyclophosphamide and phosphoramide mustard and to an inactive metabolite, acrolein. Cyclophosphamide is an alkylating agent, resulting in DNA cross-linkage. Its action is non-specific with respect to the cell cycle, and it therefore acts on cells with a low proliferative index as well as on actively proliferating cells.

*Indications.* Cyclophosphamide is usually used in conjunction with systemic corticosteroids for the treatment of severe immunobullous disorders, vasculitides, and connective tissue diseases.

*Adverse effects.* Cyclophosphamide has many potential adverse effects. There is an increased risk of hematologic malignancy, transitional cell cancer of the bladder, and cutaneous squamous cell carcinoma. Severe myelosuppression can result from high-dose cyclophosphamide. Bladder toxicity in the form of hemorrhagic cystitis is a common adverse effect, probably due to the acrolein metabolite of cyclophosphamide. Increased fluid intake and frequent voiding of the bladder should be undertaken to try to reduce this complication; mesna (sodium 2-mercaptoethane sulfonate), an agent that binds acrolein, may also be used. Irreversible infertility is a significant risk with cyclophosphamide therapy. Other possible adverse effects include gastrointestinal upset, alopecia, mucosal ulceration, cardiomyopathy, and pulmonary fibrosis.

## Cyclosporin

*Mechanism of action.* Cyclosporin inhibition of calcineurin-dependent dephosphorylation of "nuclear factor of activated T cells" is described above under topical use.

*Indications.* Cyclosporin is an effective treatment for severe psoriasis and severe atopic eczema. It is used systemically when topical therapy has failed. The usual dosage is 2.5 to 5 mg/kg/day in divided doses.

*Adverse effects.* The main serious adverse effects associated with cyclosporin are nephrotoxicity and hypertension. Other side effects include gastrointestinal symptoms, headache, hypertrichosis, and gingival hypertrophy. Long-term use of cyclosporine has been associated with lymphoproliferative malignancies in transplant patients.

## Hydroxyurea

*Mechanism of action.* Hydroxyurea inhibits ribonucleotide diphosphate reductase, an enzyme that catalyzes the conversion of ribonucleotides to their deoxyribonucleotide form. This results in inhibition of DNA synthesis.

*Indications.* The main dermatologic use of hydroxyurea is for the treatment of psoriasis.

*Adverse effects.* Hydroxyurea can cause myelosuppression. Most patients on hydroxyurea develop megaloblastic changes of the blood, which do not necessitate drug discontinuation. Cutaneous adverse reactions include lichen planus, dermatomyositis-like eruption, hyperpigmentation, leg ulcers, and photosensitivity. Hepatitis, renal impairment, hematologic malignancy, and nonmelanoma skin cancers have also been reported in association with hydroxyurea. Hydroxyurea is teratogenic, and therefore, conception should be avoided while the patient is taking the drug.

## Methotrexate

*Mechanism of action.* Methotrexate is a competitive inhibitor of dihydrofolate reductase (see Chapter 53). This results in inhibition of DNA synthesis and inhibition of T and B lymphocyte replication and function.

*Indications.* Methotrexate is used to treat moderate to severe chronic plaque psoriasis, pustular psoriasis, and psoriatic arthritis. Methotrexate is usually administered as an oral dose once weekly. Subcutaneous and intramuscular routes of administration can also be used.

*Adverse effects.* Nausea, malaise, and headache can occur on the day of methotrexate administration. Oral folic acid, 5 mg/day, usually ameliorates these symptoms. Myelosuppression, pulmonary fibrosis, and ulcerative stomatitis are rare side effects. Hepatic fibrosis occurs with high cumulative methotrexate dosages, particularly in patients with other risk factors such as high alcohol consumption and pre-existing hepatitis. Serum-based liver function tests do not accurately reflect fibrosis; therefore, liver biopsies may be indicated in patients on long-term methotrexate therapy.

## Mycophenolate mofetil

*Pharmacokinetics.* Mycophenolate mofetil (MMF) is the morpholinoethyl ("mofetil") ester of mycophenolic acid (MPA), a phenolic acid derivative obtained from a strain of *Penicillium* mould (Fig. 66-4). MMF is absorbed after oral intake and rapidly split by esteratic action to yield free MPA, which is converted to an inactive glucuronide in the liver. β-Glucuronidase, present in the epidermis and gastrointestinal tract, then converts the inactive glucuronide back to its active form.

*Mechanism of action.* MPA is a non-competitive inhibitor of inosine monophosphate dehydrogenase, thereby blocking conversion of inosine-5-phosphate and xanthine-5-phosphate to guanosine-5-phosphate. In this way, *de novo* purine synthesis is inhibited. Lymphocytes rely on *de novo* purine synthesis because they lack the purine salvage pathway and are therefore particularly susceptible to the effects of MPA.

*Indications.* MMF is usually used in conjunction with corticosteroids for the treatment of severe immunobullous diseases (e.g., pemphigus vulgaris). It has also been used in the treatment of psoriasis.

*Adverse effects.* The main adverse effects of MMF are dose-dependent gastrointestinal effects such as abdominal pain, nausea, vomiting, and diarrhea.

## Anti-malarial Agents

### Chloroquine, hydroxychloroquine, and quinacrine

Quinine is a naturally occurring compound found in the bark of the cinchona tree. Historically, quinine was used to treat fevers and malaria (see Chapter 54). After World War

FIGURE 66-4    Mycophenolate mofetil.

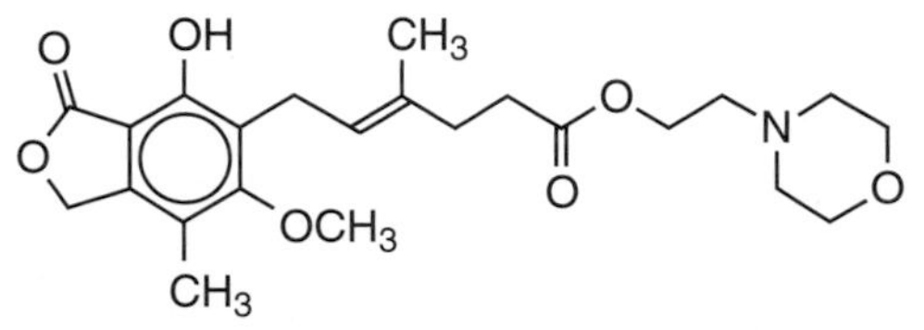

I, chloroquine, hydroxychloroquine, and quinacrine were developed as synthetic anti-malarial derivatives of quinine. The first report of the use of these drugs for dermatological conditions was in 1951, when it was noted that cutaneous lupus improved with quinacrine treatment.

*Mechanism of action.* Anti-malarial agents have been shown to have many photoprotective, anti-inflammatory, DNA binding, and immunosuppressive effects. Precisely which effects are of clinical relevance remains largely unknown.

*Indications.* The only FDA-approved dermatological indication for anti-malarial drug therapy is chronic cutaneous lupus erythematosus.

*Adverse effects.* Ocular adverse effects occur with chloroquine and hydroxychloroquine. These include corneal deposits, loss of accommodation due to depressive effects on ocular muscles, and retinopathy. Only retinopathy is potentially irreversible, but this is rare with chloroquine doses less than 4 mg/kg/day and hydroxychloroquine doses less than 6.5 mg/kg/day. Other adverse effects include gastrointestinal intolerance, bone marrow suppression (rare), blue–grey pigmentation (skin, nail beds, palate), yellowish pigmentation with quinacrine (skin, sclera, urine), bleaching of hair roots, exacerbation of psoriasis, rash (morbilliform, lichenoid, exfoliative), and neuromuscular effects (psychosis, nervousness, irritability, vertigo, tinnitus, muscle weakness).

# Miscellaneous Systemic Drugs Used in Dermatology

## Dapsone
Dapsone is a sulfone antibiotic that is used primarily to treat leprosy (see Chapter 53). Its use in dermatology is not clearly related to its primary use.

*Mechanism of action.* The precise mechanisms by which dapsone exerts its effects are not known. Inhibition of neutrophil chemotaxis, neutrophil respiratory burst, lysosomal enzyme activity, and myeloperoxidase cytotoxic system are proposed mechanisms.

*Indications.* Dapsone is used to treat dermatitis herpetiformis. This is a condition that characteristically causes small, extremely pruritic vesicles in patients. Pruritus usually resolves rapidly with dapsone use.

*Adverse effects. N*-hydroxy metabolites of dapsone are potent oxidants and can cause significant hemolysis, particularly in glucose-6-phosphate dehydrogenase (G-6-PD)–deficient individuals. These metabolites also cause elevated methemoglobin levels, which result in reduced oxygen-carrying capacity of red blood cells. Cimetidine may reduce dapsone-induced methemoglobinemia. In view of these potential hematological adverse effects, patients should have G-6-PD levels and complete blood counts checked prior to commencing dapsone treatment, followed by regular blood counts after initiation of therapy. Other rare, idiosyncratic, serious adverse effects of dapsone therapy include agranulocytosis, motor peripheral neuropathy, psychosis, hepatitis, severe hypoalbuminemia, and dapsone hypersensitivity syndrome (fever, rash, hepatitis).

## Colchicine
Colchicine is derived from the plant *Colchicum autumnale*. Its main use is for the treatment of acute gout (see Chapter 28. However, it has been used to treat numerous dermatological conditions, particularly those with evidence of neutrophilic infiltration.

*Mechanism of action.* Colchicine inhibits the polymerization of tubulin and thus prevents microtubule assembly. It concentrates in leukocytes, and its anti-tubulin action has inhibitory effects on neutrophil motility and chemotaxis.

*Indications.* Colchicine can be used in Behcet's disease, Sweet's syndrome (acute febrile neutrophilic dermatosis), and dermatitis herpetiformis. Evidence of the efficacy of colchicine is derived predominantly from case reports and case series.

*Adverse effects.* The main side effects of colchicine are gastrointestinal. Abdominal pain and diarrhea commonly occur with doses greater than 0.6 mg twice daily.

## Psoralen and ultraviolet A (PUVA)
Psoralens are a group of furanocoumarins (Fig. 66-5) extracted from various plant sources. They act as photosensitizers that increase the damaging effect of ultraviolet A radiation (320 to 400 nm wavelength) on nucleic acids. The combination of psoralens with ultraviolet A radiation (PUVA) is useful in treating several dermatological conditions.

*Mechanism of action.* The psoralen molecule is planar and therefore can intercalate between the bases of nucleic acids. When activated with UVA radiation, the furan portion of the molecule reacts covalently to alkylate the pyrimidine bases of DNA, thus suppressing DNA synthesis, interrupting the cell cycle, and inducing local cutaneous immunosuppression. Psoralens are administered orally or topically prior to irradiation in order to sensitize the skin to UVA. This regimen continues twice weekly for several weeks.

*Indications.* PUVA is used for the treatment of several skin conditions, including psoriasis, atopic dermatitis, cutaneous T-cell lymphoma, and, in some centres, vitiligo.

**FIGURE 66-5** | Therapeutically useful psoralens.

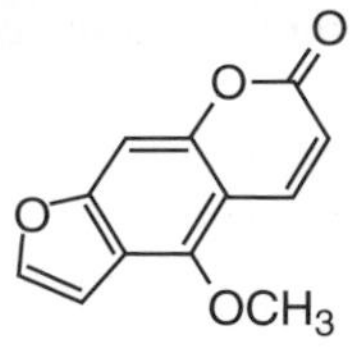

5-Methoxypsoralen

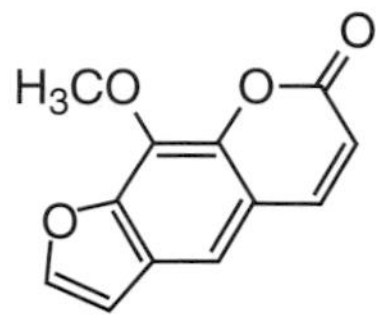

8-Methoxypsoralen

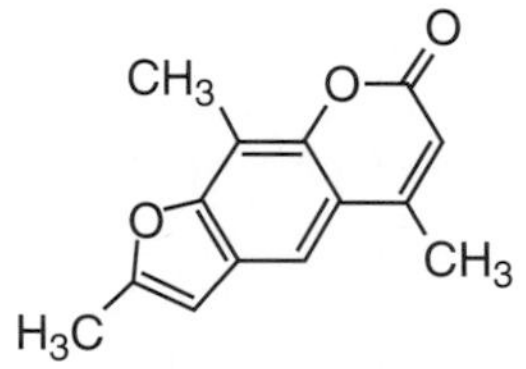

Trimethylpsoralen

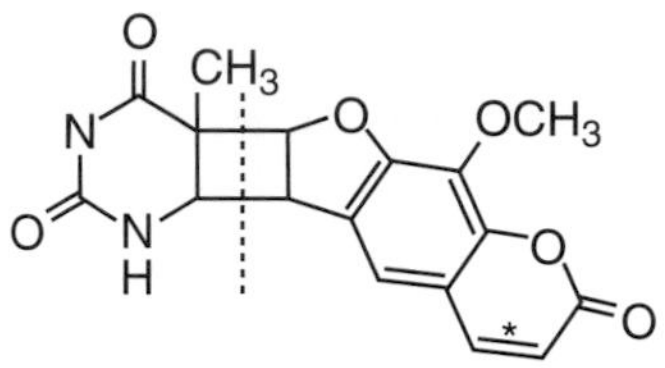

Adduct of thymine (left) with
8-Methoxypsoralen (right)
(Additional adduct can be
formed through double bond
marked with asterisk)

*Adverse effects.* Acute adverse effects include nausea (with oral psoralen), erythema, pruritus, and burning. Adverse effects associated with long-term PUVA or repeated PUVA courses include skin aging (freckling, wrinkling) and increased incidence of skin cancers.

## Biological Therapy

Biological therapy refers to the use of protein drugs derived from living organisms for the treatment of disease. Recent advances in the understanding of the pathophysiological mechanisms of psoriasis have resulted in the development of several biological therapies that target specific components of the disease process.

### Mechanism of action

Four basic strategies are employed in biological therapy for psoriasis. These are described, with examples, below:

1. Reducing the number of pathogenic/activated T cells: **Alefacept** is a fusion protein that binds to the CD2 molecule on T cells, leading to selective reduction in the number of memory T cells by apoptosis.
2. Inhibiting T-cell activation: **Efalizumab** is a humanized monoclonal antibody that blocks the interaction of leukocyte function–associated antigen 1 (LFA-1) on T cells with intracellular adhesion molecule 1 (ICAM-1) on antigen-presenting cells. This interaction is required for T-cell activation (see Chapter 40).
3. Immune deviation: This strategy involves changing the cytokine profile produced by T cells. Psoriasis demonstrates a predominantly T1 cytokine profile. Treatment with recombinant interleukin-10 (a T2 cytokine) can encourage a shift to a T2 cytokine profile and improve psoriasis.
4. Blocking inflammatory cytokines: TNFα is a proinflammatory cytokine found in elevated levels in psoriasis. Anti-TNFα agents such as **etanercept** (a protein that binds TNFα) and **infliximab** (a monoclonal antibody against TNFα) improve psoriasis.

### Indications

Most biological agents in current development for dermatological disease are for the treatment of psoriasis.

### Adverse effects

The aim in developing biological therapy for psoriasis is to target specific components of the immune system without widespread immunosuppressive effects. However, there is a risk of reactivation of latent tuberculosis with the anti-TNFα agents. Injection site reactions can occur as biological agents are administered via intravenous, intramuscular, or subcutaneous routes.

## SUGGESTED READINGS

Altman DJ. The role of the pharmaceutical industry and drug development in dermatology and dermatologic health care. *Dermatol Clin.* 2000;18:287-296.

Brazzini B, Pimpinelli N. New and established topical corticosteroids in dermatology: clinical pharmacology and therapeutic use. *Am J Clin Dermatol.* 2002;3:47-58.

Freedberg IM, Eisen AZ, Wolff K, et al, eds. *Fitzpatrick's Dermatology in General Medicine.* 6th ed. New York, NY: McGraw-Hill; 2003.

Gupta AK, Ryder JE, Nicol K, Cooper EA. Superficial fungal infections: an update on pityriasis versicolor, seborrhoeic dermatitis, tinea capitis, and onychomycosis. *Clin Dermatol.* 2003;21:417-425.

Kira M, Kobayashi T, Yoshikawa K. Vitamin D and the skin. *J Dermatol.* 2003;30:429-437.

Lin P, Torres G, Tyring SK. Changing paradigms in dermatology: antivirals in dermatology. *Clin Dermatol.* 2003;21:426-446.

Menter MA, ed. Psoriasis for the clinician: a new therapeutics era ('the biologics') beckons. *J Am Acad Dermatol.* 2003;49(2 suppl): S39-S142.

Nghiem P, Pearson G, Langley RG. Tacrolimus and pimecrolimus: from clever prokaryotes to inhibiting calcineurin and treating atopic dermatitis. *J Am Acad Dermatol.* 2002;46:228-241.

Thiers BH, ed. New and emerging therapies. *Dermatol Clin.* 2000; 18:1-200.

Thiers BH, Levine N, eds. Systemic dermatologic therapy. *Dermatol Clin.* 2001;19:1-219.

Winterfield L, Cather J, Cather J, Menter A. Changing paradigms in dermatology: nuclear hormone receptors. *Clin Dermatol.* 2003;21:447-454.

Winterfield L, Menter A. Psoriasis and its treatment with infliximab-mediated tumor necrosis factor alpha blockade. *Dermatol Clin.* 2004;22:437-447.

Wolverton SE, ed. *Comprehensive Dermatologic Drug Therapy.* 1st ed. Philadelphia, Pa: WB Saunders; 2001.

Zanolli M. The modern paradigm of phototherapy. *Clin Dermatol.* 2003;21:398-406.

# 67

# Chemical Carcinogenesis

## AB OKEY AND PA HARPER

In North America, more than one person in three will develop cancer. This can occur at any age, but the incidence and mortality rates for most types of cancer rise steeply with age. Cancer is the cause of death for about one person in four. What are its causes? From epidemiological studies, it is estimated that 60 to 90% of human cancers are primarily due to environmental factors. "Environmental factors" means all non-genetic elements, including not only environmental chemicals, but also other contributing elements such as diet and cultural and behavioural practices that are collectively termed "lifestyle."

There is little doubt that exposure to xenobiotic (foreign) chemicals (in the form of environmental substances or drugs) is a major risk factor in the overall incidence of human cancer. About one-third of cancer deaths in North America are related to the use of cigarettes and other tobacco products. Other medical, industrial, and environmental chemicals that are strongly implicated in the human cancer problem are summarized later in this chapter.

The lung cancer problem (Fig. 67-1) illustrates an important manner in which cancer differs from most other chemically induced toxic responses. That is, cancer usually appears only after a long *latent period*. Lung cancer is almost entirely attributable to cigarette smoking, but lung cancer, like other human cancers, typically is not clinically evident for as long as 10 to 20 years after exposure to the agent that caused the tumour. Obviously, this great time delay between exposure and cancer detection complicates identification of the responsible agents.

In North American males, mortality from lung cancer escalated rapidly after World War II. This rise was the result of the increased frequency of cigarette smoking that became common in the male population around the time of World War I. In the North American female population, cigarette smoking did not become common until World War II. The rise in mortality from lung cancer in females is tragically reminiscent of the escalation that began in the male population two decades earlier. Within the decade of the 1990s, lung cancer overtook breast cancer as the leading cause of cancer-related deaths in North American females.

## CHEMICAL CARCINOGENS: DIVERSITY OF ORIGINS AND CHEMICAL STRUCTURES

### "Natural" Versus "Synthetic" Carcinogens

Tables 67-1, 67-2, and 67-3 list a variety of agents that have been reported to be carcinogenic. It is important to note that these lists include both natural and synthetic chemicals. Although many of the known carcinogens are products of modern synthetic chemistry or byproducts of industrial processes, the natural world contained carcinogens long before humans developed technologically based industrial societies.

The following are examples of naturally occurring carcinogens: aflatoxin $B_1$, a potent liver carcinogen, is routinely formed by moulds that contaminate improperly stored foodstuffs; polycyclic aromatic hydrocarbons, such as benzo[a]pyrene, are universally generated by partial combustion processes, including the burning of wood and charcoal-cooking of food, as well as by internal combustion engines; safrole, a volatile oil from sassafras tea, is a carcinogen in mice and possibly in humans. Many other examples of naturally occurring carcinogens could be given. The point is that carcinogens are formed both by natural processes and by human activities.

### Prevalence of Carcinogens in the Chemical World

It is important to understand that not all chemicals have carcinogenic properties, regardless of whether they are natural products or synthetic chemicals. News reports in the popular media often give the incorrect impression that the majority of drugs and environmental chemicals cause cancer.

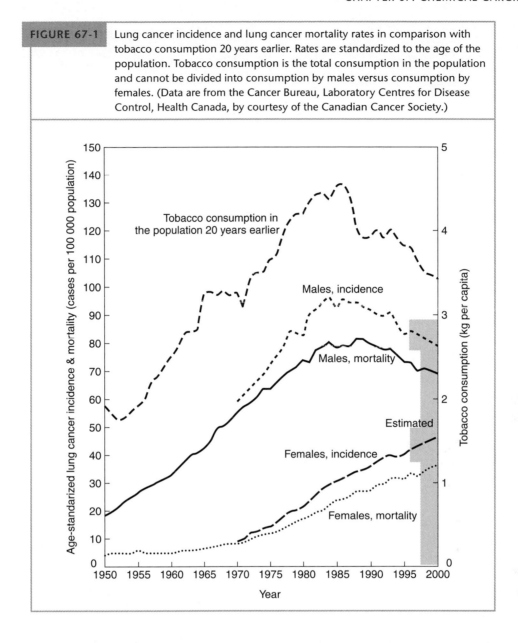

**FIGURE 67-1** Lung cancer incidence and lung cancer mortality rates in comparison with tobacco consumption 20 years earlier. Rates are standardized to the age of the population. Tobacco consumption is the total consumption in the population and cannot be divided into consumption by males versus consumption by females. (Data are from the Cancer Bureau, Laboratory Centres for Disease Control, Health Canada, by courtesy of the Canadian Cancer Society.)

Table 67-4 gives some perspective on the prevalence of carcinogens among the overall spectrum of known chemicals. It can be seen that the number of *known* carcinogens is very small when compared with the number of existing chemical structures. In truth, however, the vast majority of chemicals, even those in common use, have not been adequately tested for carcinogenicity. Thus, it is impossible to state the magnitude of total exposure to carcinogens with any degree of accuracy. The methods used to test chemicals for carcinogenicity are described later in this chapter.

## Diversity of Chemical Types

It is immediately apparent, even from just the names of the agents listed in Tables 67-1, 67-2, and 67-3, that carcinogens are found in a wide variety of chemical classes. A central theme from a pharmacological perspective is that the biological activity of a compound should be related to the compound's structure. However, there are no simple structure–activity rules by which a given compound can be designated as a carcinogen (or non-carcinogen) solely by virtue of its chemical structure.

This apparent lack of structure–activity relationship perplexed early workers in the field of experimental chemical carcinogenesis. Since carcinogens occurred in a wide variety of chemical classes, it was feared that there might be a large number of mechanisms by which these diverse chemical structures caused cancer. Later evidence has shown that this is not so. The scheme in Figure 67-2 provides a model that attempts to unify diverse chemical structures into a common pathway leading to cancer.

| TABLE 67-1 | Some Environmental Factors and Industrial Agents Implicated in Human Carcinogenesis |
|---|---|
| Ionizing radiation | |
| Ultraviolet radiation | |
| Alcohol | |
| Aromatic amines | |
| Arsenic | |
| Asbestos | |
| Aflatoxins | |
| Benzene | |
| Benzidine | |
| Cadmium | |
| Carbon tetrachloride | |
| Chromium | |
| Soots, tars, mineral oils | |
| Tobacco smoke | |
| Vinyl chloride | |

| TABLE 67-2 | Examples of Carcinogenic Anti-cancer Drugs |
|---|---|
| Adriamycin | |
| Chlorambucil | |
| Cyclophosphamide | |
| Doxorubicin | |
| Mechlorethamine | |
| Melphalan (phenylalanine mustard) | |
| Mitomycin C | |
| Procarbazine | |
| Streptozotocin | |
| Triethylene melamine (TEM) | |
| Triethylenethiophosphoramide | |
| Uracil mustard | |

## CARCINOGENESIS AS A MULTISTAGE BIOCHEMICAL AND BIOLOGICAL PROCESS

The complex diagram in Figure 67-2 provides a framework for examining the sequence of events in chemical carcinogenesis. The diagram emphasizes that cancer is the result of a progressive multistage process, and it is used for reference as the particular stages in the carcinogenic process are examined below.

### Direct-Acting Carcinogens

The common final target of most chemical carcinogens is DNA. It is possible that certain RNA species or specific proteins also might be the critical targets, but virtually all current evidence focuses on DNA as the critical site for carcinogen action. Some drugs (such as alkylating agents used in chemotherapy of cancer) are chemically reactive in the form in which they are administered. These have the ability to bind directly to nucleophilic sites on DNA, RNA, and proteins. This ability probably is responsible for both their ability to kill cancer cells (as therapeutic agents) and their ability to induce new tumours. (Cyclophosphamide, an important alkylating agent used in cancer therapy, *does* require metabolic activation in order to exert its cytotoxic effects; see Chapter 57.)

## Metabolic Activation into Ultimate Carcinogens

The term *ultimate carcinogen* refers to the chemical species that directly interacts with DNA. Most cancer-causing chemicals are not carcinogenic in the form in which they enter the body. Compounds such as polycyclic aromatic hydrocarbons (e.g., benzo[*a*]pyrene, found in cigarette smoke) are chemically unreactive in their parent form and cannot form covalent bonds with DNA. Enzyme systems within the organism biotransform unreactive procarcinogens, or pre-carcinogens, into chemically reactive products that can covalently interact with nucleophilic sites on cellular macromolecules.

As Figure 67-2 suggests, metabolic activation usually requires more than one enzymatic step. Initial activation often is carried out by various species of cytochrome P450 (see Chapter 4), but activation by reductases, peroxidases, and prostaglandin synthetic pathways also is well established. Regardless of the pathway(s) involved,

| TABLE 67-3 | Miscellaneous Drugs Classified by IARC as Carcinogenic to Humans |
|---|---|
| Azathioprine | |
| Cyclosporin | |
| Diethylstilbestrol (DES) | |
| Tamoxifen | |
| Thiotepa | |
| IARC = International Agency for Research on Cancer (IARC)/World Health Organization. | |

| TABLE 67-4 | Cancer and Chemicals: Numerical Considerations |  |
|---|---|---|
| As of November 2003: |  |  |
| Total organic and inorganic chemicals registered in Chemical Abstracts (American Chemical Society) (natural and synthetic) |  | >22 000 000 |
| Chemicals in common widespread use |  | ~70 000 |
| Chemicals demonstrated to be carcinogenic in laboratory animals |  | ~2000 |
| Chemicals classified as "carcinogenic to humans" by IARC |  | ~50 |

the final product (ultimate carcinogen) is a reactive electrophilic species.

Some specific examples of metabolic activation pathways are given in Figures 67-3 and 67-4. Figure 67-3 outlines the biotransformation processes that result in the conversion of the procarcinogen benzo[a]pyrene (BP) into an ultimate carcinogenic form capable of covalent binding to DNA. BP has been studied more than any other carcinogen. The primary activation scheme shown in Figure 67-3 is well supported by experimental evidence, but this is not the only pathway by which BP can be activated into an ultimate carcinogen.

The first step in the activation of BP is its conversion into an arene oxide, BP 7,8-oxide. This is catalyzed by a species of cytochrome P450 known as CYP1A1. BP 7,8-oxide then serves as a substrate for epoxide hydrolase, an enzyme that converts the oxide to a dihydrodiol by the addition of a molecule of water. The dihydrodiol is much more water-soluble than the parent compound, and it originally was thought that BP 7,8-oxide was effectively "detoxified" by the action of epoxide hydrolase. Subsequent investigation, however, revealed that the dihydrodiol can be further converted by CYP1A1 to BP 7,8-diol-9,10-epoxide. This diol epoxide is chemically reactive and capable of covalently binding to DNA; hence, it is an ultimate carcinogenic form of BP.

Figure 67-4 indicates that various species of P450 enzymes also are involved in the initial activation steps for such structurally diverse carcinogens as 2-acetylaminofluorene (AAF, an aromatic amine), nitrosamines, vinyl chloride, and aflatoxins. Figure 67-4 also serves to re-emphasize that metabolic activation commonly involves more than one enzymatic step before an ultimate carcinogen is formed. In the case of AAF, the initial step is formation of N-hydroxy-AAF, catalyzed by the P450 enzyme CYP1A2. The N-hydroxy intermediate may then follow one of several pathways leading to formation of a sulfate ester, an acetate ester, or a nitroxide radical. All of these pathways are contenders for the generation of an ultimate carcinogen. The specific pathway depends upon the tissue: sulfo-transferase activity predominates in liver, whereas acyltransferase activity predominates in non-hepatic tissues such as the mammary gland. Both liver and mammary gland are susceptible to tumour induction by AAF, implying that different ultimate carcinogens can be formed from the same parent compound in different tissues by different metabolic pathways. Differences in metabolic capabilities among different tissues may, in part, explain why some carcinogens are tissue-selective in inducing tumours.

The discussion up to this point might imply that cytochrome P450 isoenzymes are undesirable and are harmful to the organism. There is no question that P450 enzymes are capable of converting many classes of chemicals into reactive intermediates that are toxic or carcinogenic. It should be recalled, however, that P450-mediated reactions are the major pathways by which most hydrophobic drugs and environmental chemicals are converted into forms that can be conjugated and excreted (see Chapter 4).

Epoxide hydrolase also could be viewed as both a "beneficial" enzyme and an enzyme that is deleterious to health. The determination of whether these enzymes are beneficial or harmful depends upon many complex factors such as dose and route of administration of their drug substrates and the efficiency with which activation pathways are coupled with conjugating enzymes. The teleological goal of P450 enzymes and epoxide hydrolase is to facilitate the elimination of xenobiotic chemicals (see Chapter 4). Conversion of some xenobiotic agents into toxic or carcinogenic metabolites could be viewed as an occasional accidental byproduct of the action of generally beneficial enzymes.

## Detoxication

Metabolic activation does not invariably lead to covalent attacks on critical macromolecules such as DNA. Most cells are well equipped with mechanisms that inactivate reactive metabolites before these metabolites strike critical targets. The predominant means of "detoxication" is via conjugation with glutathione (GSH), glucuronate, acetate, or sulfate (see Chapter 4). Cells that are deficient in GSH are known to be at high risk of cell death from reactive metabolites formed in the biotransformation of many drugs (see Chapter 43). GSH-deficient cells also may be at high risk for neoplastic transformation when exposed to carcinogens. Moreover, epidemiological studies have indicated an increased risk of lung cancer in smokers with deficient glutathione S-transferase activity combined with elevated CYP1A1 activity.

In normal cells, most reactive metabolites probably are detoxified by conjugating enzymes or by reaction with non-critical protein targets. Cells at highest risk will be those that have an imbalance between the rate at which reactive metabolites are generated and the rate at which those metabolites can be conjugated and excreted. As noted above, however, there are also a number of examples whereby conjugation reactions serve to increase, rather than decrease, the reactivity of chemicals, as a consequence of the formation of chemically unstable species that spontaneously decompose to electrophilic, DNA-binding molecules.

## Covalent Interaction with Tissue Nucleophiles

Much of the progress in understanding chemical carcinogenesis has been made by tracing the route of parent compounds forward from their site of application through dis-

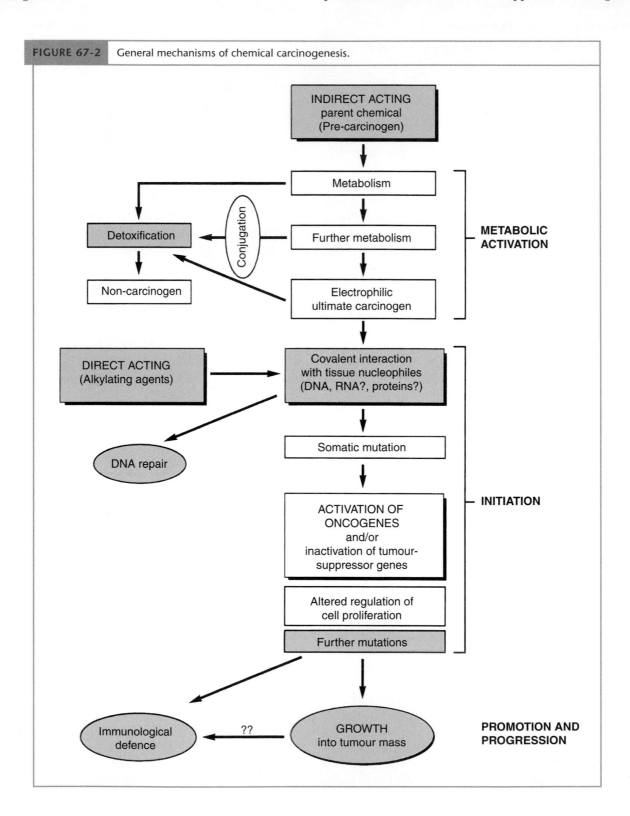

FIGURE 67-2    General mechanisms of chemical carcinogenesis.

**FIGURE 67-3** Metabolic activation of benzo[a]pyrene. Only the main activation pathway is shown; however, many other metabolic products can be formed from BP via several metabolic pathways involving P450 species or other enzymes.

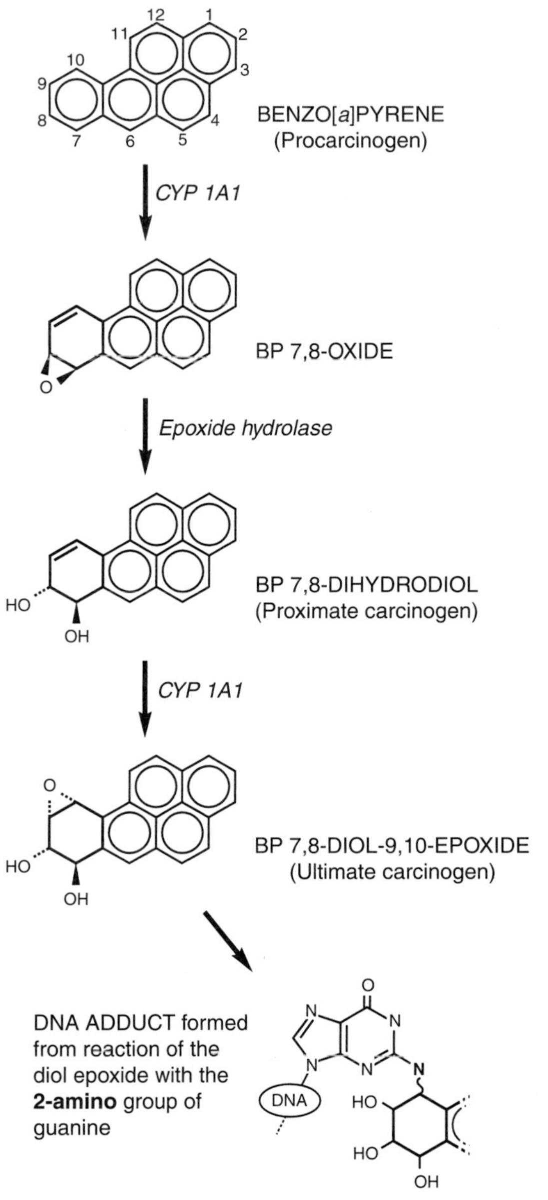

atomic sites within each base. Recent evidence indicates that major classes of chemical carcinogens, such as chemicals from cigarette smoke or aflatoxins, leave characteristic "fingerprints" consisting of specific adduct patterns on nucleotides in "hot spots" in the key genes that govern conversion of normal cells into a clinical tumour. Such patterns may allow the epidemiologist to link major forms of human cancers to the causative agents.

Some chemicals appear to be carcinogenic by non-genotoxic mechanisms. These non-genotoxic agents act via several disparate pathways, including disruption of hormonal regulation of cell growth and stimulation of oxidative stress that eventually leads to DNA damage. Although the emphasis in chemical carcinogenesis usually has focused on exogenous chemicals that are foreign to the human body, endogenous processes also may contribute to DNA damage. For example, it has been proposed by Ames and colleagues that spontaneous damage to DNA from endogenous oxidants in cells may be far more abundant than the DNA damage wrought by exogenous chemicals. It is not at all clear, however, to what extent the DNA damage from endogenous processes contributes to human cancer.

## Initiation (Neoplastic Transformation)

Covalent binding of the ultimate carcinogen to DNA alters the genetic message. If the carcinogen-adducted nucleotide in DNA is not recognized and repaired before cell division, the genetic lesion may be "fixed" as a mutation as a consequence of inaccurate DNA replication caused by the adduct. This mutation will then be inherited by progeny stemming from the altered cell. This permanent alteration is the initial cellular event in the cancer process.

Not all chemically induced mutations lead to cancer. Many DNA lesions probably are lethal to the cell bearing them. In addition, DNA-repair enzymes usually operate with high efficiency. Individuals who are genetically deficient in DNA-repair enzymes exhibit an increased risk for some, but not all, forms of cancer.

Over the past several years, considerable excitement has been generated by the prospect that the primary targets of chemicals and other carcinogens might be a limited number of *oncogenes* (literally cancer genes). As stated by Bishop (1987), "proto-oncogenes are the keyboard upon which carcinogens play." As a general model, the conversion of proto-oncogenes into oncogenes is a key event in the initiation of tumourigenesis (see Fig. 67-2). Proto-oncogenes are normal cellular genes, most of which code for cellular growth factors or growth factor receptors, for example, *erbB*. Other important oncogenes include *myc*, *fos*, and *jun*, which act as transcription factors; *bcl-1*, which acts as a cell-cycle kinase activator; and *ras*, which is a GTP-regulated molecular signalling switch. When a proto-oncogene is damaged by a carcinogen (e.g., undergoes mutation, chromosomal translocation), the resulting

tribution to various tissues and through specific biotransformation pathways that convert procarcinogens into ultimate carcinogens.

In several instances, the chemical identity of the ultimate carcinogenic form has been determined by chemical characterization of carcinogen adducts isolated from DNA. Carcinogen adducts (covalently bound forms) have been detected on all four nitrogen bases in DNA and at several

**FIGURE 67-4**   Examples of activation pathways for selected carcinogens.

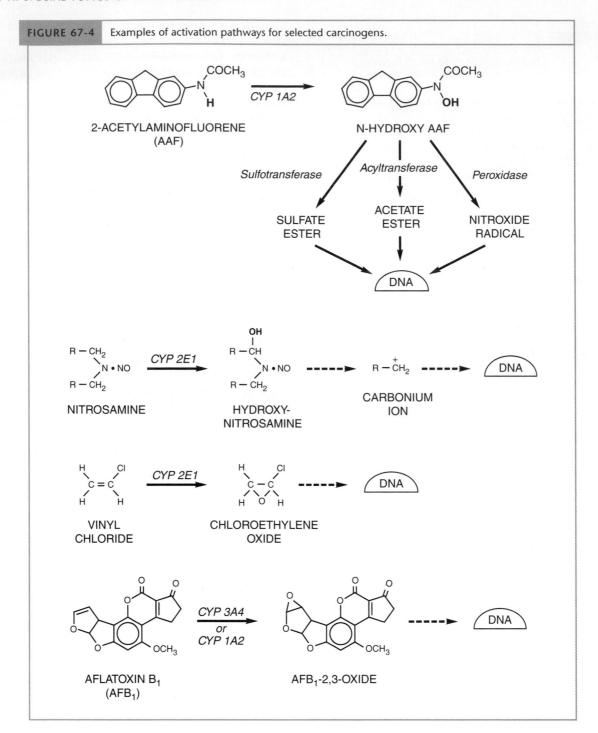

oncogene drives the abnormal cell division and abnormal cell differentiation that typify neoplastic growths.

Even more important, as shown during the last several years, is inactivation of tumour-suppressor genes. One particular tumour-suppressor gene, *p53*, is mutated in about half of all human cancers and may be the most common genetic target in human cancer. *p53* appears to play multiple roles in that it is a transcription factor that can provoke arrest of the cell cycle and also induce apoptosis (programmed cell death). The retinoblastoma (Rb) gene prod-

uct is another example of a gene product that functions as a transcription factor and that can alter the cell cycle.

## TUMOUR PROMOTION AND PROMOTERS

In its simplest form, the multistage cancer process can be thought of as two major events: initiation (described above) and promotion.

Promotion refers to a poorly defined set of circumstances that permit initiated cells to proliferate into tumour masses. Several chemicals that are not in themselves "complete" carcinogens (i.e., do not act as initiators) are able to promote the development of tumours that have been initiated by other agents. Examples of tumour promoters are listed in Table 67-5.

Generally, *initiators* are thought to be agents that are capable of forming mutagenic electrophilic metabolites, as previously described. In principle, initiation can be accomplished by a single exposure to the initiating agent. The mutationally based initiation process seems essentially irreversible.

In contrast, *promoting agents* do not appear to be mutagenic; instead, they exert their effect through non-genotoxic pathways involved with selective stimulation of proliferation of the initiated cell. In order to produce tumours experimentally, the promoting agent must be given after treatment with an initiator, and the promoter must be given repeatedly over a prolonged time period. The actions of promoters appear to be reversible, at least in early stages. This simplified picture of initiation followed by promotion is giving way to an understanding that several important human tumours—for example, colon cancer—arise as a consequence of a sequential accumulation of mutations in proto-oncogenes and tumour-suppressor genes. Each mutation pushes the cell further from the normal regulation of limits to proliferation and closer to the invasive and metastatic phenotype that typifies a serious clinical disease.

One hallmark of cancer cells is general instability of the genome. Human cancer cells contain high frequencies of chromosomal abnormalities as well as mutations. Damage to those genes that are responsible for maintaining stabil-ity of the genome is likely to be a key early event in the process of carcinogenesis. If these *stability genes* (including the genes governing DNA replication, DNA repair, and chromosomal segregation) are altered by mutation, the stage is set for a cascade of further mutations that may hit oncogenes and tumour-suppressor genes, thereby leading to unregulated cell growth, invasiveness, and metastasis.

## DETECTION OF CARCINOGENS

Table 67-6 summarizes the major methods used at present to test chemicals for potential carcinogenic activity.

### Long-Term Tests In Vivo

The ultimate "proof" that a given chemical is a human carcinogen can be obtained only by carefully designed epidemiological studies and by rigorous evaluation of clinical observations. Given the multitude of drugs and environmental agents to which humans are exposed and the long latent period between exposure and tumour appearance, it is not surprising that confirmation of carcinogenicity in humans is a protracted and difficult process.

Bioassays in laboratory animals (usually rodents) have until recently been the primary method of testing chemicals for carcinogenic potential. Rodent tests have been criticized as irrelevant to the human cancer problem because such tests frequently employ doses that are greatly in excess of probable human exposure levels for the chemical in question. At these high doses ("maximally tolerated doses"), cytotoxic effects of the test chemical might lead to increased tumour formation via mitogenesis, per se, rather than by adduct-induced mutagenesis. Recent molecular epidemiology studies in humans, however, indicate that many important human cancers are associated with adduct-driven mutagenesis rather than the secondary effects of mitogenesis. Although there are legitimate concerns about the relevance of the high doses used in rodent bioassays, experience has shown that most chemicals that induce a significant frequency of tumours at high doses also induce some tumours at lower doses.

High doses are employed in animal tests for a very practical reason—namely, to increase the sensitivity of the assay. Thorough rodent bioassays for carcinogenicity of a *single chemical* typically cost in excess of US $1 million and may require 2 to 5 years of research. High doses are used to reduce the number of animals required and the consequent cost of the assay. Usually, a maximum of a few hundred animals can be studied, and it is necessary to test with doses that potentially can produce a high frequency of tumours. On the other hand, a chemical that caused cancer in one animal out of 1000 tested (for example, at lower doses) would not be detected as a carcinogen, yet a similar increase in cancer frequency in the North American human population would afflict more than 300 000 people.

| TABLE 67-5 | Selected Examples of Tumour Promoters in Laboratory Animals |
|---|---|

Mouse skin tumours
  Phorbol esters from croton oil (e.g., 12-*O*-tetradecanoyl-phorbol-13-acetate [TPA])
  Phenol
  Anthralin
  Hexadecane
  Iodoacetic acid
  Cigarette smoke condensate
  Extracts of unburned cigarettes
  Surfactants and detergents
  Benzoyl peroxide
  Abrasions or wounding

Rodent liver tumours
  Phenobarbital
  Dichlorodiphenyltrichloroethane (DDT)
  Polychlorinated biphenyls (PCBs)
  2,3,7,8-Tetrachlorodibenzo-*p*-dioxin (TCDD, "dioxin")

| TABLE 67-6 | Methods for Detection of Carcinogens |
|---|---|

Long-term tests in vivo
  Clinical observations and epidemiology
  Bioassays in laboratory animals, including mice
    genetically engineered to be susceptible to carcinogens

Short-term screening tests
  Covalent binding of test compounds to DNA after
    metabolic activation in vivo or in vitro
  Tests for chromosome damage
  Chromosomal abnormalities by cytogenetic assays
  Sister chromatid exchange
  Micronucleus formation
  Sperm abnormalities

Mutational tests
  Bacterial (Ames' *Salmonella* test)

Neoplastic transformation of mammalian cells in culture

Carcinogenic activity in rodents does not prove that a chemical will be a carcinogen in humans, but nearly all known human carcinogens are also carcinogenic in rodents. Any chemical that is a carcinogen in laboratory animals must be considered a *potential* carcinogen in humans. Specific knowledge of the exact mechanism(s) by which cancers arise is required before any discrepancies in animal testing versus human carcinogenesis can be explained.

## Short-Term Screening Tests

As stated in the previous section, in vivo animal tests are the definitive method for demonstrating carcinogenic activity. Because in vivo tests are expensive and time-consuming, less expensive short-term tests have been developed to cope with the thousands of chemicals that must be tested for potential carcinogenic activity.

Most of the screening tests are based on the premise that carcinogens act by damaging DNA and are therefore mutagenic. *Mutagenesis tests in bacterial systems* are much quicker and cheaper than whole-animal tests for carcinogenesis. Bacterial mutational test systems (e.g., the Ames assay) are used in literally thousands of laboratories around the world and are especially valuable as an inexpensive screen in the development of compounds that may have market potential.

Early attempts to correlate mutagenesis in bacterial systems with carcinogenesis in animals were compromised because the necessity for host-mediated metabolic activation of procarcinogens was not yet recognized. Present-day tests employ a combined system using mammalian liver enzymes (to activate procarcinogens) and *Salmonella* bacterial strains (to detect mutations). This system has shown that approximately *90% of carcinogens are mutagenic* and that many mutagens are carcinogens.

The science of carcinogenesis has not yet developed to the stage where any single test is considered adequate as an all-encompassing screen for carcinogenic chemicals. Rather, a battery of tests is required both in vivo and in vitro.

## DOSE–RESPONSE CONSIDERATIONS IN CARCINOGENESIS

In general, the carcinogenic response, like other pharmacological responses, is quantitatively related to dose (or to exposure). As illustrated in Figure 67-5, the frequency of tumours in a population increases linearly with the logarithm of the dose. This linear log-dose–response relationship has been shown experimentally to hold for several carcinogenic chemicals provided that the carcinogen doses administered yield a medium level of tumour response. At very high or very low doses, linearity of the dose–response relationship is in question.

At very high doses, animals may die from toxicity before tumours have an opportunity to develop to a detectable stage.

The greatest difficulty, however, lies in *interpretation of the tumour response expected at very low doses.* Much of human exposure to potential carcinogens is of a chronic, low-dose nature. If the tumour dose–response curve is linear and originates at zero, there is no dose that will not produce a finite increase in tumour frequency. Only zero dose would yield zero increase in risk—that is, there is no totally safe dose for carcinogens.

The other potential problem is that the dose–response relationship is not linear at very low doses. This includes the possibility that a *threshold* dose may exist below which tumour risk is not significantly elevated. Alternatively, tumours that result from exposure to the test chemical may be superimposed on a background of spontaneous tumours that are present in every laboratory species. Recently, the concept of "hormesis" has gained attention. Hormetic responses involve non-linear dose–response curves in which low doses actually confer a benefit to the exposed animals rather than a risk. Much more research is required to determine whether hormesis is broadly applicable to risk assessment.

To date, there has been *no satisfactory experimental definition of the nature of the dose–response curve at very low carcinogen doses.* A few large-scale experiments involving thousands of rodents have been attempted, but these still have been inadequate to define response at very low doses, partly because this is inherent in the statistical uncertainty present when any rare event is measured. Only extremely large numbers of animals would reduce this uncertainty to a level where the nature of the response itself could be determined. It also is apparent that no laboratory animal can be treated in an environment that is totally free from contamination by trace levels of other chemicals that are

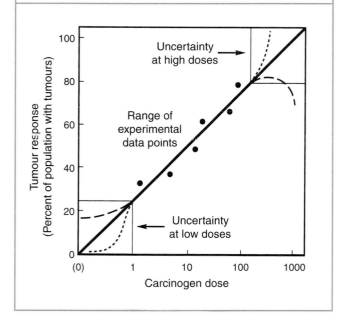

**FIGURE 67-5** Hypothetical carcinogen dose–response curves. Uncertainty at low doses may be caused by the presence of a background of spontaneous tumours in every laboratory species. The lower broken line (small dots) represents the possibility of a "sub-linear" response that is less than expected at that dose and may include a threshold below which no significant response can be observed.

unwanted in the experiment. For these and other reasons, the tumour response at very low doses may never be adequately defined by animal experiments.

Various mathematical models have been constructed in an attempt to predict the magnitude of tumour response at very low doses. Each model requires certain assumptions that have not all been experimentally validated. At present, there is no conclusive answer as to whether there is a safe dose ("threshold") for any carcinogen. Regulatory agencies must make decisions about many potential carcinogens, often without having experimental evidence that might confirm risk at very low doses. As is true in other areas of toxicology, carcinogenic risk can be determined with greater assurance when the specific mechanism by which each agent acts is well understood.

## VARIATION IN CANCER SUSCEPTIBILITY

Why does one person in three develop cancer and the other two do not? Susceptibility is determined by many factors. Chief among these is the level of exposure to potential carcinogens. But even among groups exposed to the same agents, some individuals will develop cancer and others will not. The multistage model of carcinogenesis suggests several levels at which individuals can vary in their response to carcinogens (see Fig. 67-2).

## DNA Repair and Immune Competence

Cells from individuals with genetically based deficiencies in DNA repair are more sensitive than normal cells to the induction of mutations by chemicals, ultraviolet light, and ionizing radiation. Several DNA-repair deficiencies have been described in humans, including Bloom's syndrome, Fanconi's anemia, ataxia–telangiectasia, and xeroderma pigmentosum. For some of these diseases, individuals are more susceptible to certain cancers than are individuals with normal DNA-repair capacity. It is not yet clear, however, whether DNA-repair deficiencies invariably lead to increased risk of chemically induced cancer. Nevertheless, very recent discoveries show that damage to genes that encode DNA repair enzymes plays a key role in the development of such tumours as hereditary non-polyposis colon cancer. The search for inactivation of DNA repair genes in other forms of cancer is currently of intense interest.

The importance of the immune system as a defence against cancer is illustrated by the rise in cancer risk that occurs in patients receiving intensive immunosuppressive therapy following kidney transplantation and by the susceptibility to Kaposi's sarcoma in patients whose immune system is compromised by HIV infection.

## Imbalance in Enzymes that Activate or Detoxify Chemical Carcinogens

The earliest events in the process of chemical carcinogenesis are biotransformation reactions carried out by various carcinogen-metabolizing enzymes (see Fig. 67-2). In laboratory animals, it can be shown that the risk of chemically induced cancer is strongly influenced by the activity of these enzymes. As noted previously, however, the relationship between enzyme activities and carcinogenesis is complex. Some enzymes (e.g., cytochrome P450 and epoxide hydrolase) function both to activate certain carcinogens and to detoxify them.

In laboratory animals, it generally appears that a high level of cytochrome P450 in the *liver* protects peripheral tissues from chemical carcinogens, provided that the animal is exposed to the carcinogen by a route that permits the liver to clear the carcinogen from the circulation before it is distributed throughout the body. Thus, if an animal ingests a carcinogen orally or is given an intraperitoneal injection, high hepatic P450 activities enhance first-pass clearance of the carcinogen by the liver and effectively reduce the carcinogen dose that is delivered to other tissues.

In contrast, if carcinogens are applied *directly* to tissues, such as the skin or lung surface, tumour risk generally rises with increased P450 activities in those tissues. In such cases, metabolic activation may occur locally within the tissue (by P450 and other enzymes), but this activation is not well coupled with conjugating systems or an excretory route.

Animal experiments such as these suggest that some variation in human susceptibility to chemical carcinogens might be due to variation in levels of carcinogen-metabolizing enzymes in different individuals. It would be reasonable to hypothesize that variation in the level and activity of the many enzymes that can biotransform potential carcinogens would be one contributing factor in cancer risk. Recent advances in phenotyping and genotyping of human subjects for several carcinogen-metabolizing enzymes have made it feasible to conduct epidemiological studies on the role of these enzymes in cancer risk. As mentioned earlier, smokers who possess high activity of an activating enzyme, CYP1A1, combined with deficient activity of a conjugating enzyme, glutathione S-transferase, may have a considerably elevated risk of developing certain forms of lung cancer. A polymorphism that results in high CYP1A1 gene expression in African-American women also has been reported to substantially increase the risk of breast cancer. However, the same CYP1A1 polymorphism that appears to increase CYP1A1 enzyme activity leading to elevated lung cancer risk in Japanese men and breast cancer in African-American women does not appear to be associated with increased CYP1A1 expression in eastern Mediterranean subjects or with increased lung cancer risk in Nordic males. This example again reminds us that the process of carcinogenesis is multifactorial and that factors that elevate risk in one population might not necessarily elevate risk in another population with different genetic background or environmental circumstances.

## PREVENTION OF CARCINOGENESIS/ REDUCTION OF RISK

The fact that cancer is a multiple-step process provides the opportunity for reducing cancer risk by intervention at any of several levels.

### Selective Inhibition of Carcinogen Activation and Selective Enhancement of Carcinogen Detoxication

In laboratory animals, it is possible to use *chemoprophylaxis to reduce cancer risk.* Chemical pretreatments can be given that inhibit activation pathways or stimulate detoxication pathways, thereby inhibiting tumour initiation. For example, pretreatment of rats with phenobarbital or even with the pesticide DDT partially protects them from induction of mammary tumours and leukemia when they are later exposed to benzo[a]pyrene. These agents appear to protect by enhancing liver P450 enzyme activities and increasing

hepatic clearance of the carcinogen. Certain natural products such as green tea protect from chemical carcinogens in animal models by acting at several levels, including reducing metabolic activation of precarcinogens or provoking apoptosis in cells that have become malignantly transformed. Unfortunately, as previously described, phenobarbital and DDT also can promote development of liver cancer in rats treated with nitrosamines. At this time, we do not have the ability to use chemicals to selectively switch on detoxication pathways and switch off activation pathways in such a way as to confer universal protection from chemical carcinogens.

## Antioxidants and Anti-inflammatory Agents

Several antioxidants (of synthetic origin or from plant materials) inhibit chemical induction of tumours in laboratory animals. Such chemicals include butylated hydroxytoluene (BHT), butylated hydroxyanisole (BHA), beta-carotene, and vitamin E. Antioxidants potentially inhibit cancer by "scavenging" reactive metabolites before they can bind to DNA. However, many antioxidants also can provoke increased formation of reactive oxygen species (ROS), which themselves can cause toxicity. In clinical trials, antioxidants such as retinoids and vitamin E generally have produced disappointing results as agents to reduce cancer risk.

Non-steroidal anti-inflammatory drugs (NSAIDs) such as aspirin, indomethacin, ibuprofen, sulindac, and celecoxib inhibit chemical carcinogenesis in animal models, particularly in the colon. Epidemiological studies in human populations also indicate reduced risk of colon cancer and breast cancer in people who routinely take some of these anti-inflammatory drugs. Again, however, NSAIDs are not without risk themselves since they can cause other toxic effects such as hemorrhage; such agents would need to be used with caution as cancer preventatives in large populations of currently healthy people.

## Anti-estrogens and Anti-androgens

The selective estrogen receptor antagonists tamoxifen and raloxifene significantly reduce the risk of breast cancer in laboratory animal models and in human populations as demonstrated in epidemiological studies. However, epidemiological studies also indicate that tamoxifen may slightly increase the risk of uterine cancer. Prostate cancer risk is reduced in men taking finasteride, an inhibitor of the enzyme 5-α reductase that converts testosterone to the more potent androgen, dihydrotestosterone.

## Avoidance

Many clinical trials have been completed or are underway to test the ability of various chemical agents to reduce cancer or precancerous lesions in human subjects. However, in view of the complexity of chemical carcinogenesis, it is not surprising that no "all-purpose anti-cancer pill" has yet been discovered—nor is any likely to be developed in the near future. The best method currently available for reducing cancer risk is avoiding, or reducing exposure to, known causative agents.

We can never have a completely carcinogen-free environment since carcinogens arise from both natural and human processes. We can, however, avoid high-risk situations. Elimination of cigarette smoking would reduce cancer mortality more than any other single public health measure. It is a continual source of frustration to scientists involved in cancer research that progress in this area has taken so long to be achieved among males in a few developed countries, and that these improvements are being overshadowed by the trend to increased cigarette smoking among young females in these same countries as well as the growing market for tobacco products in the large developing nations.

# SUGGESTED READINGS

Ames BN, Gold LS. Chemical carcinogenesis: too many rodent carcinogens. *Proc Natl Acad Sci USA.* 1990;87:7772-7776.

Ames BN, Gold LS. The causes and prevention of cancer: the role of environment. *Biotherapy.* 1998;11:205-220.

Bertram JS. The molecular biology of cancer. *Mol Aspects Med.* 2001;21:167-223.

Bishop JM. The molecular genetics of cancer. *Science.* 1987;235:305-311.

Calabrese EJ. Toxicological awakenings: the rebirth of hormesis as a central pillar of toxicology. *Toxicol Appl Pharmacol.* 2005;204:1-8.

Conney AH. Enzyme induction and dietary chemicals as approaches to cancer chemoprevention: The Seventh DeWitt S. Goodman Lecture. *Cancer Res.* 2003;63:7005-7031.

Galati G, Teng S, Chan TS, O'Brien PJ. Cancer chemoprevention and apoptosis mechanisms induced by dietary polyphenolics. *Drug Metabol Drug Interact.* 2000;17:311-349.

Guengerich FP. Metabolism of chemical carcinogens. *Carcinogenesis.* 2000;21:345-351.

Hecht SS. Tobacco carcinogens, their biomarkers and tobacco-induced cancer. *Nat Rev Cancer.* 2003;3:733-744.

Hengstler JG, Bogdanffy MS, Bolt HM, Oesch F. Challenging dogma: thresholds for genotoxic carcinogens? The case of vinyl acetate. *Annu Rev Pharmacol Toxicol.* 2003;43:485-520.

Ingelman-Sundberg M. Polymorphism of cytochrome P450 and xenobiotic toxicity. *Toxicology.* 2002;181-182:447-452.

Knudson AG. Two genetic hits (more or less) to cancer. *Nat Rev Cancer.* 2001;1:157-162.

Lippman SM, Hong WK. Cancer prevention science and practice. *Cancer Res.* 2002;62:5119-5125.

Luch A. Nature and nurture—lessons from chemical carcinogenesis. *Nature Rev Cancer.* 2005;5:113-125.

McLaughlin J, Gallinger S. Cancer epidemiology. In: Tannock I, Hill RP, Bristow RG, Harrington L, eds. *The Basic Science of Oncology.* 4th ed. New York, NY: McGraw-Hill; 2005:4-24.

Miller JA. Research in chemical carcinogenesis with Elizabeth Miller—a trail of discovery with our associates. *Drug Metab Rev.* 1994;26:1-36.

Nebert DW, Dalton TP, Okey AB, Gonzalez FJ. Role of aryl hydrocarbon receptor-mediated induction of the CYP1 enzymes in environmental toxicity and cancer. *J Biol Chem.* 2004;279:23847-23850.

Okey AB, Harper PA, Grant DM, Hill RP. Chemical and radiation carcinogenesis. In: Tannock I, Hill RP, Bristow RG, Harrington L, eds. *The Basic Science of Oncology.* 4th ed. New York, NY: McGraw-Hill; 2005:25-48.

Pitot HC III, Dragan YP. Chemical carcinogenesis. In: Klaassen CD, ed. *Casarett & Doull's Toxicology: The Basic Science of Poisons.* 6th ed. New York, NY: McGraw-Hill; 2001:241-319.

Seifried HE, McDonald SS, Anderson DE, Greenwald P, Milner JA. The antioxidant conundrum in cancer. *Cancer Res.* 2003;63:4295-4298.

Sills RC, French JE, Cunningham ML. New models for assessing carcinogenesis: an ongoing process. *Toxicol Lett.* 2001;120:187-198.

Silva Lima B, Van der Laan JW. Mechanisms of nongenotoxic carcinogenesis and assessment of the human hazard. *Regul Toxicol Pharmacol.* 2000;32:135-143.

Sporn MB, Suh N. Chemoprevention: an essential approach to controlling cancer. *Nat Rev Cancer.* 2002;2:537-543.

Yuspa SH. Overview of carcinogenesis: past, present and future. *Carcinogenesis.* 2000;21:341-344.

# 68

# Chemical Teratogenesis

## PG WELLS

Teratology, or the study of congenital defects, is derived from the Greek word *teras*, meaning monster. The initiation of congenital (birth) defects is termed teratogenesis. Interest in structural abnormalities in the newborn dates back to at least 5000 B.C., when Babylonian priests had a list of 62 malformations recognizable at birth. Since the 1960s, teratology has expanded as a consequence of the recognition that mutational and functional abnormalities or anomalies result from prenatal insult, sometimes in the absence of structural defects (Fig. 68-1). There are many different causes of anomalies. This chapter is limited to teratogenesis associated with maternal exposure to drugs and environmental chemicals, which are collectively termed xenobiotics.

The study of chemical teratogenesis is relatively recent, dating from 1933, when Hale showed that maternal deprivation of vitamin A in pigs produced offspring without eyes (anophthalmia). Widespread scientific interest and public concern did not develop until 1960, when the first reports surfaced of teratogenicity associated with the sedative–hypnotic drug thalidomide. Although this drug was withdrawn from the market in 1961, it recently has been reintroduced for other uses, such as the treatment of leprosy. Stringent educational requirements for patients have now been established in an attempt to avoid thalidomide use by women during pregnancy. The thalidomide tragedy stimulated an enormous growth in basic and applied research in this field, but we still know relatively little about how xenobiotics cause congenital anomalies and even less about how predisposing genetic and environmental factors interact in individual unborn children.

Each year in the United States, about 200 000 birth defects are reported (7% of all live births). Over 560 000 infant deaths, spontaneous abortions, stillbirths, and miscarriages are estimated to be due to defective prenatal development. These figures no doubt are underestimates of the problem, since an unknown percentage of known defects are not reported and many defects, particularly functional and mutational anomalies, are not recognized at all. In other instances, there may be failure to recognize that the defect is associated with exposure to a drug or environmental chemical. About 20 to 30% of reported defects are thought to result from spontaneous genetic aberrations; 6% are clearly related to drugs and chemicals, leaving the cause unknown in over 60%. Many cases of unknown causation probably result either from unrecognized exposure to drugs and chemicals or from a complex interaction between a drug effect and genetic or environmental factors. One study found that the average woman takes 10 prescription or non-prescription drugs during her pregnancy, most of them without a physician's supervision. It has been estimated that over 125 000 women of childbearing age in the United States are exposed annually to potential chemical teratogens in their jobs, and presumably all women are exposed to some extent to the enormous array of environmental chemicals.

## ASSESSMENT OF HUMAN RISK

There are a number of special problems in the detection of chemical teratogenicity and assessment of human risk that make this field of toxicology particularly difficult. Since the developmental process is complex and it takes many years to reach maturity, currently employed indices fail to detect many xenobiotic effects. In the human population, fewer than 50% of abnormalities can be detected at birth. Over 30% of early embryos are estimated to die unrecognized; 15% of recognized pregnancies abort spontaneously. In successful pregnancies, subtle biochemical or functional defects usually go unrecognized. In other cases, the defect may be detected, but the causal role of the drug may not be identified because the defect is expressed only under conditions of genetic predisposition or of certain physiological, pathological, or environmental stresses that may go unrecognized. In this case, particularly susceptible individuals will not be distinguished from the general population by epidemiological studies that cannot include sufficient detail about individual predisposing factors.

FIGURE 68-1    Consequences of chemical teratogenesis. (Modified from Neubert et al., 1980.)

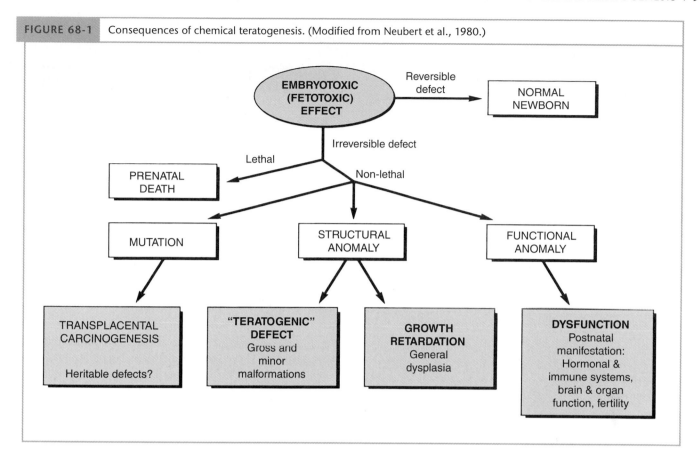

Most human teratological studies are restricted to the perinatal period and fail to evaluate the maturational process. If the children are monitored for about 5 years, the total number of defects identified during that period is more than six times greater than the number detected at birth. Some important structural defects (e.g., cardiac anomalies), subtle behavioural deficits, or mutational anomalies may not be detected until even later. For example, infants exposed in utero to the transplacental carcinogen diethylstilbestrol did not develop vaginal adenocarcinomas until puberty. Unfortunately, long-term follow-up studies are too expensive and time-consuming to be employed for all drugs. Therefore, teratological evaluation often must depend upon retrospective epidemiological studies and voluntary reporting of rare toxicities by astute physicians who have extensive records of their patients' histories.

During the clinical testing of new drugs in studies on human volunteers and patients, pregnant women are rarely included. Therefore, the fetal toxicity of most drugs can be assessed only after their use in the general population. Indeed, many drugs carry a warning that their safety during pregnancy and lactation has not been established. Once drugs are released for general use, epidemiological studies can detect potent teratogens or drug-induced anomalies that are rare in the baseline population. However, such studies are less successful in identifying weaker teratogens or drugs that are teratogenic only in predisposed patients. Such potential predisposing conditions as genetic differences, pathophysiological influences, concurrent drug use, or chemical exposure seldom are discernible. Virtually never considered, especially in relation to environmental chemical teratogens, are such factors as the precise timing and magnitude of confounding influences, individual differences and gestational variations in drug disposition, and differences in specific toxicologically critical pathways of drug elimination, bioactivation, and detoxification and associated pathways of cytoprotection and macromolecular repair.

To some extent, the teratological risks to humans can be reduced by pre-clinical studies employing in vivo animal models and in vitro tests, as discussed later. However, such methods have serious limitations. Thalidomide was found to be non-teratogenic in pregnant mice and rats, but, unfortunately, in humans it proved to be an extraordinarily potent teratogen, causing embryolethality and a wide range of congenital anomalies in over 10 000 surviving children. Retrospective teratological studies have shown the teratogenic dose in mouse and rat to be about 5000 mg/kg, compared with 0.5 to 1 mg/kg in humans.

For all these reasons, relatively little can be stated as fact in the field of chemical teratogenesis. Teratologists disagree

| TABLE 68-1 | Human Developmental Toxicants* |
|---|---|
| Androgenic chemicals | |
| Angiotensin-converting enzyme (ACE) inhibitors<br>Captopril, enalapril | |
| Antibiotics<br>Tetracyclines | |
| Anti-cancer drugs<br>Aminopterin, busulfan, cyclophosphamide, methylaminopterin,<br>mercaptopurine, methotrexate, procarbazine | |
| Anticonvulsant drugs<br>Phenobarbital, phenytoin, trimethadione, valproic acid | |
| Anti-thyroid drugs<br>Methimazole | |
| Chelators<br>Penicillamine | |
| Chlorobiphenyls | |
| Cigarette smoke | |
| Cocaine | |
| Coumarin anticoagulants<br>Warfarin | |
| Ethanol | |
| Ethylene oxide | |
| Diethylstilbestrol | |
| Iodides | |
| Lithium | |
| Metals<br>Methylmercury, lead | |
| Misoprostol | |
| Radiation (ionizing)<br>Therapeutic, radioiodine, atomic fallout | |
| Retinoids<br>13-*cis*-retinoic acid, etretinate | |
| Thalidomide | |
| Toluene abuse | |

*This list is not complete and refers primarily to drugs because of the lack of data in humans with respect to environmental chemicals.
(Primarily from Rogers and Kavlock, 2001. Reprinted with permission.)

even about the identification of "known" human teratogens. However, Table 68-1 lists some drugs and related agents that are sufficiently potent teratogens for their effects to be recognized clearly above the spontaneous incidence of human congenital malformations. This list is not complete; if occupational and environmental chemicals and additional categories of "probable" and "suspected"

human and animal teratogens were included, this list would number over 800 (Lemire and Shepard, 2004).

# TERATOLOGICAL PRINCIPLES

## Direct Fetal Susceptibility: Critical Periods

The kinds and frequencies of anomalies caused by a teratogenic agent depend critically upon the developmental stage at the time of exposure. This so-called *critical period* is illustrated for several representative human organs in Figure 68-2. The embryonic and fetal periods represent distinct developmental stages as illustrated, but the term "fetal" will be used here to describe the entire prenatal period. The fetus is more susceptible to chemical insult than at any stage in its postnatal life in part because of the high rate of cellular proliferation and differentiation, functional development, and growth taking place over a relatively brief period of time. For example, the DNA content of the mouse fetus is increased about one million times within the first 11 days of gestation (21-day pregnancy) and 1000 times during the first three days of organogenesis.

The specificity of the critical period can be illustrated by considering the formation of the palate, which involves the horizontal convergence and fusion of the two palatal shelves. In the mouse, cleft palate (failure of the palatal shelves to close) can be induced by an appropriate teratogen only when this is administered between gestational days 8 and 13. However, even this "single" process is complex. Palatal closure involves initial cellular proliferation, synthesis of intercellular substances, elevation of the two palatal shelves from a vertical to a horizontal position, midline contact and fusion of the two shelves, and finally formation of a bony plate. Thus, the critical period for any organ development actually is a continuum of discrete but interdependent processes that can be affected differentially by teratogens with different mechanisms or by the same teratogen at different times.

In the case of teratogens with different mechanisms, 6-aminonicotinamide causes cleft palate if administered at any time during palatal closure (days 8 to 13); dexamethasone is teratogenic only when given around day 13; 2,4,5-trichlorophenoxyacetic acid only around day 12; and 2,3,7,8-tetrachlorodibenzo-*p*-dioxin (TCDD, or dioxin) only between days 10 and 12 (Fig. 68-3). In the case of the same teratogen at different times, treatment of pregnant mice with 5-azacytidine on gestational day 15 produces an extreme reduction in brain size, particularly in the cerebral cortex, with abnormal layering of pyramidal cells in the hippocampus and a reduced corpus striatum. Later treatment, on day 19, produces damage in more restricted areas, with dead cells observed mainly within the subependymal and external granular layers of the cerebellum.

FIGURE 68-2　Human prenatal development and critical periods of susceptibility to teratogenic agents. Bars represent the organs, with colour indicating their most susceptible period.

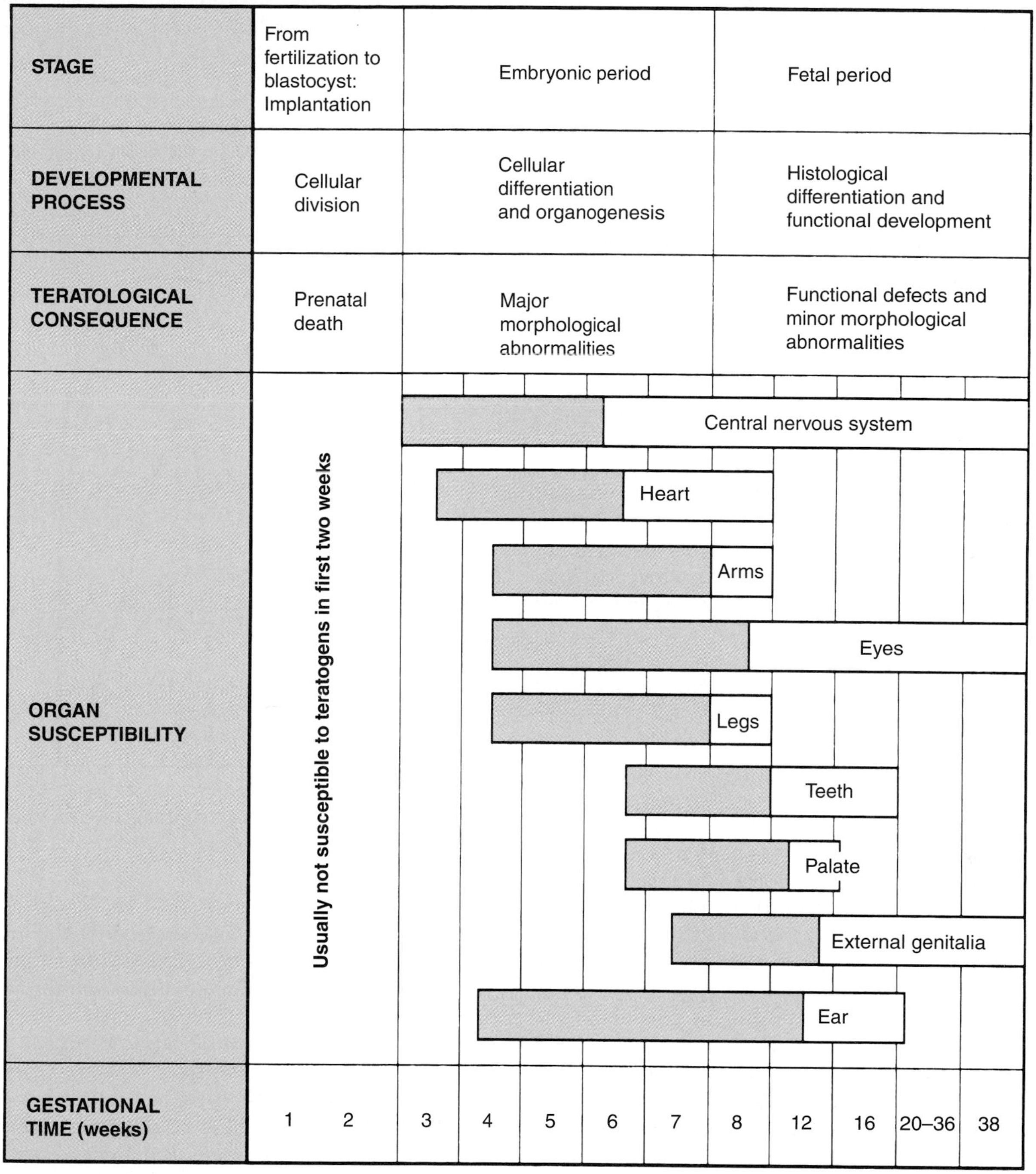

| STAGE | From fertilization to blastocyst: Implantation | Embryonic period | | Fetal period | | | | |
| --- | --- | --- | --- | --- | --- | --- | --- | --- |
| DEVELOPMENTAL PROCESS | Cellular division | Cellular differentiation and organogenesis | | Histological differentiation and functional development | | | | |
| TERATOLOGICAL CONSEQUENCE | Prenatal death | Major morphological abnormalities | | Functional defects and minor morphological abnormalities | | | | |
| ORGAN SUSCEPTIBILITY | Usually not susceptible to teratogens in first two weeks | Central nervous system / Heart / Arms / Eyes / Legs / Teeth / Palate / External genitalia / Ear | | | | | | |
| GESTATIONAL TIME (weeks) | 1　2 | 3 | 4　5　6　7 | 8 | 12 | 16 | 20–36 | 38 |

The one critical period that often is not susceptible to the production of anomalies by teratogens is the initial development from fertilization to completion of the blastocyst. Since this stage involves little cellular differentiation, the cells have not achieved specific developmental roles, and damage at this stage often either causes the death of the embryo or has no lasting effect.

Established critical periods nevertheless are not absolute since malformations occasionally have been demonstrated after chemical exposure during the preimplantation phase. This is particularly likely with highly lipid-soluble xenobiotics that persist in the mother or with DNA-damaging xenobiotics that initiate molecular lesions that may lead to mutations (permanent alterations in DNA). Such mutations are retained during cell division, producing potentially teratogenic alterations in cellular function. Similarly, severe skeletal anomalies have been induced by teratogen exposure during the third trimester after the phase of organogenesis and limb formation.

## Indirect Maternal Effects

In general, indirect insult to the fetus, mediated through effects on the mother, involves inadequate nutrient delivery secondary to either maternal malnutrition or pathophysiology, or to reduced uterine blood supply to the fetus.

Maternal blood flow through the uterus to the placenta generally can be maintained at the expense of perfusion of other maternal organs; however, the homeostatic mechanisms can be overcome by high doses of drugs or endogenous substances that are vasoconstrictors (e.g., ergotamine, serotonin, bradykinin, angiotensin) or that reduce maternal cardiac function (e.g., propranolol). In humans, the consequences appear to be mainly mild, reversible growth retardation rather than congenital malformations. In animals, treatment with vasoconstricting substances even at high doses produces resorptions (in utero death) without malformations. Thus, reduced uterine blood flow and its attendant deprivations generally do not produce measurable anomalies.

## Teratogenic Consequences

As indicated in Figure 68-1, teratogenesis can be viewed according to the major outcomes—namely, fetal death or structural, mutational, or functional abnormalities.

In the early stage of cellular division before differentiation, as discussed previously, **fetal death** usually occurs in the absence of teratogenicity. During later developmental stages, often lower doses of a drug are teratogenic while higher doses cause fetal death. However, with some teratogens, it is possible to induce a 100% incidence of **anomalies,** such as cleft palate, in the complete absence of fetal lethality (e.g., glucocorticoids in rodents), while other teratogens (possibly chloramphenicol in rodents) can induce fetal lethality without causing malformations. The latter case sometimes is difficult to establish, however, since malformed fetuses may die and be resorbed before detection. Teratogenicity cannot be estimated reliably if fetal lethality exceeds 50%. Since fetal death, teratogenicity, and growth retardation can be caused by different toxic mechanisms, the respective dose–response curves may be quite different, and their interrelation may vary at different times of gestation (Fig. 68-4). For example, dioxin induces about the same incidence of cleft palates

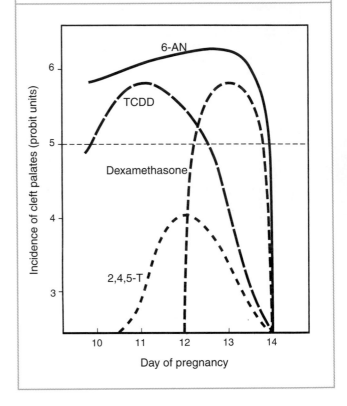

**FIGURE 68-3** Time course of the susceptibility of the NMRI strain of mice to the induction of cleft palate by various agents. Doses given: 6-aminonicotinamide (6-AN) = 12 mg/kg; dexamethasone = 40 mg/kg; 2,3,7,8-tetrachlorodibenzo-*p*-dioxin (TCDD) = 30 μg/kg; 2,4,5-trichlorophenoxyacetic acid (2,4,5-T) = 300 mg/kg. Differences in the period of maximum susceptibility suggest differences in the mode of action of the various compounds in inducing cleft palate. (From Neubert et al., 1980. Reprinted with permission.)

(teratogenicity) in mice when given throughout gestational days 6 to 15 as throughout days 9 to 13, but fetal death is induced only when dioxin is given throughout days 6 to 15.

Chemically induced **mutations** can occur in fetal somatic cells, resulting in transplacental carcinogenicity, and possibly teratogenicity. There are few data concerning chemical mutations in fetal germ cells, and consequent hereditary disorders, in humans. Perhaps the best-known human somatic mutation involves in utero exposure to the synthetic estrogen diethylstilbestrol, as a result of which female children developed a rare vaginal adenocarcinoma at puberty and male children developed a spectrum of structural and functional reproductive anomalies. While the correlation between mutagenicity, or DNA modifications, and carcinogenicity, or the initiation of cancer, is estimated to be between 67 and 90%, their relationship to teratogenicity is less clear. Teratogenicity is

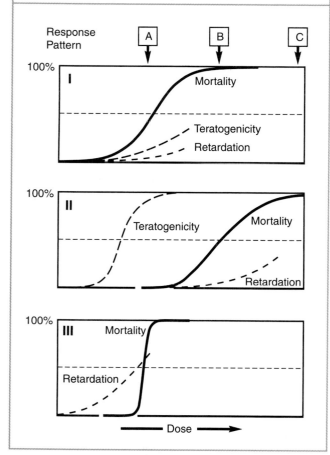

**FIGURE 68-4** Hypothetical response pattern of an embryotoxic action. The three different effects have been evaluated separately; they may show quite different dose–response relationships. The outcome varies considerably, depending on the response pattern in (I) early, (II) mid, and (III) late gestation and the dose (A, B, C). The letters A, B, and C illustrate positions along the dose–response curve where the effects differ most dramatically. (From Neubert et al., 1980. Reprinted with permission.)

tion of lipids, proteins, and DNA, thereby initiating either mutagenesis or teratogenesis. Retrospective surveys of experimental studies in animals suggest a high risk of teratogenicity (80 to 85%) from exposure to chemicals with in vivo and/or in vitro cytogenetic activity, which refers to cellular alterations resulting from modifications in gene structure and/or expression. The relationship for carcinogenic chemicals as a subgroup is more striking; 92% also demonstrate teratogenicity. Aberrations in chromosome number can be caused by chemicals that affect microtubules and interfere with the role of spindle fibres in disjunction of chromosomes at anaphase of mitosis or meiosis; 64% of such chemicals were found to be teratogenic.

**Functional anomalies** are, for many teratogens, a more sensitive indication of prenatal damage than overt structural malformations. The later fetal period is most susceptible to functional teratogenesis because of the high activities of histogenesis, or specialized cellular development, and functional maturation. The earlier embryonic period of organogenesis, which has little of these activities, is relatively insensitive to functional teratogenesis. Functional teratogenicity may include (1) permanent "imprinting" or alteration of discrete biochemical pathways; (2) changes in organ function, such as in the lungs or ears; (3) and system deficits, such as in the central nervous system (CNS) (i.e., dysfunction and learning disabilities), the hormonal or immune systems, the reproductive system (i.e., sexual function and fertility), and those that reduce life expectancy. Since detection of such functional anomalies often requires decades of follow-up and is labour-intensive as well as costly, few human data are available in this field.

Examples in humans include behavioural anomalies (low intelligence quotients and learning disabilities) in children exposed in utero to ethyl alcohol, phenytoin, or methylmercury. Examples in experimental animals include a permanently induced cytochrome P450 enzyme system in the offspring of pregnant mice treated with phenobarbital and the postnatal reduction in pulmonary oxygen consumption and respiratory rate in neonatal pups exposed in utero to excess vitamin A. Functional teratology can be produced over a wider gestational range than structural teratology, even up to the time of birth and into the neonatal period, as in the case of the developing CNS. Thus, the traditional view of the first trimester of human pregnancy as the period of greatest teratological susceptibility can no longer be considered accurate.

more complex than mutagenesis, and not all teratogens would be expected to be mutagens and carcinogens. Also, chemically induced damage to DNA can alter gene transcription, thereby dysregulating critical developmental processes and initiating teratogenesis in the absence of mutations or independent of mutational mechanisms.

Nevertheless, mutagens can initiate six of the nine teratogenic mechanisms listed in Table 68-2. Another point common to mutagens and teratogens is that many such chemicals are enzymatically bioactivated in vivo to a reactive intermediary metabolite, as discussed in subsequent sections (see also Chapters 4 and 67). These reactive intermediates or, in a few cases, the original reactive parent chemical may bind covalently or irreversibly to essential fetal cellular macromolecules or lead to irreversible oxida-

## Cellular Mechanisms

The basic biological mechanisms related to the early events in teratogenicity are listed in Table 68-2. Any given teratogen often initiates several mechanisms, and, conversely, any given mechanism may be initiated by a variety of causes separate from, or complementary to, the effects of the potential chemical teratogen.

Pathogenesis is often characterized by the appearance of demonstrable cellular and tissue damage. Increased cellular death is the most frequent sign of abnormal development, and the teratogenic process often, but not inevitably, involves some degree of focal cellular necrosis and/or alteration in physiological patterns of apoptosis. Failure of either the proper amount or sequence of cellular interaction and reduced biosynthesis of essential macromolecules such as DNA, RNA, proteins, and mucopolysaccharides can be important steps in teratogenesis. Impairment of morphogenetic movement (i.e., the migration or translocation of cells or groups of cells) is notably involved in neuronal maldevelopment. Finally, tissues can be traumatized mechanically by invasion of foreign materials or abnormal accumulation of tissue fluids or blood, resulting in anomalous development.

## Genetic and Environmental Modulation

The genetic and environmental factors modulating teratological susceptibility are poorly understood and, in many cases, likely involve a complex interdependence. For most teratogens, it is not known whether the genetic predisposition or resistance is mediated via a pharmacological mechanism, as discussed later, or via a biological response mechanism. One example of the latter case may be the difference in susceptibility of various strains of mice to the induction of cleft palates. The inbred A/J mouse has a spontaneous incidence of cleft palates and is more susceptible than outbred mouse strains to the induction of cleft palates by the anticonvulsant drug phenytoin. The palatal shelves of the relatively resistant outbred mice are oriented on a horizontal plane toward each other to start with, whereas the palatal shelves of the susceptible A/J mouse remain vertical and distant from each other until late in the closure period, thus being potentially more susceptible to developmental interferences. Other cases remain unexplained, such as resistance to thalidomide teratogenicity in rats and mice compared with exquisite susceptibility in humans and to a lesser extent in rabbits, although reduced osidative stress in the former appears to play a role. Conversely, the susceptibility of rodents and the resistance of humans to salicylate teratogenicity also is unexplained, as are a multitude of other species and strain differences in teratological susceptibility.

Environmental determinants of teratological susceptibility are just as poorly recognized and understood. Stress and nutritional deficiency by themselves can increase the incidence of cleft palates in rodents and likely can potentiate the teratogenicity of many chemicals. Ambient temperature also can be important, as demonstrated in the case of 6-aminonicotinamide, a teratogenic chemical that also blocks temperature regulation in animals. In studies at room temperature, 6-aminonicotinamide produced a fall in maternal body temperature, and the offspring were normal, while in studies conducted at 36°C, normal

| TABLE 68-2 | Successive Stages in the Pathogenesis of a Developmental Defect* |
|---|---|

**Mechanisms**
Initial types of change in developing cells or tissues after teratogenic insult:
- Mutation (gene)
- Chromosomal breaks, non-disjunction, etc.
- Mitotic interference
- Altered nucleic acid integrity or function
- Lack of normal precursors, substrates, etc.
- Altered energy sources
- Changed membrane characteristics
- Osmolar imbalance
- Enzyme inhibition

**Pathogenesis**
Ultimately manifested as one or more types of abnormal embryogenesis:
- Excessive or reduced cell death
- Failed cell interactions
- Reduced biosynthesis
- Impeded morphogenetic movement
- Mechanical disruption of tissues

**Common pathways**
Too few cells or cell products to effect local morphogenesis or functional maturation
Other imbalances in growth and differentiation

**Final defect**

*Initiation of one or more mechanisms by the teratogenic cause from the environment leads to changes in the developmental system that become manifested as one or more types of abnormal embryogenesis. This in turn leads into pathways that often seem to be characterized by too few cells or cell products to effect morphogenesis or functional maturation, but the suggestion that this is a single common pathway for all developmental defects is conjecture.

(From Wilson, 1977. Reprinted with permission.)

maternal body temperature was maintained, and there was a substantial increase in teratological anomalies. In animals, a growing number of drugs and chemicals with or without their own intrinsic teratogenic activity have been shown to modulate the fetal damage produced by known teratogenic agents, but in most cases the underlying mechanisms are not known.

# PHARMACOLOGICAL PRINCIPLES

## Placental Transfer and Fetal Chemical Disposition

Once believed to be a protective barrier isolating the fetus from harmful external influences, the placenta now is known to be more akin to a sieve, permitting chemicals with a molecular weight under 600 Da ready access to the fetus while excluding only the largest (above 1000 Da) or most highly charged molecules such as heparin. Fetal blood concentrations of many chemicals are equivalent to maternal concentrations, and even some charged quaternary ammonium compounds can cross the placenta in limited quantities, possibly facilitated by a placental active transport process (see also Chapter 2). It is likely that at least some drug transporters shown to function in many other tissues will prove to be similarly important in modulating the placental transfer of some teratogens, although this area is only beginning to be explored.

Fetal factors such as a blood pH that is 0.1 to 0.15 units below that of the mother, and occasional differences in plasma protein binding of chemicals, are theoretically important in determining chemical concentrations in fetal blood and tissues, but such factors have not been shown to have a remarkable influence on chemical teratogenicity. For complete reviews of fetal drug disposition, see Waddell and Marlowe (in Juchau, 1981).

## Fetal Chemical Biotransformation

The principles of drug biotransformation are covered in Chapter 4, as well as in a number of reviews in specific reference to chemical teratogenesis (see Suggested Readings at the end of this chapter). In general, most enzymatic pathways of drug biotransformation are at a much lower level of activity in the fetus than in adults. In animals, this activity for the most part is low or negligible until birth. In the human fetal liver, enzymatic activity for most cytochromes P450 may be measurable as early as 6 weeks, but at mid-gestation it is only 20 to 40% of that in adults, with considerable inter-individual variation. A few P450 isoenzymes, such as CYP3A7, have higher activity than that of adults, and recent evidence indicates that at least one fetal P450 isoenzyme (CYP1B1) has high activity in the fetus and low activity post-natally. In non-human primates that have mid-gestational P450 activities similar to those in humans, activity increases fourfold from 10 days before to 10 days after birth. P450 activity in fetal animals cannot be induced substantially by chemicals such as phenobarbital and 3-methylcholanthrene until about 3 days before birth, although dioxin is an effective inducer of CYP1A1, an isoenzyme measured by aryl hydrocarbon hydroxylase (AHH) activity, earlier in gestation. In human fetuses, enzymatic induction appears to occur much earlier, although still less than in adults.

The developmental activity for a number of important enzymes is shown in Figure 68-5. Within any one class of enzyme, the developmental activity for a specific isoenzyme and its substrates may vary considerably, as with the cytochromes P450 (Fig. 68-5A). One of the groups of UDP-glucuronosyltransferases demonstrates high activity during the third trimester and perinatal period and declines rapidly thereafter; the other transferase group develops after birth (Fig. 68-5B). However, sulfotransferase activity in early fetal life can be equivalent to adult levels, although this pathway is capacity-limited for chemicals. The fetus also has significant activities of prostaglandin H synthase (PHS) and lipoxygenases, which may play a role in chemical teratogenesis. In general, however, the fetus is deficient in enzymatic activities for chemical biotransformation and thus often is unable to eliminate chemicals and detoxify reactive intermediates. In addition, the fetus is deficient in most of the enzymes that protect tissues from xenobiotic-initiated oxidative stress (see "Reactive Intermediate–Mediated Mechanisms" below).

## Teratogenic Specificity

The concept of "critical period" (see "Direct Fetal Susceptibility: Critical Periods" above) can be restated here as **phase specificity**. Teratogens will cause markedly different anomalies depending on the phase of fetal development. For example, methylnitrosourea is a transplacental carcinogen in rats only if administered on gestational day 20, whereas earlier administration will cause a spectrum of structural and functional anomalies. This late susceptibility to carcinogenicity may be due to a requirement for a sufficiently developed fetal enzymatic system for bioactivation of the chemical to a carcinogenic reactive intermediate within the fetus, although other factors such as increased placental transport of a maternally produced reactive intermediate or processes involved in carcinogenic promotion cannot be excluded.

**Drug specificity** is closely linked to phase specificity. Many teratogens interfere with intermediary processes that occur only during discrete phases in development. These *specific teratogens* cause a limited number of anomalies or a characteristic syndrome of malformations. A partial exception to the principle of drug specificity is a limited group of general or *universal teratogens* that interfere with fundamental processes such as nucleic acid metabolism or protein synthesis that occur throughout the stages of cellular division and differentiation. Universal teratogens would include the cytotoxic anti-cancer drugs, such as cytosine arabinoside and 6-mercaptopurine. However, even the so-called universal teratogens may demonstrate a certain degree of specificity, as shown in Figure 68-6. Treatment of pregnant mice with 6-aminonicotinamide produces more limb defects when given on gestational day 9 than on day 10, while cytosine arabinoside is teratogenic on both days, if not more so on day 10. Furthermore, 6-aminonicotinamide preferentially affects the hindlimbs, while cytosine arabinoside affects both the forelimbs and hindlimbs.

**Dose specificity** also can affect both the type and the frequency of anomalies. For example, low doses of a number of teratogens given to pregnant mice on gestational day 10 cause polydactyly (i.e., extra phalanges or digits), medium doses of the same teratogens reduce the length of phalanges and long bones without causing polydactyly, and high doses cause amelia (i.e., the absence of entire

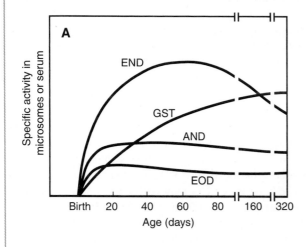

**FIGURE 68-5** Developmental changes in activities of selected drug biotransformation enzymes in the rat. (A) Hepatic cytochromes P450 and serum glutathione S-transferase. AND = aminopyrine N-demethylase; END = ethylmorphine N-demethylase; EOD = ethoxycoumarin O-demethylase; GST = serum glutathione S-transferase. (B) Glucuronidation of group I and group II substrates in males and females.

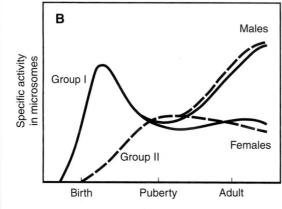

oxygen species, which can *irreversibly* alter essential cellular macromolecules.

The specific, reversible interaction of drugs with their receptors generally is responsible for the intended therapeutic effects of the drugs, as well as many of their side effects. Fetal toxicity caused by such an interaction is due to exaggeration of the pharmacological activity for which the drug is used therapeutically. However, fetal toxicity caused by the irreversible interaction of a reactive intermediate with fetal tissues in most cases is unrelated to the pharmacological mechanism by which the drug exerts its therapeutic effect. There are exceptions, however, such as the anti-neoplastic alkylating drugs, whose therapeutic effect of destroying neoplastic cells is based on their covalent binding to DNA, which also is responsible for their teratogenicity. In the case of environmental chemicals that have no therapeutic purpose, the discrimination is based only upon reversible binding to a receptor as opposed to the irreversible interaction of a reactive intermediate or reactive oxygen species with cellular macromolecules.

## Receptor-Mediated Mechanisms

Since fetal toxicity occurring via these mechanisms generally but not always represents an exaggerated therapeutic response, the toxicological sequelae (including teratogenic effects) usually are predictable and proportional to fetal and maternal blood chemical concentrations, if not to the dose assimilated. The principles underlying such

limbs). In this case, the malformation is more dependent upon the dose of the teratogen than on its mechanism of action. The lowest dose is thought to act by causing limited focal necrosis in the apical region of the developing limb bud, which responds with a compensatory overproduction of phalangeal cells, leading to polydactyly.

## Chemical Mechanisms

Chemical mechanisms of teratogenesis can be classified into two general categories: (1) those related to the classical, *reversible* interaction of a stable chemical or its active metabolite(s) with a receptor; and (2) those involving highly reactive chemicals, their respective reactive intermediary metabolites, or resultant reactive

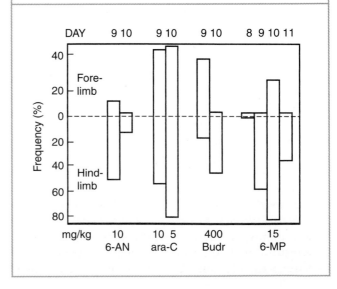

**FIGURE 68-6** Frequency of limb abnormalities produced by various agents applied at different stages of pregnancy in the NMRI strain of mice, showing the great variability with different chemicals. 6-AN = 6-aminonicotinamide; ara-C = cytosine arabinoside; Budr = 5'-bromouracil deoxyriboside; 6-MP = 6-mercaptopurine. (From Neubert et al., 1980. Reprinted with permission.)

mechanisms are discussed in Chapter 59; this discussion will be limited to teratogenesis.

The induction of cleft palates and limb anomalies in rodents by high doses of corticosteroids is an instructive example. This does not constitute an exaggerated therapeutic response, but it is an exaggeration of the physiological role of endogenous corticosteroids in palatal development and is dependent upon reversible binding of the corticosteroid to its receptor. In general, the amount of glucocorticoid administered to pregnant mice and taken up by the fetus correlates with the degree of inhibition of DNA and protein synthesis and with teratogenic susceptibility. The A/J strain of mice, which is highly susceptible to glucocorticoid teratogenicity, has the same endogenous maternal and fetal concentrations of corticosterone as the C57BL/6J strain, which is resistant. However, A/J mouse facial mesenchymal cells have two to three times more cytoplasmic glucocorticoid receptors than those from C57BL/6J mice, and this is reflected in an increased inhibition of growth and DNA synthesis in A/J compared with C57BL/6J mice.

The teratogenicity of opioid analgesic drugs likely constitutes another example of a receptor-mediated mechanism, since the incidence of most anomalies in animals can be reduced by pre-treatment with opioid antagonists (see Wells, 1988).

## Reactive Intermediate–Mediated Mechanisms

Drugs that themselves are not teratogenic ("proteratogens") can be enzymatically converted, or bioactivated, to two types of teratogenic reactive intermediates: electrophiles and free radicals. Teratological susceptibility to such proteratogens depends upon the balance of competing pathways of elimination, bioactivation, detoxification, cytoprotection, and repair (Fig. 68-7).

For **electrophiles,** a representative scheme for the enzymatic formation (bioactivation) of a potentially toxic, electrophilic reactive intermediary metabolite (often an epoxide) and its various detoxification pathways is presented in Figure 68-8. This type of bioactivation is only one of several kinds reviewed in detail in some of the works cited. Glutathione *S*-transferases and epoxide hydrolases are critical enzymes for the direct detoxification of reactive intermediary metabolites. In a limited number of cases, however, these so-called detoxifying enzymes can be involved in the subsequent formation of an even more reactive and toxic intermediary metabolite. UDP-glucuronosyltransferases and similar transferase enzymes, while not directly involved in detoxifying reactive intermediates, can be quantitatively major pathways of drug elimination, thereby preventing much of a chemical from being metabolized via a bioactivating pathway.

Under normal conditions, a reactive intermediate is evanescent—it is immediately detoxified and excreted.

However, if bioactivation exceeds detoxification, the highly reactive electrophilic site on the chemical intermediate will bind covalently to nucleophilic sites on essential fetal cellular macromolecules. If fetal repair mechanisms are inadequate, covalent binding of the chemical is thought to initiate a process, as yet poorly understood, that ends in cellular death or functional alterations. In a few cases, such as the anti-neoplastic alkylating drugs, the parent compound is sufficiently reactive to bind covalently without need for bioactivation. Chemicals believed to be bioactivated to a teratogenic electrophilic reactive intermediate include cyclophosphamide, thalidomide, phenytoin, and benzo[*a*]pyrene, although other mechanisms may be involved in their teratogenic effects.

With some chemicals, bioactivation or certain detoxifying pathways may constitute a quantitatively minor route of metabolism and yet have major teratological importance. For example, while only about 5 to 10% of the reactive arene oxide intermediate of phenytoin is hydroxylated and thereby detoxified by epoxide hydrolase, specific inhibition of this enzyme will increase the teratogenicity of phenytoin. The bioactivation of most if not all proteratogens likely occurs within the fetus or its associated tissues, rather than in maternal tissues, since reactive intermediates are too unstable to be transported across several membranes and over a considerable distance to the fetus. For example, the enzymatic bioactivation and embryopathic effects of many teratogens have been demonstrated in whole embryo culture, which excludes maternal tissues. In humans, fetal activities of P450 isoenzymes, while generally relatively low, nevertheless may be sufficiently high for teratologically relevant bioactivation. In rodents, fetal P450 activities are substantially lower and are less likely to contribute substantially to bioactivation. Alternatively, activities of other potential bioactivating enzymes such as PHS may be relatively high in both human and rodent fetuses.

PHS, formerly known as prostaglandin synthetase, is an enzyme system which also possesses cyclooxygenase (COX) activity, and it is involved in the bioactivation of many drugs, primarily to reactive **free radical** intermediates. The fetus has significant activity of both the I and II isozymes of this enzyme system, and the hydroperoxidase component of PHS may oxidize some drugs to a teratogenic reactive intermediate, as postulated for a number of proteratogens, including benzo[*a*]pyrene, thalidomide, phenytoin, and related anticonvulsant drugs (Fig. 68-9). PHS knockout mice are partially protected from the embryopathic effects of benzo[*a*]pyrene, and PHS inhibitors like acetylsalicylic acid (Aspirin) reduce the teratogenicity of phenytoin in mice, and of thalidomide in rabbits. Drug radicals may react directly with fetal tissues or may react with oxygen to produce toxic reactive oxygen species (ROS), such as superoxide anion radicals, hydrogen peroxide, and hydroxyl radicals. In a process known as **oxidative stress,** these ROS can oxidize fetal molecular tar-

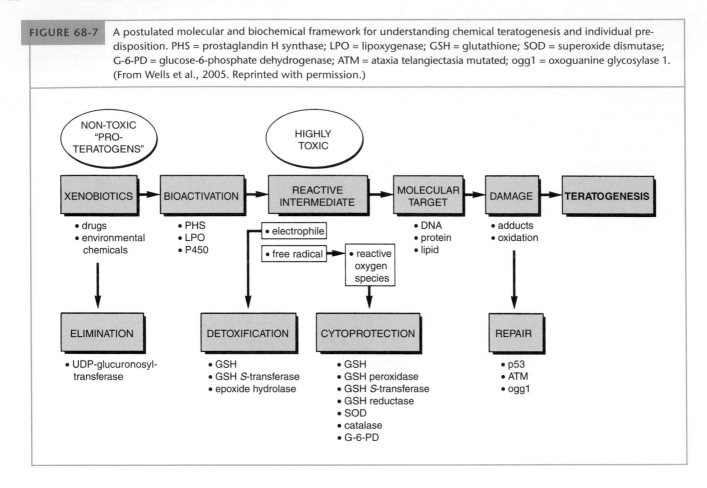

**FIGURE 68-7** A postulated molecular and biochemical framework for understanding chemical teratogenesis and individual pre-disposition. PHS = prostaglandin H synthase; LPO = lipoxygenase; GSH = glutathione; SOD = superoxide dismutase; G-6-PD = glucose-6-phosphate dehydrogenase; ATM = ataxia telangiectasia mutated; ogg1 = oxoguanine glycosylase 1. (From Wells et al., 2005. Reprinted with permission.)

gets such as DNA, protein, and lipid. These oxidative lesions are thought to play a role in teratological initiation.

A similar bioactivation of proteratogens to a teratogenic, free radical intermediate may be catalyzed via the lipoxygenase pathway, which is involved in the synthesis of leukotrienes and related hormones. In addition, by acting as the cofactor for reduction of prostaglandin $G_2$ (PGG$_2$) to prostaglandin $H_2$ (PGH$_2$), and via a similar role in leukotriene synthesis, drugs may perturb the physiological balance among the fetal synthesis of prostaglandins, prostacyclin, thromboxanes, and leukotrienes, with potential teratological consequences.

ROS also can be produced via redox cycling of some hydroxylated chemicals (Fig. 68-10), which may include some stable drug metabolites formed in maternal liver and transferred across the placenta into the fetus. In addition, some drugs reducing fetal cardiovascular function have been implicated in ROS production via the same reperfusion reaction that occurs in the adult heart and brain during heart attacks and stroke (see Halliwell and Gutteridge, 1999).

Although ROS likely must be formed within the embryo, maternal factors other than drug metabolism theoretically may modulate the relevant embryonic processes of ROS formation and detoxification and DNA repair, among other pathways, thereby altering risk. For example, knockout mice deficient in inducible nitric oxide synthase

(iNOS) are partially protected from the embryopathic effects of benzo[a]pyrene and phenytoin, even though embryos do not express iNOS. This suggests that soluble nitric oxide can diffuse from the maternal and/or embryonic tissues into the embryo, where it reacts to enhance ROS formation and related forms of macromolecular damage. Little is known about whether and how diffusible maternal factors may affect embryonic risk from ROS.

The fetus has low concentrations of glutathione and low activities of most cytoprotective enzymes such as glutathione reductase, glutathione peroxidase, superoxide dismutase (SOD), and catalase, all of which are critical for cellular protection against free radical damage (see Fig. 68-10). The only exception is glucose-6-phosphate dehydrogenase (G-6-PD), for which embryonic and fetal levels equal or exceed those in the mother. The generally low level of cytoprotective pathways in the fetus likely increases its risk for free radical–mediated toxicity. In rodent models, inhibition of these cytoprotective enzymes enhances susceptibility to phenytoin teratogenicity, as does the use of a mouse strain with a hereditary deficiency in G-6-PD. Conversely, in a rodent embryo culture model, addition of SOD or catalase to the culture medium enhances embryonic anti-oxidative activity and completely inhibits the embryopathic effects of phenytoin and benzo[a]pyrene. Similarly, in vivo, maternal administration of stabilized catalase

FIGURE 68-8    Postulated role of proteratogen bioactivation and detoxification of electrophilic reactive intermediates in chemical teratogenesis.

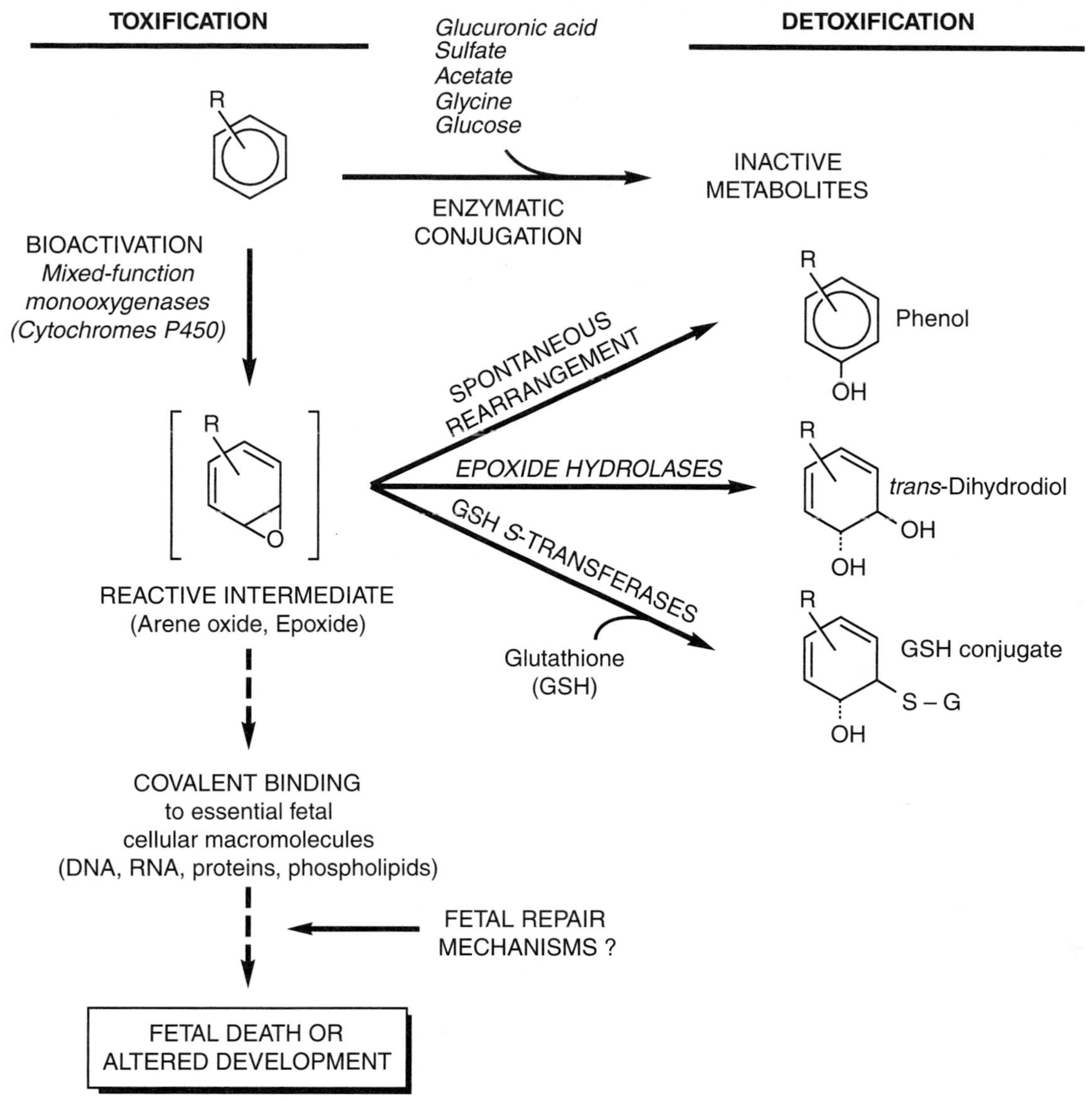

enhances embryonic catalase activity and reduces pheny-toin teratogenicity. The embryopathic contribution of ROS is further implicated by studies showing that free radical spin trapping agents (e.g., phenylbutylnitrone) and antiox-idants (e.g., vitamin E), which neutralize ROS, can block the teratogenicity of phenytoin and related drugs in mice, and of thalidomide in rabbits.

In addition to causing oxidative damage to cellular macromolecules, ROS also are involved in physiological reactions via the activation of several signal transduction pathways, and this latter effect may be particularly impor-tant to fetal development at lower levels of ROS produc-tion (Fig. 68-11). For example, the ROS-initiating terato-gen phenytoin enhances the activation of Ras and NF-κB,

and its embryopathic effects can be reduced by inhibitors of either of these processes, suggesting an important tera-tological role for ROS-mediated signal transduction. Con-versely, the teratological contribution of ROS via oxida-tive DNA damage, as distinct from signal transduction, is suggested by the enhanced embryopathic effects of the ROS-initiating agents benzo[a]pyrene and gamma radia-tion in knockout mice deficient in p53 or ATM (ataxia telangiectasia mutated), which are important in detecting and repairing DNA damage.

Since many proteratogens are bioactivated to both elec-trophilic and free radical reactive intermediates, it is diffi-cult to determine their relative teratological contributions, particularly in humans. Interestingly, however, at least for rodents, the ability of SOD and catalase to block the embryopathic effects of phenytoin and benzo[a]pyrene suggests an important teratological role for oxidative stress as distinct from the covalent binding of the chemical. A secondary principle illustrated by phenytoin is the potential contribution of more than one chemical mech-anism to the teratogenicity of drugs—namely, a reversible, receptor-mediated interaction as well as irreversible inter-actions of reactive electrophilic and free radical interme-diates. This can be further complicated by the ability of ROS to both oxidatively damage cellular macromolecules and enhance signal transduction. Human studies suggest

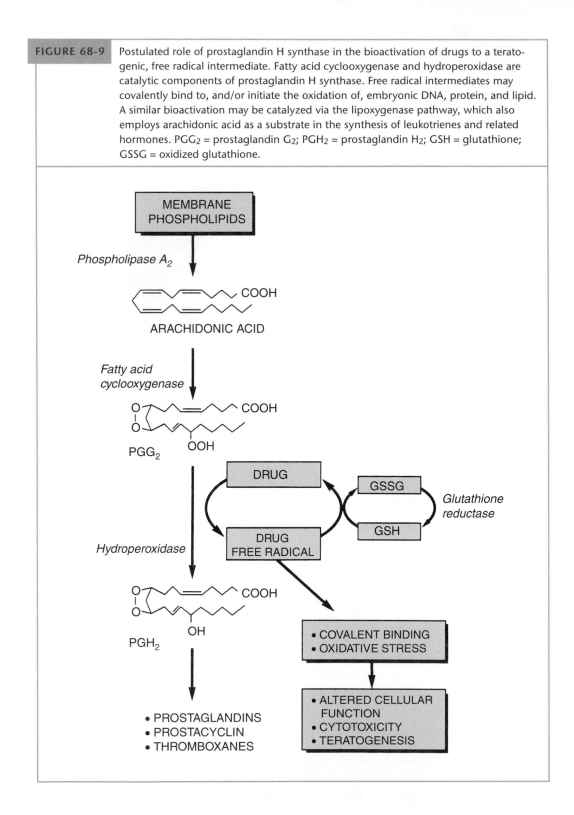

**FIGURE 68-9** Postulated role of prostaglandin H synthase in the bioactivation of drugs to a terato-genic, free radical intermediate. Fatty acid cyclooxygenase and hydroperoxidase are catalytic components of prostaglandin H synthase. Free radical intermediates may covalently bind to, and/or initiate the oxidation of, embryonic DNA, protein, and lipid. A similar bioactivation may be catalyzed via the lipoxygenase pathway, which also employs arachidonic acid as a substrate in the synthesis of leukotrienes and related hormones. $PGG_2$ = prostaglandin $G_2$; $PGH_2$ = prostaglandin $H_2$; GSH = glutathione; GSSG = oxidized glutathione.

**FIGURE 68-10** The role of cytoprotective pathways in detoxifying reactive oxygen species initiated by xenobiotic free radical intermediates. GSH = glutathione; GSSG = oxidized glutathione. (From Kappus, 1986. Reprinted with permission.)

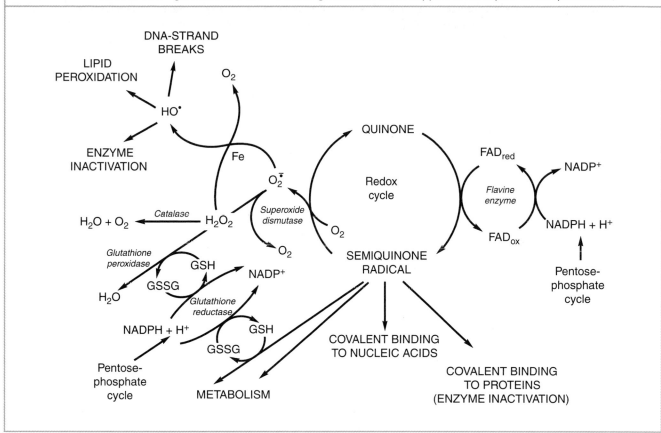

that some particular types of birth defects caused by phenytoin may be due to a reactive intermediate, while others may be due to a receptor-mediated mechanism resulting from excessive maternal plasma concentrations of phenytoin. The relative teratological contributions of these mechanisms may well vary with gestational age, strain, species, and environmental conditions.

## Genetic and Environmental Modulation

Modulatory influences, particularly in the case of toxicological mechanisms involving reactive intermediates, generally are complex and poorly understood. In addition to the complicating effects of the maternal and placental systems, modulating factors tend to affect multiple pathways of drug elimination, bioactivation, and detoxification, and associated pathways of cytoprotection and macromolecular repair, with unpredictable teratological consequences. A number of **genetic determinants** of chemical teratogenesis have been evaluated, primarily on rodent models, and benzo[a]pyrene provides a useful model for discussion. The non-constitutive P450 isoenzyme CYP1A1, often measured as aryl hydrocarbon hydroxylation (AHH; formerly hydroxylase)), is controlled genetically by the Ah locus and is involved in the bioactivation of aryl hydrocar-

bons such as benzo[a]pyrene to teratogenic reactive intermediates. Different people, and different strains of mice, are genetically either non-responsive or responsive to CYP1A1-inducing agents, and only the responsive ones show an increase in CYP1A1. In mouse strains bred to produce both CYP1A1-responsive and -non-responsive fetuses in the same litter, there is a five- to fifteenfold variation in the induction of AHH activity among individual littermates following maternal pre-treatment with the CYP1A1 inducer 3-methylcholanthrene. Littermates that are responsive to AHH induction are more susceptible to benzo[a]pyrene-initiated malformations, and they have an increased amount of covalent binding of radiolabelled benzo[a]pyrene to fetal tissues compared with the AHH-non-responsive littermates.

In other studies using pregnant inbred B6 mice, which produce only AHH-responsive offspring, benzo[a]pyrene causes an incidence of fetal resorptions, stillbirths, and malformations that is fourfold higher than that in inbred AK mice, which produce only AHH-non-responsive offspring.

In summary, the teratological susceptibility to some chemicals appears to be genetically determined, the determinant can reside within the fetus rather than the mother, and this fetal determinant can be active early in

**FIGURE 68-11** Postulated complementary roles of reactive oxygen species (ROS)-initiated signal transduction and oxidative macromolecular damage in teratogenesis. This is a composite scheme based primarily upon results from studies of the ROS-initiating teratogens benzo[a]pyrene, phenytoin, methamphetamine, and gamma radiation. The protective role of DNA repair, implicating the teratological importance of oxidative DNA damage, was shown in knockout mice deficient in p53, ataxia telangiectasia mutated (ATM), or oxoguanine glycosylase 1 (ogg1), which detect and/or repair DNA damage. The signal transduction proteins Ras and NF-κB were implicated by the respective protective effects of a farnesyl-protein transferase inhibitor (blocks Ras activation) and NF-κB antisense oligonucleotides in reducing phenytoin embryopathies. These pathways should be considered as representative components—it is likely that additional repair proteins, oxidative damage to other cellular macromolecules (i.e., proteins, lipid), and other proteins involved in ROS-dependent signal transduction pathways contribute to the risk of such embryopathies. (See Wells et al., 2005 for background information.) (Modified from Kennedy JC, et al. Antisense evidence for nuclear factor-κB-dependent embryopathies initiated by phenytoin-enhanced oxidative stress. *Mol Pharmacol.* 2004;66:404-412, with permission.)

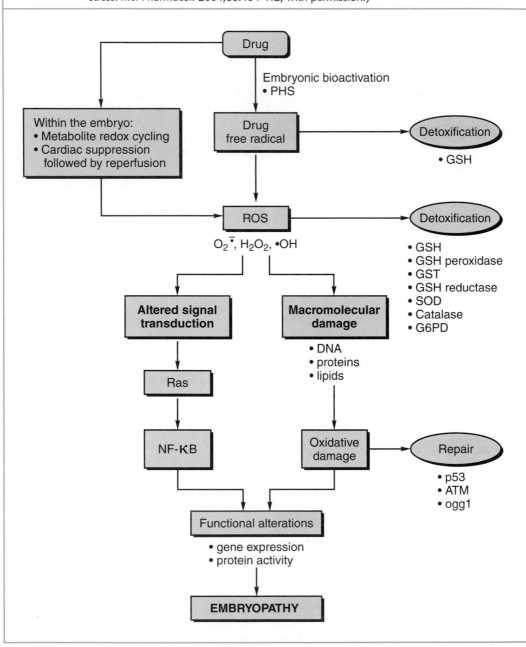

development. This also might explain why, in humans, it is possible that only one of fraternal (dizygotic) twins may be afflicted with a drug-induced anomaly or how only one of several children from the same mother may demonstrate a teratological response following exposure in utero to a drug that had been taken by the mother in the same doses during all her pregnancies.

The observations above for the Ah locus likely apply to genetic systems that regulate other enzymatic pathways of elimination, bioactivation, detoxification, cytoprotection, and repair. For example, there have been rare cases reported involving patients who are deficient in epoxide hydrolases or enzymes involved in glutathione synthesis who have experienced life-threatening hepatotoxicity due to their inability to detoxify the reactive intermediates of certain drugs. Such genetically determined deficiencies would be expected to have serious teratological consequences for the fetuses of pregnant women exposed to potential teratogens that are normally detoxified via these pathways. Evidence in humans suggests that a lower activity of fetal epoxide hydrolase may predispose such fetuses to phenytoin teratogenicity. The potential importance of maternal UDP-glucuronosyltransferases in chemical teratogenesis has been demonstrated for benzo[a]pyrene, which can be eliminated via glucuronidation prior to its bioactivation to the reactive 7,8-diol-9,10-epoxide intermediate. More importantly, maternal glucuronidation prevents the hydroxylated metabolites of benzo[a]pyrene from crossing the placenta into the fetus. The embryotoxicity of benzo[a]pyrene is significantly increased in Gunn rats, which have a genetic deficiency in UDP-glucuronosyltransferases. With respect to cytoprotection, pregnant mice with hereditary deficiencies in G-6-PD are more susceptible to phenytoin teratogenicity.

Finally, repair of DNA damage is facilitated by a number of pathways, including those involving the p53 tumour suppressor gene, ATM, and oxoguanine glycosylase 1 (ogg1). Teratogenicity of the DNA-damaging agents benzo[a]pyrene and gamma radiation is enhanced respectively in p53-deficient and ATM-deficient pregnant knockout mice, and the deficient fetuses have a higher incidence of in utero death (see Fig. 68-11). Similarly, ogg1 knockout fetuses are more susceptible to neurodevelopmental deficits caused by the ROS-initiating drug methamphetamine. Conversely, for a few target tissues or other teratogens, a deficiency in p53 in a limited number of cases actually may protect the fetus, although the underlying mechanisms remain to be established. Overall, however, deficiencies in fetal DNA repair, particularly with respect to oxidative damage, may be an important teratological risk factor.

Relatively little is known about the **environmental determinants** that modulate chemical teratogenicity, particularly with teratogens that are bioactivated to a toxic reactive intermediate. Such determinants could include individual physiological differences, concurrent pathophysiological conditions, and exposure to other drugs or environmental chemicals. For example, in pregnant mice, the teratogenicity of phenytoin and similar drugs is potentiated by pre-treatment with the epoxide hydrolase inhibitor trichloropropene oxide, the glutathione depletors diethyl maleate and acetaminophen, the glutathione synthesis inhibitor buthionine sulfoximine, the glutathione reductase inhibitor bis-chloroethylnitrosourea (BCNU), and the phospholipase $A_2$ activator tetradecanoylphorbol acetate. Phenytoin teratogenicity also is enhanced in pregnant mice fed a selenium-deficient diet, which decreases the levels of glutathione peroxidase, a cytoprotective enzyme that detoxifies hydrogen peroxide and lipid hydroperoxides initiated by free radicals (see Fig. 68-10). Conversely, phenytoin teratogenicity in mice is reduced by pre-treatment with the prostaglandin cyclooxygenase inhibitor acetylsalicylic acid, the dual cyclooxygenase/lipoxygenase inhibitor eicosatetraynoic acid, the antioxidants caffeic acid and vitamin E, the free radical spin-trapping agent phenylbutylnitrone, and, under some conditions, the glutathione precursor N-acetylcysteine.

A variety of physiological and pathological reactions in the body can produce superoxide, which is converted via an iron-catalyzed reaction to highly toxic hydroxyl radicals; hence, iron has been implicated in a number of free radical–related diseases. In pregnant mice, phenytoin teratogenicity is reduced by pre-treatment with the iron chelator deferoxamine. Drug radicals also can react directly or indirectly with oxygen to produce superoxide. As discussed earlier, addition of SOD or catalase, which detoxify superoxide and hydrogen peroxide, to a mouse embryo culture system, or maternal treatment with these agents in vivo, blocks the embryopathic effects of benzo[a]pyrene and phenytoin. Environmental factors with such effects on pathways of xenobiotic elimination, membrane drug transporters, bioactivation, and detoxification and on associated pathways of cytoprotection and molecular repair, similarly would be expected to modulate the risk of teratogenesis in pregnant women exposed to certain potential teratogens. However, such possibilities have only recently been recognized in animal studies, and there are few data in humans on which to base any estimate of actual risk. In some cases, knowledge of such modulatory effects ultimately may be employed to therapeutic advantage.

In addition, the complexities of developmental processes and maternal–placental–fetal interdependencies often preclude the straightforward predictions that are possible in other fields of toxicology. For example, in nonpregnant animals, induction of the P450 system generally will increase, while inhibition will decrease, the toxicity of chemicals that are bioactivated to a reactive intermediate. However, in pregnant mice, the teratogenicity of phenytoin and cyclophosphamide paradoxically is *decreased* by P450 induction and *increased* by inhibition.

Thus, it appears that enzyme induction and other environmental perturbations have complex effects in vivo relating both to simultaneous effects on multiple pathways of xenobiotic elimination, bioactivation, and detoxification and to confounding maternal effects. The underlying mechanisms for the most part are not understood, and more studies will be necessary to identify and characterize the environmental determinants of teratogenesis, particularly with regard to human risk.

## EXPERIMENTAL TERATOLOGY

The thalidomide tragedy clearly demonstrated the need for improved methods to detect potential chemical teratogens and elucidate their teratological mechanisms. In vivo studies employing more non-rodent animal species are now combined with a battery of in vitro tests. In vivo studies of pregnancy are time-consuming and expensive, however, and are not practical for screening large numbers of drugs and chemicals. Furthermore, the chemical and biological complexities of the maternal–placental–fetal interactions encountered in vivo generally preclude the elucidation of discrete teratological mechanisms. Thus, in vivo studies are most useful for the ultimate teratological testing of chemicals that have been pre-screened in vitro and for applied aspects of teratological research.

For the above reasons, a large number of in vitro teratological screening methods have been devised, as exemplified in Table 68-3. This discussion will consider briefly four major categories: cells in culture, embryonic organs in culture, whole embryos in culture, and artificial embryos.

Embryonic **cells** in culture are used to study potential teratogens at various developmental stages, including cellular differentiation, cell–cell interactions, and cellular migration. This method is valuable particularly as a rapid pre-screen for chemical teratogenicity and can provide mechanistic information as well.

Numerous types of **organs and tissues** in culture have been used in teratological studies, including palate, limbs, kidneys, sex organs, and skin. This method adds more dimensions to the developmental processes tested in cellular cultures. The explanted organ primordium consists of heterogeneous tissue components that progress through the organogenetic stages, thereby providing a measure of several developmental processes.

**Whole embryos** from mice, rats, or rabbits can be removed from the uterus at various developmental stages and cultured in vitro. This method permits a more comprehensive evaluation of the developmental process than the other in vitro systems. However, substantial facilities are required and the technique is labour-intensive and time-consuming. The embryo culture technique is suited ideally for mechanistic studies of chemical teratogenesis, but it is not readily applicable to general teratological screening of large numbers of chemicals.

A number of non-mammalian life forms, such as *Hydra attenuata,* have been developed as **artificial embryos.** The adult *Hydra* are sheared into small pieces of tissue and compressed by centrifugation into an artificial "embryonic pellet." This pellet "embryo" will develop into multiple adults within 1 week, undergoing a remarkable range of complex developmental processes somewhat analogous to mammalian prenatal development. Such model systems are useful in detecting teratogenic potential for large numbers of chemicals in a fairly quick and inexpensive manner.

## CLINICAL APPLICATION

There are several textbooks or chapters dealing with the clinical approach to maternal and fetal toxicology, including teratogenesis (Koren, 2001; Schardein, 2000; Lemire and Shepard, 2004), some of which are updated regularly. In the clinical setting, often the major dilemma is to determine whether the drug or environmental chemical to which the pregnant woman is or was exposed is potentially teratogenic in humans and, if so, the likelihood of having an abnormal child. Unfortunately, despite the substantial teratological database for animal models, the human risk is established for only a relatively small number of teratogens that are highly potent in humans and/or cause abnormalities rarely observed in the general population. For less potent human teratogens, which likely include most xenobiotic exposures, little is known about the human determinants of susceptibility that may render a relatively small number of fetuses highly susceptible.

However, journal reports of individual associations of a xenobiotic with fetal anomalies often are published as case reports or letters to the editor. While useful in identifying important areas requiring more intensive human research, including the use of essential controls, such unsubstantiated reports may be used erroneously as proof of teratogenicity, resulting in unnecessary abortions and lawsuits claiming improper practices of clinicians or the pharmaceutical or chemical industries and in the unwarranted withdrawal of safe drugs from the market.

During a pregnancy, the decision of a family is further complicated by the fact that, even with exposure to a known human teratogen, not all pregnant women will give birth to an abnormal child. Unfortunately, as with weaker teratogens, the determinants of susceptibility in humans are unknown, and hence there are no prenatal tests to guide family decisions. The scientific and practical complexities underlying such decisions, together with a growing public interest in this information, have led to the establishment of several centres around the world composed of multidisciplinary teams of clinicians and

| TABLE 68-3 | In Vitro Tests for Screening Teratogenic Chemicals |
|---|---|
| **Biological Unit** | **End Points Measured** |
| Virus | Plaque-forming units |
| Bacteria | Growth rate |
| Tumour cell | Number attached to surface |
| Prechondrocytes (chick, rodent) | Colonies formed and staining with Alcian blue |
| Neural crest cells (chick) | Morphogenesis of cell |
| Embryonic stem cells (mouse) | Differentiation and cytotoxicity |
| Palate mesenchyme (human) | Morphogenesis of cell |
| *Hydra attenuata* | Regeneration of adults from tissue fragments |
| Planaria | Regeneration of organ systems from fragments |
| *Drosophila* | Maturation of larvae or colonies formed from disrupted embryo |
| *Xenopus laevis* eggs | Malformations in embryos grown from eggs |
| FETAX (frog embryo teratogenesis assay) | Midblastula stage *Xenopus* embryos assessed for viability, growth, morphology |
| Fish eggs | Malformations in free-swimming hatchlings |
| Limb bud | Morphological and biochemical increments |
| Whole embryo (rodent) | Increase in somites, crown length, protein, DNA, and malformations |
| Chick embryo | Malformation |

(From Shepard TH, et al. Teratology testing: I. Development and status of short-term prescreens. II. Biotransformation of teratogens as studied in whole embryo culture. In: MacLeod SM, Okey AB, Spielberg SP, eds. *Developmental Pharmacology*. New York, NY: AR Liss; 1983:147; and Rogers JM, Kavlock RJ. Developmental toxicology. In: Klaassen CD, ed. *Toxicology: The Basic Science of Poisons*. 6th ed. New York, NY: McGraw-Hill; 2001:351-386.)

biological and social scientists who can provide comprehensive and up-to-date advice to both families and clinicians on the reproductive effects of xenobiotics and physical dangers such as radiation (Koren, 2001).

# SUGGESTED READINGS

Halliwell B, Gutteridge JMC. *Free Radicals in Biology and Medicine.* 3rd ed. New York, NY: Oxford University Press; 1999.

Juchau MR, ed. *The Biochemical Basis of Chemical Teratogenesis.* New York, NY: Elsevier/North-Holland; 1981.

Juchau MR, Boutelet-Bochan H, Huang Y. Cytochrome P450-dependent biotransformation of xenobiotics in human and rodent embryonic tissues. *Drug Metab Rev.* 1998;30:541-568.

Kappus H. Overview of enzyme systems involved in bioreduction of drugs and in redox cycling. *Biochem Pharmacol.* 1986;35:1-6.

Kavlock RJ, Daston GP, eds. *Drug Toxicity in Embryonic Development.* Handbook of Experimental Pharmacology. Vol 124. Pts I and II. Heidelberg, Germany: Springer-Verlag; 1997.

Korach KS, ed. *Reproductive and Developmental Toxicology.* New York, NY: Marcel Dekker; 1998.

Koren G, ed. *Maternal-Fetal Toxicology: A Clinician's Guide.* 3rd ed. New York, NY: Marcel Dekker; 2001.

Lemire RJ, Shepard TH. *Catalog of Teratogenic Agents.* 11th ed. Baltimore, Md: Johns Hopkins University Press; 2004.

Manson JM, Kang YJ. Test methods for assessing female reproductive and developmental toxicology. In: Hayes AW, ed. *Principles and Methods of Toxicology.* 3rd ed. New York, NY: Raven Press; 1994:989-1037.

Marnett LJ. Prostaglandin synthase mediated metabolism of carcinogens and a potential role for peroxyl radicals as reactive intermediates. *Environ Health Perspect.* 1990;88:5-12.

Neubert D, Barrach HJ, Merker HJ. Drug-induced damage to embryo or fetus. In: Grundmann E, ed. *Drug-Induced Pathology.* New York, NY: Springer-Verlag; 1980:242-331.

Rogers JM, Kavlock RJ. Developmental toxicology. In: Klaassen CD, ed. *Casarett & Doull's Toxicology: The Basic Science of Poisons.* 6th ed. New York, NY: McGraw-Hill; 2001:351-386.

Schardein JL. *Chemically Induced Birth Defects.* 3rd ed. New York, NY: Marcel Dekker; 2000.

Wells PG. Analgesics: direct embryopathic effects, and indirect biochemical effects modulating the teratogenicity of other drugs and chemicals. In: Kacew S, Lock S, eds. *Toxicologic and Phar-*

930 | PART X: SPECIAL TOPICS OF PHARMACOLOGY

*macologic Principles in Pediatrics.* New York, NY: Hemisphere Publishing Corp; 1988:127-166.

Wells PG, Bhuller, Y, Chen CS, et al. Molecular and biochemical mechanisms in teratogenesis involving reactive oxygen species. *Toxicol Appl Pharmacol.* 2005;207(2 suppl):s354-s366.

Wells PG, Kim PM, Nicol CJ, Parman T, Winn LM. Reactive intermediates. In: Kavlock RJ, Daston GP, eds. *Drug Toxicity in Embryonic Development.* Handbook of Experimental Pharmacology. Vol 124. Pt I. Heidelberg, Germany: Springer-Verlag; 1997:451-516.

Wells PG, Winn LM. Biochemical toxicology of chemical teratogenesis. *Crit Rev Biochem Mol Biol.* 1996;31:1-40.

Wilson JG. Current status of teratology. In: Wilson JG, Fraser FC, eds. *Handbook of Teratology.* Vol 1. New York, NY: Plenum Press; 1977:47-74.

## ONLINE RESOURCES

Motherisk (Toronto Hospital for Sick Children, Canada):
http://www.motherisk.org

Society of Toxicology (United States):
http://www.toxicology.org (see Resources > Sites of Interest)

Teratology Society (United States):
http://teratology.org (see Links > Toxicology and Teratology Databases and Literature)

# 69

# Behavioural Pharmacology

## LA GRUPP AND H KALANT

Behavioural pharmacology refers to the study of the changes in behaviour produced by a drug and the mechanisms by which the drug produces those changes. Such research draws on the knowledge and techniques of a number of different disciplines, including anatomy, biochemistry, pharmacology, physiology, and psychology. Since human behaviour differs in important ways from that of laboratory animals, new behaviourally active drugs must ultimately be tested in humans. However, initial screening is done in various species, including rats, mice, cats, dogs, monkeys, and others. This chapter gives an overview of the types of procedures used in such screening studies. More detailed descriptions of the experimental procedures can be found in a behavioural pharmacology handbook such as that by van Haaren (see Suggested Readings at end of chapter).

The study of drug effects on learned behaviours and on certain instinctive or naturally occurring ones, such as locomotion, food and water intake, and aggressive and sexual behaviour, requires accurate and reliable methods for quantifying the rates and patterns of these behaviours and sufficient control over the environment to minimize disturbing influences. All these measures are first carried out in the absence of drugs in order to provide a stable control or baseline level of performance, against which drug effects can be compared and quantified. The following two sections identify some of the behaviours referred to later and describe the techniques used to measure them.

## TYPES OF BEHAVIOURS STUDIED

### General Central Nervous System Screening

Before experimental drugs are put through exhaustive testing for therapeutic efficacy, they are run through a series of general tests to explore the range of their effects. This series typically includes tests of sensory and motor functions, reflexes, and cognitive functions. For example, in the rota-rod motor test, a laboratory rat is placed on a slowly rotating wooden rod. Untreated animals are easily able to maintain their balance on the rod, but some behaviourally active drugs can make the animals unable to maintain balance. Similarly, the moving belt is an apparatus that resembles a moving walkway on which the animal must pace at the right speed to avoid being pushed off on to a shock grid; thus, it tests motor coordination. Startle threshold tests measure the minimum intensity of a sudden noise or electrical stimulus required to startle the animal and cause it to jump or flinch. Anxiety in laboratory rats can be measured by seeing whether they avoid entering the unwalled (i.e., unprotected) arms of an elevated runway from which it would be possible to fall (see "Elevated plus maze" below). Similarly, if presented with an anxiety-provoking object, rats will attempt to hide, cover, or bury the object when given the opportunity to do so. Such "defensive burying" will also occur in response to anxiogenic medication and be reversed when anxiolytic drugs are given. Cognitive functions (e.g., learning, memory) are examined by such tests as the ability of the animals to learn to solve a maze problem in order to win a food reward or avoid a punishment.

There are many different types of maze tests used for this purpose, such as the Y- or T-maze, the series of Hebb mazes of graded difficulty, and the Barnes escape maze, but one of the most widely used is the Morris water maze, which is a test of learning and spatial memory. In this test, a rat is placed into a tank of water in which it must swim. It can rest by locating and climbing on to a small platform placed just below the surface of the water. Over the course of repeated trials, it learns to locate the platform rapidly by using spatial reference points. Memory is then tested after a period of time by seeing how rapidly and directly it heads for the platform. The test can then be extended by changing the location of the platform and forcing the animal to re-learn it. The effects of various drugs on this whole process can then be evaluated.

## Instinctive Behaviour

### Locomotion and exploration

Locomotion refers to simple motor activity that forms part of exploratory behaviour or other acts of general movement. It is measured by such means as counting the number of revolutions an animal makes in a running wheel, or the number of sectors traversed during a measured time period in a large open field that has been marked off in a grid pattern. Locomotion might be a goal-oriented behaviour, but exploration invokes a motivational component related to curiosity and, as such, can be used to study mood states.

### Sensory function

Since the execution of any behaviour requires the use of one or more senses, drugs that affect sensory function can also affect behaviour. For example, the sensation of pain has been extensively studied by means of the hot-plate and tail-flick tests. Typically, a rat or mouse is placed with its paws on a metal plate warmed to about 50°C, or the tail is immersed in very warm water, and the latency to retract a paw or the tail, respectively, is measured. The test drug is given, and the procedure is repeated at various times after the dose. The drug effect is measured as the difference in latency between the pre-drug baseline and the post-drug tests.

### Food and water intake

Food selection and total amount of food and water consumed, either per day or per meal, are measured. With the aid of computer programs, the pattern of consumption can be analyzed in much finer detail. Again, the drug effect is measured as the change in food consumption patterns from pre-drug baseline.

### Aggressive behaviour

This can be measured by placing two or more animals together in a cage and counting the number of spontaneous attacks or the number of times an animal assumes a dominant or submissive posture. However, most laboratory animals tend to be bred for docility, so that aggressive behaviour needs to be elicited. For example, one can induce animals to fight by placing them on a grid that delivers an irritating but non-damaging electrical current to the paws. In this shock-induced aggression model, one can measure posturing and the number of attacks and bites. Alternatively, isolation for periods of more than 2 to 3 weeks produces a hypersensitivity to physical stimuli that leads to attack and fighting. Finally, aggressive behaviour towards a particular target (usually another male of the species) can be elicited by certain drugs such as the dopamine agonists apomorphine and amphetamine or by electrical stimulation of certain limbic brain regions such as the septum or amygdala. Most aggressive behaviour occurs in males and is modulated to a large degree by testosterone.

### Sexual behaviour

Receptive females are made available to their male counterparts, and the frequency of sexually related behaviours of both the female (the lordosis posture) and the male (mounting, intromission, ejaculation) is measured. Drug-treated animals can be compared with placebo-treated animals with respect to the frequency of these behaviours.

### Ethological methods in behavioural pharmacology

Ethology is the evolutionary study of behaviour in different species in natural environmental contexts. Although most behavioural studies of drug action monitor changes in learned behaviours, much can be gleaned from the study of drug effects on the species-specific manifestations of instinctive behaviours related to sex, maternal behaviour, aggression, foraging for food, and social interactions. For example, the bonding of newborn mice or ducklings to their mothers or the species-specific patterns of aggressive and defensive behaviours between males can be studied in the presence and absence of drugs. The administration of mood-altering drugs will produce a variety of changes in these behaviours that can be documented and related back to the central actions of the drugs. The quantitative measurement of these behaviours is usually done by analysis of audio and video records of the events that occurred so that the patterns will not be altered by direct intervention of the experimenter.

## Learned Behaviours

Many types of learning tasks have been used to test the effects of drugs. For example, the effect of cannabis has been tested in rats learning to find their way through a series of mazes of increasing complexity to earn a food reward at the exit from each maze. However, two special types of learning that have been very extensively used in drug studies are classical conditioning and operant conditioning.

### Classical conditioning

This kind of training or learning procedure is best illustrated by reference to a well-known experiment with dogs by the Russian physiologist I.P. Pavlov. A tuning fork was sounded, followed seconds later by the presentation of some powdered food. Dogs salivate when food is presented to them. Initially, the sound did not elicit any salivation; however, after a number of pairings, the sound came to elicit salivation. The dog had learned that the sound predicted the presentation of food and had learned to salivate at the sound in preparation for the food. In the language of learning theory, the sound was the **conditional stimulus (CS)**, which initially did not elicit an **unconditional response** (UCR, salivation), but which, through repeated association with the food (**unconditional stimulus, UCS**), came to elicit the salivation as a **conditional response (CR)** in the absence of food. The effect of drugs on the acquisition and maintenance of this conditional response can be studied.

### Operant conditioning

This type of learning involves a procedure whereby the probability of occurrence of some particular behaviour can be either increased or decreased, depending upon the consequences of the behaviour. For example, if a food pellet is presented to a hungry animal every time it presses a lever, it is highly likely that the animal will repeat its lever-pressing behaviour and thereby obtain food pellets until its hunger is satisfied. The lever press is termed an **operant response** because the animal operates on its environment to change it in some biologically significant way; the food pellet is termed a **positive reinforcer** because it reinforces or strengthens the behaviour that resulted in its presentation (i.e., the lever-press response). The whole process is termed **positive reinforcement**. Similarly, if a lever press *prevents* the presentation of an *unpleasant* stimulus (e.g., an air blast), the lever press is again termed an *operant;* the air blast is termed a **negative reinforcer** because it strengthens the response that prevents the unpleasant event. The whole process is termed **negative reinforcement**. Finally, if the lever press results in the delivery of a painful stimulus (e.g., a foot shock), the animal is reluctant to perform the response again. The process is called **punishment,** and the foot shock is the **punisher.** Both positive and negative reinforcement refer to processes that *increase* the probability of the behaviour, whereas punishment *decreases* it.

The animal may be required to make the response according to a specific **schedule of reinforcement**. For example, reinforcers can be presented or avoided either after a specified or variable number of lever-press responses (fixed ratio and variable ratio, respectively) or after a specified or variable period of time has elapsed (fixed interval and variable interval, respectively) since the last presentation of the reinforcer. For example, a fixed-interval 60-second (FI 60) schedule of food reinforcement indicates that a food pellet will be delivered as a result of the first response that occurs at least 60 seconds following the last food delivery. A fixed-ratio 10 (FR 10) schedule indicates that one food pellet will be delivered for every 10 presses of the response lever. These formulae, which specify the relationship between the response and the delivery of the reinforcer, generate very stable and reliable patterns of responding. Drug effects are easily and effectively measured against such stable control levels of behaviour.

The following sections examine (1) the behavioural effects of drugs that alter neurotransmitter function, (2) some of the behavioural factors that determine drug action, (3) the effects of drugs on the processes of learning and memory, (4) the stimulus properties of drugs, (5) behavioural models of mental disorders, and (6) the reinforcing properties of drugs.

## DRUGS, NEUROTRANSMITTERS, AND BEHAVIOUR

When a drug enters the central nervous system (CNS), it alters the ongoing activity of the neurotransmitter systems in different ways that produce behavioural effects. The drug action may take various forms, such as a direct effect on ionic permeability; a change in the release, synthesis, or reuptake of a neurotransmitter; or a direct action on receptor sites. Since different neurotransmitter systems coexist in many brain areas, drug-induced changes in the activity of one system may, by shifting the balance of activity, affect behaviour as much by altering activity in the other systems as by acting directly on its own target system. Thus, in order to establish a causal relationship between behaviour and a particular neurotransmitter system, a number of complementary experimental approaches must be taken.

For example, if a change in behaviour follows a reduction in the level of a neurotransmitter, then (1) blocking the receptor sites for that transmitter should have a similar effect on behaviour, and (2) replacing that neurotransmitter should cause behaviour to return to normal. The remainder of this section examines the relationships between some neurotransmitter systems and behaviour, examines how drugs that modify neurotransmitter function also modify behaviour, and examines how similar behaviours can sometimes be related to the activity of a number of different neurotransmitters.

### Serotonin (5-HT)

Over the past 20 years, seven distinct families of 5-HT receptors have been identified ($5\text{-HT}_1$ to $5\text{-HT}_7$), and at least 15 subpopulations have now been cloned. Specific agonists and antagonists have been developed for many of these receptors, and their use allows a better understanding of the different behavioural effects in which 5-HT is involved. Serotonergic activity is decreased by a number of agents, including synthesis inhibitors (e.g., *p*-chlorophenylalanine, or PCPA), receptor blockers (e.g., ketanserin), agents that interfere with storage (e.g., MDMA), and neurotoxins that selectively destroy serotonin-containing cell bodies (e.g., 5,7-dihydroxytryptamine). In general, **when serotonergic activity is decreased,** a number of behavioural changes occur, including the following examples:

1. Sensitivity to a number of different painful stimuli is increased, as shown by a decrease in the threshold stimulus required to make a rat or mouse escape a hot plate or jump in response to an electric shock.
2. The increased sensitivity to painful shock leads to faster acquisition of an avoidance response by animals.
3. Decreasing 5-HT levels by the administration of reserpine or PCPA, or damaging the serotonin-containing

cell bodies of the entire brainstem raphe nucleus, leads to a suppression of the electroencephalographic (EEG) signs of both slow-wave and paradoxical sleep and produces insomnia. This state may last as long as 2 weeks before compensatory mechanisms restore a more balanced sleep function.

4. When two rats are placed on an electrified grid, they tend to approach, attack, and bite each other (shock-induced aggression). When a mouse is introduced into a rat's cage, the rat may suddenly attack the mouse and kill it by breaking the neck (muricide). These are both considered to be experimental models of aggression. Serotonin depletion, produced by PCPA or by raphe lesions, leads to an increase in these aggressive behaviours.

5. In male rats, serotonin depletion leads to an increase in sex-related behaviours such as mutual grooming, scratching, and sniffing of the genitalia. Castrated males will show a temporary increase in sexual behaviour after injection of PCPA. After serotonin depletion, males will increase the frequency with which they engage in heterosexual activities if a female rat is present or with which they mount other males if no female is present.

In general, agents that **increase serotonergic activity** (such as the monoamine oxidase [MAO] inhibitors or the precursor 5-hydroxytryptophan) antagonize the effects described above and produce analgesia, activation of reward pathways (see "Neurobiology of Reinforcement" below), and facilitation of some types of learning. However, drugs that produce a marked increase in serotonergic activity give rise to a set of abnormal behaviours known as the *serotonin behavioural syndrome*, which includes head-weaving, forepaw-treading, spreading of the hind limbs, flattening of the body against the floor, and rigidly erecting the tail.

In addition, **5-HT agonists** have a marked effect on eating and drinking. They reduce food intake, especially in the form of non-protein calories, and increase water intake. Serotonin reuptake inhibitors, which increase 5-HT concentration at the receptor, have been used clinically to help obese patients lose weight by inhibiting appetite. Finally, agents such as fluoxetine (Prozac), which inhibit the reuptake of serotonin back into the cell, are known to be effective in treating depression and other mood disorders (see Chapter 25).

## Acetylcholine

Two major subtypes of acetylcholine (ACh) receptor, muscarinic and nicotinic, are found in the CNS. Modification of central cholinergic function by agonists (e.g., nicotine, arecoline, carbamylcholine), cholinesterase inhibitors (e.g., physostigmine), and antagonists (e.g., mecamylamine, atropine, scopolamine) (see Chapters 11 and 12) produces a number of characteristic effects on behaviour:

1. Both atropine and physostigmine produce a dissociation between behaviour and the apparent state of consciousness indicated by the EEG pattern. After atropine, the animal is behaviourally awake, but its EEG shows a sleeping pattern. Physostigmine, on the other hand, causes the animal to appear to be sleeping, but its EEG is that of an awake animal.

2. Anticholinergic agents usually increase spontaneous locomotor activity, unless this is already elevated prior to drug administration. In that case, either no change, or a decrease in activity, results. Conversely, agents such as physostigmine, which increase cholinergic activity by inhibiting cholinesterase, lead to a decrease in general motor activity.

3. Stimulation of cholinergic synapses in the hypothalamus and limbic system has profound effects on feeding and drinking. Direct application of a cholinergic agonist to these areas produces rapid and copious drinking in water-satiated animals and increases drinking by thirsty animals. These effects can be blocked by the administration of atropine.

4. Physostigmine can disrupt the performance of a previously acquired shock avoidance response, and this disruption can be prevented by pre-treatment with the receptor blocker atropine.

## Catecholamines (Dopamine and Noradrenaline)

As with serotonin, both dopamine (DA) and noradrenaline (NA) receptors have been categorized into distinct families—five for DA and two for NA, each with its own subtypes. Catecholamine levels can be altered by drugs that inhibit synthesis (e.g., $\alpha$-methyl-$p$-tyrosine, or AMPT) or degradation (e.g., MAO inhibitors) of DA and NA, block their reuptake (e.g., cocaine), interfere with their storage (e.g., reserpine), or destroy catecholamine-containing cell bodies (e.g., 6-hydroxydopamine, or 6-OHDA). Additionally, a large variety of selective DA and NA antagonists (e.g., pimozide and phenoxybenzamine, respectively) and agonists (e.g., apomorphine and clonidine, respectively) are also available (see Chapters 11, 13, 14, and 24). The behavioural effects of alteration of catecholamine systems in the brain include the following:

1. Both DA and NA play a role in **locomotor activity**. A decrease in catecholamine levels, as a result of the administration of reserpine or AMPT, leads to a profound decrease in spontaneous locomotor activity, which can be reversed by the administration of their

common precursor, L-dopa. L-Dopa given alone produces an increase in locomotor activity. The relative contribution of DA and NA systems to this behaviour is the subject of much research.

2. Reduction of catecholamine levels by the administration of 6-OHDA decreases the level of **aggression** in animals tested in the shock-induced fighting paradigm. The decrease can be antagonized by the DA agonist apomorphine. The functional relation between catecholamines and 5-HT in the control of aggressive behaviour is not yet known.

3. The application of NA directly to certain areas of the hypothalamus elicits **feeding** in a totally satiated animal. Other α-adrenergic agonists also increase feeding, whereas β-adrenergic agonists decrease it, and each effect can be blocked by the corresponding receptor blocker. It is believed that the α system inhibits satiety and thus turns feeding on, while the β system directly inhibits feeding control centres. DA also plays a primary role in feeding: the selective destruction of DA-containing cell bodies in the striatum can result in both **aphagia** and **adipsia,** to the point where the animals must actually be force-fed to ensure their survival. The relationship among these two neurotransmitter systems and cholinergic and serotonergic systems in the control of food and water intake is not yet fully understood.

4. A variety of drugs that decrease catecholaminergic activity, including inhibitors of synthesis and those that interfere with storage, attenuate the performance of a previously acquired **shock-avoidance** response. This attenuation can itself be reduced by the administration of the precursor L-dopa.

The foregoing lists of behavioural changes produced by modification of neurotransmitter activity merely scratch the surface. They are intended only to illustrate the wide range of behavioural alterations that have been studied and to indicate the complexity of behavioural interactions among the known neurotransmitter systems.

## EFFECTS OF DRUGS ON BEHAVIOUR CONTROLLED BY SCHEDULES OF REINFORCEMENT

One way to examine the effects of drugs on behaviour is to administer a test drug to an animal that is performing a simple, discrete, and easily measurable task and then observe the change in its performance from a pre-drug placebo baseline. The procedures of operant conditioning afford stable behavioural baselines against which drug effects can be meaningfully assessed. Figure 69-1 illustrates this point. Hungry pigeons were trained to peck a key in order to receive brief access to a hopper of grain. The presence of a red light indicated that an FR 30 was in effect, whereas a green light signalled the operation of an FI 5-minute schedule. The appearance of the red and green lights alternated, and the pigeons learned to tailor their response pattern to fit the particular schedule of reinforcement that was signalled by each visual stimulus. They were then tested after an injection of saline and after four different doses of d-amphetamine. Under the FI 5-minute schedule, all four doses of amphetamine increased the response rate, but under the FR 30 schedule, these same doses all reduced responding. Thus, the same dose of d-amphetamine produced opposite effects on responding in the two schedules of reinforcement.

The interpretation of such findings depends upon the type of hypothesis from which one starts. The behavioural mechanisms hypothesis states that drugs act on behaviour by influencing processes involved in either the learning of a new behaviour (such as motivation or memory) or the ability to perform it once it has been learned (e.g., stimulus perception or response output capability). In contrast, the rate-dependency hypothesis states that the *direction* of effect of a drug on the rate of responding (i.e., either increase or decrease) depends on the pre-drug (i.e., saline-tested) rate of occurrence of the behaviour and is independent of the mechanism of action of the drug. If the rate of responding is low before drug, a post-drug increase in the rate is likely to ensue at low and intermediate drug doses. If the pre-drug response rate is high, a post-drug decrease in rate will be found even at low and intermediate doses. Rate-dependent effects occur under schedules of both positive and negative reinforcement and have been seen with barbiturates, benzodiazepines, antipsychotics, and stimulants. As it applies to human psychopharmacology, rate dependency is a viable explanation for the paradoxical sedating effects of amphetamine-like stimulants such as Ritalin in the treatment of attention deficit hyperactivity disorder (ADHD) in children and adolescents.

Although rate of responding is an important determinant of drug action, it is not the only operative factor and therefore should be considered to *modulate* rather than totally determine the effects of drug action. This is highlighted best by a number of studies on the role of anti-anxiety agents in punished responding. Specifically, if rate of responding were the sole determinant of the effect of a benzodiazepine such as diazepam, then at equivalent pre-drug response rates, this agent should increase responding to the same extent, regardless of whether the responding is being punished or not. However, it reliably increases low rates of punished responding more than correspondingly low rates of unpunished responding. Presumably other factors, such as the drug action on the emotional motivational state of the animal, are operating to produce this result.

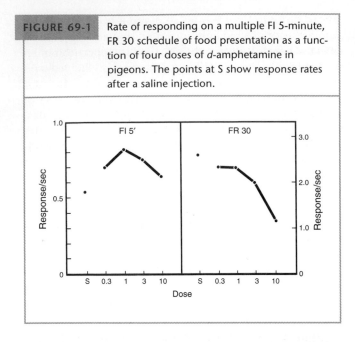

**FIGURE 69-1** Rate of responding on a multiple FI 5-minute, FR 30 schedule of food presentation as a function of four doses of *d*-amphetamine in pigeons. The points at S show response rates after a saline injection.

# DRUG EFFECTS ON LEARNING AND MEMORY

The ability of the brain to modify its output as the result of some previous experience is one of the most important yet least understood of its functions. This modification involves learning and memory. Learning refers to the process by which experiences produce changes in the CNS, ultimately leading to a change in behaviour. The changes in the CNS are collectively referred to as memory and involve registration of information in some manner that permits its later recall into consciousness. Memory involves three separate steps: registration of the information in a transitory short-term memory, its consolidation into a more durable long-term trace, and the eventual retrieval from long-term storage when necessary. Learning involves the selective strengthening or reinforcing of specific neural connections by the presentation of rewarding or aversive stimuli. This effect of a reward involves the activation of a so-called "reward" circuit connecting DA neurons in the ventral tegmentum of the midbrain to the nucleus accumbens in the forebrain via the bundle of axons known as the medial forebrain bundle (MFB). In addition to the dopaminergic axons, the MFB also contains noradrenergic, serotonergic, and other axons, which modulate release of DA from the axon terminals and the sensitivity of the "target" neurons on which the released DA acts. Hence, drugs that block or otherwise alter the actions of these various neurotransmitters can profoundly affect learning. Some agents that influence the processes of learning and memory are considered briefly below.

## Pituitary Peptides

Hypophysectomized animals, which lack adrenocorticotropic hormone (ACTH), show deficits in learning a shock-avoidance response and in inhibiting the response once the shock is discontinued (extinction). The administration of ACTH to these animals normalizes both their learning and extinction of the avoidance response. This effect is not necessarily related to the endocrine action of ACTH, since the effect is obtained with fragments of ACTH (α-melanocyte-stimulating hormone and β-lipotropin) that do not act on the adrenal glands (see Figs. 19-3 and 48-2). These peptides are thought to work by modulating neurotransmitter activity in the brain in such a way as to increase arousal and heighten attention to motivationally relevant stimuli.

Vasopressin acts to *delay* extinction of a learned behaviour such as a shock-avoidance response. This action can also be dissociated from its pressor and antidiuretic effects (see Chapter 44) and is exerted through specific vasopressin $V_1$ receptors in the brain.

## Proconvulsants

Strychnine, which at high doses produces convulsions, acts by blocking postsynaptic inhibition (see Chapter 18), thereby enhancing neuronal transmission. Both pre-trial and post-trial injections of low doses of this drug facilitate the acquisition of a visual discrimination task as well as a maze-learning task. Other proconvulsant drugs, such as picrotoxin, bemegride, and pentylenetetrazol, have similar effects.

## Amphetamine

Amphetamine acts by promoting the release and blocking the reuptake of both DA and NA from nerve endings. Injections of this drug have been reported to improve learning, perhaps through its effects on attentional mechanisms. Yet, its ability to reduce fatigue and increase arousal raises the possibility that the improvement is related more to sustained ability to perform the task than to a real effect on the learning processes. Large doses actually impair learning by causing rapid flight of ideas and an inability to focus the attention on the task at hand.

## Cholinergics and Anticholinergics

The turnover of acetylcholine in the rat hippocampus is increased while the animal is learning a new task to obtain a food reward. Conversely, anticholinergic drugs such as atropine and scopolamine impair learning. Drugs that increase cholinergic activity, such as physostigmine, have been reported to facilitate learning. These effects are of central origin, since the quaternary derivatives that do not pass the blood–brain barrier (e.g., atropine methylbromide) are ineffective. As with amphetamine, the facilitation is presumed to be related to improved attention.

## Protein Synthesis Inhibitors

Memories appear to be encoded partly by changes in the composition, quantity, or concentration of RNA in nerve cells. In turn, these changes in RNA would direct the synthesis of different amounts or types of protein. The changes in both RNA and protein may be important for memory processes. Indeed, RNA synthesis and metabolism are both increased in trained animals compared with untrained ones. Modern subcellular labelling techniques have shown that during the course of learning a new task, there is an increase in protein synthesis in the specific synapses that are involved in the performance of the task. Much evidence suggests that associative learning (Pavlovian conditioning) involves, among other things, increased production of protein kinase C in the cell body and its transport to the specific synapses at which the conditional and unconditional stimuli coincided. Administration of protein synthesis inhibitors (e.g., **puromycin, anisomycin,** and **cycloheximide**) can produce amnesia and impaired retention of a previously learned task. Further research is needed to elaborate fully the role of RNA in memory.

## STIMULUS PROPERTIES OF DRUGS

## Meaning of "Stimulus Properties"

Discriminative stimuli enable an animal to distinguish (discriminate) between two or more situations in which a particular response will have different outcomes. For example, a rat may be trained in an operant chamber to press one of two levers to obtain a small food pellet as a reward. A signal light can then be added as a discriminative stimulus; for example, when the light is on, the rat will be rewarded only for pressing the left-hand lever, but when the light is off, it will be rewarded only for pressing on the right-hand lever. The rat soon learns to discriminate correctly according to the presence or absence of the signal light. Responding is then deemed to be under stimulus control. A mundane example in everyday life is the traffic signal: a green light is the discriminative stimulus for removing one's foot from the brake and placing it on the accelerator to proceed through the intersection in relative safety.

Drugs may also be thought of as stimuli that have some properties in common with visual and other sensory stimuli. For example, each acts on specialized stimulus-specific receptors and causes biochemical reactions that initiate or modify a neuroelectrical response in the CNS. Both an exteroceptive stimulus, such as a light, and an interoceptive stimulus, such as a drug, can act as (1) unconditional stimuli that elicit unconditional reflex responses, (2) conditional stimuli (see "Classical conditioning"), (3) reinforcing stimuli (see "Operant conditioning"), or (4) discriminative stimuli that set the occasion for a response. The sections below deal with drugs in their role as discriminative stimuli.

## Methods of Study

Discriminative stimulus properties of drugs are usually studied by means of the two procedures described below.

### State-dependent learning

In this procedure, one group of animals is trained to perform a response in the non-drugged condition, while a second group is trained to make this response while under the influence of a certain drug. Once training is complete, the groups are subdivided. Half of the animals in each group are tested in the drugged condition and the other half in the non-drugged condition. If state-dependent learning has occurred, the animals will perform the task correctly only when tested under the same condition (either drugged or non-drugged) as during training. If the drug simply impaired the animal's ability to perform the response, animals of both groups would do worse when tested under drug than when tested without drug.

In a typical experiment, one group of animals is trained to escape a shock by making a right turn in a T-maze while under the influence of pentobarbital, while a second group is trained to turn left when the saline vehicle is given. Upon testing, the first group is observed to make the correct response under pentobarbital but to respond randomly under saline, while the second group responds randomly under pentobarbital and correctly under saline. State-dependent learning has been demonstrated with a wide variety of drugs, including ethanol, pentobarbital, scopolamine, morphine, amphetamine, cannabis, and mescaline.

Similar experiments can be carried out with human subjects using test behaviours that are within the normal human repertoire, for example, pressing one button to earn a cash reward under the influence of a drug and a different button under the influence of placebo.

### Drug-discrimination procedure

In this procedure, animals are trained to make one response after a drug injection and a different response after an injection of either the drug vehicle or a different drug. In effect, the subjective state produced by the effects of the injection is the stimulus that gains control over behaviour.

In an experiment typical of this procedure, an animal pressing a lever while under the influence of a given drug obtains food, but if it presses the lever after getting the saline vehicle, it receives electric shock. Animals given such differential training eventually learn to press under drug and to withhold pressing under saline. Drug discrimination has been shown with the same drugs as state-dependent learning. The difference between drug-discrimination and state-dependent learning lies in the objectives and the training techniques. In drug-discrimination studies, the purpose is to see whether the subjective effects produced by one drug are similar to, or different from, those produced by another drug. Therefore, animals are trained to associate different responses with the different effects of two drugs (or a drug and its vehicle). In state-dependent learning, the purpose is primarily to see how a specific drug interacts with the learning process; therefore, the animals are trained under the influence of only one drug and then tested either with the same drug or its vehicle. However, drug-discrimination information can also be obtained by testing with a drug other than that used in training; if it also elicits the same response as the training drug, it is assumed to have produced a state similar to that caused by the training drug.

## Generalization Gradients

One way to examine the control exerted by drug stimuli is to determine the drug-generalization gradient associated with that drug. Typically, a discrimination based on a certain drug and dose is established, and testing is then carried out with a number of different doses of the same drug or with a number of different doses of a different drug. In the former case, the purpose is to find out how strong the drug test stimulus has to be for the animal to react to it in the same way as to the training stimulus. In the latter case, the purpose is to see whether the test drug stimulus is perceived as qualitatively similar to, or different from, the training drug stimulus. The results yield a drug-generalization gradient that indicates the strength of responding to different values of a drug stimulus.

Figure 69-2 illustrates a typical generalization gradient for groups of rats trained to press one lever under the influence of a 1.0-mg/kg dose of *d*-amphetamine and to press a second lever under saline. Typically, drug-generalization gradients show a progressive decrease in responding the lower the test dose is in relation to the training dose. At test doses higher than the training dose, response gradients do not drop off but tend to plateau. Figure 69-3 gives drug-generalization gradients for animals trained to discriminate alcohol from saline and then tested with alcohol, a barbiturate, and a benzodiazepine. These gradients illustrate that even drugs of different classes can share

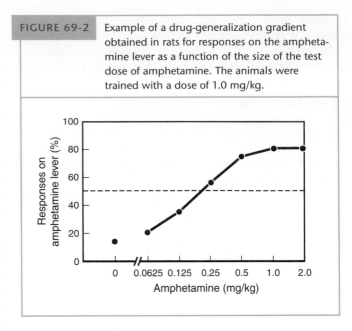

FIGURE 69-2  Example of a drug-generalization gradient obtained in rats for responses on the amphetamine lever as a function of the size of the test dose of amphetamine. The animals were trained with a dose of 1.0 mg/kg.

certain stimulus properties when care is taken to use equivalent doses.

## Discriminability

Drug discriminability is defined operationally as those properties of a drug that render it an effective discriminative stimulus. It can be measured in terms of (1) the speed of acquisition of discrimination and (2) the maximum degree of control of behaviour attained by a drug as the dose is increased (i.e., if drug A at any dose does not exert

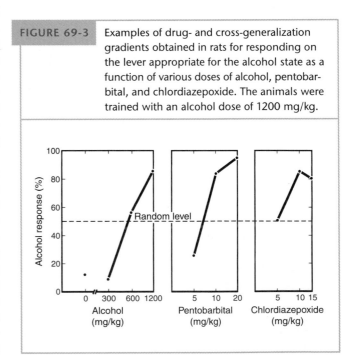

FIGURE 69-3  Examples of drug- and cross-generalization gradients obtained in rats for responding on the lever appropriate for the alcohol state as a function of various doses of alcohol, pentobarbital, and chlordiazepoxide. The animals were trained with an alcohol dose of 1200 mg/kg.

as great a degree of stimulus control as a second drug, B, after similar training histories, then drug B is a more effective discriminative stimulus). Drugs may differ in their discriminability, just as in other effects, in terms of both potency and efficacy (see Chapter 7).

## Mechanisms of Stimulus Control Exerted by Drug Stimuli

A drug must act centrally in order to be readily discriminable. Thus, amphetamine and atropine provide effective discriminative stimuli, but their peripherally acting analogues hydroxyamphetamine and atropine methylbromide do not.

Sensory stimuli may be perceived very differently under the influence of a drug than in its absence or than under the influence of a different drug. These changes may form the basis of drug discrimination.

In order to determine the pharmacological systems involved, animals that have been well trained to discriminate a particular agonist may be tested after pre-treatment with a general antagonist and with a series of specific antagonists for different receptor subtypes. For example, if morphine has been established as a discriminative stimulus, the performance of the animal can be compared after pre-treatment with naloxone and then with specific antagonists of μ, δ, and κ receptor subtypes (see Chapter 19). A difference in the effects of the various antagonists will indicate which receptor subtype is involved in the development of the discrimination. An alternative method is to prevent the acquisition of drug discrimination by interfering with the presumed neurotransmitter mediating the drug effect. For example, if the acquisition of stimulus control by amphetamine is blocked by pre-treatment with the catecholamine-depleting drug AMPT, this would confirm that the discriminative stimuli produced by amphetamine arise from its action of releasing the catecholamines DA and NA from nerve endings.

## BEHAVIOURAL MODELS OF MENTAL DISORDERS

In the development of new drugs for treating disorders in humans, it is usually advantageous to have animal models of those disorders. This applies equally to drugs used for treating emotional disorders and psychoses. Examples of the animal models used for screening potential new drugs of these types are described below.

## Anxiety

A number of animal models are available that generate anxiety-like behaviour and are used to test the anxiolytic properties of drugs.

### Elevated plus maze

An elevated plus maze is an apparatus with four long, narrow arms in the shape of a plus or cross, mounted on a pedestal about 3 to 5 feet above the floor. Two of the arms are completely open; the other two have side walls high enough to block the subject's view of the drop to the floor. Rats instinctively explore their environment, but they are normally reticent to "walk the plank" by entering either of the open arms because of the obvious risk of falling. Instead, they prefer to enter the arms that have protective sides. Anxiolytic compounds, such as the **benzodiazepines,** considerably increase the amount of time that animals will spend exploring the open arms; this effect indicates a reduction in fear or anxiety, and it appears to be specific since other types of psychoactive drugs do not produce this effect.

### Conditioned emotional response

Differences in dimensions of the elevated plus maze can produce different results. Therefore, other behavioural models are also used. One of these is the conditioned emotional response, or CER. In this model, a hungry animal is placed in a small chamber and trained to press a lever to obtain a food pellet. Once this response is learned and reliably performed, a tone or other sensory stimulus is turned on for a short period (usually 2 to 5 minutes) at the end of which one brief foot shock is delivered. Initially, the animal does not associate the stimulus with the imminent foot shock, but after several sessions, it shows a consistent pattern of vigorous lever-pressing in the absence of the stimulus and marked reduction of pressing in the presence of the stimulus. The animal has learned to associate the stimulus with the shock, and the resultant "anxiety" deters it from active lever-pressing. In this model, the administration of benzodiazepines (but not other psychoactive agents) results in a re-emergence of lever-pressing during the stimulus, which indicates a decrease in the animal's state of anxiety.

A variant of the CER procedure is used to study **conflict.** In this situation, the onset of the stimulus indicates that shocks will be delivered each time a food pellet is obtained. The conflict arises because lever-pressing in the presence of the stimulus brings the inseparable combination of food and foot shock. Under these circumstances, the rate of lever-pressing is diminished when the stimulus appears, but anxiolytic agents tend to lessen the conflict and enhance lever-pressing.

## Depression

### Behavioural despair (Porsolt test)

A rat that is placed in a small glass cylinder partly filled with water will attempt to escape by climbing up the sides but is unsuccessful because the glass is smooth and the top of the cylinder is out of reach. After a period of intense effort, the animal appears to "give up" and curls up and floats on the surface of the water. Antidepressant medications, but not other types of psychoactive drugs, reinstate the escape behaviour. This finding led to the use of the test as a screening procedure for new antidepressant medications. The reappearance of the escape behaviour following treatment with the antidepressant does not occur immediately but, as in recovery from depression in humans, is seen only after a period of chronic dosing (see Chapter 25).

## Olfactory bulbectomy

Bilateral removal of the olfactory bulbs produces a constellation of behavioural, associative, and neurochemical changes that resemble some aspects of human depression (Richardson, 1991). Bulbectomized animals are irritable, aggressive, and even hyperactive at times. Their cognitive abilities are impaired, as indicated by difficulty in learning to avoid a foot shock by withholding a response (passive avoidance). These deficits can be significantly attenuated by chronic treatment with antidepressant drugs, but not by other classes of psychoactive drugs. While the olfactory bulbs have obvious important sensory functions, it is thought that their involvement in affective functions is related to their direct synaptic connections with a number of important limbic structures such as the hippocampus, amygdala, and septum (see Chapter 16). These areas are known to modulate the development and expression of emotional behaviour. Furthermore, bulbectomy reduces the levels of a number of important neurochemicals in these structures, including DA, NA, serotonin, and acetylcholine. These transmitters are known to be involved in the elaboration of emotional behaviour and are important targets for antidepressant medication.

## Chronic mild stress

Animals that are continuously exposed to a series of changing and unpredictable low-level stressors develop behavioural deficits that resemble some of the symptoms of endogenous depression. Such stressors include periods of deprivation of food, water, or sleep; cage tilting; introduction of a strange animal; and periods of loud noise or unpredictable mild electric shock. The behavioural deficit is best described as a state of *anhedonia,* or flatness of affect, marked by a relative indifference to stimuli that are normally rewarding. For example, rats normally prefer and seek out highly palatable substances such as sucrose or saccharin, or they will learn to press a lever to obtain delivery of a low-level electric stimulus to the reward system of the brain (see "Neurobiology of Reinforcement" below). Animals exposed to chronic mild stress no longer respond as avidly to these stimuli. However, their responses return toward normal during chronic treatment with antidepressant drugs.

## Schizophrenia

Of all mental disorders, schizophrenia is undoubtedly the hardest to model in animals because it is an illness marked by disordered thought, delusions, hallucinations, ambivalence, and incongruous affect. These symptoms appear to be uniquely human and would be very difficult to model in other species. However, the paranoid ideation and hallucinations produced in humans by high doses of amphetamine or cocaine have led to a closer examination of the effects of high-dose **psychostimulants** in animals. One of the most frequently observed effects is stereotypic behaviour, defined as the focused and continuous repetition of apparently purposeless behaviours such as licking, sniffing, gnawing, and repetitive circling activity. These appear to be analogous to certain repetitive behaviours produced by high doses of psychostimulants in humans. In general, antipsychotic drugs that control many of the schizophrenic symptoms in humans also block these stimulant-induced stereotypic behaviours in animals. This finding is the basis for the use of this model to screen potential new antipsychotic drugs.

# GENETICALLY ALTERED ANIMALS AS BEHAVIOURAL MODELS

Genetic techniques can be applied to the study of behavioural actions of drugs. For example, molecular biology technology now permits the genetic code of specific genes to be altered by inserting foreign DNA into the cell, thereby deactivating genes and blocking production of their products. Animals with this "gene knockout" can then be bred, and their offspring studied. Alternatively, a gene from one species can be transferred into a different species that does not normally express the gene, thus producing "transgenic" species. This approach has been used primarily with mice, and very little with rats. Careful examination of the behavioural consequences of these procedures can lead to better understanding of the functions of the gene and its biochemical products. For example, the serotonin transporter is a regulator of serotonin uptake by the cell. Knockout mice lacking both copies of this transporter gene will have an excess of serotonin in the synaptic cleft and thus an increase in serotonergic activity. Behavioural tests pertaining to serotonergic drugs can then be conducted in these animals.

A related procedure is the selective breeding of behavioural traits. For example, male and female animals that have a propensity to consume large amounts or small amounts of alcohol can be selectively mated. After a number of generations of selective breeding, the offspring will differentially display high or low levels of alcohol consumption. The two lines can then be tested for the effects of drugs that modify the respective drinking behaviours and the interaction of drugs and selected environmental factors. In the same way, other genetic selections such as selectively bred high- and low-anxiety mice, or animals prone or resistant to alcohol withdrawal seizures, can be used to investigate drug actions on these behaviours.

## DRUGS AS REINFORCERS

As seen in the previous sections, psychoactive drugs have stimulus properties of their own, can alter ongoing behaviour maintained by positive and negative reinforcement, and can influence basic biological functions such as eating, drinking, sleeping, and learning. However, drugs can also modify behaviour by acting as reinforcers or punishers in their own right. If a certain behaviour (e.g., pressing a lever) results in the intravenous infusion of a psychoactive drug, the consequences of that drug exposure may reinforce the preceding behaviour (i.e., increase the probability that the animal will go back and press the lever again) or may punish it (i.e., decrease the probability of pressing the lever again, or stop it altogether). Psychomotor stimulants (e.g., cocaine, amphetamine), opioids (e.g., heroin, morphine), and some CNS depressants and anxiolytics (e.g., pentobarbital, diazepam) are positive reinforcers and can generate avid self-administration by animals and humans. The reinforcing properties of these drugs are believed to contribute to their risk of generating drug dependence or abuse (see Chapter 70).

In contrast, neuroleptics (e.g., chlorpromazine, haloperidol), tricyclic antidepressants (e.g., amitriptyline), opioid antagonists (e.g., nalorphine), and hallucinogens (e.g., LSD, mescaline, THC) are not self-administered by animals and can act as punishers (i.e., cause avoidance of the behaviour that results in self-administration) or negative reinforcers (i.e., strengthen behaviour that results in removal of the drug). Caffeine, nicotine, and ethanol act as positive reinforcers under certain circumstances, but also act as punishers under other conditions, especially in nonhuman subjects.

These latter examples illustrate an important limitation of the assessment of drug abuse potential in animals: *All drugs that are readily self-administered by animals also show dependence or abuse potential in humans, but not all drugs that generate such problems in humans are readily self-administered by animals.* Ideally, therefore, one would wish to study dependence liability directly in humans, but this is difficult for various reasons, including ethical concerns about administering potentially dangerous or addicting drugs to humans and the presence of confounding variables such as uncontrolled differences in nutritional status, cultural and psychological background, and previous drug experience. For these reasons, studies of drug self-administration in experimental animals are still important in the investigation of abuse and dependence liability of a drug. Various methods have been developed for this purpose.

In the experimental analysis of drug-taking behaviour, drug-taking is viewed as an operant response that is reinforced by the effects of the drug. These reinforcing effects may then motivate further drug-taking behaviour by themselves, independently of the reasons for the initial drug-taking. However, most drugs also have some unpleasant, punishing (aversive) effects, even in the same range of dosage that produces reinforcement. The strength of reinforcement by a drug in a given individual therefore depends on the balance between reinforcing and punishing effects.

Drugs differ in the strength of their direct positive reinforcing properties. It is much more likely for experimental animals to acquire a high level of self-administration of cocaine, amphetamine, or heroin than of alcohol or cannabis, and they are extremely unlikely to acquire such behaviour toward LSD or mescaline. Such differences may account for the common but misleading distinction between "hard drugs" and "soft drugs."

There are a number of theories pertaining to the development of drug addiction or the transition from drug-taking to drug addiction. The *Pleasure, Withdrawal, and Opponent Theory* emphasizes that drugs are first taken because their effects are pleasant but that repeated drug use leads to tolerance and dependence such that unpleasant withdrawal symptoms ensue upon the cessation of use. Compulsive drug-taking is therefore maintained to avoid unpleasant withdrawal symptoms. The *Aberrant Learning Theory* suggests that drugs produce abnormally strong or aberrant associations involved in reward learning, more powerful than natural reward associations. Finally, the *Incentive-Sensitization Theory* focuses on how drug-related cues trigger excessive incentive motivation for drugs, leading to compulsive drug-seeking, drug-taking, and relapse. The central idea is that addictive drugs alter brain systems, which become enduringly hypersensitive (or "sensitized") to specific drug effects and to drug-associated stimuli. The drug-induced brain change is called neural sensitization and leads psychologically to excessive attribution of salience to stimuli related to drug presentation, causing a pathological "wanting" to take drugs.

## Methods of Studying Drug Reinforcement

**Oral self-administration** can be produced quite simply by putting the drug in the food or the drinking water so that the animal is forced to consume the drug while satisfying its physiological need for food or water. However, such obligatory consumption tells us nothing about the reinforcing properties of the drug and is not relevant to the human situation in which a choice is almost always available. Therefore, the appropriate animal models include a choice between drug solution and water, and consumption is measured in terms of both absolute amount of drug ingested and relative volumes of drug solution and water consumed.

**Intravenous self-administration** involves the implantation of an indwelling venous catheter, connected via a motor-driven infusion pump to a reservoir of drug solution. When the animal presses a lever that closes the pump circuit, the pump is activated and delivers a preset dose from the reservoir. Programmable equipment allows the experimenter to control the number and spacing of lever presses required to activate the pump. This setup is illustrated in Figure 69-4. One advantage of the intravenous route is that the taste of the drug, which is often aversive to animals, is no longer a problem. A second advantage is that the drug effect is usually very rapid in onset, so that if the drug has primary reinforcing properties, they can be demonstrated more easily. It is not necessary to have a second catheter and pump for water, since the animal can drink water normally.

Both oral and intravenous methods can be used to study the factors that control drug self-administration.

Intravenous studies are particularly useful for investigating primary reinforcing properties of drugs (i.e., their ability to generate repeated self-administration without the need for other external inducements). This is often referred to as their abuse potential. Central stimulants, such as cocaine and amphetamine, are the most potent in this regard. Morphine and heroin are quite effective, but the newer agonist–antagonist opioids (see Chapter 19) are not. Some barbiturates, benzodiazepines, nicotine, and methaqualone are moderately effective, but alcohol is only weakly and unreliably reinforcing in this type of experiment. Cannabinoids and hallucinogens such as LSD and mescaline are aversive; after experiencing their effects, the animal will not press the lever again.

It is common practice to train the animals to self-administer cocaine and then to substitute a test drug that is under study. If the animal continues to self-administer this drug with a response rate greater than for saline, the drug is considered to be reinforcing. The relative abuse potential of different drugs (i.e., their relative strengths of reinforcement) can be assessed by the **progressive-ratio method.** After a stable response rate has been established

---

**FIGURE 69-4** Schematic representation of the apparatus for investigating reinforcing properties of drugs by the self-administration model in experimental animals (monkeys). Similar set-ups have been used with rats and other species.

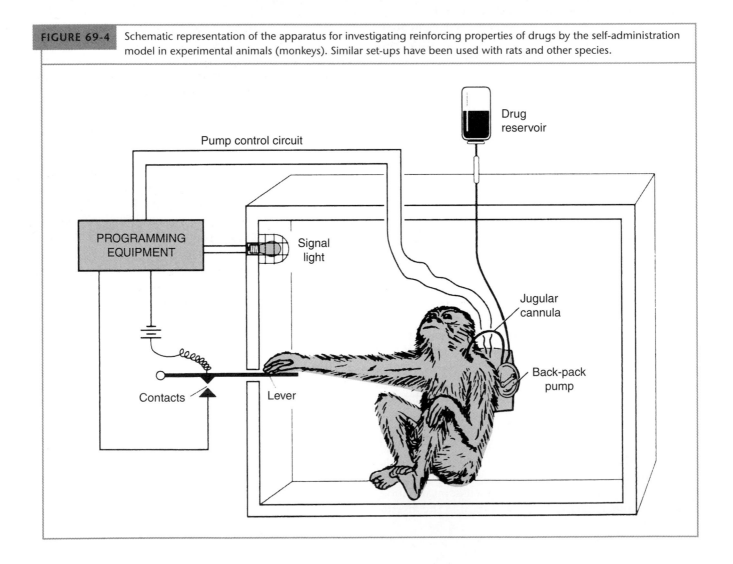

on a fixed-ratio schedule, the ratio (i.e., the number of lever-presses required to obtain one reward) is systematically increased in logarithmic steps. This makes the subject work progressively harder for the same amount of drug. The break point—the ratio value at which drug self-administration ceases or falls below some defined criterion—is a measure of the reinforcing strength of that drug under those particular experimental conditions: the higher the break point, the greater the reinforcing strength. The break points for different drugs under the same conditions provide a ranking of the relative reinforcing strengths of the drugs.

## Neurobiology of Reinforcement

The anatomy of the reinforcement system was first uncovered in 1954 by James Olds and Peter Milner, who were researchers at McGill University in Montreal. They observed that animals would learn to press a lever to self-administer brief trains of low-intensity electric current to the hypothalamic area. At times, the rate of lever pressing was so robust that only exhaustion would interrupt it. Subsequent research identified the *medial forebrain bundle* (MFB) as the most effective site for this "self-stimulation" and as one of the neural circuits involved in reinforcement.

The MFB is a bundle of axons running from the midbrain to the basal forebrain and connects many limbic, hypothalamic, and midbrain structures with one another. It contains ascending catecholaminergic (i.e., DA- and NA-releasing) and serotonergic neurons. The midbrain dopaminergic system has been closely linked to the mechanism of reinforcement, particularly the dopaminergic axons that arise from cell bodies in the *ventral tegmentum* near the substantia nigra and synapse with cells of the *nucleus accumbens* located just in front of the hypothalamic preoptic area. A variety of studies have shown that reinforcement produced by food, water, drugs of abuse, and even sexual behaviour can be modulated by pharmacological manipulation of this tegmental–accumbens dopaminergic pathway. However, though the different reinforcers all activate this pathway, there is clear selectivity in that they activate different populations of DA neurons within it. Thus, cocaine, for example, inherently activates different DA neurons acting on different accumbens targets than water does.

Pharmacological manipulation is possible because the dopaminergic pathway is subject to a wide variety of facilitatory and inhibitory influences exerted by other neurotransmitters that act upon it. Among the most clearly identified are opioid, GABA, and noradrenergic fibres that form

---

**FIGURE 69-5** Schematic representation of the main known elements of the brain "reward system." GABA = γ-aminobutyric acid; − = inhibitory action; unmarked synapses are excitatory. (Adapted from Koob, 1992 and McBride et al., 1993.)

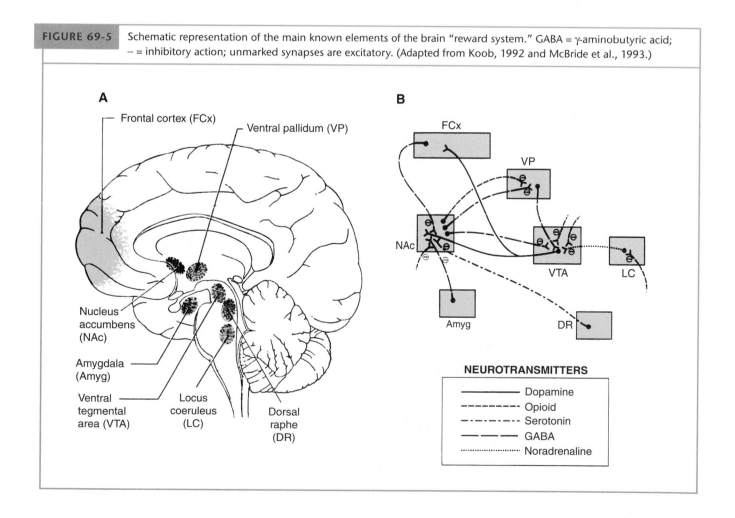

synapses at various points in the dopaminergic pathway. Knowledge about this complex interplay of neurotransmitters in the reinforcement process is growing rapidly, and the picture is changing accordingly. A schematic representation of present knowledge is shown in Figure 69-5.

The tegmental pedunculopontine nucleus (TPP) is a brainstem structure that has been identified as an important mediator of drug reward. Lesions of the TPP have been shown to block the rewarding properties of nicotine and opiates as well as the rewarding properties of natural stimuli, including food and sex. It is thought that the TPP influences drug reward through its connections to the ventral tegmental area in the midbrain. It also plays an important role in differentiating between positive drug reinforcement and negative reinforcement by drug withdrawal in the dependent subject (see Chapter 70).

## SUGGESTED READINGS

Bechara A, van der Kooy D. A single brain stem substrate mediates the motivational effects of both opiates and food in non deprived rats but not in deprived rats. *Behav Neurosci.* 1992; 106:351-363.

Berridge KC, Robinson TE. What is the role of dopamine in reward: hedonic impact, reward learning, or incentive salience? *Brain Res Rev.* 1998;28:309-369.

Carelli RM, Wondolowski J. Selective encoding of cocaine versus natural rewards by nucleus accumbens neurons is not related to chronic drug exposure. *J Neurosci.* 2003;23:11214-11223.

Crawley JN. Behavioral phenotyping of transgenic and knockout mice: experimental design and evaluation of general health, sensory functions, motor abilities, and specific behavioral tests. *Brain Res.* 1999;835:18-26.

Deadwyler SA, Hayashizaki S, Cheer J, Hampson RE. Reward, memory and substance abuse: functional neuronal circuits in the nucleus accumbens. *Neurosci Biobehav Rev.* 2004;27:703-711.

Grabowski J. *Psychopharmacology: Basic Mechanisms and Applied Interventions.* Washington, DC: American Psychological Association; 1993.

Katz RJ. Animal model of depression: pharmacological sensitivity of a hedonic deficit. *Pharmacol Biochem Behav.* 1982;16: 965-968.

Koob GF. Drugs of abuse: anatomy, pharmacology and function of reward pathways. *Trends Pharmacol Sci.* 1992;13:177-184.

Koob GF, Heinrichs SC, Britton K. Animal models of anxiety disorders. In: Schatzberg AF, Nemeroff CB, eds. *Textbook of Psychopharmacology.* 2nd ed. Washington, DC: American Psychiatric Press; 1998:133-144.

Landgraf R, Wigger A. High vs. low anxiety-related behavior rats: an animal model of extremes in trait anxiety. *Behav Genet.* 2002;32:301-314.

Leonard BE. *Fundamentals of Psychopharmacology.* Chichester, United Kingdom: John Wiley; 1993.

McBride WJ, Murphy JM, Gatto GJ, et al. CNS mechanisms of alcohol self-administration. *Alcohol and Alcoholism.* 1993;(2 suppl): 463-467.

Olds J, Milner P. Positive reinforcement produced by electrical stimulation of the septal area and other regions of rat brain. *J Comp Physiol Psychol.* 1954;47:419-427.

Palanza P, Morellini F, Parmigiani S, vom Saal FS. Ethological methods to study the effects of maternal exposure to estrogenic endocrine disrupters: a study with methoxychlor. *Neurotoxicol Teratol.* 2002;24:55-69.

Porsolt RD, Anton G, Blavet N, Jalfre M. Behavioural despair: a new model sensitive to antidepressant treatments. *Eur J Pharmacol.* 1978;47:379-391.

Richardson JS. The olfactory bulbectomized rat as a model of major depressive disorder. In: Boulton A, Baker G, Martin-Iverson M, eds. *Neuromethods, Vol 19: Animal Models in Psychiatry, II.* Clifton, NJ: Humana Press; 1991:61-79.

van Haaren F, ed. *Methods in Behavioral Pharmacology.* Amsterdam, Netherlands: Elsevier; 1993.

Wahlsten D, Metten P, Phillips TJ, et al. Different data from different labs: lessons from studies of gene-environment interaction. *J Neurobiol.* 2003;54:283-311.

White NM, Franklin KBJ, eds. The neural basis of reward and reinforcement: a conference in honor of Peter M. Milner. *Neurosci Biobehav Rev.* 1989;13:59-186.

# 70

# Drug Abuse and Drug Dependence

## H KALANT AND LA GRUPP

### CASE HISTORY

Mrs. R.J., a 49-year-old bookkeeper, was referred by her family physician to a drug dependence program for assessment of her heavy use of analgesics and anxiolytics. Five years earlier, she was stopped for a traffic light when her car was hit from behind by a truck. She suffered mild whiplash injury and considerable bruising of her shoulder and knees, but the injuries healed rapidly, and she recovered almost complete function by 2 months later. However, she remained nervous and apprehensive about driving, had difficulty sleeping, and complained of persistent headaches and muscular pains. She gradually became more preoccupied with her symptoms, stopped working, and began to spend more and more time in bed. Her physician had initially prescribed lorazepam for relief of her anxiety and insomnia and acetaminophen with codeine (30 mg) for relief of pain. She had used these in steadily increasing amounts and was now taking the lorazepam four to six times a day and up to 25 tablets of the acetaminophen/codeine combination daily. He strongly urged her to cut down her intake, but she said that she could not, because of severe muscle tension, tooth-grinding, and pounding of her heart if she decreased the doses.

The examining physician at the drug dependence centre did a systematic drug history and learned that she had previously taken AC&C tablets (acetaminophen, caffeine, and 8 mg of codeine) at a rate of up to 50 tablets a day for almost 20 years. Several years before the motor vehicle accident, she had been hospitalized for a suspected suicide attempt with acetylsalicylic acid. She had started smoking cigarettes in her late teens and was currently smoking about 30 a day. She had a chronic cough and respiratory wheezing that was heard on examination, but she denied that these were connected with her smoking habits. A urine screening test carried out at the clinic was also positive for traces of THC, the psychoactive component of marijuana. A family history revealed that her father, one brother, and a maternal uncle had all had problems with excessive drinking of alcohol.

She agreed to take part in a drug withdrawal program but stopped attending after 5 weeks, and her husband found new bottles of acetaminophen–codeine pills in the medicine chest at home. Her physician and her husband are currently seeking advice about alternative methods of convincing her to accept treatment.

## DEFINITIONS OF ABUSE, ADDICTION, AND DEPENDENCE

Since the beginning of the twentieth century, the term "addiction" has been applied to certain patterns of heavy use of psychoactive drugs (e.g., opioids, cocaine, alcohol) that are used primarily for their effects on consciousness, mood, and perception of the internal and external environments. One rarely, if ever, hears of addiction to digitalis, sulfonamides, or warfarin. No fully satisfactory definition of drug addiction has ever been achieved. An Expert Committee of the World Health Organization (WHO) made repeated attempts to define it and differentiate it from "habituation" but was unable to produce definitions that were fully consistent with clinical experience.

For various reasons, it became clear that both terms were unsatisfactory, and the WHO committee recommended that they be replaced by the single term **drug dependence**, which would include varying degrees of intensity of desire for the drug, all degrees of damage to both the individual and society, and all degrees of both physical and psychological need to continue using the drug.

In recent years, there has been a widespread adoption of the term **substance dependence**, in which "substance" is really an abbreviation of *psychoactive substance*. The purpose is to avoid the artificial distinction between alcohol and other drugs, since the major features of dependence are found in all types of drug dependence. The revised fourth edition of the *Diagnostic and Statistical Manual of the American Psychiatric Association (DSM-IV-TR)* defines substance dependence as a maladaptive pattern of substance use, leading to clinically significant impairment or distress, as manifested by three or more of the criteria shown in Table 70-1, occurring at any time in the same 12-month period.

The term *addiction* continues to be widely used, however, both by professionals and by the general public. Because of excessive preoccupation with heroin and other morphine-like drugs, and with the dramatic (but not life-threatening) withdrawal reaction to which they can give rise, there has been a tendency to equate addiction with physical dependence, and even with physical dependence of the opioid type.

In an effort to avoid the confusion caused by these various definitions and concepts, the term **hazardous use** was introduced. This is an operational term based purely on empirical epidemiological considerations, with no implications regarding dependence. It means use of a drug in such amounts and frequency as to carry a significantly greater risk of physical, mental, or social harm than would be expected in the general population of the same age, sex, and socio-economic status. This is a useful term for public health considerations, but there is still a need for mechanistic terms to describe the processes leading to such levels of consumption.

## Drug Abuse

In contrast to the terms "dependence" and "hazardous use," both of which can be defined operationally, drug abuse is essentially a value-judgement term, with different uses and meanings for different people. Some consider it to be synonymous with non-medical use—any use of a drug for other than recognized therapeutic purposes being considered abuse. Yet, even though alcohol is rarely employed therapeutically in modern medicine, most use of alcohol is not considered abuse. Others equate the term with heavy or excessive use, but there is no generally accepted definition of "heavy" or "excessive," and in any case it is not clear how these terms differ from "hazardous use." Still others apply the term "drug abuse" to illicit use, including *any* use of an illicit drug (such as cannabis or LSD) or non-approved use of a licit but restricted drug (such as amphetamine or cocaine).

In reality, *drug abuse means any drug use that the speaker, or society at large, does not approve of.* Because of the subjectivity and vagueness of this concept, many experts in this field believe that the term is useless and should be abandoned. However, like "addiction," "drug abuse" continues to be widely employed even in scientific and clinical publications, and the reader must usually guess what the writer meant by it. Perhaps the best definition (Jaffe, 1985) is the following:

| TABLE 70-1 | *DSM-IV-TR* Criteria for Diagnosis of Substance Dependence* |
|---|---|
| 1. | Tolerance: need for increased amounts of the substance to achieve the desired effect, or markedly decreased effect with the same amount of the substance |
| 2. | Withdrawal: occurrence of a withdrawal syndrome characteristic of the substance in question, or use of the same or a closely similar substance to prevent or relieve this syndrome |
| 3. | Use of larger amounts, or over longer periods, than intended |
| 4. | Persistent desire to cut down or control use, or unsuccessful efforts to do so |
| 5. | Spending of a great deal of time getting and using the substance, or recovering from its effects |
| 6. | Giving up, or reducing, important social, occupational, or recreational activities because of substance use |
| 7. | Continuing use despite knowledge of having persistent or recurrent physical or psychological problems that are likely caused or exacerbated by the substance use |

*Specifiers, that is, items 1 and 2 in the table, indicate whether the dependence is or is not accompanied by physiological dependence. (Based on American Psychiatric Association. Washington, DC; 2000:197-198.)

Drug abuse refers to the use, usually by self-administration, of any drug in a manner that deviates from the approved medical or social patterns within a given culture. The term conveys the notion of social disapproval, and it is not necessarily descriptive of any particular pattern of drug use or its potential adverse consequences.

The term *abuse potential* is used to describe the degree of risk that a drug will be used for non-medical purposes. Its operational measurement and significance are described in Chapter 69.

Regardless of whether one talks of addiction or dependence, the essential feature is not tolerance or physical dependence, but compulsive drug-taking (i.e., an observable behaviour rather than a postulated metabolic alteration). The affected individual, whether human or experimental animal, spends inordinate amounts of time and effort seeking the drug even when it is known not to be available, will work much harder to get the drug when it *is* available, and persists in drug use even when this causes harm to health, personal relations, or function in society, and when the user would want to stop using. This behaviour pattern is often referred to as *psychological dependence*. A somewhat more descriptive term, which will be used in this chapter, is **behavioural dependence**, or stimulus-controlled self-administration of drugs, as explained in the section on behavioural dependence. Many people consider this unimportant because one can be "psychologically" dependent on chewing gum, work, television, and so forth. This is totally wrong. It cannot be emphasized enough: *Behavioural dependence is the central problem in drug addiction, while tolerance and physical dependence are secondary features—consequences of the drug-taking.*

If we accept this concept, the terminology becomes a matter of relatively little importance, and classification of drugs as "addictive" or "non-addictive," or "hard" or "soft," is an oversimplification. It is the interaction among the drug, the user, and the environmental context that determines whether or not dependence arises in a given case. The questions of real concern to the patient and the physician, as well as to society at large, are the following:

1. Why does the user experience a desire or a need to use the drug? In other words, what initiates use, and what keeps it going?
2. How does use turn into dependence?
3. How intense is the dependence and to what extent does it control the user's lifestyle?
4. What are the consequences of this behaviour to the user, to the user's family and immediate associates, and to society at large?
5. How can it be prevented or be reversed if it has already developed?

In order to understand abuse and dependence, it is necessary to examine normal or socially accepted patterns of use of psychoactive substances and then see what differentiates these normal patterns from unacceptable or harmful ones.

# SOCIALLY APPROVED USE OF PSYCHOACTIVE DRUGS

## History of Drug Use

Virtually every society in human history has had at least one psychoactive drug that was used in ways approved by that society and was incorporated into its customs and traditions. The type of drug used was originally a matter of chance, depending on what natural products with suitable pharmacological properties were discovered in the vicinity. The drugs used in pre-industrial societies covered the whole spectrum of psychoactive drug categories. A few examples are given in Table 70-2.

With the development of travel and trade between regions and nations, drugs native to one part of the world have become accepted and highly appreciated in other areas. Common examples are coffee, tea, and tobacco. The development of chemistry and industrial technology led to the isolation of pure active ingredients from natural products and the synthesis of highly potent derivatives, analogues, and substitutes. These are generally much less bulky and more stable than the natural products, and

their use has spread around the world as a function of travel, commerce, education, communication, and availability of money for non-essentials.

Usually, the first members of a society to adopt new drugs from another society are those whose activities bring them into contact with other cultures. Originally, these were often sailors, traders, and explorers. In modern times, business people, diplomats, performing artists, athletes, and university students on foreign fellowships are frequently involved. If they are prestigious figures in their own societies, their new patterns of drug use tend to be quickly imitated by others.

## Social Functions of Psychoactive Drug Use

The universality of drug use and the ease with which one society adopts the drugs of another suggest that drug use must have important social functions. The earliest known role was a **religious** or magical one. The red colour of wine has made it a symbolic substitute for blood in the religious sacraments of many societies, both ancient and modern. The feeling of warmth, due to alcohol-induced vasodilatation, has made it symbolic of the spirit of life itself, as indi-

| TABLE 70-2 | Examples of Psychoactive Substances with Socially Accepted Uses in Various Parts of the World | |
|---|---|---|
| Society | Preparation | Pharmacological Agent or Category |
| Arabia, East Africa | Khat (ĝat) | Cathinone—central stimulant |
| Bolivian Indians | Coca | Cocaine—central stimulant |
| North American Indians | Tobacco | Nicotine—ganglionic cholinergic agonist |
| Indonesia | Betel | Arecoline—like nicotine |
| Southeast Asia | Opium | Morphine and other opioids |
| India, North Africa | Cannabis | Tetrahydrocannabinol (THC)—sedative |
| Amazon Indians | Kaapi, epena | Indole derivatives—hallucinogens |
| Southwest Amerinds | Mescal | Mescaline—hallucinogen |
| Oceania | Kava | Kavapyrones—sedative, anticonvulsant |
| Universal | Beer, wine, etc. | Ethanol—sedative |
| Universal | Coffee, tea | Caffeine—central stimulant |

cated by such names as spirits, eau de vie, akvavit (a Scandinavian rendition of *aqua vitae),* and even whiskey (from the Gaelic for "water of life"). The hallucinogenic effects of peyote, epena, kaapi, and ololiuqui are used in the religious rites of various South and Central American populations to attain an otherworldly state in which contact with the gods or spirits is sought.

At a later stage, drugs were incorporated into **secular ceremonies,** such as passing around the kava bowl at the start of a Polynesian council meeting, smoking the pipe of peace among North American Indians, passing the "joint" at early marijuana parties before its use became widespread, and drinking toasts with alcohol at weddings or other special events.

Such practices led to drugs being used to induce **conviviality** in social gatherings, to increase pleasure, and to facilitate social interaction. In general, the drugs favoured for this type of use have been either stimulants (khat, coffee, coca) or low doses of sedatives that produce disinhibition of behaviour and emotional expression (alcohol, cannabis).

With increasing secularization of a society and progressive loosening of social controls over individual behaviour, drug use for individual **private pleasure** became steadily more common. Drinking wine with meals, smoking a cigarette at coffee break, and drinking caffeine-containing soft drinks as refreshments are among the many examples of such use.

The last stage in the evolution of socially accepted drug use is **utilitarian,** at both individual and corporate levels. Individual utilitarian use is illustrated by the use of alcohol by salesmen who entertain clients during business negotiations or by tense, nervous, depressed, or angry people who drink to feel better or to be able to release sentiments that they are unable to express when sober. Corporate utilitarian use is illustrated by commercial enterprises that create employment and profits from the manufacture, advertising, and sale of alcohol, tobacco, and other drugs and by the governments that gain large revenues from the sale of, and customs duties and taxes on, these items.

## Factors Governing the Extent of Use

The most important factor is the **degree of social acceptance or rejection** of a drug. For example, orthodox Muslims and Mormons do not use alcohol on religious grounds, even though societies around them use large amounts. Muslim society accepted the use of cannabis, whereas European and North American societies still reject it officially, even though large numbers of people use it.

**Social upheaval** or rapid reorganization may suddenly weaken the conventional attitudes that control alcohol or drug use in stable times. If these substances are readily available, major epidemics of excessive use may occur at such times of crisis and disappear when stability

returns. Examples include the "gin epidemic" during the Industrial Revolution in England, the methamphetamine epidemic in Japan after its defeat in 1945, and the heroin epidemic among American troops in Vietnam in the 1960s and 1970s.

Despite common assertions to the contrary, **legal controls** do affect the extent of drug use, but they work most effectively when they are in harmony with the prevailing social values and attitudes. For example, the move to enact Prohibition of alcohol in the United States (by a variety of state and federal measures beginning in 1916 and by constitutional amendment in 1920) was in keeping with popular sentiment before and during World War I. The female suffrage movement and the temperance movement both saw alcohol-related problems as a major factor working against the well-being of women and children and as a threat to young recruits just entering the U.S. armed forces. Therefore, Prohibition was, at first, strongly supported and highly effective in reducing both alcohol consumption and the death rate from alcoholic cirrhosis and other alcohol-related illnesses. Similarly, restriction of hours of sale in pubs in the United Kingdom during World War I produced a sharp reduction in alcohol-related accidents and an increase in industrial productivity.

The law also works as an effective deterrent to drug use if it provides severe penalties, is seen to be strictly enforced, and is enforced with a high degree of probability that offenders will be caught and punished. Alcohol rationing was enforced strictly by the German occupation forces in France during World War II, and this brought about a sharp fall in the death rate from cirrhosis, which rose rapidly again after the liberation of Paris in 1944.

In contrast, the law is not an effective deterrent when it is not in keeping with prevailing attitudes or when it is seen to have a low probability of being applied successfully against the majority of offenders. The eventual failure of alcohol Prohibition in the United States was due largely to public disillusionment with the apparent lack of uniformity, fairness, and effectiveness of enforcement, and the constitutional amendment was repealed in 1932. American and Canadian laws prohibiting the use of cannabis have continued to be supported by the majority of public opinion, and there has been no widespread push for complete legalization of cannabis by outright repeal of these laws as there was for repeal of Prohibition, although the majority of Canadians now favour removing criminal sanctions against possession of small amounts for personal use.

Another important factor is **price,** in *real* or *constant* units, corrected for inflation and expressed in relation to average income and cost of living. In California, Ontario, Trinidad, and other jurisdictions in which studies have been done, there is almost a mirror-image relationship between the time courses of changes in the cost of alcohol (expressed in these terms) and the per capita consumption (Fig. 70-1) and the frequency of various alcohol-related problems, such as the cirrhosis death rate or the

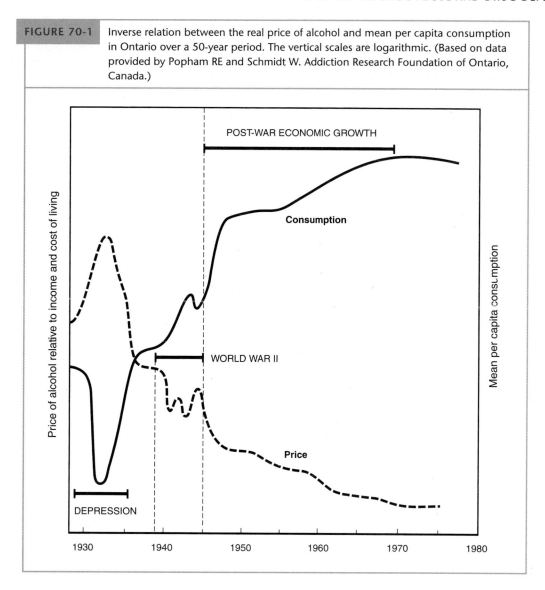

**FIGURE 70-1** Inverse relation between the real price of alcohol and mean per capita consumption in Ontario over a 50-year period. The vertical scales are logarithmic. (Based on data provided by Popham RE and Schmidt W. Addiction Research Foundation of Ontario, Canada.)

frequency of alcohol-related driving accidents. The relatively slow increase in alcohol consumption and cirrhosis death rate in the United States after the repeal of Prohibition in 1933 probably reflects the influence of the severe economic depression at the time. The same inverse relationship between unit price and consumption has been observed for tobacco and for several illicit drugs, including cocaine and heroin.

A closely related factor is **ease of availability.** When liquor stores in Ontario were changed to the self-service type, with all the goods displayed and available in open racks rather than held in a stockroom and brought to the counter by the clerk, the volume of sales rose quite substantially.

Occupational factors often relate to ease of access. For example, employees of breweries, distilleries, wineries, and drinking establishments are at higher risk of alcoholism, and physicians, nurses, and pharmacists are at increased risk of dependence on licit opioids, anxiolytics, and other psychoactive drugs.

**Travel and mass communication** facilitate the spread of drug use by giving large numbers of people the chance to learn about new drug practices. The methamphetamine ("speed") epidemic in Japan was brought to North America by American occupation troops stationed in Japan after 1945. The popularization of cocaine in North America and Western Europe in the past three to four decades has probably been greatly assisted by the enormous publicity and initial glamorization that the drug received in the mass media.

## Relation to Individual Use

It is very important to know how the extent of use of a drug by a whole population is related to the level of use by individual members of that population. Theoretically, for example, the average per capita consumption could increase even if the number of heavy users decreased; this would occur if large numbers of former non-users all began to use small amounts while the smaller numbers of heavy users all used less. In that case, an increase in average per capita consumption might not be a cause for worry. Alternatively, increased per capita consumption might mean that all users, including the heavy users, were consuming more, and this would probably mean a major increase in drug-related problems.

This question is studied by examining the **distribution-of-consumption curve.** If the user population is surveyed and the percentage of users is determined for each interval in a scale of average daily consumption, the results can be plotted in a histogram or on a continuous curve. Conceivably, one might find a bimodal curve, with the large majority of moderate users grouped around one mode near the low end of the consumption scale and a small number of heavy users clustered around a second mode near the high end. This would be the case if heavy users were qualitatively different from moderate users and responded to different controlling factors. In reality, however, the distribution-of-consumption curves for different drugs and populations all prove to be unimodal but skewed, with a large majority of users in the lower range of the scale and smaller and smaller numbers at progressively higher levels of intake (Fig. 70-2).

Even more important, when there is a change in the mean per capita consumption of the whole population, it comes about through a corresponding displacement of the entire curve. Thus, an increased mean consumption reflects an upward shift of the modal level of use, a decrease in the numbers of users below the modal level, and an increase in the numbers above it. This is accompanied by an increased incidence and prevalence of drug-related problems of health, behaviour, and economic function. The opposite happens when the mean per capita consumption falls.

This means that heavy users respond in the same direction as light users do to changes in price, legal status, availability, and social attitudes. This has been demonstrated experimentally in a study employing alcoholic and non-alcoholic volunteers. Half of each group was allowed to buy alcoholic drinks at half price during a "happy hour"; the other half were not. Overall, the alcoholics drank much more than the non-alcoholics, but within each group, the "happy hour" subgroup drank at least twice as much as the regular-price group (Table 70-3).

The conclusion is that *heavy or harmful use of drugs cannot be clearly separated from "normal" drug use.* In other words, the individual and social functions that make psychoactive drug use so universally prevalent carry with them the risk that some individuals or some societies may use too much and encounter the problems resulting from these higher levels of use. Social policy on drugs must take this into account when deciding what level of harm is acceptable in return for what level of social pleasure or functional benefit. At the same time, the goal of research and education is to find ways of reducing the width of the

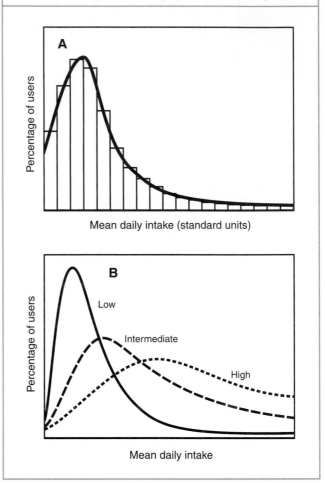

FIGURE 70-2 Schematic representation of distribution of consumption of alcohol and other psychoactive drugs in a population. (A) Distribution shown as a histogram and as a smooth unimodal skewed curve. (B) Relation between shape of the curve and mean per capita consumption by three different populations with low, intermediate, and high per capita consumption.

distribution-of-consumption curve so that a given modal value will be accompanied by fewer individuals in the upper part of the consumption range.

## BEHAVIOURAL DEPENDENCE

Although social, legal, economic, and other factors mentioned above appear to have comparable effects on the level of alcohol and other drug use by light users and heavy users, there are nevertheless important quantitative and qualitative differences between dependent and non-dependent users. An understanding of these differences is essential for the development of effective means of preventing and treating drug dependence.

| TABLE 70-3 | Effect of Purchase Price on Consumption of Alcohol by Volunteer Subjects in a Long-Term "Model Economy" Experiment | |
|---|---|---|
| | **Mean Number of Drinks Consumed** | |
| Subjects | "Happy Hour" in Effect* | No "Happy Hour" in Effect |
| Moderate drinkers | 20.9 | 10.1 |
| Alcoholics | 117.6 | 49.6 |

*In the "happy hour" condition, drinks were available at half price for 3 hours each day.
(Data from Babor et al., 1978.)

## Drug-Taking as Reinforced Behaviour

People use psychoactive drugs for many different reasons. Some may use alcohol, cannabis, or opioids for relief of boredom, frustration, tension, anxiety, or pain. Others may use them for a more positive type of pleasure associated with feelings of relaxation, joviality, "euphoria," or even physical visceral sensations that they find intensely gratifying. Still others use amphetamines or other stimulants to achieve feelings of heightened alertness, endurance, and power (also referred to as "euphoria," a rather unspecific word). Others use drugs because their social group does and there is pressure on them to conform. The only thing common to all these motives is that the use of drugs is somehow **rewarding** to the user, whether by producing pleasure, by relieving displeasure, or by winning approval of the user's peers.

Some of the reward is the result of the direct pharmacological action of the drugs on the "reward system" of the brain, described in Chapter 69. This action is responsible for what is termed direct, or primary, positive reinforcement of drug-taking behaviour. Methods for studying and quantifying this type of reinforcement are also described in Chapter 69. It is important to recognize that reinforcing properties of drugs do not by themselves explain drug dependence. They are an important factor in the acquisition of drug-taking behaviour, but the majority of individuals who try psychoactive drugs, and who find the effects pleasing ("rewarding"), do not become dependent. Moreover, though the intrinsic reinforcing properties of heroin are much greater than those of alcohol, far more people are dependent on alcohol than on heroin.

In behaviourist terms, drug dependence is the consequence of frequently and strongly reinforced drug-taking behaviour so that this behaviour becomes a dominant response that increasingly replaces other possible responses that are less effective in satisfying the individual's drives. It is implicit in this concept that the drug effects must be experienced as a consequence of actively taking the drug. Receiving the drug passively will not give rise to behavioural dependence. Animals or humans can easily be made physically dependent on a drug (e.g., an opioid given by a nurse or physician for relief of severe chronic pain) by being given repeated doses of sufficient size to give rise to withdrawal symptoms if the drug is suddenly stopped. Yet, if they have played no role in the drug administration, they will go through the withdrawal reactions without later making any efforts to obtain more drug. For drug-seeking activity to occur, they must experience reinforcing effects produced by taking the drug themselves.

In addition to the requirement for self-administration, it is also necessary to examine a number of other internal and external factors that contribute to the differing degrees of risk of dependence in different persons.

### Time relations

For the effects of a behavioural response to be reinforcing, those effects must be experienced quite soon after the response is made. Therefore, a drug that produces its reinforcing effects rapidly is more likely to give rise to repeated drug-taking than one that has a slow onset of action. Thus, heroin is much more addictive than, for example, methadone (see Chapter 19).

### Route of administration

It follows from the preceding point that the route of administration will have an important effect on the speed of reinforcement and therefore on the probability of producing dependence. For example, heroin is much more likely to produce dependence if taken intravenously than if taken by mouth. The same is true of cannabis and of cocaine when they are smoked rather than swallowed.

### Sources of drugs used

The existence of a dependent or harmful pattern of use does not imply that the drugs used are necessarily illicit. Dependent use is seen with prescribed drugs, over-the-counter drugs, as well as "street" drugs. Thus, they may be obtained in the illicit market, purchased in a pharmacy, given by a friend, or obtained by prescription. Those purchased in the illicit market may be illegally imported from other countries (e.g., heroin, cocaine, khat), synthesized in illegal laboratories here (e.g., amphetamines, "ecstasy," designer drugs), or deviated from the licit to the illicit market (synthetic opioids, benzodiazepines). One of the problems related to prescriptions is "doctor-shopping" by the user, that is, obtaining independent prescriptions for the same drugs from several physicians and often having these filled in different pharmacies. This is becoming easier to detect because of the existence of a computerized central registry of prescriptions. A second problem is forgery of prescriptions using prescription pads stolen from the physician's office. It is important for the physician to keep the pads in a securely locked drawer when not in use.

## Genetic predisposing or protective factors

In rats and other experimental animals, selective breeding over a number of generations has yielded lines that will voluntarily consume high or low amounts of a drug or that will show high or low sensitivity to some of the drug-induced changes in behaviour. Such genetic selection experiments have been carried out repeatedly with alcohol, and similar genetic selection has been carried out for high and low intake of opioids and other drugs.

Similarly, in humans, genetic factors may influence the sensitivity of an individual to either the reinforcing or the punishing effects of a drug, or both. The sons of alcoholic fathers, even when adopted in very early infancy by non-alcoholic families, are three to four times more likely to become alcoholics themselves than the similarly adopted sons of non-alcoholic fathers. What is inherited is almost certainly not a biological *need* for alcohol, but either a greater sensitivity to its reinforcing effects or a greater resistance to its punishing effects, or both. Studies of the non-alcoholic children of alcoholic parents are providing a growing body of evidence that both reinforcing and aversive effects of alcohol are under genetic control and that high-risk and low-risk individuals differ in the intensity of these effects.

The evidence for a genetic influence is greater in those alcoholics with an early onset of heavy drinking, a history of juvenile anti-social behaviour, rapid progression of the level of alcohol intake, and a high frequency of problems associated with intoxication. However, it is important to recognize that *the inheritance of these genetic factors does not inevitably make the person become an alcoholic.* Environmental factors play an essential role; genetic factors affect the degree of susceptibility to them.

The dopamine $D_2$ receptor is thought to be implicated in the genetic vulnerability of the type of alcoholic just described. The $D_2$ receptor exists in at least two allelic forms, and the A1 allele is reported to be significantly more common in these patients. However, there is strong evidence that the risk of alcoholism is determined by multiple genes rather than by a single gene. As a result, there are numerous so-called genetic markers (see Chapter 10) of increased risk of alcoholism, such as monoamine oxidase and adenylyl cyclase activities. A great deal of current research is devoted to identifying gene variants associated with greater or lesser risk of dependence on different drugs. For example, a mutant gene encoding a variant of the α4 subunit of nicotinic cholinergic α4β2 receptors is reported to be associated with increased sensitivity to the locomotor stimulating and reinforcing effects of nicotine.

Some of these genetic variants are currently being investigated for their possible usefulness in detecting those individuals at greatest risk of becoming dependent on alcohol or other drugs in adult life so that they may be given the benefit of early application of preventive measures.

Conversely, a high proportion of Chinese, Japanese, and Korean people have genetic variants of alcohol dehydrogenase and acetaldehyde dehydrogenase that result in faster oxidation of ethanol to acetaldehyde and slower oxidation of acetaldehyde to acetate (see Chapter 22). Therefore, the ingestion of ethanol produces a high steady-state level of acetaldehyde that causes them very unpleasant effects (flushing, tachycardia, nausea, and dizziness) that greatly decrease the likelihood of further drinking, or at least of heavy drinking. However, if other factors mentioned above are conducive to the development of alcohol dependence, it is possible for people with the atypical form of acetaldehyde dehydrogenase to become dependent in spite of their initially aversive reaction to alcohol.

It must be emphasized that genetic factors simply affect the *degree of risk*; they are not the sole cause of dependence, and the majority of drug-dependent individuals do not have an identifiable genetic predisposition.

## Motivational factors

In experimental animals, the existence of an aversive motivational state (e.g., fear or approach–avoidance conflict; see Chapter 69) can increase the intake of ethanol and other sedative or anxiolytic drugs (see Chapters 22 and 23). Food restriction, leading to chronic weight reduction, can increase the intake of a wide range of drugs of different pharmacological classes, even those that do not provide calories or directly reduce appetite. In humans, periods of heavy drinking or drug use are often triggered by situational changes that produce worry, fear, disappointment, anger, or frustration. Such states presumably increase the reinforcing effect of those drugs that are capable of relieving the discomfort.

Numerous studies have shown that situational and personality factors of various kinds are associated with heavy use of psychoactive drugs. Though there is no single pattern of "dependence-prone personality," adolescents with drug problems frequently have histories of parental abuse, long-standing alienation from family and friends, reduced impulse control, and emotional distress beginning in childhood and preceding the start of drug use. Again, the drugs appear to act as "negative reinforcers" by giving temporary relief from the subjective distress caused by these preceding difficulties.

## Stimulus control

Environmental stimuli that are regularly associated with the availability and use of a drug can become discriminative stimuli (see Chapter 69), in the presence of which the drug-seeking behaviour occurs. The drug-taking is then said to be under stimulus control, rather than being a voluntarily initiated act. Such stimuli, by their repeated association with the reinforcing effects of the drug, can become conditioned reinforcers that produce brief drug-like reinforcing effects. For example, if a light is used regularly to indicate to a rat that it can obtain a drug injection by pressing a lever, the rat will later press the lever just to obtain the signal light. Similarly, humans who repeatedly experience the "rush" on self-injecting heroin or amphetamine into a vein often come to feel a brief "rush" on simply inserting a needle into the vein, even if the syringe is empty.

These conditioned responses are eventually extinguished if the conditioned stimuli do not continue to be paired with the drug from time to time. However, as long as they are present, they may contribute to the phenomenon of **drug-craving** and the risk of **relapse** into drug use. Addicts who have been in hospital or prison for months or years, without any craving for drugs, can feel a compulsion to take drugs within hours of returning to the environment in which they had regularly taken drugs before.

## Neurobiological Mechanisms of Transition from Non-dependent to Dependent Use

As described in the preceding sections, all repeated drug use implies that the drug effects are reinforcing, but some major change is involved in the transition to dependence. Many different neurobiological changes have been described in animals that have passed from non-dependent to dependent drug use. These changes affect a large variety of transmitters, receptors, second-messenger systems, gene expression mechanisms, and effector mechanisms. It is not yet clear, however, how they are related to the onset of dependence, and whether they are all independent adaptive changes or different parts of an integrated mechanism. Accordingly, there are different theories, none of which has yet gained general acceptance.

For example, one theory states that repeated heavy drug use causes desensitization of the reward circuitry so that, in the absence of the drug, the person is in a state of dysphoria and requires the drug in order to feel more or less normal. This implies that negative reinforcement underlies the dependence. A different theory holds that repeated use results in sensitization of the reward circuitry so that the drug becomes more intensely rewarding and takes over from the normal reinforcers that operate in non-dependent individuals. This implies that intensified positive reinforcement underlies dependence. These opposing views would have different implications for approaches to treatment.

Such conflicting theories are not necessarily mutually exclusive. Recent research indicates that chronic heavy drug use may produce a change in the actions of the GABA$_A$ receptors on γ-aminobutyric acid (GABA) interneurons in the ventral tegmental area (VTA) that tonically inhibit the dopaminergic neurons (see Chapter 69). In the changed state, the GABA$_A$ receptor is reported to be converted from an inhibitory receptor (by influx of Cl$^-$ ions) to an excitatory receptor (by efflux of HCO$_3^-$ ions). As a result, the reinforcement mechanism is said to switch from a dopaminergic pathway for positive reinforcement to a non-dopaminergic one for negative reinforcement. This field of study is extremely active at present and is undergoing rapid evolution of concepts.

## Intensity and Significance of Behavioural Dependence

Since many different factors, as noted above, can enter into the creation of conditioned drug-taking behaviour, and each can vary widely in degree, it is not surprising that the resulting behavioural dependence can also vary greatly in degree from relatively minor to an overwhelming compulsion that dominates all other behaviour. It may be directed toward a drug or substance that is intrinsically rather harmless or to one that is toxic and gives rise to serious physical consequences. The drug selected may be inexpensive and legally available, so the drug use per se does not cause social harm, or it may be expensive or illegal, so simply obtaining the drug may give rise to serious problems. The cost of the drug may deprive the user or the user's family of other necessities, or the user may obtain more money by theft, drug trafficking, or other illegal means and thus risk arrest and prison. In other words, behavioural dependence is neither harmful nor harmless in itself; the degree of harm depends on what consequences it brings in the individual case.

## TOLERANCE AND PHYSICAL DEPENDENCE

Many drugs give rise to the phenomenon of increase in tolerance when they are taken repeatedly or chronically. In other words, it becomes necessary to take progressively larger doses to achieve the same degree of drug effect. This may be illustrated graphically as a shift in the dose–response curve (Fig. 70-3). It may be produced in two quite different ways, referred to as *metabolic* (or *dispositional*, or *pharmacokinetic*) *tolerance* and *functional* (or *target tissue*, or *pharmacodynamic*) *tolerance*.

### Metabolic Tolerance

The reactions by which the drug is detoxified, in the liver in most instances, may become more active as a result of enzyme induction (see Chapter 4) following repeated use of the drug. It is then necessary to take a larger dose in order to maintain effective concentrations of the drug in the blood and brain for the same length of time as before. This form of tolerance is not likely related to physical dependence, because it is really equivalent to taking smaller doses of drug. Common examples include tolerance to numerous anxiolytic and sedative drugs and, to some extent, alcohol.

Metabolic cross-tolerance is also important for drugs that are biotransformed by hepatic microsomal enzymes. Induction of the cytochrome P450 system by barbiturates,

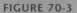

**FIGURE 70-3** (A) Shift in the *dose*–response curve illustrates tolerance but gives no indication of the mechanism. (B) Metabolic tolerance does not alter the concentration–response curve, but target tissue tolerance shows a shift in the *concentration*–response curve similar to that in the dose–response curve.

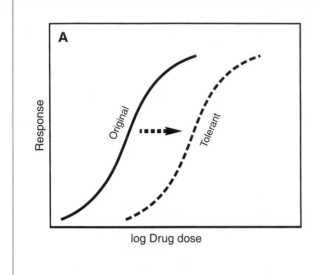

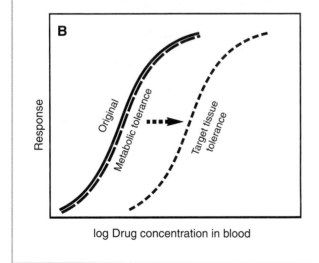

alcohol, or phenytoin, for example, can cause increased rates of biotransformation of many other drugs (see Chapters 4 and 22).

## Functional Tolerance and Physical Dependence

### Tolerance as adaptation

The brain or other tissues on which the drug acts may undergo adaptive changes that tend to offset the effect of the drug. For example, if ethanol, barbiturates, or benzodiazepines cause depression of neuronal excitability,

changes in ion fluxes, and impairment of neurotransmission, the adaptation might consist of changes in the cell membrane that facilitate both passive and active ion fluxes and neurotransmitter release and increase the excitability of the neuron. These changes would tend to compensate for the effect of the drug and produce an apparently normal functional state while the drug is present (tolerance).

Such adaptive changes have been found in virtually every type of neuronal function examined, including energy metabolism, spontaneous and evoked electrical activity, neurotransmitter turnover, numbers and affinities of neurotransmitter receptors, intracellular signal transduction systems, and expression of various genes and oncogenes. In most cases, however, it is impossible to know whether the observed changes are necessary for the production of tolerance or are merely manifestations of tolerance.

### Relation to physical dependence

When the drug is withdrawn, the same changes that resulted in tolerance now give rise to a "drug-opposite" effect that is recognized as a withdrawal reaction. For example, the hyper-excitability that produced tolerance to ethanol, barbiturates, or benzodiazepines now forms the basis of a **withdrawal syndrome**, which may range from sleeplessness, tremor, and irritability to hallucinations and tonic–clonic seizures. The severity depends upon the degree of adaptive change in the nervous system, which, in turn, depends on the degree and duration of exposure to the drug. Since the withdrawal reaction is abolished by a fresh dose of the drug, it constitutes evidence of **physical dependence** on the drug.

### Drug-specific withdrawal patterns

The particular characteristics of the withdrawal syndrome depend on the adaptive changes induced by the drug, which depend on the pharmacological actions of the drug. Thus, morphine suppresses gastrointestinal motility and constricts the pupil, and the morphine withdrawal syndrome includes intestinal hypermotility, cramps and diarrhea, and pupillary dilatation. Cocaine or amphetamine causes hyperactivity and euphoria, and the withdrawal reaction is characterized by profound fatigue, lethargy, and depression. It is a common misconception to think that a drug does not cause physical dependence if it does not cause a morphine-type withdrawal reaction. This is obviously quite illogical; there is no reason why a central stimulant such as cocaine should produce a withdrawal reaction similar to that of morphine.

### Intensity

The intensity of withdrawal reaction is also related to the time course of drug action. For example, a drug that acts for a relatively long time, because of high plasma protein binding and slow biotransformation or excretion, frequently gives rise to less intense withdrawal symptoms than a drug that acts quickly, intensely, and briefly. Presumably, the slow elimination of the drug permits some measure of physiological re-adaptation to occur while the drug concentration is slowly falling. This probably explains the less intense withdrawal reaction experienced after methadone than after heroin or morphine.

### Non-drug factors in tolerance

Tolerance is not simply a physiological adaptive response to the physical presence of the drug. Rather, it is a response to the functional disturbance produced by the drug. This depends not only on the kind and amount of drug but also on the sensitivity of the individual, the type and level of the person's ongoing activity at the time the drug is taken, the environment in which it is taken, and the user's previous drug history.

Individuals, strains, and species with greater **initial sensitivity** to a drug will experience greater functional disturbance upon their first use of the drug than more resistant subjects do, and, therefore, they will have a greater stimulus to the development of tolerance.

The same dose of a drug produces tolerance more rapidly if the subject is alert and **performing some task** under the influence of the drug than if the drug is taken at rest. This is particularly true if the drug effect causes the **loss of some reinforcer** that the subject is working to obtain.

Tolerance, especially to relatively low doses of a drug, may also be in part a **conditional response.** For example, an animal that receives a dose of morphine every day in the same environment and that has its body temperature taken each time to monitor the hypothermic effect of the drug shows much greater tolerance in that environment than it does if the drug administration and temperature measurement are then carried out in a different environment. The environmental stimuli that are repeatedly associated with drug administration become conditional stimuli; they bring on tolerance more rapidly by eliciting a conditional response that resembles the unconditional adaptive response to the drug itself (i.e., that is opposite in effect to the action of the drug).

A subject who has a **history of drug tolerance,** and who has then reverted to normal sensitivity after stopping the drug, re-acquires tolerance and physical dependence more rapidly upon resuming drug use than on the first time around.

These observations show that tolerance is not a simple process, but a complex phenomenon with many components. The same dosage of the same drug can therefore give rise to wide inter-individual differences in the degree and rate of development of tolerance and physical dependence, and even within the same individual at different times and with respect to different effects of the drug. Many different biochemical mechanisms have been proposed to explain tolerance; so far, none can account for all the behavioural complexities of the process.

### Role of physical dependence in maintaining drug dependence

Physically dependent subjects whose drug use is interrupted for any reason may, upon feeling withdrawal symptoms, learn that by taking more drug they obtain rapid relief from these symptoms. This results in a corresponding negative reinforcement that contributes to the strengthening and maintenance of drug-taking and behavioural dependence.

The conditioning of behaviour (i.e., learning to take more drug in response to certain stimuli arising during the withdrawal syndrome) may also help to explain the high relapse rate among drug-dependent people. Since these stimuli are not really specific (e.g., intestinal hypermotility, muscle tension, tremor, hyper-irritability), they can also be produced by other causes, such as physical illness or emotional disturbance. When they are produced, even though the person has not been using drugs for some time, these stimuli can evoke the conditioned drug-taking response just as if they were part of a true withdrawal reaction.

## CROSS-TOLERANCE AND TRANSFER OF DEPENDENCE

If two drugs cause essentially similar pharmacological effects via essentially the same mechanism, one might anticipate that adaptive changes that arise from the use of one drug will also confer tolerance to the other; that is, there will be **cross-tolerance.** In fact, it has been noted clinically for many years that alcoholics are unusually resistant to general anaesthetics, barbiturates, and other hypnosedatives. In one study, the minimum alveolar concentration of halothane required for anaesthesia (see Chapter 20) rose from 0.76% in normal subjects to 1.31% in a group of alcoholics. The same transfer of tolerance is seen from one opioid analgesic to another and from alcohol and barbiturates to other hypnosedatives and anxiolytics.

Conversely, when one drug in a cross-tolerance group is withdrawn, another in the same group can be used to decrease or abolish the withdrawal symptoms; that is, there is a **transfer of physical dependence** (cross-dependence). In fact, new synthetic opioid analgesics are tested for dependence liability by testing their ability to prevent withdrawal symptoms in heroin addicts or in heroin-dependent monkeys. When one treats delirium tremens or other alcohol withdrawal symptoms by giving a benzodiazepine, one is really making therapeutic use of this transfer of dependence. However, it is still necessary to gradually reduce the dosage of the substitute drug, or nothing will have been accomplished except to replace one drug problem with another.

## POLYDRUG ABUSE

As noted at the beginning of this chapter, the term "drug abuse" is poorly and variably defined, but it usually carries the connotation that the pattern of use is likely to give rise to harm. The term *polydrug abuse* refers to the concurrent use of two or more drugs in a similarly potentially harmful way. Among the common examples are combined use of heroin and cocaine, ketamine and "ecstasy," and alcohol and cannabis. Such polydrug abuse is more common among young users than among older ones, and it is becoming increasingly common in North America and many other parts of the world.

Polydrug use appears to carry a higher risk of physical and mental damage than use of a single drug. Several possible reasons for this include the following: polydrug users generally have a higher total drug use than single-drug users, thus increasing the total risk of adverse events; drug interactions among the multiple drugs used may give rise to adverse events that are less likely with a single drug; use of several drugs usually carries the likelihood that multiple routes of administration (oral, smoking, parenteral injection) are being used, each of which carries its own risks; and since polydrug use is commoner among young users, including adolescents, there is additional vulnerability because of immature emotional, cognitive, and physiological functions. Clinical surveys suggest that polydrug abuse carries an increased risk of neurocognitive impairment and psychiatric morbidity.

## TREATMENT OF DRUG DEPENDENCE

From the nature of dependence, it is obvious that the goal of treatment is to stop the undesired drug-taking response from continuing to be self-reinforcing. Psychological and social therapy, in the form of counselling and individual and group psychotherapy, are aimed at building up other behavioural responses for problem solving that are, at the same time, reinforced by social approval and that increase the patient's self-esteem. In other words, long-term treatment of drug dependence requires more than just getting the patient through a withdrawal period with the aid of a tranquillizer—it requires a process of behavioural retraining to enable the patient to make different and more helpful responses to the stimuli that have habitually elicited drug-taking behaviour.

Pharmacological agents can help in various ways, as outlined below.

### Specific Receptor Blockers

Specific blockers can be used to prevent the drug from producing its usual effects, including its reinforcing effect. The first efforts to do this were directed toward a few drugs for which specific transmitter or receptor mechanisms were known (e.g., naltrexone to block μ-opioid receptors and thus prevent all actions of heroin, including its reinforcing action; see Chapter 19). Similarly, α-methyl-*p*-tyrosine, an inhibitor of catecholamine synthesis (see Chapter 13), has been used to block the "high" produced by cocaine or amphetamine. In theory, failure of the drug-taking behaviour to provide the anticipated reward should lead to **extinction** of this conditioned behaviour. In opioid-dependent persons, opioid receptor blockers are not used in this way until withdrawal from the opioid is complete; if used too soon, the blockers will precipitate a severe withdrawal reaction. Blockers of benzodiazepine receptors (e.g., flumazenil; see Chapter 23) are not used in treating benzodiazepine dependence because they would also precipitate a dangerous withdrawal reaction.

### Non-specific Blockers

Non-specific blockade of reinforcement can also be used. With increasing recognition of the complexity of the neuronal circuits involved in the reward system (see Chapter 69), which appears to be shared by quite diverse psychoactive substances, it seemed possible that reinforcement by a variety of different drugs might be prevented non-specifically by the use of agents that interfere with the reinforcement mechanism per se without being specific antagonists of those drugs.

In view of the important role of dopamine in the reinforcement circuits (see Chapter 69), efforts were first made to block reinforcement by administering dopamine receptor blockers such as butyrophenones and phenothiazines (see Chapter 24). These were found to decrease alcohol intake but not opioid intake, and the side effects make them unsuitable for treating drug-dependent humans. However, selective dopamine receptor *agonists* such as bromocriptine and lisuride appear to have some value in reducing alcohol consumption, although the mechanism is not clear.

Serotonin, apparently acting on 5-HT$_2$ and 5-HT$_3$ receptors, is believed to prevent reinforcement by inhibiting the activity of the dopaminergic pathway from the VTA to the nucleus accumbens (see Fig. 69-5). Therefore, a number of serotonin reuptake inhibitors (e.g., fluoxetine, citalopram, trazodone) and 5-HT$_{1A}$ receptor agonists (e.g., buspirone) have been tested in the expectation that they would increase the level of 5-HT inhibitory activity on the VTA dopamine neurons and thus reduce reinforcement by alcohol, nicotine, and other drugs. These agents did produce large and dose-dependent decreases in intake of alcohol and amphetamine by rats. Rather surprisingly, however, some *blockers* of 5-HT$_2$ receptors (e.g., ritanserin) and 5-HT$_3$ receptors (e.g., ondansetron) were equally effective in rats, but the effects of all these drugs in humans were rather modest. It is not yet clear whether they will be more useful when combined with other blockers of reinforcement or as accessory agents in a program that includes psychosocial and other types of treatment.

Opioid receptors in both the VTA and the nucleus accumbens also play an important role in reinforcement, either by modulating the activity of dopamine neurons or by an independent mechanism (see Chapter 69). Alcohol intake by rats is increased by administration of low doses of centrally acting μ-opioid receptor agonists and is markedly decreased by opioid receptor blockers such as naloxone and naltrexone. These findings led to clinical studies that have demonstrated a significant beneficial effect of **naltrexone** in reducing the risk of relapse in recovering alcoholics and in reducing the amount of alcohol consumed if relapse does occur. The use of naltrexone for this purpose has been approved in Canada, the United States, and many other countries.

**Acamprosate** (calcium acetylhomotaurinate) is an analogue of taurine, an amino acid that is normally present in the brain and that has actions similar to those of ethanol on GABA$_A$, *N*-methyl-D-aspartate (NMDA), and glycine receptors and on voltage-gated calcium channels. Acamprosate differs from naltrexone in that it has a more selective effect on motivation for alcohol consumption than for other drugs. It reverses the changes in glutamatergic transmission at NMDA receptors in the brain that are found during chronic heavy drinking. How this results in decreased motivation to drink is not yet well understood, but numerous clinical studies have demonstrated that acamprosate prolongs periods of abstinence and decreases the amount of alcohol consumed during relapses. The effect is more prolonged than that of naltrexone and may persist for up to a year after drug treatment is stopped. The side effects of both drugs are minor, except that naltrexone can have significant interaction with non-steroidal anti-inflammatory drugs. The possible benefit of combining naltrexone and acamprosate in the treatment of alcoholism is currently under investigation.

## Drug Substitution

A less reinforcing and legally available drug can be substituted for a more reinforcing and illicit one (as in **methadone** or **buprenorphine maintenance** treatment for heroin addicts). Note that these agents do not constitute, *by themselves,* a treatment of the dependence. They simply permit the patient to satisfy the drug need legally, under medical supervision and control. The real treatment component is the social and psychological rehabilitation that should be going on while the patient comes to the clinic regularly to receive the methadone. Since this rehabilitation, when it occurs, usually requires a long time to change the patient's behaviour significantly, methadone maintenance treatment is often carried on for many years.

Substituting a less reinforcing drug is also done in preparation for withdrawal. The second drug can then be gradually reduced in dosage to avoid a major withdrawal reaction (e.g., methadone withdrawal therapy in heroin dependence, benzodiazepines for withdrawal from alcohol).

## Aversive Agents

Aversive agents interact with the drug to produce an unpleasant instead of a rewarding effect (e.g., **disulfiram** or **calcium carbimide** in the treatment of alcoholics; see Chapter 22).

While reinforcement blockers and aversive agents are sound in theory, they have had rather limited success. This is because many patients are unwilling to take them and thus cut themselves off from the possibility of deriving the desired effects from their drug of dependence. Others may agree to take the blocker or aversive agent but then simply stop taking it if they change their mind. Therefore, the effectiveness of these drugs depends very heavily on the patient's motivation.

**Counter-conditioning** is a behavioural counterpart of this approach, aimed at eliminating stimulus control of drug self-administration. Stimuli that are associated with drug-taking are repeatedly paired with a very aversive stimulus such as an electric shock or apomorphine-induced nausea. Unfortunately, this technique is also not very successful. It reduces drug self-administration while the aversive conditioning is in progress, but the benefit seldom lasts after the course of conditioning is finished.

## Treatment of Underlying Problems

This involves pharmacotherapy of emotional disturbances that may be contributing to the problem drug use. In many individual cases of alcoholism or sedative dependence, lithium or antidepressants may prove helpful by treating an underlying depression that may be causing or aggravating the dependence.

## SUGGESTED READINGS

Babor TF, Mendelson JH, Greenberg I, Kuehnle J. Experimental analysis of the "Happy Hour": effects of purchase price on alcohol consumption. *Psychopharmacology.* 1978;58:35-41.

Brady JV, Lukas SE, eds. *Testing Drugs for Physical Dependence Potential and Abuse Liability.* NIDA Research Monograph Series No 52. Rockville, Md: National Institute on Drug Abuse; 1984.

deLint J, Schmidt W. Alcoholism and mortality. In: Kissin B, Begleiter H, eds. *The Biology of Alcoholism, Vol 4: Social Aspects of Alcoholism.* New York, NY: Plenum Press; 1976: 275-305.

Di Chiara G. Nucleus accumbens shell and core dopamine: differential role in behavior and addiction. *Behav Brain Res.* 2002;137:75-114.

Efron DH, Holmstedt B, Kline NS, eds. *Ethnopharmacologic Search for Psychoactive Drugs.* Washington, DC: US Department of Health, Education and Welfare; 1967.

Fishman J, ed. *The Bases of Addiction: Report of the Dahlem Workshop on the Bases of Addiction, Berlin 1977, September 26-30.* Berlin: Abakon-Verlagsgesellschaft; 1978.

Goldstein A. *Addiction: From Biology to Drug Policy.* New York, NY: Freeman; 1994.

Hogg RC, Bertrand D. What genes tell us about nicotine addiction. *Science.* 2004;306:983-985.

Jaffe JH. Drug addiction and drug abuse. In: Gilman AG, Goodman LS, Rall TW, Murad F, eds. *Goodman & Gilman's The Pharmacological Basis of Therapeutics.* 7th ed. New York, NY: Macmillan; 1985:532-581.

Jaffe JH, Naranjo CA, Bremner KE, Kalant H. Pharmacological treatment of dependence on alcohol and other drugs: an overview. In: *Approaches to Treatment of Substance Abuse.* Geneva, Switzerland: WHO Programme on Substance Abuse; 1993:75-101.

Kalant H, Kalant OJ. *Drugs, Society and Personal Choice.* Toronto, Ontario: Addiction Research Foundation; 1971.

Kalant H, LeBlanc AE, Gibbins RJ. Tolerance to, and dependence on, some non-opiate psychotropic drugs. *Pharmacol Rev.* 1971;23:135-191.

Kauer JA. Learning mechanisms in addiction: synaptic plasticity in the ventral tegmental area as a result of exposure to drugs of abuse. *Annu Rev Physiol.* 2004;66:447-475.

Kissin B, Begleiter H, eds. *The Biology of Alcoholism, Vol 4: Social Aspects of Alcoholism.* New York, NY: Plenum Press; 1976.

Koob GF, Ahmed SH, Boutrel B, et al. Neurobiological mechanisms in the transition from drug use to drug dependence. *Neurosci Biobehav Rev.* 2004;27:739-749.

Laviolette SR, Gallegos RA, Henriksen SJ, van der Kooy D. Opiate state controls bi-directional reward signaling via GABA$_A$ receptors in the ventral tegmental area. *Nat Neurosci.* 2004;7:160-169.

Mason BJ. Acamprosate and naltrexone treatment for alcohol dependence: an evidence-based risk-benefits assessment. *Eur Neuropsychopharmacol.* 2003;13:469-475.

Morgan D, Roberts DC. Sensitization to the reinforcing effects of cocaine following binge-abstinent self-administration. *Neurosci Biobehav Rev.* 2004;27:803-812.

Nestler EJ, Hyman SE, Malenka RC. Reinforcement and addictive disorders. In: *Molecular Neuropharmacology: A Foundation for Clinical Neuroscience.* New York, NY: McGraw-Hill; 2001: 365-382.

Popham RE, Schmidt W, deLint J. The effects of legal restraint on drinking. In: Kissin B, Begleiter H, eds. *The Biology of Alcoholism, Vol 4: Social Aspects of Alcoholism.* New York, NY: Plenum Press; 1976: 579-625.

Popham RE, Schmidt W, deLint JE. The prevention of alcoholism: epidemiological study of the effects of government control measures. *Br J Addict.* 1975;70:125-144.

Robinson TE. Perspectives: addicted rats. *Science.* 2004;305:951-953.

Tabakoff B, Hoffman P, eds. *Biological Aspects of Alcoholism. Implications for Prevention, Treatment and Policy.* Seattle, Wash: Hogrefe & Huber; 1995.

# 71

# Principles of Toxicology

## C WOODLAND AND PG WELLS

Toxicology is the scientific discipline concerned with the adverse effects of chemical and physical agents and radiation on biological systems. It is a multidisciplinary field of study that draws from a number of related disciplines, including biology, chemistry, physiology, immunology, pathology, pharmacology, and public health. Because of the vastness of the subject and the specialized approaches to its study, only a general survey of pharmacotoxicological principles can be presented here. Further information on clinical toxicology and the management of poisonings can be found in Chapter 72.

Various classification systems are used to designate specialized areas of interest within the field of toxicology. One such classification is based on the purpose or application to which the results of the research are to be applied (e.g., forensic toxicology, clinical toxicology, occupational toxicology, environmental toxicology). Another classification is made on the basis of the organ system primarily affected by the toxic reaction (e.g., cardiovascular toxicology, renal toxicology, neurotoxicology). A third classification is based on the research methods used to study the toxicity (e.g., biochemical toxicology, molecular toxicology, behavioural toxicology).

Similarly, the toxic agents themselves are classified in different ways, reflecting different special interests. Technically, a toxin is a toxic substance that is derived from a biological source (i.e., plants, animals, bacteria, or fungi), whereas a toxicant is derived from an anthropogenic (i.e., human-made) source. However, these terms are now sometimes used interchangeably. One toxicological system classifies agents according to their relative potential for causing poisoning (Table 71-1). Another system, relating specifically to the study of toxic materials of biological origin (toxinology), is based on the source of the toxin (e.g., snake, spider, or bee venoms; plant or marine animal toxins). Still other classifications go by the chemistry of the toxic agents (e.g., aromatic amines, halogenated hydrocarbons) or by the mechanism of toxic action (e.g., sulfhydryl enzyme inhibitors, methemoglobin producers).

Despite these numerous areas of special attention, the objectives are fundamentally the same in all: to understand the mechanisms by which exogenous substances give rise to toxicity in living subjects, to define the quantitative relationships, to identify factors that increase or decrease susceptibility in individuals or populations, and to develop methods for preventing or treating the toxic reactions.

## DOSE–RESPONSE RELATIONSHIPS

When investigating the adverse effects of an agent on a biological system, the toxicologist must determine the relationship between the dose and the response. The dose–response concept is defined as a correlative relationship between exposure and effect (see Chapter 7). Three important assumptions are implicit in this definition: (1) the observed response is, in fact, due to the chemical administered, (2) the degree of response is related to the magnitude of the dose, and (3) the response in question is precisely defined and quantifiable.

A typical log-dose–response curve is shown in Figure 71-1 and is explained in detail in Chapter 7. The dose (e.g., mg/kg) is plotted on a logarithmic scale along the horizontal axis, and the response is plotted on an arithmetic scale along the vertical axis. The dose–response curves for *therapeutic dose, toxic dose,* and *lethal dose* are generally independent of each other. Concentration–response curves are also commonly used in toxicology.

The ratio of body weight to surface area differs between species, as illustrated in Table 71-2, so blood concentrations of chemicals will differ between species depending upon which parameter is used to standardize the dose. Of these two parameters, surface area generally reflects more accurately the metabolic factors that control chemical disposition, which can lead to substantial discrepancies in chemical blood concentrations depending upon whether the dose is standardized by body weight or surface area. For example, as shown in Table 71-2, if a mouse were given the same dose as a human standardized on a per kilogram

| TABLE 71-1 | Classification of Toxicants According to Poisoning Potential | |
| --- | --- | --- |
| **Toxicity Rating** | **Example** | **LD$_{50}$ (mg/kg)\*** |
| Slightly toxic (5–15 g/kg) | Ethanol | 8000 |
| Moderately toxic (0.5–5 g/kg) | Sodium chloride | 4000 |
| | Ferrous sulfate | 1500 |
| | Malathion | 1300 |
| | Methanol | 1000 |
| Very toxic (50–500 mg/kg) | Acetylsalicylic acid | 300 |
| | Acetaminophen | 300 |
| | Diazinon | 200 |
| | Phenobarbital | 150 |
| | Imipramine | 65 |
| Extremely toxic (5–50 mg/kg) | Theophylline | 50 |
| | Diphenhydramine | 25 |
| Super toxic (<5 mg/kg) | Potassium cyanide | 3 |
| | Methotrexate | 3 |
| | Strychnine | 2 |
| | Nicotine | 1 |
| | Digoxin | 0.2 |
| | *d*-Tubocurarine | 0.05 |
| | Tetrodotoxin | 0.01 |
| | TCDD (dioxin) | 0.001 |
| | Botulinum toxin | 0.00001 |

\*LD$_{50}$ is the lethal dose (mg/kg of body weight) for 50% of exposed animals. This list is an approximation, and the relative rank of each chemical may vary substantially depending upon the species tested, as well as other parameters such as strain, age, sex, and route of exposure.

body weight basis rather than by surface area, the resulting chemical blood concentration in the mouse might be only about one-tenth of that achieved in the human.

Two important dose–response parameters are the no observed adverse effect level (NOAEL) and the lowest observed adverse effect level (LOAEL). The NOAEL is the highest dose at which no adverse effects are seen, while the LOAEL is the lowest dose that does evoke an adverse response (see Fig. 71-1). The NOAEL represents the **threshold** where toxic effects begin (i.e., **threshold dose**). How the response is defined will influence the determination of the threshold dose. For example, for acetylsalicylic acid (ASA, Aspirin), the threshold dose that causes gastrointestinal bleeding (one to two tablets of ASA in an adult) is different from that which results in tinnitus (20 to 30 tablets), or that which is associated with systemic acidosis (40 to 50 tablets). On the other hand, some chemicals evoke a non-threshold response, where even one molecule can theoretically evoke a response. These chemicals, including some agents that cause cancer, are represented by a non-threshold dose–response line as illustrated in Figure 71-2.

Responses to chemicals may develop over a period of time, so it is important to establish a fixed observation period. Some toxic effects develop quickly and are reversible (e.g., inebriation and acidosis due to methanol poisoning), while others develop over several days and are irreversible (e.g., blindness resulting from methanol poisoning). Similarly, the toxic effects resulting from single (i.e., acute) exposures may differ from those resulting from repeated, long-term (i.e., chronic) exposures.

Another commonly determined dose–response function is the LD$_{50}$ (the dose causing the death of 50% of the exposed test animals; see Chapter 7). This parameter should be used with caution for several reasons. First, the LD$_{50}$ often varies substantially depending upon such factors as the species, strain, age, sex, and route of exposure. For example, the LD$_{50}$ for TCDD (a dioxin) can vary over 1000-fold between the guinea pig and the hamster, and TCDD does not cause acute lethality in humans, at least at exposure levels encountered to date. Second, some chemicals with relatively negligible acute toxicity, such as the environmental chemical benzo[*a*]pyrene, nevertheless may initiate other or delayed toxicities, such as cancer or birth defects, and may do so at doses much lower than those necessary to cause lethality or other less drastic acute toxicities. Finally, the target tissue can vary from strain to strain and species to species, as it does for TCDD, and a particular toxicity, such as acute lethality, determined in one animal model often is not predictive of the

| FIGURE 71-1 | Features of the semi-logarithmic dose–response curve (see also Chapter 7). The log-dose–response relationship is typically represented by a sigmoidal curve. The NOAEL (no observed adverse effect level) is the highest dose or concentration examined at which no toxicity is observed. The LOAEL (lowest observed adverse effect level) is the lowest dose examined at which an adverse effect is observed. The NOAEL is also referred to as the threshold dose. |
| --- | --- |

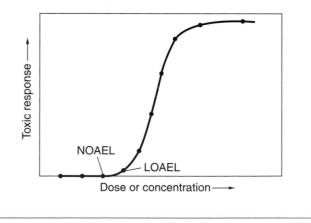

| TABLE 71-2 | Species Differences in Dosages Adjusted by Weight and Body Surface Area* | | | | |
|---|---|---|---|---|---|
| **Species** | **Body Weight (g)** | **Dosage (mg/kg)** | **Dose (mg/animal)** | **Surface Area (cm²)** | **Dosage (mg/cm²)** |
| Mouse | 20 | **100** | 2 | 46 | **0.043** |
| Rat | 200 | 100 | 20 | 325 | 0.061 |
| Guinea pig | 400 | 100 | 40 | 565 | 0.071 |
| Rabbit | 500 | 100 | 150 | 1 270 | 0.118 |
| Cat | 2 000 | 100 | 200 | 1 380 | 0.145 |
| Monkey | 4 000 | 100 | 400 | 2 980 | 0.134 |
| Dog | 12 000 | 100 | 1 200 | 5 770 | 0.207 |
| Human | 70 000 | **100** | 7 000 | 18 000 | **0.388** |

*In the highlighted examples, one would have to give a mouse approximately a tenfold higher dose corrected for surface area to get roughly the same dose as a human dosed per kilogram.
(From Klaassen and Watkins, 2003. Reprinted with permission.)

spectrum, let alone the severity, of toxicities expressed in other animal models or humans.

The $LD_{50}$ is sometimes used with the $ED_{50}$, or effective therapeutic dose for 50% of the population, to calculate the therapeutic index (TI; see Chapter 7):

$$TI = LD_{50} / ED_{50}$$

The TI provides a rough approximation of the safety of a chemical, bearing in mind both the above limitations and the absence of information on the slopes of the curves for either of the two components of this index. The larger the TI value, the safer the drug—an index of 10 indicates a relatively safe drug. In any event, an acceptable index is relative. In the case of rapidly lethal diseases, such as some cancers, potentially helpful drugs are tolerated with higher incidences and severities of toxicity than would be acceptable for a drug used to treat headaches.

Parallel dose–response curves for two substances indicate that the agents have different $LD_{50}$ values but that this difference is proportional over the whole scale of responses. However, intersecting dose–response curves of two substances may give one substance a lower $LD_5$ but a higher $LD_{50}$, analogous to the principle underlying the *certain safety factor* in Chapter 7. The *potency* of a toxin is defined by the position of its dose–response curve along the dose axis. Thus, a substance with an $LD_{50}$ of 8 g/kg is less potent than one with an $LD_{50}$ of 5 g/kg.

While dose- and concentration–response curves typically illustrate increasing toxicity as the dose or concentration is increased, this is not always the case. For many substances, particularly trace elements and vitamins necessary for physiological processes, the response curve may be shaped like a "U," reflecting adverse effects at both low and high doses or concentrations (Fig. 71-3). For example, iron is an essential element in humans. If iron concentra-

tions are too low, deficiency disease (e.g., anemia) will result. At moderate concentrations, homeostasis is maintained and no toxicity is observed. However, as the concentration of iron escalates, toxicity (e.g., cardiovascular toxicity) begins to appear.

Another deviation from the common dose–response presentation is exhibited when low doses of a chemical are protective to human health while higher doses are

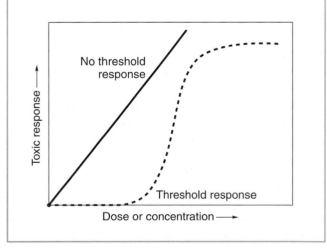

FIGURE 71-2    A comparison of the dose–response curves for chemicals with threshold or non-threshold responses. Most chemicals exert a threshold response such that toxicity results only after a minimum, or threshold, dose or concentration is reached. On the other hand, for some chemicals, one molecule theoretically is sufficient to cause toxicity. The latter is particularly true with agents that cause cancer.

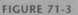

FIGURE 71-3 | Biphasic responses at low and high concentrations. For chemicals such as vitamins and minerals involved in physiological processes, adverse effects may be observed when concentrations are either too low or too high, whereas concentrations in between these extremes are associated with normal physiological function. For example, when plasma iron concentrations are low, anemia may result. At high plasma iron concentrations, cardiac and other toxicities may result.

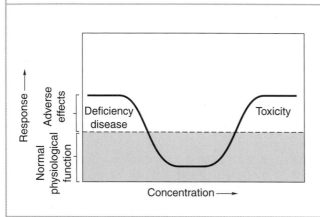

time of puberty. Similarly, children with leukemia who are successfully treated with DNA-damaging anti-cancer drugs may in later life develop other forms of cancer initiated by the anti-leukemic drug therapy given in childhood.

## MECHANISMS OF TOXICITY

In general, chemicals initiate adverse effects by one of two mechanisms: (1) reversible binding of the parent molecule and/or a stable metabolite to a cellular receptor (see Chapter 8), or (2) bioactivation of a relatively non-toxic chemical to a highly toxic electrophilic or free radical reactive intermediate that irreversibly (covalently) binds to or oxidizes cellular macromolecules such as DNA, protein, and lipid (see Chapter 68; Fig. 68-7). These two mechanisms differ in several basic and clinically important ways that are summarized in Table 71-3. Toxicities initiated by reversible, receptor-mediated binding usually are relatively predictable, occurring as a result of drug overdose or exposure to excessive amounts of environmental chemicals, and they can be confirmed by detecting a high plasma or tissue concentration of the chemical. However, toxicities initiated via irreversible macromolecular lesions caused by

toxic. For example, routine consumption of small doses of alcohol appears to reduce the incidence of certain cardiovascular diseases such as coronary heart disease and stroke, ostensibly by affecting lipid levels and endothelial function, while routine consumption of large doses is associated with a variety of toxicities including liver disease and cancer. As shown in Figure 71-4, the optimal dose of ethanol is found at the intersection of the curves, corresponding to the lowest overall morbidity and mortality. Many chemicals have been shown to be beneficial or protective in very low doses, resulting in a J-shaped dose–response curve (Fig. 71-5B). The mechanisms involved in these conflicting beneficial and toxic effects may or may not be the same. Conversely, an inverted U- or J-shaped dose–response curve can be exhibited if the endpoint is health or longevity (Fig. 71-5A), as in the case of some potential carcinogens that protect against cancer in very low doses. This concept of a toxicant in low doses having beneficial actions is often referred to as **hormesis**, which is defined as the stimulatory effect of subinhibitory concentrations of a toxic substance on an organism.

Variants on this theme include dose–response curves that are reversed with respect to time so that a beneficial effect is noted at first and a contrasting response develops at a later date. For example, in utero exposure of the developing embryo and fetus to the synthetic estrogen diethylstilbestrol (DES) can protect against miscarriage in some high-risk pregnancies, but the offspring may subsequently develop rare cancers and other abnormalities around the

FIGURE 71-4 | Dose-dependent protection versus toxicity. For some potentially toxic chemicals, low doses or concentrations may exert a protective effect for sustaining health or reducing certain diseases, while higher doses or concentrations are associated with toxicity or increased risk of other diseases. For example, the dashed line indicates that low doses of ethanol are associated with a reduction in coronary heart disease and stroke, while the solid line indicates a dose-dependent increase in the toxic effects of ethanol, such as liver disease and cancer. The point where the two lines cross corresponds to an optimal ethanol dose for a decrease in overall morbidity. This biphasic effect is sometimes referred to as hormesis, as shown in Figure 71-5.

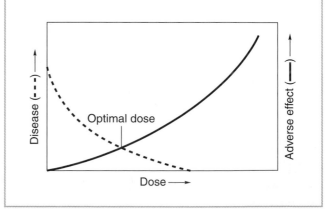

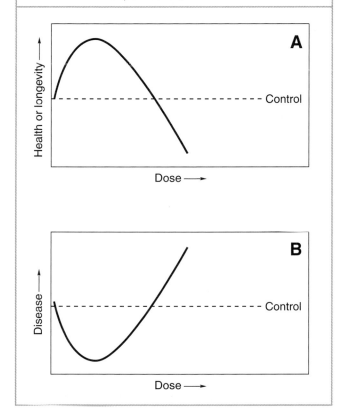

**FIGURE 71-5** Dose–response curves indicating hormesis. This phenomenon refers to the stimulatory or beneficial effects observed with some xenobiotics at low doses. (A) Low doses of a chemical may increase health or longevity compared with no chemical exposure, whereas high doses decrease health or longevity relative to controls. (B) Low doses of a chemical may decrease the risk of disease relative to controls, while higher doses increase the risk of disease. (Adapted from Calabrese EJ. Hormesis: a revolution in toxicology, risk assessment and medicine. *EMBO Reports*. 2004;5(1 suppl):S37-S40, with permission.)

Most drugs and environmental chemicals can initiate reversible, receptor-mediated toxicities if the exposure level is sufficiently excessive. In the case of drugs, the toxicological sequelae usually will include a predictable exaggeration of the pharmacological effect for which the drug is employed therapeutically, for example, severe hypotension from an overdose of a β-adrenergic blocker, which is given in therapeutic doses to lower blood pressure. In contrast, bioactivation to a toxic reactive intermediate occurs with a smaller but still substantial number of chemicals, including the analgesic drug acetaminophen, some organophosphate insecticides, and the herbicide paraquat. Many chemicals that cause cancer (carcinogens), birth defects (teratogens), tissue necrosis, neurodegenerative disorders, and immunologically mediated hypersensitivity reactions (allergens or immunogens) are believed to initiate their toxicity at least in part via bioactivation to a reactive intermediate. The target tissue often is determined by the site of bioactivation because the reactive intermediate is too reactive to travel across membranes to distal tissues without first reacting with more proximal targets. Hence, tissue necrosis caused by high doses of acetaminophen occurs predominantly in the liver and kidney, while that caused by inhalation of the pesticide paraquat occurs in the lung.

## MODIFIERS OF TOXICITY

In analogy to the sources of variation in drug response (see Chapter 58), a number of factors can modify the manifestations of toxicity. These modifiers may alter toxicity via a variety of mechanisms, most often altering chemical biotransformation or disposition. For example, the toxicity of a compound can by enhanced by decreased activity in pathways of elimination (allowing the accumulation of excessive concentrations), increased activity in pathways of bioactivation to a toxic reactive intermediate, or decreased activity in detoxifying or cytoprotective pathways for removing reactive intermediates or reactive oxygen species. For chemicals like aminoglycoside antibiotics that are eliminated by renal excretion without being biotransformed, reduced renal filtration or secretory functions can lead to chemical accumulation and toxicity. For drugs such as the anticoagulant warfarin that are rapidly toxic, have a narrow therapeutic index, and are highly bound (over 90%) to plasma carrier proteins such as albumin, exposure to other chemicals or conditions that displace the drug from its carrier protein, or diseases that result in a decreased level of carrier protein in the plasma, will increase the free (active) drug concentration. In the case of warfarin, this leads to internal bleeding. Other potential mechanisms of toxicological enhancement include reduced pathways for repair of cellular macromolecules damaged by reactive intermediates (see Chapter

reactive intermediates may occur at therapeutic plasma drug concentrations or presumably safe exposure levels of environmental chemicals. This toxicological predisposition usually results from individual biochemical imbalances involving one or more of the following: decreased chemical elimination, enhanced chemical bioactivation, decreased detoxification of reactive intermediates, decreased cytoprotective pathways that remove reactive oxygen species, or decreased repair of damaged cellular macromolecules (see Chapter 68; Figs. 68-7 to 68-10). In most people, in the absence of excessive exposure levels, bioactivation does not exceed the capacity of the multiple protective pathways, and reactive intermediates are formed and removed with no toxicological consequence.

| TABLE 71-3 | Characteristics of Xenobiotic Toxicity Initiated by Reactive Intermediates Compared with Reversible, Receptor-Mediated Interactions | |
|---|---|---|
| | **Mechanism of Tissue Interaction** | |
| **Characteristic** | **Reactive Intermediate** | **Receptor-Mediated** |
| Initiating species | Reactive intermediary metabolite (highly unstable): electrophile or free radical<br>Often a minor metabolite amounting only to 1–10% of total xenobiotic/metabolites | Parent compound and/or a stable major metabolite |
| Molecular target | Multiple sites within different cellular macromolecules (DNA, protein, lipid, and carbohydrate) | Specific receptor on one type of macromolecule (usually a protein) |
| Target interaction | Irreversible<br>    Covalent binding (arylation/alkylation)<br>    Oxidation | Reversible binding (usually) |
| Duration of target interaction | Cumulative | Transient |
| Toxic effects* | Unrelated to therapeutic effect[†] | Generally an extension of the therapeutic effect |
| Toxic dose/concentration | Toxicity can occur at therapeutic plasma drug concentrations or "safe" concentrations of environmental chemicals | Toxicity occurs when therapeutic or safe plasma concentrations are exceeded |
| Onset of toxicity | Toxicity occurs well after the time of the peak plasma xenobiotic concentration, and usually after the xenobiotic no longer is detectable in plasma or urine<br>Depending upon both the xenobiotic and the toxicity, this delay can be hours, days, months, or years | Toxicity usually increases with rising plasma xenobiotic concentration, and decreases with or shortly after declining concentrations |

*Effect in this case refers to the effect of therapeutic drugs and is not relevant to environmental chemicals.

[†]There are some exceptions, such as alkylating anti-cancer drugs, where drug toxicity does result from the same mechanisms by which tumour cells are killed.

(From Wells PG, Winn LM. Biochemical toxicology of chemical teratogenesis. *Crit Rev Biochem Mol Biol.* 1996;31:1-40. Reprinted with permission.)

68). With receptor-mediated effects, toxicity may be altered by the number of receptors and their functional state, particularly in the fetus, neonate, and elderly, and by concomitant exposure to receptor agonists and antagonists, including the often unconsidered accumulation of active metabolites that bind to the same receptor as the parent compound.

## Route of Administration

The route of administration may affect the observed toxicity of a given substance. Routes commonly used for toxicity testing and their influence on the degree of toxicity are shown in Table 71-4. Procaine toxicity depends on the rate and completeness of absorption compared with the rate of hydrolysis by plasma esterases. In most cases, it is probably the variation in bioavailability that accounts for the differences in the $LD_{50}$ found with different routes of administration. Pentobarbital toxicity is related to peak tissue concentrations. Because pentobarbital is primarily absorbed from the intestinal tract rather than from the stomach, absorption is slow and may result in relatively lower tissue levels compared with dosing by the parenteral routes.

## Duration and Frequency of Exposure

Another aspect to consider when assessing the toxicity of a substance is the duration and frequency of exposure. In toxicology, **acute** exposure is defined as exposure lasting less than 24 hours, during which time the substance may have been administered as a single, repeated, or continuous dose. **Subacute** exposure means exposure for 1 month or less. **Subchronic** exposure means a duration of 1 to 3 months, and **chronic** means more than 3 months. However, these terms are often used loosely; for example, chronic salicylate toxicity is said to develop after use of the drug for more than 2 days.

Different durations of exposure may result in different manifestations of toxicity. For example, acute exposure to benzene results in central nervous system depression, but chronic exposure may be associated with hematological malignancy.

| TABLE 71-4 | Effect of Route of Administration on $LD_{50}$ in Rats, Relative to Intravenous Injection | | |
|---|---|---|---|
| Route | Procaine | Isoniazid | Pentobarbital |
| Intravenous | 1.0 | 1.0 | 1.0 |
| Intraperitoneal | 5.0 | 0.9 | 1.6 |
| Intramuscular | 14.0 | 0.9 | 1.5 |
| Subcutaneous | 18.0 | 1.0 | 1.6 |
| Oral | 11.0 | 0.9 | 3.5 |

(Based on data from Loomis TA. *Essentials of Toxicology.* Philadelphia, PA: Lea & Febiger; 1968.)

## Age

The age of the subject can have an important impact on toxicity. For instance, newborn infants with immature thyroid glands are more susceptible to iodine toxicity than adults. Age differences can often be accounted for by the levels of activity of drug receptors, drug metabolizing enzymes, and drug transporters, in addition to differences in the size and volume of body compartments. Table 71-5 shows the degree of toxicity resulting from the exposure of newborn, pre-weaning, and adult rats to three different insecticides. The variability in toxic response to insecticides in rats of different ages may depend on age-related variations in relative organ size, maturation of enzyme systems, and distribution patterns of the toxin. For example, the relative toxicity of malathion in different species is inversely related to the rate of biotransformation of malathion by the hepatic cytochrome P450 system (see Chapter 4). Since this system is markedly hypofunctional in the neonatal rat, this may explain the much higher toxicity of malathion in the newborn. β-Adrenergic receptors are also hypofunctional in newborn rats and humans. Death by overdose of dichlorodiphenyltrichloroethane (DDT) in the rat is usually attributable to ventricular fibrillation, and immaturity of the β-adrenergic response system may protect the newborn against the increase in myocardial irritability caused by DDT.

| TABLE 71-5 | Effect of Age on Acute Toxicity in Rats* | | |
|---|---|---|---|
| Age | Malathion | DDT | Dieldrin |
| Newborn | +++ | + | + |
| Pre-weaning | ++ | ++ | +++ |
| Adult | + | +++ | ++ |

*+, ++, +++ = increasing degrees of toxicity.

At birth, human newborns typically have lower renal function and levels of anti-oxidative and drug metabolizing enzymes. These generally increase with age, but the newborn or young child may be at greater risk of toxicity due to greater toxin exposure. Children are more susceptible than adults are to severe toxicity from antihistamines, lead, salicylates, and some anti-cancer agents. In some cases, children may be more susceptible to toxicity due to multiple mechanisms. On the other hand, young children appear to be protected from the toxicity induced by acetaminophen compared with older children and adults. Neonates and young infants have lower levels of the particular P450 isoenzymes necessary to bioactivate acetaminophen to a toxic reactive intermediate.

Since both neonates and the elderly have reduced renal function, they are more susceptible to the accumulation and toxicity of chemicals such as aminoglycoside antibiotics (e.g., gentamicin) that are predominantly removed via renal elimination. With human drug exposures such as these, toxicity can often be prevented by dosing adjustments. On the other hand, the toxicity resulting from environmental exposures is less controlled. Children generally consume more food per kilogram of body weight than adults do, and they also tend to place more things (such as dirt) in their mouths, thus potentially exposing them to a greater number of environmental chemicals. Aging may result in the bioaccumulation of some chemicals (particularly those that are hydrophobic) and may also increase the risk of toxicity.

The timing of exposure during in utero development also affects toxicity. For instance, the critical period of exposure to thalidomide that is associated with birth defects is generally the first trimester of pregnancy (see Chapters 61 and 68). Once an organ or tissue is formed, teratogens generally do not cause structural malformations.

## Sex Differences

Many instances of differences in chemical-induced toxicity have been noted between male and female animals, although these sex differences are less clear in humans. Both pharmacokinetic and pharmacodynamic differences exist between the sexes. Initial gastric emptying time has been shown to be significantly slower (by approximately 10%) in females compared with males. Women also have a higher percentage of body fat than men, resulting in larger volumes of distribution ($V_d$) for hydrophobic compounds and lower $V_d$ for hydrophilic compounds such as ethanol (see Chapter 22). In addition, plasma protein binding to $\alpha_1$-acid glycoprotein is lowered by estrogen and its equivalents, while levels of some serum drug-binding globulins increase. During pregnancy, the concentration of albumin and other proteins decreases, resulting in higher free drug concentrations (see Chapter 61). Sex differences in the activity of drug metabolizing enzymes have also been reported in humans, although the differences in plasma concentrations are typically relatively minor, and the data are conflicting.

Fewer differences in receptor-mediated toxicity are apparent. Differences in responses to analgesics between the sexes have been attributed to differences in the density of receptors, drug–receptor affinity, or signal transduction pathways. The extent to which sex differences and the hormonal changes associated with oral contraceptive use, pregnancy, and menopause contribute to clinically significant toxicity needs further study.

## Nutrition

The role of nutrition in toxicology is complex but must be considered when evaluating the toxicity of a given substance. Variability in nutrition may affect the toxic response through alterations in absorption, distribution, biotransformation, and excretion of drugs and environmental chemicals.

The presence of food in the stomach may enhance the absorption of some drugs (e.g., β-adrenergic receptor blockers, hydralazine, diazepam, lithium, and carbamazepine) but may reduce the absorption of others (e.g., penicillins, isoniazid, and rifampin). Malnutrition appears to reduce the absorption of tetracyclines and rifampin.

The biotransformation of drugs and chemicals is affected by nutrition in various ways. Rats that were fasted for 24 hours had a decreased rate of glucuronidation of 7-hydroxycoumarin, which returned to normal after a glucose infusion. Rats fed a diet low in polyunsaturated fats and high in saturated fats had lower than normal activity of cytosolic glutathione $S$-transferase. Animals fed a low-fat, high-protein diet had lower than normal elimination half-lives for antipyrine and theophylline; this observation suggests that substitution of dietary protein for fat may accelerate some drug transformations. Conversely, children with kwashiorkor (a form of liver damage due to dietary deficiency of certain amino acids) appear to have delayed biotransformation of tetrachloroethylene, which has led to the development of toxicity from this substance when it was used as an antiparasitic agent.

Some dietary components have been shown to interact with medications and other chemicals. For instance, taking therapeutic medications that are substrates for the drug metabolizing enzyme CYP3A4 (e.g., calcium-channel antagonists) with grapefruit juice can lead to toxicity because components of grapefruit juice (e.g., furanocoumarin derivatives) demonstrate competitive and mechanism-based inhibition of this isoenzyme, generally resulting in higher drug concentrations (see Chapter 4). Drug transport mediated by P-glycoprotein and some organic anion-transporting polypeptides (OATPs) is also inhibited by grapefruit juice. Diets high in garlic, which contains allyl sulfides, may increase the activity of phase one and phase two enzymes (see Chapter 4) as a result of enzyme induction by allyl sulfides. Rats given allyl sulfides show decreased toxicity from carbon tetrachloride exposure because of increased detoxification by enzymatic pathways.

Maternal diet has also been shown to affect in utero exposure to potential toxins. For instance, the incidence of birth defects induced by the anticonvulsant drug phenytoin is increased in the embryos of selenium-deprived mice with reduced selenium-dependent glutathione peroxidase activities, which protect against the increase in reactive oxygen species brought about by phenytoin. An important example in humans is folic acid supplementation by pregnant women. Folic acid reduces the incidence of neural tube defects in infants born to women with no known risk factors, as well as in those born to women with established risk factors for neural tube defects, such as exposure to anticonvulsant drugs.

## Genetic Variability

A frequent cause of exceptional predisposition to chemical toxicities involves genetic differences in one or more critical biochemical pathways (see Chapters 10 and 68). For receptor-mediated toxicities, this often involves lower levels, or even complete absence, of enzymes or enzymatic activities necessary for drug elimination, such as isoforms or isozymes of the cytochromes P450, UDP-glucuronosyltransferases, and $N$-acetyltransferases, resulting in the accumulation of a drug and/or its stable metabolite to toxic concentrations. Such deficiencies usually must be great enough to account for the loss of a major component of the xenobiotic elimination in order to substantially decrease clearance and increase plasma and tissue concentrations.

For toxicities produced by reactive intermediates, toxicological predisposition may result from genetically high activity and/or inducibility of bioactivating pathways such as cytochromes P450 (e.g., CYP2D6, CYP1A1) or from lower activities of enzymes that detoxify reactive intermediates (e.g., epoxide hydrolases, glutathione $S$-transferases). Unlike the situation with receptor-mediated toxicity, these pathways often constitute only a minor component of the total elimination of the xenobiotic. However, due to the extraordinary potency of reactive intermediates, pathways that control their formation and detoxification nevertheless have a dramatic effect on toxicological susceptibility, often without measurably affecting plasma concentrations of the parent compound.

For example, while epoxide hydrolase contributes to only about 10% of phenytoin elimination, a genetic deficiency in this enzyme renders such individuals highly susceptible to an otherwise rare but potentially fatal liver necrosis. In another rare case, a genetic deficiency in the enzyme γ-glutamylcysteine synthase results in a marginal ability to synthesize glutathione (GSH), which is essential for the detoxification of both electrophilic and free radical reactive intermediates, as well as reactive oxygen species. Toxicologically relevant genetic deficiencies in enzymes involved in cytoprotective pathways against reactive oxygen species and oxidative stress also have been reported, including GSH peroxidase, GSH reductase, superoxide dismutase, catalase, and glucose-6-phosphate dehydrogenase. Recent evidence suggests that genetic deficiencies in enzymes and other proteins involved directly or indirectly in the repair of cellular macromolecules damaged by reactive intermediates also may enhance toxicological susceptibility. For example, in knockout mice deficient in proteins like p53 and ATM (ataxia telangiectasia mutated), which are involved in DNA repair, developing embryos are more susceptible to the embryopathic effects of DNA-damaging agents like benzo[a]pyrene and gamma radiation.

Genetic susceptibility also can play a further role in immunologically mediated hypersensitivity reactions (see also Chapter 59). For example, everyone taking the antibiotic penicillin has some of this drug covalently bound to their proteins, yet only a relatively small number of these people experience true hypersensitivity reactions. In this case, individual differences in such pathways as antigen recognition and processing and control of the immunological cellular response of T and B cells are the critical determinants of susceptibility.

## Environmental Modifiers

All of the toxicologically relevant pathways discussed above in relation to genetic variability, at least theoretically, can be either increased or decreased by a multitude of environmental modifiers, including other drugs (e.g., prescription, over-the-counter, herbal products), environmental chemicals (industrial and natural), and microbial agents (e.g., viruses, bacteria). Most of these modifiers alter at least one pathway, and typically more than one. The consequences usually are difficult, if not impossible, to predict because not all, if any, of the effects of most modifiers are known. Toxicity depends upon the net alteration in the balance of several pathways, and the full complement of environmental modifiers to which a patient is exposed is not usually appreciated. Even the relatively circumscribed area of drug interactions often is quite complicated, particularly since the effect of a modifier on a given pathway may be completely opposite in acute compared with chronic exposure. For receptor-mediated and reactive intermediate–mediated toxicities, alterations also can result, respectively, from coexisting agonists/antagonists and macromolecular damage.

## Disease

Coexisting diseases often can alter susceptibility to the toxicity of drugs and environmental chemicals. These effects may be readily anticipated, such as in some liver diseases that impair drug metabolism and elimination and in renal diseases that impair the elimination of drugs that are cleared by the kidney. In either of these cases, the disease would result in excessive drug accumulation. Effects of other diseases may be less apparent. For example, cardiovascular diseases can result in decreased liver blood flow, which inhibits the metabolism of so-called high-clearance drugs such as lidocaine, and decreased renal blood flow, which reduces the elimination of drugs that are cleared without metabolism via the kidney. Gastrointestinal diseases also can alter drug metabolism, particularly for chemicals that are extensively metabolized in the intestinal wall during absorption. Infection and inflammation have also been shown to inhibit drug metabolism catalyzed by some cytochrome P450 isoenzymes due to the production of cytokines. Via a number of mechanisms, diseases of the kidney, liver, and gastrointestinal system can alter the amount or binding capacity of carrier proteins in the plasma, thereby altering the free, and potentially toxic, concentration of the chemical. Numerous other effects of these and other diseases in modifying toxicological susceptibility have been reported, and in many cases, the underlying mechanisms remain to be fully characterized. An optimal appreciation of even the known possibilities requires extensive knowledge of the disposition and potential toxicological mechanisms for all drugs and chemicals to which a patient is exposed.

## RISK ASSESSMENT

The process of risk assessment involves identifying whether or not a chemical causes adverse effects, assessing whether there is a relationship between the dose or concentration of the chemical and its toxicity, and determining whether there will be sufficient exposure to cause harm. Risk characterization in humans is particularly challenging because it generally requires extrapolation from animal or in vitro models. While epidemiological data are sometimes available, hazards are generally identified from structure–activity analyses, in vitro toxicity tests, or animal bioassays, where doses and study conditions can be strictly controlled. The interpretation of human exposures often is confounded by a variety of complicating factors (including the interactions of several agents and inter-subject differences) and by the fact that the duration, route, and level of exposure to chemicals are often difficult to define. Inter-subject differences include environmental and genetically determined differences in receptors, drug metabolizing enzymes, drug transporters, and enzymes that repair DNA.

Two values that are particularly important in risk assessment are the LOAEL and the NOAEL. Increasingly sophisticated analytical techniques have steadily lowered the limits of detection and quantification for an increasing number of chemicals. Measurable amounts of metals, aflatoxins, dioxins, pesticide residues, and chlorinated hydrocarbons are now found where none were previously detected, perhaps only because our ability to detect and measure them has improved. Similarly, the degree to which we can detect and observe an effect also depends on the sensitivity of the tests. For example, acceptable levels of lead in the blood of young children have dropped steadily over the past 30 years: 40 µg/dL in 1974, 30 µg/dL in 1978, 25 µg/dL in 1985, 15 µg/dL in 1991, and 10 µg/dL in 1993 (respectively, 1.92, 1.44, 1.20, 0.72, and 0.48 µmol/L). This reduction in acceptable blood concentrations has occurred as a result of the improved ability of complex, sensitive neuropsychological tests to detect subtle defects produced by lower concentrations of lead.

Different mathematical approaches may be utilized in risk assessment. It is difficult to extrapolate, for predictive purposes, from high-dose, high-frequency responses to low-dose, low-frequency responses given the shape of the log-dose–response curve (see Fig. 71-1). Once an acceptable risk is defined, the "virtually safe dose" may cover a range of doses depending on the nature of the dose–response curve at the low end of the scale. A reference dose (RfD) or reference concentration (RfC) is defined as an estimate of the daily exposure to a chemical that is assumed to be without an adverse health impact.

Those who believe that very low levels of chemicals in the environment pose significant risks may support a very cautious approach to determining the reference dose. Because of the imprecision implicit in measurements at the low end of the dose–response scale, arbitrary safety factors may have to be used. For example, when setting a virtually safe dose of a chemical for which definitive human data and experience of predictive value are available, the NOAEL determined in animals may be reduced by a safety factor of 10 for humans. In the absence of human data, however, the NOAEL in animals might have to be reduced by a safety factor of 1000 to be considered virtually safe in humans, especially in children. In general, a safety factor of 100 is applied to the NOAEL to account for inter-species and inter-individual differences. In other words, the population should be exposed to 100-fold less of the chemical than its value for the NOAEL.

Sometimes, a "benchmark dose response" (BMR) is calculated, which utilizes the entire dose–response curve instead of a single dose by replacing the NOAEL with a value derived from the extra step of fitting the entire dose–response data set to a mathematical model for the toxic response of interest. The benchmark response is defined by the risk assessor and is often specified at 1%, 5%, or 10% (i.e., toxicity in 10% of animals). A measure of the variability within the data set can be accounted for by using the lower 95% confidence limit of the benchmark dose. This BMR is thought to be more appropriate than the use of the NOAEL and allows for the application of lower uncertainty factors.

In addition to toxicological data, other factors may need to be considered in establishing acceptable risk levels. The beneficial effects of a chemical (in terms of economics, employment, standard of living, quality of life, taxes generated, etc.) must be weighed against its known detrimental effects (health effects, loss of environmental resources, loss of work, lawsuits, etc.). For example, the application of toxic pesticides has been credited with reducing morbidity and mortality in countries with endemic malaria. Toxicological risk assessment, therefore, is concerned with promoting the safety of the individual without simultaneously reducing the benefits to contemporary society.

## SUGGESTED READINGS

Klaassen CD, ed. *Casarett & Doull's Toxicology: The Basic Science of Poisons.* 6th ed. New York, NY: McGraw-Hill; 2001.

Klaassen CD, Watkins JB, eds. *Casarett & Doull's Essentials of Toxicology.* New York, NY: McGraw-Hill, 2003:14.

Lu FC, Kacew S. *Lu's Basic Toxicology: Fundamentals, Target Organs and Risk Assessment.* 4th ed. London, United Kingdom: Taylor and Francis; 2002.

Timbrell, JA. *Principles of Biochemical Toxicology.* 3rd ed. Philadelphia, Pa: Taylor and Francis; 2000.

## ONLINE RESOURCES

Environmental Health and Toxicology, U.S. National Library of Medicine:
http://sis.nlm.nih.gov/enviro.html

EXTOXNET, The Extension Toxicology Network:
http://extoxnet.orst.edu

MedWatch, U.S. Food and Drug Administration:
http://www.fda.gov/medwatch

Motherisk (The Hospital for Sick Children):
http://www.motherisk.org

Society of Toxicology:
http://www.toxicology.org (see Sites of Interest)

The Teratology Society:
http://teratology.org (see Links > Toxicology and Teratology Databases and Literature)

TOXNET, Toxicology Data Network, U.S. National Library of Medicine:
http://toxnet.nlm.nih.gov

# 72

# Poisonings and Antidotal Therapy

## C WOODLAND

### CASE HISTORY

A 47-year-old woman weighing about 60 kg (132 lb.) was brought to the emergency department by ambulance with a verbal history of having ingested about 60 regular-strength acetaminophen tablets (325 mg each) in a suicide attempt approximately 6 hours earlier. The patient was awake and alert on arrival. In the interval, she had vomited twice and was now complaining of nausea. There was no significant past medical history and no medications had recently been used. Her temperature was 37°C, pulse 88 beats/min, respirations 20/min, and blood pressure 110/70 mmHg. The rest of the physical examination revealed only mild sweating and slight epigastric distress.

Since the patient had already vomited twice and there was a significant time delay between acetaminophen ingestion and arrival at the hospital, activated charcoal was not administered. Laboratory investigations included determinations of aspartate aminotransferase (AST), alanine aminotransferase (ALT), alkaline phosphatase, bilirubin, and international normalized ratio (INR; prothrombin). In addition, blood samples were sent to the laboratory for plasma acetaminophen and salicylate levels.

The results of the laboratory analyses were all within normal ranges. Salicylate was not detected. However, the acetaminophen level was 1200 μM (180 μg/mL) at approximately 6 hours post ingestion. When this value was plotted on an acetaminophen nomogram, it fell in the "probable hepatic toxicity" range.

In order to prevent hepatic injury, the patient was started on an intravenous infusion of N-acetylcysteine, which lasted for 21 hours, after which time the hepatic laboratory tests were repeated. The results were normal, and the patient was transferred from the emergency department to the psychiatry service.

## POISONINGS

Poisons are substances that, by their chemical or pharmacological actions, disturb the structure or function of organisms to cause injury, illness, or even death. While the word "poisoning" sometimes conjures up images of an intentional malicious act, the majority (85%) of human poisonings are unintentional. In the 1500s, Paracelsus, an alchemist–physician considered to be the father of modern toxicology, stated, "All substances are poisons; there is none which is not a poison. The right dose differentiates a poison from a remedy."

Exposures to poisons can be classified as acute, chronic, or acute on chronic; the latter refers to a significant single-episode exposure to a compound to which one is already chronically exposed. The 2004 Annual Report of the American Association of Poison Control Centers Toxic Exposure Surveillance System documented 8.3 reported human exposures per 1000 population, with a mortality rate of 0.05%. The incidence of poisonings is highest in children, with children under 6 years of age accounting for over 50% of human poison exposures, but only 2% of all human fatalities. In individuals over 13 years of age, most ingestions involve an intentional component, with suicides accounting for over 50% of poisoning fatalities.

The substances that are most frequently reported in human exposures are shown in Table 72-1. Drugs account for over one-third of all reported human poison exposures, with the largest numbers of fatalities occurring from exposures to analgesics, sedatives/hypnotics/antipsychotics, antidepressants, stimulants and street drugs, cardiovascular drugs, and alcohols, in descending order of frequency.

The reader should refer to Chapter 71 for a discussion of the principles of toxicology, including potential mechanisms of toxicity and factors that affect toxicity.

# PRINCIPLES OF TREATMENT

Regardless of the agent or agents suspected in a poisoning, physicians should exercise good medical judgement and treat the patient and not just the poisoning. Therefore, establishing or maintaining the airway, breathing, and circulation should be the physician's first priority. In order to treat poisonings optimally, the physician must have a clear understanding of some basic toxicological principles and should consider the following therapeutic goals:

- Reducing the systemic bioavailability of the toxin
- Inhibiting the biotransformation of the ingested compound to toxic metabolites and increasing the biotransformation to non-toxic metabolites
- Enhancing the excretion of the toxin
- Minimizing the adverse effects of the absorbed toxin (e.g., by pharmacological antagonism, chelation)

While some interventions make theoretical sense, in clinical practice their benefits are sometimes limited. Initial treatment should focus on preventing or decreasing the absorption of a poison. Once the poison is absorbed and distributed in the body, the use of antidotal therapy and efficient ways of increasing its elimination should be considered. More than one method of decontamination may be utilized. However, the medical approach that is taken generally depends on the suspected degree of poisoning, the time that has elapsed between the ingestion and the medical intervention, and the availability of antidotes. Laboratory results do not always dictate the course of treatment in poisonings, and they are sometimes not available in time to be of use.

# MODIFICATION OF ABSORPTION AND DISTRIBUTION

## Measures for Decreasing the Absorption of Toxins

The treatment of a poisoning often depends on the route of exposure to the poison. Most poisonings result from the oral ingestion of chemicals, but poisonings can also occur by inhalation; dermal, rectal, or vaginal exposures; and parenteral exposures including intravenous, intramuscular, and subcutaneous routes. The route of absorption dictates the initial therapy.

### Oral ingestion

Therapeutic interventions aimed at minimizing the absorption of an ingested material include removing the unabsorbed toxins from the gastrointestinal tract and preventing the absorption of any remaining substances.

| TABLE 72-1 | Substances Most Frequently Involved in Human Poison Exposures |
|---|---|
| **Substance** | **Percent of Cases** |
| Analgesics | 11.5 |
| Cleaning substances | 9.4 |
| Cosmetic and personal care products | 9.2 |
| Sedatives/hypnotics/antipsychotics | 5.3 |
| Foreign bodies | 5.0 |
| Topicals | 4.7 |
| Cough and cold preparations | 4.5 |
| Antidepressants | 4.2 |
| Pesticides | 4.2 |
| Bites/envenomations | 4.0 |
| Plants | 3.1 |
| Alcohols | 3.0 |
| Antihistamines | 3.0 |
| Cardiovascular drugs | 3.0 |
| Food products, food poisoning | 2.9 |
| Antimicrobials | 2.7 |
| Vitamins | 2.6 |
| Hydrocarbons | 2.2 |
| Chemicals | 2.0 |
| (From Watson et al., 2005. Reprinted with permission.) | |

*Activated charcoal.* The administration of activated charcoal (AC) is the most common therapeutic intervention in severe poisonings resulting from ingestion. AC is an inert, non-absorbable, odourless, tasteless, fine black powder that has a high adsorptive capacity by virtue of its large surface area for binding. It binds most toxins within the lumen of the gastrointestinal (GI) tract and markedly reduces absorption when administered orally or by orogastric or nasogastric tube. The charcoal-bound toxin then passes through the GI tract and is eliminated in the feces.

For optimal binding, a charcoal to toxin ratio of at least 10:1 should be used, if possible. When the ingested dose of a toxin is a matter of speculation, a single dose of 1 g of AC per kilogram of body weight is recommended. The success with which AC prevents absorption of a substance depends not only on the substance itself but also on the time between ingestion of the substance and administration of the charcoal. As an example, the values in Table 72-2 illustrate the progressive decrease in efficacy against acetylsalicylic acid (ASA, aspirin) with increasing delay in administration of AC.

| TABLE 72-2 | Efficacy of Activated Charcoal (AC) as a Function of Time | |
|---|---|---|
| **Time of AC Dosing Relative to ASA Ingestion** | **ASA Adsorbed to AC (%)** | |
| Simultaneous | 59 | |
| +30 minutes | 48 | |
| +60 minutes | 21 | |
| +180 minutes | 9 | |

When the gastrointestinal absorption of a drug is delayed (e.g., after ingestion of a large quantity or ingestion of a sustained-release or enteric-coated formulation), the beneficial effects from the use of AC are more significant. Multiple doses of AC are sometimes recommended for compounds with long half-lives, small volumes of distribution, and low protein binding. Repeated administration of AC is generally recommended for life-threatening ingestions involving carbamazepine, dapsone, phenobarbital, quinine, or theophylline.

While AC is useful in most poisonings by ingestion, it is not effective in removing polar compounds with low molecular weights (e.g., methanol, ethylene glycol), metals (e.g., iron, lead), and highly ionized salts (e.g., those of lithium, cyanide). The use of AC is contraindicated when there is a gastrointestinal obstruction or an unprotected airway.

*Gastric lavage.* Gastric lavage is another method of decontamination that is occasionally still used to reduce the absorption of a poison. It involves inserting a long tube through the mouth or nose into the stomach. Water or a similar fluid is instilled through the tube into the stomach and is then withdrawn by aspiration in the hope that the ingested substance has been dissolved in the fluid or is being withdrawn with it. This process is often repeated many times until the recovered contents are clear. Gastric lavage is usually reserved for liquid substances or highly toxic medications, when the patient is seen soon after the ingestion. On the other hand, large tablets or clumps of tablets (concretions) may not be able to pass through the tube. The potential risks of the procedure and of tracheal aspiration, coupled with the variable and often ineffective removal of poison, limit the use of this procedure in most poisonings.

*Emesis.* Historically, the induction of vomiting was commonly used as a method of reducing the absorption of a poison. Emesis was commonly induced with syrup of **ipecac,** which stimulates the chemoreceptor trigger zone and also causes local irritation of the gastrointestinal tract. Ipecac is a plant material containing a mixture of alkaloids that generally induces vomiting within 5 to 20 minutes after ingestion of a single dose. Ipecac should only be administered to alert, conscious patients within 60 minutes following the ingestion of a potentially toxic amount of a poison. However, there are many contraindications to its use, and both experimental and clinical studies have found the administration of ipecac to be of little benefit in most poisonings. Therefore, its use is no longer recommended.

*Whole bowel irrigation.* For large ingestions of sustained-release or enteric-coated preparations or compounds that do not bind to AC, an electrolyte solution of polyethylene glycol can be used to flush the GI tract, even when a relatively long time (up to 6 to 8 hours) has elapsed since ingestion. This is also an approach that is sometimes considered for "body packers," who have purposely swallowed plastic or latex packages of illicit drugs.

### Other routes of exposure
The absorption of toxic gases or vapours by the pulmonary route can be minimized by rapidly removing the victim from the place of exposure. The absorption of poisons through the skin can usually be lessened by removing contaminated clothing and gently washing the skin with mild soap and cold water. Abrasion of the skin (i.e., removing the keratin barrier) by overly vigorous rubbing and the use of hot water (i.e., increasing local circulation) should be avoided, as they may enhance the absorption of the toxin. When the toxin is injected, as is the venom of a snake bite, restricting the movement of the affected limbs is often recommended to slow the systemic distribution of the poison; however, the application of constricting bands or wraps proximal to the site of injection is not indicated in many countries because few individuals are able to safely and effectively utilize such techniques.

## Techniques for Altering Distribution of Toxins

### Limiting recirculation
One of the approaches to the therapy of a poisoning involves interruption of gastrointestinal (enteroenteric or enterohepatic) recirculation of the substance. Some lipid-soluble drugs (e.g., phenobarbital) have long plasma half-lives, perhaps in part because they undergo significant recirculation between the gastrointestinal tract and the portal blood. Repeated oral administration of AC will bind these drugs within the gut lumen, cause them to be excreted in the feces, and thus enhance their clearance from the body. For example, administration of repeated oral doses of AC has reduced the serum half-life of phenobarbital from 110 hours to 45 hours and has shortened the duration of phenobarbital-induced coma.

### Limiting distribution and recirculation by manipulation of pH

The distribution of some drugs is partially pH-dependent, since uncharged molecules usually cross membrane barriers more easily. When the p$K_a$ of a drug is below the pH of the surrounding fluid, acidic drugs will be more ionized and basic drugs will be less ionized than when the p$K_a$ is equal to the pH. The opposite is true when the p$K_a$ of a drug is higher than the pH. Therefore, appropriate modification of the pH can increase the degree of ionization of the drug and thus minimize its distribution (see Chapter 2). This process is called ion trapping. Weak acids are less ionized in acidic environments, allowing them to be easily absorbed from the GI tract and reabsorbed in the kidneys. Moreover, when taken in excess, acidic drugs may lower the pH and thus increase their own absorption. For example, the acidemia (e.g., plasma pH = 7.0) that may occur in a salicylate poisoning facilitates the entry of salicylate (p$K_a$ = 3.2) into the central nervous system (CNS). Normalizing the plasma pH to 7.4 reduces the amount of unionized salicylate, thus limiting the distribution of this toxin into cells.

By the same principle, the diffusion of weak bases can be lessened by lowering the pH, thus increasing the ratio of ionized to unionized molecules. For example, the non-ionized form of morphine can diffuse from the blood into the lumen of the stomach, where gastric acid ionizes it and prevents back-diffusion into the blood (ion trapping). Therefore, repeated oral doses of AC can help to remove morphine even after it has been administered parenterally, although this is not a common practice.

In severe poisonings involving acidic drugs, bicarbonate may be given in bolus doses or by intravenous infusion. Attempts to lower the pH in the treatment of overdoses involving basic drugs are less common in practice, but may be used.

## MODIFICATION OF ELIMINATION

The liver and the kidneys are the major organs responsible for the elimination of most drugs. While the biotransformation of chemicals occurs primarily in the liver, it may also occur in the kidneys (acetaminophen, carbon tetrachloride), lungs (paraquat), plasma (succinylcholine), or gastrointestinal wall (orally ingested adrenaline). In general, the products of biotransformation are more water-soluble than the original compounds and can be eliminated more readily by the kidneys. Though the transformation products are usually less toxic than the original compounds, in some cases the metabolites are more toxic than the parent compound (see Chapter 4). By manipulating the pathways of biotransformation and excretion, elimination can be enhanced. As noted earlier, elimination of toxins in the gastrointestinal tract can be accomplished by interrupting gastrointestinal recircula-

tion by the use of repeated doses of AC. However, most techniques used to enhance elimination of toxic substances from the body involve increasing renal excretion or extracorporeal clearance.

## MANIPULATION OF METABOLIC PATHWAYS

Therapeutic interventions in metabolic processes have concentrated on preventing the development or accumulation of toxic metabolites, because there is no safe, effective way to enhance the biotransformation of a toxic substance to non-toxic metabolites rapidly enough to make a clinically important difference in an acute intoxication. Examples of compounds that are biotransformed into pharmacologically active or toxic metabolites include imipramine, parathion, methanol, and acetaminophen.

**Acetaminophen** (*N*-acetyl-p-aminophenol) is the most commonly ingested pharmaceutical in poisonings. In therapeutic doses, acetaminophen is mainly conjugated with glucuronic acid or sulfate and is eliminated in the urine. Only a small percentage of the parent compound undergoes oxidation by cytochrome P450 enzymes (mainly CYP2E1, but also CYP3A4) to form a reactive metabolite, commonly called NAPQI (*N*-acetyl-p-benzoquinoneimine). Normally, this metabolite is detoxified through combination with glutathione (Fig. 72-1). However, when an overdose of acetaminophen is taken, the conjugation pathways are saturated and more acetaminophen is biotransformed to NAPQI. The increased amount of this metabolite exhausts the reserves of glutathione, the reactive metabolite accumulates, and hepatocyte damage results (see Chapters 4 and 43).

Treatment of acute acetaminophen intoxication currently involves the administration of the thiol donor *N*-acetylcysteine (NAC). NAC binds to NAPQI and helps to prevent the accumulation of toxic intermediates by a variety of mechanisms, including facilitation of glutathione formation. However, the exact mechanism of action of NAC is unclear. NAC is most effective if given within 10 hours of acetaminophen ingestion. For single acute doses of acetaminophen, a nomogram is available to aid physicians in predicting the occurrence of toxicity as a function of blood acetaminophen level and time post-ingestion (Figure 72-2).

**Methanol** (found in windshield washer fluid) and **ethylene glycol** (found in engine antifreeze) are alcohols that are biotransformed by alcohol dehydrogenase to toxic metabolites. Poisonings with these alcohols are accompanied by an increase in the osmolal gap, which is calculated by subtracting the expected plasma osmolality from the measured osmolality. Methanol itself is of relatively low toxicity, but when it is metabolized by the enzyme alcohol dehydrogenase to formaldehyde, which is, in turn, oxidized to formic acid, severe metabolic acidosis (due to the

FIGURE 72-1 Biotransformation of acetaminophen. In therapeutic doses, most of the acetaminophen follows the conjugation pathways to form sulfate and glucuronic acid esters. At higher doses, the conjugation pathways become saturated, and more of the toxic metabolite is formed, leading to hepatocyte damage. (From Gossel TA Jr, Bricker D. *Principles of Clinical Toxicology.* 3rd ed. New York, NY: Raven Press; 1994:278. Reprinted with permission.)

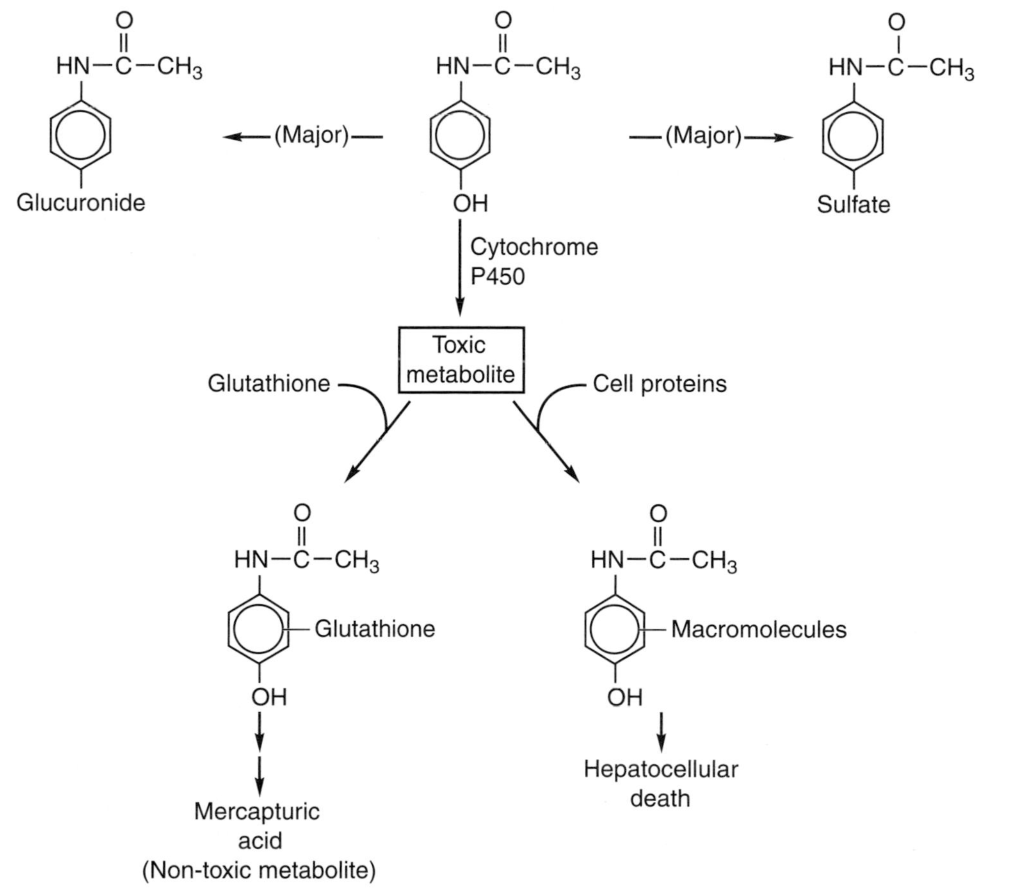

formation of formic, lactic, and α-ketobutyric acids) and blindness (formic acid causes optic nerve demyelination) may result. Similarly, ethylene glycol is oxidized by alcohol dehydrogenase to glycolic acid and oxalic acid, the latter causing toxicity following precipitation in the kidneys, heart, and brain.

To reduce the biotransformation of these alcohols to toxic metabolites by alcohol dehydrogenase, ethanol or fomepizole (4-methylpyrazole) is commonly administered. Both ethanol and fomepizole have higher affinity for alcohol dehydrogenase than methanol or ethylene glycol do, and, therefore, they markedly reduce the rate of oxidation of methanol and ethylene glycol and the consequent development of toxicity (see Chapter 22). The remaining methanol or ethylene glycol can be removed by hemodialysis (see "Dialysis" below) before it can be converted to toxic metabolites. In the case of methanol poisoning, folic acid is given, in addition, to facilitate the breakdown of any formate to carbon dioxide and water.

## ENHANCED EXCRETION

### Renal Excretion

Attempts to enhance the renal excretion of a toxic substance will be successful only if that substance is excreted to a significant degree in an unchanged or toxic form in the urine (i.e., if a substantial portion of the total body clearance of the substance occurs normally through the kidneys). In order to judge this accurately, it is necessary to know the renal clearance as well as the total body clearance of the substance in the toxic or overdose state. Relatively few substances encountered in clinical poisonings have a significant renal excretion following an acute overdose.

These compounds are listed in Table 72-3. Although the major part of a dose of amphetamines, phencyclidine, or phenobarbital undergoes biotransformation in the liver, significant portions are excreted unchanged through the kidneys. Enhanced renal excretion is accomplished by the systemic administration of compounds that alter the pH of

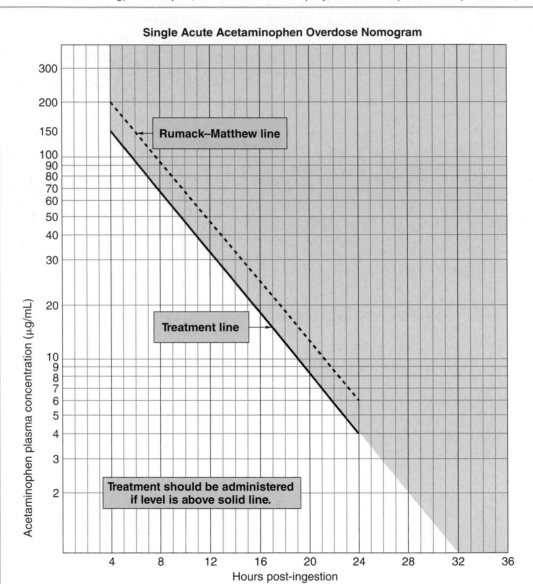

**FIGURE 72-2** Nomogram of serum acetaminophen concentration vs. time since ingestion, in cases of acute acetaminophen poisoning. The use of the treatment line or the Rumack–Matthew line varies between countries. (From McNeil Pharmaceuticals as copied from Ford et al., eds. *Clinical Toxicology.* Philadelphia, Pa: WB Saunders Company; 2001:268. Reprinted with permission.)

The nomogram has been developed to estimate the probability of whether a plasma acetaminophen concentration in relation to the interval post-ingestion will result in hepatotoxicity and, therefore, whether acetylcysteine therapy should be administered.

**Cautions for use of this chart:**
1. Time coordinates refer to time post-ingestion.
2. Graph relates only to plasma concentrations following a single acute overdose ingestion.
3. The Treatment Line is plotted 25% below the Rumack–Matthew Line to allow for potential errors in plasma acetaminophen assays and estimated time from ingestion of an overdose.

the urine ("ionized diuresis"), including alkalinization of the urine with sodium bicarbonate or acidification of the urine with ammonium chloride, depending on the drug to be eliminated. By the appropriate raising or lowering of the urine pH, the degree of ionization of acidic and basic drugs, respectively, is increased. Because the ionized drug in the urine is less able to cross cell membranes and be reabsorbed, it is excreted. Alkalinization of the urine may increase the excretion of salicylates and phenobarbital, whereas acidification of the urine may increase the excretion of amphetamines and phencyclidine. In practice, however, acidification of the urine is not routinely recommended in overdoses with these two drugs because they may cause rhabdomyolysis, which is accompanied by leakage of myoglobin into the blood. Acidification of the urine allows the myoglobin to precipitate in the renal tubules and cause renal failure.

## Extracorporeal Clearance

Extracorporeal clearance of toxins commonly takes two forms: dialysis or hemoperfusion. Both of these require the availability of trained specialists, but they are often of great benefit in poisonings by drugs that can be removed by these methods.

### Dialysis (peritoneal dialysis, hemodialysis)
Based on the principle of diffusion of a solute from a more concentrated to a less concentrated solution, dialysis brings body fluid containing a toxin into contact with a permeable membrane that separates it from a toxin-free dialysis fluid into which the toxin can diffuse. For dialysis to be effective, certain conditions must be met. The dialyzing membrane must be permeable to the toxic molecule, and the toxin should equilibrate rapidly between the circulating plasma and the dialysis fluid. The toxin should be removed in significant quantities compared with the total body burden of toxin or to spontaneous clearance. In addition, ideally, the degree of toxicity from the poison should be a function of its concentration within the body and the length of time that this concentration is maintained. If a toxin produces prompt and irreversible damage, removal of the remaining toxin by dialysis is not likely to be of great therapeutic value. From a clinical perspective, dialysis may be considered in severe intoxications (e.g., deep and pro-

longed coma) or in the presence of potentially lethal blood concentrations of the toxin. Decreased renal and hepatic clearance and deterioration in the clinical state due to the toxin are also indications for dialysis.

Hemodialysis is usually much more effective than peritoneal dialysis. In practice, the toxins that respond best to hemodialysis include ASA, lithium, methanol, and ethylene glycol.

### Hemoperfusion
Hemoperfusion consists of passing blood from a blood vessel over a resin or charcoal column and then back into the circulation, leaving the toxin bound to the column. Although less widely available, this technique has essentially the same conditions and criteria for use as dialysis, with the advantage that lipophilic and highly protein-bound drugs are cleared more efficiently.

## PHARMACOLOGICAL MEASURES FOR TERMINATING EFFECTS

An antidote may be defined as a remedy for counteracting a poison. Some examples of classical antidotes are given below, classified by their mechanisms of action.

## Antagonism

**Naloxone** (Narcan) antagonizes the sedation, respiratory depression, and miosis associated with an overdose of a morphine-like analgesic by reversibly competing with the opioid for μ- and κ-opioid receptors (see Chapter 19). A critical concentration of naloxone must be achieved and maintained at the receptor site in order for a reversal of narcotic effects to occur and persist.

Naloxone often is administered as an intravenous bolus, and the effects it produces are often of brief duration. This occurs for two reasons: (1) the relatively high CNS concentration of naloxone produced by the combination of bolus injection and high blood flow to the brain is rapidly reduced through redistribution of the drug, and (2) the half-life of naloxone is short, approximately 30 minutes. Hence, naloxone is often given by repeated dosing or by continuous intravenous infusion. Alternatively, an analogue with a longer half-life, such as naltrexone or nalmefene, may be used.

**Oxygen** may be considered a competitive antagonist to carbon monoxide, and **flumazenil** (a selective GABA$_A$-receptor antagonist) is a competitive antagonist to benzodiazepines.

**Atropine** therapy for carbamate or organophosphate insecticide poisoning is an example in which the antagonist (atropine) competes with the *effects* of the agonist (insecticide), not with receptor binding of the agonist itself. Both carbamate and organophosphate insecticides pro-

| TABLE 72-3 | Renally Excreted Substances | | |
|---|---|---|---|
| **Weak Acids** | **Ions** | **Weak Bases** | **Others** |
| Phenobarbital | Br⁻ | Phencyclidine | Arsenic |
| Salicylates | I⁻ | Quinidine | |
| | Li⁺ | Amphetamine | |

duce clinical effects by inhibiting the enzyme acetylcholinesterase. Because acetylcholine is no longer being degraded, its concentration in nerve synapses increases, producing excessive and persistent stimulation. Clinically, this is a picture of acetylcholine excess, or "cholinergic syndrome." A sufficiently high concentration of atropine will block the action of acetylcholine on postsynaptic receptors and will reverse the clinical effects (see Chapter 12). Thus, atropine competes with the *effect* of the insecticide but does nothing against the insecticide itself.

**Diazepam** can be considered a non-competitive antagonist of strychnine, and **pyrimidine** is a non-competitive antagonist of isoniazid.

## Chemical Neutralization

**Cyanide** poisoning occurs primarily in the industrial setting, but it may also result from exposure to residential fires, pharmaceuticals (e.g., sodium nitroprusside), or plant materials containing amygdalin (prussic acid glycoside), which can be hydrolyzed to yield free cyanide. Cyanide combines strongly with ferric iron in various proteins, including cytochrome oxidase, and prevents oxidative metabolism in the mitochondria of all tissues.

In the treatment of acute cyanide poisoning, the administration of sodium nitrite creates a large circulating pool of ferric iron (methemoglobin), which attracts the cyanide ion away from the cytochrome oxidase, permitting the resumption of oxidative metabolism. The next step in therapy is to supply the mitochondrial enzyme (rhodanese, or sulfur transferase) that normally detoxifies cyanide with its substrate (sodium thiosulfate) so that the enzyme can "neutralize" the cyanide ion by converting it to the non-toxic sodium thiocyanate.

Supplemental oxygen and sodium bicarbonate are also useful in the treatment of cyanide poisoning.

## Oxidation–Reduction

Excessive amounts of certain compounds (e.g., benzocaine, nitrites, phenazopyridine, dapsone) will oxidize hemoglobin ($Fe^{2+}$) to methemoglobin ($Fe^{3+}$), resulting in decreased oxygen delivery by the blood. Administered methylene blue (tetramethylthionine) acts as a cofactor to accelerate the conversion of methemoglobin to hemoglobin by methemoglobin reductase. Within 1 hour of administration of methylene blue, most of the methemoglobin will be reduced, and tissue oxygenation will be restored.

## Chelation

Chelators are agents that complex with metals (e.g., lead, zinc, iron, arsenic) to inactivate them and facilitate their elimination. This type of therapy is used to treat metal intoxication. An ideal chelating agent should be able to tightly bind a specific metal and form a non-toxic chelate that can be excreted readily from the body. Chelating agents should be administered as soon as possible following exposure to the toxic metal because the agents are more efficient at preventing enzyme inactivation by the metal than they are at reactivating the metal-poisoned enzyme. Among the chelators used in clinical practice are deferoxamine, ethylenediaminetetraacetic acid (EDTA), dimercaprol (BAL), succimer (DMSA), and penicillamine.

### Deferoxamine

Acute **iron poisoning** is one of the most common metal intoxications. Following ingestion of excessive amounts of iron, plasma iron concentrations exceed the iron-binding capacity of transferrin, and free (unbound) iron is distributed into cells, where it causes disruption of the mitochondria. Patients with iron intoxication are given **deferoxamine,** which binds circulating free and loosely bound iron and enhances its elimination in the urine. It does not bind iron strongly enough to detach it from cytochromes and other essential molecules containing tightly bound iron. Deferoxamine reduces the mortality rate in acute iron poisoning. It is relatively non-toxic; the adverse effects include occasional acute allergic reactions and cardiac and nervous system toxicity with prolonged administration.

### Dimercaprol and succimer

Dimercaprol (BAL, British anti-Lewisite) is used to treat patients with **arsenic or mercury poisoning.** It is administered so as to form a chelate with a ratio of two molecules of BAL to one molecule of metal. The chelate complexes are excreted in the urine and bile. BAL increases the urinary excretion of arsenic in the first 24 hours. The magnitude of the increase depends on the body load of arsenic and the adequacy of renal function. Dimercaprol is an oily liquid and must be given intramuscularly. Moreover, it has numerous adverse effects at therapeutic dosage. Therefore, it has been replaced to a considerable extent by water-soluble analogues, such as **succimer,** which have a higher therapeutic index and greater flexibility of administration. Succimer (dimercaptosuccinic acid, DMSA) is usually given by mouth, is well absorbed, and, if given within a few hours after poisoning, is an effective chelator of arsenic, mercury, and lead, forming complexes that are rapidly excreted in the urine. Gastrointestinal upset and rashes are the most common adverse effects.

### Calcium disodium EDTA

Ethylenediaminetetraacetic acid (EDTA, edetate) is an effective chelator of many di- and trivalent cations. Calcium disodium edetate (versenate), rather than EDTA itself, is used clinically as a chelating agent because EDTA and sodium EDTA would also chelate calcium. Calcium disodium EDTA does not cause hypocalcemia because it chelates on metals that have a higher affinity for EDTA than calcium does (e.g., lead, zinc). It is now used primarily to treat lead poisoning. Following the administration of calcium disodium EDTA, lead from soft-tissue depots displaces the calcium ion and forms a stable lead–disodium EDTA complex that is excreted in the urine. Urinary lead levels reach a maximum 6 hours after administration of the calcium disodium EDTA, and excretion is nearly complete in 18 hours. Lead excretion decreases with subsequent doses. A "rest period" is often recommended between courses of therapy to allow for redistribution of the metal within the body and to prevent zinc depletion.

## Antigen–Antibody Reactions

Serum globulins with specific activity against a given substance have been used in the form of antitoxins (to treat *Clostridium botulinum* poisoning) and antivenins (to treat envenomations from poisonous snakes or spiders). More recently, the development of antigen-binding fragments (Fab) derived from specific anti-digoxin antibodies has improved the treatment of poisoning from the digitalis glycosides. Patients with life-threatening digoxin poisoning who receive intravenous digoxin antibody fragments demonstrate an immediate decrease in free digoxin serum concentrations; favourable changes in cardiac arrhythmias and reduction of hyperkalemia occur within 30 minutes of administration (see Chapter 32).

## SUMMARY

A comprehensive understanding of the principles of medicine, pharmacology, and toxicology is essential to the management of poisoned patients. Each patient must be treated as an individual, taking into consideration the medical history, exposure to other agents (e.g., chronic medications), circumstances of the exposure to the poison, and time between exposure and presentation for treatment. In many countries, regional poison information centres exist and are the best sources for current and accurate information on poisonings.

## SUGGESTED READINGS

American Academy of Pediatrics. *Handbook of Common Poisonings in Children.* 3rd ed. Elk Grove Village, Ill: Amercian Academy of Pediatrics, Committee on Environmental Health; 1994.

Barceloux DG, McGuigan MA, Hartigan-Go K. Position statement: cathartics. *Clin Toxicol.* 1997;35:743-752.

Cartilena LR Jr. Clinical toxicology. In: Klaassen CD, ed. *Casarett & Doull's Toxicology: The Basic Science of Poisons.* 6th ed. New York, NY: McGraw-Hill; 2001:1109-1122.

Chyka PA, Seger D. Position statement: single-dose activated charcoal. *Clin Toxicol.* 1997;35:721-741.

Dart RC, ed. *Medical toxicology.* 3rd ed. Baltimore, Md: Lippincott, Williams & Wilkins; 2003.

Goldfrank LR, Flomenbaum NE, Lewin NA, et al, eds. *Toxicologic Emergencies.* 7th ed. Norwalk, Conn: McGraw-Hill Professional; 2002.

Klaassen CD. Principles of toxicology and treatment of poisoning. In: Brunton L, Lazo J, Parker K, eds. *Goodman & Gilman's The Pharmacological Basis of Therapeutics.* 11th ed. New York, NY: McGraw-Hill; 2006:1739-1751.

Krenzelok EP. New developments in the therapy of intoxications. *Toxicol Lett.* 2002;127:299-305.

Krenzelok EP, McGuigan MA, Lheureux P. Position statement: ipecac syrup. *Clin Toxicol.* 1997;35:699-709.

Krenzelok EP, Vale JA. Position statement: gut decontamination. *Clin Toxicol.* 1997;35:695-697.

Olson KR, ed. *Poisoning and Drug Overdose.* 4th ed. New York, NY: Lange Medical Books/McGraw-Hill; 2004.

Rumack BH. Acetaminophen hepatotoxicity: the first 35 years. *Clin Toxicol.* 2002;40:3-20.

Tenenbein M. Position statement: whole bowel irrigation. *Clin Toxicol.* 1997;35:753-762.

Vale JA. Position statement: gastric lavage. *Clin Toxicol.* 1997;35: 711-719.

Vale JA, Krenzelok EP, Barceloux GD. Position statement and practice guidelines on the use of multidose activated charcoal in the treatment of acute poisoning. *Clin Toxicol.* 1999; 37:731-751.

Watson WA, Litovitz TL, Rodgers GCJr, et al. 2004 annual report of the American Association of Poison Control Centers Toxic Exposure Surveillance System. *Am J Emerg Med.* 2005;23: 589-666.

Page numbers followed by *f* denote figures; those followed by *t* denote tables

Retinol, 844, 891-892, 893f
Retinyl esters, 843
Retrobulbar neuropathy, 687
Reverin. See Rolitetracycline
Reverse pharmacology, 77
Reverse transcriptase inhibitors
    non-nucleoside, 754-755
    nucleoside and nucleotide
        adverse effects of, 751-752
        chemical structure of, 751f
        mechanism of action, 751
        types of, 752-754
Reversible antagonists, 81
Reversible cholinesterase inhibitors,
    124-125
Rheumatrex. See Methotrexate
Rh$_0$D immune globulin, 552
Rhodopsin, 76
Rhubarb, 576
15R-hydroxyeicosatetraenoic acid, 366
Ribavirin, 742t, 744f, 748-749, 760
Riboflavin
    chemical structure of, 854f
    dietary reference intake for, 845t
    properties of, 855
    tolerable upper intake levels for, 848t
Ricinoleic acid, 576, 576t
Rickets, 851-852
Ridaura. See Auranofin
Rifadin. See Rifampin
Rifampin
    description of, 712, 715
    enzyme induction by, 817
    minimum inhibitory concentration
        for, 715t
    receptor for, 76t
    resistance mechanisms of, 665t
Riluzole (Rilutek), 221
Rimactane. See Rifampin
Rimantadine, 742t, 745
Rimonabant, 347
Risedronate, 886f, 886-887
Risk assessments
    during pregnancy, 823-824
    teratogens, 912-914
    toxicity, 967-968
Risperidone (Risperdal)
    chemical structure of, 309f
    description of, 306, 394
    hyperprolactinemia caused by, 307,
        313, 314f
Ritalin. See Methylphenidate
Ritonavir, 743t, 756
Rituximab (Rituxan), 550, 779t, 790
Rivastigmine, 125
Rivotril. See Clonazepam
Rizatriptan, 392t, 393
Ro 151788. See Flumazenil
Rocuronium, 178
Rofecoxib, 358, 372t-373t, 380, 809t
Roflumilast, 489
Rogitine. See Phentolamine
Rolaids, 561t
Rolitetracycline, 702
Rondomycin. See Methacycline

Ropinirole, 217f, 219
Ropivacaine
    biotransformation of, 272-273
    chemical structure of, 267f
    description of, 274
    properties of, 268t
Rosiglitazone, 645, 646f
Rosuvastatin, 475-477, 476t, 477f, 478t
Rough endoplasmic reticulum, 188, 193
Roundworms, 736t
Routes of administration
    concentration–time curve, 13f
    gastrointestinal tract, 12
    inhalation, 12
    injection, 11-13
    oral, 12
    percutaneous, 11
    pulmonary epithelium, 12
    rectal, 12
    selection criteria for, 13
    sublingual, 12
    topical, 11
    toxicity affected by, 964
Rovamycine. See Spiramycin
Roxatidine, 564
Roxithromycin, 707
R-Smads, 90
RU-486. See Mifepristone

**S**
S19014, 150
Sabril. See Vigabatrin
Saccharin, 20t
Safrole, 900
Salazopyrin. See Sulfasalazine
Salbutamol, 144, 150, 150f, 487
Salicylamide, 369
Salicylates
    acetylsalicylic acid. See Acetylsalicylic
        acid
    antipyresis uses of, 367
    cyclooxygenase inhibition by, 366
    description of, 365
    drug interactions, 368-369, 836
    fetal toxicity of, 826
    gastrointestinal system affected by,
        367-368
    hematologic uses of, 368
    inflammatory bowel disease treated
        with, 579-581
    methotrexate toxicity affected by, 368
    oxidative phosphorylation inhibited
        by, 368
    pharmacological effects of, 367-368
    properties of, 372t-373t
    respiratory system affected by, 367
    therapeutic uses of, 369-370
    toxicity of, 369
    uricosuric effect of, 367
    urinary clearance of, 66t
Salicylic acid
    chemical structure of, 366f
    description of, 369
    serum binding of, 31t
Salicylism, 369

Salicylsalicylic acid. See Salsalate
Salivary glands, 119t
Salmeterol, 150, 487
Salmonella, 676t, 680t, 700t, 704t-705t,
    707t, 715t
Salofalk. See Mesalazine
Salsalate, 369
Salvarsan. See Arsphenamine
Salvinorins, 339, 340f
Sandimmune. See Cyclosporine A
Sandomigran. See Pizotifen
Sandopril. See Spirapril
Sandostatin. See Octreotide
Sansert. See Methysergide; Methysergide
    maleate
Saquinavir, 742t, 751f, 756
Saralasin, 385
Sarcoplasmic reticulum, 174, 412
Sargramostim. See
    Granulocyte–monocyte colony
    stimulating factor
Sarin, 126f
Sativex, 348
Saw palmetto berry, 869t, 872-873
Scatchard plot, 70, 71f
Sch, 89
Schistosoma spp.
    S. haematobium, 728t
    S. japonicum, 728t
    S. mansoni, 728t
Schistosomiasis, 728t
Schizonticides
    blood, 733-734
    tissue, 732-733
Schizophrenia
    behavioural models of, 940
    description of, 304
    glutamate in, 314
    re-hospitalization rates for, 309f
Schwann cells, 190
Scientific journals, 10
Scopolamine
    chemical structure of, 131f
    description of, 133
    general anaesthesia premedication
        use of, 255
Scurvy, 860, 864
S-Demethylation, 37f
Secobarbital, 19
Secoisolariciresinol diglucoside, 874
Second messengers
    adenylyl cyclases as, 86-87
    cAMP as, 86-87
    phospholipase C, 87
    phospholipid, 87
    receptor-activated, 281
    termination of signalling by, 88
Secondary hemostasis, 507
Secretory glands, 122
Sedation
    amnesia with, 298-299
    antihistamine-related, 400
    antipsychotic drug-induced, 313
    intravenous, 265
    morphine, 243